COLLEGE INSTRUMENTAL TECHNIQUE SERIES

GUIDE TO

TEACHING WOODWINDS

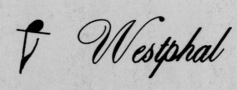

Westphal

GUIDE TO
TEACHING WOODWINDS

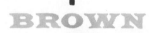

BROWN

COLLEGE INSTRUMENTAL TECHNIQUE SERIES

Edited by FREDERICK W. WESTPHAL, PH.D.
Sacramento State College, Sacramento, California

BARTLETT: *Percussion Ensemble Method*

EDWARDS: *String Ensemble Method*

HUNT: *Brass Ensemble Method*

WESTPHAL: *Woodwind Ensemble Method*

WESTPHAL: *Guide to Teaching Woodwinds*

COLLEGE INSTRUMENTAL TECHNIQUE SERIES

GUIDE TO
TEACHING
WOODWINDS

FLUTE • OBOE • CLARINET • BASSOON • SAXOPHONE

FREDERICK W. WESTPHAL, Ph.D.

Professor of Music
Sacramento State College
Sacramento, California

Photography by **Donald L. Gerhauser**
Music Consultant, El Dorado County Schools
Placerville, California

WM. C. BROWN COMPANY PUBLISHERS
135 SOUTH LOCUST STREET • DUBUQUE, IOWA

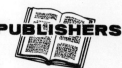

Manufactured by WM. C. BROWN CO. INC., Dubuque, Iowa

Printed in U. S. A.

For Hinda, Rick and Carl

PREFACE

This book is written primarily for the college student who is preparing for instrumental teaching in the schools and secondly as a general reference book for those interested in the teaching and study of the woodwinds. Preparation for teaching the woodwind instruments is normally a very small portion of the total requirements for a teaching credential, and in the typical teacher education program only a minimum amount of time is available for this purpose. For this reason it is necessary that the essential instructional material be carefully organized to present down-to-earth practical information as clearly and concisely as possible. Further, if the woodwind portion of the school instrumental program is to flourish, it is necessary to provide information which will support skilled instruction not only in the beginning stages of study, but which is of sufficient depth that the teacher can provide genuine assistance and instruction to his more advanced students.

Only a very small portion of the woodwind students in the schools are fortunate enough to be able to study with a skilled specialist on their instrument. All teachers are expected to be highly skilled specialists on one instrument, but cannot reasonably be expected to be equally skilled on all the instruments of the orchestra and band. This specialized skill in musicianship and performance, in performance standards and general know-how can be successfully applied to other instruments, however, if the teacher has sufficient specific detailed information about the other instruments. It is the purpose of this book to provide this detailed information.

Preparation for teaching the woodwind instruments is a two-part study. First, the study of one or more of these instruments to gain at least a minimum personal proficiency in performance in order to develop a feel for the way in which the woodwinds accomplish their musical expression, an understanding of the mechanical basis of the instrument which all the woodwinds share, and to provide the basis for empathy with future students which is so necessary for the most effective teaching. This personal proficiency provides the basis for the second phase of the study—that of completely understanding the problems of each instrument beyond the level of personal performing ability so that effective instruction can be given on all levels of advancement. The author's *Woodwind Ensemble Method* provides the material for the first phase of this preparation and the present volume the material for the second phase. The two portions of this preparation may be studied either together or successively with equal success.

The detailed material for teaching the entire family of woodwind instruments has never before been gathered and organized into a single source of sufficient scope and depth to accomplish the desired aim. Several fine books on teaching the beginning levels are available, but the additional information necessary for carrying the students to the more advanced levels is available only in scattered sources such as methods books and an occasional book on a specific instrument. It has been necessary for the instructor to present this material in lectures or other forms, or for the student to gather the material for himself. The success of this procedure is dependent upon the amount of time available for this purpose, which is rarely sufficient to do a thorough job.

This book is based on many years of research which included all available printed material, a detailed study of the widest variety of methods books for all instruments, the expressed needs of teachers on all educational levels, the performance abilities of thousands of school musicians, and teaching experiences in the East, Midwest, South and West coast. In this way the standard practices and procedures of a wide variety of skilled teachers, as well as professional players on each instrument, were discovered and the information correlated and organized into a single body of information consistent with the needs of teachers.

The primary problem in presenting such information is found in the semantics used to describe and explain a particular facet of performance. Each teacher has his own vocabulary and few agree on the exact terms to be used even though each is explaining the same thing, intend the same meaning, and hopes to produce an identical response in the student. Much of the difference of opinion in how a particular thing should be achieved on an instrument comes from the words used to describe it rather than the intended result. In this book an attempt has been made to resolve these semantics into standardized procedures, making use of the most commonly used and understood terms. This will provide the student with a standard vocabulary upon which he can build with confidence.

Where there are several prevailing points of view on a particular procedure, all are presented and described. Every experienced teacher is fully aware that there is considerable diversity of opinion among authorities on many facets of woodwind technique and performance. The very fact that there is such a variety of successful approaches to the various problems is a clear indication that there are several ways in which each of these problems can be solved. In presenting the various points of view, the reader is left free to choose that which he prefers based on his own concepts, desires and experience, as well as those of his instructor. In each instance the point of view presented first is the personal choice of the author, but the reader may use any of them with confidence in success and with the weight of authority behind the choice.

In organizing the material for maximum practical use and understanding, the step-by-step method of presentation with liberal utilization of photographs is employed for many sections. In each instance a professional player using a typical standard approach was used as a model for that instrument. In all instances where the embouchure is visible in the photograph, the player was performing on the instrument when the photograph was taken.

Other features of the book include check lists for various aspects of performances; identification of commonly found faults in each aspect of performance together with causes, results and suggestions for correction; identification of technique problems unique to each instrument and with the correct procedures suggested; discussions of alternate fingerings and when and how to use each; a bibliography of study material for each instrument; a consideration of mouthpieces for clarinets and saxophone; the selection and adjustment of single and double reeds; study and achievement questions for each chapter; and finally, complete fingering charts for each instrument and special charts of trill fingerings for each, making use of a standardized nomenclature in an easy to read format.

Each chapter is complete in itself. Readers interested in a particular subject or in a particular instrument may refer to that chapter for complete information without cross references. For this reason it is felt that the book will be a useful permanent reference when the student enters the teaching profession, and also for those teachers who may feel the need for additional information of this type.

The author is indebted to many fine teachers and professional musicians who, over a number of years, contributed generously of their time and knowledge; to his own graduate students who forcefully brought the need for this book to his attention; to his own teachers who provided models of inspiration; and to his friends and colleagues who have given generously of their time.

The author is especially indebted to Donald L. Gerhauser for the photographs in the book. He is a highly skilled public school music teacher and supervisor, a versatile and artistic performer on woodwind instruments, and an experienced photographer who combines great technical skill with an unusual sense of composition and proportion. In bringing this unique combination of knowledge and skill to the complex problems involved in this type of photography, he has made an invaluable contribution for which the author is most grateful.

A special vote of thanks is due Maury Silverman and his staff of the California School Music Service for their courtesy and genial cooperation in making music, instruments and material of various kinds available for examination and photography. To the men who successfully combine the jobs of professional musicians and teachers for the tedious job of posing for the photographs, the author is most grateful. These include Robert Klump, flute; Norman Gillette, oboe; Dennie Green, clarinet; Daniel McAullife, bassoon; William Wood, saxophone, and my colleague, Robert Humiston, for the sequence on making and adjusting oboe reeds. And finally, to my wife, who not only willingly assumed full responsibility for managing the household during the time this book was being prepared, but most capably performed above and beyond the call of duty in preparing the final manuscript, I wish to publicly express my sincere appreciation.

TABLE OF CONTENTS

CLARINET

The clarinet is considered the basic instrument of the woodwind family and it is the appropriate instrument with which to begin the study of teaching the woodwinds. In the schools there are probably more clarinet students than all the other woodwinds combined. It is by far the most common beginning woodwind instrument and countless thousands of youngsters begin the study of the clarinet each year. Some to continue on the clarinet, others to transfer to another woodwind instrument, and unfortunately many to discover that they have too little interest, motivation or talent to continue.

For these reasons as well as to insure continued development of more advanced players the basics of teaching clarinet must be thoroughly understood. While it is desirable for all teachers to have as much experience on all the woodwinds as possible, the greatest experience should be on the clarinet. The basics learned on it can be successfully applied to all the other woodwinds.

THE CLARINET FAMILY

From the high E-flat to the B-flat Contra-Bass the clarinet family forms a choir whose pitch range and tone color more nearly approximates that of the string family than any other family of woodwind instruments. A full compliment of instruments in the clarinet family forms the basis of the modern concert band. Late nineteenth and twentieth century orchestral composers have taken advantage of the variety of clarinet sounds and have used all the intsruments except the Contra-Bass.

Fingerings for all the instruments are identical except for minor adjustments on the lower pitch instruments made to help tonal control. The basic embouchure is the same for all instruments with adjustments made according to the size of the mouthpiece of the instrument.

Since the B-flat instrument is the most commonly used of the family, the discussions in this chapter will center around it, with special problems and differences between it and the other instruments in the family noted in the course of the discussion.

All the instruments in the family have the same theoretical *written* playing range:

but all are transposing instruments and *sound* in different ranges.

The transpositions and ranges in which each instrument sounds is as follows:

1. *E-flat Clarinet*: Sounds a minor third higher than written.[1]

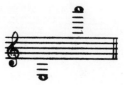

Written   Sounds

Range of actual sounds[2]

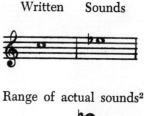

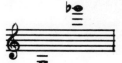

---

[1]As an aid in remembering transpositions of instruments a written "C" sounds the designated pitch of the instrument. A written "C" for any E-flat instrument sounds E-flat; a written "C" for any B-flat instrument sounds B-flat. The octave in which the sounding note is heard is determined by whether it is a soprano, alto, tenor, bass or contra-bass member of the family.

[2]In the range of actual sounds for each of the instruments the highest note is the limit of the intermediate playing range given in this chapter, rather than the theoretical upper limit.

2. *B-flat Clarinet*: Sounds a major second lower than written.

Written   Sounds

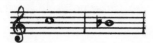

Range of actual sounds

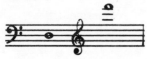

3. *E-flat Alto Clarinet*: Sounds a major sixth lower than written.

Written   Sounds

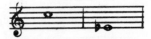

Range of actual sounds

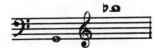

4. *B-flat Bass Clarinet*: Sounds an octave plus a major second lower than written.

Written   Sounds

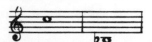

Range of actual sounds

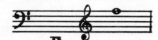

5. *E-flat Contra-Bass Clarinet*: Sounds an octave plus a major sixth lower than written.

Written   Sounds

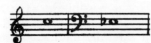

Range of actual sounds

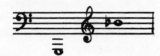

6. *B-flat Contra-Bass Clarinet*: Sounds two octaves plus a major second lower than written.

Written   Sounds

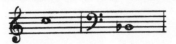

Range of actual sounds

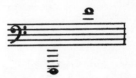

In addition to the preceding instruments which are in common use today there are three obsolescent instruments in the clarinet family which are found in orchestral scores. They are the D clarinet, another version of the E-flat soprano; the C clarinet which has been replaced by the modern B-flat instrument; and the Basset Horn, actually an Alto Clarinet in F. Even though music for these instruments is rarely found it is well to be acquainted with their transpositions.

7. *D Clarinet*: Sounds a major second higher than written.

Written   Sounds

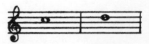

8. *C Clarinet*: Sounds as written.

Written   Sounds

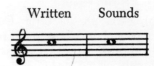

9. *Basset Horn*: Sounds a perfect fifth lower than written.

Written   Sounds

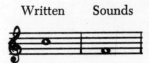

PLAYING RANGES

As indicated previously all the instruments in the clarinet family have the same theoretical written playing range, but in practice this complete range is rarely if ever called for. Certain portions of the playing ranges of the various instruments are technically easier than others for students in various stages of development, and on the lower pitched instruments notes in the extreme high register are rarely used because the tone quality produced is not really satisfactory and contributes little to the sonority of an orchestra or band.

There are generally accepted playing ranges for each of the instruments which are useful in teaching situations so that one may know what to expect from students. For convenience these have been designated as *Beginning*, the range a typical elementary school player should have by the end of his first year of study; *Intermediate*, the range which can be expected from the average good high school player; and *Advanced*, the range in which the professional player is called upon to perform. The differences in these ranges for clarinets are primarily in the upper limits, since the lowest notes do not present major difficulties either in tone production or fingering. As in any technical skill great variation in accomplishment from individual to individual can be expected, and these playing ranges are given simply as general indications.

The E-flat and A clarinets are not generally considered beginning instruments, but are usually assigned to players with previous experience on the B-flat clarinet. Students transferring to these instruments from the B-flat clarinet would not be considered beginners on these instruments and can be expected to have a much greater range than that indicated for beginners. The beginning range is, however, that which students transferring will be able to play easily and with good tone quality without too much experience on the new instrument.

1. *B-flat Clarinet (E-flat, and A)*

Beginning   Intermediate   Advanced

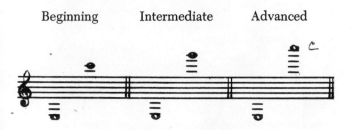

The Alto, Bass and Contra-Bass instruments, like the E-flat and A, are usually given to players who have developed a basic facility on the B-flat clarinet. As the fundamental pitch of the instrument gets lower the higher notes are increasingly unsatisfactory in quality, and for this reason most arrangers write for the Bass and Contra-Bass instruments primarily in the range indicated below as *Intermediate*. Neither the Alto nor the Contra-Bass instruments are used in orchestra. Orchestral composers and orchestrators normally use a much wider

range for the Bass clarinet than that used in band, approximately that range indicated below as *Advanced*, since the tone quality of the instrument in the upper portion of the range blends well with the string tone. All three of these instruments demand special attention to the fingering for those notes above the Intermediate range.

2. *Alto, Bass, Contra-Bass Clarinets.*

Intermediate

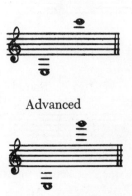

Advanced

ASSEMBLING THE INSTRUMENT

Proper assembly and disassembly of the instrument is of the utmost importance, and must be taught to students from the very first lesson. Probably more damage—bent keys, rods, bent connecting levers, etc.— is done to instruments in putting them together and taking them apart than by all other means combined. Instruments with damaged and out-of-line mechanism do not respond properly, and a great deal of the difficulty students, especially beginners, have in playing their instruments can be traced to damaged mechanism. For this reason, as well as for the simple necessity of keeping the instrument in perfect mechanical condition, proper habits of assembly must be firmly established.

The assembly of an instrument must be accomplished without putting pressure on any key or rod which will bend it in any way. It is obviously impossible to put the clarinet together without touching the keys, so in selecting the way in which the parts are held the hands and fingers must be against posts or keys and rings which are not affected by the pressure put upon them. There are, of course, various possibilities. The following step-by-step procedure is given in detail, and every student should practice it carefully until each procedure is correct and automatic. Before starting the process make sure that all cork joints are well greased with prepared cork grease so that undue pressure will not have to be applied. Study the photograph and directions for each step carefully and repeat the operation several times before proceeding to the next.

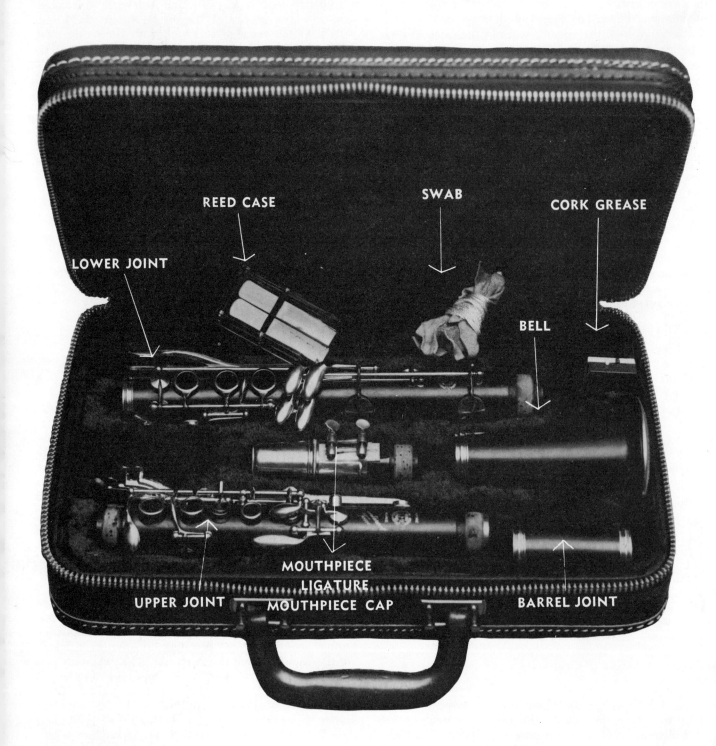

Figure C-1.

Assembling the B-flat Clarinet (E-flat and A)

A. Lower Joint and Bell Assembly

1. Figure C-2. Grasp the lower joint with the left hand, palm of the hand against the wood of the instrument beneath the keys, and with the flesh between the thumb and the forefinger against the thumb rest.

2. Figure C-3. With the palm in position, the first and second fingers cover and press the second and third rings holding the joint firmly in the palm of the hand. The other two fingers are free, and do not press on the keys. The base of the thumb is held firmly against the wood at the side of the instrument, but there must be no pressure against the rod underneath it. Students with small hands may need to press on the key covering the tone hole on the side of the instrument. There is no

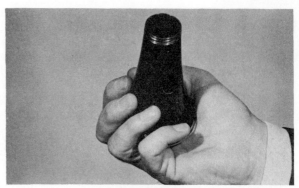

Figure C-4.

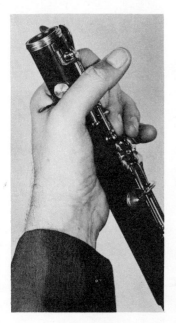

Figure C-2.

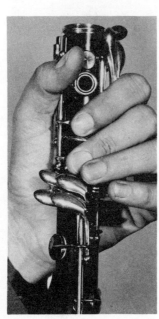

Figure C-3.

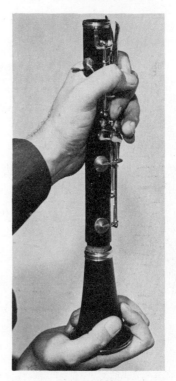

Figure C-5.

danger of bending it since it is normally in a closed position.

3. Figure C-4. The right hand graps the bell with the large end of the palm of the hand with the fingers holding it securely.

4. Figure C-5. The bell is then pushed on the lower joint with a twisting motion until it rests solidly against the joint.

B. Lower Joint to Upper Joint Assembly

1. Figure C-6. The upper joint is held in the left hand with the palm of the hand against the wood on the under side of the instrument.

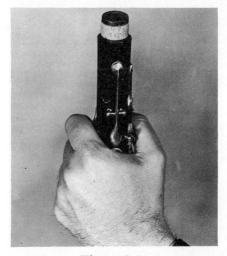

Figure C-6.

2. Figure C-7. The first finger of the hand presses on the first tone hole, and the remaining three fingers fall naturally over the remaining tone holes and the one key on the top of this joint. Pressure down on this key will not bend it as it fits solidly against the the body of the instrument when pressed down.

The ring of the second hole must be held completely down throughout the assembly of these two sections as it raises the connecting lever between the upper and lower joints so that they may be fitted together without bending. Bending this connecting lever out of line is the most common fault of improper assembly.

3. Figure C-8. The thumb rests against the lever keys on the side of the instrument. It may exert some pressure against these keys since they are not subject to bending if the pressure is downward in their normal plane of movement against the body of the instrument.

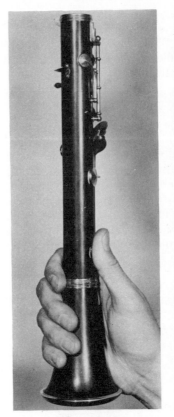

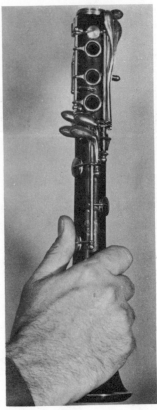

Figure C-9.   **Figure C-10.**

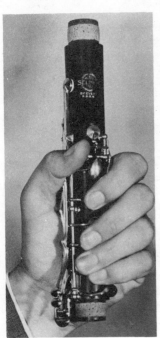

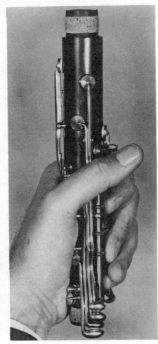

Figure C-7.   **Figure C-8.**

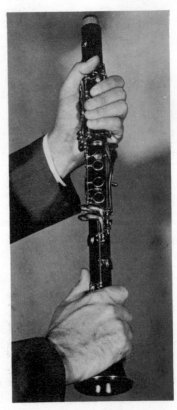

Figure C-11.

4. Figure C-9. The previously assembled lower joint and bell are held in the right hand. First finger on the wood of the lower joint, the remaining three fingers on the bell pressing the instrument against the palm of the hand.

5. Figure C-10. The ball of the thumb presses down on the key covering the bottom tone hole on the side of the instrument to add stability and control to the procedure.

6. Figure C-11. With the left hand and right hand holding the two sections properly, they are pushed together with a slight rotary motion back and forth. They must not be twisted too far from their normal alignment or the overlapping keys on either side will be bent.

7. Figure C-12. If the ring covering the second hole of the upper joint is closed, the connecting lever is raised to allow connection on the lower joint to move freely under it.

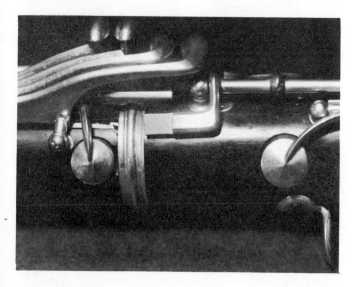

Figure C-12.

8. Figure C-13. When the two sections are firmly together line up the two sections of the connecting lever.

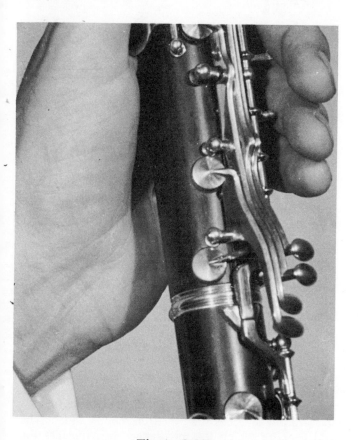

Figure C-13.

C. Adding the Barrel Joint

1. Figure C-14. Hold the barrel joint in the palm of the right hand with the thumb over the upper end and the fingers curled around it.

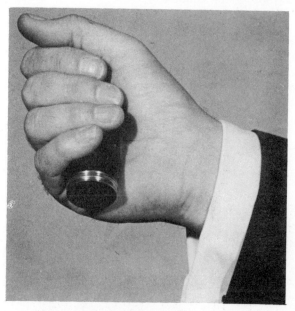

Figure C-14.

2. Figure C-15. Rest the end of the bell on the leg with the left hand holding the upper joint the same way the upper joint was held when it was connected with the lower joint. Slide the barrel joint on with a twisting motion.

D. Adding the Mouthpiece

1. Figure C-16. Hold the mouthpiece in the palm of the right hand with the tips of the fingers over the flat portion. With the clarinet resting on the leg, and the left hand holding the upper joint as before, insert the mouthpiece with a twisting motion until it is firmly seated.

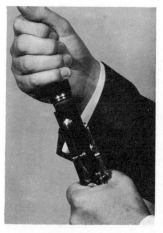 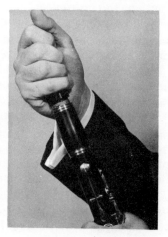

Figure C-15.   **Figure C-16.**

2. Figure C-17. Line up the flat part of the mouthpiece so that it is centered exactly on the register key on the bottom of the clarinet. The final step in the process is to add the reed. This is discussed at the end of this section of the chapter.

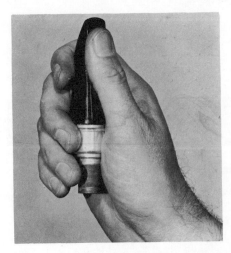

Figure C-18.

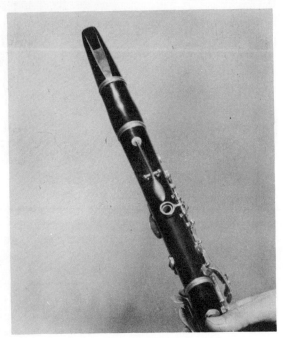

Figure C-17.

5. Figure C-20. Line up the flat portion of the mouthpiece so that it is centered exactly on the register key on the bottom of the instrument. The mouthpiece is now ready for the reed. Placement of the reed is discussed later in this chapter.

Assembling the Metal B-flat Clarinet

The metal B-flat clarinet which is widely used for young beginners has the upper joint, the lower joint, and the bell constructed as a single unit which greatly simplifies assembly. Only the barrel joint and the mouthpiece are involved in the assembly, but even so it is possible to bend keys when adding them to the body of the instrument if it isn't done properly. Young students using this model instrument should be taught the following procedure from the very beginning of their study of the instrument.

1. The mouthpiece and barrel joint are stored assembled together in the case. Remove the cap, ligature and reed from the mouthpiece.

2. Rest the clarinet in a vertical position on the leg, holding the upper joint with the left hand as described in sections B 1, 2 and 3 above.

3. Figure C-18. Hold the barrel joint and mouthpiece in the right hand, thumb on the flat part of the mouthpiece, first and second fingers around the mouthpiece pressing it against the thumb. The third and fourth fingers are not used unless the student has a small hand.

4. Figure C-19. Push the barrel joint on so it fits firmly. No twisting motion will be needed with a cork of this small diameter if it is properly fitted and well greased.

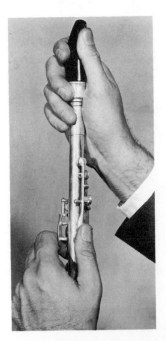

Figure C-19.

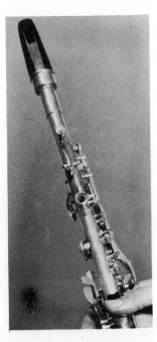

Figure C-20.

Assembling the Alto and Bass Clarinet

The way in which the Alto and Bass Clarinet are assembled differs from the procedure for the soprano instruments in only one major way. Because the bell extends up and over some of the key mechanism on the lower joint when it is in place, the upper and lower joints are put together first, then the bell is added. The metal neck on which the mouthpiece fits, replaces the tuning barrel of the soprano instruments and poses no difficulty in assembly. Because the keys and rods on these instruments are longer they are even more susceptible to the danger of being bent than the smaller intruments and must be handled with great care. Be sure all cork joints are well greased before starting the assembly. In the photographs a Bass Clarinet is used, but the procedures for the Alto and Contra-Bass instruments are identical.

A. Lower and Upper Joint Assembly

1. Figure C-21. The upper joint is held in the left hand with the palm of the hand against the wood on the underside of the instrument.

2. Figure C-22. The first finger of the hand presses on the first tone hole, and the remaining three fingers fall naturally over the remaining tone holes and the one key on the top of this joint. Pressure down on this key will not bend it as it fits solidly against the body of the instrument when pressed down. The cover of the second hole must be held down firmly throughout the assembly of these two sections as it raises the connecting lever between the upper and lower joints so that they may be fitted together without danger of bending.

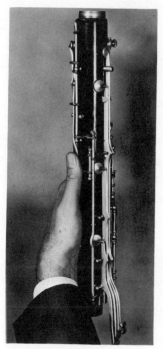

Figure C-21.   Figure C-22.

3. Figure C-23. The lower joint is held in the right hand, with the long rods of the keys operated by the right little finger protected against pressure by the palm of the hand cupped over them.

4. Figure C-24. The ball of the thumb presses the upper pad of the two tone holes on the right side, and the base of the thumb presses the lower. Avoid any pressure against the rods of these keys.

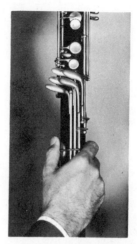
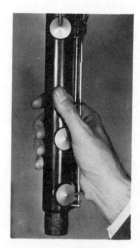

Figure C-23.   Figure C-24.

The second finger of the right hand covers and presses the pad on the left side of the instrument, and the remaining three fingers grasp the wood of the joint. Make slight adjustment in hand position if necessary to avoid any pressure on the long rods of these keys.

5. Figure C-25. With the left and right hands holding the two sections properly, they are pushed together with a slight rotary motion back and forth. They must not be twisted too far from their normal alignment or the overlapping keys on either side will be bent. When the two sections are firmly together line up the connecting lever or levers.

B. Adding the Bell

1. Figure C-26. The lower joint of the two sections already assembled is held in the left hand, with the palm of the hand against the wood of the instrument beneath the keys, and with the flesh between the thumb and forefinger near or against the thumb rest.

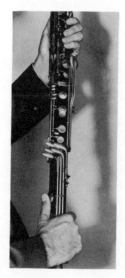
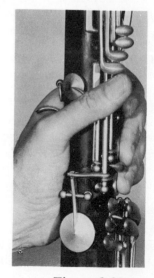

Figure C-25.   Figure C-26.

2. Figure C-27. With the palm in position, the first and second fingers cover and press the second and third rings, holding the body of the instrument firmly in the palm of the hand. The other two fingers are free and do not press on the keys bneath them.

3. Figure C-28. The base of the thumb is held firmly against the wood at the side of the instrument, but there must be no pressure against the rod under the finger.

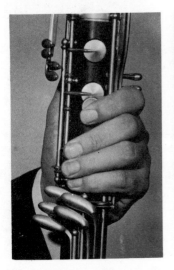
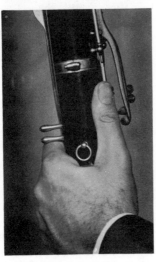

Figure C-27. **Figure C-28.**

4. Figure C-29. The right hand grasps the bell with the lower part of the front firmly placed in the crotch of the thumb. The thumb and forefinger hold the bell firmly on either side. The thumb presses the key on the bell so that it will clear the operating lever on the lower joint.

5. Figure C-30. The bell is pushed on the lower joint with a slight rotary motion from right to left to properly connect the key on the bell. Center the bell on the tone holes of the lower joint, and test keys to see that pad or pads on bell close firmly.

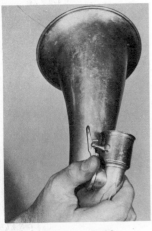
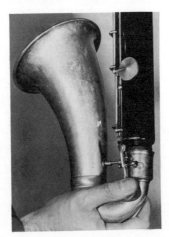

Figure C-29. **Figure C-30.**

D. Adding the Neck

1. Figure C-31. Grasp the neck with the right hand fingers, the little finger just above the cork joint. Holding the upper joint with the left hand as described in section A above, and the instrument across the legs, push on the neck section and center it on the register key beneath the instrument.

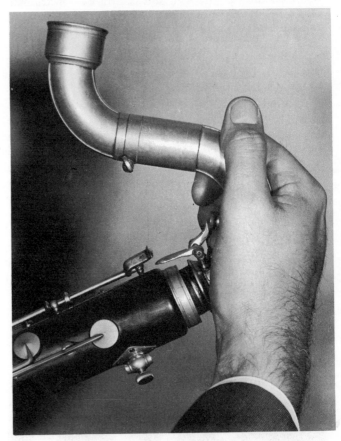

Figure C-31.

E. Adding the Mouthpiece

1. Hold the mouthpiece in the palm of the right hand with the tips of the fingers over the flat portion. With the clarinet resting across the legs, and the left hand holding the wood of the upper joint near the neck push on the mouthpiece and align the flat table with the body of the instrument. Avoid any pressure against a rod with the left hand while performing this operation. Placement of the reed on the mouthpiece is discussed later in this section of the chapter.

Placing the Reed on the Mouthpiece

Placement of the reed on the mouthpiece is highly critical since the way in which it is fitted to the mouthpiece determines its response and tone quality to a considerable degree. Placement and procedure is the same for all instruments in the clarinet family. If the reed is put on the mouthpiece and the ligature slipped over it there is danger that the ligature will chip or split the reed if it touches it. Many reeds are damaged this way by students, and even professionals have been known to ruin a good reed by hitting it with the ligature. To avoid the slightest chance of damage, and as a matter of efficient procedure it is recommended that the ligature be put on first and the reed slipped under it. The following step by step outline should be followed assiduously by all clarinetists from the beginning to the most advanced stage of development.

1. Figure C-32. Place the ligature over the end of the mouthpiece about half way down, holding it away from the flat portion of the mouthpiece with the left forefinger. (Screws on the double-screw model ligature are on the flat side of the mouthpiece, while the screw of the single-screw model is on the side away from the flat portion.) Tension type ligatures without screws are not recommended.

2. Figure C-33. Holding the reed with the thumb and forefinger of the right hand slip it under the ligature.

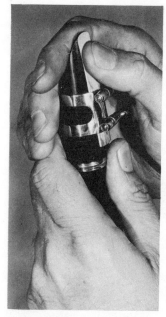
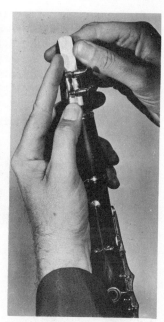

Figure C-34A   **Figure C-34B**

4. Figure C-35. The reed is the proper distance from the tip when a hair-line of black can be seen when the tip is pressed against the lay.

5. Figure C-36. Holding the reed in place with the thumb and forefinger of the left hand tighten the two screws just to the point at which they are holding the reed firmly. Avoid getting the screws too tight, which restricts the vibration of the reed.

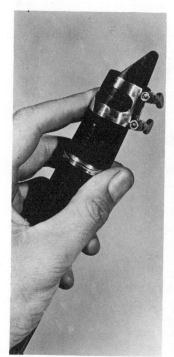
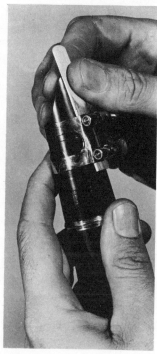

Figure C-32.   **Figure C-33.**

3. Figure C-34A. Slide the ligature down so that the edges are over the guide lines etched in the mouthpiece. Figure C-34B. Center the reed exactly at the butt so an equal amount of reed extends over each side of the flat table and at the tip so that it exactly matches the curvature of the mouthpiece.

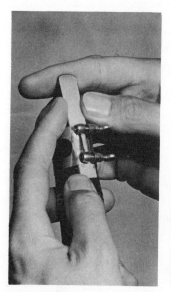
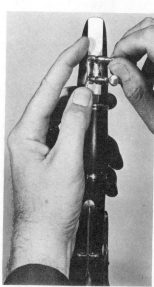

Figure C-35.   **Figure C-36.**

6. Figure C-37. When the instrument is not in use the mouthpiece cap should be in place. In order to avoid chipping the end of the reed with the cap, the upper portion of the cap should be placed lightly against the curved portion of the mouthpiece and slid into position keeping contact with the mouthpiece.

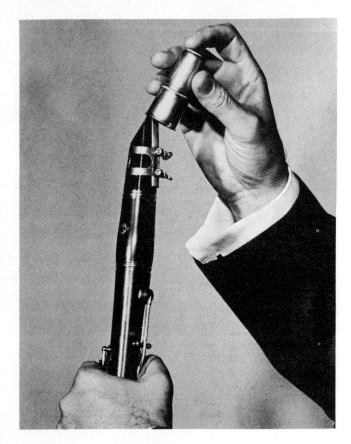

Figure C-37.

Common Faults in Assembly

There are incorrect procedures in assembling a clarinet which are commonly seen among students. The younger the student and the less experienced he is the more often he violates the best procedures. Advanced players have learned through experience the value of careful assembly, and rarely, if ever, deviate from an accepted method of preparing his instrument for playing. If the opportunity arises, observe carefully how a professional clarinetist takes his instrument from the case and puts it together, the care and detail with which the reed is put on the mouthpiece, and the way in which the instrument is tested to assure that everything is operating properly.

The following items are the most frequent faults:

1. *Holding the joints improperly.* This puts undue pressure on keys and rods which eventually forces them out of adjustment. Bent keys rub against each other and

move sluggishly or stick; bent rods cause the key to stick against its pivot screw. Some keys, especially those operated by the little finger of the left hand, are bent so that it is difficult for the fingers to reach them. Key 4x on the upper joint, operated by the first finger of the right hand, is especially vulnerable.

2. *Failure to grease cork joints.* A small container of prepared cork grease is a must for every clarinet case, and every case has a place for it. Teachers should make sure that every student has it in his case. Assuming that the cork fits properly a small amount of grease applied once a week or oftener if necessary and spread evenly over the cork will make the joints slide together easily. Excess grease must be wiped off with a soft cloth. Corks which are too large, or which are not greased make it difficult to assemble the instrument causing excess pressure against the mechanism of the instrument and possible damage. If any cork is excessively tight after being greased it may be rubbed down to the proper size with very fine sand paper.

3. *Connecting lever out of line.* The small connecting lever or levers between the upper and lower joints are the most vulnerable pieces of the clarinet mechanism. An examination of the typical elementary school beginning clarinet class would reveal that at least fifty per cent of the instruments have this lever bent out of line to a lesser or greater degree (except, of course, those students using the one piece metal instrument). This is caused by failure to hold down the ring of the second hole of the upper joint which raises the lever so that the connecting portion on the lower joint can slide under it easily. This point must be repeatedly emphasized with young or beginning students. An out of line or bent connecting lever does one of two things to the mechanism of the instrument. (1) The rings for the keys of the lower joint are kept from going down far enough for the pad connected with them on the same rod to close completely. If this happens notes which call for the fourth or fifth finger to be down either play with difficulty, squeak, or do not respond at all. If students are having difficulty in producing notes involving the fourth or fifth fingers the connecting lever is the first place to check. (2) If the portion of the lever on the upper joint is bent upward, there is no difficulty in playing notes with the right hand, but alternate fingerings for the B-flat above the staff (100 400 and 100 050) do not respond. If, when these important alternate fingerings are introduced, they are difficult to play check first the condition of this lever.

4. *Bent keys or rods.* Bent keys or rods are most frequently the result of improper assembly of the instrument. The clusters of keys played by the left and right little fingers, and the first finger of the right hand are very carefully arranged to fit under these fingers for the most efficient operation. It is possible to play with one of them bent even though the pad does not leak, but this builds in the technique of the player an improper relationship between the keys which frequently

makes technique rough and uneven. Bent keys or rods should be realigned by a repairman as soon as they are discovered. They must be removed from the instrument for straightening—never attempt to straighten a key while it is on the instrument. This puts tremendous pressure on the small posts and can easily break them or the key, making a major repair job out of a minor one.

5. *Reed improperly placed on the mouthpiece.* The way in which the reed is placed on the mouthpiece determines to a large degree how the instrument responds. Inexperienced players do not understand the importance of perfect reed placement, and teachers must check constantly to see that it is done properly. Check first to see that it is properly centered both at the tip and at the butt. A reed which is crooked is hard to blow, squeaks, or does not respond properly. If the reed is centered properly, check the distance of the tip from the tip of the mouthpiece. When looking directly across the tip of the reed toward the mouthpiece just a hair-line of black of the mouthpiece should be seen. Reeds which are too far down from the tip or which extend past the tip of the mouthpiece require greater wind pressure to produce a tone than when they are properly placed. There are minor deviations from this rule of placement which can be used in emergencies.

Check List for Assembly

Observe the student in the operation of assembling and disassembling the instrument and check the following items. Incorrect items for older students should not be called to their attention until the entire process is completed; younger students should be corrected immediately. If any mistake is made the entire process should be repeated until perfect.

	Yes	No	Comments
1. Were corks examined to see if they were well greased?			
2. Upper joint held properly?			
3. Lower joint held properly?			
4. Bell joint held properly?			
5. Barrel joint or neck held properly?			
6. Mouthpiece held properly?			
7. Connecting lever(s) perfectly aligned?			
8. Flat part of mouthpiece aligned?			
9. Ligature placed over mouthpiece before reed?			
10. Reed correctly placed on mouthpiece?			
11. Ligature tightened to proper degree?			
12. Parts assembled in the right order?			
13. Parts disassembled in the right order?			
14. Parts properly placed in case?			

HOLDING POSITIONS FOR THE CLARINETS

The manner and position in which the clarinet is held affects both directly and indirectly such important musical items as tone quality, intonation and technical facility. The proper position is one in which the body is in a comfortable erect position, in which the hands and arms fall naturally into position, and which permits the formation and development of the best embouchure. Authorities are in virtually unanimous agreement on what the proper playing positions are for all the instruments in the clarinet family, and the ones given here follow this standard. Basic seated, standing and rest positions are given here, with details of hand and finger positions following in the next section.

The B-flat, E-flat or A Clarinet is held directly in the center of the front of the body. The instrument is at about a 40 degree angle with the body, and is balanced between the right thumb and the mouth, assisted by the left thumb. Head erect, chin up, eyes straight ahead, with shoulders up but relaxed. Elbows hang free from the body. Both feet flat on the floor. Shoulders and back must not touch the back of the chair when playing. Adjust the height of the music stand so that music can be easily read in this position. When two students are playing from the same music, angle the chair slightly toward the center of the stand so that the position of the body and instrument can remain correct.

B-flat, E-flat and A Clarinets

Seated Position

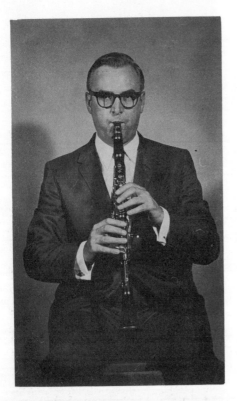

Figure C-38. Front View.

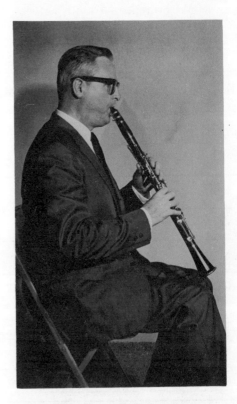

Figure C-39. Side View.

The position of the instrument when the player is standing should be identical with the seated position. Only the position of the body itself is changed. Stand erect with feet slightly apart, one foot ahead of the other to help maintain balance. Head remains erect, with chin up and eyes straight ahead. Shoulders up but relaxed, and elbows free from body. Raise the music stand, if one is being used, so that head does not tilt downward. Every player should regularly spend a portion of his practice time standing to become at ease playing in a standing position.

Standing Position

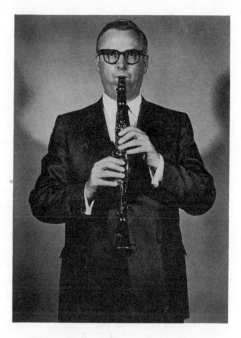

Figure C-40. Front View.

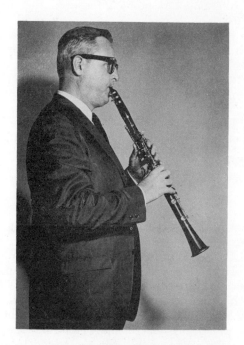

Figure C-41. Side View.

Rest Position

In the standard rest position, the clarinet is placed diagonally across the legs with the tone holes down. Some players prefer to turn the instrument so the tone holes are up. From either position it can be quickly picked up and returned to playing position. If the instrument is to be left in this position any length of time

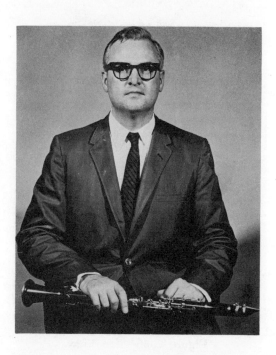

Figure C-42. Standard Rest Position.

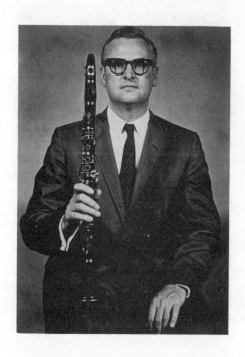

Figure C-43. Semi-Rest Position.

the cap should be put over the reed to protect it from possible damage.

The alternate rest position for these instruments is one which is used effectively by many band directors because it looks well from the audience. It is actually a semi-rest position, since the right hand remains in contact with the instrument. The bell is rested on the right leg with the clarinet in a vertical position with the right hand remaining in playing position. The clarinet can be returned to playing position quickly. This position is most effectively used during rests when the entire clarinet section of the band arrives at this position and returns to the playing position simultaneously.

Alto and Bass Clarinets

Seated Position

The Alto or Bass Clarinet (shown in photograph) is held between the legs of the player directly in front of the body. In a vertical position the bell is slightly closer to the player's body than the top of the instrument in order to put the mouthpiece at the best angle for correct embouchure formation. The weight of the instrument is held by the neck strap, with the right thumb carrying practically none of the weight, but simply controlling the position of the instrument, and balancing it in the mouth with the aid of the left thumb. Head erect,

chin up, eyes straight ahead, with shoulders up but relaxed. Elbows hang free from the body. Both feet flat on the floor. Sit forward so the instrument does not touch the chair, and shoulders and back do not contact the back of the chair. Adjust the height of the music stand for easy reading. When two players are using the same music, angle the chairs slightly toward the center of the stand so that the position of the body and instrument can remain correct.

The preceding position is the standard one for these instruments and it is mandatory that boys use it. However, girls who play these instruments frequently find it necessary, because of clothing styles, to hold the instrument to their right resting the instrument against their right leg rather than between the legs. This position is widely used, and is accepted in most sections of the country as a necessary alternative. There are some disadvantages to this position, however, since the long keys which are against the leg do not have guards to protect them from the pressure which results. For this reason they are subject to being bent either by the pressure or by catching on the clothing, and frequently operate sluggishly. Use this alternate holding position for the instruments only in case of necessity, and impress on the player the importance of protecting the keys. If this position is used then the neck and mouthpiece must be adjusted so that the proper embouchure can be formed.

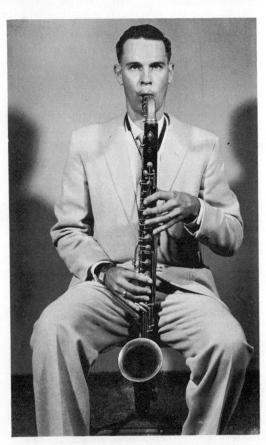

Figure C-44. Front View.

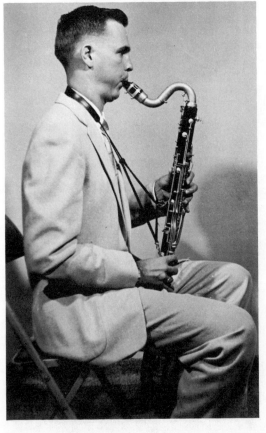

Figure C-45. Side View.

Standing Position

The Alto Clarinet is shown in these photographs. When the player is standing the position of the instrument itself and its relationship to the body should be identical with the seated position. Only the position of the body itself is changed. Stand erect with feet slightly apart, one foot ahead of the other to maintain balance. Head remains erect, with chin up and eyes straight ahead. Shoulders up but relaxed, and elbows free from the body. A certain amount of regular practice time should be spent standing in order to develop ease playing in this position.

Rest Position

In the rest position for the Alto and Bass clarinets, the neck strap is lengthened or unhooked and the instrument laid diagonally across the legs with the tone holes down. From this position it can be quickly picked up and returned to playing position, although players must allow sufficient time for adjusting or hooking the neck strap. If the instrument is to be left in this position for any length of time, the cap should be put over the reed to protect it from possible damage.

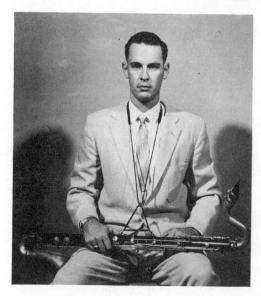

Figure C-48. Rest Position.

If the rest position is to be held for a very brief time, many players prefer to leave the neck strap hooked and rest the bell against the leg as in the photograph or simply lay the instrument across the legs with the lower joint resting against the right leg.

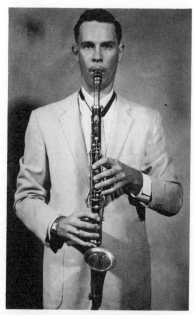

Figure C-46. Front View.

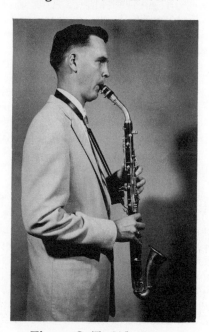

Figure C-47. Side View.

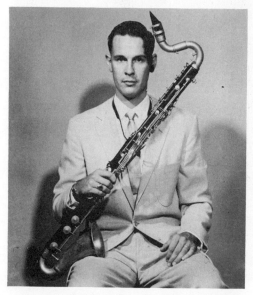

Figure C-49. Alternate Rest Position.

Contra-Bass Clarinet

Seated Position

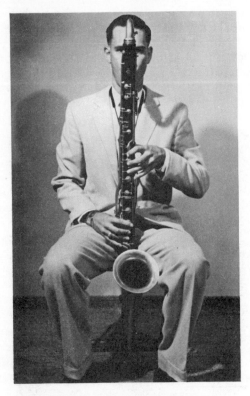

Figure C-50. Front View.

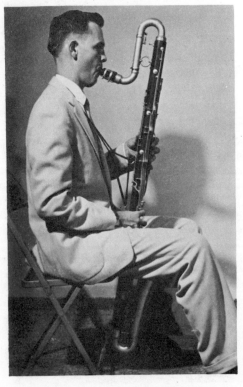

Figure C-51. Side View.

The E-flat Contra-Bass is pictured. The position for the B-flat Contra-Bass instrument is similar. The Contra-Bass is held between the legs of the player directly in front of the body. The instrument is slightly out of perpendicular with the bell closer to the player's body in order to put the mouthpiece at the best angle for the correct embouchure formation, and to allow for a comfortable position of the right hand. The weight of the instrument may be held by a neck strap as in the photographs or by an end-pin which may be added to the instrument. In either case none of the weight of the instrument is supported by the right thumb. Head erect, chin up, eyes straight ahead, with shoulders up but relexed. Elbows hang free from the body. Both feet on the floor. Sit forward on the chair so that the instrument does not touch the chair.

Common Faults in Holding Positions

The proper holding position for an instrument can further rapid musical development, or it can make progress difficult. Teachers must continually check students positions for it is important that any deviations be corrected immediately before they develop into habits. Once an incorrect position is established, it is extremely difficult to correct. Students themselves must learn to *feel* the right position, and should be encouraged to check their positions daily in front of a mirror both at school and at home. A full-length mirror is an integral part of the well-equipped instrumental room of every school.

The following are the most commonly found faults in holding positions, and most apply to all the instruments in the clarinet family.

1. *Instrument Not Centered on Body.* Some students allow the instrument to point toward one knee or the other rather than straight ahead. This is sometimes found when two students are reading from the same music and direct the instruments toward the center of the stand rather than turning their chair and their entire body, but most of the time there is no discernible reason at all. This position affects the embouchure, and thereby tone quality and control, since more of the reed is in the mouth on one side than the other thus making the line of support by the lip slightly diagonal across the reed rather than straight across. This adds a roughness or edge to the tone quality since the reed is vibrating unevenly. The slightest unevenness is magnified many times in the tone which is produced.

2. *Bell Resting on Leg.* This is a common fault with the B-flat Clarinet, and is done by the student to take the weight of the instrument off of his right thumb, or perhaps simply because he is tired or lazy or both. Some students compensate by turning their head in the direction of the leg on which the bell is resting, but even this does not correct the adverse effect on the embouchure. Sometimes the head is tilted slightly back, putting the mouthpiece into the mouth at a too small angle, which in turn puts too much pressure against the reed

restricting its vibration as well as changing the direction of the breath entering the instrument. All of these have an influence on the tone quality being produced. With some students it is possible to hear the tone quality improve if they will sustain a tone while moving the instrument from their leg into the proper position. Resting the instrument on a leg is an easy habit to fall into and should be corrected promptly every time it is seen.

3. *Fingers Assisting Thumbs in Holding the Instrument.* At the beginning stage of experience on a clarinet many students do not feel secure in holding and balancing the instrument between the right thumb and mouth, and add other fingers to secure and stabilize the instrument. This feeling is by no means restricted to very young students. Various fingers are found out of position to help hold the instrument—little fingers under the instrument or under keys, first finger of the right hand pressing on the rod on which the rings of the lower joint operate, etc. Any deviation from the standard holding position will affect smoothness of technique, or make some notes difficult to play, and in general impede progress on the instrument. Beginners will need continual checking and correction, but even more advanced students will sometimes fall rather quickly into a bad habit.

4. *Head Inclined Downward.* This problem is encountered in students at all stages of development. When the head is inclined downward, the effect on the embouchure is the same as if the clarinet were being held straight out. The angle at which the reed enters the mouth is so great that the lips cannot control the reed, and the tone which results is reedy and open in quality, and the intonation is inevitably poor. Some advanced players drift into this position when the music stands which they use are too low. This is especially true in a standing position. One remedial measure which can be taken is to put the music stand higher than it would normally be, forcing the student to raise his head, but at the same time keep the instrument at its normal 40 degree angle with the body. More often than not a decided change for the better in tone quality can be heard if the student will sustain a tone (open G, for example) while moving the head and instrument into the proper relationship. An advanced player can clearly demonstrate why this position is poor by sustaining a tone while moving the clarinet from its proper position to the straight position and back again. Even when demonstrated by a good player the change in tone quality is easily noticeable.

5. *Slouched Body.* Varying degrees of poor posture occur almost universally—shoulders slumped or curved forward, leaning against the back of the chair with spine curved, feet crossed or hung over a rung on the chair or various combinations of these. Poor posture affects breathing and breath control to the point the students may find it impossible to support the tone adequately. It pulls the arms, and consequently the fingers out of

position making technique rough. Poor posture is contagious in an instrumental group and a good teacher will see that it never starts. Emphasize to the students in as many ways as possible that good posture minimizes fatigue while poor posture increases it, and at the end of a long rehearsal players with good posture might not be physically tired at all while those with poor posture might well be physically exhausted even though their contributions to the rehearsal were not their best because of the poor posture.

6. *Moving the Body while Playing.* Nothing is more distracting to other members of the group or to the director than a player who beats time with his instrument, or who makes grandiose movements of body and instrument to emphasize a phrase or a difficult technical spot. An audience is also distracted and frequently amused by these movements. Moving the instrument up and down or back and forth changes the position of the reed in the mouth, moving the body itself alters the coordination of the muscles involved in breath support. Both the body and the instrument must be held in the proper position without any undue motions if the best musical results are to be achieved.

7. *Alto and Bass Clarinet Angle.* The most prevalent violation of a good position on the Alto and Bass clarinets involves having the bell of the instrument pushed too far forward or pulled too far back. With the bell out of poistion in either direction the angle of the mouthpiece and reed in the mouth and consequent control by the embouchure is changed. The proper relationship between mouthpiece and embouchure is built into the instruments through the shape of the neck if the instruments are almost perpendicular. Slight deviations from the exact perpendicular come naturally to players as they gain experience on the instruments and is to be expected.

8. *Adjustment of Neck Strap.* The adjustment of the neck strap on the Alto, Bass, and Contra-Bass instruments allows little deviation from the ideal if it is to be used to the best advantage. The standard adjustment of the neck strap is one in which the mouthpiece falls naturally into the embouchure without tilting the head up or down and with the weight of the instrument supported by the neck strap rather than the right thumb. An adjustment which is too high or too low forces the student to raise or lower his head which is not only a muscular strain if continued over a period of time, but also forces the embouchure formation into an unnatural shape. Because of the weight of these instruments it is virtually impossible for the right thumb to support it without cramping the right hand and forcing the fingers out of position. When a student transfers to the Alto or Bass clarinet it is well worth the time spent to help him find the proper adjustment of the neck strap since the correct and natural playing position for the instrument is so dependent on it.

HAND POSITIONS

The same basic hand position is used on all instruments in the clarinet family, the only difference being the slightly increased space between the fingers on the larger instruments. This position may be defined as one in which the fingers fall naturally into place and are completely relaxed without any muscular tension in the fingers, wrists, arms or shoulders. It is only in this perfectly relaxed condition that it is possible to develop rapid, accurate and dependable facility.

Proper position and shape of the hands on the instrument must be stressed from the very beginning of clarinet study, and checked in detail regularly until it is habitual. Even the youngest students can achieve this correct position, and indeed, progress much faster with the correct placement than with one which deviates even slightly. Almost all the difficulties beginners have in playing across the break, in playing the throat tones with facility, and in playing the lowest tones on the instrument can be traced to faulty hand and finger positions and placement. It is very easy for beginners who have not acquired a feel for the instrument to deviate to a position which temporarily feels better or gives them a greater sense of security. But the fact remains that the proper placement of the hands develops both a faster sense of security and feeling right than an incorrect one. Perhaps the greatest service a teacher can be to a student is to insist that he establish and maintain this correct position.

The following step-by-step procedure for establishing the hand position should be studied thoroughly, preferably with an instrument with which to experiment. Study both the text and the photographs carefully until they are perfectly clear. The "Guide Position" which is given is the fundamental position for hands and fingers and should be maintained at all times except when the fingering for a note involves moving a finger to another location. This position on the instrument may be compared to the guide position on the typewriter which makes it possible to develop speed and accuracy so quickly on that machine. It is used on the clarinet for the very same reason.

A. Right Hand Position

1. Figure C-52. The right thumb contacts the thumb rest on the flesh to the side of and at the base of the nail. The ball of the thumb is against the body of the instrument.

2. Figure C-53. The right little finger touches lightly Key F, and the remaining fingers are no more than an inch above the three tone holes. When closing the holes the tips of the fingers overlap the rings slightly so that the ball of the finger directly beneath the fingernail is in the center of the tone hole. The fingers fall into a natural curve without tension which allows maximum control and accuracy of movement.

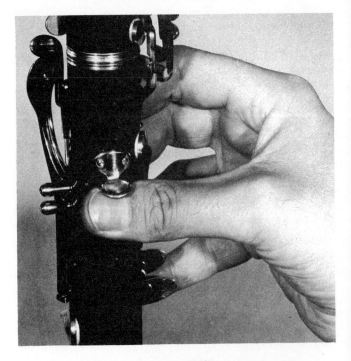

Figure C-52.

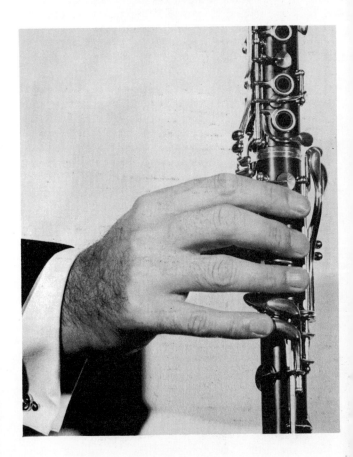

Figure C-53.

B. Left Hand Position

1. Figure C-54. The left thumb has the double duty of closing the tone hole and operating the register key beneath the instrument either independently or together. It is placed at a diagonal angle across the instrument so that the fleshy part of the ball is closing the hole, and the side of the tip just touching, but not pressing the register key. The register key is controlled by vertical movements of the first joint of the thumb.

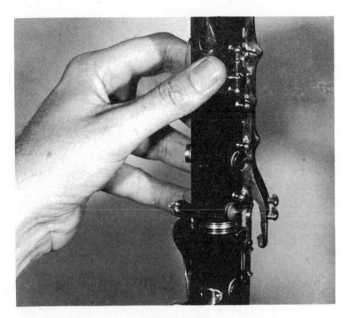

Figure C-54.

2. Figure C-55. The left little finger touches lightly Key E, and the remaining fingers cover the tone holes.

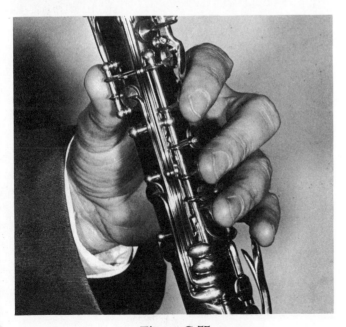

Figure C-55.

3. Figure C-56. The tips of the fingers overlap the rings slightly so that the ball of the finger directly beneath the fingernail is in the center of the tone hole. The fingers are in a natural curve.

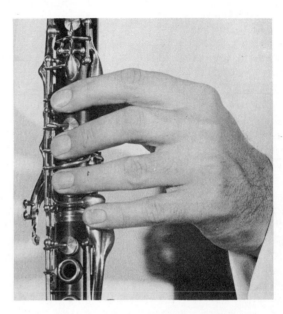

Figure C-56.

C. Guide Position

1. Figure C-57. With the thumbs and little fingers in place as described above and the remaining fingers over the tone holes a guide position is established which should be maintained constantly. Note that the fingers are at approximately a ninety degree angle to the instrument, and the wrists flat. The entire finger moves from the knuckle and closes the tone holes with a snap or click, pressing just hard enough to close the holes. Avoid too much pressure against the holes with the fingers. Fingers are kept no more than an inch directly above their hole.

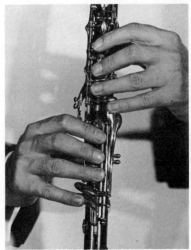

Figure C-57.

Movement of Fingers from Guide Position

Fingerings for certain notes on the instrument tend to pull the hands out of position unless fingers are moved efficiently and with minimum motion. These movements do not seem to come naturally to all students, but can be readily developed if they are understood and the teacher provides music which isolates the problem. A constant check on finger positions for these notes is necessary until the movements become habitual.

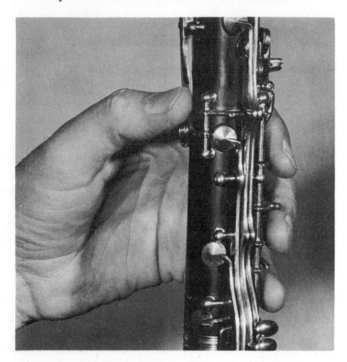

Figure C-58.

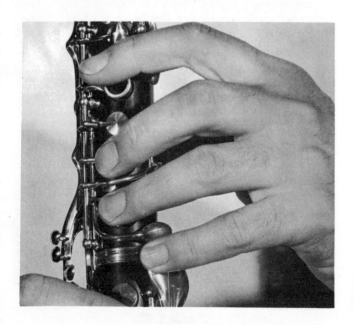

Figure C-59.

1. Figure C-58.
The left thumb fingering B-flat:

The hole is opened and the register key is opened by a vertical motion of the first joint of the thumb. The thumb contacts the register key at the side of the tip. The register key is opened with the same motion while the hole is kept closed for notes in the upper register.

2. Figure C-59.
Left hand fingering A:

The first finger is rolled toward the A key pressing it with the side of the first joint. The little finger must remain touching the E key and the other two fingers directly over their tone holes.

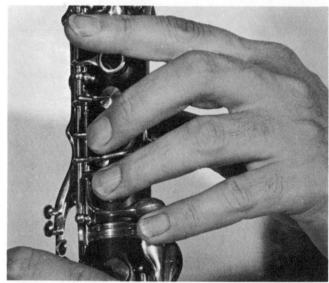

Figure C-60.

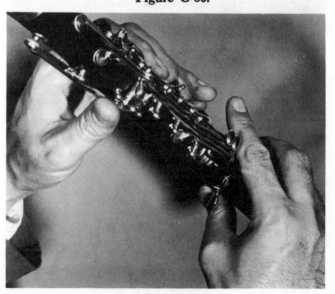

Figure C-61.

3. Figure C-60.
Left hand fingering G-sharp:
The first finger is straightened and brought directly down to contact the G-sharp key on the bottom of the finger between the first and second joints. The remaining fingers must remain in the guide position.

4. Figure C-61.
First finger right hand fingering E-flat-B-flat: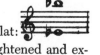
The first finger of the right hand is straightened and extended to open key 4x with a downward motion. The remaining fingers must remain in the guide position.

The same motion is used for the chromatic fingering of F-sharp: which involves the use of two of the side keys rather than one.

Common Faults in Hand and Finger Position

A clarinetist with perfect hand position both at rest and in playing is a rare individual, but at the same time a player whose hand and finger positions are poor develops facility slowly and seldom if ever becomes what would be considered a good performer. A beginning student who persists in quickly establishing the proper positions makes rapid progress in acquiring technical facility. There is a direct relationship between how the instrument is held, hand and finger positions and success on the instrument. The closer to the standard position the faster the rate of progress, and conversely the poorer the position the slower the rate of progress. Extremely poor positions make any progress on the instrument virtually impossible and quickly discourages the student.

It is of the utmost importance that proper positions be established from the very beginning of clarinet study, through careful continuous checking by the teacher who must insist on the proper position. Some teachers take the attitude that positions are not important for elementary school beginners, and that poor positions can be corrected when they become more advanced. Nothing could be more unfortunate than this attitude since many students are discouraged from continuing, and even those who do continue with the instruments have great difficulty in correcting non-standard positions once the muscular pattern is established incorrectly. It is so easy and simple to do it correctly in the beginning and so difficult to correct that every teacher who is truly interested in his pupil's progress will do everything possible to establish the proper habits from the very beginning.

The common faults which are listed here occur over and over again in students. All of these faults have an adverse affect on facility and technique—making some progressions rough, some difficult, and others impossible.

1. *Right Thumb.* There are two common faults with the position of the right thumb:

(a) Pushing the thumb too far under the instrument so that it contacts the thumb rest away from the nail, some students contacting at the first joint of the thumb and some even higher. This condition can frequently be detected by merely looking at the student's thumb since an incorrect position will cause a callous on any player who spends enough time playing the instrument to be considered an average performer. No callous will develop if the thumb is in the proper position. When the thumb is too far under the instrument the fingers are forced into an unnaturally acute angle so that the fingers must cover the tone holes toward the tip or even with the tip rather than with the natural pad on the finger beneath the nail. Younger students especially have difficulty in covering the tone holes at or toward the tip since their fingers are small, and the result is squeaks or difficulty in producing a tone at all. Further, when the fingers are at an acute angle which approaches the tone hole directly, there is considerable muscular tension which makes rapid movement difficult. When this condition is corrected with intermediate or advanced students there is a noticeable improvement in facility and smoothness of technique in the space of a few days.

Figure C-62. The right thumb must contact the thumb rest in the natural hollow on the side near the base of the nail as indicated in the photograph.

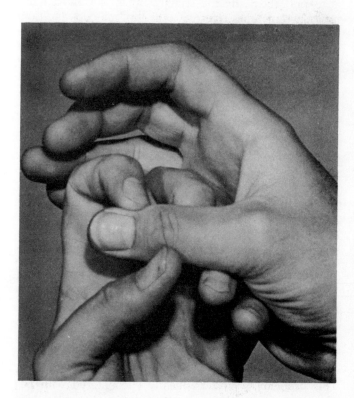

Figure C-62.

(b) The second fault is that of contacting the thumb rest with the nail itself so that the side of the finger rather than the ball is against the body of the instrument. This condition is more prevalent in beginners than it is with intermediate and advanced students, since if the condition persists advancement on the instrument is virtually impossible and the student does not continue playing. This puts the weight of the instrument on the thumb in such a way that a tremendous amount of muscular tension is needed to support the instrument and the student tires quickly. It also turns the hand slightly downward making it difficult for the fingers to contact the holes and keys in the correct way. Fortunately this faulty position is easy to correct if discovered before it becomes habitual. Students are grateful for the correction since they are immediately more comfortable playing the instrument.

2. *Little Fingers.* The guide position calls for each little finger to be in contact with a key so that they will be in a position to move rapidly and easily to other keys which they operate. If they are not on the guide keys, then there is a slight delay in putting the finger in place making for rough technique. Beginners whose little finger position has not been established frequently go so far as to take their instrument out of the mouth to look at the keys to see exactly where the little finger should go. If the fingers are on the proper key then they soon move naturally to the desired location. The most frequently found fault in the placement of the little fingers is to find them sticking straight up in the air—a tense position sometimes referred to as the "tea-cup" position. From this position they must feel for the proper key. The right little finger is frequently found hooked under the keys, apparently to help support the instrument. The left little finger frequently is placed entirely underneath the instrument for the same reason. The best, and perhaps the only, remedial measure is to insist that the fingers remain in the guide position actually touching their respective keys.

3. *Fingers Over Tone Holes.* There are several commonly found faults in the position of the fingers over the tone holes, each of which affects technical facility.

(a) Lifting the fingers too high, i.e., more than an inch above the tone holes. This is extremely common, even among advanced players, and causes unevenness in rapidly moving passages. Since the fingers usually are unequal distances above the holes it takes a slightly longer space of time for the finger highest above the holes to close the hole than it does for the finger which is closest. This space of time is frequently microscopic, but it is enough that unevenness can be heard. It is significant to note that this fault is never found among the finest players or among the professionals.

(b) Closing the holes with the tips of the fingers. This problem is most frequently encountered with beginners or inexperienced players, but also occurs with more advanced students. It happens when the fingers

do not fall in the natural curve, and may occur even though the remainder of the hand position is correct. It is frequently the result of a faulty position of the right thumb (see above), and if this is the case is easily corrected by correcting the placement of the thumb. Using the tips of the fingers to close the holes causes the fingers to fall into an unnatural position which creates muscular tension and stiff movements. Younger students with small fingers have difficulty in closing the holes entirely and get squeaks or no tone at all. The remedial action for this problem is to insist that the pad of the finger close the tone hole with the tips of the fingers lapping over and touching the ring. Figure C-63 shows a pencil pointing at the center of the natural pad on the finger. Most fingers have a natural bump which can be easily seen by looking at the fingers in profile. This natural bump must fit exactly in the center of the tone hole. This determines the amount of the overlap at the tip of the finger which varies according to the size and shape of the fingers. Check also to be sure that the wrists are flat.

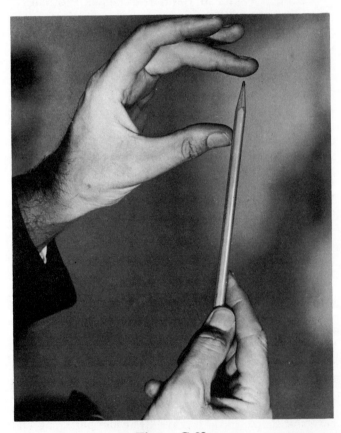

Figure C-63.

4. *Fingers Not Curved.* This problem is directly related to the preceding discussion, since a proper curve will normally result in the tone holes being closed by the pad of the finger. However, it is almost always the result of a greater or lesser degree of misplacement of

the thumb. If the thumbs and first fingers of both hands are properly placed they will form a "U." Figure C-64 shows the position of the right thumb and forefinger. That of the left is similar. The other fingers follow exactly the same curve as the forefinger. Figure C-65 shows the curve of the fingers in position on the instrument.

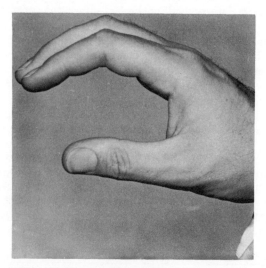

Figure C-64.

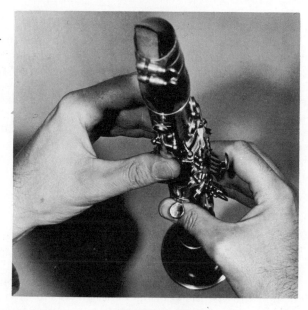

Figure C-65.

5. *Left Thumb.* The left thumb must be positioned so that it can open and close both the tone hole and

the register key singly or together. The diagonal angle described in the holding position, with the tone hole covered by the pad of the thumb, and the corner of the finger operating the register key is the position which produces the best results, and which is almost universally accepted as correct. There are several common deviations from this standard position: *, at right angles*

(a) The thumb is held almost parallel with the body of the instrument rather than diagonal. While it is possible to operate the register key properly from this position, the fingers are pulled out of position on the top of the instrument sometimes to the point that the student cannot reach the keys with the left little finger, and there is general difficulty in technique involving the left hand. Remedial measures include changing the direction of the thumb to the diagonal so that the thumb and forefinger form the "U" as pictured above, and insisting that the left little finger remain in contact with its guide key.

(b) The thumb slides back and forth over the tone hole to open and close the register key rather than operating it with a vertical movement of the joint. This will not normally happen if the thumb is in the proper relation to the body of the instrument, but it does occur and must be checked. The best remedial measure is to position the thumb properly and then have the student play intervals of the twelfth from the chalameau to the clarion register which involve only opening the register key. It should be noted that intervals of the twelfth can not be slurred down over the break. The following example is typical of the material which can be used for this purpose.

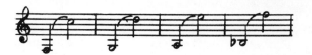

(c) The thumb is removed from the tone hole and put on the body of the instrument when playing the throat tones G, G-sharp, and A which do not involve the use of the left thumb. The thumb should be no more than an inch directly below the tone hole just as the fingers on the tone holes above the instrument are kept within an inch. Beginning students are especially susceptible to this difficulty, and frequently have trouble replacing the thumb for the following note. Practicing a pattern such as the following will impress on the student the correct use of the thumb in this connection, although persistent effort is necessary to make the correction if it has become habitual.

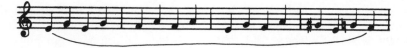

6. *Angle of Hands.* The standard placement of the hands on the instrument places the fingers of both hands at an almost perfect right angle to the instrument. This right angle is relatively easy to achieve with the right hand once the placement of the thumb is correct, but there is frequently a problem with the left hand. One well known and accepted approach to hand position which can be described as a standard deviation from the position given previously calls for the left fingers to approach the instrument at a slightly downward angle so that the edge of the first finger touches the "A" key. The little finger remains in contact with the "B" key for the guide position. Figure C-66 illustrates this posi-

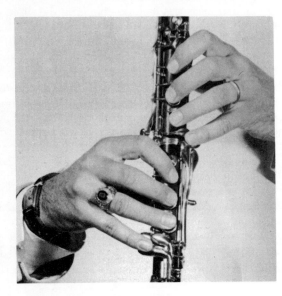

Figure C-66.

tion. This position shortens the amount of roll the first finger must do in order to play "A." But it does have the disadvantage, and it is a serious one, of pulling the little finger away from the keys it operates, making the finger stretch into a flat positon to reach them with the resulting undesirable muscular tension. This is not a problem for the player who has long fingers, but it is a problem for the player with short fingers, and a serious problem for the young beginner. A student with short fingers who uses this left hand position will have to roll his entire hand in order to reach the keys with the little finger, and some students have been observed rolling their entire left shoulder to put the little finger into position. The slight advantage of shortening the amount of roll of the first finger for "A" is greatly outweighed by the disadvantages and this hand position is not recommended, although many fine teachers will not agree. The right hand fingers angle downward so that the side of the first finger is directly above the first side key.

7. *First Finger Left Hand.* The first finger of the left hand is involved in covering a tone hole and operating two keys, and as a result is constantly changing position. There are two common faults in the way in which this finger is used:

(a) The finger hops from the tone hole to the "A" key rather than rolling, and the result is an unwanted "G" grace note preceding the "A" unless the tone is completely stopped. The rolling motion of the finger is controlled from the knuckle and involves a rather wide movement of the second joint. The movement can be seen and understood by the student making use of a pencil. Put four fingers on the pencil and hold it against them with the thumb, lining up the four fingers as if on the instrument. Hold the end of the pencil with the other hand and move the second joint of the first finger from side to side, so that none of the other fingers move. The rolling motion of the tip of the finger is exactly that used on the instrument. A musical example such as the following one applies this movement to the instrument. In practicing it the left little finger should press down firmly on its guide key closing it completely so that the hand will be held in the correct position.

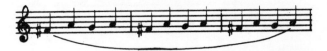

(b) The finger presses the G-sharp key with the side of the finger by rolling the entire hand over rather than by straightening the finger and pressing the key with the bottom of the finger at the second joint, or the curve of the finger will be increased and the key pressed with the tip of the finger. Both of these draw the hand out of position and cause technical difficulties with the note or notes which follow. The following exercise makes use of notes which will illustrate the correct usage of the finger.

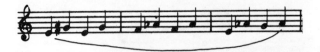

8. *First Finger Right Hand.* In addition to covering a tone hole the first finger of the right hand operates four keys on the side of the instrument, but is primarily concerned with the first one of the group which produces E-flat and B-flat in the two registers of the instrument, and it is with this fingering that we are concerned in the first of the two problems presented:

(a) The first finger presses the key with the side of the finger by turning the entire hand rather than stretching the finger and playing it with the bottom of the finger. Turning the hand pulls the rest of the fingers

Check List for Holding and Hand Positions

The following list of items provides a thorough check of holding positions and hand positions, and is limited to the seated positions for the instruments. The check should be performed while the student is playing and perferably when he is not aware that the check is being made. Any items which are checked "No" should be corrected with the deviation explained to the student, what effect it has on his playing, and why the correct position is important. Students make a more serious effort to correct mistakes if they thoroughly understand the reasons for them.

A. Holding Position

	Yes	No	Comments
1. Instrument in center of body?			
2. Angle with body correct?			
3. Head up?			
4. Shoulders up and relaxed?			
5. Elbows free from body?			
6. Height of music stand correct?			
7. Body posture good?			
8. Feet in place?			
9. Neck Strap (if any) adjusted properly?			

B. Hand Positions

1. Right thumb contacting thumb rest properly?			
2. Left thumb at diagonal across instrument?			
3. Tip of left thumb touching register key?			
4. Fingers curved?			
5. Fingers across instrument at proper angle?			
6. Right little finger touching guide key?			
7. Left little finger touching guide key?			
8. Thumbs and forefingers form a "U"?			
9. Wrists flat?			
10. First finger roll to "A" key?			
11. Register key operated by vertical movements of the first joint?			
12. Side G-sharp played with bottom of straight finger?			
13. Right hand kept in position when forefinger plays a side key?			
14. Guide position consistently maintained?			
15. Balls of fingers closing holes?			

out of position which in turn creates technical problems. In correcting this make sure that the little finger is kept firmly in place on the guide key. Practice the following exercise with the little finger pressing and closing the guide key so that the hand will be kept in place, and making sure that the key is pressed with the bottom of the finger near the second joint.

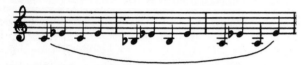

(b) A second, and fortunately less common, fault in the use of the first finger of the right hand is found when the bottom of the finger underneath the second joint is pressed against the rod to which the rings of the tone holes are connected. Beginners do this to help steady the instrument, and if not corrected immediately it becomes habitual. If this finger is pressing the rod it is immobilized and the tone hole is opened and closed by movements of the second joint of the finger, an intolerable condition which hinders technical development. Remedial action is to insist on the "U" shape formation between the thumb and forefinger, and the proper curve on all the fingers.

EMBOUCHURE FORMATION

"The embouchure is the interpreter of our sensations and of our musical ideas. A good embouchure is therefore indispensable, and all our labours must tend to this result."—H. Klose

An embouchure may be defined as the formation of the performer's lips with supporting muscles, teeth and jaws in relation to the mouthpiece and reed which have to do with tone production. The criteria for a good embouchure may be stated as follows:

A good embouchure is one which over the entire range of the instrument:

1. Produces (or has the potential of producing) a rich, full bodied, clear tone.

2. Plays perfectly in tune.

3. Allows the player to use the full scope of articulations from a hard short staccato to the smoothest legato at all dynamic levels and without adverse effect on tone quality.

4. Allows the player to use the full range of dynamics from the very softest to the very loudest under complete control and without affecting either pitch or tone quality.

5. Plays and is controlled with a minimum amount of physical exertion.

6. Once developed can be maintained with a reasonable amount of practice.

Conversely a poorly formed embouchure is one in which:

1. The tone quality is reedy, thin, nasal, or which changes quality from register to register on the instrument.

2. Plays upper register, lower register or throat tones out of tune consistently, or with which it is difficult or impossible to adjust the pitch of individual tones.

3. Produces staccato notes which are hard, with mechanical noises, or which have poor tone quality.

4. Has a restricted dynamic range in which tonal body is lost at soft levels, and very loud levels impossible to produce.

5. Requires an undue amount of physical exertion.

6. Deteriorates rapidly without an undue amount of daily practice.

Among fine clarinet teachers there is considerable difference of opinion on exactly how the best embouchure should be formed, but at the same time there are many points on which there is unanimous agreement. Much of the difference of opinion can be traced to the semantics with which the formation is explained, since it is difficult to write and talk about something which is physical and musical. However, it becomes clearly apparent that there are basically only two clarinet embouchures in general use today. Each is subject to minor differences from teacher to teacher but the fundamental and basic formation is the same. The major difference between the two is found in the shape of the lower lip, one embouchure bunches the lower lip to a greater or lesser degree, the other stretches it to a lesser or greater degree. Both descend from a long line of illustrious performers and teachers and both meet the criteria for a good embouchure when properly developed. Historically, the first is an Americanized version of the old French school of playing, while the second is an Americanized version of the old German school of playing. Both can be traced back through generations of students and teachers to fine emigrant clarinetists who came to this country around the turn of the century as principal clarinetists in major symphony orchestras and whose teachings have been modified and refined to fit the demands of the contemporary American musical scene.

For convenience and clarity the bunched lower lip formation is called a "Soft Cushion" and the stretched lower lip a "Hard Cushion." The words "hard" and "soft" are relative and must not be taken literally. Those familiar with embouchure formation on other instruments will recognize immediately that the same dichotomy exists not only in the other woodwind instruments but on instruments in the brass family as well.

The Soft Cushion Embouchure

The basic formation of the soft cushion embouchure can be achieved through the following step-by-step procedure: Check each step with a small mirror on the music stand.

1. Keeping the lips lightly together drop the lower jaw so that the teeth are about three-eighths of an inch apart.

2. Shape the lips as if saying the letter "O." The corners of the mouth are slightly compressed and there are wrinkles in the lips, especially the lower one.

3. With the teeth dropped and the lips in the "O" position the rim of the lip which divides it from the chin should be directly in front of the top edge of the front teeth. Feel this with a finger and raise or lower the jaw until this relationship is correct.

4. Maintaining this position insert the mouthpiece of the clarinet into the mouth allowing the reed to push the lower lip over the teeth. If the wrinkles in the lower lip are maintained, the line dividing the lip from the chin is directly over the front edge of the lower teeth. Students with thicker than average lips will probably adjust so that less lip is over the teeth. Contract the lips and especially the corners of the mouth inward and around the mouthpiece so that no air can escape.

5. The end of the reed must be clear of any contact with the lip for three-eighths to a half-inch in order to vibrate freely. Feel this with the tongue.

6. The upper teeth rest, but do not press, on the top of the mouthpiece about a half inch from the end.

7. The lower teeth remain in the open position established in step three above, and must not bite or exert pressure against the lower lip.

8. The chin is held in a firm flat position with a slight downward pull of the muscles.

9. The first efforts at tone production should be with the mouthpiece alone. Check the embouchure formation in the mirror, and using standard breath support produce a tone by blowing without using the tongue. Continue practicing with the mouthpiece alone until a steady natural tone of the higest pitch (approximately C, second line above the treble clef) can be sustained for at least ten seconds. Check constantly in the mirror to be

certain that the effort of blowing and producing a tone does not change the shape of the embouchure. When this is accomplished the student is ready to proceed with tone production on the entire instrument.

The following illustrations show a typical soft-cushion embouchure formation. As in all photographs in this book where the embouchure is visible the photographs of the mouthpiece in the embouchure were taken during performance on the instrument. Figure C-67 shows the shape of the lips as described in steps two and three of the step-by-step procedure. Notice the wrinkles in the lips which are produced when the corners of the mouth are pushed toward the center. Support of the reed and mouthpiece by this inward pressure from the corners is basic to this type of formation. Figure C-68 and Figure C-69 show the front and side views of this embouchure in action. Observe how much of the mouthpiece is in the mouth and the angle of the mouthpiece in relation to the chin. Notice the shape of the chin in the side view where the chin muscles are firm and pulling down.

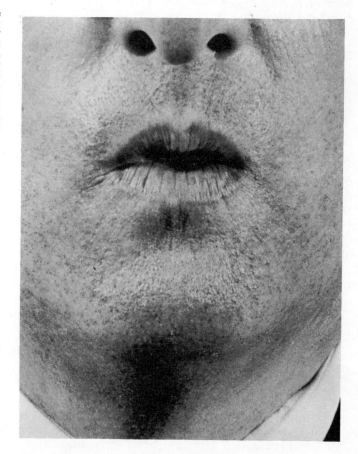

Figure C-67.

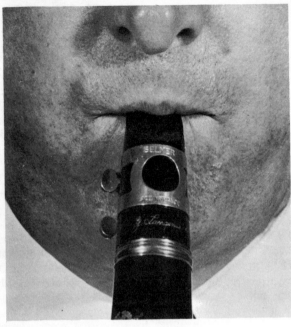

Figure C-68. Front View.

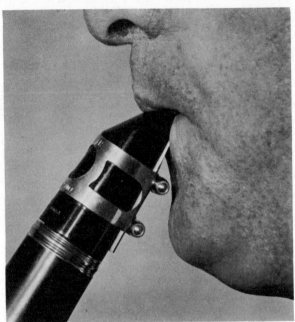

Figure C-69. Side View.

Any experienced teacher will verify the fact that while it is fairly simple to explain and form the embouchure in the manner given above, maintaining it in perfect condition over a period of weeks and months while the student is struggling with tone production and fingering problems is an entirely different matter. For this reason it is suggested that every student who is working on embouchure formation, whether he is at the beginning, intermediate, or advanced level, have a small mirror on the music stand for constant reference.

The teacher will have to check frequently to catch any deviations from the standard. Students, especially beginners of any age, are not always capable of discovering their own mistakes, or of actually knowing when they are right and when they are wrong. The embouchure must be established by how it feels in the mouth and how the tone sounds, as well as how it looks in the mirror. The teacher must tell the student when he is right so he can discover the right feel, hear the right sound, and see the right shape.

1. Perhaps the most frequent mistake in the formation of the soft cushion embouchure is indicated by the presence of a dimple in one or both cheeks. These are caused when one muscle is pulling back the corner of the mouth, while at the same time another muscle is attempting to contract the lower lip. This situation is much easier to discover than it is to correct, and the only solution is long sustained tones while the student watches himself in a mirror to see that the dimple doesn't return. This is a serious problem since the pulling back of the corners lessens the support of the lip against the

reed with a consequent loss of tone quality. Students with this condition tire easily since two sets of muscles are pulling against each other.

2. A second problem which must be checked is the amount of lower lip over the teeth. Too much lip over the teeth produces an open tone with many squawks but too much mouthpiece in the mouth produces the same symptoms so a visual check and experimentation with the amount of mouthpiece in the mouth is necessary. Too little lip over the teeth produces a cushion which is too small to control the vibrations of the reed and produces a very nasal reedy tone quality which is usually quite flat in pitch, especially in the upper register. But again, too little mouthpiece in the mouth produces much the same sound so a visual check for this is also necessary. It is virtually impossible to produce a smooth pleasing tone which is in tune if there is too little mouthpiece in the mouth, or too little lip over the lower teeth. The ensemble quality of many school bands which is objectionable because of the clarinet section sound could often be remedied by simply adjusting distance of the mouthpiece in the mouth and/or amount of lower lip. These adjustments are relatively easy to make, requiring a minimum amount of attention to establish by intermediate and advanced students.

3. Biting the reed with the lower teeth to a greater or lesser degree is a frequently found condition. This pressure against the reed restricts the amount of vibration possible, and produces a thin stuffy tone with little body, and requires considerably more breath pressure to produce a tone than the correct pressure. Reducing

this pressure by dropping the jaw back into the open position immediately frees the tone and improves both body and quality. Students with this excess pressure find it difficult to produce tones above high "C" and this difficulty is usually a sure sign of excess pressure. The position of the lower jaw in relation to the lip remains the same throughout the entire range of the instrument. As an aid in getting this open position the student may play low "E" as loudly as he can which forces the lower jaw down and demands quite a relaxed condition if the note is to be played very loudly. He can then be directed to play over his entire range with this same embouchure adjustment. While this position is much too open for high notes, it does put across the point.

4. The amount of mouthpiece to put in the mouth is dependent on several variables—facial characteristics, mouthpiece, and reed—and the final determination is made by ear, moving the mouthpiece back and forth slightly, to secure the best tone quality. The physical characteristics of the student's dental-facial formation are an important factor. Students with thicker lips will use less of the lower lip over the teeth than the average given in the step-by-step procedures, while students with thin lips will need the entire red of the lip over the teeth. Students with mouth formation wider than average will use fewer wrinkles in the lower lip. The adjustments are made to secure a firm but not hard cushion for the reed to rest on, which has sufficient area to control vibrations of the reed with a minimum of effort.

5. The type of mouthpiece being used is a second factor to be considered in shaping the embouchure. The length and amount of curvature of the lay, and the size of the opening at the tip help determine the exact location of the mouthpiece. The lower teeth must be slightly forward, i.e., toward the tip of the mouthpiece, of the point at which the lay starts breaking away from the reed in order that the cushion may control its vibration. A mouthpiece with a slight curvature and small opening at the tip requires that the lower teeth be fairly close to the break-away point, while a mouthpiece with a larger curvature and wide opening at the tip requires that the lower teeth support the cushion closer to the tip of the mouthpiece farther away from the break-away point. The exact placement can be determined only by hearing the student play and adjusting the distance of the mouthpiece into the mouth to achieve a tone with the best body which is well in tune and which is easily controlled.

6. The third variable—the reed—is directly related to, and must be chosen for a particular mouthpiece and an individual student. However a general observation concerning the strength of the reed used on a mouthpiece and embouchure formation is possible. Stiffer reeds require more pressure of the cushion against them for control than do softer ones, and a reed which is too stiff tends to encourage biting. If less mouthpiece is used for stiff reeds than for soft ones the tendency to bite with the lower teeth is reduced.

7. Puffing cheeks is a problem with many beginners as well as with some more advanced students. They indicate a lack of support by the cheek muscles which may or may not affect the support corners of the mouth are giving the mouthpiece. It always indicates that breath support necessary to produce the tone is not properly focused and directed into the mouthpiece. This problem must be corrected if the student is to achieve his goal of becoming a fine player. Frequently the student does not realize that the cheeks are puffed, and the use of the mirror to check embouchure formation is valuable. When the student can see that the cheeks are not puffed he can feel the muscular support which is necessary to keep them in place and make the correction. It is sometimes useful to have him feel the cheeks with one hand while playing open "G."

8. Some students will achieve a good embouchure except for the fact that the upper lip is somewhat relaxed which either allows a little air to escape or which puts too much pressure by the upper teeth against the mouthpiece. If this occurs the student may be told to push down with the upper lip to push the mouthpiece entirely away from the upper teeth while playing so that he can feel the muscular movement. The amount of downward pressure can then be relaxed to the proper amount.

9. Escaping air from one corner of the mouth while playing is another clear indication that something is wrong with the embouchure formation. Normally it means that the lips are not being kept in a circle with pressure against the mouthpiece from all directions, but are being relaxed at that corner. The imagery of suggesting that the lips act as a draw-string closing around the mouthpiece is frequently helpful. This is described as the "laundry-bag" concept by one teacher, and seems to have real and effective meaning to many students.

10. A very commonly found problem with beginners is their failure to keep the chin muscles firm. Instead of pulling downward the chin is pushed upward and the muscles bunched under the reed. This carries with it an excess of pressure agains the reed both with the lip and in association with the lower jaw. Only a minimum amount of success is possible for the student who has this condition, and unless it is corrected the student will soon drop the instrument. This condition is extremely difficult to correct once it has become fixed, and for this reason must be observed and corrected and measures taken to keep it from occurring from the very first day of study. A mirror will help the student check himself while practicing. *Stop*

The Hard Cushion Embouchure

The hard cushion embouchure is formed in virtually diametric opposition to the soft cushion, and like the soft cushion is subject to many slight variations.

The basic formation of this embouchure can be achieved through the following step-by-step procedure. Use a mirror on the music stand to check each step.

1. Drop the lower jaw so that the teeth are about three-eighths of an inch apart, allowing the lips to open also.

2. Draw the lower lip over the teeth so that approximately one-half of the red of the lip is covering the teeth. Test by putting a finger against the lip to see that the front edge of the upper teeth is in the center of the lip.

3. Using the "smile" muscles pull the corners of the mouth back in a smiling position.

4. The chin is held firm in a flat and pointed position pulling the lower lip against the teeth, forming a smooth hard cushion upon which the reed rests.

5. Put the mouthpiece in the mouth so that the upper teeth are resting approximately a half-inch from the lip. This distance is adjusted in or out for students with a greater than normal underbite or with an over-bite.

6. The corners of the mouth are pushed together to prevent air from escaping while maintaining the smiling position.

7. A slight downward pressure of the upper lip and a slight upward pressure of the lower lip provide the support for the mouthpiece and reed.

8. First efforts at tone production should be made with the mouthpiece alone as described in step 8 of the soft cushion formation. Continue to check constantly with the mirror to maintain the proper shape.

Common Faults in Hard Cushion Embouchure Formation

Problems encountered forming the proper hard cushion embouchure may be summarized as follows:

1. The amount of lip over the lower teeth is dependent on the size and thickness of the lips of the individual student. Students with very thin lips may need to put the entire lip over the lower teeth, while students with thick lips may need to use as little as one-third of the lower lip. The correct distance can be determined by a visual check and by the tone quality produced.

2. The amount of mouthpiece in the mouth is determined by the nature of the teeth of the individual student. The position described above is satisfactory for the average or normal formation, and is suggested as a means of putting the lower teeth at the proper supporting point under the lower lip against the reed. This distance is determined in the same manner as described for the soft cushion formation. Students with protruding upper teeth will need to place them farther than a half inch on the mouthpiece. If the lower teeth or jaw

protrude he will need less than a half inch distance from the tip of the mouthpiece.

3. The chin must be kept pointed at all times as it is this muscular tension in a downward direction which maintains the hard cushion over the lower teeth. If the chin is relaxed or pushed up the cushion is lost and there is too much pressure against the reed which restricts its vibration resulting in a poor tone quality. A stretched flabby hard cushion formation produces the poorest imaginable tone quality on the instrument.

4. The corners of the mouth should maintain the smile position and the most frequently encountered problem in this connection is that they are pulled back too far into a position similar to the make-up on a happy circus clown. This exaggerated position makes control difficult and often causes air leakage around the mouthpiece. This condition can be corrected by pushing the corners of the mouth slightly toward the mouthpiece, while relaxing the tension on the smile muscles.

5. Biting or excess pressure of the lower teeth against the reed is as frequent with this embouchure formation as with the soft cushion formation. Excess pressure restricts the reed vibration, demands excess breath pressure to produce a tone, makes high tones difficult to play in tune, and inhibits the development of a good tone quality. Insist that the teeth remain apart as described. If there is too much pressure the student can feel well-defined indentations on the inside of his lower lip with his tongue and will complain of a "sore" lip.

The problems involving the mouthpiece, the reed, and puffing cheeks are similar with those encountered with soft cushion formation and need not be repeated here.

Comparison of the Soft and Hard Cushion Embouchures

Both the soft cushion and the hard cushion type of embouchure are subject to infinite variation, all of which are slight, depending on the training of the person using them. None of these variations affect the basic formation, but primarily involve the semantics used in describing them. No two teachers will agree exactly on how to describe the correct formation. The production of pleasing musical sounds as the end product of developing an embouchure is the goal of every teacher and performer, and is the same no matter what road is taken to get there. The final judgment of whether an embouchure is good or bad cannot be made on how it is described or how it is formed but how it actually sounds.

The decision on whether to use the soft cushion or the hard cushion approach is dependent on the ultimate type of tone quality desired. Both styles produce musically pleasing sounds. A comparison between fine players using both styles will reveal that generally speaking the soft cushion embouchure produces a dark full-bodied tone quality capable of great shading, while the hard cushion produces a clear flute-like quality somewhat less

Check List for Embouchure Formation

The following check on embouchure formation must be made while the student is playing and preferably when he is not aware that a check is being made. Any errors should be carefully explained to the student, the correction worked out with him while he is observing the embouchure in a mirror. Remedial exercises can be assigned on the basis of this list.

A. Soft Cushion Embouchure	Yes	No	Comments
1. Lips rounded with wrinkles?			
2. Mouthpiece proper distance in mouth?			
3. Corners of lips pushed inward?			
4. Sufficient lip over lower teeth?			
5. Are lower teeth biting?			
6. Cheeks puffed?			
7. Dimples in cheek?			
8. Air escaping?			
9. Chin firm and down?			

B. Hard Cushion Embouchure			
1. Mouthpiece proper distance in mouth?			
2. Proper amount of lip over lower teeth?			
3. Chin firm and pointed?			
4. Cheeks in proper smiling position?			
5. Lower lip smooth and firm?			
6. Corners pushed in slightly?			
7. Are lower teeth biting?			
8. Cheeks puffed?			
9. Air escaping?			

full-bodied but capable of a variety of shading. Few teachers or students have the opportunity of making direct comparisons between the two approaches, but should take advantage of the opportunity if it arises. People like the sound with which they are most familiar which is as it should be.

Other Embouchure Formations

The Double Embouchure. This embouchure formation, sometimes referred to as the "French Embouchure," calls for the upper lip as well as the lower lip to be over the teeth, hence the designation "double embouchure." Except for the upper lip over the teeth this embouchure is formed using either the soft cushion or the hard cushion shape, or a formation between the two.

This type of embouchure is rarely used today and when it is used is justified on the basis that it is the official "French" style. But an investigation reveals that it is no longer widely used in France. In fact when the question on the use of the double embouchure was put to the principal clarinetist of a famous French musical organization touring the United States the reply was a hearty laugh, and the statement that he knew no one who used it.

The few teachers in this country who still play with the double embouchure do not always insist that their students use it. It is a very difficult embouchure to develop since only those players with a longer than normal upper lip can pull it over the teeth easily, those with normal length upper lip have some difficulty, and a short upper lip makes it impossible. Strength and control is achieved very slowly with this embouchure, but its most serious drawback, and one which a player who uses it admits, is that constant daily practice is necessary to maintain it, since strength and control is lost rapidly if the instrument is not played. For this reason alone this formation is undesirable, and for all practical purposes can be considered obsolescent since only players of the older generation continue to use and teach it. Experience has shown that students who change from the double embouchure to either the soft or hard cushion formation have little desire to return to it.

The German Embouchure. This embouchure differs from all the previous embouchures in that neither the upper lip nor the lower lip is over the teeth. With this embouchure the clarinet is pushed firmly against the upper teeth by the right thumb, and the lower lip is placed against the reed from a position in front and beyond the front edge of the lower teeth. The upper teeth contact the top of the mouthpiece almost an inch from the tip—twice as far as other embouchures. This

embouchure is infrequently used and taught in this country, since it demands a mouthpiece with a long lay and preferably reed with the German cut which are not commonly available.

This is the most difficult of all embouchure formations to develop. Considerable lip pressure is required for control, and this is acquired slowly since so few muscles, compared to other embouchures, can be involved. One authority mentions the fact that it is difficult to make the delicate shadings required by contemporary standards of interpretation with this embouchure.

In order to reduce the amount of lip pressure and to gain a greater control of the tone, the embouchure is modified considerably when used in this country. These modifications include the use of a shorter lay on the mouthpiece which allows the use of a less stiff reed and requires a little less mouthpiece in the mouth. But the fact remains that even with these modifications this embouchure formation is much more difficult to develop, lacks flexibility, and is much more difficult to develop a fine tone than either of the standard formations.[3]

Old Italian Embouchure. This embouchure formation is mentioned as a curiosity rather than as having any practical value, since it has not been used for many, many years. The formation of this embouchure calls for both lips to be over the teeth as in the French formation, but with the mouthpiece turned over with the reed against the *upper* teeth. This formation is said to have required a very soft reed which made intonation a real problem, and variety in articulation was obviously impossible. It is interesting to speculate on how players using this embouchure actually sounded!

TUNING

All clarinets must be carefully and regularly tuned to the standard international pitch of A-440. Tuning for them as for all wind instruments is best done with an electronic aid which provides a visual check on pitch. Tuning bars and tuning forks are useful for checking single notes through the use of "beats" or direct comparisons, but are not as useful as an instrument which could check the pitch of all the notes on the instrument. The piano is perhaps the poorest source of tuning notes that it is possible to imagine, unless it has been tuned by an expert tuner within the previous few days. Piano pitch is affected by temperature changes which cause the string to stretch or contract, raising and lowering the pitches, and over a period of time the over-all pitch of the instrument sinks lower than the standard A-440. Temperature affects the piano and wind instruments

---

[3]Those interested in greater details about the German Embouchure should consult Eby, W. M. *The Clarinet Embouchure* pp. 11-16. Copyright 1927 by W. M. Eby New York: Walter Jacobs, Inc.

in reverse directions. A low temperature raises the pitch of the piano and lowers the pitch of wind instruments, while a high temperature lowers the pitch of the piano and raises the pitch of wind instruments. Obviously, a player who is playing a solo with piano accompaniment, or in an ensemble which includes a piano must tune and play in tune with it. But other than this the piano should not be used for tuning purposes. Use tuning bars, tuning forks, or preferably an electronic instrument.

On woodwind instruments the pitch of a given note is determined by the distance from the tip of the mouthpiece or double-reed to the first open hole. Thus, the pitches of two successive notes on a clarinet—say C and B-flat which are one tone hole apart in fingering—is not determined by the distance between the two tone holes involved, but by the ratio of the distance from each of the tone holes to the tip of the mouthpiece. For this reason the ratios between the tip of the mouthpiece and the various first open holes must be maintained as close to the original as possible when tuning adjustments are made. A B-flat clarinet when tuning to an A-440 tuning bar plays B-natural on the third line. If the tuning barrel is pulled a quarter of an inch or more to bring the clarinet pitch down to A-440, it will be found that the throat tones are quite flat. In changing the ratio of the distance for the B-natural, the ratios for the throat tones was made out of proportion and they respond by being flat. The further out the tuning barrel is pulled for the B-natural to be in tune, the flatter the throat tones will be. A similar situation prevails on the other instruments in the clarinet family.

For this reason, if the intonation of the clarinet is to remain good over its entire range, tuning adjustments must be made in *three* places on the instrument: at the barrel joint, at the middle joint and at the bell joint. The three tuning notes for each instrument of the clarinet family and the corresponding concert pitch is given below. They must be used in the order given tuning the barrel joint, middle joint, and bell joint in that sequence. If all three notes cannot be tuned perfectly distribute the difference between them. Once the instrument itself is accurately tuned, the remainder of the intonation on the instrument is dependent on the player.

1. *E-flat Clarinet*

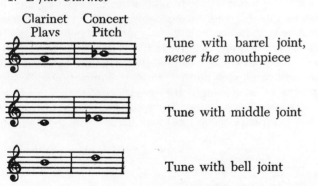

2. *B-flat Clarinet*

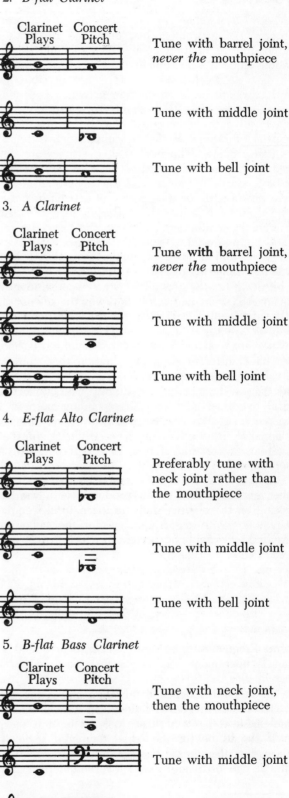

3. *A Clarinet*

4. *E-flat Alto Clarinet*

5. *B-flat Bass Clarinet*

INTONATION

Natural Tendencies of the Instrument. The process of tuning the instrument just described produces the best possible foundation upon which to build good intonation, since the instrument is as nearly in tune with itself as it is possible to get. It is not possible for a manufacturer to build an instrument which is absolutely perfectly in tune throughout its entire range. On clarinets all notes above third line B-flat are products of partial vibrations of the air column or overtones of the pitches below. The pitches of overtones are determined by the natural acoustical laws of vibration. The first harmonic is an octave, and the second harmonic an octave plus a fifth, or the interval of a twelfth. Because of the acoustical properties of the clarinet, the octave and other even numbered notes in the harmonic series cannot be produced. Hence the clarinet overblows a twelfth, or to put it simply when the register key is added to a fingering of a tone in the chalameau register the resulting tone is a twelfth. Other woodwind instruments overblow an octave, which is why the key operated by the left thumb is called a register key on the clarinet, and an octave key on the oboe and saxophone.

Notes produced as overtones in the natural harmonic series have different rates of vibration than the same interval in the tempered scale.[4] The higher in the harmonic series the greater the discrepency between the natural overtones and the corresponding note in the tempered scale. The first harmonic, or octave above the fundamental, is perfectly in tune, while the next—the twelfth—is slightly out of tune in comparison with the tempered scale.

The following example shows a comparison of the pitches of three notes when produced with the same fingering on the clarinet showing the natural frequency of the tones with the frequencies of the same notes demanded by equal temperament in which the clarinetist plays.[5]

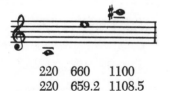

Natural Frequency	220	660	1100
Equal Temperament	220	659.2	1108.5

The "A" is the fundamental vibration and is the same. The "E" a twelfth above is the third note in the harmonic series and is eight-tenths of a vibration sharper than it should be for the equal tempered scale. The C-sharp, two octaves and a major third above the fundamental is the fifth note in the overtone series, and is

eight and one-half vibrations flat. This extreme flatness of the C-sharp is compensated for by raising the first finger of the left hand. If a stroboscope is available a clarinetist in the class can demonstrate this relationship on these notes as well as other similar series of notes using different fundamentals.

The clarinet, using the twelfth for notes in the clarion register, has greater intonation problems than the oboes or saxophones which use the octave for their second register. However, instrument manufacturers have made the most effective compromises possible to bring the entire range into tune with the tempered scale and as players devolop the continual process of adjusting the embouchure to accommodate the slightly out-of-tuneness becomes a natural response, and playing in tune becomes automatic. As a result of this situation, the clarinet has natural tendencies in intonation with which every teacher and player should be familiar. These natural tendencies are for the chalameau register to be sharp and for the degree of sharpness to increase as the pitch gets lower in this register. The clarion register has a natural tendency to be flat with the degree of flatness increasing as the pitch gets higher in the register.

The natural tendency of the notes above the high C is to be flat in pitch if played as true harmonic with the exact same fingering as their fundamental. However, none of these notes uses the exact same fingering, the natural out of tuneness being compensated for by opening additional tone holes—most obviously the first finger of the left hand being up for these notes, and the G-sharp key with the right little finger being added to most of them. These standard fingerings reduce the natural tendencies of these notes to be flat, and make it possible to play them perfectly in tune.

Reed and Intonation. A reed which is too hard tends to make the instrument sharp while a reed which is too soft tends to make the instrument flat. A soft reed emphasizes the natural tendencies of the notes and does not respond to embouchure adjustments, so in addition to a general flatness the instrument is out of tune with itself. A student who consistently plays flat, but whose embouchure formation is correct, is playing on a reed which is too soft. If he is given a harder reed the overall flatness disappears rather quickly, although he will probably protest that it is too hard to blow, which simply means that he is not accustomed to supporting the tone as much. Most students make the adjustment to slightly stiffer reeds quite readily. If the student has been playing on an extremely soft reed he should be gradually brought to playing on the proper strength through a succession of increasingly stiff reeds.

The student who has been using a reed which is too hard compensates for the over-all sharpness by pulling

---

[4]Refer to the appendix on acoustics of woodwind instruments for details of this harmonic structure.

[5]Stuffer, Donald W. *Intonation Deficiencies of Wind Instruments in Ensemble* Washington, D. C.: Catholic University of America Press, 1954. page 77. This is the most complete study of intonation of wind instruments available.

out the barrel joint and other joints of the instrument. Unfortunately the instruments do not permit pushing in an equal amount to compensate for the habitually flat player. Providing the embouchure formation is correct, a student who has to pull the instrument out an excessive amount to play at the standard pitch is playing on a reed which is too stiff. This tuning habit is frequently the best clue to an overly stiff reed. If he is given a softer reed the pitch will be lowered, although he will complain about the tone quality he is producing, although no change in quality will be apparent to the listener.

Embouchure and Intonation. The embouchure is the primary controlling factor in intonation as well as tone quality, two aspects of performance which must be well done if the musical effect is to be pleasing. It is for this reason that so much emphasis is given to proper embouchure formation, and justly so. Too little mouthpiece in the mouth emphasizes the flatness of the clarion and high registers. It is virtually impossible to play the high register in tune without sufficient mouthpiece in the mouth no matter how hard the student bites—and he will. Too much mouthpiece in the mouth tends to make the general ptich a little flat, but even more important makes pitch control of individual notes difficult.

The angle at which the clarinet is held determines the way in which the embouchure can control it. If the bell is too far out from the body—i.e., farther than a forty degree angle—the embouchure cannot support the reed and there is an over-all flatness in pitch. If the bell is held closer to the body than normal the over-all pitch is sharpened. This can be verified by having a student sustain an open G while moving the bell of the instrument back and forth. There will be a marked change in both pitch and tone quality.

Mouthpiece and Intonation. Mouthpieces with a close lay tend to be sharper than mouthpieces with an open lay, although through proper reed selection and embouchure formation the player can compensate for these natural tendencies of the mouthpiece. All mouthpieces do not have the same internal dimensions—i.e., throat and bore size and shape—and the same type of mouthpiece does not fit all instruments. If the size of the bore does not match the bore of the clarinet itself the instrument is difficult to play in tune with itself. If a student is having serious intonation problems and other possible causes have been checked, have him try other mouthpieces of different brands. If the mouthpiece con-

struction is the problem some quite serious intonation difficulties can be solved by changing mouthpieces, although the student will not suddenly cease playing out of tune and start playing in tune because of the automatic adjustments his embouchure has been making to accommodate the out-of-tune mouthpiece. However, the mouthpiece has its greatest influence on tone *quality*, and is not to be blamed for poor intonation until all other causes have been checked and corrected.

Dynamics and Intonation. There is an unfortunate tendency for the clarinetist to play flatter as he gets louder and sharper as he gets softer, the degree of flatness or sharpness increasing as the degree of dynamics approaches the extremes. This must be compensated for by embouchure adjustments. The student has the tendency to increase the pressure of the lower lip when playing softly and to decrease the pressure as he gets louder. This tendency is especially apparent in students who do not use the proper abdominal breath support. To overcome sharpness when playing softly relax the embouchure slightly, decrease the velocity of the air through the instrument but maintain the same firm support of the breath with the diaphragm and abdominal muscles that is used when playing loudly. To prevent becoming progressively flatter and flatter as the loudness of a tone increases, drop the lower teeth slightly but increase the pressure of the lips around the mouthpiece, especially the pressure of the lower lip against the reed.

Relaxing the embouchure when playing softly allows a greater length of the reed to vibrate which lowers the natural pitch of the reed itself and hence the pitch of the tone being played. Dropping the lower jaw and increasing the pressure around the mouthpiece when playing loudly allows the maximum length of the reed to vibrate in order to produce a loud tone with the increased pressure of the lower lip against it raises its natural rate of vibration to maintain the proper pitch. The dynamic levels between a normal mezzo piano and mezzo forte usually require little or no adjustment for intonation. Dynamic levels of piano, pianissimo and softer, and forte, fortissimo and louder demand increasing compensation.

The following tone exercises are excellent practice in control of pitch through wide dynamic levels. Practice them slowly enough to use an entire breath. Maintain constant firm breath support while controlling the dynamics by changing the velocity of the breath through the instrument.

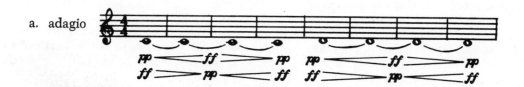

a. adagio

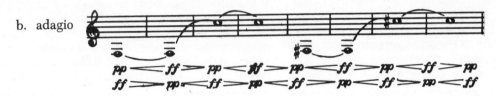

b. adagio

$pp <\!\!\!-\!\!\!ff\!\!\!-\!\!\!> pp <\!\!\!-\!\!\!ff\!\!\!-\!\!\!> pp <\!\!\!-\!\!\!ff\!\!\!-\!\!\!> pp <\!\!\!-\!\!\!ff\!\!\!-\!\!\!> pp$

$ff\!\!\!-\!\!\!> pp <\!\!\!-\!\!\!ff\!\!\!-\!\!\!> pp <\!\!\!-\!\!\!ff\!\!\!-\!\!\!> pp <\!\!\!-\!\!\!ff\!\!\!-\!\!\!> pp <\!\!\!-\!\!\!ff$

Practice exercise "a" in major or minor scale patterns to include the range of the instrument in which the student is proficient. Exercise "b" is best practiced chromatically from low E to F in the staff as indicated. This is also a good exercise for developing register crossing, and it is well to check to see that the student is operating the register key by vertical movements of the joint of the thumb and not sliding the thumb.

Intonation in Ensemble. The ability to tune the clarinet to the standard pitch and to play the instrument in tune with itself is essential. However, very few woodwinds other than practicing do much playing alone, but rather with other instruments in ensembles of two or three up to a full orchestra or band. Hence playing the instrument in tune with itself is only the starting point for good intonation. The student must listen to other instruments and make slight adjustments so that he is exactly in tune with the other players. The worst possible situations intonation-wise are the result of not listening to the others, or when a player insists that his pitch is right and everyone else is wrong.

Other woodwind instruments have natural tendencies toward out of tuneness which are different than those on the clarinet, brass instruments have different problems, and strings still others. The musically intelligent player will recognize these different problems, and will compromise his intonation for the sake of perfect ensemble intonation. Training in listening and hearing intonation is a valuable contribution which an instrumental teacher can make to his students. But it must be emphasized that the basis for good intonation must be the ability to play an instrument in tune with itself at the standard pitch.

Deviations from the Standard A-440 Pitch. There is an unfortunate tendency for some groups to use as a standard tuning note a pitch which is higher than A-440. One large university even went so far as to have its tuned percussion retuned to the standard of A-445. Even if groups don't deliberately tune to note higher than A-440 they have a tendency to drift to a higher pitch while playing. The result of a higher pitch is a multiplicity of intonation problems. Clarinets and other woodwind instruments, as well as the brasses are manufactured so that they play in tune at A-440. They are simply not in tune with themselves at higher pitches and the players must force the pitch higher, biting on the reed, and make constant adjustments. Some of the poor intonation in school bands and orchestras can be attributed to this situation. If a group which has been playing high is brought down to the A-440 standard and held at this pitch there is an amazingly rapid improvement in intonation.

The use of a stroboscopic device is extremely valuable in checking and developing correct intonation. It should be a part of every well equipped instrumental program and used regularly. It should be available for students to use individually for personal checks—indeed, this should be insisted upon. Serious use of such a device will develop intonation rapidly and efficiently. And, since it is built to the A-440 standard will help maintain the proper pitch level.

TONE

Basically the tone quality on a clarinet must be the same over the entire range of the instrument. It must not vary greatly from note to note, nor from register to register. In developing a good tone a great deal of attention must be given to this problem of matching quality. The better the balance of quality over the instrument the better the musical results and the better the response of the listeners.

In the preface of his method for clarinet Gustave Langenus makes the following statement regarding tone on the clarinet:

> "Everything should be sacrificed for a beautiful tone. No amount of technic, when the tone is coarse, will give such pleasure as a simple phrase played with a clear and pleasing tone quality. A beautiful voice is expected from a singer; if he does not possess this, his high notes and vocalisms do not charm, but leave us cold. The same is true of the clarinetist. No instrument can emit such a rough, disagreeable sound as the clarinet, and, on the other hand, no wind instrument can equal it in golden tones. The tone of the lower register resembles the contralto in richness and mellowness, while the clarion register possesses the sweet and tender qualities of the soprano."[6]

The range of the clarinet is divided into four registers, which should be memorized since so much of the literature about the instrument makes reference to them:

[6]Langenus, Gustave. *Complete Method for the Boehm Clarinet*, Part I. New York: Carl Fischer. 1923. page X.

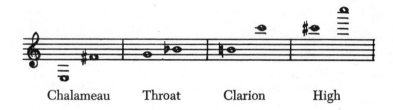

Chalameau   Throat   Clarion   High

The chalameau register got its name from the instrument from which it developed whose playing range was limited to these notes. The clarion register was added during the course of the development of the instrument for when these notes were added to the clarinet it was used to replace a primitive valveless brass instrument called the clarion. The throat tones are so labeled because in the early development their pitch was primarily controlled by the player's throat. The reason for the designation *high register* is obvious.

Referring back to the use of harmonics on the clarinet we find that notes in the chalameau register and the throat tones are produced as fundamentals of the vibrating column of air; those in the clarion register by the third notes in the overtone series; and those in the high register by either the fifth or seventh tone in the overtone series.

There is no single standard for a good tone on instruments of the clarinet family. The two basic embouchures described for the instruments produce different qualities, both fulfilling all the criteria for a good tone, and both equally pleasing when fully developed. Deviations from these two basic embouchures produces slightly different qualities. But no matter what the differences a clarinet still sounds like a clarinet and if the tone is pleasing it is a good tone.

Every teacher and clarinetist should avail themselves of every opportunity to hear live performances of fine instrumentalists. Or if this is not possible study the recorded performances of repertoire for the clarinet listed in an appendix on a high quality phonograph where realistic reproduction can be heard. Compare the tone qualities of the various artists in so far as it is possible to separate quality from phrasing, technique, and general musicianship. A comparison of the recorded performances of French artists, German artists, English artists, and American artists will be quite revealing. All will be quite different, all will be pleasing, and in spite of the inter-mingling of cultures national differences will be readily discernible.

A good tone is the product of all the elements involved in playing: instrument, mouthpiece, reed, embouchure and breath support. If any of these is defective then tone quality suffers accordingly.

Problems of tone production and quality are many and varied, but may usually be traced to their source, and should be corrected immediately. Refer also to the sections on mouthpiece, reed, and embouchure.

Following are some of the most prevalent problems or faults in tone:

1. *Small, pinched, or muffled tone.* Assuming a proper mouthpiece and reed, a small, pinched, or muffled tone may be caused by too much pressure on the reed with the lower jaw, or by having too little mouthpiece in the mouth. Adjust the distance in the mouth by experimentation to the point of optimum quality and fullness, yet avoiding the tendency of the tone to break into the next upper partial which is caused by too much mouthpiece in the mouth. Too much pressure against the reed can be remedied by asking the student to play flatter. This will cause him to relax the pressure of the lower jaw and free the reed. Unless he also relaxes the support of the lip against the reed, he will not actually play flatter in pitch, the effect will simply be a freer tone quality.

2. *Squawky tone.* The squawky tone which can be described as lacking in body and focus, generally uncontrolled, and commonly flat in pitch is caused by one of three things. Not enough support for the reed with the lower lip; poor embouchure formation evidenced by not enough pressure around the mouthpiece with the upper lip, the corners of the mouth, as well as the lower lip; or by a poor reed. Corrections for these have been discussed in previous sections.

3. *Hard, cold tone.* A tone which is inflexible and which lacks the intangible quality of vitality is described as hard and cold. This is caused by a mouthpiece which has a lay which is too open and too long, or by a reed which is too hard.

4. *Squeaking.* Squeaking on a clarinet is usually caused by a hole not being completely covered by one of the fingers, a condition most common with beginners; by a leaky pad which must be identified and replaced; by the reed; or by an incorrect embouchure which is putting pressure unequally on the reed.

5. *Weak, colorless tone.* A tone which is otherwise smooth in quality, but is lacking in body, quality, and carrying power is most often due to lack of proper breathing and breath support.

6. *Loud, racous tone.* This quality is always the result of too much breath support which overblows the instrument and presses it beyond its true dynamic range. Insisting on a full dynamic range, and limiting the volume the student is allowed to produce will correct this problem. This condition is also associated with a mouthpiece which has a longer lay with an open tip,

and with the use of reeds which are too stiff. In school bands, it is never one clarinet which has this problem but the entire section which indicates clearly that the director is responsible for letting it develop.

7. *Control of soft tone.* Difficulty in producing and controlling a soft tone is principally due to the inability of the player to project a steady concentrated small stream of air into the instrument. Check breathing and breath support, and have the student practice focusing a steady stream of air into the palm of his hand. Other possible causes may be a reed which is too stiff, a mouthpiece which is too open, or a poorly shaped embouchure. Check all three if breath support is not the solution.

8. *Dynamics and tone quality.* Some students will loose their tone quality when playing at extremes of loudness and softness. This is normally due to an undeveloped embouchure. Keep the volume of tone within the ability of the embouchure to retain control, and concentrate on embouchure development through the use of the proper exercises.

TONGUING

Tonguing refers to the manner in which the tongue operates in relation to the reed and breath support in order to articulate the tones. This placement and action must be rapid and under complete control at all speeds. It must, in coordination with breath support, be able to produce on the clarinet all varieties of articulation from the hardest staccato to the softest legato. In short, the clarinetist must be able to match sound for sound the entire gamut of bow strokes used on the violin.

The manner in which the tongue touches the reed, the place it touches, and how it moves is dependent somewhat upon the embouchure formation. There are several points of view on how this is done and each is effective, but there is one point upon which all authorities are agreed and that is that *the tongue never touches the tip of the reed.* No matter which style of tonguing is used the tongue must contact the reed away from the tip.

In essence the tongue acts as a valve to control the flow of breath through the mouthpiece, stopping the breath and vibration when it touches the reed, and allowing the vibration to begin again when it is removed and the air flow begins again. Effective articulation is entirely dependent upon the flow of air, and hence upon proper breath support and control. The interrelationship between breath pressure and tongue pressure against the reed allows the production of every conceivable kind of attack from the hardest marcato-staccato to the very smoothest legato within the widest dynamic range. The amount of pressure of the tongue against the reed determines the hardness of the attack, the amount of wind pressure against the tongue determines the loudness of the attack.

There are three basic methods of tongue placement used on the clarinet, each subject to variations according to the personal desires of the teachers using them.

They have several things in common however: (1) the tongue is relaxed. A tongue under tension cannot move rapidly enough, nor can it be controlled; (2) Tongue movement is confined to the forward part of the tongue; and (3) The tongue acts as a valve for the air and is dependent on good breath support. The three methods may be outlined as follows:

First Method. This method is used with the soft cushion embouchure previously described and is the method taught by many fine clarinetists. It produces maximum flexibility and facility, and is adaptable to solo, chamber music, band, and orchestra performance. This method in combination with the soft cushion embouchure is recommended by the author.

With the mouthpiece in playing position, and the embouchure correctly formed, feel with the tip of the tongue the junction of the reed and the lower lip. The reed and lip form a small "V" shaped pocket. The tongue should be in this pocket with the top of the tip of the tongue curved up and touching the reed lightly about three-eighths of an inch from the tip.

To start the tone put the tongue in place on the reed and build up wind pressure against it. Release the air into the instrument with tongue action similar to that in pronouncing the syllable "too." The center of the tongue is depressed slightly so that the tongue will not lie flat on the reed. Figures C-70A and C-70B below shows this tongue position.

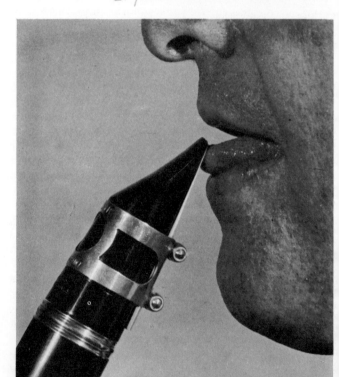

Figure C-70A.

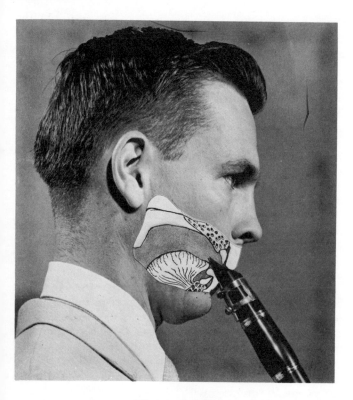

Figure C-70B.

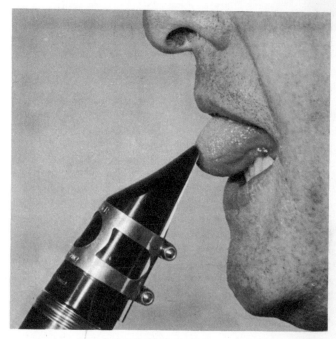

Figure C-71.

Second Method. This method is used with the hard cushion embouchure previously described, and is recommended by many fine clarinet teachers. It produces great flexibility and is adapted to all types of performance.

With the mouthpiece in place and the embouchure properly formed, the tongue is drawn up and back with the tip pointed. The center of the tongue is arched and the throat kept open. Action of the tongue is foward contacting the reed an eighth or sixteenth of an inch from its tip with the top of the tongue about an eighth of an inch from its tip. Pressure of the tongue against the reed may be light or heavy depending on the type of articulation desired. To start the tone place the tongue against the reed, build up air pressure against it, and release the air with a tongue action similar to that in pronouncing "du" to start the tone. Figure C-71 shows the tongue in position on the reed for this type of articulation.

Third Method. This method is used with either the soft cushion or the hard cushion embouchure. With the mouthpiece in place and the embouchure properly formed, the tip of the tongue is anchored against the base of the lower teeth. Keeping the tongue anchored against the teeth the tongue moves up and forward to contact the reed an eighth to half inch from its tip. The point on the tongue which contacts the reed is found naturally and is determined by its natural placement. Experience with advanced students who use this method has indicated that this technique of using the tongue

does not have the potential of as great a variety of articulations as either of the previous methods, nor is speed and control developed as rapidly or to as great an extent. Unless there is a strong personal preference for this method, it should be used with caution.

The reader may compare the placement and action of the tongue for the three methods by forming an embouchure using the thumbnail or a pencil to replace the reed. Compare the ease, natural feeling, and rapidity of motion possible on each of the three. The method which feels most comfortable and which provides the most rapid movement will probably be the one which you as a clarinetist would develop fastest. Experience on other woodwinds, or on a brass instrument will help determine the result.

Alto, Bass, and Contra-Bass Clarinets. Any of the three methods of tongue placement and action described can be successfully used on the Alto, Bass, or Contra-Bass clarinet. Normally these instruments are played after some experience on the B-flat clarinet and the same system should be used as on that instrument. The difference between these instruments and the soprano instruments will be found in the point at which the tongue contacts the reed. Since there is more reed in the mouth because of the larger mouthpiece, the point of contact is further away from the tip of the reed. But the placement of the tongue in relation to the lower lip and teeth remains essentially the same. It may be found that additional pressure of the tongue will be needed to close the reed if the mouthpiece has an open lay. Because of the larger reed its response is slower and it becomes increasingly difficult to produce a short staccato or to articulate as rapidly as we go from Alto to Bass to Contra-Bass. A short staccato on the Contra-Bass instrument is not only difficult to produce but is not musical in sound. Staccato on this instrument should more nearly reproduce the pizzicato sound of the string bass.

Developing Tongue Action. For the purposes of developing articulation on the clarinet the position of the tongue *against* the reed is considered the normal (home, or rest) position. For it is from this position that it starts the tone. There is no forward movement preceding the beginning of the tone since the breath support is against the tongue. One writer has compared this concept with a pipe organ. There is wind pressure against the opening into the pipe before a key is pressed. When a key is pressed electrical contacts open the pipe, the air is released through it and a tone produced. When the key is lifted the pipe is closed, the tone stops but wind pressure against the pipe remains. So it is on the clarinet—tongue against the reed, and breath pressure against the tongue before the tone is started.

The commonly used word "attack" to describe the articulation of a tone is most unfortunate since it implies, if only subconsciously, both violence and forward movement. It has come into use in the English language as a mistranslation of the Italian word "attacca" which means *begin* and not attack. The words articulate and articulation are more meaningful in English, and the word attack should not be used when discussing articulation with students.

The first step in developing correct tongue action is to develop the starting and stopping of a tone. This is accomplished by a continual pressure of air against the mouthpiece with standard abdominal support. The tongue acts as a valve, releasing and stopping the flow of air through the instrument with the pressure remaining constant, much as the flow of water through a faucet is turned on and off. The water pressure doesn't fall to zero when the faucet is closed, and neither must the breath pressure when the tongue closes the reed against the mouthpiece.

Breath support and articulation are inseparable, so proper breath support must be developed before articulation is started. Almost all teachers insist that beginning clarinetists establish the beginnings of a good embouchure and breath control through developing a satisfactory tone in the chalameau register before using the tongue against the reed. This is done by simply blowing to start the tone and stopping the air flow to end the note. If this is done then favorable conditions are set up for beginning the learning of articulation.

The following exercises are widely used to establish tongue action. They are mechanical exercises for tongue action and not music. If the students play them musically they are not deriving the full benefits. They must be played fortissimo and very slowly. No movement of the breathing mechanism is involved, diaphragm and abdominal muscles remain in tight support from beginning to end and *must not* move either at the beginning or end of the notes. Breath pressure against the tongue and mouthpiece remains the same during the rests as it is during the time the notes are sounding. After breath pressure is built up against the mouthpiece the tongue moves away quickly with a motion similar to pronouncing the syllable "Too," or "Du" depending on placement of the tongue, and the note will start fortissimo and with an accent. Without diminishing the loudness of the one the tongue returns to its position on the reed with a motion like saying the letter "t." Thus the action of the tongue during the exercise is "T-o-o-o-o-o-t" or "D-u-u-u-t." If the notes were short the tongue action would be a simple "toot" or "duut." Mechanical noise of the tongue leaving and returning to the reed must be heard. If it is not, then the pressure of the tongue is too light. These exercises should be practiced at least five minutes a day until the tongue action is secure.

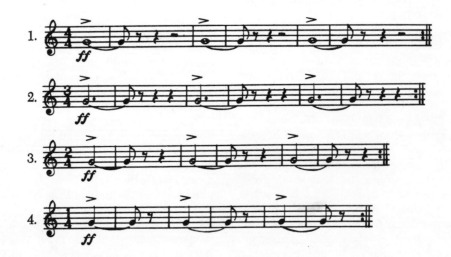

When these have been established on the open G, practice them also on the following notes:

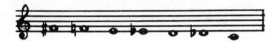

Having established the loudest and hardest articulation, it is necessary to establish the pianissimo with a soft articulation. Tongue action is the same. Support from the diaphragm and abdominal muscles remains the same, but the velocity of the air is reduced so that the loudness level of the tone is pianissimo. Sustain the open G as softly as possible. When it is established return the tongue to the reed quickly and with only enough pressure to stop the vibration of the reed but so that the tip of the reed does not close the mouthpiece, and air continues to go through the instrument. The same amount of air moves through the instrument during the rests as during the time the note is sounding! Hence breath pressure and velocity remains constant throughout. Play the exercise very softly and very slowly. Both beginnings and ends of the note are slow to respond. Include it in the daily practice routine until facility is established.

When this exercise is performed successfully on the open G practice also the following notes:

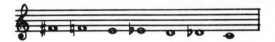

When both the fortissimo and pianissimo tongue actions are established, further development can be applied to melodic figures through the use of the "45 exercises upon different combinations of articulation, etc." in Part I of the Klose Method for Clarinet, Carl Fischer Edition. So that the articulation patterns will move slowly enough to develop security and accuracy in tongue action and breath support the speed must be greatly decreased. Sixteenth notes are played as half-notes at a slow speed. The following examples indicate the manner in which they are played. Follow the dynamic markings exactly. All notes are started with the tongue. All notes at ends of slurs and all staccato notes are stopped with the tongue. Breath support remains constant throughout, with dynamics controlled by changes in velocity. Breath pressure against the reed continues during the rests. Careful practice of these will establish complete control of tognue action in a few weeks.

The basic principles illustrated by these four examples can be applied to all the 45 exercises: First notes under slurs are forte and a diminuendo is made for the durtaion of the slur mark so that the last note under the slur is piano. The final note is stopped by the tongue. All staccato notes are

adagio

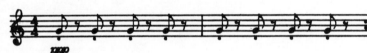

No. 2. Written:

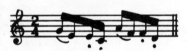

Played:

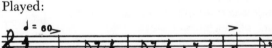

No. 5. Written:

Played:

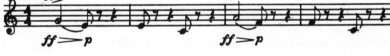

No. 7. Written:

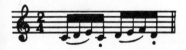

Played:

No. 10. Written:

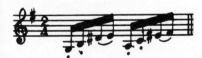

Played:

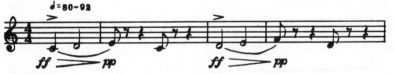

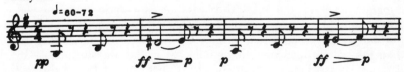

piano and started and stopped by the tongue. Eliminate all movements of any portion of the abdominal muscles or the diaphragm, support remains constant. These principles may also be applied to the Joseph Küffner "Fifty Progressive Duets" in the Klose Method Part I, but also published separately in several editions. These are technically easy and can be used by the students in the lower intermediate stage of development to begin musical application of articulation. More advanced students find ready adaptation of these principles of articulation in the C. Rose "Forty Studies for Clarinet" Books I and II, and the C. Rose "32 Studies for Clarinet," all published by Carl Fischer.

Variety in articulation. Once correct tongue action is established according to the method selected, variety in articulation can be developed. The exact sounds desired are determined by musical taste and style. A tremendous variety of articulations is possible on the clarinet through the use of varying degrees of pressure of the tongue against the reed combined with varying amounts of breath support and velocity of wind through the instrument. This can be illustrated by a member of the class playing in the following ways:

1. Sustain an open G at a good solid forte level. While maintaining this dynamic level and keeping the lengths of the notes the same start with maximum tongue pressure against the reed and play a series of notes with gradually diminishing pressure of the tongue.

2. Do the same maintaining a piano level for the open G, but starting with minimum pressure against the reed and play a series of notes with gradually increasing pressure of the tongue. It will be found that tongue pressure beyond a certain point will introduce an objectionable amount of mechanical noise.

3. Starting with an open G softly play a series of staccato notes simultaneously increasing both loudness of the tone and pressure of the tongue against the reed. Be sure to eliminate any movement of the breathing mechanism. Experimentation will show that the louder the staccato note the greater the tongue pressure needed to control it and if the result is to be musically pleasing the louder the staccato the longer duration it must have. Staccato at loud dynamic levels automatically become marcato notes.

The success of these experiments depends on the degree of advancement of the player performing them. An advanced player will be able to carry the illustrations much farther and show a greater variety of articulated sounds.

Accents, Sforzando, Forte-piano. Accents, sforzando, and forte-piano notes must be played in relation to the dynamic level of the musical phrase. A sforzando is not a note played as loudly as it is possible to play, but simply an isolated note one or two degrees louder than the notes which precede or follow it in the phrase. It demands assistance from the breath so that the breathing mechanism supplies additional support and velocity

simultaneously with the release of the reed by the tongue.

The forte-piano requires immediate relaxation of support and velocity by the breathing mechanism, coupled with whatever degree of simultaneous support at the instant the tone starts demanded by the music itself. Accents indicated above or below the notes must be only one dynamic level above the notes which precede or follow them. Many accents may be accomplished by only increased tongue pressure against the reed, others demand slight movements of the breathing muscles. It must be clearly understood that there are no rapid movements of any breathing muscles in support of tongue action except for accents, sfzorando, and forte-piano note.

Common Articulation Problems. There are a multitude of problems connected with articulation on members of the clarinet family, and the following are the most common:

1. *Movement of the jaw in tonguing.* This is the result of too large or too violent movements of the tongue. Rather than confining the movement to the front portion of the tongue the student is moving the entire tongue. The solution is to ask the student, no matter what his technical advancement, to practice the basic exercises for developing articulation constantly checking in a mirror on the music stand to eliminate all movement. Jaw movements can occur with all methods of correct tongue placement, as well as with incorrect tongue placement.

2. *Sluggish tongue.* Assuming that placement of the tongue is correct this can be corrected only by hard practice. The use of major and minor scales, scales in the third pattern, major and minor arpeggios using various patterns of slurred and tongued notes will provide the most rapid cure for a sluggish tongue. The playing of staccato chromatic octaves up and down is excellent. The student should use a metronome while doing this practice in order that the beat can be kept constant, or he will slow down and speed up according to the technical difficulty of the note patterns.

3. *Hard attack.* This is the result of too much tongue pressure against the reed in relation to the amount of breath support, or because too much tongue is in contact with the reed. Review the fundamental pianissimo exercises suggested for developing tongue action and continue practice until it can be done successfully. The hard attack is frequently associated with movements of the lower jaw which must also be eliminated. Use a mirror constantly for checking.

4. *Poor Staccato.* A poor staccato or no staccato at all, if tongue placement is otherwise correct, is caused by lack of sustained, continuous breath support. The support is being relaxed between staccato notes and then tightened simultaneously with the beginning of the note by the tongue. Check breathing carefully, since if this is the case the air is most frequently being inhaled with a chest movement rather than by the diaphragm

and abdominal muscles. A good staccato is rarely possible with incorrect breath placement.

If a check reveals that all is well with placement of breath and the support is continuous, then a poor staccato is the result of incorrect tongue placement or movement. Frequently the cause is simply that the student is not returning the tongue quickly enough to its place on the reed to stop the vibration. This can be developed by practicing slow repeated notes at a very soft dynamic level, increasing the dynamic level as proficiency is attained. Many students are simply afraid to stop a note with their tongue and need encouragement.

5. *Lack of coordination between tongue and fingers.* This is the result of practicing and playing too fast without the essential slow working out process. Slow down the tempo until the tongue and fingers are perfectly coordinated, and increase speed gradually. Do not allow the student to exceed the maximum tempo at which there is perfect coordination between tongue and fingers. Use of a metronome to maintain a constant tempo is mandatory. Often there are gaps in the speeds at which the tongue and fingers can be coordinated, i.e., coordination is perfect at slower speeds and at faster speeds, but impossible at that particular speed. These gaps can be located with the use of the metronome, and the same exercises suggested for the correction of a sluggish tongue used for correction.

In developing tonguing action, facility and variety a constant check must be kept on placement and use of the tongue, and especially on maintaining the proper breath support. Students at all levels of advancement can lapse into incorrect procedures which will become habitual if not caught and Corrected promptly. Good articulation is simple and easy to develop correctly if the proper attention is given to it.

Flutter Tonguing. The flutter tongue is produced by rolling the tongue rapidly against the reed as in rolling the letter "r" in "b-r-r-r," producing a very rapid tremolo. There is no set speed for the roll, but the more rapid the tongue movement the more effective. Flutter tonguing technically is not an articulation but a special tonal effect. It is used occasionally in music by twentieth century composers. While this effect can be executed on a single reed instrument, it is not as effective on clarinet or saxophone as it is on the flute and brass instruments. There is no standard designation for flutter tonguing, and when it is required written directions are given in the printed music.

Double and Triple Tonguing. The standard technique of double or triple tonguing used for very rapid articulations on the flute and on brass instruments is not practical on the clarinet, although some professional players profess to make use of them. The double tongue is executed by rapid movements of the tongue as in pronouncing the syllables "tu-ku." The "tu" syllable is pronounced with the tongue against the reed, the "ku" syllable with the tongue stopping the flow of air by striking the roof of the mouth. The alternation of the tongue against the reed and against the roof of the mouth produces two entirely different sounds which are impossible to match. Triple tonguing, is produced by the syllables "tu-ku-tu" or a similar set, and is impractical on the clarinet for the same reason.

TECHNIQUE PROBLEMS

In the course of acquiring a technical proficiency on the instrument which is accurate, under control, and facile, certain out of the ordinary problems are encountered which will slow the progress of the student unless they are approached in logical ways. The importance of solving the technical problems in the correct way must be impressed on the student, as well as the reasons for a particular solution. Many technical problems on the clarinet demand that the player make a choice between two or more alternatives. Each alternative must be practiced until it becomes an involuntary part of his technique and how each alternative is used must be made so much a part of his technique that the correct choice becomes involuntary and instantaneous. The following problems are those which are most frequently found.

1. *Use of left and right little fingers.* The mechanism of the standard Boehm system clarinet has some notes which can be played with either the right or left little fingers, others only with the right or left little finger. These are as follows:

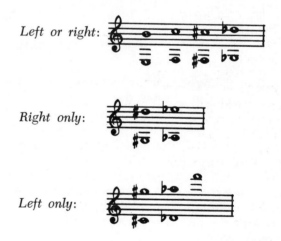

Using the basic rule of good fingering choice which says that the same finger is not used in two different places for successive notes, the little fingers are used alternately when two or more consecutive notes involving their use occur. Following are examples of how this selection is made: "L" indicating left and "R" indicating right little finger. Students should be encouraged to put either an L or an R under the first note in a pattern involving the little fingers. Even professionals do this occasionally to assure smoothness and accuracy. It is necessary to read ahead to see if a G-sharp-D-sharp or a note in the high register involving the use of this key

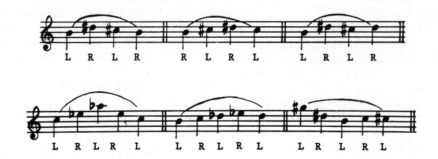

is in the pattern and plan ahead so that the correct little finger is free to contact this key without sliding.

2. *Sliding the little fingers.* There are instances where even the best finger choice will not eliminate the necesity for sliding a little finger from one key to another for consecutive notes. If a student is sliding a finger, first make sure that no alternative pattern is possible. If sliding is called for then be sure he follows the correct procedure.

Sliding is done from one key to another which is lower so that the finger slides down toward the body of the instrument. With the right little finger slide from the F or G-sharp key to the E or F-sharp key but not in the reverse. With the left little finger slide from the E key to the F, C-sharp, or F-sharp keys but not the reverse. Most students find it better to do the necessary sliding with the right little finger since the keys are better arranged for this purpose than those on the left, and it is almost always possible to arrange the fingering pattern so this is possible.

The proper sliding is done by increasing the curvature of the finger and pressing down so that it slides off of the top key onto the lower one. If the finger does not slide easily an old professional trick is to rub the finger beside the nose where the skin is oily and the finger picks up enough of this oil to slide easily. Rubbing the finger in the hair works equally well.

Following are some examples showing correct sliding. L and R indicate left and right little fingers while the notes marked ʌ indicate that the finger slides from the first to the second.

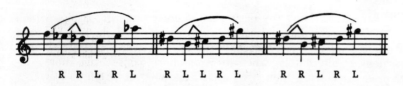

3. *Crossing the break.* The "break" on the clarinet occurs between the third-line B-flat throat tone and B-natural in the clarion register where the production of the tone changes from the fundamental vibration to the third harmonic. The fingering pattern starts dupli-

cating that for notes a twelfth lower. Developing facility in crossing the break is one of the major problems for beginning students, although the problem is considerably simplified if the proper procedure is used. Above all never tell the student that it is going to be difficult since this automatically sets up a psychological block and makes it difficult even though that particular student would otherwise have little difficulty.

Crossing from the chalameau to the clarion register must not be introduced until the student is secure in the chalameau register, playing with a reasonable good tone and with accurate fingerings. The process of crossing should then be introduced by slurring an interval of a twelfth from the chalameau register which demands only the opening of the register key with the left thumb. Check to see that the left thumb is opening the register key by vertical movements of the first joint and not by sliding it onto the register key.

Exercises similar to the following are used in several methods books to introduce the clarion register.

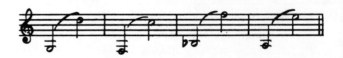

Once the student is playing the clarion register notes, he should establish some security in this register before attempting to cross back and forth between the chalameau range or throat tones to the clarion register. Finger positions must be perfect so that they cover the tone holes accurately or the student will squeak. If finger placement is accurate crossing from chalameau notes to clarion notes can be developed without too much difficulty. Crossing from throat tones to clarion register develops more slowly since, for example, the interval open G to third line B-natural involves closing six tone holes and a key with one of the little fingers—coordination which beginners acquire slowly. Even more advanced students have difficulty playing this interval smoothly.

Here is a most useful device for both developing facility in crossing from a throat tone to notes in the clarion register. The right hand portion of the fingering for any of these notes:

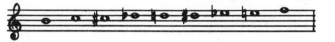

can be kept down while playing any of these notes:

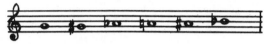

This means that fingers in the right hand are down and in place before the note in the clarion register is played thus eliminating the problem of placement, and making a smoother interval. This is especially useful in passages which cross back and forth over the break. Keeping the fingers of the right hand down when playing the throat tones does not affect the pitch of the throat tones. In fact, many clarinetists feel that the right hand fingers down improves the sonority of the throat tones.

Following are some examples of how this is used. Fingers of the right hand are kept down for the duration of the brackets. All clarinetists on all levels of advancement should develop facility with this device for the sake of smooth technique.

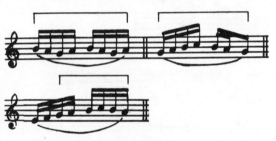

4. *Slurs into the high register.* Even though the notes in the high register can be played well many, if not all, clarinetists have difficulty in slurring from the clarion register to a note in the high register. The notes in the higher register seem to pop when they start. This is due to acoustical properties of the instrument since a different series of overtones produce the high tones than produce the clarion tones. Some of the roughness in slurring to the high tones can be corrected through adjusting breath support. High notes require less breath support for the same dynamic level than do notes in the clarion register. This difference can be demonstrated by playing octaves into the clarion register using the same amount of breath support for each note. The upper note will be considerably louder than the lower. The necessary adjustments in breath support can be readily made once the player is conscious of their need.

A second technique, and one which is mandatory if perfect slurs from clarion to high registers are to be achieved, is the use of the half-hole with the first finger.

This use of the first finger half-hole is part of the standard fingering for oboe and bassoon, and can be effectively put to a similar use on the clarinet. Most fingerings for notes in the upper register call for the first finger to be up to open the hole. If instead of being lifted off the hole, the first finger is rolled down toward the second finger so that half of the hole is opened we have the half-hole position for the tone hole. It is important that the finger roll and not slide if facility is to be achieved. In order to make a perfect slur from a note in the clarion register to one in the high register roll the first finger into the half-hole position instead of lifting it off and reduce the amount of breath support. Figure C-72 shows the half-hole position on the B-flat clarinet and Figure C-73 the position on Bass clarinet.

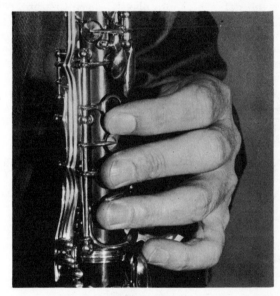

Figure C-72.

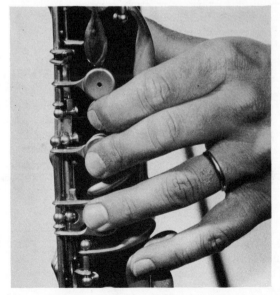

Figure C-73.

In the following example the half-hole is used to slur to each of the upper notes:

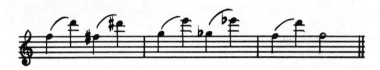

The half-hole technique is used only for slurring to the notes. Do not use a half-hole if the note is tongued. Do not keep the finger to the half-hole position for notes in the clarion register other than the one slurred to. The Bass clarinet uses the half-hole position as part of the standard fingering for all notes in the clarion register.

5. *Articulated G-sharp key.* Some model clarinets have an articulated G-sharp key (G-sharp first space above the staff which also plays C-sharp first line below the staff). Advantages and disadvantages of this mechanism are discussed in the section of selection of instruments. This key facilitates certain passages. It makes easy trills and shakes on these notes:

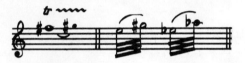

since the little finger can be kept down on the G-sharp—C-sharp key and the trill or shakes made with the right hand alone. Passages such as the following are easier since the little finger can be kept in position and there are no movements in the left hand.

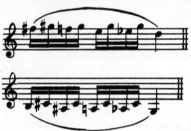

If the instrument has an articulated G-sharp key take full advantage of it. The articulated key is standard on all saxophones and oboes.

6. *Use of 7th. ring.* Some models of B-flat, E-flat, and A clarinets have seven instead of six rings. It is the ring for the tone hole of the third finger, so it is simple to see whether a particular instrument has it or not. It is not found on Alto, Bass, or Contra-Bass clarinets because of the covered tone holes on these instruments.

The seventh ring adds an important and most useful alternate fingering for:

which are fingered with only the first and third fingers down. The seven ring model instrument is highly recommended since it facilitates such passages as the following:

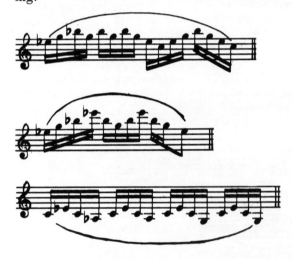

7. *Selection and use of alternate fingerings.* There are alternate fingerings for many notes on the clarinet, and if the smoothest and most useful technique is to be acquired it is necessary that they be learned and that the best choice of fingering be made each time there is a choice. The choice should be the one which gives the smoothest progression and the best facility and intonation. The notes on the following staff have standard alternate fingerings. Each quarter note indicates a fingering for that pitch. Special trill fingerings are not included, but are given in a special trill fingering chart following the regular fingering chart.

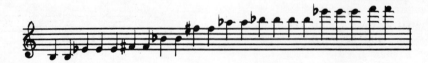

Choice of fingerings which involve using either the left or right little fingers has already been discussed. Review this if necessary. Following are some of the more common usages for certain fingerings. Study them carefully and try them, or have some clarinetist illustrate the correct choice and other possible choices to determine the reason for using this particular fingering.

B-natural: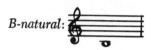

Two Fingerings: (1) T 123 050   Diatonic
(2) T 123 406x   Chromatic

Typical uses for each fingering are illustrated below:

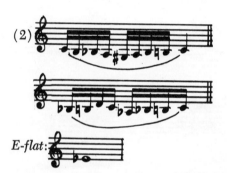

E-flat:

Three Fingerings: (1) T 120 4x00
(2) T 123x 000
(3) T 100 400

The first is the normal fingering which must be used unless there is a partciular reason for using one of the others. The second keeps the fingering for the note entirely in the left hand and is recommended for chromatic passages and for trilling. The third fingering is quite sharp and is used only for rapid arpeggiated passages where the duration is so short that the out-of-tuneness is not heard. Following are typical uses for each fingering.

(1)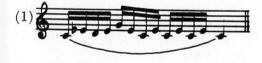

(2)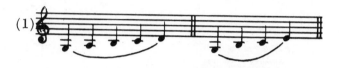

(3)

F-sharp: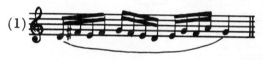

Two Fingerings: (1) 0 100 000   Diatonic
(2) T 000 4xy00 Chromatic

The first is the normal diatonic fingering. The second is mandatory in chromatic passages, and is frequently the best choice when the F-sharp is approached or left chromatically. Following are typical uses of each:

(1)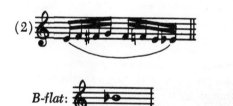

(2)

B-flat:

Two Fingerings: (1) R A00 000
(2) A00 4z00

The first is the normal fingering which is used both in diatonic and chromatic passages. The second is useful only in slow moving passages where maximum sonority is desired, since its sound is much bigger than the normal fingering and it is perfectly in tune. It cannot be used where the note which follows uses fingers of the right hand, since the hand must be out of place in order to reach key 4z. Following are typical uses of each:

(1)

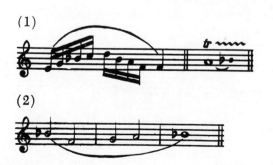

(2)

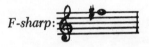

F-sharp:

Two Fingerings: (1) TR 123 050   Diatonic
                (2) TR 123 45x0   Chromatic

The first is the normal diatonic fingering, the second mandatory in chromatic passages. The second is also frequently the choice when the F-sharp is approached or left chromatically, or to lead smoothly to a fingering for a note in the high register.

Following are typical uses of each:

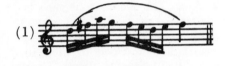

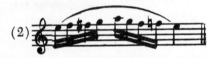

A-flat:

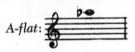

Two Fingerings: (1) TR 123C-sharp 000
                (2) TR 120 450

The first is the normal fingering for both diatonic and chromatic passages. Since it involves the use of the left little finger its use must be properly prepared for in any pattern involving the little fingers. The second is used only in rapid arpeggiated passages since its quality does not normally match perfectly the other notes of the clarion register, and on some instruments it is slightly out of tune. The following illustrate typical uses of each:

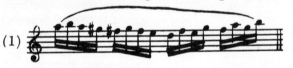

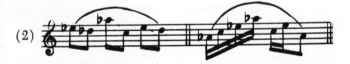

B-flat:

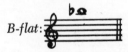

Four Fingerings: (1) TR 120 4x00
                 (2) TR 123x 000
                 (3) TR 100 400
                 (4) TR 100 050

The first is the normal fingering and is a safe choice for any passage. The second is suggested, but not mandatory for chromatic passages, and trills, but has limited usefulness because the third finger must not slide to or from its tone hole; misuse of this fingering is very common. The third fingering produces a tone of excellent quality well in tune and is used in either slow or fast arpeggiated passages. The fourth produces a good quality of tone, but is slightly sharp and its use is restricted to rapid arpeggiated passages. The following illustrate typical uses of each.

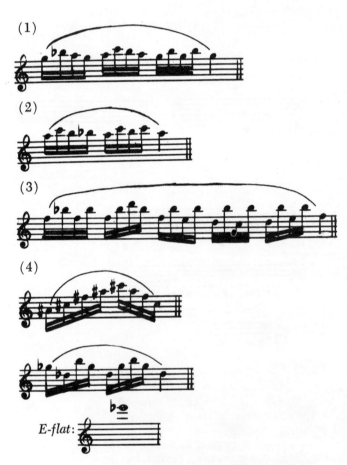

E-flat:

Three Fingerings: (1) TR 023 45x0   G-sharp
                  (2) TR 023 006   G-sharp
                  (3) TR 023 050   G-sharp

The first is the normal fingering used for either diatonic or chromatic passages, and should be the choice unless there is a particular reason for not using it. The second is an excellent alternate fingering of good quality and well in tune and is particularly useful when slurring from the lower portion of the clarion register to the high E-flat. The third choice is quite flat in pitch, although the tone quality is good. It is used in rapid passages in the high register where facility is more important than tone quality. Over use of this third fingering, frequently as first choice, is a common fault among inexperienced clarinetists. The following illustrate typical uses of these fingerings.

(1)

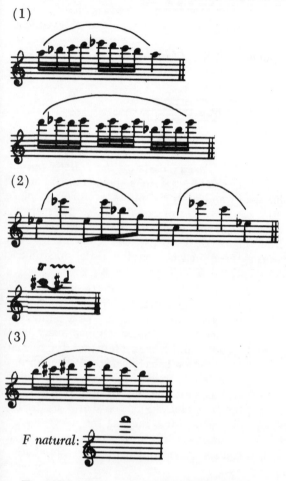

(2)

(3)

F natural:

Two Fingerings: (1) TR 023C-sharp 000 G-sharp
(2) TR 123C-sharp 456 (no G-sharp)

The first is the normal fingering used for both diatonic and chromatic passages. The second is a special fingering which is useful for slurring from the clarion or lower registers to this note, or when playing softly in the high register and there is the slightest chance that the other fingering will not speak, or when it is played in a long diminuendo. The second finger is of good tone quality and well in tune (provided the G-sharp key is not used) and will produce only this F. When it is used there is no chance of getting another note by mistake—it either plays F or nothing, and will not squeak. The following illustrates typical uses of these fingerings.

(1)

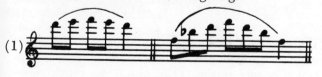

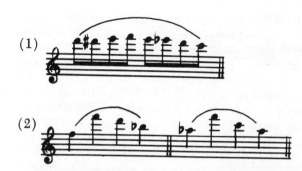

(1)

(2)

TRANSPOSITIONS FOR THE CLARINETIST

The clarinetist is frequently expected to transpose and play on this instrument from parts written for an instrument in a different key. The professional must be able to do this, and advanced school players should develop some facility, at least on the more common transpositions. This ability is acquired only by doing it, slowly at first, and then with increasing speed. These transpositions, many of which are encountered even on the high school level include:

1. *Playing Piano, Violin, or "C" Clarinet on the B-flat Clarinet.* The need for this transposition is so frequent that every clarinetist past the lower intermediate stage of development should begin to acquire facility. This is the transposition from the concert key to the B-flat clarinet. Playing from piano music is frequently recreational in nature which helps encourage development. Parts for "C" clarinets are frequently found in the original editions of symphonic music from the classic period, although modern school editions transpose them to the B-flat instrument. The process of making the transposition from the concert pitch to B-flat clarinet involves adding two sharps or subtracting two flats from the key signature and reading the notes a tone higher than written. The following example illustrates the interval and key signature transpositions.

Piano   B-flat Clarinet
Key: C   Key: D

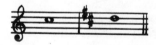

Piano   B-flat Clarinet
Key: A-flat   Key: B-flat

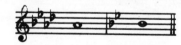

Piano   B-flat Clarinet
Key: G   Key: A

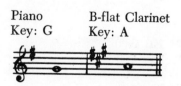

2. *Playing "A" clarinet parts on the B-flat clarinet.* Much of the orchestral literature includes parts written for the "A" clarinet as well as for the B-flat. While the "A" instruments are common enough, frequently being owned by the school and loaned to the student, this transposition is so frequent that facility should be acquired. To play "A" clarinet parts on the B-flat clarinet transpose each note down one-half step either through changing the key signature or simple reading down. The "A" instrument is chosen by the composer in order to avoid asking the clarinets to play in a large number of sharps or flats, so when an A part is being played on the B-flat the technical demands on the player are greater than if it were being played on the A instrument. The following example ilustrates the interval and key signature transpositions.

A Clarinet   B-flat Clarinet
Key: C   Key: B

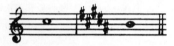

A Clarinet   B-flat Clarinet
Key: B-flat   Key: A

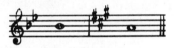

A Clarinet   B-flat Clarinet
Key: A-flat   Key: G

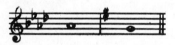

3. *Playing Alto Saxophone parts on the B-flat Clarinet.* It is mandatory that a player who doubles on Alto saxophone and clarinet be able to transpose and play the saxophone parts on the clarinet. There are other occasions where this facility is needed as well. To play the E-flat Alto saxophone parts on the B-flat clarinet transpose a perfect fifth lower, or add one flat or subtract one sharp from the saxophone key signature and play a fifth lower making the proper adjustments for accidentals. The following illustrates the interval and key relationships.

Alto Saxophone   B-flat Clarinet
Key: C   Key: F

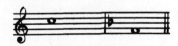

Alto Saxophone   B-flat Clarinet
Key: D   Key: G

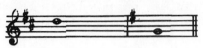

Alto Saxophone   B-flat Clarinet
Key: B-flat   Key: E-flat

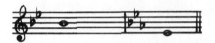

4. *Playing "D" Clarinet parts on the E-flat Clarinet.* The high D clarinet is used in some orchestral music of the nineteenth and early twentieth centuries in place of the E-flat clarinet. In this country these parts are almost invariably played on the E-flat instrument. The transposition involved is exactly the same as that for playing music for A clarinet on the B-flat intsrument. Each tone is played a half-step lower.

5. *Playing String Bass or Tuba Parts on the E-flat Contra-Bass Clarinet.* The E-flat Contra-Bass clarinet is coming more and more into general use as a permanent member of the concert band. Since a great many band arrangements do not publish a printed part for this instrument, a string bass or tuba part is substituted, and the player is expected to make a direct transposition. This is a purely mechanical transposition. Substitute a treble clef for the bass clef, add three sharps to the key signature and play as written, making the necessary adjustments for accidentals. School musicians rapidly gain facility in this transposition until it becomes automatic.

Tuba   Clarinet
Key: C   Key: A

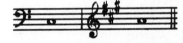

Tuba   Clarinet
Key: A-flat Key: F

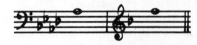

Tuba   Clarinet
Key: G   Key: E

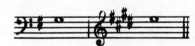

SELECTION OF INSTRUMENTS

The system of fingering used on present day instruments was adapted from the principles first applied to the flute by Carl Boehm. This mechanical system, called the Boehm System clarinet, was developed in Paris between 1835 and 1845 by Klose who was professor of clarinet at the Paris Conservatory and whose method is still widely used, and by Auguste Buffet, founder of the Buffet company. The Boehm system is now the standard for all clarinets, although it took over fifty years after its introduction for it to be accepted.

The fingering mechanism which preceded it is known as the Albert System, an instrument with thirteen keys and two rings. It had many deficiencies, among them poor intonation, and it was virtually impossible to play in all keys. This mechanical difficulty in playing in all keys with the Albert System and the models which preceded it, made it necessary for composers to use the B-flat, A, and C instruments according to the key of the music, and all professional clarinetists used all three. Albert System clarinets were widely distributed in this country up until about 1925, and many of the instruments are still for sale in loan shops. Needless to say, no student should be handicapped by starting to play an Albert System even though the instrument would be inexpensive.

Models of the Boehm System Clarinet. Various models of clarinets are available and are usually designated by two numbers indicating the number of keys and the number of rings:

1. 17-6, seventeen keys and six rings. This is the standard model of the instrument, and a fair estimate would indicate that probably over 85% of all instruments in use are this model. Few if any Class II or Class III instruments are available in anything other than this model.

2. 17-7, seventeen keys and seven rings. This model differs from the preceding model in that a ring is added to the one hole covered by the third finger. This ring operates an additional small tone hole covered by a pad and makes possible an extremely useful alternate finger-

ing for E-flat and B-flat: 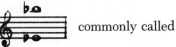 commonly called

the "Fork B-flat" fingering, since the B-flat is produced by closing the first and third tone holes. This additional ring adds no complication to the mechanism of the instrument, but improves intonation of certain notes, and makes certain technical passages smoother and easier. It adds very little to the cost of the instrument, and it is this model which should be purchased for a student past the intermediate level of instruction, or who aspires to becoming a fine clarinetist.

3. Articulated G-sharp. This key is found both on the 17-6 and 17-7 models and although it is designated as the articulated G-sharp key it also produces C-sharp:

 An articulated G-sharp key is one which

is connected to the rings operated by the fingers of the right hand so that if the G-sharp key is being held open by the left little finger it is automatically closed when the rings on the lower joint are down. This facilitates trills involving G-sharp or C-sharp, as well as certain other passages. The addition of this key has two disadvantages: it adds complicated mechanism to the instrument involving two springs working against each other which seem to get out of order frequently, and it eliminates the use of the alternate fingering for F in the high register. For these reasons an instrument with the articulated G-sharp is not recommended.

4. Full Boehm. A full Boehm clarinet has twenty keys, seven rings, and an articulated G-sharp. It is rarely seen, and never recommended for use, being more of a curiosity than anything else. The three additional keys are added to those already operated by the little fingers and create a very heavy and complicated mechanism on the lower joint. The disadvantages of this model far outweigh its advantages.

Metal and Plastic Instruments. The one-piece metal or plastic clarinets on which the lower, and upper joints (and sometimes the bell as well) are manufactured as a single piece have some advantages for use with young beginners. When they were first introduced their principal advantage was in their low cost as compared to instruments made of wood. Even today their cost is less than one-third that of the artist quality wooden instrument. The metal instruments are less susceptible to damage in the hands of youngsters than are wood or plastic instruments, and easier and more economical to maintain. Their principal disadvantage is their poor musical quality. Since they are production line instruments most of the work is done by machines, there is not the accuracy of intonation nor the careful fitting of moving parts found on Class I wood instruments.

In the early 1930's at least two fine instrument manufacturers were producing metal clarinets of a musical and mechanical quality comparable to the finest metal flutes. These instruments permitted the highest quality of musical performance, but failed to be accepted since the workmanship on them put them into the same price class as the fine wooden instruments, and prejudice against metal clarinets on the artist level could not be overcome. It took over fifty years before the prejudice against metal flutes was overcome and professionals began using them instead of wood instruments. It is a proven scientific fact that there is no difference in tone quality between a wood instrument and a metal instrument *provided* the quality of workmanship is the same. Perhaps the future will see a return of fine metal clarinets.

The use of various plastic materials for clarinets has been a post World War II development. Most plastic clarinets look like wooden instruments, although at least one manufacturer makes them in colors other than black. Plastic has the advantage of being moulded into shape rapidly and economically, and some plastics approach the hardness of wood. Not only are B-flat clarinets made of plastic, but also Alto and Bass instruments. The chief advantage of plastic instruments lies in their cost. Since they are inexpensive to make their cost is considerably lower than wood instruments. As with the one-piece metal instruments, a minimum of hand work and attention seems to be given to plastic instruments. There is a tremendous range from good to bad in plastic instruments—they are not all the same by any means. Choose critically between various brands when purchasing. Disadvantages of plastic clarinets include the danger of the body of the instrument breaking when dropped, something which does not happen to wood or metal instruments, and the plastic is difficult if not impossible to repair. Damaged joints on plastic instruments are usually replaced by a new one, with mechanism of the broken joint transferred to the replacement. Posts knocked loose on a plastic instrument pose a more difficult repair job than on wooden instruments.

Plastic clarinets seem to be gradually replacing metal clarinets, and it is possible that the metal instruments will disappear from the scene in time. Avoid purchasing imported metal clarinets. Historically the quality of such instruments has been so poor that they rapidly deteriorate beyond practical usage, and have not been of particularly musical quality.

STUDENT QUALIFICATIONS AND APTITUDES

A certain amount of innate musical talent is necessary to play any instrument successfully, and the fact that the student does not possess this necessary minimum of talent may be determined either by testing or by permitting experiment on the instrument.

Standards of physical aptitudes for the clarinet are not always reliable. It goes without saying that the student must be physically large enough so that he may hold the instrument with the proper hand position and cover the holes properly. Students who are too small to play the instrument develop poor hand positions which are extremely difficult to correct, make slow progress, and tend to become discouraged because of the physical handicap. Any student with normal teeth, lip and chin formation can play the clarinet successfully. Thick lips and thin lips, overbite and underbite, crooked teeth and straight teeth can all be compensated for the embouchure formation without any adverse results on future development.

A natural aptitude for the clarinet may be determined by the success of the student in producing a steady natural tone of the highest pitch (approximately concert "C" above the staff) with the mouthpiece and reed alone after some instruction on embouchure formation.

The student should be able to produce strong clear tones in this manner and sustain them five to ten seconds before preceding with the complete instrument. Some students will accomplish this quickly, others may fail for some time but with instruction and guidance may develop an equal facility.

The clarinet is the best and most common beginning instrument of the woodwind family, and large numbers of students should be started on the instrument in the elementary school. Once facility is developed on the clarinet, the student can easily transfer to flute, oboe, bassoon, or saxophone with little loss in facility, and will pick up his musical progress on the new instrument without difficulty.

In selecting students for any instrument it must be remembered that interest and persistence are the greatest of all aptitudes.

CARE OF THE CLARINET

Assemble and disassemble with care. Keep the instrument in its case when not in use. It is most important that the instrument be thoroughly dried after each playing. The process of drying it and putting it into the case does not take much time, and is well worth the time spent. The habit of thorough drying should be established from the very beginning of clarinet study. The suggested step-by-step process is efficient and should be checked regularly by the instructor until it is easily accomplished by the student.

1. *Drying the Clarinet*. Take the instrument apart in the reverse order of assembly. Shake moisture out of each end of each joint and place the parts carefully in the case. Then swab each piece using a chamois swab made of a single piece of chamois with a strong cord long enough to reach through the length of the upper and lower joints and with a weight on the end of the string. The weight should be absolutely smooth so as not to scratch the bore of the instrument. Swabs of this type in sizes to fit the B-flat, Alto, and Bass clarinets are available commercially and are inexpensive. Or a B-flat clarinet swab can be made of a well tanned piece of chamois four inches by six inches. Tie a heavy nylon cord eighteen inches long to one corner, and tie a smooth weight like a small lead fishing weight to the end of the cord. Swabs for Alto, Bass or Contra-Bass instruments may be similarly made in increasingly larger sizes. An old linen handkerchief which is lint free may be substituted for the chamois if desired as it is equally efficient.

2. The mouthpiece must be cleaned from both ends. Place the forefinger in the center of the chamois and wipe out tone chamber. (Figure C-74.) Twist chamois and clean bore. (Figure C-75.) Wipe outside of mouthpiece. The chamois must not be pulled through the mouthpiece as the metal weight may scratch the lay or chip the tip.

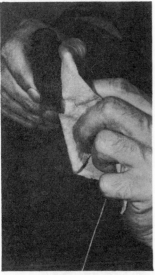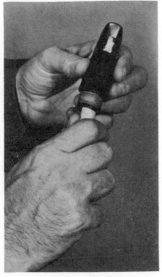

| Figure C-74. | Figure C-75. |

3. The barrel joint is cleaned by drawing the swab through once or twice. (Figure C-76.) Then fold the chamois over the forefinger and carefully wipe all moisture out of both of the connecting sleeves. (Figure C-77.)

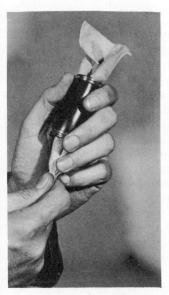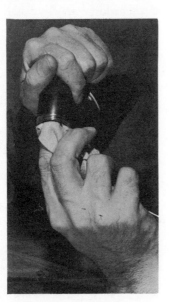

| Figure C-76. | Figure C-77. |

4. The upper joint is cleaned by dropping the weight from the top (Figure C-78) and drawing it through several times. (Figure C-79.) Then wipe moisture off the cork end. The swab must be dropped from the top down as the bore of the instrument increases gradually toward the bottom of the joint. A swab put in from the larger end frequently sticks and is difficult to remove.

Teachers of beginning classes will save them many hours of time spent in removing stuck swabs from the upper joint if they will insist on always starting the process from the top of each joint.

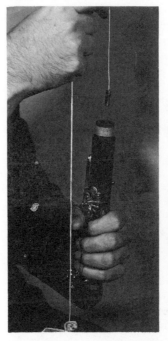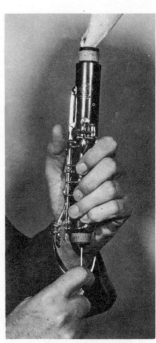

| Figure C-78. | Figure C-79. |

5. The lower joint is cleaned by dropping the weight on the swab from the top (Figure C-80) and drawing

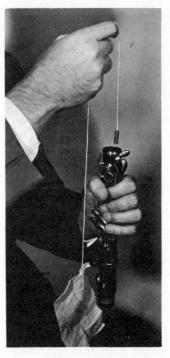

Figure C-80.

it through several times. (Figure C-81.) Put the fore-finger in the center of the chamois and wipe out the upper end. (Figure C-82.) Then wipe off cork end as before.

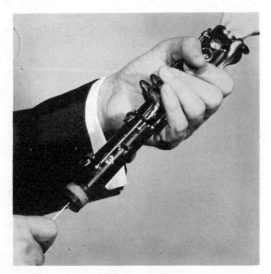

Figure C-81.

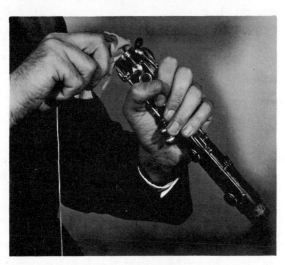

Figure C-82.

6. The bell should be wiped out from the large end with the chamois as shown in Figure C-83. Clean the upper end in the same fashion as on the lower joint.

Parts are replaced in the case as they are dried. Beginners cases must be checked to be sure that the parts are properly in place. Tone holes up, side keys on both joints fitted exactly into the space provided in the case, ligature and mouthpiece cap in place on the mouthpiece. Cases must never be forced closed. If they do not close easily check the placement of the parts. The photograph earlier in the chapter identifying parts of the clarinet shows a typical arrangement of parts in the case.

The reed must be removed from the mouthpiece, carefully dried, and placed in the reed case so that it will dry flat without warping.

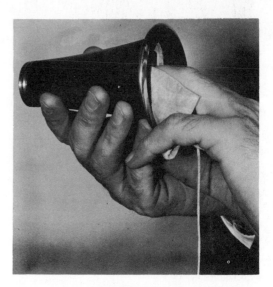

Figure C-83.

Regular Maintenance of the Instrument

1. *Oiling the Bore.* Even though they are made of the hardest wood available—Grenadilla—wood instruments are subject to cracking. Careful drying after each playing will help avoid this but authorities recommend that the bore of a wood instrument be oiled with specially prepared bore oil. New instruments should have the bore oiled once a week for three months, once every two weeks for the next three months, once a month for the next six, and then five or six times each year.

This must be done with care so that no oil gets on the pads, since it dries out and hardens the pads and they no longer cover the holes without leaking. The oiling can be done with a commercial oiler, or with a swab kept for this purpose. The swab should be lightly oiled, not saturated, and drawn through the parts of the instrument once or twice so as to coat the inside very lightly. The outside of the instrument is not oiled as a rule, although it may be given a very light coat of oil occasionally where temperature and humidity extremes are common.

2. *Dusting the Instrument.* After an instrument has been in use over a period of time, dust collects under the key mechanism. This can and should be removed with a soft watercolor brush. (Figure C-84.)

3. *Oiling the Mechanism.* The mechanism, if it is to remain in the best playing condition, must be oiled regularly four or five times a year. Special oil for this purpose is commercially available. A drop of oil on the end of a toothpick should be put at each pivot point of each key. (Figure C-85.) Do this carefully so that no oil can get onto the pads.

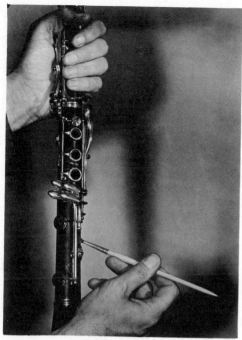

Figure C-84.

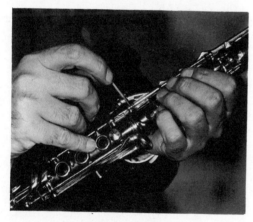

Figure C-85.

4. *Shining the Keys.* Silver polish should never be used on the keys. If keys become excessively dull they must be polished by a repairman who will remove them from the instrument. They are never polished while they are on the instrument. Keys may be kept in good condition if they are wiped regularly with a soft cloth or a chamois to remove perspiration and dirt. Using silver polish on the keys while they are on the instrument will foul pivot points on the mechanism, and damage pads so that they will leak. It is well to caution students against polishing the keys.

5. *Bent Keys.* In spite of the best of care keys become bent out of line. No attempt should be made to straighten them while they are on the instrument. This puts excessive pressure on both the keys and their posts and the instrument may be damaged even more. Keys

must be removed from the instrument by a repairman who has the tools to straighten and align them. Bent keys will cause unevenness in technique, since some of them stick, or become out of line so that the fingers do not fall on them naturally.

6. *Sticking Pads.* If the instrument is not thoroughly dried before it is put into its case, or if the humidity is excessive even temporarily, some pads on the instrument will stick tightly, or will stick momentarily before opening. Moisture can be removed from them by placing a cigarette paper between the pad and the tone hole, pressing down on the key firmly. Then release the key and repeat the process until the key no longer sticks. If this does not relieve the sticking, put the cigarette paper in place, press on the key, and pull it slowly from under the pad. Repeat the process several times. If the condition reoccurs regularly have the pad replaced. Never use powder on pads to stop sticking.

7. *Water in Tone Holes.* Some instruments tend to collect water in certain tone holes under pads that are normally closed, producing a bubbling tone when these keys are opened. This may be removed by opening the key and blowing firmly into the hole. If time permits take the instrument apart and swab the joint on which this occurs thoroughly. If a particular hole collects water regularly it may frequently be corrected by removing the key and coating the inside of the tone hole lightly with vaseline. Avoid a heavy coat of vaseline as it will soak into the pad.

8. *Leaky Pads.* Pads on an instrument wear out with use. Some wear out more rapidly than others and begin to leak causing the instrument to respond with difficulty on certain notes or if the leak is a large one to squeak on certain notes. To test for leaks take the instrument apart. Plug the lower end of the joint with a cork or with the palm of the hand. Cover the tone holes and close all keys as if playing, avoiding using more pressure against the holes or keys than is used when playing. Blow through the other end with as much pressure as possible. Leaky pads can be identified by leaking air. If a tone hole normally covered by a key and pad held closed by a spring leaks when maximum wind pressure is applied the spring on that key must be strengthened or replaced. A joint in perfect condition will not leak air no matter how much breath pressure is applied.

If the leak cannot be located by the above method, an alternative method which assures positive seating of all pads is to use cigarette papers (or feeler papers if purchased commercially). The cigarette paper should be cut or torn into strips about a quarter inch wide. Slide one end of the paper under the pad, put the normal amount of pressure against the pad if the key is not held closed with a spring, and slowly draw the paper out. As long as the pressure against the paper remains constant there is no leak. If the pressure suddenly lessens the pad is not properly seated. Repeat the process completely around the pad so that all edges are tested.

The process of blowing cigarette smoke through the instrument to identify a leak through seeing the cigarette smoke coming out of the leak is not recommended. The nicotine in the smoke coats the pads and if this is done frequently will damage them so that they harden and leak.

Pads may leak because they are not seated properly, or because they are worn. A loose membrane on the bottom of the pad indicates that it should be replaced immediately, even though it is not leaking at that time. It soon will be, and if the condition persists it will produce a buzz when that particular key is used to play a note.

9. *Regular Overhaul.* The condition of every instrument must be checked at least once a year by the instructor or by a repairman. Regular maintenance keeps an instrument in playing condition over a period of years, rather than allowing it to gradually deteriorate becoming increasingly difficult to play. Every instrument must have a complete overhaul every three to five years depending on amount of usage. If fine instruments receive a yearly checkup and regular overhauls they will last in virtually perfect condition for many years. The services of a competent repairman is invaluable and an asset to any program of instrumental instruction.

BIBLIOGRAPHY OF STUDY MATERIALS

The wealth of musical material for the study of clarinet is so extensive that it is impossible to include a complete survey of what is available. Information on music for clarinets is available from several sources, among them the following:

1. Opperman, Kalmen. *Repertory of the Clarinet.* New York: Ricordi 1960. This book lists texts, methods of all sorts, solos, ensemble music of all types which includes clarinet, concerti, etc. It is the most complete listing available, but does not evaluate nor grade the material.
2. Thurston, Frederick. *Clarinet Technique.* London: Oxford University Press, 1956, pp. 51-98. A list of solos, concerti, and ensembles involving clarinet. No texts, methods, etudes, etc., are included. The lists are not graded nor evaluated.
3. *Selective Music Lists: Instrumental and Vocal Solos and Ensembles.* Published by the National Interscholastic Music Activities Commission, 1201 Sixteenth St., N.W. Washington 6, D. C. Selective and graded lists of solos and ensembles using clarinets.
4. Catalogs of retail stores specializing in woodwind music which list currently available publications of all publishers both foreign and domestic.[7] An examination of such a catalog will reveal that an astounding quantity of excellent material for all purposes is available.

In the sections which follow, beginning methods, the standard methods, and additional materials, are listed with comments about each. Lists of materials without personal contact with them are of little value, and the reader is urged to examine as many of these as possible. Actual use for the purpose of evaluation is essential, since many books do not give the results in practice that a visual examination would indicate.

Except for the very beginners, a student should be studying in several books at the same time in order to get a well rounded experience, to maintain interest, and provide stimulation to the study of the instrument. The following types of materials for simultaneous study are suggested:

1. *A Method Book.* These are basic and provide continuity, and can be selected to fit the needs of the student at any stage of his progress.
2. *Technical Studies.* By this is meant the study of major and minor scales, arpeggios, etc. in various forms. These are on various levels of difficulty and should be studied in this order: (a) Klose—pages 123-135 in the Klose-Bellison published by Carl Fischer but published in other standard method books as well; (b) J. B. Albert— Twenty-four Varied Scales and Exercises; (c) Fritz Kroepsch— 416 Progressive Daily Studies Book III; and (d) Carl Baermann—Complete Method for Clarinet, Part III. Various other similar studies are available and may be inserted at appropriate stages if needed.
3. *A Book of Etudes or Studies.* A number of these are listed in the section on additional study materials. Typical of these books are those by Lo-Presti, Rose, Perier, and Jean-Jean. It is important to include a variety of these books in order to provide an opportunity to study various musical styles.
4. *Duets or Other Ensemble Music.* Ensemble experience is an integral part of the learning process on every level.
5. *Solos.* A great variety of solo material is available for every level and it is important to begin this type of experience as early in the student's study as possible. Many solos are available for the beginning level and the potential number increases rapidly as the technical development of the student increases.

As examples of how materials can be grouped for study the following are typical. The groups are not progressive but simply illustrative of what can be used at various stages of development.

Group I. Suitable for a Beginning Student
  a. Bodegraven, Paul Van. *Adventures in Clarinet Playing*, Book I.
  b. Collis, James. *Modern Course for the Clarinet,* Book I.

---

[7]See appendix IV for a list of these.

c. Endresen, P. *Supplementary Studies for Clarinet.*
d. Kueffner, J. *Fifty Progressive Duets, op. 80.*
e. Appropriate solo material.

Group II.   Suitable for an Intermediate Student
a. Langenus, Gustave. *Method for Clarinet*, Part I.
b. Klose, H. *Method for Clarinet*, p. 123-135. Technical Studies.
c. LoPresti, Ronald. *20 Melodic Studies for Clarinet*
d. Voxman, H. *Selected Duets for Clarinet*, Vol. I.
e. Appropriate solo material.

Group III.   Suitable for an Upper-Intermediate Student
a. Baermann, Carl. *Complete Method for Clarinet*, Part II.
b. Albert, J. B. *Twenty-four Varied Scales and Exercises.*
c. Rose, C. *40 Studies for Clarinet.*
d. Bach-Langenus. *J. S. Bach Clarinet Duos.*
e. Appropriate solos.

Group IV.   Suitable for an Advanced Student
a. Langenus, Gustave. *Method for Clarinet*, Part III.
b. Baermann, Carl. *Complete Method for Clarinet*, Part III.
c. Perier, A. *Etudes De Gener Et D'Interpretation*, Vol. I.
d. Mozart, W. A. *Three Duos.*
e. Appropriate solos.

It should be emphasized that these groups are suggestive and are not progressive. They are not a course of study. Indeed, a course of study which would be applicable to all students would be impossible. Study materials must be selected to fit the needs of a particular student or class. The best teacher is one who not only knows a large repertoire of materials, but chooses carefully and makes use of it.

The sections which follow list typical materials in various classifications. The use of the words beginning, intermediate, and advanced to indicate levels of difficulty are simply general indications since the words have different meanings to different people. Experience with the materials will soon classify and identify exact grade of difficulty.

Beginning Methods

In the beginning study of the clarinet authorities are almost unanimous in agreement on at least two points: that a reasonable good tone and facility should be developed in the chalameau register before the clarion register is introduced, and that articulation, or tonguing, must not be started until the chalameau tone is established and in the process of developing. Many beginning methods books violate the second of these by introducing articulation with the first or second lesson through the attempt to teach rhythmic reading, simultaneously with tone production. This sets up almost insurmountable problems for the student who must learn to hold the instrument, form an embouchure, establish breath support, learn to articulate, and learn fingerings for the notes.

With all these problems presented at the same time it is a wonder that any student succeeds, and accounts for the very slow progress of many classes. Taking the student into the clarion register before the chalameau register is well established causes serious problems in embouchure development, since an unsettled embouchure will make incorrect adjustments in order to play the clarion register. If the problem of crossing the break is introduced at the same time the difficulties are multiplied many fold. Some beginning methods do this.

In selecting a method book for the beginning clarinet all these things must be taken into account. Several standard beginning method books are listed below. As many of these as possible should be examined before making a selection for actual use.

Group I. These books present the technical problems in good order, establish the chalameau register first, delay articulation, and have material of musical interest. Two or more of them may be used simultaneously with good results. Paul Van Bodegraven's "Adventures in Clarinet Playing" and the method by James Collis are an excellent pair.

Bodegraven, Paul Van. *Adventures in Clarinet Playing.* Book I, Book II. Staff Music Publishing Co.

Bodegraven, Paul Van. *A Clarinet Method for Grade Schools.* Carl Fischer.

Collis, James. *Modern Course for the Clarinet.* Book I, Book II. Henri Elkan Music Publishers.

Phillips, Harry I. *The Clarinet Class.* Summy-Birchard Publishing Co.

Stubbins, William H. *The Study of the Clarinet.* George Wahr Publishing Co.

Waln, George. *Elementary Clarinet Method.* Belwin.

Group II. Many of these books use the rhythm approach and introduce articulation from the very beginning. Others present problems without sufficient foundation for solving them, or lack musical interest. All have many assets, and may be preferred as the beginning text. Any of them can be used with one of the Group I books after the student is established. Some of them progress faster and farther than others, approaching the technical level of those in Group III.

Anzalone, Valentine. *Breeze-Easy Method for Clarinet.* Book I, Book II. M. Witmark & Sons.

Dalby, Cleon E. *All Melody Method for Clarinet.* Book I, Book II. Pro-Art Publications.

Herfurth, C. Paul. *A Tune A Day for Clarinet.* Book I, Book II. Boston Music Company.

Hetzel, Jack. *Hetzel's Visual Method for the Clarinet.* Oliver Ditson Company.

Hovey, Nilo W. *Belwin Clarinet Method.* Vol. I, II, & III. Belwin, Inc.

Hovey, Nilo W. *Rubank Elementary Method for Clarinet.* Rubank, Inc.

Liegel, Leopold. *Carl Fischer Basic Method for the Clarinet.* Carl Fischer.

Manring, Ernest. *Elementary Method for Clarinet*. Mills Music, Inc.

Lindeman, Ben. *Melodious Fundamentals for Clarinet*. Charles Colin, Inc.

Group III. These books progress farther or faster or both than either of the previous groups. The second volume of these in both the first and second group would fall into this classification as well. These books can be used to follow those previously considered, or picked up before they are completed.

Hendrickson, Clarence V. *Hendrickson Method for Clarinet*. Belwin, Inc.

Hovey, Nilo W. *Daily Exercises for Clarinet* (compiled from the works of Albert and Pares). Belwin, Inc.

Langenus, Gustave.[8] *Complete Method for the Boehm Clarinet*. Part I. Carl Fischer.

Lindeman, Ben. *Melodious Fundamentals for Clarinet. Intermediate Series*. Charles Colin, Inc.

Mitchell, Albert G. *Mitchell's Class Method for the Clarinet*. Oliver Ditson.

The Standard Methods

There are four standard methods for the clarinet which are widely used, and all except one, that by Langenus, are about a hundred years old. None of them are suitable for the beginning student according to present day pedagogy since methods of instruction have undergone many changes in the years since they were written. A thoroughly schooled clarinetist will have studied portions, or all of each of them at one stage or another in his development. All are quite different in their content, unlike the present day beginning methods which seem to have been cast from the same mold, and all have valuable contributions to make. The four are discussed below in some detail, and should be examined carefully.

I. Langenus, Gustave. *Complete Method for the Boehm Clarinet*. Part I, Part II, Part III. Carl Fischer, Inc.

This is the only one of the standard methods which was written in the twentieth century, and which makes use of contemporary teaching techniques. Gustave Langenus was a distinguished New York clarinetist who has had tremendous influence on the clarinet through his teaching and his many publications of original works and arrangements for the instrument. Parts I and II are progressive, and Part I can be started after completion of a beginning method, or toward the end of the beginning method, depending on which one is selected. Part II is a continuation of Part I. Part III is Virtuoso Studies and Duos and represent a wide jump in technical requirements over the end of Part II and is for advanced students.

Part I of this method is without doubt the best organized and presented method for any of the woodwind instruments. It presents and develops the various technical problems for the instrument logically and musically. Any student who thoroughly studies Parts I and II will have both an excellent technical as well as musical foundation upon which to build his performance. Any teacher who is responsible for the development of clarinetists on any level should study these books thoroughly, and should be able to play Part I in order to thoroughly understand the instrument.

All three volumes make extensive use of duets which add interest to the study of the instrument. All are carefully edited in the most musical fashion, and contain written comments and instructions which clarify the purpose of the study.

II. Baermann, Carl. *Complete Method for Clarinet, Op. 63*. Two editions. Revised and edited by Gustave Langenus. Carl Fischer, Inc. Parts I, II, III complete or Parts I and II in a single volume and Part III in a single volume. No piano accompaniments. Cundy-Bettoney Co., Inc. Revised by Harry Bettoney and published as follows: Parts I & II in a single volume; Piano accompaniment to Part II; Part III; Part IV; Piano accompaniment to Part IV; Part V.

Carl Baermann (1820-1865) was the most noted German clarinetist of his day, and a prolific composer for the instrument. His father was also a noted clarinetist and it is probable that father and son collaborated on this method. Both Baermanns worked toward the technical improvement of the mechanism of the clarinet at the same time Theobald Boehm was working on the improvement of the flute. They developed a Baermann system clarinet which was similar to the Albert system clarinet, but which was never widely used outside of Germany, having been superceded by the Boehm system clarinet which was developed in France at about the same time. The Cundy-Bettoney edition indicates fingering choices for the Albert-Baermann system as well as for the Boehm system.

Part I, or the 1st Division, is purely theoretical introductory material which is interesting but of little practical value. In the Carl Fischer edition it is eleven pages long, and in the Cundy-Bettoney edition the complete general instructions by Baermann are reprinted along with additional technical information by the editor to the extent of 52 pages.

Part II is useful for the upper intermediate level of study. It develops gradually and thoroughly the facility for different fingerings through occasional pages of one measure mechanical studies, but primarily through a series of very musical studies, some of them given names to indicate that they are solos, progressively through major and minor keys up to and including three flats. All facets of nineteenth century musical style are developed, with emphasis on the development of a sense of phrasing as well as technical development. A piano

---

[8]By far the best choice to follow any beginning method, or to be introduced after the student is past the easy beginning stage.

accompaniment is available for all the fifty studies in Part II except for the mechanism and scale studies. The use of the piano accompaniment is recommended, and is quite valuable in giving the student continual experience playing with accompaniment and all the values inherent in this experience. The accompaniments are not pianistically difficult and can be played easily by a pianist with average technique. This piano accompaniment is published only by Cundy-Bettoney, but the rehearsal letters are identical with those in the Carl Fischer edition so that it can be used with either edition.

Part III is designated as daily studies and are for advanced players. All studies are in all keys, and encompass the entire professional range of the instrument. These include scales, chromatic scales, major and minor arpeggios, diminished seventh chords, interrupted scales, broken major and minor chords, returning scales, dominant seventh chords, scales in thirds, scales in sixths, and four general studies on octaves and staccato. Mastery of this volume is a must for the advanced clarinetist, for it provides a technical facility in all keys which forms the basis for much of the music he will be playing.

Part IV is a continuation of Part II of this method, and is Opus 64 of Baermann's works. It is published in this country only by Cundy-Bettoney and a piano accompaniment is available. It does not continue progressively through the keys from where Part II left off, but is devoted to certain technical problems. Many of the studies in this part as well as in Part II would make interesting and satisfactory solos for public performance.

Part V is published by Cundy-Bettoney and is a collection of excerpts from the works of Baermann other than Opus 63 and 64. It is for the advanced student, and if the previous four parts have been covered, there is little need for studying this volume as it will add little to the advancement of the student. The music is repetitious and boring.

III. Klose, H. *Celebrated Method for the Clarinet.* Revised and Enlarged by Simeon Bellison. Carl Fischer, Inc. Published complete or Parts I and II separately.

This is perhaps the most widely used of the standard methods for clarinet, for it contains much valuable material. Klose was professor of clarinet at the Paris Conservatory around 1850, and with August Buffet is credited with the development of the Boehm system clarinet. His method was the first written for this system, and the mechanism studies were intended to introduce the various uses of this new system.

The Klose method is not a beginning method, nor is it progressive in difficulty. In order to use it effectively the teacher must skip around through the volume. Excerpts designed for the advanced beginner and intermediate level students are published by the Carl Fischer company under the title "Klose-Prescott" method. It is less expensive, and although it is not progressive it contains essential material from both parts I and II of the complete edition.

Use of the Klose method can start with the advanced beginner. The 68 and 141 mechanical exercises present in capsule form fingering problems which can be mastered and put to use by the beginner who has a basic facility in the chalameau and clarion registers of the instrument, and who has learned to cross the break without too much difficulty. The "Fifty Progressive Duets" by Joseph Kuffner, Op. 80 are useful on this stage of development and are reprinted in this edition of the Klose mehod. These duets are also published separately by Carl Fischer, for those who don't wish to purchase the method, and are very useful in the young clarinet class since both parts of the duet are written for the student, rather than the student-teacher pattern used in some methods.

The Klose "Scales and Exercises" are in duet form and take the student through major keys only, and are more difficult than those by Kuffner. The scale and arpeggio exercises at the beginning of Part II are basic to the study of the clarinet, and should be studied by the intermediate student as the first of a series of progressively more difficult studies of this type.

The "Fifteen Grand Duets" pages 136-201 of Part II are for the advanced student, and are widely used, although they require considerable editing by the teacher in order to bring them into line with contemporary performance styles. The "Twenty Studies" on pages 216-255 are quite advanced technically and present various technical problems. These too require considerable editing since these, as well as the entire book, are basically a reprint of the 1898 edition with very minor additions to the original plate by the editor in order that a new copyright could be secured.

The present edition concludes with a reprint of Book II of the Kroepsch "416 Progressive Daily Studies for the Clarinet," which starts with exercises in three flats and progresses through the keys to six flats. The Kroepsch studies are considered in detail later.

IV. Lazarus, Henry. *Method for Clarinet in Three Parts,* available complete, or each part singly. Cundy-Bettoney, Revised by Gustave Langenus. Carl Fischer, Revised by Simeon Bellison.

Henry Lazarus (1815-1895) was the most famous English clarinetist of his time. From 1858 he was professor at Kneller Hall, the great English school of music. His method was written for use with his students at Kneller Hall, and the duets it contains are among the most interesting and challenging in clarinet literature.

In addition to the original method by Lazarus each edition includes certain works by other composers. The Cundy-Bettoney edition includes: Berr—Fifteen Progressive Duets, Kuffner—Fifty Progressive Duets, Albert—Twenty-Four Varied Scales, Schmidt—Twenty-Four Technical Exercises, Klose—Scale Studies, Blancou—Forty Studies from the works of Mazas, Cavallini—Thirty Caprices. The Carl Fischer Edition adds: Kuffner—Fifty Progressive Duets, Klose—Scale Studies, Albert—

Twenty-Four Varied Scales, and Kroepsch—416 Exercises for the Clarinet, Book I.

The range of difficulty in this method is from lower intermediate to quite advanced. The Cundy-Bettoney edition has a greater variety of material in both the intermediate and advanced range of difficulty and would be the better choice.

Summary

The methods by Baermann, Klose and Lazarus were all written at about the same time—the middle of the nineteenth century. The danger in using these methods to the exclusion of all other material lies in the fact that the musical style is exclusively that of the mid-nineteenth century. Limiting the experience of the student to this style is not the best procedure, and although these either singly or in combination must be used, care should be taken to include material of other styles from Baroque to Contemporary.

The Langenus method, unlike the other three, does include a wide variety of musical styles in the three volumes from baroque to the early twentieth century. It should be the basic method for the student, and can be supplemented by Baerman, Klose and sections of Lazarus in order to get a wide variety of material on approximately the same level of technical difficulty. None of these methods could be considered a beginning method, and must be preceded by one of the standard beginning methods books.

Additional Study Materials

The supply of study materials for the clarinet is practically inexhaustible, and it is impossible to make an exhaustive analysis of the entire scope. Particular attention should be paid to the materials printed in France. The major development of the study of clarinet and other woodwind instruments has been in France through the influence of the Paris Conservatory which has been in continuous existence for over a hundred years. There have been a series of outstanding artist-teachers at this institution from Berr and Klose to the present day. Each has made significant contributions to the study literature for the instrument, in particular Perier and Jean-Jean whose works have become classics for the instrument.

The following list of material represents a typical cross section of that which is most useful in varying situations, but is by no means all inclusive. These and others should be examined and put into use to determine what results will be obtained. Different teachers will obtain different results from the same material, so it is necessary to adapt material not only to the individual student, but to the pedagogy and concepts of the teacher.

Albert, J. B. *Twenty-Four Varied Scales and Exercises.* Carl Fischer. Intermediate. Goes through the circle of keys in major and minor scales in three forms, thirds, tonic arpeggios, and chromatic scales. Basic to the development of good technique.

Bitsch, Marcel. *Twelve Rhythmical Studies for Clarinet.* Alphonse Leduc. Extremely difficult rhythmically, these studies present and develop the complex rhythmic structure of meter changes and cross rhythms of the more advanced twentieth century style. Excellent for the advanced clarinetist to develop and establish facility in these styles.

Blancou, V. *Forty Studies from the Works of Mazas.* In Two Books. Cundy-Bettoney. Excellent studies in the intermediate range of difficulty arranged from the violin studies of Mazas. They are in the nineteenth century idiom and help develop basic facility. Mostly easy keys.

Delecluse, U. *Quinze Etudes from the Works of J. S. Bach.* Alphonse Leduc. Difficult. Excellent transcriptions of fifteen Bach works. An important item in the study of style.

Endresen, P. *Supplementary Studies for Clarinet.* Rubank, Inc. Beginning. A most useful collection of studies which can be used on the beginning level after the student is well started on his study of the instrument.

Jean-Jean, Paul. *Progressive and Melodic Studies for Clarinet.* Vols. I, II, III. Alphonse Leduc.

Volume I. Twenty Fairly Easy Progressive and Melodic Studies. While they are progressive and melodic, they are not fairly easy as the title indicates, but fall into the upper intermediate or lower advanced levels. These are excellent musically and are extremely well edited. They provide basic concepts in phrasing and style which is not obtainable elsewhere and should be a part of the study of every clarinetist who has reached a fairly advanced stage of development.

Volume II. Twenty Average Progressive and Melodic Studies. Numbered 21 to 40 in the series, these are not average but advanced level of difficulty. Keys used are three, four and five sharps and three and four flats, major and relative minor. These are useful to follow the first volume for those students who are seriously studying the instrument.

Volume III. Twenty Rather Difficult Progressive and Melodic Studies. Numbered 41 to 60 in the series, these are very difficult, completing the circle of keys through seven sharps and seven flats. They are only for the most advanced clarinetist who is interested in a real technical challenge.

Jean-Jean, Paul. *Twenty-five Technical and Melodic Studies. Alphonse Leduc.* While technically difficult, these studies are excellent musically. They carry the musical style into the twentieth century, especially from a rhythmic standpoint and should be studied by all advanced clarinetists. Some of them are with the accompaniment of three B-flat clarinets. A second volume has the second and third clarinet parts, while the fourth part is printed with the solo part. While useful in a clarinet class of more advanced students these do not make good program material.

Jean-Jean, Paul. 18 *Etudes de Perfectionnemen*. Editions Musicales Andrieu Freres. These eighteen studies are intended by the author to follow the preceding volumes. They are technically difficult, and for some reason, less musically interesting than the composer's other works. They are useful for the more advanced student who is consuming material at a rapid rate, but not essential in the normal progression of study.

Jean-Jean, Paul. 16 *Etudes Modernes pour Clarinette*. Buffet-Crampon & Cie. These extremely difficult studies are perhaps the only studies available which are built on strictly twentieth century harmonic progressions—whole tone scale, various types of triads and seventh chords other than the nineteenth century usage. These are essential to complete the study of any serious student of the clarinet.

Jean-Jean, Paul. *Vade-Mecum du Clarinettiste*. Alphonse Leduc. A unique book in clarinet literature designed for the use of the advanced clarinetist in maintaining his technical development when lack of time does not permit regular practice. The aim of the six studies according to the author "is to prepare instrumentalists in a very short space of time (about one-half hour) when, due to their occupations, they are not able to devote the time necessary for developed exercises and must nevertheless be ready to execute difficult passages from the standpoint of lips, tongue and fingers." These are skillfully written and accomplish their aim.

Kroepsch, F. *416 Progressive Daily Studies*. In Four Volumes. Carl Fischer or International Music Co. Books I and II, lower advanced, go through the circle of keys with two or three line exercises developing various facets of technique. The exercises are challenging and interesting. Basic to the development of good technique. Book III, lower advanced. Is in three sections, each going through the circle of keys in the form of scales and arpeggios. The same key in each of three sections should be studied simultaneously. Follows the Albert Scale studies in the sequence of basic scale and arpeggio studies. Book IV. Advanced level. Goes through the circle of keys with an etude in each. Difficult and not too interesting to most students.

Langenus, Gustave. *Clarinet Cadenzas*. Carl Fischer. Subtitled "How to Phrase Them" this book has 52 cardenzas selected from symphonic literature, chamber music, and solo repertoire written and phrased to indicate exactly how each is actually performed as contrasted to how they are notated. A very useful collection.

Langenus, Gustave. *Fingered Scale Studies*. Carl Fischer. Major and minor scales over the entire range of the instrument with alternate fingerings indicated for the most rapid execution. Very useful in developing proper selection of fingerings.

Langenus, Gustave. *Practical Transposition*. Carl Fischer. The only book available which teaches transposition for the clarinet. The procedures indicated in the book can be carried on through application to standard study material.

Lester, Leon. *Melodious Studies for Clarinet Solo*. Henri Elkan Music Publisher. An excellent collection of material for middle to advanced beginners, to be used after the student has developed facility crossing the break and the clarion register. One of the few good books on this level it should be given serious consideration. Concludes with a collection of familiar song melodies which the student will enjoy playing.

LoPresti, Ronald. *20 Melodic Studies for Clarinet*. Luverne Publications. Written by a talented young American composer especially for clarinet, and edited by William F. Osseck of the Eastman School of Music faculty, this is an outstanding collection of studies for the lower intermediate level. It is musically and technically sound and will help musical as well as technical development. A must for every intermediate student.

Mueller, Ivan. *22 Easy Studies*. Vols. I, II. International Music Co. Intermediate grade. Interesting and useful.

Pares, G. *Daily Technical Exercises for Clarinet*. Carl Fischer. *Foundation Studies for Clarinet*. Rubank, Inc. Two editions of the same material, of intermediate level of difficulty, these studies have been revised by Harvey S. Whistler (Rubank edition). Almost exclusively devoted to scale patterns in major and minor keys through four sharps and four flats. The scales appear in more different forms and patterns than in any other scale book, and for this reason add interest to their study.

Perier, A. *Le Debutant Clarinettiste*. Alphonse Leduc. While titled "The Beginning Clarinetist" this is not a beginning method book. It is however, an excellent, if not the best, choice of material for the lower intermediate level of difficulty. It lies well for the clarinet and is most musical, and combines well with Book II of the Langenus Method to provide additional material on this stage of development. Highly recommended.

Perier, A. *Vingt Etudes Faciles et Progressives*. Alphonse Leduc. Intended by the composer to follow the preceding book, these twenty studies are somewhat more difficult than that book and fall into the lower advanced level of technical difficulty. They are excellent studies of approximately the level of difficulty as the Rose 40 Studies and are recommended for use with them.

Perier, A. *Etudes De Genre Et D'Interpretation*. Vols. I, II. Alphonse Leduc. Fairly difficult studies in various styles for the development of interpretation of various kinds. Excellent material for the advanced student.

Perier, A. *Trente Etudes*. Alphonse Leduc. Selected from works of Bach and Handel and the nineteenth century violin school of Paganini and Dont these studies are quite difficult, but develop a sense of style and technical facility.

Perier, A. *Recueil De Sonates*. Vols. I, II, III. Alphonse Leduc. This collection of sonatas is "For the study of the classic style" and contains arrangements of compositions by J. S. Bach, Corelli, LeClair, Vivaldi, Geminiani, etc. Because the emphasis is on the study of the style, the technical range is wide within the general classification of advanced. Since the study of this particular style is often neglected by clarinetists, these volumes are invaluable, and at least one volume should be on the study list of every advanced clarinetist.

Rose, C. *26 Etudes for Clarinet*. Alphonse Leduc.
40 Studies for Clarinet. Vols. I, II. Carl Fischer.
32 Studies for Clarinet. Carl Fischer.
20 Studies from the Works of Rode. Cundy-Bettoney. The Rose studies are as much a standard part of the study of the clarinet as the Klose method, being included on the study list of practically every clarinetist. The four sets of studies are arranged above in the order of technical difficulty. The 26 Studies, which are available only in the French edition, are suitable for students on the upper intermediate stage of study; the 40 Studies and the 32 Studies on the lower advanced level of study; and the 20 Studies on the middle advanced level. All these editions require considerable editing by the teacher to make them meet contemporary standards of performance technique, but they are most rewarding, and some if not all of these books should be used.

Voxman, H. & Wm. Gower. *Advanced Method for Clarinet*. Vol. I, II. Rubank, Inc. Designed to fill the gap between the usual beginning methods and the time the student is ready to begin the study of one of the standard methods and its correlated material, the word "Advanced" in the title is not to be taken seriously. These are excellent books for the intermediate student. The material is selected from a wide variety of sources, arranged in progressive order, and carefully edited. Should be studied simultaneously with the books by LoPresti and Lester for a wider variety of experience.

Endresen, P. *Supplementary Studies for Clarinet*. Rubank, Inc.

Purseglove, A. *Crossing the Register*. Belwin. To supplement a beginning method when this problem is involved.

Voxman, H. *Classical Studies for Clarinet*. Rubank, Inc. Arrangements of music of Bach and Handel. *Selected Studies for Clarinet*. Rubank, Inc.

STUDY AND ACHIEVEMENT QUESTIONS

1. What is the theoretical playing range of the clarinet?
2. Select a band arrangement scored for a full compliment of clarinets. Transpose the clarinet parts to the pitches they actually sound and make a two-line piano score of these parts.
3. Indicate on a staff the beginning, intermediate, and advanced playing ranges of the Soprano clarinets. The Alto and Bass clarinets.
4. Identify the various parts of a clarinet making use of an instrument for illustration.
5. Perform the correct assembly process for the B-flat clarinet showing the correct holding position for each step. Do the same with an Alto or Bass clarinet.
6. Demonstrate the correct procedure for placing a reed on the clarinet mouthpiece. Add the protective cap.
7. Observe one or more beginning clarinet students assemble their instrument and fill out the check list for assembly. Do the same for intermediate and advanced level students. Correct any improper procedures if there is an opportunity to do so. This observation may be done in the college class, but is especially valuable if it can be done in an actual public school situation.
8. Demonstrate the correct holding position for the B-flat, Alto or Bass, and Contra-bass instruments.
9. Consider the advantages and disadvantages of holding the Alto or Bass clarinet to the right of the right leg rather than between the legs.
10. Describe and demonstrate the basic guide position of the hands on one or more instruments in the clarinet family.
11. Using a student who is unfamiliar with the clarinet give him complete instructions on the holding position and detailed instructions on establishing the correct hand position.
12. Describe and demonstrate the position and movements of the left thumb in playing from the lower to the upper register. In playing the third-line B-flat.
13. Describe and demonstrate the positions and movements of the first finger in playing second-line G-sharp. In playing second space A. Do the same for first finger right hand in fingering first-line E-flat or first-space F-sharp.
14. Observe one or more beginning players and fill out the check list for holding and hand positions. Do the same for intermediate and advanced players. If there is an opportunity to do so correct any improper procedures suggesting remedial measures. Make this observation in the public school situation if possible.

15. Describe and discuss the various types of clarinet embouchure formations. Indicate your choice and reasons for it. Then describe and demonstrate the step by step procedure for its formation. Do the same with a student who is unfamiliar with the instrument.

16. Observe one or more beginning, intermediate and advanced players and fill out the check list for embouchure formation for each. Suggest corrections and remedial measures.

17. Describe and perform the tuning process for one or more instruments in the clarinet family using intermediate or advanced players and an electronic tuning device if available.

18. What are the factors which will make a clarinet flat? sharp? Instruct an advanced player on how to demonstrate some of them.

19. Identify the four registers of the clarinet's range.

20. Listen to beginning, intermediate, and advanced clarinet players. Diagnose any problems in tone quality and suggest corrections.

21. Discuss various ways of placement and use of the tongue in articulation. Select the one you prefer and describe it in detail. Discuss various ways of developing articulation.

22. Select a musical example which has successive notes making use of the little fingers. Mark the sequence of left and right.

23. Indicate a procedure for making "crossing the break" easier. For slurring into the high register.

24. List the notes which have alternate fingerings, demonstrate each, and illustrate how each is used.

25. Identify the various transpositions which may be required of a clarinetist and describe how each is done.

26. Discuss the selection of an instrument for various purposes, and the basis for each. Discuss the brands available and make recommendations for various levels of performance.

27. Discuss student qualifications and aptitudes. If there is an opportunity, observe the process of selection, and discuss it with a public school teacher.

28. Perform the process of disassembly and swabbing. Discuss regular maintenance of the instrument. Test an instrument for leaks. Examine one or more instruments for needed repairs or adjustments.

29. Make a comparative analysis of as many beginning methods as you have available. Select and rank them in order of preference.

30. Examine available standard methods and additional study materials for clarinet and list them with comments.

31. Prepare a suggested list of material to include all five types of materials suggested for simultaneous study for an upper beginner, an intermediate, and an advanced student.

32. Listen to several phonograph records of clarinet literature, comment on and compare tone quality, phrasing, articulation, and general facility.

33. Attend a woodwind event in a solo and ensemble festival. Observe the players and make a detailed critique of as many as possible on details of holding positions, hand positions, embouchure formation, tuning, intonation, tone quality, articulation, and technique. Describe any faults found in any of these, the symptoms, possible causes, and corrections for each.

CHAPTER TWO

FLUTE

Flutes are the most ancient of the woodwind instruments since their tone production is simple as it is produced by an edge tone rather than a vibrating reed. Flutes have appeared historically in many forms from the earliest civilizations. The present-day family of instruments include the C flute, the piccolos in C and D-flat, and the Alto Flute. The Alto Flute is frequently mis-labled and called a bass flute. A true bass flute would sound an octave lower than the C flute, but the alto flute is in G and sounds only a perfect fourth lower than the C instrument. Many experiments have failed to produce a truly satisfactory bass flute sounding an octave lower than the C instrument, primarily because of the difficulty in producing and controlling the tone on an instrument of this size.

All the instruments in the flute family currently in use are built in the Boehm system and have identical fingerings for the same written notes. All but the C flute are transposing instruments. The transpositions and ranges in which each instrument sounds is as follows:

1. *C Flute*

Written   Sounds   Range of actual sounds

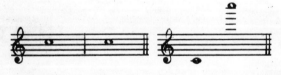

2. *C Piccolo*

Written   Sounds   Range of actual sounds

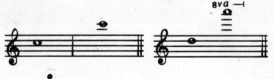

3. *D-flat Piccolo*

Written   Sounds   Range of actual sounds

4. *Alto Flute*

Written   Sounds   Range of actual sounds

Note that the piccolo lacks a foot-joint in its construction, so that the low C and C-sharp are missing from its range. These are omitted because an instrument of this size cannot produce them with satisfactory tonal body. The D-flat flute which was widely used in bands for many years seems to be gradually disappearing from the musical scene.

PLAYING RANGES

With the exception of the two lowest notes which are omitted from the piccolo, all the instruments in the flute family have the same theoretical written playing range. There are commonly accepted playing ranges for the flute which for convenience may be designated as *Beginning*, the range a typical young beginner can be expected to play by the end of his first year of experience; *Intermediate*, the range commonly required for the average good high school player; and *Advanced*, the range in which the professional is expected to perform. These ranges are very flexible with some beginning students achieving tone production in the Intermediate range rather quickly. The piccolo is not a beginning instrument and should be played by a student who has had experience on the flute.

1. *Flute*

Beginning   Intermediate   Advanced

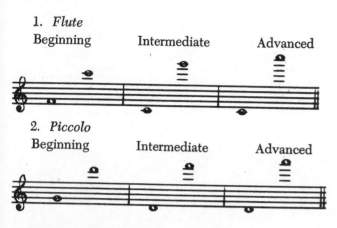

2. *Piccolo*

Beginning   Intermediate   Advanced

ASSEMBLING THE INSTRUMENT

Although in comparison with the oboe and clarinet the mechanism of the flute is sturdy, it must neverthe-less be assembled and disassembled with care. The assembly of the instrument must be accomplished without putting pressure on any key or rod which will bend it in any way. Before starting the process of assembly check to see that connecting sleeves are clean and smooth. If they fit together with difficulty, wipe with a very small amount of prepared cork grease, although this is not necessary for an instrumnet in good condition.

The way in which the flute is assembled is subject to some variation according to the desire and experience of the teacher. No matter what procedure is used students must be taught from the very first lesson to perform the process correctly. The following step-by-step process of assembly is a standard one which can be understood and performed easily by beginners. Study the photograph and directions for each step carefully and repeat the operation several times before proceeding to the next.

PARTS OF THE INSTRUMENT

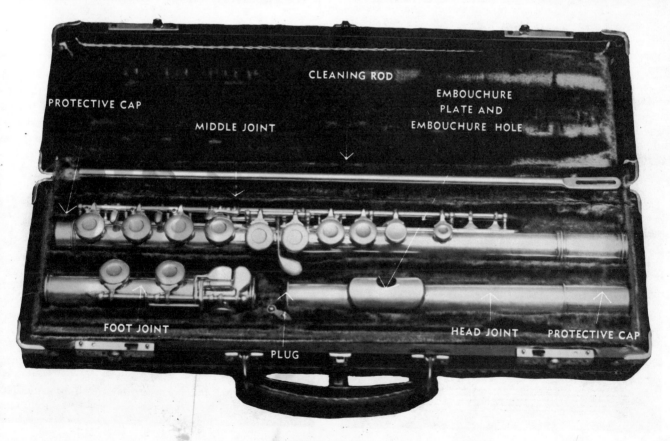

Figure F-1.

1. Figure F-2. Hold the open flute case in the lap. Take the head joint out of the case with the right little finger in the end. Parts of the instrument fit tightly in the average case and removing them in this way avoids picking them up by the keys and puts the hand into a good position for grasping the joint.

3. Figure F-4. Holding the joint in the left hand remove the protective cap and return it to the case. Teachers must insist that the protective caps be kept on the instrument when it is in the case to avoid bending or damaging the connecting sleeves. Students have an unfortunate tendency to lose these caps.

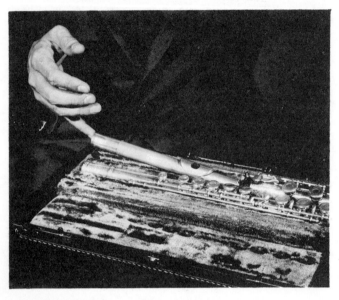

Figure F-2.

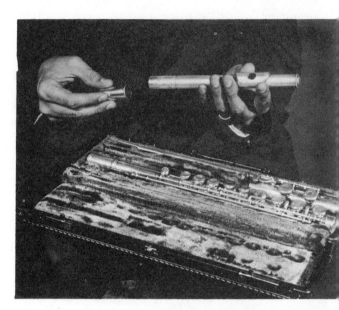

Figure F-4.

2. Figure F-3. With the joint partially out of the case, roll the hand over as shown and pick up the joint, transferring it to the left hand.

4. Figure F-5. Take out the middle joint with the little finger of the right hand in the same way the head joint was removed, holding the middle joint at the end away from the keys. Remove the protective cap and return it to the case.

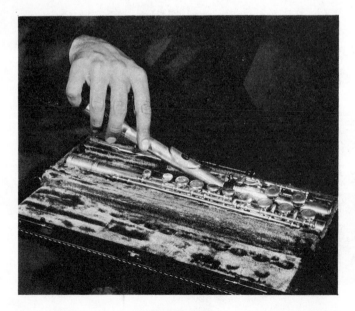

Figure F-3.

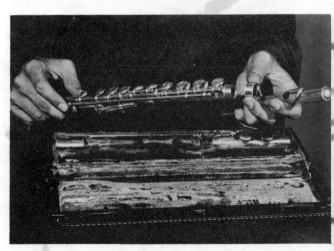

Figure F-5.

5. Figure F-6. To assemble the head and middle joints, hold the middle joint in the right hand at the end away from the key mechanism. The palm of the hand is on the top of the instrument, fingers are curled around the body, and the joint is held firmly by the thumb and forefinger. With this holding position there is no pressure against key mechanism.

6. Figure F-7. Hold the head joint in the palm of the left hand, with the thumb over the embouchure plate and the fingers firmly around the pipe.

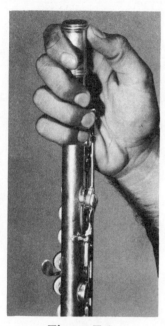 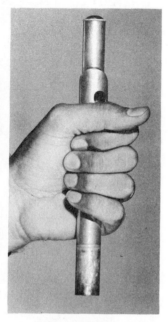

Figure F-6.   Figure F-7.

7. Figure F-8. Holding the head and middle joints as described push the parts together with a twisting motion. Line up the hole in the embouchure plate so that it is centered on the tone holes on the top of the instrument in their *closed* position.

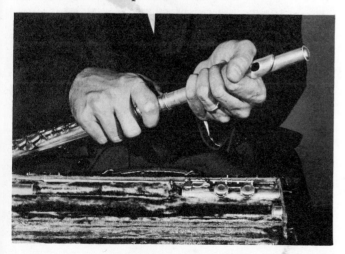

Figure F-8.

8. Figure F-9. Take the foot joint from the case again using the end of the little finger. Place the thumb against the rim at the end which fits on the middle joint below the keys operated by the right little finger. The joint fits loosely in the palm of the hand, held firmly by the thumb and forefinger with the remaining fingers around the pipe.

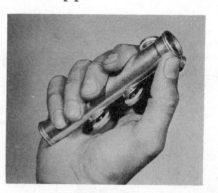

Figure F-9.

9. Figure F-10. Hold the assembled head and middle joints in the palm of the left hand near the lower end for their connection with the foot joint. Fingers are over the tone holes and thumb over the connecting rods on the left side of the instrument. The joint is held by pressure of the base of the thumb pushing the flute against the palm. Avoid pressure against the rods. This particular holding position is the most critical of all because of the possibility of bending the rods. Check this position carefully.

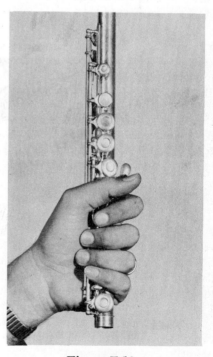

Figure F-10.

10. Figure F-11. and F-12. Holding the foot joint and the middle joint as described put on the foot joint with a twisting motion to the right. Figure F-11. shows the beginning of this process and Figure F-12. the conclusion. The foot joint is in the correct position when the rod on which the keys pivot is centered on the closest tone hole. This puts the keys on the foot joint in the best position for efficient operation by the little finger.

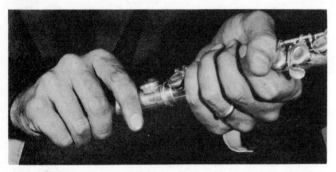

Figure F-11.

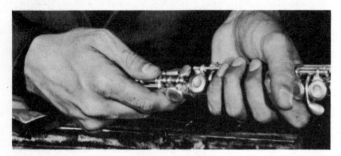

Figure F-12.

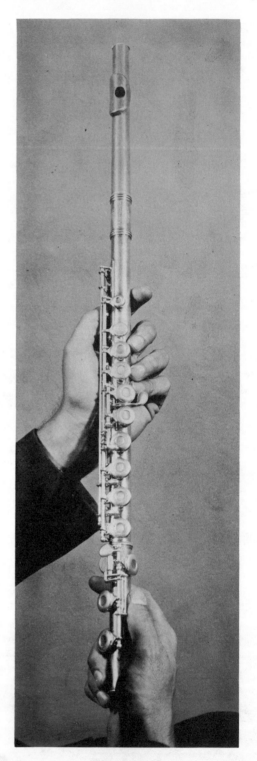

Figure F-13.

Figure F-13. This photograph shows the assembled flute with the head and foot joints properly positioned. Check the head joint to see that the tone hole is centered on the tone holes on the top of the instrument, and that the pivot rod on the foot joint is centered on the bottom tone hole. This is the basic position of the parts. Experienced students will vary this position slightly to accommodate shape and size of hands, and embouchure formation. Avoid wide deviations from this standard.

Common Faults in Assembly

There are, of course, several ways in which the flute may be assembled, and various teachers will have different procedures and methods. The only criteria for a good procedure is that no pressure is put on rods, plates or keys during the process. The procedure outlined above is a common standard one and may be safely used for beginners. As familiarity with the instrument increases, students may change the procedure to suit themselves. The following items are the most common faults or inaccuracies in the assembly of the flute.

1. *Failure to Clean Connecting Sleeves.* All connecting sleeves both inside and out must be kept absolutely clean and smooth if the instrument is to be assembled easily. With a soft lint-free cloth wipe the outside and inside of the connecting portions thoroughly and regularly. No lubrication of these connecting parts is necessary on an instrument in good condition. However, if they fit together with difficulty even though they are clean a very light coating of petroleum jelly or prepared

cork grease will make them slide together easily. Avoid a heavy coating, and wipe off excess. When the connecting sleeves do not slide together easily the alignment of the parts is difficult and excess pressure is put on keys and rods.

2. *Failure to Align Head Joint.* The center of the embouchure hole must be lined up exactly with the tone holes on the top of the instrument. As a convenient and accurate way to insure proper alignment some authorities recommend scratching lines on the side of these two parts of the instrument once the exact correct alignment is established. When this is done it is simple to match the lines. If the head joint is not properly aligned the holding position of the instrument becomes somewhat unnatural resulting in unsteady hand positions which in turn make holding and fingering the instrument more difficult than necessary. Improper alignment of the head joint does not normally affect the embouchure placement of the flutist, except early beginners, as the student will almost invariably turn the instrument to put the embouchure plate in the proper position sacrificing the most comfortable holding position of the instrument.

3. *Failure to Align Foot Joint.* The foot joint must be aligned so that the rod on which the keys pivot is centered on the nearest tone hole. The most common mistake which inexperienced flute students make is to align the rod on the foot joint with the rod on the middle joint. The purpose of the correct alignment is to put the three keys on the foot joint in the best position for the little finger of the right hand to operate them. Improper alignment will pull the right hand out of position so that holding the instrument is unsteady and will make development of finger technique in the right hand difficult, as well as affecting embouchure development. If the foot joint is turned too far up the student will of necessity put the fingers of the right hand too far over the tone holes so that the little finger can reach the keys. If the foot joint is too far down the little finger must push forward or punch the keys rather than depressing them in the proper fashion.

4. *Holding the Joints Improperly.* In the preceding section on assembly, the exact holding position of each section for each operation was described in detail. If this is not done properly there is undue strain on rods and keys which will bend them out of alignment. This will cause leaks in the pads covering holes which in turn make some notes impossible or difficult to produce, and these leaks are difficult to locate and correct. Mechanism which is seriously bent will cause sluggish movement of keys to the point where technical development is adversely affected.

Check List for Assembly

Observe the student in the operation of assembling the flute and check the following items. Incorrect items for older students should not be called to their attention until the entire process is completed; younger students should be corrected immediately. If any mistake is made the entire process should be repeated until perfect.

	Yes	No	Comments
1. Were parts removed from case carefully and in approved manner?			
2. Were protective caps in place on instrument in the case?			
3. Middle joint held properly in assembly with head joint?			
4. Head joint held properly in assembly with middle joint?			
5. Embouchure hole properly aligned with middle joint?			
6. Foot joint held properly in assembly with middle joint?			
7. Middle and head joints held properly with assembly of foot joint?			
8. Rod of foot joint properly aligned with middle joint?			
9. Were final checks and adjustments of alignment of head and foot joints made after completion of assembly?			

HOLDING POSITION FOR THE FLUTE

The way in which the flute is held influences both directly and indirectly the type of tone quality produced, the embouchure formation, intonation, and the development of technical facility. The proper position is one in which the head and body is in a comfortable relaxed position, in which the hands and arms fall naturally into position, and which permits the formation and development of the best embouchure as well as the efficient development of accurate and useful technical facility. There is almost unanimous agreement among authorities on what the best playing position for flute is. The description and illustrations given here follow this standard. Seated, standing, and rest positions are given with details of hand and finger positions following in the next section.

The flute is held to the right of the body with the left hand closest to the head. The instrument angles slightly downward with the head tilted so that the line of the lips is parallel with the line of the flute. The head is turned slightly to the left to bring the instrument into a more comfortable position for the right arm and hand. The instrument is held firmly in position through three points of contact with the body: (1) the base of the left forefinger, (2) the right thumb, and (3) the right little finger depressing the E-flat key. Head erect except for a slight tilt to the right, chin up, eyes straight ahead, with shoulders up but relaxed. Elbows are free from the body in a relaxed position. Both feet flat on the floor. Shoulders and back must not touch the back of the chair when playing. Turn the chair slightly to the right so that the back corner will not interfere with the right arm or shoulder. Adjust the music stand so that music can be easily read in this position. When two students are playing from the same music, angle the chairs slightly toward the center of the stand so that the position of the body and instrument can remain correct.

Seated Position

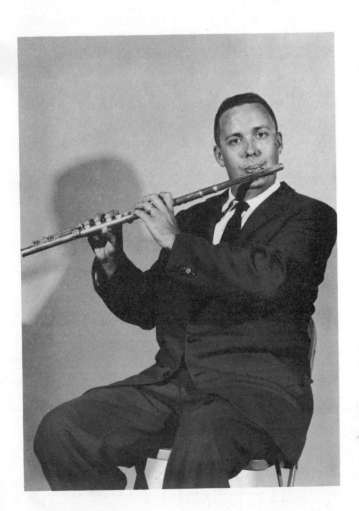

Figure F-14. Front View

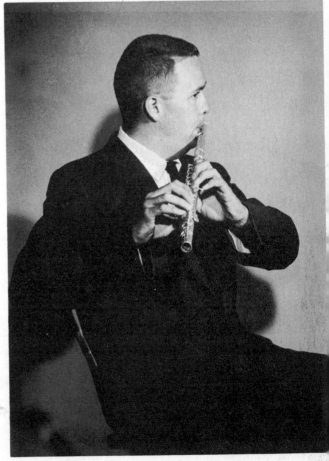

Figure F-15. Side View

The position of the instrument itself when the player is standing should be identical with that in the seated position. Only the position of the body itself is changed. Stand erect with feet slightly apart, one foot ahead of the other to help maintain balance. Head remains erect, with chin up and eyes straight ahead. Shoulders up but relaxed, and elbows free from the body. Raise the music stand, if one is being used, so that the head does not tilt downward. Every player should regularly spend a portion of his practice time standing to become at ease playing in a standing position.

Standing Position

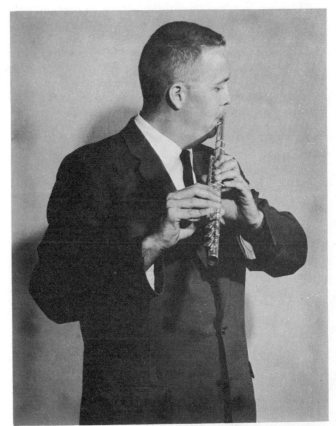

Standing Position

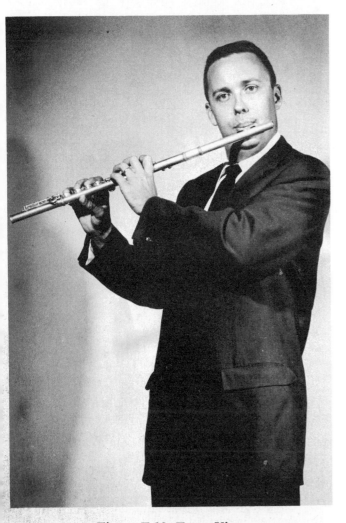

Figure F-17. Side View

Figure F-16. Front View

Rest Position

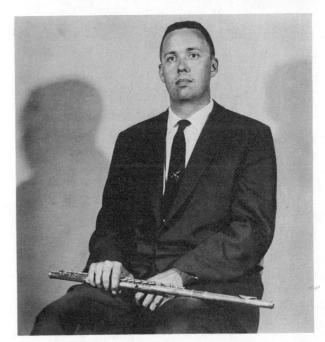

In the standard rest position the flute is placed squarely across the legs with the tone holes up to keep moisture off of the pads. From this position the instrument can be quickly picked up and returned to playing position.

Figure F-18. Standard Rest Position

HOLDING POSITION FOR THE PICCOLO

The holding position for the piccolo is identical with that for the flute, except for the adjustments in hand position which are necessary because of the small size of the instrument. The instrument angles slightly downward with the head tilted so that the line of the lips is parallel with the line of the piccolo. Elbows must be kept free of the body in a relaxed position. Head erect except for a slight tilt to the right, chin up, eyes straight ahead, with shoulders up but relaxed.

Seated Position

Seated Position

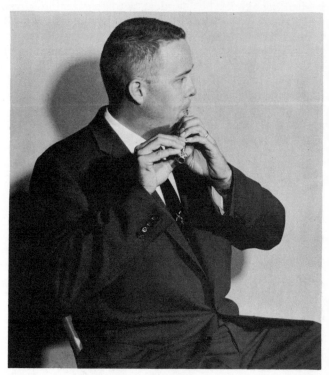

Figure F-20. Side View

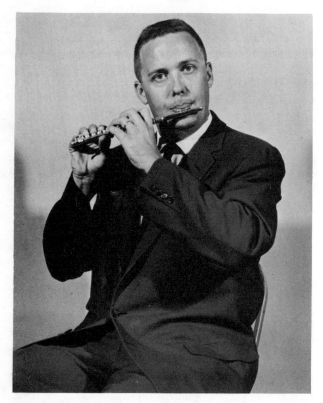

Figure F-19. Front View

Standing Position

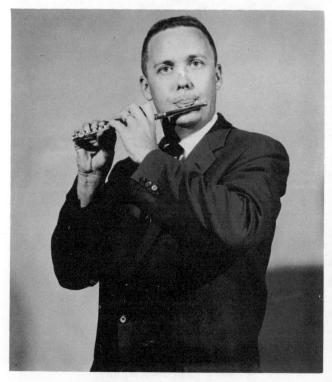

The position of the piccolo when the player is standing should be identical with its position when the player is seated. The smallness of the instrument tends to encourage a cramped position of the arms with the shoulders rolled forward. Check especially this portion of the standing position. Stand erect with feet slightly apart, one foot ahead of the other to help maintain balance. Head remains erect, with chin up and eyes straight ahead. Every player should spend a portion of his regular practice time standing to become at ease playing in a standing position.

Figure F-21. Front View

Common Faults in Holding Position

The way in which the flute and piccolo are held influences the rate and potential degree of musical progress on the instrument. Progress can be facilitated by a perfect holding position or it can be drastically slowed or even made impossible by a poor position. The instructor must check continually, especially during the first few months of study on the instrument, to correct any deviations before they become habitual. The player must learn to feel the correct position, and a continual check will help him achieve this. Every player should be encouraged to check his position daily in front of a mirror, either at home or at school.

The following are the most commonly found faults in holding positions for the flute, and to some extent the piccolo. Since the piccolo is normally played by a flutist, any deviations from the standard will be transferred to that instrument. The effect of certain deviations is greatly magnified when the player transfers to the piccolo resulting in poor intonation, restricted range, and poor tone quality.

1. *Angle of Flute.* Two angles are involved in the relationship between the flute and the embouchure: the horizontal or up and down illustrated in the front view of the holding position, (how far down from parallel is the end of the flute),; and the front to back relationship illustrated in the side view of the holding position, (is the end of the flute forward or backward from a right angle with the body). A check of photographs of the holding position given in various flute methods and texts reveals that the recommended horizontal angle of the instrument is between ten and twenty degrees from parallel with the floor. An angle of less than ten degrees puts an undue strain on the right arm since it must be held up higher for the correct hand position to be achieved. An angle of more than twenty degrees demands an unnatural tilt of the head to the right if the proper relationship of the embouchure plate and the lips is maintained with consequent difficulty in breath support and control. This angle is all-important in the success which the student will have in forming and developing an embouchure, tone control, and in achieving the optimum hand positions. Remember the line of the lips must be parallel with the flute. Have the student check frequently with a large mirror.

The front to back angle of the instrument is also highly critical as it affects primarily the formation and function of the embouchure. The flute should be held at a ninety-degree angle with the head, or to put it another way the end of the flute in playing position must be parallel with the lips. If the flute is pushed or pulled back from this parallel relationship, the angle of the embouchure hole with the lips is changed causing inefficient use of the breath which would then be directed toward a corner of the blow hole rather than directly across it. This situation results in a thin breathy tone, in difficulty in playing the lowest notes with full

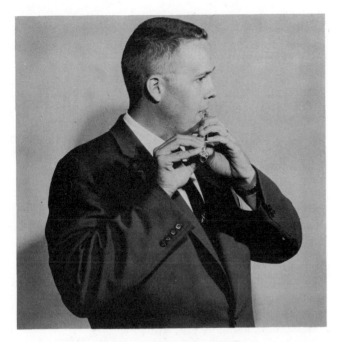

Figure F-22. Side View

Rest Position

Since the piccolo is physically small in size, there is no rest position across the legs of the player in which the instrument can be placed with any safety at all. It must be held in a hand as shown in the photograph. If the player is a boy and is wearing a coat the instrument may be safely tucked into the outside breast pocket. Do not put the instrument on the music stand for it is not safe.

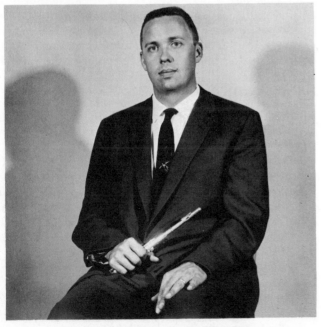

Figure F-23. Piccolo Rest Position

volume, in playing at all in the highest register, as well as multiplying intonation problems.

2. *Head Inclined Downward.* This problem is encountered in students at all stages of development, and is frequently encouraged by the habit of playing with a music stand which is too low, or by practicing at home with the music on a chair or table. When the head of a flute student is inclined downward one of two undesirable things happens: (1) the lower jaw is thrust out and held in a rather rigid position in order to produce an acceptable tone, or (2) the flute is rolled forward to help shape the embouchure putting hands in a cramped position. Frequently these happen together. A rigid lower jaw prohibits accurate control of intonation and makes intervals difficult and inaccurate, as well as reducing the potential tone quality. The cramped hand position tires the young student quickly and encourages poor posture, frequently to the extent of encouraging him to drape the right arm over the back of the chair. A cramped hand, usually caused by a bent wrist, makes technical advancement slow and inaccurate. The inclined head is easy to detect and should be corrected immediately. Have the student check frequently in a mirror to establish the proper position.

3. *Slouched Body.* Varying degrees of poor posture occur in almost every student, especially the younger ones. Good posture must be stressed from the very first lesson, in every lesson, and in every rehearsal until good posture becomes a habit. Degrees of poor posture include shoulders slumped or curved forward, leaning against the back of the chair with the spine curved, feet crossed or hung over a rung on the chair, or unique with the flute, hanging the right arm over the back of the chair to help support the instrument. More often than not these occur in combination. Poor posture affects breathing and breath control to the point that the students may find it impossible to support the tone adequately. This is especially important with the inexperienced flutist where problems of breath control are more acute than on other woodwinds. Poor posture pulls the arms, and consequently the fingers out of position making technical advancement slow, and technique rough and inaccurate. Emphasize to the students in as many ways as possible that good posture minimizes fatigue while poor posture increases it. Frequent checks by the student in a large mirror are invaluable in establishing the best posture.

4. *Arms and Elbows.* The position of the arms and elbows in playing the flute tend to tire the beginning student more than on any other woodwind instrument, just as beginners tire quickly when studying the violin or viola. Good body posture and absolutely correct holding position of the instrument will help minimize this fatigue. Because of the physical discomfort of playing the instrument for long periods of time in the early stages of study, beginners should be instructed to practice no more than twenty minutes at a time without a break of a half hour or more. As the students become physically tired poor posture and holding position is greatly encouraged. It is at this point that the right arm begins to be hung over the back of the chair and the body to slouch.

5. *Moving the Body While Playing.* Excessive body movements while playing is more frequently found in advanced players than in beginners because the instrument itself does not restrict these movements in any way. Beating time with the end of the instrument, swaying back and forth in time with the music, grandiose flourishes of the instrument at the end of difficult passages, etc., are extremely distracting to the conductor of a group and to the other players, and frequently humorous to an audience. All movements have a tendency to change the position of the embouchure plate on the lips, interfere with the coordination of the muscles controlling breath support and in general make for a poorer performance. The habit of body movement during performance is very difficult to correct once it becomes ingrained, since the player frequently doesn't realize he is doing it. Any such movements must be corrected immediately and firmly.

6. *Use of Crutch.* A crutch on the flute is a device similar to the right hand-rest used on the bassoon, which is fitted into a socket on the body of the flute and rests in the crotch of the left thumb and index finger. Use of the flute crutch has virtually disappeared, and instruments being manufactured today are not equipped with the device, although some older instruments will still have the socket on them. The crutch was intended to assist in holding the flute, and to keep the right hand fingers in the best playing position. That it ever succeeded is doubtful, and its disappearance causes no regrets. No authority of today recommends its use, and if an older instrument which was provided with a place for the crutch is used, the socket into which it fitted should be removed from the body of the instrument. The socket, if allowed to remain will interfere with the establishment of the proper contemporary hand position.

HAND POSITIONS

The flute is supported at the base of the left forefinger, the right thumb and right little finger, and steadied with a slight pressure of the embouchure plate against the lower lip. If all of these are in the right place the instrument is held firm and steady and there is no feeling of insecurity on the part of the student. It is easier to achieve a good hand position on the flute than on any other woodwind because of the way in which the key mechanism is arranged. There is no need for any muscular tension in the fingers, wrists, arms or shoulders. A comfortable relaxed position allows facility to develop rapidly.

The exact placement of the hands and shape of the fingers on the instrument will vary slightly from student to student according to the length of the fingers, especially the thumbs, but the basic procedure must be the same. The following step-by-step procedure for establishing the hand position on the flute should be studied thoroughly, perferably with an instrument so that a feel for the right position can be developed. Study both the text and the photographs carefully until they are perfectly clear. The "Guide Position" which is given is the fundamental position for hands and fingers and should be maintained at all times except when the fingering for a note involves moving a finger temporarily to another location—a situation which is less frequent on the flute than on other woodwinds. This guide position puts all fingers into the best position for developing speed and accuracy.

A. Left Hand Position

1. Figure F-24. The body of the flute rests at the base of the index finger between the knuckle and first joint. The structure of the finger provides a small shelf for the instrument.

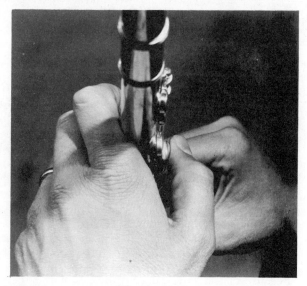

Figure F-24.

2. Figure F-25. The thumb of the left hand is curved slightly to contact the B-natural lever with the ball of the finger.

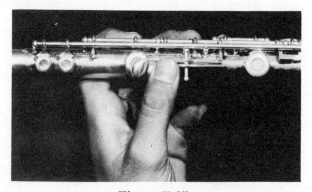

Figure F-25.

3. Figure F-26. The remaining fingers are curved to contact the proper plates with the flesh beneath the nail. The index finger has considerable curve, the other fingers less and less curve, with the little finger only slightly curved and touching lightly the G-sharp key.

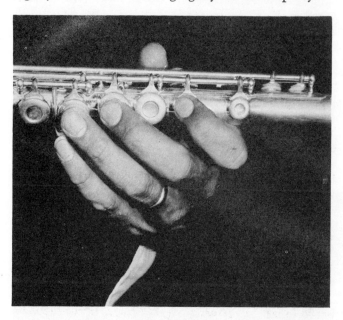

Figure F-26.

B. Right Hand Position

1. Figure F-27. The body of the flute is supported on the cushion of the right thumb contacting the tube opposite the space between the first and second fingers.

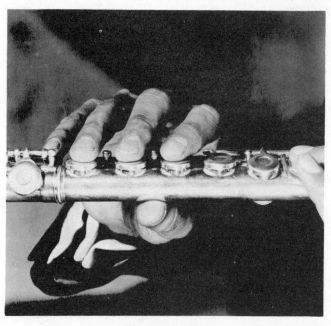

Figure F-27.

2. Figure F-28. The little finger helps balance the instrument by depressing the D-sharp key (on all except four notes in the normal playing range). Cushions of the remaining fingers contact the center of the indentations of their keys. Fingers are at a right angle with the flute.

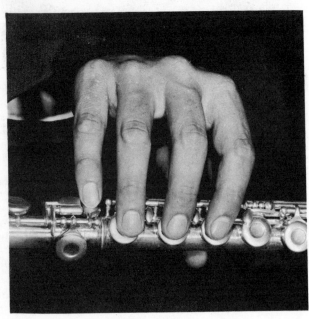

Figure F-28.

C. Guide Position

1. Figure F-29. With the thumbs and little fingers in position there will be a definite "U" shape between the thumb and index finger of each hand. This is important if the fingers are to lie in a natural curve and not cramped. Keeping the little fingers in place adjust the position of instrument on the left index finger and the point of contact of the right thumb to achieve this shape.

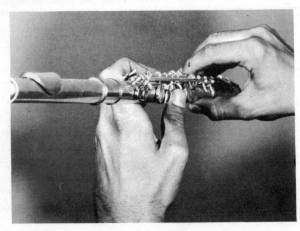

Figure F-29.

2. Figure F-30. The photograph shows the guide position as observed by the teacher. Note the curve on the fingers of the left hand, and that the fingers of the right hand are at a right angle with the instrument. Little fingers are touching their keys. This position should be kept at all times while playing except when a finger of the right hand is moved to a trill key, or the little finger to a low C or C-sharp. Maintaining this guide position will help facilitate rapid progress. Check the guide position often until it becomes established and is automatic.

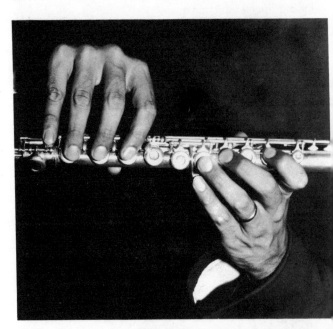

Figure F-30.

Because of the physical construction of the flute in the Boehm system, the hand position is more comfortable and the fingerings less complicated than on any other woodwind instrument. There are no complex fingerings to pull the hand out of position to reach a side key, and the guide position can be established and maintained somewhat more easily and efficiently than on the other woodwinds. There is no excuse at all for a poor hand position on the flute.

The only alternate placement of fingers involves the use of the B-flat lever with the left thumb, three trill keys in the right hand, and the keys for low C and C-sharp with the right little finger. These are discussed in the following.

1. *Use of B-flat Lever.* The left thumb may be as conveniently placed on the B-flat lever as on the B-natural lever. Figure F-31 shows the thumb in position on the B-flat lever. The normal position is on the B-natural lever. There is considerable confusion on the part of non-flutists as to the use of these two levers. Contemporary professional teaching treats this B-flat

as a trill or special fingering, to be used only on special occasions with the 100 400 fingering used as the standard fingering in both diatonic and chromatic passages. Keep the thumb on the B-natural lever except when the music clearly calls for the use of the B-flat lever. Never slide the thumb from the natural to the flat lever. The thumb

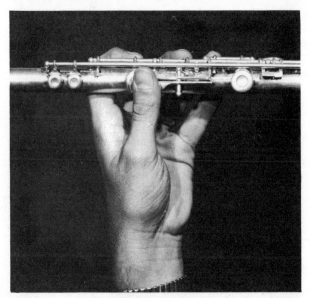

Figure F-31.

does not slide easily and technique will be rough and uneven if this is done. The student will eventually learn to use both fingerings with equal facility and apply them according to the demands of the music. Refer to section on Technique problems for a fuller discussion.

2. *Right Hand Trill Keys*. The three trill keys operated by the three fingers of the right hand are: (1) the side B-flat key operated by the fourth finger; (2) the D-natural trill key operated by the fifth finger; and (3) the D-sharp trill key operated by the sixth finger. In operating these keys the hand must stay in the guide position with only the finger or fingers being used on these keys moved out of position. Figure F-32 shows the first finger moved out of guide position to operate the side B-flat lever. Keeping the little finger in place depressing the E-flat key helps maintain the correct position. Trills on which these keys are used are given in the trill fingering chart.

3. *Right Little Finger*. The previous discussion of finger position indicated that the right little finger should depress the E-flat key on all except a very few tones. It is important that the habit of using the E-flat key correctly be developed from the very beginning of flute study to help steady the instrument as well as to assist intonation and tone quality.

The right little finger is involved in the fingering for the low C and C-sharp. In playing these notes the little finger must be kept in a curved position and the

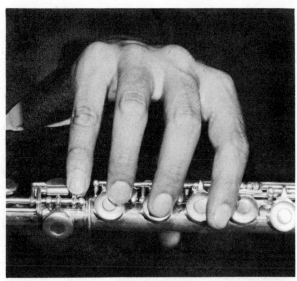

Figure F-32.

key depressed with the ball of the finger. If necessary adjust the foot-joint so that those students with short fingers can reach these keys easily with the correct finger position. The low C key is provided with a roller on most flutes so that the finger can be rolled from the C to the C-sharp key and vice versa in a slurred chromatic passage. This rolling must be practiced at the time these low notes appear in the course of study in a chomatic relationship—normally after the student has been playing several months.

Common Faults in Hand and Finger Positions

A good hand position is a great asset to the study of the flute, and is relatively easy to achieve. It will help develop facility and control, while a poor hand position retards this development. The first experiences with the instrument must emphasize hand position, and it must be continually checked until the best position for that particular player is established. Physical differences among students must be taken into account, but allow as little deviation from the standard as possible. The small hands of the grade school student frequently forces compromises, but he should gradually change into the most desirable position as he grows physically. Some students lo this naturally, while others must have constant reminders from the instructor.

A beginning player who persists in quickly establishing the proper positions makes rapid progress. The use of a mirror of sufficient size so that the student can see the entire length of the instrument is an asset in establishing position.

The items which are listed here are those with which problems occur most frequently, and are those to which the instructor should be alerted. Deviations in any of these will have an adverse affect on facility and technique and a combination of several will be a severe handicap to progress.

Check List for Holding and Hand Positions

The following list of items provides a means of quickly checking holding positions and hand positions. The check should be performed while the student is playing and preferably when he is not aware that the check is being made. Any items which are checked "no" should be corrected with the deviation explained to the student, what effect it has on his playing, and why the correct position is important. Students make a more serious effort to correct mistakes if they thoroughly understand the reason.

A. *Holding Position*

	Yes	No	Comments
1. Correct horizontal angle with body?			
2. Correct vertical angle with body?			
3. Head tilted to follow line of flute?			
4. Shoulders up but relaxed?			
5. Elbows free from body?			
6. Body posture good?			
7. Feet well placed?			
8. Height of music stand correct?			
9. Uses correct rest position?			
10. Excessive body movements?			

B. *Hand Positions*

1. Left index finger contacting flute at proper place for best support?			
2. Right thumb correctly placed?			
3. Left little finger touching G-sharp key?			
4. Right little finger depressing D-sharp key?			
5. Left thumb contacting key properly?			
6. Balls of fingers contacting keys			
7. "U" shape between thumbs and index fingers?			
8. Basic guide position maintained?			
9. Wrist flat?			
10. No muscular tension?			
11. Left thumb kept on B-natural lever?			
12. Fingers no more than one inch above tone plates?			
13. Fingers curved?			

1. *Left Thumb.* The point at which the left thumb contacts the B-natural lever is highly critical in achieving the best position of the left hand. The most common error is to put the thumb too far up on the plate. This pulls the wrist down and forces the other fingers into a cramped position—especially the first finger which must have considerable curve under normal circumstances. This upward extension of the thumb is sometimes caused by having the flute too far down on the index finger. Check this first of all. The normal position calls for a "U" shaped opening between the thumb and index finger, and achieving this, with the little finger in position on its key, will usually put the thumb in the proper place. In the correct position the wrist is virtually flat. An upward hump in the wrist will pull the thumb too far down on the plate, pulling the first finger over the instrument so that it is no longer curved, but in a right angle at the first joint.

2. *Left Little Finger.* The normal position for the left little finger is a natural curve, touching but not pressing the G-sharp key. Common errors in this position include the habit of putting the finger beneath the key to help support the instrument, or extending it upward in a stiff position. Both errors cause muscular tension in the entire hand, and must be avoided. Check frequently in the early stages of development for once this habit is established it is difficult to correct. The student should be encouraged to check himself in a mirror frequently until the proper position is achieved.

3. *Right Thumb.* The exact position for the right thumb for an individual player is determined by the length of his thumb in relation to the other fingers. The body of the flute must rest on the ball of the thumb normally orientated between the first and second fingers above the flute. This position usually gives the most security to the holding of the instrument. However, it can be moved closer to the first or to the second finger if necessary to put the other fingers at a right angle with the instrument. The thumb can be moved forward or backward on the instrument to the place where the fingers fall in a natural curve over the top. There is considerable fluctuation in the exact place on the ball of the finger contacting the instrument. Some authorities, and these are in the minority, recommend that the thumb contact the side of the flute with the tip of the thumb. While an experienced player can hold the flute in this way, an inexperienced student will have a strong feeling that the instrument is not being held securely with the result that the embouchure plate moves on the lower lip. If the thumb is too far under the instrument, contacting it near or on the joint, the fingers are forced into a sharp curve and contact the keys with the tips rather than the ball of the fingers. This tense and cramped position is a decided handicap to technical development.

4. *Right Little Finger.* The most common fault with the right little finger is the failure to keep the D-sharp key depressed. This is especially prevalent in those students who have transferred from the clarinet or another woodwind as a continually depressed key is unique with the flute. This depressed key is quite important as it is one of the points of support and control of the instrument, and if not used gives the student a feeling of insecurity in holding the instrument. In addition the open key adds resonance to the tone, and must be open if all tones on the instrument are to be perfectly in tune. Check carefully and continually from the very beginning of study on the instrument on the use of this finger.

5. *Sliding Left Thumb.* Use of the left thumb on the B-natural and B-flat levers has been discussed. Some students develop the unfortunate habit of using only the thumb B-flat which forces them to slide the thumb from one lever to the other. The instrument is not constructed to facilitate this procedure, and as a result technique is uneven, and in fact, many incorrectly inflected B's result from this habit. Most authorities agree that the 100-400 fingering for B-flat should be the only fingering used in the beginning stages of flute study, with the thumb B-flat introduced after some facility is attained. If a student has developed the habit of sliding the thumb, introduce the other fingering for B-flat and insist that he use it exclusively until facility is developed.

6. *Right Hand Trill Keys.* While these keys are not used to a great extent, it is nevertheless necessary that they be used properly. Insist that the hand be kept in the full guide position except for the finger concerned Most students will be well into the intermediate stage of development before encountering the need to use these keys, and hand position will be well established. For this reason it is not difficult to maintain the correct position of all fingers.

EMBOUCHURE FORMATION

An embouchure may be defined as the formation of the performer's lips with supporting muscles, teeth and jaws in relation to the embouchure hole which have to do with tone production. A good embouchure may be defined as one which, over the entire range of the instrument, produces (or is capable of producing) a rich, full bodied, clear tone; plays perfectly in tune; allows the full scope of articulations with minimum effort; allows the full range of dynamics to be played with complete control; plays and is controlled with a minimum of physical exertion. A poor embourchure is one in which any one of these criteria is lacking or is deficient in any way.

The flute is unique among the woodwinds in that there is no vibrating reed for the performer to contend with. Embouchure formation and development, lies entirely within the physical control of the player who does not have to be involved with the complexities of mouthpieces and/or reeds. Unlike those instruments which produce a tone with a reed which is constantly changing and having to be replaced, the embouchure plate and hole on the flute remains constant and unchanging. This is an advantage, but the flute has the disadvantage, since the entire control does lie with the player, of requiring a more flexible and accurate embouchure development.

The flute tone is technically described as an "edge-tone" in the study of acoustics. Briefly this means that the stream of air is concentrated and directed toward a sharp edge where it is set into turbulence. In the instance of the flute, part of the turbulent air is going into the flute and part escaping into the open air. This concept of splitting the air stream into two parts is basic to understanding how the flute embouchure works. The function of the embouchure is to direct the air stream toward the far edge of the embouchure hole in such a way as to produce the desired quality and pitch of tone.

There is probably more unanimity of opinion on the desirable embouchure for the flute than on any other woodwind instrument. The wide divergence of opinion on the proper formation found with the other woodwinds simply doesn't exist for the flute, although there are slight differences which occur because of physical differences in the players themselves. The following is the standard procedure for shaping the embouchure. Use the head joint alone until the student's embouchure is set.

1. Hold the head joint with the embouchure hole against the lips. Feel with the tongue so that the hole is centered on the lips.

2. Roll the joint forward until the embouchure hole is parallel with the floor, and so that the lower lip covers one-fourth to one-third of the hole.

3. Keeping the lower lip relaxed, pull the corners of the mouth back slightly to firm the upper lip.

4. Allow the center of the upper lip to relax to produce an opening no more than one-sixteenth of an inch high and one-half inch long. This opening desirably should be more of a diamond shape than an oval. It is never circular. Figures F-33, F-34, and F-35 show three views of the properly formed embouchure.

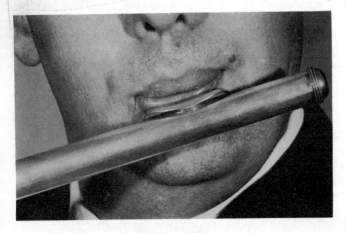

Figure F-33.

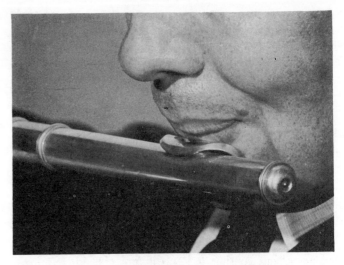

Figure F-34.

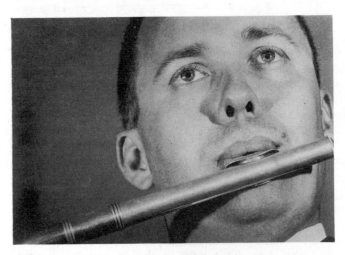

Figure F-35.

Setting the Embouchure

The following should be done in front of a mirror. Using the head joint alone, form the basic embouchure as described. Hold the joint with the left hand and stop the open end with the right. Using standard abdominal breath support, blow a gentle concentrated stream of air through the hole in the lips directed toward the opposite edge of the embouchure hole rather than down into it. Move the lower jaw and lips slowly back and forth until a tone which approximates the pitch of second space "A" is produced. Continue to experiment with the speed of air through the lips and the adjustment of the lower jaw and the lips until a rather full steady tone can be sustained for at least ten seconds.

Open the end of the head joint and repeat the process, this time producing a pitch which approximates the "A" first time above the treble clef. It will be found that to produce this pitch requires a slightly greater pressure of the breath, and a change in its direction achieved by pushing the jaws and lips slightly more forward to direct it more across the hole rather than down. Continue to experiment with wind velocity and direction until a full steady tone on this pitch can be sustained for at least ten seconds. When these tones produced by the closed and open head joint can be produced easily the student is ready to assemble the complete instrument and proceed with the regular course of instruction.

However older students and students with a strong natural aptitude for the flute can experiment further with the head joint alone to produce harmonics in addition to the two fundamentals. With the end of the head joint closed a pitch of approximately "E" third line above the staff can be produced, and with the end of the head joint opened a pitch approximating "A" fifth space above the clef can be produced. These are produced by using a greater velocity of air and by adjustments of the lower jaw and lips. They are not easily produced by many students, and it is not wise to insist that all students be able to produce them before continuing with the complete instrument. Those students who are able to produce these harmonics easily will be able to make more rapid progress in tone production in the early stages of instruction than those who cannot. These approximate pitches are produced with the head joint closed and open.

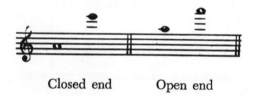

Closed end   Open end

Success in producing a clear full tone on the flute is determined by: (1) the amount of embouchure plate covered by the lower lip, (2) the direction of the stream of air, (3) the focusing of a concentrated stream of air determined by the size and shape of the aperture formed by the lips; and (4) the use of standard abdominal breathing and breath support. Each of these factors is closely related with all others and cannot be altered without changing another factor. The problem in achieving a fine flute embouchure is to bring all these factors into the proper relationship with each other. These factors are not static in performance but constantly changing to control pitch, intonation, dynamics, and tone quality. The influence of each is considered separately in the following:

1. *Standard Abdominal Breathing and Breath Support.* This procedure is standard for all wind instruments, and without it no great progress on an instrument is possible. The flute is especially critical in respect to breathing as the production of an edge tone is inherently wasteful of breath. Beginning flutists are notoriously short of breath because they have not learned to use the embouchure and instrument efficiently. Dizziness is a common complaint of the beginning flutist. It is the result of more than normal breathing both in amount and frequency of breaths taken which puts too much oxygen into the blood stream. The body soon adjusts to this and the dizziness will pass. However, when a student becomes dizzy he should stop playing until the dizziness is gone. Breathing exercises, combined with regular and brief practice sessions on the flute will soon eliminate the dizzy spells. Some students become alarmed at the dizziness and it is well to explain its cause and how it can be eliminated.

2. *Aperture Shape and Size.* The size and shape of the aperture formed by the lips is of prime importance to control the amount, direction and shape of air being directed across the embouchure plate. The exact size and shape can be seen only when the student is producing a sound. It should be roughly diamond shaped as shown in Figure F-36. The exact size of the aperture varies directly with the octave being played: larger for the first octave, smaller for the second octave, and still smaller for the third octave: larger for softer dynamic levels and smaller for louder ones within the basic size for the octave being played.

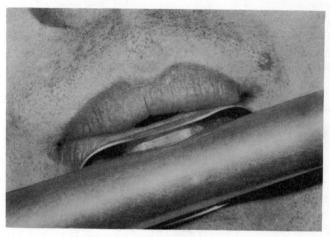

Figure F-36.

The function of this aperture is to first, shape the stream of air into a concentrated and well focused flow, and secondly to control the amount and intensity of the flow. The shape of the air stream must be wide enough from side to side to strike the entire width of the embouchure hole and narrow from top to bottom to avoid wasting air. This shape can best be achieved when the corners of the lips are pulled back slightly with the upper lip firm and the lower lip relaxed. Avoid a pucker in the lips which shapes a round aperture. The round shape of the air stream produced strikes only a portion of the opposite edge of the embouchure hole and produces a breathy noisy tone quality.

The air stream coming from the lips must be centered in the side to side relationship with the embouchure hole. Move the flute from side to side on the lower lip until this hole is centered. Many normal lips do not naturally form the aperture exactly in the center of the lips, and the flute must be adjusted to the student's lip formation. This adjustment is basic, and must be done at the very beginning of flute study.

3. *Amount of Embouchure Plate Covered by Lower Lip.* In the first octave of the flute range in which the beginning student first plays approximately one-fourth to one-third of the embouchure hole is covered by the lower lip. The exact amount to be covered varies from individual to individual depending on the other factors involved, and must be the subject of considerable experimentation. A good starting position for this experimentation is to put the inner edge of the embouchure hole at the lower edge of the lip on the line where the lip and the chin meet. The exact adjustment is then done by ear. More of the hole may be done by: (1) moving the flute down on the lip, or (2) rolling the flute in slightly; and conversely less of the hole may be covered by: (1) moving the flute up on the lip, or (2) by rolling the flute out slightly. The exact adjustment is strongly affected by the size and shape of the aperture in the lips and by the direction of the stream of air. The first experiments in determining the amount of hole to be covered are best done by rolling the flute back and forth, then if a major adjustment is necessary moving the flute up or down on the lip.

If too little of the hole is covered by the lower lip: (1) the air stream is used inefficiently and too much is required to produce a tone, (2) very little dynamic range is possible and the general amount of tone produced is small, (3) a tone of poor quality—uncontrolled and breathy—is produced, and (4) the range is limited and notes in the third octave will be difficult to produce and control.

If too much of the hole is covered by the lower lip: (1) a small thin tone quality is produced, (2) very little dynamic range is possible—the tone will disappear entirely when the student attempts to play softly, (3) articulation is limited and slow in response, (4) a true legato is difficult in certain passages. Covering too much of the embouchure hole is a great temptation for beginners as it requires less than the normal amount of air to produce a tone. Watch this closely in the beginning stage.

Once the basic amount of hole to be covered is discovered and established the small adjustments in this amount which are required for playing in the various octaves of the instrument, for controlling dynamics, and for controlling intonation, are made by a slight back and forth movement of the lower jaw and lips. The lower jaw and lips are pulled back for the low tones and forward for the high ones. This movement of the lower jaw and lips also controls the direction of the air stream, and it must be emphasized again that the

amount of hole covered and the direction of the air stream are very closely interrelated. In a performance by an advanced flutist these movements of the jaw and lips are quite noticeable and almost constant as he adjusts for tone placement, intonation, and dynamics. Avoid at all costs making these adjustments in amount of hole covered and direction of the air stream by rolling the flute in and out or by moving the head up and down. Such movements hinder rather than help progress on the instrument; it is not possible to make the rapid and delicate adjustments necessary for fine performance in this way.

4. *Direction of the Stream of Air.* The tone of the flute is produced by a stream of air which is blown toward the opposite edge of the embouchure hole, part of it going into the flute and part into the open air. Contrary to the unfortunate popular opinion blowing a flute is *not* the same as making a sound on a jug or pop bottle. The size, shape, and location of the flute embouchure plate and hole are the result of the most careful acoustical calculations and it resembles only slightly the acoustical conditions of a jug. A student who begins his study of the flute with the concept that blowing a flute is like blowing a pop bottle begins with a severe handicap which is difficult to overcome.

The direction of the air stream determines how much air will go into the instrument and how much into space, producing corresponding changes in the turbulence of the air which in turn control both pitch and volume. The actual direction is controlled by forward and backward movements of the corners of the lips working with corresponding movements of the lower jaw. While for the purposes of this discussion we are isolating the direction of the air stream, in actual practice it is closely interrelated to and is inseparable from breath support, intensity of the air stream, and amount of embouchure hole covered by the lower lip.

The actual direction of the air must be determined by considerable experimentation, and control established by experience and practice. As a guide to the effect of the direction of the air stream some general statements may be made. The more downward the air stream: (1) the lower in pitch the flute will respond, and (2) the louder the volume of sound produced. Conversely the more outward the air stream is directed: (1) the higher in pitch the flute will respond, and (2) the softer the volume.

In performance, then, the direction of the air stream is used with extremely small adjustments to control the intonation on individual notes, and with somewhat greater adjustments to control the octave in which a note will sound. Octave skips, for example, will result in quite noticeable movements of the lips and lower jaw changing the direction of the air stream, as well as the amount of embouchure hole covered by the lower lip. The movement of the lips has many similarities to the movements of a brass instrument player as he changes pitch on his instrument.

Check List for Flute Embouchure Formation

The following check on flute embouchure formation must be made while the student is playing and preferably when he is not aware that a check is being made. Any errors should be carefully explained to the student, and the correction worked out with him while he is observing the embouchure in a mirror. Remedial measures can be assigned on the basis of this list.

	Yes	No	Comments
1. Flute parallel with line of lips?			
2. Aperture in lips centered in side-to-side relationship with embouchure hole?			
3. Proper amount of embouchure hole covered by lower lip?			
4. Size and shape of aperture in lips correct?			
5. Air stream properly directed?			
6. Corners of mouth pulled back slightly?			
7. Direction of air stream controlled by lips and lower jaw?			
8. Produces clear, full-bodied tone?			

TUNING

As a non-transposing instrument, the flute sounds the pitch written for it. The instrument is designed so that it will sound A-440 when the head joint is pulled about an eighth of an inch from the middle joint. This allows some margin of safety so that the instrument can be played slightly sharper than standard pitch if necessary. For the proper development of temperament and intonation on the instrument it is important that all students tune regularly to A-440, making use of a tuning bar or an electronic tuner, and practice with the instrument adjusted to this pitch. If the instrument is in tune with the head joint pulled out an eighth of an inch, all practice which the student does should be done with it in this adjustment.

The pitch adjustment of the instrument in basic tuning is made only at the head joint-middle joint juncture. If the instrument is being played so flat that it is still low in pitch with the head joint all the way in, or conversely if it is being played so sharp that the head joint must be pulled out more than a quarter of an inch the problem lies in the embouchure formation and not in the instrument. If the head joint is pulled out more than three-eighths of an inch in order to bring the instrument down to pitch, intonation on the instrument suffers and it is virtually impossible to play the instrument in tune with itself.

Cork in Head Joint. The cork, (plug or stopper) in the end of the head joint is there simply to close the end of the pipe. The exact location of this cork is highly critical for tuning and intonation, and once it is properly located must not be moved. The end of the cork must be exactly seventeen millimeters from the center of the embouchure hole. So that this distance can be checked, the cleaning rod which is provided with the instrument has a line etched in the metal at this distance from one end. To check the distance, insert the cleaning rod carefully into the end of the head joint until it is touching the stopper. The etched line, as shown in Figure F-37, should be exactly in the center of the embouchure hole. If it is too far toward the closed end, unscrew the cap on the end, and push the plug into place. If it is too

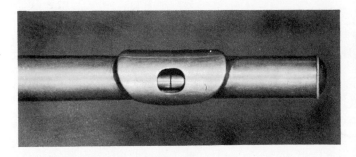

Figure F-37.

far toward the open end tighten the cap slowly until it is pulled into place. If it is necessary to unscrew the cap tighten it so that it moves gently into place. Screwing the cap firmly will pull the cork out of place. In the absence of an etched cleaning rod, the plug can be adjusted by tuning the three octave "D's" to as close to perfect octaves as possible.

Beginning students should be warned rather early in their study about keeping the plug in place. Frequently it is pulled out of place by the student who will loosen or tighten the cap without thinking or who will push it out of place inadvertently when the instrument is being cleaned after use. Should it ever be necessary to remove the plug from the instrument, remove the screw cap and push the plug out the end of the head joint which fits into the middle joint of the instrument. The head joint of the instrument is slightly conical with the closed end appreciably smaller than the open end. Forcing the plug out the small end could damage the cork so that it will leak. This plug should be removed only under the most urgent circumstances, and preferably by an expert repairman. Students who are curious about the construction of their new instruments must be warned not to remove or tamper with the plug.

INTONATION

The basic mechanical design of the flute as developed by Boehm produced an instrument which is inherently as well in tune as it is possible to produce an instrument which plays in the tempered scale. While there are small differences from manufacturer to manufacturer the temperament of the instrument is such that, with the proper embouchure formation and control, it can be played perfectly in tune. With modern manufacturing techniques and research in the production of instruments, any serious intonation problems can be traced to their source and corrected.

Natural Tendencies of the Instrument. The first octave of the flute is produced by the fundamental vibrations of the pipe, the second octave by the first (or octave) overtone, the third octave by the second or third overtone (the twelfth and double octave above the fundamental). Since the frequencies of the natural overtones do not correspond exactly with the corresponding frequencies demanded by the tempered scale, the intonation of the flute is compromised somewhat by the design in order that all notes in all octaves can be played in tune with the average good embouchure. The result of this compromise is that the first octave has a natural tendency to be flat with the notes C through E being flatter than the rest and somewhat more difficult to bring up to pitch than the others. The second octave is sharp in comparison to the first octave, but close to the standard pitch, except for the third space C-sharp which is quite sharp in comparison to the second octave and considerably sharp to the first octave, with the highest B and C being quite sharp even in comparison with the rest of the third octave.

The notes in the first and second octaves may, with some experience and a well controlled embouchure, be easily adjusted to play in tune. The third octave requires more adjustment, although fingerings have been selected which overcome to some degree the natural tendencies of the instrument. Because of the embouchure adjustments needed to produce and play tone in the third octave in tune, it is well to delay extending the range of the student into this area until he is playing and controlling notes in the first and second octave with ease and precision.

Effect of Embouchure on Intonation. The all-important role of the embouchure on intonation has been alluded to several times. In reality all intonation problems other than mechanical ones with the instrument, can be traced to and corrected by the embouchure. It is for this reason that so much stress must be placed from the very beginning of study on accurately forming and developing the embouchure. The embouchure controls the pitch of the notes by altering the direction of the air stream across the embouchure hole. The pitch is flattened by pulling the lips and lower jaw back so the air stream is directed more downward into the hole. The pitch is raised by pushing the lips and lower jaw forward so that the air stream is directed more across the hole. Minor adjustments in pitch needed to put the tones in tune are accomplished most efficiently by small movements of the lips, with jaw movements reserved for large adjustments and changes in the octave in which the notes appear. These adjustments are the product of critical listening on the part of the player, whose attention must be called to the necessity of making them very early in beginning study. The use of an electronic aid is highly recommended for establishing normal intonation in the student's mind. With experience these embouchure adjustments become automatic.

The placement of the embouchure plate on the lower lip affects overall pitch and intonation. If the plate is too low the pitch will be generally flat, if the plate position is too high on the lip the pitch will be generally sharp. This is one of the first things to look for when a student is playing consistently flat or sharp over the entire range of the instrument. This low or high placement has an adverse effect on tone quality as well, and limits the changes in air stream direction which it is possible for the player to make and still produce a tone.

Dynamics and Intonation. Dynamics—loudness or softness—on the flute are controlled by the velocity of the air stream striking the embouchure hole. The greater the velocity the louder the tone. The pitch of the flute and other instruments, such as the tonette and song flute, on which the sound is produced by an edge-tone, is directly affected by the velocity of the air stream. The greater the velocity the sharper the pitch. Thus, in making a diminuendo the pitch will get flatter and flatter and in a crescendo the pitch will get sharper and sharper unless the embouchure compensates. This compensation is done by simultaneously changing the direction of the air stream striking the embouchure hole. As the velocity of the air diminishes and the tone becomes softer the direction of the air stream is gradually raised by a forward movement of the lips and lower jaw so that it is directed more across the hole. In a crescendo as the velocity of the air increases to make the tone louder the direction of the air stream is gradually changed so that it is directed more and more into the embouchure hole. This delicate and demanding relationship between velocity and direction of the air stream must be consciously developed, and progresses simultaneously the development of the embouchure only if attention is devoted to it. The regular practice of long tones with crescendo and diminuendo should be a part of every flutist's daily schedule.

Playing Position and Intonation. A playing position which is incorrect in any aspect can have an adverse effect on intonation. A slouched position which makes breath support inadequate makes control of wind velocity difficult or impossible with the consequences usually being flatting in pitch. The angle at which the instrument is held is important and becomes a problem in intonation if the angle of the flute doesn't follow the line of the lips. This deficiency results in the air stream striking the embouchure hole at an angle rather than directly and accentuates the natural tendencies of the instrument toward being out of tune. Tilting the head down or up changes the direction of the stream of air, and will produce an overall flatness or sharpness in pitch.

Mechanical Factors and Intonation. If a player is to achieve the very best intonation the instrument upon which he is playing must be in perfect mechanical condition. On the flute two mechanical factors influence intonation: leaky pads and the height of the pads above the tone holes. Leaky pads are caused by bent rods of keys, or by simple deterioration of the covering of the pad. Pads deteriorate so slowly that frequently the student is not aware of any change at all, so a regular inspection of their condition is called for. A leaky pad will cause a note or notes to respond with difficulty and somewhat sharp in pitch. Leaky pads caused by bent rods or keys seem to occur most frequently on the lower end of the instrument especially the foot joint. Many students cannot produce low C or C-sharp because of leaks, and if they can the pitch is impossible to control. These notes are naturally quite flat in pitch and do not respond to adjustments when there is a leak.

The height of pads above the tone holes is highly critcal for perfect intonation. Frequently the pad cups are bent up or down by various kinds of accidents, or through careless assembly. A pad which is too close to the tone hole tends to flatten the pitch, while a pad which is too far above the tone hole will sharpen the pitch. An out of adjiustment pad will have the greatest effect on the note on which it is the first open hole down the pipe from the head joint, as well as other notes to a lesser degree. It does not, of course, affect a note when it is in the closed position. Inspect the instrument regularly for height of the pad cups. All of them should be the same distance above their tone holes. If any of them are out of line the correction should be made by an expert repairman. Do not attempt to bend keys on the instrument yourself unless you have the proper tools.

Alternate Fingerings and Intonation. The flute has fewer alternate fingerings than any other woodwind instrument except perhaps the saxophone. Except for an alternate fingering for the third line B-flat which does not affect pitch, and an alternate fingering for fourth-line F-sharp which does, all the alternate fingerings are found for notes in the third register. The alternate fingerings in this register provide one means of controlling intonation both with the instrument itself and in ensemble playing. Different instruments and different players will produce slightly different pitches with alternate fingerings in this register. The standard fingering provided in the fingering chart is the one which the greatest percentage of players will find to be closest in tune. If, for some reason it is not, then try another fingering. The player should be aware of the alternate fingerings for the various notes, and should be able to use them with facility. He should check the pitch relationships between the fingerings for the same note and be aware of them. The pitch differences between alternate fingerings will vary from player to player and it is impossible to make a positive statement on what these differences will be. It is frequently necessary to select a fingering for the sake of perfect intonation rather than the fingering which offers the best facility. The player should never hesitate to put intonation before facility.

TONE

The most valuable asset of any flutist is a beautiful tone, and it is to this purpose that the student must direct his constant attention. The quality of the tone must be the same over the entire range of the instrument and at all dynamic levels. The better the balance of quality over the instrument the better the musical results and the more favorable the playing is to the listener.

The range of the flute is divided into three registers commonly called the first octave, the second octave, and the third octave:

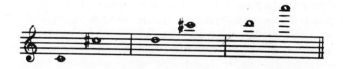

First Octave   Second Octave   Third Octave

Notes in the first octave are produced by the fundamental vibration of the air column, those in the second octave by the column of air vibrating in two segments (the first partial), and the notes in the third octave produced by the column of air vibrating in three, four or possibly five segments (the third, fourth, and fifth partials of the overtone series).

Beginners on the instrument tend to have a discernibly different tone quality in each of the three octaves as they extend their playing range. In addition to the details of tone production much of the student's attention needs to be directed to the problem of matching quality over the entire instrument.

There is no single standard for determining what is a good tone on the flute, although there tends to be less difference in tone qualities of the best professionals than on any of the other woodwind instruments. Every teacher and flute student should take advantage of every opportunity to hear live performances of fine instrumentalists. If this is not possible, study the recorded performances of the flute repertoire on a high quality phonograph. Compare the tone qualities of the various artists. With the universality of the phonograph record, it is quite possible to study the sounds of fine musicians from France, Germany and other nations as well as our own artists. A careful comparison of tone qualities produced by artists from other nations will reveal some differences, although these differences are not as easily detected via the phonograph recording as they are in personal performance. In spite of the differences all the tone qualities will be pleasing as they will have in common the essential elements of a good tone: clarity, body, and perfect intonation.

A good tone is the product of all the elements involved in performance: instrument, embouchure and breath support. If any of these is defective then the tone quality suffers accordingly. Problems of tone production and quality are many and varied, but may usually be traced to their source and must be corrected immediately. Following are some of the most prevalent problems or faults in tone:

1. *Small or Weak Tone.* This is a common fault with beginning flutists, but is found among more technically advanced students as well. In most instances it can be traced directly to poor breathing habits and lack of support. Check the inhalation process of the student to see that the breathing is diaphragmatic rather than in the chest, and that the student has the proper concept of support with the diaphragm and abdominal muscles. Remedial measures should be assigned. If breathing appears to be correct, it is possible that the throat is tight restricting the flow of air at this point. Work for an open relaxed throat so that the air can get out. The second condition which could produce a small, weak tone is the placement of the embouchure plate on the lower lip. If the plate is too far down on the lower lip, too much of the embouchure hole is covered and not enough air is entering the instrument

to produce the desired tonal body. Move the plate on the lower lip so that no more than one-fourth of the embouchure hole is covered.

2. *Hollow Tone.* The hollow unfocused sound is a typical problem in tone for a great many students. It, like other tonal problems, is caused by the lack of a mental standard of sound on the part of a student who doesn't know that this particular quality is undesirable in the instrument. This sound is achieved when too little of the embouchure hole is covered, and is usually accompanied by a chronic shortage of breath. This sound is also achieved by those students who have the concept of, and form the embouchure for a pop bottle or jug. And if the student is allowed to progress in this fashion without correction the flute begins to sound like a chromatic jug band. Students with the hollow tone sound will always have difficulty in playing in the third octave of the instrument. The correction for this sound is simply to move the embouchure plate to the correct position on the lower lip and to correct the direction and control of the air stream. Since major changes in embouchure formation and control are increasingly difficult to achieve as the student's technical facility and experience increases, this type of tone quality must be detected early in the beginning stage and remedial measures taken immediately.

3. *Shrill High Register.* The tones of many players who have acceptable quality in the first two octaves tend to thin out and become shrill in the third octave. Theoretically, if the student is achieving an acceptable quality in the lower octaves this should not happen. If it does it usually means that he simply isn't listening to his tone and attempting to match the quality over the entire range of the instrument. This condition sometimes exists when the extension of the student's range into the third octave is delayed too long, or when the tone studies—long tones, crescendo, diminuendo—are not applied to this octave with regular practice. This tone quality is frequently found when too little of the embouchure hole is covered by the lower lip which, in the third register, emphasizes the upper partials in the tone produced. When this shrill quality exists in a student, check first the amount of embouchure hole covered and the forward movement of the lips and lower jaw necessary to close more of the embouchure hole and to redirect the air stream in a more upward direction for this register. If this situation is correct, assign tone studies of various kinds in the third register. Octave studies from the second to third register in crescendo and diminuendo as shown at the top of p. 89 are excellent if the student is listening critically to both the tone quality and intonation.

4. *Control of Soft Tone.* Difficulty in producing and controlling a soft tone is principally due to the inability of the player to project a steady concentrated stream of air in the proper direction across the embouchure hole. Check breathing and breath support, and have the student practice focusing a steady stream of air into

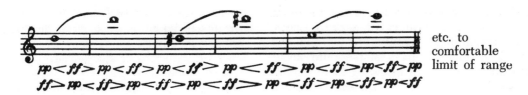

etc. to
comfortable
limit of range

the palm of his hand. Other possible causes are an aperture in the lips which is too large and which permits an air stream which is too large. This is causing the student to reduce support to make the tone soft, which in turn makes him lose control of the tone. A third possible cause is that the air stream is directed too far down into the embouchure hole. As softer and softer dynamic levels are reached, the size of the opening in the lips must be slightly and gradually decreased, and the direction of the air stream gradually raised by a forward movement of the lips and lower jaw. There is a very close interrelation between the amount of air being used and the direction of the air stream which must be discovered and used by the player.

5. *Dynamics and Tone Quality.* Students with otherwise good tone quality will lose it when playing at extremes of loudness or softness. This is caused by an undeveloped, poorly formed or inadequately controlled embouchure, or by lack of proper breath control or a combination of both. If tone quality and intonation are to be maintained in a crescendo the amount of opening in the lips must gradually be increased, and the direction of the air stream gradually lowered through pulling back the lips and lower jaw while increasing the intensity of the air stream. To maintain tone quality in a decrescendo gradually decrease the size of the opening in the lips, change the direction of the air stream by a forward movement of the lips and lower jaw. Briefly, the louder the tone the greater the intensity of the air stream, the larger the aperture in the lips, and the less of the embouchure hole covered. Conversely, the softer the tone the less the intensity of the air stream, the smaller the aperture in the lips, and the more embouchure hole covered. Good control is a combination of these three factors, and if they are in the proper balance both tone quality and intonation will remain good.

Recommended Material for Tonal Development. For the more advanced flutist whose tone quality and control has not kept pace with his technical development, and for the flutist who wishes to further improve his playing, two books by Marcel Moyse are highly recommended. His *De La Sonorite: Art et Technique* (published by Alphonse Leduc) lays out an organized plan for tonal development and is considered the standard text for this purpose, although in general the technical requirements of the book are on a fairly advanced grade. A new book of Mr. Moyse *Tone Development Through Interpretation* (published by McGinnis and Marx) provides additional material in this field including a consideration of vibrato on the instrument. A phonograph record, the "Moyse Study Record No. 1" illustrates the principles laid down in this book. The record is also available from McGinnis and Marx.

TONGUING

Tonguing refers to the manner in which the tongue operates in relation to the aperture in the lips and breath support in order to articulate the tones. The placement and action of the tongue must be rapid and under complete control at all speeds, and at all dynamic levels. It must, in coordination with breath support, be able to produce on the flute all varieties of articulation from the hardest staccato to the softest legato. By skillful use of the tongue and breath the flutist is able to reproduce the sound and effect of the multitude of bow strokes used by a fine string player, plus the effects of double tonguing, triple tonguing, and flutter tonguing.

The absence of a mouthpiece and reed or a double reed to contend with makes articulation on the flute considerably simpler than on other woodwinds, for the tongue can physically act as a valve in controlling the flow of breath into the instrument. There is considerable unanimity of opinion among authorities on the placement of the tongue in flute articulation, although there are small differences in the imagery used to achieve this placement.

Fundamental Articulation. Fundamental articulation is the basic movement of the tongue used to start a note in the absence of any other marking on the music such as a staccato and for the first note under a slur. This articulation and the legato style must be thoroughly mastered by the beginning student before proceeding to any other type of articulation. To start a note with fundamental articulation the tip of the tongue is placed against the front teeth at the base of the gums in such a way that no air passes through the lips. To start a tone, build up air pressure against the tongue using standard abdominal support, and release the air by using a movement of the tongue as in pronouncing the syllable "tu", "ta" or "du." When the air is released the tone should start cleanly without a sudden increase or decrease in loudness. When a series of articulated notes is played the tongue moves as in pronouncing the syllable selected to start each tone. The process of starting the next tone automatically cuts off the preceding tone. The tone is never stopped by the tongue except in such a series, and the student in practicing such a series of articulated notes must concentrate his attention solely on the beginnings of the notes. If the beginnings are correct the endings of the preceding notes will also be correct. Sustain each note for its full value.

An open throat for a free flowing stream of air is absolutely necessary for any type of articulation. Check the student visually for any sign of tenseness in the throat muscles. The syllables "tu," "ta," and "du" have become standard to provide the imagery for the tongue action because when the tongue movement is correct they force an open throat and a low tongue. With some experience the student will notice a difference in the type of articulation produced by "tu" or "ta" and "du"— the "du" movement producing a softer attack than the other syllables. More advanced flutists will take advantage of this difference to produce the exact sound demanded by the musical style. Beginners may find it helpful to try all three syllables to discover which works best for them at this stage.

The exact placement of the tip of the tongue is subject to some variation from teacher to teacher, but depends primarily on the length of the players tongue and the exact concept of the sound to be produced. Some authorities suggest that the tongue, in this type of articulation, be placed on the gum above the teeth, others suggest that it be placed somewhat down on the teeth so that the tip does not touch the gum at all. The placement of the tip against the teeth at the gum line is without a doubt the most common and the safest for the beginning student, who will automatically make adjustments of the placement up or down to suit his own physical characteristics as his facility is developed.

In the hands of experienced flutists the placement of the tongue varies directly with the loudness of the attack and with the octave, or pitch range, in which the note appears. As a general rule the tongue moves downward on the teeth as the notes get louder or as the pitch range gets lower, and moves higher on the teeth and onto the gum itself as the notes get softer or as the pitch range gets higher. These changes in location of the tongue for the attack are very slight, but are necessary if the sound of the attack is to remain the same over the entire dynamic range and pitch range of the instrument. Most students will make these adjustments automatically, although if they are having problems it is well to discuss the procedure with them.

In developing fundamental articulation keep the following points in mind:

1. The tongue touches the front teeth at the gum line to stop the flow of breath.

2. The breath is released, after being built up in pressure, by tongue action using "tu," "ta," or "du."

3. Support of the breath by the diaphragm and abdominal muscles remains constant throughout a series of articulated notes. Supporting muscles do not and must not move in conjunction with the tongue.

4. Position of tongue is higher for lower pitch range and lower for high pitch range.

5. Position of tongue is lower for loud dynamic levels and higher for soft dynamic levels.

6. Avoid starting notes with an accent, or increasing or decreasing the volume of the tone after the attack.

Legato and Staccato Articulation. Once the fundamental articulation is established the student may easily progress to other types of articulation of which those described as legato or staccato are basic. Various types of articulations demand varying lengths of silence between successive notes, and in combination with dynamic variations will produce a variety of effects required for various musical styles. Basically the legato articulation is one in which the action of the tongue makes a minimum interruption in the flow of sound. In developing this type of articulation there must be a continuing emphasis on a steady flow of air, unchanged by movements of the breathing muscles, with rapid and gentle strokes of the tongue. Using the syllable "du" rather than "ta" or "tu" will produce the soft articulation usually associated with the music in which this type of articulation is demanded. The following is a typical example of legato articulation.

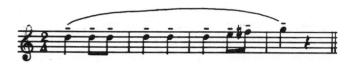

Staccato articulation should not be introduced until both the fundamental and legato styles of articulation have been mastered. The same tongue movement and placement and the same steady stream of air is used in staccato articulation. The only difference is that in staccato articulation the tongue returns to its place on the teeth or gums to stop the flow of air, but the air pressure against the tongue remains the same during the period of silence as during the production of tone. Staccato articulation is the only type in which the tongue is used to stop the tone. Because of the longer period of silence between notes in this type of articulation students are frequently tempted to relax breath support during the silence. If this is done, then the breathing muscles come into operation simultaneously with tongue action, resulting in an accent, and making it virtually impossible to develop a fast staccato. The following is a typical beginning staccato exercise.

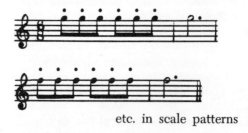

etc. in scale patterns

Multiple Tonguing. Because on the flute the tongue acts as a true valve in the control of breath double tonguing and triple tonguing are possible and fairly commonly used just as they are on the brass instruments. These multiple tonguings are virtually impossible on the other woodwinds and their use is exceptional. Almost all advanced flute methods include material for developing facility in these articulations. A third type of multiple tonguing which the flute has in common with the other woodwinds is flutter tonguing. Introduction of any type of multiple tonguing on the flute must be delayed until the fundamental, legato and staccato articulation styles are virtually mastered, and considerable technical facility has been achieved on the instrument. Double and triple tonguing are used only on the most rapidly moving passages where normal single tonguing is impossible.

Double Tonguing. Double tonguing is achieved by "tu-ku" (or "ti-ki," or "doo-goo"). The first syllable is pronounced with the tongue in the same position as for single tonguing, and the second syllable with the tongue striking the palate to stop the flow of air. The two syllables flow together in rapid succession in what is essentially a single movement of the tongue—hence the designation double tonguing. Needless to say this type of tonguing is restricted to use where the notes are grouped in two's. The alternation of the syllables allows the tongue to move much more rapidly, and to articulate the notes much faster than is possible in using single tonguing. Double tonguing is used in rapid repetitions of the same note, or for rapidly moving passages in which there are pitch changes. These two types of usages are illustrated in the following.

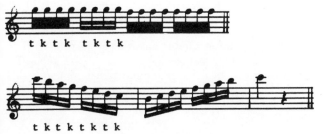

Because the second of the two syllables tends to be a little weaker in sound than the first (although the differences can be almost completely eliminated with practice) it is common practice to have the "tu" fall on the metrically strong notes and the "ku" on the metrically weak ones. The following illustrates this procedure:

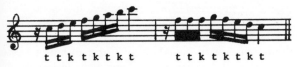

Double tonguing may be used with notes of uneven value if they move so rapidly that single tonguing does not give the right effect. The same syllables are used with this unequal rhythm. The following illustrates a typical use of this technique.

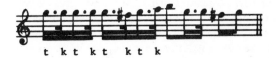

Triple Tonguing. Triple tonguing is used for rapidly moving passages where the notes are grouped in three's. The same two syllables used for double tonguing are utilized in order to alternate impulses between the tip and middle of the tongue, except that in the most common procedure one syllable is repeated. The syllables most commonly recommended and certainly those with which triple tonguing should begin are "tu-ku-tu," or its closest relation "doo-goo-doo." Using either of these it is possible to develop complete facility. An alternate method sometimes recommended for use on flute, as well as for use on brass instruments, is to simply use double tonguing but grouping the notes in three's as: "tu-ku-tu," "ku-tu-ku," "tu-ku-tu," "ku-tu-ku," etc. Triple tonguing is used for articulating rapidly repeated notes of the same pitch, or rapidly moving passages with pitch changes. The following shows a typical usage.

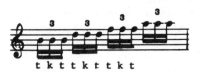

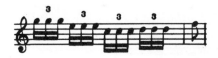

If the passage calling for triple tonguing begins on the second of the group of three notes, the first two notes are articulated with the syllables "tu-ku." If the passage begins with the third note of a group it is articulated with the syllable "tu."

Triple tonguing can be used in groups of three notes of unequal rhythmical value, just as double tonguing can be used with groups of two notes of unequal value, in passages where the music is moving so rapidly that single tonguing is difficult or doesn't give the proper effect. The same sequence of syllables is used for the unequal rhythm as for the patterns of equal rhythm. Following is a typical example for this technique.

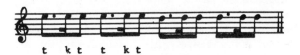

Flutter Tonguing. Technically speaking flutter tonguing is not an articulation but a special tonal effect which has come into use in twentieth century music, and first used by Richard Strauss. Darius Milhaud uses it in the first movement of his Sonatine for Flute as well as in several orchestral compositions. Contemporary composers are making even more extensive use of the unusual effect flutter tonguing gives, not only on the flute but on all other wind instruments.

The flutter tongue is produced by rolling the tongue rapidly against the roof of the mouth as in rolling the letter "R" in "b-r-r-r,' producing a very rapid tremolo. There is no set speed for the roll, but the more rapid the tongue movement the more effective the sound. Some students have considerable difficulty in producing a satisfactory roll of the tongue, and some few will find it impossible as the rolled "R" is not natural to English speaking people. Some flutists resort to using the gutteral "R" in the manner of the German language where the "R" can be rolled by vibrations of the soft palate at the back of the throat. This does not produce a true flutter tongue sound, but is better than nothing.

There is no standard notation to indicate flutter tonguing, and notes or passages to be flutter tongued have directions in a language. Some of the words used in other languages to indicate this effect include: *flatterzung, coupe de langue roule, en roulant la langue, tremolo dental,* and *frullante.* Sometimes, on isolated long notes, a rapid tremolo is indicated by four or five strokes across the stem of the note. The following illustrates typical notations.

Flutter

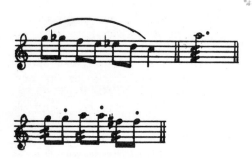

Common Problems in Articulation

1. *Articulation too Heavy.* In this type of sound each note starts with an accent, and is normally caused by too much pressure of the tongue against the teeth accompanied by too great a pressure of the breath against the tongue. The best solution is to have the student practice articulation at the pianissimo level, correcting first the legato articulation, then the fundamental articulation, and finally the staccato. A second cause of this type of sound is found when the student is pushing his breath simultaneously with the beginning of the at-

tack, and is normally accompanied by the inability to develop much speed in articulation. This condition is rather difficult to correct as it involves basic principles in breath support which require the student to begin at the beginning of this process and redevelop his responses. Practice in front of a mirror where the student can detect movements of the breathing mechanism is mandatory as students are not always aware of these movements. Slow practice and much patience is required to correct this condition.

2. *Sluggish Tongue.* Inability to tongue rapidly should not be a major concern with beginners, since time and practice is necessary to develop speed in articulation, but in more advanced players where technique has developed past articulation ability, it is a matter of considerable concern. Sluggish tonguing in most instances, where tongue placement and breath support are correct, is a simple matter of insufficient practice devoted to developing speed and accuracy. Special articulation exercises should be assigned to these students, with specific instructions on how many times each day to practice them, to use a metronome, and with specific metronomic speeds to use. Any player can develop satisfactory speed and control if he is using his tongue and breath support properly and if he will spend enough time on the problem.

Some students lack speed in articulation because they are moving the back of their tongue as well as the front portion. Movements in articulation are confined to the forward portion of the tongue, with the center and back remaining static, and the primary concept of this motion is of the tip moving up and down rather than forward and backward. Movement of the back portion of the tongue almost invariably carries with it movements of the throat which can easily be seen. To correct, the entire process of tongue placement and development of articulation must be gone through from the very beginning to allow new muscular habits to be formed. Some students make the correction quickly while others are never able to completely overcome the problem.

3. *Lack of Coordination Between Tongue and Fingers.* This is frequent among more advanced students who have developed a fair amount of facility on the instrument without detailed attention to articulation. It is purely and simply the result of practicing too fast without first working out notes and tonguing slowly and carefully. These students must practice slowly, at whatever tempo perfect coordination between fingers and tongue is possible, and gradually increase the speed. The use of a metronome on such exercises is invaluable to maintain a steady tempo and to help in the gradual increase in speed. Major and minor scales and arpeggios, making use of various articulation patterns, are good media of practice for this purpose.

4. *Slow Staccato.* Some players have difficulty in executing a true staccato rapidly. Other things being

correct, this problem can be traced to the lack of breath support and maintaining continuous breath pressure against the tongue or through the aperture in the lips. Some players will be found to be relaxing abdominal support of the air at the end of each note, or cutting off the stream of air in the throat. The concept of the tongue stopping staccato notes as well as starting them with the breath pressure continuing against the tongue during the space of silence will help correct this situation. Once this is corrected, speed and control can be readily developed.

5. *Movement of the Jaw in Tonguing.* This is the result of too large or too violent movements of the tongue, which are frequently accompanied by changes in pitch of the tone as the embouchure is moved. Rather than confining the movement to the front part of the tongue, the student is moving the entire tongue. The solution is to ask the student, no matter what his technical advancement, to practice the basic exercises for developing articulation constantly checking in a mirror to eliminate all movements.

TECHNIQUE PROBLEMS

A good technical proficiency on the flute is one which is accurate, under complete control, and facile. In developing this proficiency the flutist must be aware of certain mechanical or technical problems peculiar to the instrument which must be approached logically. While in the training of the flutist some of the devices which will be discussed are not introduced until the student is quite advanced, many of them will be quite valuable to students who are still in the intermediate stage of their development. For this reason the school teacher as well as the private teacher must be fully aware of the various potentials and introduce them whenever the problem arises in the day to day work with the student, and even to provide an opportunity to include them in the instruction of the players. The best organized and most logical presentation of all the problems connected with flute playing is found in the "Altes Method for Flute" (in two volumes) as revised by Caratge and published in 1956 by Alphonse Leduc, Paris. The text is printed in English as well as French, and every instructor who is seriously interested in the welfare of his flutists past the beginning stage should study the contents of this method thoroughly. Much of the material is quite difficult technically and the method itself is suitable for study only by advanced students.

Approached logically and with full information on available choices technical problems on the flute are neither complex to solve, nor complex to use. Intelligent selection and use of alternate fingerings and other procedures will simplify technical problems to an extent undreamed of by the uninformed. Both the importance of the correct solution and the reasons for a particular solution must be impressed on the student. Each alterna-

tive must be practiced until it becomes an involuntary part of the player's technique and how each alternative is used must be made so much a part of his technique that the correct choice becomes involuntary and instantaneous. Both players and teachers should not hesitate to mark instructions on the printed pages as reminders.

Following are problems which occur frequently and their solutions:

1. *B-flat Fingerings.*

There are three fingerings for the B-flat in the first and second octaves: T 100 400, TB-flat 100 000, and T 100 4x00. In establishing the correct hand position for the flute it was emphasized that the left thumb should be placed on the B-natural lever, that the T 100 400 fingering was the basic fingering and the only fingering which the student should use in the beginning stages of development. Early introduction of the use of the B-flat lever with the left thumb leads to sliding the thumb back and forth between the B-natural and B-flat levers. This sliding is one of the worst habits a flutist can develop as the keys do not lend themselves to convenient sliding. Sliding makes technique rough, and the students play wrong notes because they don't remember which lever the thumb is on. The basic rule for fingering on all woodwinds must be applied: "Never use the same finger in two different places on successive notes if an alternate fingering is possible." The third fingering for this note, the use of the side B-flat lever is a trill fingering and its use is limited to this function.

With the T 100 400 fingering the one to use except in special situations, and the side B-flat lever reserved for trills, the problem arises as to exactly when the thumb B-flat should be used. The thumb *must* be on the B-natural lever to play B-natural—C-flat in the first and second octaves and F-sharp—G-flat in the third octave. Except for these notes the thumb may be placed on either lever. When the B-flat is preceded or followed by one of these notes either directly or in a sequence of tones the basic fingering must be used. The rule to apply is simply that the thumb must not be used on the B-flat lever when the sequence of notes would require that the finger slide to the natural lever.

The B-flat lever is however extremely useful in many situations, and the student must learn when to use it to facilitate technical smoothness. Theoretically, as well as in actual practice in most music, the thumb can be placed on the B-flat lever when playing in the keys of F major, d minor, B-flat major, g minor (the presence of an F-sharp in the third octave would present a problem), E-flat major, A-flat major, and f minor. Its use in keys with more than four flats would be contingent on making adjustments in the thumb position for the G-flats in the third octave. The following illustrates a passage in which the thumb B-flat would be used.

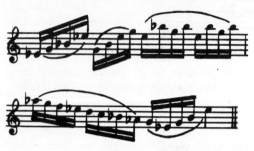

2. D-sharp Key. The D-sharp key played by the right little finger has three important functions in flute technique: (1) it acts as a point of support and control in holding the instrument, (2) it acts as a vent key to improve tone quality and intonation in all three octaves, and (3) it plays the note D-sharp and E-flat. In performing these functions the key is depressed into its open position on all except a very few tones on the instrument. The notes on which the D-sharp key is *not* depressed are indicated in the following:

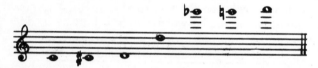

Failure to keep the D-sharp key depressed is one of the most common deficiencies of the beginning flutist. Unless the importance of this is continually stressed, difficulties first of all in holding the instrument securely and later in intonation present themselves. There is a tendency on the part of the player to omit depressing the D-sharp key in passages involving the low C and C-sharp where these notes are combined with notes on which the D-sharp key should be depressed. The D-sharp key has a considerable effect on the right hand notes in the first octave, and must be used. This is one instance where it is necessary to slide a finger from one key to another, and the instruments are constructed in such a way to make this possible even if not convenient. If the finger will not slide the old professional trick of rubbing the ball of the little finger at the side of the nose or in the hair to pick up lubrication can be resorted to. The example below illustrates a sequence in which it is necessary to slide the little finger from one key to another. Gaining facility in the sliding is a matter of considerable practice and effort, but it must be done.

3. F-sharp Fingering. 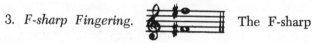 The F-sharp in the first and second octaves are two fingerings: T 123 006, and T 123 050. The first of these is the basic, standard fingering while the second is trill fingering only, and its use must be limited to this function. There is widespread misunderstanding about the use of the fifth finger rather than the sixth finger for this note. This is probably because the fifth finger in the right hand is the basic standard fingering for F-sharp on the saxophone and in the clarion register of the clarinet and this fingering has been transferred to the flute by instructors who have not made a thorough study of the instrument. Let it be understood once and for all that T 123 006 is the fingering for F-sharp on the flute which *must* be used at all times except where circumstances demand the use of the trill fingering for technical reasons. These circumstances will occur when the notes are moving at a rapid rate of speed, where the use of the sixth finger for F-sharp would make the passage rough or impossible ot play. The illustration on top of page 95 is a typical passage in which the T 123 050, or trill fingering must be used.

4. Special Fingerings. A few special fingerings in addition to the normal trill fingerings are useful in certain circumstances. These are required because of the acoustical response of the instrument, and while the regular fingerings will respond, these will improve the response.

a. When slurring from "A" in either the second or third octave to third octave "E," play the "A" with the regular fingering and the "E" with the regular fingering but without the D-sharp key.

b. The "F-sharp" and "A" in the third octave can be played, controlled and kept in tune better if the low C-sharp key is used instead of the D-sharp key.

c. The "E," "F-sharp" and "G-sharp" in the third octave, respond with some difficulty and are quite sharp on some instruments when they are attacked at the fortissimo level, although they will be in tune and respond at lower dynamic levels. The use of special fingerings for these notes which correct this type of response. Special fingerings to be used in the fortissimo attack level are: (1) E—T 120 450 without D-sharp key; (2) for F-sharp—T 103 050 D-sharp; (3) G-sharp—O 023 G-sharp 056 D-sharp.

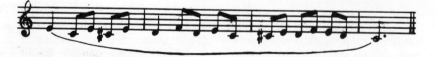

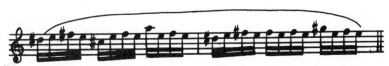

5. *D and E-flat Fingerings.* The fingerings for the "D" and "E-flat" in the first, second and third octaves are all slightly different. The beginning flutist has a tendency to play them all with the same fingerings, and the instructor must check carefully to see that the proper fingerings are being used. The fingering for the fourth line D and fourth space E-flat differs from that in the first octave in that the first finger must be up in order to vent the pipe at the proper place. Unless this finger is up on these notes, the sound is that of a pure harmonic and will be different from other tones in the second octave. The "D" above the staff poses no problem as the basic fingering is quite different from those of the other two octaves. The "E-flat" above the staff is fingered like the lowest D plus the G-sharp key. This is the only note on the instrument for which all fingers are used.

6. *Selection and Use of Alternate Fingerings.* There are alternate fingerings for some notes in the first and second octaves, and for almost all the notes in the third octave of the flute. If the smoothest and most useful technique is to be developed it is necessary that these alternates be learned, when and how they are to be used, and the best choice made each time there is a choice. This choice should be the one which gives the smoothest progression and the best facility and intonation. Some of the alternate fingerings are not exactly in tune. They can be used only when the sequence of notes in which they appear is moving so rapidly that the note is not sufficiently exposed for the ear to get an exact impression of the pitch. If the notes are moving slowly enough that the faulty intonation can be heard, the alternate fingering must not be used. Some of these alternate fingerings have already been discussed. Others will appear in the complete fingering chart for the instrument.

Trill fingerings are a special type of alternate fingerings intended for trilling but which may also be used in certain other circumstances. These fingerings sacrifice intonation for facility and some are noticeably out of tune. The use of trill fingerings in other than trills is most useful, even mandatory if technique is to be smooth, and their other uses clearly understood and developed. Where they would improve the technical facility trill fingerings can be substituted for basic fingerings on grace notes, mordents, turns, and for upper neighbor tones in diatonic passages. But as with any alternate fingering, trill fingerings must not be used when the ear can hear faulty intonation.

7. *Leaving Down One or More Fingers Throughout a Passage.* Rapidly moving passages involving some tones can frequently be made smoother if certain fingers in the right hand which are not a part of the basic finger-

ings for all notes are kept down throughout. This device is used on the clarinet first as an aid to crossing the break and then for the sake of smoothness in facility, and the basic principle can be applied to the flute. Advanced players frequently make use of this technique without being conscious of it, but it is frequently a great aid to less experienced flutists if they can be directed to make use of it. In some combinations of player and instruments leaving fingers down will affect the pitch of the other notes in the passage, while in other instances having the fingers down will have little or no effect. Use of this technique is limited to those places where there is no appreciable change in intonation of any of the notes, but is always usable where the notes are moving so rapidly that the ear does not perceive an incorrect intonation. In order to use this device learn the following.

The right hand position of any of these notes may be kept down.

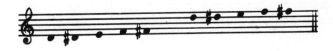

While playing any of these notes.

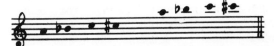

In the following musical example "A" illustrates a passage in which the first finger of the right hand is kept down throughout, "B" a passage where the first and second fingers of the right hand are kept down throughout, and "C" a passage where all three fingers of the right hand are kept down throughout. The same principle may be applied to other patterns as well as to groups of only three or four notes, and may be expanded to include other note combinations with experience.

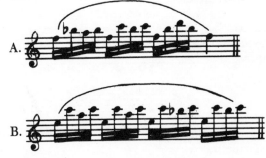

A.

B.

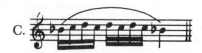

C.

HARMONICS

Acoustically it is possible to produce harmonics on any woodwind instrument. Indeed the second octave of the flute is the normal first harmonic of the notes in the first octave, and a portion of the normal fingering for all the other woodwinds makes use of either the first harmonic (oboe, bassoon, saxophone) or the second harmonic (clarinet), and these instruments are spoken of as overblowing an octave or in the case of the clarinet of overblowing a twelfth.

As indicated in the discussion of acoustics, the harmonic series falls in a regular pattern above the fundamental, and is produced by forcing the column of air to vibrate in two, three, four or more equal segments, rather than as a single segment which produces the fundamental. Harmonics are relatively simple for a competent flutist to produce, and many teachers recommend the regular practice of harmonics as a means of developing flexibility and control of the embouchure.

Harmonics on the flute can be produced on all notes in the first octave, although the lower the pitch of the fundamental the easier it is to produce a greater number of notes in the series. They are produced by decreasing the size of the aperture in the lips, increasing the intensity of the air stream, and altering the direction of the air flow as the increasingly higher overtones are produced. Considerable practice is necessary to accomplish this with facility, and the student should practice on the lowest three or four notes first until they come easily before practicing on the remaining fundamentals.

Harmonics are notated with a small circle above the note to indicate that it is played as a harmonic. Sometimes, as in notation for string instruments, the fundamental is written beneath the harmonic in a smaller note size. The following musical example gives the harmonic series on the lowest three notes of the instrument. Although the series of harmonics can be extended for ten or twelve notes above the fundamental, four notes above the fundamental as in the illustration are those most practical and most commonly used on the flute. With experience the number may be increased, especially on these lower notes.

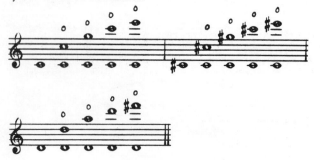

Special fingerings for harmonics for A-flat (first line above staff) and above have been derived and accepted as standard. These appear in a special section at the end of the fingering chart, and should be learned and used by advanced students. Harmonics are used at the pianissimo level only. They are especially useful for this purpose as many of the tones in the third octave are difficult to sustain on pitch at the pianissimo level when the regular fingerings are used. Harmonics, on the other hand, will not drop in pitch when played softly. Their primary use is for sustained notes, but they may also be used for moving passages in the third octave which must be played pianissimo.

Contemporary composers are making more and more frequent use of harmonics on the flute for special effects, and the skilled flutist will make use of them on older music to facilitate its performance. The following are typical examples of the use of harmonics.

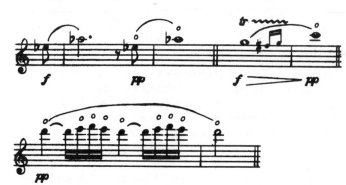

TRANSPOSITION FOR THE FLUTIST

As the flute is a non-transposing instrument, the flutist is not required in the normal course of events to do any transposition. Advanced flutists, however, like advanced players on any instrument are expected to be able to transpose parts, etudes, and various exercises to different keys and should take advantage of any opportunity to develop this facility. Teachers must see to it that the more advanced flutists are assigned problems in transposition as a part of their regular course of study.

The most frequent occasion for transposition, and this is rare, is found in older band arrangements where the flutist who does not have a D-flat piccolo available is expected to transpose the part and play it on a C piccolo. This is a relatively simple transposition. Every note is played a half-step higher than written. The following example illustrates this process.

Written for D-flat piccolo

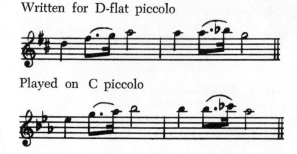

Played on C piccolo

SELECTION OF INSTRUMENTS

The modern flute was developed by Theobald Boehm (1794-1881), and the basic principles of key mechanism have been adapted and applied to the modern clarinet described as the Boehm system, and formed the basis for the development of the conservatory system for the Oboe and the mechanism of the saxophone. Attempts to apply his principles to the bassoon produced an instrument called the Sarrusophone which has never been widely adopted. All modern woodwind instruments are indebted to Boehm for their high degree of development.

Theobald Boehm was a professional flutist who became dissatisfied with the tone quality and imperfect mechanism of the old style conical bore flute. He made his first instrument in 1832 based on the old system, and did no further study of the problems until 1846 when he resumed his work on perfecting the instrument. In his own words: "I finally called science to my aid and gave two years (1846-1847) to the study of the principles of acoustics. After making many experiments, as precise as possible, I finished a flute in the later part of 1847, founded upon scientific principles, for which I received the highest prize at the World's Expositions, in London in 1851 and in Paris in 1855."[1] He continued to refine his instrument and the present cylindrical bore instrument was perfected between the years 1870-1880. Only the most minor improvements have been made since that time.

Because of the almost universal acceptance of the Boehm System modern flutes have been standardized into a single mechanical model. There is not the wide variety of models such as are available for clarinet or oboe, although certain options described below are available. Primary differences in flutes within a wide price range are in the metal used in the body and finish, and in the amount of precision hand-work used to refine the mechanism and temperament of the instrument. The basic mechanism is identical in all models. By virtual common consent of professional flutists in this country the finest instruments are those made in Boston by Powell whose instruments have become the standard of comparison by which all other instruments are measured.

Various options available for flute are as follows:

1. *Closed Tone Holes.* This is the standard model instrument on which all tone holes are covered by pads in the same fashion that the plateau system for oboe is constructed. This model used in the photographs accompanying this chapter, is recommended for students on all levels except the most advanced, and is available in a wide price range.

2. *Open Tone Holes.* Most, if not all, professional flutists use the open hole model flute. In this model the keys operated by the second, third, fourth, fifth and sixth fingers are partially covered by a ring with a circular pad. The fingers themselves act as pads just as they do on the clarinet. Professionals and advanced students prefer this model because it gives a somewhat greater control over the tone quality, and permits certain alternate fingerings which are not available with the closed tone holes.[2] The difficulty in covering the open holes accurately makes it inadvisable for use except by the most advanced players. Figure F-38 is a Powell flute with open tone holes, and a low B-natural key.

3. *Open G-sharp Key.* On the standard instrument the pad of the G-sharp key operated by the little finger of the left hand is held in a closed position by a spring. On the model instrument with the open G-sharp the pad of the key is held in an open position by a spring, which means that the key must be depressed by the little finger on all notes except where the open position of the pad is needed. Over a period of years it was discovered that the use of the open G-sharp key had many disadvantages and this model has completely disappeared from the market except for instruments made on special order. In a school situation the open G-sharp key may appear on older instruments, and the teacher should be aware of their existence.

4. *Low B-natural Key.* The only choice one has on the number of keys on the Boehm flute is the option of the low B-natural key. This key is added to the instrument by lengthening the foot joint so that the length of the tube produces B-natural rather than C-natural, and adding a key for the new note operated by the right little finger. This additional key is rarely called for in solos or orchestral literature of contemporary composers, and for this reason is not recommended for student use. Professional flutists, and the most advanced students who might be purchasing a new instrument should seriously consider a model instrument with this key. In addition to adding a half-step to the low range of the instrument, the additional length of the tubing adds resonance to the tone quality of the lower notes

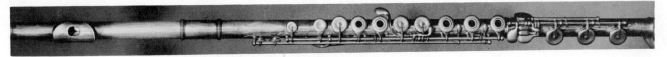

Figure F-38.

[1]Boehm, Theobald. *The Flute and Flute Playing.* Originally published in German, 1871. English translation by Dayton C. Miller 1922. p. 12.

[2]Altes. *Complete Method for Flute.* Revised by F. Caratge. Paris: Alphonse Leduc. 1956 has a table of the most useful of these fingerings on page 92 of Volume I followed by material to develop their use.

of the first and second octaves which makes it most desirable for professional calibre performance.

STUDENT QUALIFICATIONS AND APTITUDES

The flute is an excellent beginning instrument. The closed tone holes make it possible for a student to begin study as soon as he is physically large enough to achieve a reasonably accurate holding and hand position. This can be tested by observing the left hand position. If, after some instruction, he can hold the instrument with his left hand in the proper position with the little finger touching the G-sharp key he can begin study of the instrument. The right hand poses no particular problem if the left hand is satisfactory.

Other than size of the hands, standards of physical aptitudes for the flute are not always reliable. Generally speaking a student who has even teeth and lips that are firm and not too large may have an advantage over those who do not possess these attributes. The rare individual who has a pronounced underbite will probably have difficulty in achieving much success on the flute.

Advisability of flute study may be determined by success in producing tones on the head joint alone after some instruction in embouchure formation. These tones should be strong and clear and produced with the end of the head joint closed and open in the manner described in the section on embouchure. When he can sustain them for ten to fifteen seconds he is ready to proceed with the complete instrument. The student who can immediately produce a satisfactory tone on the head joint may be said to have a natural aptitude for the flute. Others may fail for some time, but with instructive guidance may develop an equal aptitude. In the final analysis, it is not natural aptitude but desire and persistence which determines future success on the instrument.

The piccolo is not a beginning instrument, as tone production and control are much more difficult than on the flute. The piccolo should only be played by those who have been successful in their accomplishments on the flute.

CARE OF THE FLUTE

Assemble and disassemble with the greatest of care. Review the instructions on assembly of the instrument until they are thoroughly understood and the students are performing the operation easily. Keep the instrument in its case when not in use. It is mandatory that the inside of the flute is thoroughly dried after each playing, and the habit of doing this thoroughly should be developed from the very first. Some flute players have the unfortunate habit of neglecting this process. Swabbing the instrument does not take much time, and will prevent the accumulation of dirt and grime inside the instrument, as well as helping to maintain sanitary conditions for playing. Disassemble the instrument in reverse order

of assembly and put in the case carefully before starting the cleaning process.

1. *Use of Cleaning Rod.* Every flute case is, or should be, equipped with a metal cleaning rod. It is to be used with a soft lint-free cloth such as an old linen handkerchief. A corner of the cloth is put through the opening near one end of the rod, drawn over the tip of the rod and wound down the length of the rod so that all except an inch or so of the length is covered. The end of the cloth is held firmly in place by a finger or fingers.

2. *Head Joint.* Shake the water out of the head joint. Insert the cleaning rod carefully so as not to move the end plug. Draw it back and forth several times so that all the inside area is wiped dry. (Figure F-39.) Put on the protective cap and replace the head joint in the proper place in the case.

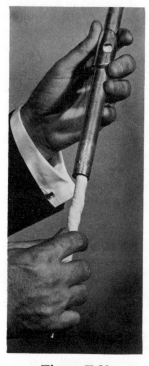
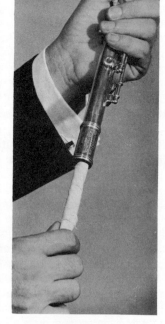

Figure F-39.   **Figure F-40.**

3. *Middle Joint.* Shake the water out of the upper end of the middle joint. Holding the joint as in the process of assembling the head joint, insert the swab and draw back and forth several times to clean the inside thoroughly. (Figure F-40.)

To clean the other end of the middle joint hold it near the other end as in assembling the foot joint and repeat the swabbing process. (Figure F-41.) Put the protective cap on the end and return joint to case.

4. *Foot Joint.* While very little moisture reaches the foot joint, it is well to clean it regularly. Hold it carefully so as not to put undue pressure on the key mechanism. (Figure F-42.)

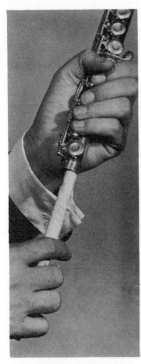

Figure F-41.

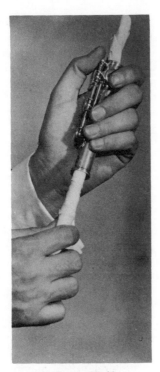

Figure F-42.

5. With a soft cloth wipe clean the inside and outside of all the connecting joints so that they will remain in good condition for assembly.

6. Using a chamois or different cloth, preferably of flannel, wipe the entire outside of each joint carefully to remove finger prints and dust. If this is done regularly and thoroughly the instrument will never need polishing.

Regular Maintenance of the Instrument

If the flute receives good care and a regular schedule of maintenance is followed it will remain in the best playing condition over a long period of time. Instruments which are in poor condition are difficult to play and result in poor players. Observing the following suggestions will help keep the flute in the perfect mechanical condition so necessary for success on the instrument.

1. *Oiling the Mechanism.* The mechanism must be oiled regularly three or four times each year. A special oil, called key oil, is available under various brand names for this purpose. A drop of oil on the end of a needle or toothpick should be put at each pivot screw of each key. Do this carefully so that no oil can get onto the pads. This regular oiling keps pivot screws from excessive wear and from rusting into place, making any repairs and adjustments on the instrument easier to accomplish.

2. *Adjusting Screws.* Most flutes have several adjusting screws, and in general the better the flute the more of these screws. The adjusting screws control the action and clearance of the various keys and pads which act together. These must be perfectly adjusted if the instrument is to respond as it should. Poor adjustment of these makes some notes difficult or impossible to play, and others to play out of tune or with poor tone quality. Every student past the beginning stage should have a small screwdriver for making these adjustments. These screws can be adjusted visually and tested by playing. When a note does not respond, check immediately to see if any adjusting screws are involved in the mechanism for that note. In addition to the adjusting screws, the pivot screws for each key should be checked regularly and tightened if necessary. New instruments are especially susceptible to developing loose pivot screws.

3. *Dusting the Instrument.* If the instrument is wiped carefully after each use as suggested above, very little dust will accumulate. However, over a period of time some dust will be found beneath the key mechanism where the regular wiping does not reach. This dust can be removed with a soft watercolor brush. If a cloth is used, it must be handled very carefully so as not to snag on the needle springs which break under pressure.

4. *Shining the Instrument.* The body and key mechanism of the flute will remain in good condition if wiped regularly. This will not only keep the keys and tube from tarnishing, but will prevent corrosion of the plates and keys in the event the player perspires excessively. Silver polish must never be used on the instrument, nor should the instrument ever be polished while the keys are in place. Using silver polish while the keys are on the instrument will foul pivot screws in the mechanism, and damage pads so they will leak. Leave polishing up to a competent repairman. Caution students against polishing the instrument, but give them careful and repeated instruction to keep the instrument clean by wiping it regularly.

5. *Bent Rods or Keys.* In spite of the best of care, keys or rods sometimes become bent out of line. Bent keys or rods occur with alarming regularity on the instruments of young players, and cause unevenness in technique, or even prevent some tones from responding at all. No attempt should be made to straighten keys or rods while they are in place on the instrument. This puts excessive pressure on both the keys and their posts and the instrument may be damaged even more. Keys must be removed from the instrument by a repairman who has the proper knowledge and tools to straighten and align them. Caution students against trying to do it themselves.

6. *Sticking Pads.* The flute is especially susceptible to sticking pads. If the instrument is not thoroughly dried before it is put into the case, or if the humidity is excessive even temporarily, some pads on the instrument may stick tightly, or will stick momentarily before they open, making technique uneven. If this happens, the first measure to take is to make sure that the student is doing a thorough job of cleaning the instrument each time it is put into the case.

Moisture can be removed from sticking pads by placing a cigarette paper between the pad and the tone hole, and pressing down on the key firmly. Release the key, move the paper and repeat the process until the key no longer sticks. If this does not relieve the sticking, put the cigarette paper in place, press the key, and pull the paper slowly from under the pad. Repeat the process several times.

If the cigarette paper does not relieve the sticking, dip the end of a pipe cleaner into a cleaning fluid such as carbon tetrachloride, benzine, or denatured alcohol. Wipe the pad with this fluid, and dry thoroughly with another pipe cleaner. Since this removes the natural oil from the pad, replace the oil by putting a very light coat of key oil over the pad with a pipe cleaner. Dry off excess key oil with another pipe cleaner.

If none of these procedures relieves the sticking, the pad should be replaced. Never use powder on pads in an attempt to stop sticking. It is rarely successful and damages the pad so that it begins to deteriorate.

7. *Leaky Pads.* Pads on an instrument wear out with use. Some wear out more rapidly than others and begin to leak, causing the instrument to respond with difficulty on certain notes. The pads on the foot joint of the flute are especially susceptible to leaking, with the result that the student has difficulty in producing these notes, if he is able to produce them at all. If a student cannot produce low C or C-sharp suspect a leaky pad. Some pads which are in good condition may leak because they are improperly seated over the tone hole. Pads deteriorate so slowly that the player is frequently not aware that the condition exists. For this reason a close inspection of the condition of the pads on every instrument should be made every three or four months.

If some notes respond with difficulty, with a change in tone quality and intonation in comparison with surrounding notes, there is a strong possibility of a leak in the instrument. Finding the exact source of a leak on a flute is a somewhat more awkward process than on some other woodwinds. To test for leaks take the instrument apart. Close the bottom end of the middle joint with a cork, close all tone holes with the six fingers using no more than the normal amount of pressure against them, and blow through the open end of the tube. Leaky pads can be identified by the air leaking through, although the assistance of a second person is sometimes necessary to find the exact location of a leak. If a tone hole which is normally covered by a key and a pad held closed by a spring leaks (the G-sharp key or a trill key for example) when maximum wind pressure is applied during the test, the spring on that key must be strengthened or replaced by a repairman. The joint should not leak no matter how much breath pressure is applied if it is in the best playing condition. The foot joint can be tested for leaks in the same manner.

If the leak is located an examination of the pad will determine whether it should be replaced or simply reseated. Accuracy in seating pads is determined best by the use of commercial feeler papers or strips of cigarette paper about a quater inch wide. Slide one end of the paper under the pad, put the normal amount of pressure against the pad if the key is not held closed by a spring, and slowly draw the paper out. As long as the pressure against the paper remains constant there is no leak. If the pressure suddenly lessens the pad is not properly seated. Repeat the process completely around the pad so that all edges are tested.

The process of blowing cigarette smoke through the instrument to identify a leak by seeing the smoke come out of the leak is not recommended. The nicotine in the smoke coats the pads and if this is done frequently will damage them so they harden and leak. Repairmen use a small light in the bore of the instrument to find leaks, as the light will shine through the open space of the leak.

8. *Regular Overhaul.* The condition of every instrument must be checked at least once each year by the instructor or by a repairman. Regular maintenance keeps an instrument in playing condition over a period of years, rather than allowing it to gradually deteriorate becoming increasingly difficult to play. Every instrument must have a complete overhaul every three to five years depending on the amount of usage. If instruments receive a yearly checkup, a regular overhaul, and proper daily maintenance they will last in virtually perfect condition for many years. The service of a competent repairman are invaluable and a great asset to any program of instrumental instruction.

BIBLIOGRAPHY OF STUDY MATERIALS

The amount of teaching material available for the flute is quite extensive once the student is past the beginning stage of his development. The further along in his studies the greater variety of music available. In order to have a well-rounded and interesting course of study it is recommended that all students past the very beginning stage be studying simultaneously from each of the following classifications of material: (1) a method book for continuity; (2) technical studies such as major and minor scales, arpeggios, etc. in various forms and keys; (3) a book of etudes or studies; (4) duets or other ensemble experience; and (5) solos with piano accompaniment.

In the sections which follow a cross-section of the most widely used material (exclusive of solo and ensemble music) available for flute is listed. It is by no means all inclusive as such a list would fill an entire volume. Additional information on all classifications can be found in the catalogs of retail stores specializing in woodwind music,[3] in the Selective Music Lists of

---

[3]See Appendix IV for a list.

Instrumental Solos and Ensembles published by the National Interscholastic Music Activities Commission; pages 31-84 of F. B. Chapman's "Flute Technique" published by Oxford University Press, etc.

A listing of composers, titles and publishers is only the starting point for acquiring teaching materials. Only personal acquaintance with the music itself can give the answer to the quality of music, and how and when it could be used. The reader is urged to examine as many of these titles as possible, and to evaluate them whenever possible through actual use. Many books do not give the results in practice that a visual examination would indicate.

Beginning Methods

Anzalone, Valentine. *Breeze-Easy Method for Flute*. Two Volumes. M. Witmark.

Bodegraven, Paul Van. *Adventures in Flute Playing*. Two Volumes. Staff Music Publishing Co.

Buck, Lawrence. *Flute Elementary Method*. Kjos Music Co.

Dalby, Cleon E. *All Melody Method for Flute*. Two Volumes. Pro Art Publications.

Eck, Emil. *Eck Method for Flute*. Two Volumes. Belwin, Inc.

Fair, Rex Elton. *Flute Method*. Two Volumes. M. M. Cole Publishing Co.

Gekeler, Kenneth. *Belwin Flute Method*. Three Volumes. Belwin, Inc.

Herfurth-Stuart. *A Tune A Day for Flute*. Two Volumes. Boston Music Co.

Hetzel, Jack. *Hetzel's Visual Method for Flute*. Oliver Ditson.

Petersen, A. C. *Rubank Elementary Method for Flute*. Rubank, Inc.

Skornicka-Petersen. *Rubank Intermediate Method for Flute*. Rubank, Inc.

Voxman, H. *Rubank Advanced Method for Flute*. Two Volumes. Rubank, Inc.

Van Vactor, David and Kitti, Arthur. *Carl Fischer Basic Method for Flute*. Carl Fischer.

Standard Methods

Altes, Henry. *Method for the Boehm Flute*. Two editions. Carl Fischer, Inc. Two Volumes; edition wtih English text published by Alphonse Leduc. The Leduc edition revised and augmented by Caratge (1956) is the finest and most complete flute method available, and is recommended for study and reference. The Carl Fischer edition, published in 1918 has the original contents of the method, but is poorly edited and has very little explanatory material. Many duets in both editions.

Berbiguier. *Flute Method*. Two Volumes. Salabert. French Text.

Brooke, Arthur. *Modern Method for Boehm Flute*. Cundy-Bettoney. Available in two volumes, or complete edition. Published in 1912, this method is no longer "modern" but does have considerable useful material on both the intermediate and advanced technical levels.

DeLorenzo, Leonardo. *L'Indispensabile. A Complete Modern School for the Flute*. Two volumes. Carl Fischer, Inc. Text in English and Italian.

Langey. *Tutor for Flute*. Carl Fischer.

Soussmann, H. Revised by W. Popp. *Complete Method for Flute*. Carl Fischer, Inc. Three volumes. Volume two contains 12 duets, and volume three has 24 studies in major and minor keys which are quite advanced in technical difficulty.

Taffanel & Gaubert. *Methode Complete de Flute*. Alphonse Leduc. French text only. Contains much excellent material on an upper intermediate and advanced level. A few duets. There is very little text and the absence of an English translation will not be a handicap to its use.

Wagner. *Foundation to Flute Playing*. Carl Fischer. Suitable for the first intermediate book.

Additional Study Materials

Andersen. *24 Etudes, Op. 15*. International, Southern Music Co., or Carl Fischer.
24 Studies in All Major and Minor Keys, Op. 21. McGinnis & Marx.
24 Instructive Studies, Op. 30. McGinnis & Marx.
24 Studies, Op. 33. International, Southern Music Co., or Carl Fischer.
26 Little Caprices, Op. 37. McGinnis & Marx.
18 Studies, Op. 41. International, Schirmer.
24 Virtuosity Studies, Op. 60. Southern Music Co.
24 Technical Studies, Op. 63. (with Op. 30, Southern Music Co.)

Andraud. *Modern Flutist*. Southern Music Co.
Has etudes by Donjon, Caprices by Karg-Elert and a number of orchestral studies, including some for piccolo and alto flute.

Berbiguier. *18 Studies*. Schirmer, International or Carl Fischer.

Boehm, T. *12 Studies for Flute, Op. 15*. Carl Fischer.
24 Caprices and Etudes, Op. 26. Carl Fischer.
24 Melodious Studies, Op. 37. Carl Fischer.

Camus. *42 Etudes*. Salabert. Piano accompaniment available.

Cavally. *Melodious and Progressive Studies for Flute*. Three volumes. Southern Music Company. Selected from the works of Andersen, Garibaldi, Koehler, Terschak, Boehm, Kronke, Kohler, and Mollerup. Volume one is suitable for lower intermediate level instruction. Studies are only generally progressive. An excellent collection. When in doubt use this series.
Original Melodious and Progressive Studies for the Beginning Flutist. Southern Music Co.

Eck, Emil. *Tone Development for Flute*. Belwin. Intermediate level. Excellent studies.

Endresen, R. M. *Supplementary Studies for the Flute*. Rubank.

Furstenau. *26 Studies for Flute, Op. 107*. Two Volumes. Fillmore or Leduc.
Studies, Op. 125. Edited by Eck. Belwin.
12 Grand Studies for Flute. Cundy-Bettoney.

Garibaldi. *Little Studies, Op. 131*. Leduc.
20 Little Etudes, Op. 132. International or Leduc.
20 Etudes Chantantes, Op. 88. Leduc.

Hovey, Nilo W. *Daily Exercises for Flute*. Belwin. Selected from works of Albert and Pares.

Hughes, L. *40 Studies, Op. 101*. International.

Jean-Jean, Paul. *16 Modern Etudes*. Leduc.
Difficult, but outstanding studies using modern idioms.

Karg-Elert. S. *30 Studies, Op. 107*. International.

Koehler. *Progress in Flute Playing, Op. 33*. Three Volumes. Carl Fischer or International. Volume one, easy studies. Volume two, studies of medium difficulty. Volume three, studies of greater difficulty.

Kummer. *24 Melodic Etudes, Op. 110*. Associated Music Publishers.

Marquee, Andre. *Daily Exercises for Flute*. G. Schirmer.

Moyse, Louis. *La Grande Velocity* (Progressive Technical Studies on Scales and Arpeggios). Southern Music Company.

Moyse, Marcel. *Tone Development Through Interpretation*. McGinnis & Marx.
De La Sonorite: Art et Technique. Leduc.
Marcel Moyse, professor of flute at the Paris Conservatory, has made great contributions to the study literature for flute. To date more than thirty volumes of original works and arrangements have been made available most by Alphonse Leduc, Paris. With the exception of his edition of the *Demersseman Studies, Op. 4*, his material is in the upper intermediate and advanced levels.

Pares, G. *Technical Exercises for Flute*. Carl Fischer.
Modern Pares for Flute. Rubank.
Two editions of the same music. The Rubank edition has been edited by Harvey Whistler.

Platonov, V. *30 Studies*. International.
24 Studies. International.

Reichert. *Daily Exercises, Op. 5*. Associated Music Publishers.

Terschak. *Daily Exercises, Op. 71*. Vol. I. Associated Music Publishers.

Voxman. *Selected Studies for Flute*. Rubank.

Wood. *Studies for the Execution of Upper Notes*. Boosey & Hawkes.

STUDY AND ACHIEVEMENT QUESTIONS

1. Identify the beginning, intermediate and advanced playing ranges of the flute and piccolo.
2. Assemble the flute, identifying each part and describing and demonstrating each step.
3. Observe one or more beginning, intermediate and advanced flute students in the process of assembly and fill out the check list for assembly. Describe corrections for any faults found.
4. Describe and demonstrate the holding and hand positions for the flute. Instruct a student unfamiliar with the instrument in how to achieve the correct positions.
5. Observe one or more, beginning, intermediate and advanced flute students and fill out the check list for holding and hand positions. Suggest corrections for any faults.
6. Discuss and demonstrate embouchure formation, setting the embouchure, and the effect of the four items which influence tone production on the flute.
7. Observe one or more beginning, intermediate and advanced flute students and fill out the check list for embouchure formation. Suggest corrections for any faults.
8. Discuss how the flute is tuned and the influence of the cork in the head joint on pitch and intonation.
9. What factors will make the over-all pitch of the instrument flat? sharp? What factors influence the pitch of individual notes?
10. Identify the three registers of the flute. Indicate those notes produced by the fundamental vibration of the air column, and by the first overtone.
11. List the most frequently found deficiencies in tone quality together with their causes and corrections.
12. Describe placement and movement of the tongue in fundamental, legato and staccato articulation. Describe how multiple tonguing is achieved and used.
13. List the notes on the flute for which there are standard alternate fingerings. Give the fingering for each alternate and an example of how and when it is used.
14. What are the uses of harmonics on the flute?
15. Discuss the advantages and disadvantages of closed and open tone holes on the flute.
16. Discuss student qualifications and aptitudes for flute study. Demonstrate the use of the head joint in this respect.
17. Perform the process of disassembly and cleaning. Discuss the regular maintenance of the instrument.
18. How may sticking pads be corrected? How may leaky pads be discovered?
19. Make a comparative analysis of as many beginning flute methods as you have available. Select and rank them in order of preference.

20. Examine available standard methods and additional study materials for flute and list them with comments.

21. Prepare a suggested list of material to include all five types of material suggested for simultaneous study for an upper beginning level student. An intermediate level student. An advanced student.

22. Discuss the use of vibrato on the flute. When and how is a vibrato developed?

23. Listen to several phonograph records of flute literature. Comment and and compare tone quality, phrasing, articulation and general facility.

24. Attend a festival event which includes flute solos. Observe the players and make a detailed critique of as many as possible on details of holding positions, hand positions, embouchure formation, tuning, intonation, tone quality, articulation and technique. Describe any faults found in any of these, the possible causes, symptoms, and corrections for each.

CHAPTER THREE

OBOE AND ENGLISH HORN

The oboe and English horn have virtually the same written range and the fingering on the two instruments is identical. The discussions in this chapter will be concerned with both instruments, although the oboe specifically will be mentioned, and unless otherwise noted all comments apply equally to both instruments.

The oboe is a non-transposing instrument, sounding the note as written. The English horn is in F, sounding a perfect fifth lower than written. The transposition for the English horn, and the range of actual sounds produced by both instruments is as follows.

1. *Oboe*

Written   Sounds   Range of Actual Sounds

2. *English Horn*

Written   Sounds   Range of Actual Sounds

PLAYING RANGES

The playing ranges for the oboe are fairly generally accepted, and are classified as *Beginning*, the range a typical young beginner can be expected to play by the end of his first year of experience; *Intermediate*, the range commonly required for the average good high school player; and *Advanced*, the complete range of the professional caliber player. These ranges are determined not so much by the fingering problems involved, but in the development of a good strong standard embouchure plus the ability to make and/or adjust reeds which

will respond both on the lowest and highest notes. The highest tones in the advanced range are rarely called for but are necessary in order to cover the range written in contemporary music of a difficult nature. The upper limits of an oboist's playing range should not be forced, but allowed to develop naturally as embouchure control grows. Forcing the upper notes before a player is ready causes serious embouchure problems since the student will make unnatural adjustments in order to reach the notes. The natural development of these tones comes when the student can play them without shifting or changing his embouchure except for the increased support necessary to control intonation.

Since the English horn is played by a competent oboist, the three stages of range development are given only for the oboe. Only the complete advanced range is given for the English horn. All ranges are as written for the instrument.

1. *Oboe*

Beginning   Intermediate

Advanced

2. *English Horn*

Playing Range

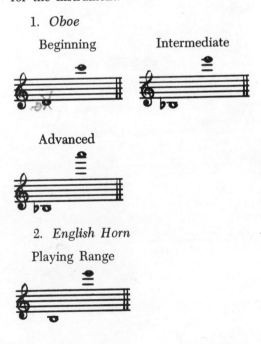

ASSEMBLING THE INSTRUMENT

Of all the woodwind instruments the oboe is the most susceptible to damage to the mechanism through careless handling in assembly or disassembly. The mechanism is extremely complicated and close fitting tolerances are necessary for certain keys to work properly. The slightest bent key or lever will cause difficulties in performance. For this reason care in handling must continually be emphasized. Beginners on the instrument have a tendency to assemble and disassemble the instrument without sufficient care or to handle the instrument as if it were ruggedly built. The proper method of putting the instrument together and taking it apart must be taught from the very beginning.

The following procedure is a standard one. Practice it until it is comfortable and natural. Before proceeding make sure that both corks are well lubricated with prepared cork grease, and that the metal lined joints into which the corks fit are wiped clean and smooth.

PARTS OF THE INSTRUMENT

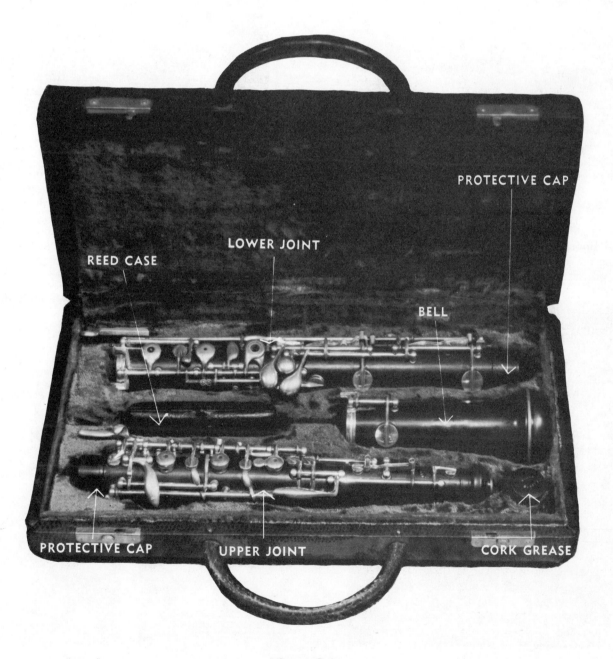

Figure O-1.

A. Lower Joint and Bell Assembly

1. Figure O-2. Grasp the lower joint with the right hand, palm of the hand on the wood beneath the instrument, with the thumb around the thumb rest.

3. Figure O-4. The left hand grasps the bell firmly in the palm, with the forefinger pressing on the key to raise the connecting lever so that it will slide over the portion of the lever on the lower joint.

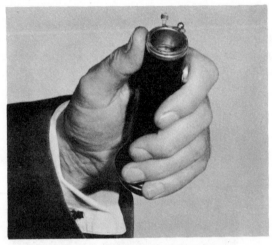

Figure O-4.

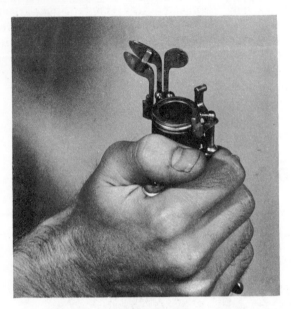

Figure O-2.

2. Figure O-3. With the palm in position, the tips of the fingers press the plates over the tone holes in holding the joint firmly. Fingers are cupped so that there is no pressure against the rods on the side of the joint.

4. Figure O-5. The bell is then pushed on the lower joint and the two portions of the connecting lever aligned. The bell should be pushed with only the slightest back and forth motion keeping the connecting lever in view constantly. If the bell is twisted on it will hit against the posts on the lower joint and be bent out of alignment.

B. Upper Joint and Lower Joint Assembly

1. Figure O-6. Grasp the upper joint with the left hand, palm of the hand on the wood beneath the instrument, with the thumb on the wood beside Octave Key A.

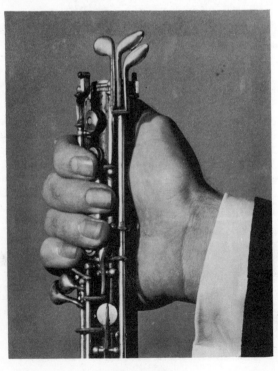

Figure O-3.

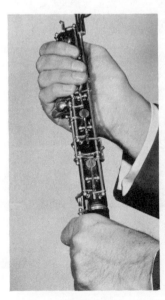
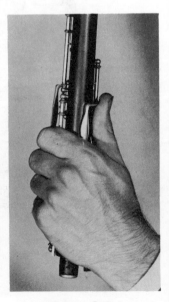

Figure O-5.   **Figure O-6.**

2. Figure O-7. The index finger depresses the top trill key (if this key is on the instrument) to raise the connecting lever. Observe the connecting lever on the left side of the instrument to see that it is lifted as the key is pressed. The remaining three fingers cover the tone holes with the second finger over the second tone hole and press to hold the joint firmly. The heel of the thumb presses the B-flat-C rocker mechanism to raise the connecting lever. Observe the connecting lever on the right side of the instrument to see that it is raised.

is identical with that used for assembling the bell, except that the thumb is moved from around the thumb rest to hold down the connecting lever on the left side of the instrument.

4. Figure O-9. Lower joint second alternate holding position. The right hand grasps the assembled lower joint and bell with the bell held in the fingers. The forefinger is on the metal band of the bell, and the thumb presses firmly on the lower key of the upper joint. This section is held securely in this position so that the two joints can be pushed together.

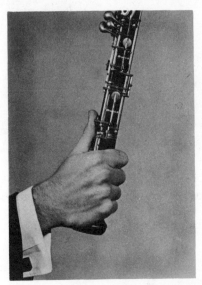

Figure O-9.

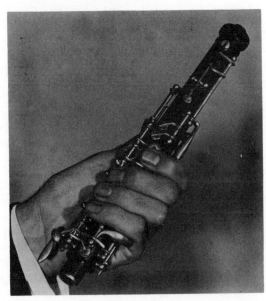

Figure O-7.

3. Figure O-8. Lower Joint First Alternate holding position. The grasp of the right hand on the lower joint

5. Refer back to Figure O-2. There are three connecting levers between the lower and upper joints. The placement of the hand on the upper joint raises two of these—the third on the top of the instrument is normally in a raised position. Keep your eyes on these while putting the two parts together so that there is no possibility of bending them.

6. Figure O-10. With the right hand in the first alternate position the two sections are pushed together. There must be no winding or twisting motion or one of the levers will be bent. Rest the bell against the body if necessary to hold the instrument firmly. If the cork is the right size and well greased the sections can be pushed together without applying too much force. Check the alignment of the connecting levers.

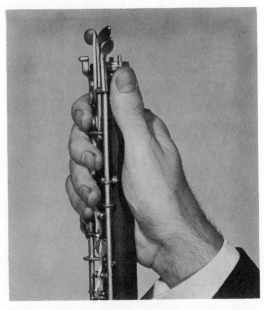

Figure O-8.

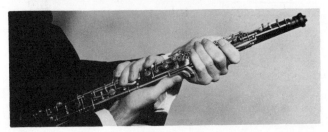

Figure O-10.

7. Figure O-11. With the right hand in the second alternate position the two sections are pushed together. There must be no winding or twisting motion or one of the levers will be bent. If the joints slide together with some difficulty, use only the very slightest back and forth motion with the lower joint, keeping the eyes on the connecting levers. Check the alignment of the connecting levers.

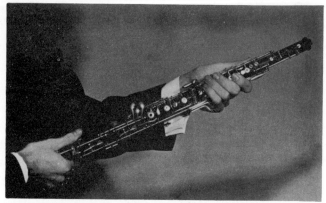

Figure O-11.

8. Figure O-12. Push the reed into the socket as far as it will go and adjust to playing position. Grease the cork on the reed if necessary to make it fit easily.

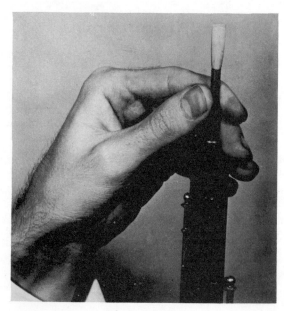

Figure O-12.

English Horn.

The assembly of the English horn is identical with that of the oboe, except that the bocal on which the reed fits is added to the end. A neck strap is helpful in holding the instrument and students should be encouraged to use it, although some professionals do not feel that it is necessary.

Common Faults in Assembly

There are, of course, several possible ways in which the oboe may be assembled, the only criteria for a good procedure being that no pressure is put on rods, plates, or keys during the process. The procedure outlined above is a common standard one and may be safely used for beginners who should practice putting the instrument together and taking it apart until the correct routine becomes comfortable and accurate. The following items are the most commonly found faults or inaccuracies in assembly of the oboe.

1. *Failure to Grease Corks.* A container of cork grease is a must for every oboe case, and the cork joints of the instrument and the reed staple must be kept well greased so that the connections may be made with ease. If the corks are not greased the instrument is assembled with difficulty and a great deal of pressure is necessary. This excessive pressure can easily cause the hand to grip the insturment too tightly and bend keys, rods, etc. If, after the corks are well greased, a joint is still assembled with difficulty, then the cork is too large. It may be fitted to the right size by sanding with fine grain sand paper either by the student or by taking the instrument to a repairman. If sanding is done, care must be taken not to sand any of the wood of the instrument, only the cork. Since the joints of many brands of oboes are metal lined, the instrument can be assembled with ease if the corks are properly fitted and well greased.

2. *Improper Sequence of Assembly.* Some students will assemble the upper and lower joints before putting the bell on the lower joint. While this procedure is quite satisfactory for experienced players, the inexperienced player will find it awkward to hold the assembled upper and lower joints without putting pressure on the mechanism when adding the bell. A further advantage of putting the bell on the lower joint first is that it provides an alternate holding position which gives the student a firm and safe place to hold the lower joint while the extremely critical connections are made between the lower and upper joints.

3. *Bending Connecting Levers.* A bent connecting lever is perhaps the most common result of improper assembly which makes some fingerings difficult or impossible to use. Unfortunately the younger players who should have the instrument in perfect playing condition are most frequently at fault. The connecting lever between the bell and the lower joint controls the closure of the pad which plays the low B-flat—the bottom of the oboe range. Young players have difficulty in producing this tone even under the best conditions and if the lever is bent or not centered properly in assembly the pad will not close completely and the student cannot produce the tone at all. If the student can play the low C and B-natural, but not the low B-flat it is almost inevitable that this pad is leaking.

Between the upper and lower joints there are three connecting levers on most instruments, two on others, which must be in perfect adjustment and perfectly aligned if the instrument is to respond properly on certain fingerings. These levers are bent during the process of assembly by twisting the joints so that the levers hit a post or key or the other portion of the lever. Insist that the students keep their eyes on these levers while these two joints are being assembled. The lever on the right side of the instrument connects the plate or ring operated by the first finger of the right hand with two small pads between the first and second tone holes of the upper joint. Both of these pads must be opened for the basic fingering for third space C and the second for the third line B-flat. If this lever is bent so that these pads do not open sufficiently these notes will be flat, if it is bent so they open too far the notes will be sharp, if it is bent too much or not aligned these notes will not respond at all.

The connecting lever on the top of the instrument is part of the articulated G-sharp mechanism, and its function is to close the pad of the tone hole which produces G-sharp when the fourth finger is down even though the G-sharp key is being held down by the left little finger. The articulated G-sharp is a very useful device in smoothing technique and is discussed later in this chapter. If this lever is bent so that it will not close

the pad, then the articulation of this key is ineffective and can readily be detected. If, however, this lever is bent down so that it is too close to the pad, then the tone hole operated by the fourth finger will not completely close, and notes involving fingers down in the right hand will not respond or will respond with difficulty. If the student can play down to second line G, but has difficulty with the F-sharp or E-natural below the chances are that this pad is leaking and the cause of the leak may be this connecting lever.

The connecting lever on the left side of the instrument controls an alternate fingering for a trill key on the upper register, and is not on all models of the instrument. If this lever is bent down so that there is space between the two portions, no problem is involved, except that the rarely used trill fingering will not respond properly, and the student will resort to the identical key operated by the left hand. If however, this lever is bent up, the trill key will be held open and the instrument will not respond or will respond with difficulty.

Correcting the adjustment on any of these bent connecting levers, or indeed on any key on the instrument, must be done by a repairman who has the proper tools and uses the proper procedure to avoid putting excess pressure on the posts which hold the keys to the instru-

Check List for Assembly

Observe the student in the operation of assembling the instrument and check the following items. Incorrect items for older students should not be called to their attention until the entire process is completed; younger students should be corrected immediately. If any mistake is made the entire process should be repeated until perfect.

	Yes	No	Comments
1. Were corks examined to see if they were well greased?			
2. Bell held properly?			
3. Lower joint held properly?			
4. Connecting lever between bell and lower joint carefully aligned?			
5. Upper joint held properly?			
6. Lower joint and bell assembly held properly for joining upper joint?			
7. Eyes on connecting levers during this process?			
8. Upper and lower joints pushed together without twisting motion?			
9. Connecting levers between these two joints carefully aligned and tested?			
10. Reed pushed firmly into socket?			

ment. Putting pressure on the keys to straighten them may well cause more serious damage to the instrument.

4. *Holding the Joints Improperly.* Holding the parts of the instrument as described and illustrated in the assembly process avoids any pressure of any kind on the mechanism which would bend any portion of it. Any other manner of holding the parts which accomplishes the same thing would be equally satisfactory. Holding the parts improperly puts pressure on the delicate mechanism of the instrument and soon bends keys or rods out of line. An instrument which is not in perfect alignment plays with difficulty, has certain notes out of tune, or simply doesn't respond at all. Beginners on the instrument must be taught to hold the parts correctly during the assembly and disassembly and checked frequently to see that they are doing so.

5. *Bent Keys or Rods.* The result of improper assembly, rough handling, or putting the instrument in its case carelessly is bent keys or rods. The keys and rods most frequently bent are those operated by the left little finger which makes certain notes difficult or impossible to produce. The cluster of three keys all operating on

the same rod must operate smoothly and accurately. I the rod is bent, realignment is difficult and complicated and must be done by a repair man. The second octave key operated by the first finger is frequently bent down so that the pad is not opened sufficiently. This cause difficulty in producing the notes in the upper part of the second octave, and frequently makes them flat in pitch

HOLDING POSITION FOR THE OBOE

The way in which the oboe is held has a direct effect on the type of tone quality produced, the embouchure intonation, and the development of technical facility The proper position is one in which the body is in comfortable relaxed position, in which the hands and arms fall naturally into position; and which permits the formation and development of the best embouchure There is virtually unanimous agreement among authorities on what the best playing position is, and the description and illustrations given here follow this standard Seated, standing and rest positions are given here, with details of hand and finger positions following in the nex section.

Seated Position

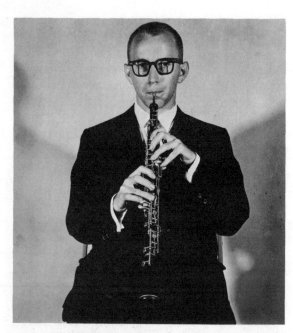

Figure O-13. Front View.

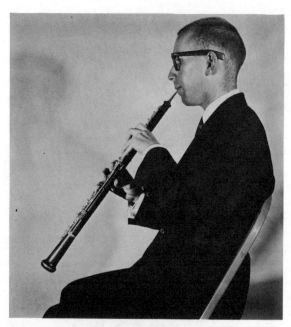

Figure O-14. Side View.

The oboe is held directly in the center of the front of the body. The instrument is at a forty degree angle with the body, with the weight of the instrument on the right thumb and balanced between the right and left thumbs and the mouth. Head erect, chin up, eyes straight ahead, with shoulders up but relaxed. Elbows, hands free from the body. Both feet flat on the floor.

Shoulders and back must not touch the back of the chair when playing. Adjust the height of the music stand so that the music can be easily read in this position. When two students are playing from the same music, angle the chairs slightly toward the center of the stand so that the position of the body and instrument can remain correct.

Standing Position

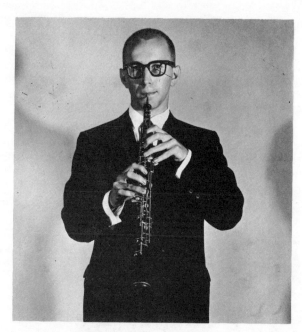

Figure O-15. Front View.

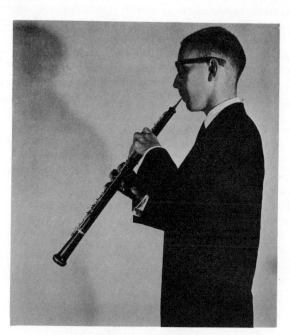

Figure O-16. Side View.

The position of the instrument when the player is standing should be identical with the seated position, only the position of the body itself is changed. Stand erect with feet slightly apart, one foot ahead of the other to help maintain balance. Head remains erect, with chin up and eyes straight ahead. Shoulders up but relaxed, and elbows free from the body. Raise the music stand, if one is being used, so that the head does not tilt downward. Every player should regularly spend a portion of his practice time standing to become at ease playing in a standing position.

Rest Position

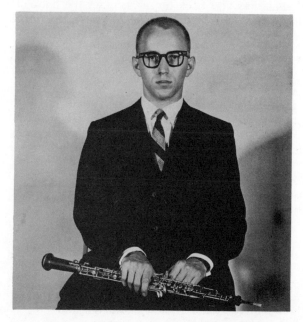

Figure O-17. Standard Rest Position.

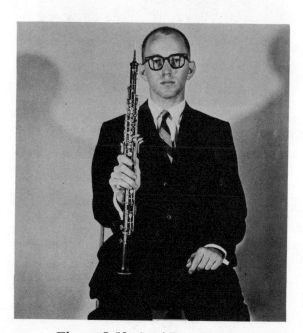

Figure O-18. Semi-Rest Position.

In the standard rest position, the oboe is placed diagonally across the legs with the tone holes up to keep moisture from running into the tone holes. From this position it can be quickly picked up and returned to playing position. Protect the reed from damage while the instrument is moving to and from this rest position, and while it is in the rest position. The semi-rest position is used during short rests in a composition when the player must be ready to resume playing immediately. This position permits some physical relaxation and helps prevent fatigue when performing over a period of time.

HOLDING POSITION FOR THE ENGLISH HORN
Seated Position

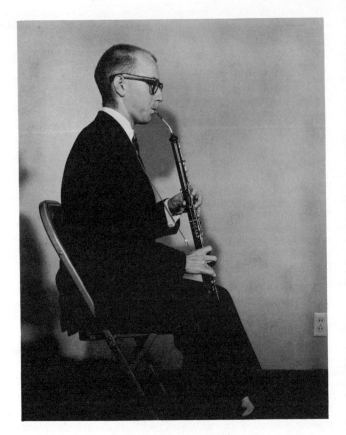

Figure O-20. Side View.

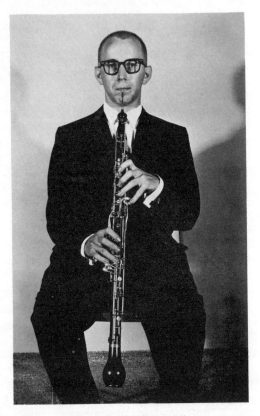

Figure O-19. Front View.

The English horn is held between the legs of the player directly in front of the body. The position of the instrument is adjusted with the bell back or forward from the absolute vertical according to the physical size of the student so that the right hand is in position comfortably, and the reed enters the embouchure at the best angle for the correct embouchure formation. Most students prefer to have the weight of the instrument held by a neckstrap. The right thumb supports none of the weight, but simply controls the position of the instrument, and balances it in the mouth with the aid of the left thumb. Advanced students may dispense with the neckstrap if they desire. Head erect, chin up, eyes straight ahead, with shoulders up but relaxed. Elbows, hands free from the body. Both feet flat on the floor. Sit forward so the instrument does not touch the chair, and shoulders and back do not contact the back of the chair. Adjust the height of the music stand for easy reading.

Standing Position

When the player is standing the position of the instrument itself and its relationship to the body should be identical with the seated position, only the position of the body itself is changed. Stand erect with feet slightly apart, one foot ahead of the other to maintain balance. Head remains erect, with chin up and eyes straight ahead. Shoulders up but relaxed, and elbows free from the body. A certain amount of regular practice time should be spent standing in order to develop ease playing in the standing position.

Rest Position

In the rest position, the neckstrap is unhooked and the instrument laid diagonally across the legs with the tone holes up. From this position the instrument can be quickly picked up and returned to playing position, although players must allow sufficient time for hooking the neckstrap. If the instrument is to be left in this position for any length of time, perhaps the bocal and the reed should be removed from the instrument for protection.

Common Faults in Holding Positions

The way in which the oboe and English horn are held has a great influence on the way in which the student progresses on the instrument. Progress can be facilitated or it can be hindered. For some reason the oboe holding position is subject to greater and more serious deviation from the normal by a greater percentage of students than those on any other instrument. The teacher must check continually, especially during the first few months of study on the instrument, to correct any deviations before they become habits. The players must learn to feel the right position, and a continual check will help them achieve this. Every player should be encouraged to observe his position daily in front of a mirror either at home or at school.

The following are the most commonly found faults in holding positions for the oboe, and to a great extent on the English horn. Since the English horn is normally played by an oboist, any deviations from the standard will be transferred to that instrument.

1. *Head Inclined Downward.* This is the most serious deviation from the normal because of the extreme effect it has on tone quality, and is, unfortunately, found in students at all stages of development. When the head is inclined downward the reed enters the embouchure at a right angle rather than the forty degree angle unless the oboe is brought corespondingly closer to the body. This virtually eliminates effective control of the reed with the lips, puts the angle at which the breath enters the reed directly into the reed, and makes delicate tonguing impossible. The tone quality produced with this position is reedy, nasal, and lacking in body. It is, as well, extremely difficult to play in tune with the head in this position. This habit must never be allowed to start. Correct it immediately and firmly to the forty degree angle. Raise the music stand so that the student will have to hold the head erect, and insist on regular practice in front of a mirror until the position is corrected. Students should see themselves, since they frequently cannot feel this incorrect position.

2. *Instrument Not Centered on Body.* Students will point the bell of the instrument toward one knee or the other rather than straight ahead. This is sometimes caused by not pointing the chair and the body toward the center of the music stand when two students are reading off of the same music. It may be caused by muscular tenseness in the arms, or by an incorrect hand position on the instrument. Whatever the cause it should be located and corrected immediately. An instrument which is not centered puts the reed into the embouchure at a slight angle, making the lip support on the reed on a diagonal rather than a right angle on the blades. While the consequences of this may not be especially noticeable in the middle range of the instrument it produces a coarse tone quality on the lowest notes, and in the high register the tones will be thin. Any problem in intonation will be magnified.

3. *Bell Resting on Leg.* This, fortunately, is not too common, and is caused by the student's desire to take the weight of the instrument off the right thumb, or because he must turn his head to read the music on the music stand. Most students, if the bell rests on a leg, will have to adjust their head up or down from the normal position in order to have the reed in the mouth. This causes changes in the way in which the embouchure controls the reed, with the resultant problems this situation leads to. If allowed to continue, this position becomes habitual and extremely difficult to correct. Locating the music stand and chair properly helps, and the use of a mirror helps the student establish the right feeling for position.

4. *Fingers Assisting Thumbs in Holding the Instrument.* During the earliest experience with the oboe, the student may feel insecure in holding the instrument and in gaining confidence in the balance between the thumbs and embouchure. This is especially true of students transferred from the clarinet to the oboe since the oboe is smaller and lighter in weight, and the finger spread is wider. Fingers will be found under the instrument, against the instrument, or moving back and forth from their proper guide position to the incorrect positions on the body of the oboe. Correct through insistence on maintaining the guide positions for the fingers both through feeling the keys and through use of the mirror. Fingers which remain habitually out of position cause roughness in technique, and even make certain passages impossible to play.

5. *Slouched Body.* Many different degrees of poor posture are found—spine curved against the back of the chair, shoulders curved forward, feet crossed or hung over a rung on the chair, etc. Poor posture affects breathing and breath control to the point that students may find it impossible to support the tone properly, and will become physically tired rather quickly while playing. It pulls the arms out of position making technique rough. Poor posture in any degree must be corrected immediately and firmly. Use of a mirror is helpful.

6. *Moving the Body While Playing.* Beating time with the bell of the instrument, swaying back and forth in time with the music, grandiose flourishes with the instrument at the end of difficult passages, etc., are extremely distracting to the conductor of a group and to the other players, and frequently humorous to an audience. All movements change the position of the reed in the mouth to a degree, interferes with the coordination of the muscles controlling breath support and in general makes for a less effective performance. The habit of bodily movement during the performance is very difficult to correct once it becomes ingrained, since the player frequently doesn't realize he is doing it. Any

such movements must be called to the attention of the player for immediate correction.

7. *English Horn Neck Strap.* While some advanced players prefer not to use a neckstrap on the English horn, it is well to insist that younger students use one. It must be adjusted so that the reed falls naturally into the embouchure. A rule of the thumb is to adjust the strap so that the reed is in the center of the lower lip when the head is erect and the lips together. From this point the player will make slight adjustments up or down in order to accommodate his particular embouchure formation. The strap must be adjusted so that the right thumb is not holding the weight of the instrument, but controlling the angle at which the instrument is held. An adjustment which is too high or too low forces the player to raise or lower his head into an unnatural position with consequent alterations of embouchure formations. The strap adjustment should enable the player to form and use exactly the same embouchure formation on the English horn that he uses on the oboe.

HAND POSITIONS

Since the oboe is usually played by a student with previous training on another woodwind instrument—usually clarinet—hand position may not be as much of a problem if the hand position on the previous instrument was good. Hand positions on all woodwind instruments are quite similar, i.e., the position in which the fingers fall naturally into place on the instrument, and in which there is no muscular tension in fingers, wrists, arms or shoulders. This naturally relaxed position allows facility to develop rapidly.

The following step-by-step procedure for establishing the hand position on the oboe should be studied thoroughly, preferably with an instrument so that a feel for the position can be developed. Study both the text and the photographs carefully until they are perfectly clear. The "Guide Position" which is given is the fundamental position for hands and fingers and should be maintained at all times except when the fingering for a note involves moving a finger to another location. The guide position puts all fingers into the best position for developing speed and accuracy. If the proportions of finger lengths to hand size is on the large side, the student may have to raise his hand position to enable his fingers to cover holes and contact keys at the proper spots.

A. Right Hand Position

1. Figure O-21. The right thumb contacts the thumb rest on the flesh to the side of and at the base of the nail. The ball of the thumb is against the body of the instrument.

2. Figure O-22. The right little finger touches lightly the C key, and the remaining fingers fall naturally into position no more than an inch directly above the three tone holes. The tips of the fingers overlap the plates

slightly so that the ball of the finger directly beneath the finger nail is in the center of the plate. This is especially important if the tone hole for the sixth finger is open, or if an open key model instrument is being used.

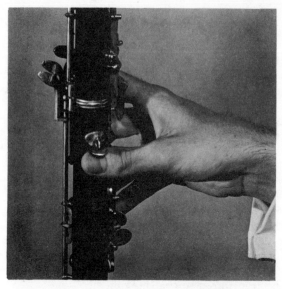

Figure O-21.

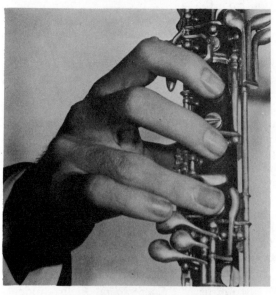

Figure O-22.

3. Figure O-23. The fingers fall into a natural curve without tension to permit maximum control and accuracy of movement.

B. Left Hand Position

1. Figure O-24. The left thumb assists in balancing the instrument and controlling the first octave key. It is placed at almost an angle across the instrument so that the fleshy part of the ball is against the wood of the instrument, and the side just touching, but not pressing

the octave key. The octave key is controlled by vertical movements of the first joint of the thumb. The ball of the thumb never loses contact with the wood of the instrument.

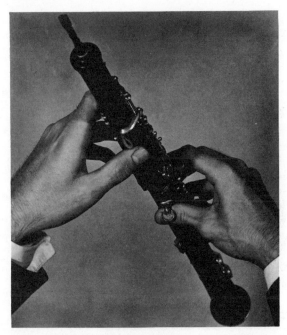

Figure O-23.

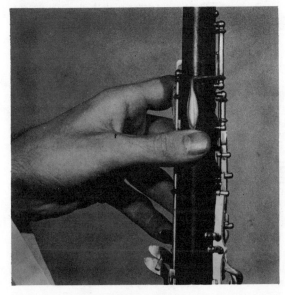

Figure O-24.

2. Figure O-25. The left little finger touches lightly the B key, and the remaining fingers fall naturally into position not more than an inch directly above the three tone holes. The tips of the fingers overlap the plates slightly so that the ball of the finger beneath the finger nail is in the center of the tone hole to close the vent holes in the plates. The fingers are in a natural curve as shown for the right hand in Figure O-23.

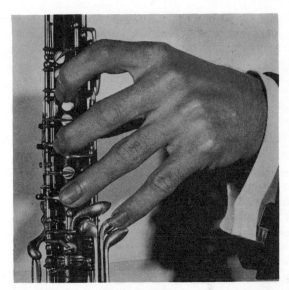

Figure O-25.

C. Guide Position

Figure O-26. With the thumbs and little fingers in place as described above and the remaining fingers over the tone holes, a guide position is established which should be maintained constantly. Note that the fingers are approaching the instrument from a slight upper angle, and that the wrists are flat. The entire finger moves from the knuckle and closes the tone holes with a snap or click, pressing just hard enough to close the holes. Avoid too much pressure against the plates with the fingers.

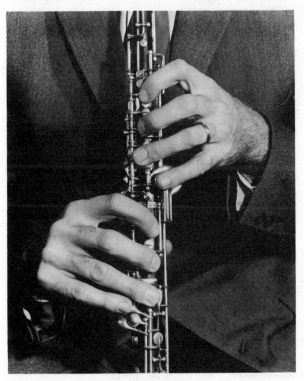

Figure O-26.

The oboe has certain fingerings which tend to pull the hands out of position unless the fingers are moved efficiently and with minimum motion. If the correct guide position is established and maintained, these finger movements will come naturally and can be readily developed. A constant check on the use and position of the fingers in these situations is necessary until the movements become habitual.

1. *Half-Hole Position for the First Finger.* The half-hole position for the first finger functions as an octave key for the first three notes in the second octave;

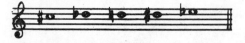

The normal position for the finger is over the plate with the vent hole covered by the ball of the finger. For the half-hole position the finger is rolled downward—not slid—with a movement of the second joint of the finger so that the vent hole is open and the finger is on the extension plate of this key. Figure O-27 shows the first finger in the half-hole position. Notice that the remainder of the fingers are kept in the guide position.

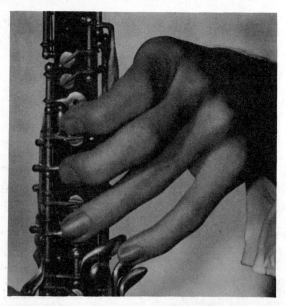

Figure O-27. First finger in half-hole position.

The following example illustrates a typical use of the half-hole:

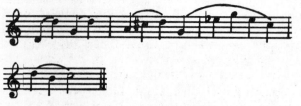

2. *The First Octave Key.* This key (Octave key A on the fingering chart) is operated by the left thumb and is used for E-natural to A-flat inclusive in the second octave:

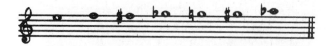

This key is opened by a vertical movement of the first joint of the thumb, with the corner of the thumb pressing the key. The thumb must not slide or roll. While this thumb is normally at a slight oblique angle with the body of the instrument, a player with short fingers will require a position more nearly straight across the body of the instrument. The position of the remainder of the fingers must be established first, and the thumb placed as close to the recommended angle as possible. No matter what angle is determined, it must be such that the octave key can be operated by the vertical movements of the first joint. The following musical example illustrates a typical use of this octave key.

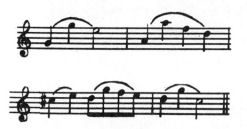

3. *The Second Octave Key.* The second octave key (octave key B on the fingering chart) is operated by the first finger of the left hand and is used for the notes A through C in the second octave:[1]

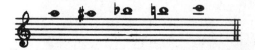

For the notes on which it is brought into use the first finger also covers the tone hole. The second octave key is operated by rolling the second joint of the finger upward, contacting the key between the first and second joints.

Figure O-28 shows the first finger in the normal position and Figure O-29 the first finger pressing the second octave key. Note carefully the point at which the finger contacts the key and that the remainder of the fingers maintain the guide position. The exact point of contact between the first finger and the second octave key varies slightly according to the length of the player's fingers.

---

[1]On some English horns the A-flat must also be played with the second octave key.

Some instruments with a fully automatic octave key do not have this side octave key, while others will have the key there in the event the player wishes to use it even though the mechanism is fully automatic. On instruments with the semi-automatic octave key it is not necessary to remove the thumb from the first octave key when using the second octave key as this key is automatically closed when the second octave key is opened. This is the reason for the designation of semi-automatic for this model. Instruments without this automatic arrangement require that the thumb release the first octave key when the second octave key is used to avoid having both keys open simultaneously.

The following example makes use of both the first and second octave keys:

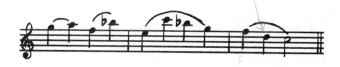

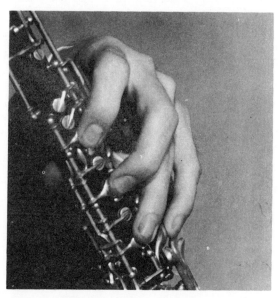

Figure O-28. First finger in normal position.

Common Faults in Hand and Finger Position

A good hand position is a great asset to the study of the oboe. It will develop facility and control, while a poor hand position handicaps this development. The first experiences with the instrument must emphasize hand position, and it must be continually checked until the best position for that particular player is established. A beginning player who persists in quickly establishing the proper positions makes rapid progress. The use of a mirror of sufficient size so that the student can see the entire length of the instrument is actually mandatory in establishing position.

The common faults which are listed here are those which occur most frequently and are those which the instructor should look for. All of these faults have an adverse effect on facility and technique and a combination of several will be a severe handicap to progress.

1. *Right Thumb.* The position of the right thumb against the thumb rest determines to a great extent the placement of the fingers over the tone holes. If the thumb is pushed too far under the instrument so that the thumb contacts the thumb rest away from the nail, the fingers are forced into an unnatural curve and cover the tone holes with the tips of the fingers rather than with the natural pad of the finger. This puts muscular tension on the fingers making them less flexible, and if an open hole instrument is being used the fingers will not properly close the tone holes. When this condition is corrected with advanced students an immediate improvement in right hand facility can be observed.

A second common fault in right thumb position is that of contacting the thumb rest with the nail itself so that the side of the finger rather than the ball is against the body of the instrument. This puts the weight of the

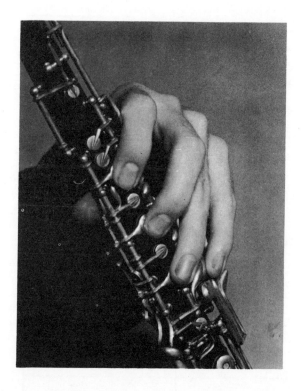

Figure O-29. First finger operating second octave key.

Check List for Holding and Hand Positions

The following list of items provides a means of quickly checking holding positions and hand positions in the seated position for the oboe. The check should be performed while the student is playing and preferably when he is not aware that the check is being made. Any items which are checked "no" should be corrected with the deviation explained to the student, what effect it has on his playing, and why the correct position is important. Students make a more serious effort to correct mistakes if they thoroughly understand the reason for them.

	Yes	No	Comments

A. Holding Position

	Yes	No	Comments
1. Oboe in center of body?			
2. At forty degree angle with body?			
3. Head erect with chin up?			
4. Shoulders up but relaxed?			
5. Elbows free from body?			
6. Body posture good?			
7. Feet well placed?			
8. Height of music stand correct?			
9. Uses proper rest position?			
10. Excessive body movements?			

B. Hand Positions

	Yes	No	Comments
1. Right thumb correctly placed?			
2. Left thumb correctly placed?			
3. Fingers in proper curve?			
4. Right little finger on guide key?			
5. Left little finger on guide key?			
6. Fingers covering holes with their natural pad?			
7. "U" shape between thumbs and forefingers?			
8. First octave key operated correctly?			
9. Second octave key operated correctly?			
10. First finger moving properly to half-hole position?			
11. Basic guide position maintained?			
12. Wrists flat?			
13. Muscular tension?			
14. Fingers no more than one inch above tone holes?			

instrument on the thumb in such a way that it is difficult to support, and the student tires quickly. Correct by insisting that the ball of the thumb be against the wood of the instrument, and a "U" shape formed by the thumb and first finger.

2. *Left Thumb.* Two common faults in the use of the left thumb are removing it from contact with the instrument when it is not in use, or when the second octave key is being used, and in sliding the thumb to open the octave key rather than using the vertical movement of the first joint. A less common problem with the left thumb is found when the student places it parallel with the body of the instrument rather than at the right angle.

Removing the thumb from the instrument removes the support which holds the instrument into place in the mouth, and frequently puts additional pressure against the lower lip with the reed which has the same unfortunate result as biting the reed with the lower teeth. It also destroys the balance of the fingers of the left hand, leaving them free in the air rather than pivoting against the support of the thumb. In inexperienced students this causes the fingers to fall out of position on the tone holes and the notes do not respond. Correct this condition as soon as it is discovered, since most players will not be aware that they are doing it.

Sliding the thumb to open the first octave key produces sluggish, erratic, and undependable operation. In inexperienced players sliding the thumb will pull the fingers out of position over the tone holes, or even pull the third finger off of its plate. Practicing the study suggested for the use of this key, and similar studies while being aware of the movement of the thumb will help correct this condition. Students transferred from clarinet to oboe do not have this trouble as a rule if their use of the left thumb was correct on the clarinet.

Placing the thumb parallel with the wood of the instrument pulls the hand so far out of position that the development of any appreciable amount of facility is extremely difficult. This position is sometimes encouraged by the improper use of the first finger of the left hand in the operation of the second octave key. Correcting the way in which this octave key is opened, developing the relationship between the thumb and first finger to approximately a "U" shape, and insisting on the correct guide position for the hand will correct the condition, although slowly and with effort if it has been long established.

3. *Little Fingers.* In the suggested guide position the little fingers are touching a key from which it is easy to move rapidly to another key when needed. If the little fingers are not in the guide position, then assurance in this movement is lost. Deviation of the little fingers from the guide position frequently puts the remainder of the fingers out of position as well. Beginners on the instrument will frequently take the instrument from the mouth and look at the keys to see which one they should use if the guide position is not maintained.

Some students take the little fingers off of the instrument and put them under the keys on the side, or even under the body of the instrument itself. All of these deviations cause problems in technical development, and the best remedial measure is to insist that the guide position be maintained. The use of a mirror, with slow practice will help establish the correct position.

EMBOUCHURE FORMATION

An embouchure may be defined as the formation of the performer's lips with supporting muscles, teeth and jaws in relation to the reed which have to do with tone production. The criteria for a good oboe embouchure may be summarized as follows: A good embouchure is one which over the entire range of the instrument produces a rich, full bodied, clear tone; plays perfectly in tune; allows the full scope of articulations; allows the full range of dynamics; plays and is controlled with a minimum amount of physical exertion when used in connection with a good reed. Conversely a poor embouchure is one which violates one of these criteria: produces a thin, reedy nasal tone quality; plays certain notes out of tune; does not allow the full scope of articulation in all ranges; has a restricted dynamic range; or requires an undue amount of physical exertion. Embouchure is inseparable from the reed and is entirely dependent on having a good, responsive reed. The best embouchure formation cannot play a poor reed, nor will an excellent reed respond properly with a poorly formed embouchure.

There are among authorities on the instrument, two basic types of embouchure formation recommended, although the differences between the two are not as great as those found between the two types of clarinet embouchure. Each of the formations is subject to infinite variation in small ways according to the teacher, and depend primarily upon the type of reed being used and the exact concept of tone quality desired. The basic difference between the two points of view is found in whether the cheek muscles and the corners of the mouth are pushed in toward the reed, or whether the cheek muscles are pulled back into a slight "smile" position while at the same time the corners of the mouth are pushed in around the reed. For convenience and clarity the first is called a "Soft Cushion" and the second a "Hard Cushion," although these terms are relative and not to be taken literally.

The Soft Cushion Embouchure

The soft cushion embouchure seems to be the most widely used formation in many sections of the country, being taught by the teachers in many of the leading universities and schools of music and by many of the fine professionals. The basic formation of the soft cushion embouchure may be achieved through the following step-by-step procedure. Check each step with a small mirror on the music stand.

1. Keeping the lips relaxed, drop the lower jaw so that the teeth are about a half inch apart. Place the tip of the reed in the center of the lower lip as in Figure O-30.

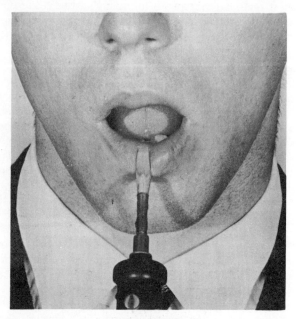

Figure O-30.

2. Roll the lower lip over the teeth until the tip of the reed is just sticking past the lip as in Figure O-31. Keeping the lower jaw down; bring the upper lip barely over the teeth. Only a very little of the lip is over the teeth—just the skin in front of the rope muscle in the lip. No muscle is over the teeth.

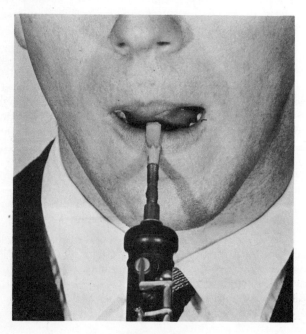

Figure O-31.

3. Bring the lips together, pushing the corners of the mouth slightly toward the reed so that the reed is supported with slight pressure from all directions. The lower jaw must be kept open so that there is no pressure against the reed with the lower teeth. Just enough reed, about an eighth of an inch, protrudes past the lips in the mouth so that it can be touched with the tongue. Figure O-32 is in front view of this embouchure formation and Figure O-33 a side view. Both photographs were taken while the instrument was being played.

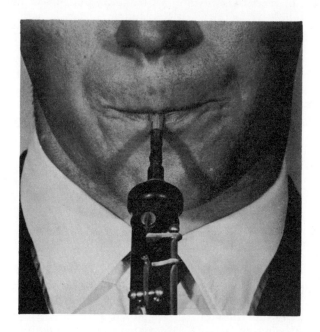

Figure O-32. Front View.

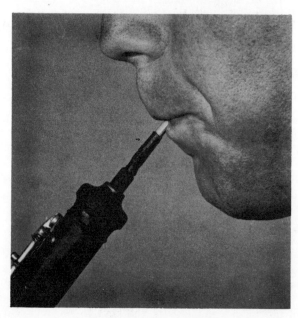

Figure O-33. Side View.

The embouchure used on the English horn is identical with that used on the oboe. Students playing both oboe and English horn must not change their basic embouchure when playing the English horn. Figures O-34 and O-35 are the front and side views of the same player taken while the English horn was being played.

The most common alternative formation for the soft cushion, and one which is perhaps used just as often as that just described is the formation which puts the entire red of both lips over the teeth but which is otherwise identical. Using the entire lip over the teeth provides a larger cushion on which the reed can vibrate, and a greater amount of lip to control the reed. This formation when used with the proper reed produces a tone quality somewhat fuller and darker in color than that when a small amount of lip is used. For this reason it is preferred by many teachers.

The following step-by-step procedure illustrates this formation.

1. Figure O-36. Relax the lower lip and place the tip of the reed slightly past the center of the lip.

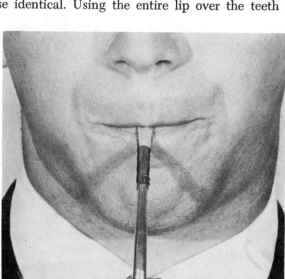

Figure O-34. Front View.

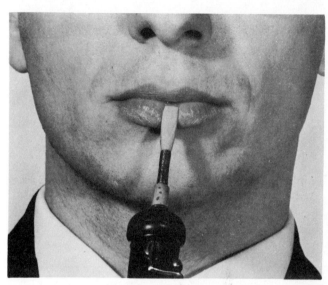

Figure O-36.

2. Figure O-37. Drop the lower jaw and roll the lower lip over the teeth until the edge of the lip is over the front edge of the teeth. Note the amount of reed extending past the lip.

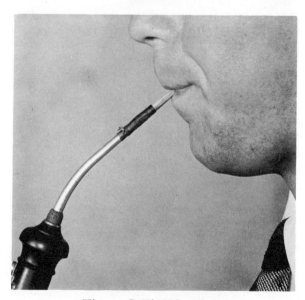

Figure O-35. Side View.

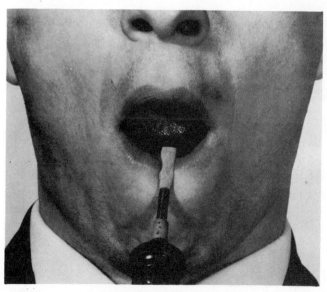

Figure O-37.

3. Figure O-38. Draw the upper lip over the teeth so that no red is showing. Bring the lips together so that no air can escape. The corners of the mouth are pushed slightly toward the reed so that it is supported with slight pressure from all directions. The lower jaw must be kept open so there is no pressure against the reed with the lower teeth.

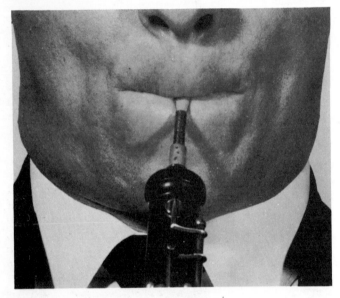

Figure O-38.

The amount of reed varies with the octave which is being played, less reed for the lower octave more for the third octave. Figure O-39 shows this embouchure position playing the low B-flat, and Figure O-40 third octave G (4 lines above staff). Note the difference in the amount of reed in the mouth.

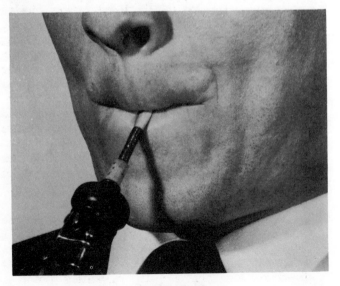

Figure O-39.

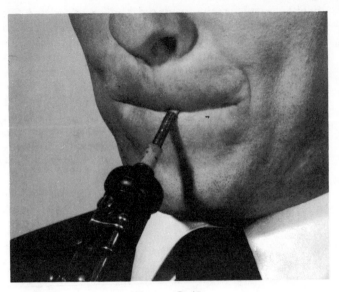

Figure O-40.

The Hard Cushion Embouchure

The hard cushion embouchure for the oboe is less widely recommended than the hard cushion formation for the clarinet, although some fine performers make use of it. The basic formation of the hard cushion embouchure for the oboe may be achieved through the following step-by-step procedure. Check each step with a small mirror on the music stand. Continue to use the mirror constantly until the embouchure is established.

1. Drop the lower jaw until the teeth are about a half-inch apart. Pull back the corners of the mouth so that the lower lip is stretched. Place the reed on the lower lip, pushing it into the mouth so that none of the red of the lower lip is showing.

2. Pull the upper lip over the teeth so that about half the lip is covering the teeth.

3. Close the lips around the reed, maintaining the stretch positions of the lips. The cheek muscles are pulled back slightly into the "smile" position, and dimples are formed in the cheeks of most students. About a quarter-inch of the reed extends past the lips so that the tongue can touch it. The lower jaw must be held open away from the lip. There must be no upward pressure or biting with the teeth against the lower lip. Chin is held flat so that the lower lip will not bunch against the reed, and the lips closed or pushed around the reed so that no air escapes.

Setting the Embouchure

Before producing a tone on the instrument, practice with the reed alone. With a properly moistened reed (this is described under the section on reeds), form the embouchure as described, checking continually in a mirror to see that it is correct. Using a little more reed in the mouth than will be used in playing on the instrument, produce a tone using standard abdominal breath support. Continue blowing until the characteristic "double crow" can be produced and sustained for five to ten seconds, before putting the reed on the instrument and adjusting the amount of reed in the mouth to the proper playing position.

Since many oboists have had previous experience on clarinet the same type of embouchure formation—soft cushion or hard cushion, will come quite naturally. A further advantage of a student with previous experience on the clarinet is that there is considerably less problem with holding the instrument and with fingering thus giving an opportunity to concentrate on embouchure formation and tone production.

A beginning student on the oboe should be given a softer reed at the start than will be used after he has developed. Such a reed will produce a rather reedy tone, but has the advantage of being easier to blow thus permitting the formation of the proper embouchure. As the embouchure develops the strength of the reed can be increased gradually. A mirror should be used constantly to check this formation until the embouchure is formed and developed.

Common Faults in Embouchure Formation

The teacher will have to check frequently to catch any deviations from the standard. Students are not always capable of discovering their own mistakes, or of actually knowing when they are right and when they are wrong, since it is just as easy for them to develop the wrong muscular formation as it is the correct one. The embouchure must be established by how it feels in the mouth and how the tone sounds, as well as how it looks in the mirror. The teacher must tell the student when he is right so he can discover the right feel, hear the right sound, and see the right shape.

Minute variations in embouchure formation are sometimes required to accommodate the physical characteristics of the student. The lower jaw should be adjusted so that the front of the lips are in a vertical line while playing. The lower lip must be neither forward or back of the upper lip. Players with thick lips will cover more of the reed than players with thin lips. The amount of reed in the mouth—just enough for the tongue to touch it—is the criteria for the proper embouchure, not the amount of reed covered by the lips. Players with uneven teeth—especially the lower ones— may need to turn the reed slightly to avoid more pressure against one side than the other, as it is necesasry that the pressure against the flat of the reed by the same across its width and equal on both the upper and lower blades. If this is necessary the amount the reed is turned is extremely slight, and care must be taken that the instrument itself is not turned but kept in position so that the hand position will be absolutely correct.

1. While the presence of dimples in the cheeks when using the soft cushion formation on the clarinet is considered an indication of a poorly formed embouchure, this is not true of the soft cushion embouchure on the oboe. Because the reed is so small, and the teeth considerably closer together on the oboe embouchure, dimples need not be avoided as they will form naturally with some students when the corners of the lips are pressed together and inward to prevent air from escaping. For almost every student using the hard cushion formation dimples are virtually inevitable and should be considered a normal result of the formation. They have no effect directly one way or the other on the type of tone quality being produced.

2. The amount of lip over the upper and lower teeth should be checked carefully until established. If the first soft cushion embouchure is being used only enough of the upper lip is over the teeth to cover them. In the usual formation of this type none of the rope muscle in the upper lip is over the teeth, although a common variation is to put enough of the upper lip over the teeth so that the rope muscle itself is against the inner edge of the upper teeth. Students with thin lips often need this amount of lip in order to provide sufficient cushion for the reed, and the tone quality produced is the only criteria to determine the exact amount of lip to be used. The lower lip normally has more of the red over the teeth in order to get enough surface to control the vibration of the reed in optimum fashion. The step-by-step suggestion of putting the tip of the reed in the center of the lower lip and rolling the lip is the best starting point for determining the exact amount. The player himself will make minor deviations as the embouchure develops in order to produce the best tone quality on the type of reed being used. When using the alternate soft cushion formation check to see none of the red of the lip can be seen.

3. The amount of pressure against the reed with the lower teeth is frequently difficult to adjust. The reed is supported by the lower lip, and biting with the lower teeth must be avoided. The lower teeth control to a degree the amount of support of the lip against the reed increasing the support for the upper and high registers and decreasing for the lower octave, making small adjustments to control intonation, and assisting in the control of dynamics. If the lower teeth are biting, excessive breath pressure is necessary to produce a tone, the tone quality is rough, and the lower notes of the instrument difficult to produce. Evidence of biting can be seen by examining the inner part of the lips for imprints of the teeth. Temporarily using a very soft reed at the expense of tone quality will discourage biting since the reed will close up completely under excess pressure. Asking the player to play flatter will cause him to drop the lower jaw and gives him the feeling of playing flatter although little or no change in pitch will be apparent to the listener.

4. Puffing cheeks is sometimes a problem with oboe players as well as with other woodwind players. This is inevitably an indication of an embouchure problem since it indicates that the muscles involved in the proper embouchure formation are not supporting properly. Players with puffing cheeks virtually always have a

Check List for Oboe Embouchure Formation

The following check on oboe embouchure formation must be made while the student is playing and preferably when he is not aware that a check is being made. Any errors should be carefully explained to the student, and the correction worked out with him while he is observing the embouchure in a mirror. Remedial measures can be assigned on the basis of this list.

A. Soft Cushion Embouchure

	Yes	No	Comments
1. Reed proper distance in mouth?			
2. Corners of lips pushed inward?			
3. Proper amount of upper lip over teeth?			
4. Proper amount of lower lip over teeth?			
5. Are lower teeth biting?			
6. Cheeks puffed?			
7. Air escaping?			
8. Instrument held at correct angle?			

B. Hard Cushion Embouchure

1. Reed proper distance in mouth?			
2. Cheek muscles pulled back?			
3. Corners of mouth closed around reed in correct position?			
4. Proper amount of upper lip over teeth?			
5. Proper amount of lower lip over teeth?			
6. Are lower teeth biting?			
7. Cheeks puffed?			
8. Air escaping?			
9. Instrument held at correct angle?			

very open tone quality which is more often than not reedy, because the breath is not properly focused and directed into the reed. Frequently the players do not realize that the cheeks are puffed, especially if the amount of air between the teeth and cheek is small, and the use of a mirror is necessary. When the student can actually see that the cheeks are in the right position, and the embouchure formation itself is correct, he can then feel the muscular support that is necessary to keep the cheeks in position. Playing a note on the instrument with one hand while feeling the cheeks with the other is useful in helping the player feel the right position.

5. The angle at which the instrument is held has a great effect on the embouchure formation. Any deviation from the recommended forty degree angle of the instrument with the body will be magnified in the embouchure. If the angle of the instrument is too wide, either because the head is dropped down or the instrument held too far out, much of the support of the lower lip is removed from the reed and the tone quality is open, rough, and difficult to control. Students with this problem automatically compensate by biting with the lower lip which brings on additional problems. Checking the angle with the use of a full length mirror until the student feels the right position is an excellent method of correction. If the angle is too great because the head is dropped, the same method may be used, or the music stand raised higher so that he will have to raise his head in order to see the music. If the angle of the instrument with the body is smaller than forty degrees additional pressure is put against the reed with the lower lip, making the tone difficult to control, the lower notes difficult to produce, and results in a general sharpness in pitch in the higher notes. Players who habitually use this smaller angle usually make their reeds in such a way as to compensate for it in order to produce a pleasing tone quality. Unless adjustment is made in the reed the tone is small in body and frequently nasal. This problem of the angle at which the instrument is held with the body is extremely difficult to correct once it has become habitual, and· for this reason it is essential that the proper holding position be established at the beginning of oboe study.

6. Air escaping from one corner of the mouth while playing is clear indication that something is wrong with the embouchure formation. With the soft cushion embouchure this means that the lips are not being pushed around the reed, but that the corner where the air is escaping is released. With the hard cushion embouchure escaping air is the result of too much pulling back of the corner of the mouth, and is corrected by tightening the corner of the mouth and pushing slightly toward the reed.

Comparison of Soft and Hard Cushion Embouchure

It must be repeated that the words soft and hard are merely relative and not to be taken literally. The soft cushion uses a thick firm support and the hard cushion a thin and slightly harder base upon which the reed rests. Each of these formations is subject to infinite variation, all of which are slight, depending upon the training and experience of the teacher using them, and upon the physical characteristics of the student. No two teachers will agree exactly on how to describe the correct formation, nor will two students respond exactly to the same type of instruction in their formation. A variety of explanations making use of various kinds of imagery is necessary to put across the idea of exactly what is desired. The production of pleasing musical sounds is the goal of every teacher and student, and the final judgment of whether an embouchure is good or poor cannot be made on how it is described or explained but on the results obtained.

The decision on whether to use the soft cushion or the hard cushion formation is in the end, dependent upon the ultimate type of tone quality desired. Some teachers prefer a tone which is dark in color and full-bodied without a reedy edge, others prefer a clear smooth tone with a slight edge on it. Both are equally pleasing when fully developed and used musically. Generally speaking the soft cushion formation produces the dark full-bodied tone with little or no edge; while the hard cushion produces a clear smooth tone of less body with a slight edge. The soft cushion formation is the more flexible since the firmness of the cushion can be altered with very slight movements of the muscles which control the lower lip, while the stretched muscles used with the hard cushion are more difficult to alter without losing control of the tone. The more flexibility in an embouchure the more shadings of tone are possible, the better the control of intonation and dynamics. Many embouchures take a middle ground between the two formations described.

Any opportunity which arises to make direct comparisons of the two formations should be taken advantage of in order to hear the differences. Comparisons between the tone qualities of professional level performers are difficult, since it is virtually impossible to isolate the one element of performance—tone quality—from all the other elements such as phrasing, articulation, and general technique. Teachers who do not have a strong personal preference for the hard cushion formation are urged to make use of the soft cushion embouchure since experience of many teachers has indicated that this embouchure is capable of more rapid development and achieves a more musical sound more quickly when used by school players of all ages than does the hard cushion.

TUNING

The problems of correct tuning for the oboe and English horn are discussed extensively in the chapter on reeds since it is the reed rather than the instrument which is tuned. Unlike the clarinets which are tuned by adjusting the various joints, the pitch of the oboe is subject to only the slightest alteration by using this device.

Refer to the chapter on reeds for information on tuning the reed.

In the orchestra the oboe has traditionally been the instrument to which all other instruments are tuned, and this practice has been carried over to some extent into the band field. The reason for this is the fact that professional oboists have always made their own reeds, and as a part of this process tune the reed and the instrument to a standard A-440 tuning fork. Thus the orchestra was reasonably sure of a standard pitch for tuning. In the hands of a professional oboist the pitch can be expected to be accurate. Most advanced student oboists who make their own reeds, or who have developed the process of adjusting a reed to a fine point will also supply a reliable reference pitch provided the instrument and reed have been properly warmed up and prepared for playing. However, less experienced oboists cannot be relied upon to provide an accurate A-440 pitch for tuning, and most conductors prefer to use an electronic tuner which sounds a constant pitch or which operated on the stroboscopic principle providing a visual check of intonation.

As the oboe is a non-transposing instrument, music written for it sounds as written. The usual tuning notes of A for orchestra and either B-flat or A for band are used.

Oboe Plays Concert Pitch   Oboe Plays   Concert Pitch

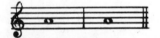   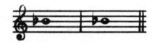

The English horn is a transposing instrument sounding a perfect fifth lower than the written note, tuning to a written E which sounds A-440, or for bands which use B-flat as the pitch reference, plays F sounding B-flat. Most players prefer to check tuning by comparing both the upper and lower octaves of the tuning note.

English horn   English horn
  plays   Concert Pitch   plays   Concert Pitch

The pitch of the English horn, as that of the oboe, is primarily dependent on the reed itself which must be adjusted and tuned to a particular instrument and embouchure formation. The pitch of the instrument may be slightly flattened by pulling the bocal a very little from its socket in the instrument, but this must be done with caution as both tone quality and intonation are susceptible to change by this procedure. Many instruments are supplied with two bocals as are the bassoons, and larger pitch adjustments can be made by choosing

the proper bocal. These bocals are of slightly different lengths, the shorter one raising the overall pitch of the instrument somewhat over the pitch produced by the longer one. Some experimentation with the two will soon indicate which of these a particular student should normally use.

INTONATION

The nature of the typical oboe tone quality seems to make the listener more acutely aware of slight deviations in intonation on this instrument than any of the other woodwinds. This is especially true of student oboists when tone quality has not progressed to the smooth quality of the professional, but tends toward a slight reediness. For this reason intonation on this instrument frequently becomes a major problem, although the oboe is no more difficult to play in tune than any other woodwind.

Natural Tendencies of the Instrument. Acoustically the first two octaves of the instrument, in which most of the playing is done, are produced by the fundamental frequency of the vibrating pipe and the first overtone. The example below gives those tones produced by the fundamental vibration and those which are the product of the first overtone (or partial vibration) when basic fingerings are used.

Fundamental   First Overtone

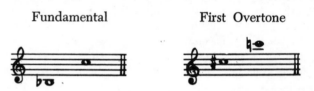

Theoretically the first overtone has exactly twice the number of vibrations as the fundamental, or exactly a perfect octave. Therefore, from the standpoint of pure theory, if the lower octave is in tune the upper octave will also be in tune. Thus the oboist has fewer acoustical problems to overcome in achieving perfect intonation than does the clarinetist.

Unfortunately the achievement of perfect intonation is not this simple. In the manufacturing of instruments certain mechanical problems will cause the instrument to respond slightly off the natural acoustical response. Each manufacturer has his own solutions to the problems of construction, and there is considerable variation from brand to brand in the temperament of the scale. A player who plays well in tune on one instrument will have intonation problems on one of a different brand. The reeds have considerable influence on intonation and one which is well in tune on one brand will not play in tune on another. The oboist must learn to control and adjust to the particular instrument he is playing, and to adjust reeds to fit it.

Each brand, or even each model, of instrument will have certain notes which have a tendency to be flat or sharp to a greater or lesser degree. These notes will be quickly discovered by the experienced player and the necessary adjustments made. Many of these tendencies for being slightly out of tune will be the product of embouchure, reed, or breath support rather than the acoustical properties of the instrument as an isolated factor. Stauffer[2] gives the following tendencies as a result of his experimentation, and they are generally, but not universally, accepted as the norm.

Notes tending to be flat

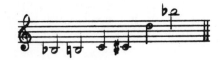

Notes tending to be sharp

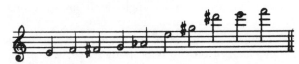

Reed and Intonation. The nature of the reed being used is of primary importance in intonation. The way in which it is cut, the type of cane used, and how well it fits the player's embouchure all have major effects on pitch. Thus the way in which the final adjustments are made on a reed will determine not only whether the instrument is properly tuned to A-440, but how well the instrument will play in tune with itself. Generally speaking a reed which responds well in all registers with a good tone quality will also play well in tune over the instrument. Consult the chapter on reeds for details of reed adjustment.

A reed which is too soft will play flat over the range of the instrument and minor adjustments in intonation will be difficult to make. Notes in the highest register will be quite flat in pitch, and the lowest four or five notes even flatter. Such a reed cannot be controlled by even the best players.

A reed which is too hard will play generally sharp over the range of the instrument. The natural tendencies for sharpness and flatness will be emphasized because the amount of control by the embouchure is limited. This condition can easily be corrected by properly adjusting the reed.

Many beginning students are deliberately started on the instrument with reeds which are too soft and pitch and intonation are intentionally made secondary to tone production and basic technique. These students should not be kept on a soft reed too long, but the strength of the reed they are using gradually increased with each new reed until the proper strength is reached. Most students will make this adjustment easily if it is brought about gradually. As an incentive to make this change there will be a parallel development toward a better

tone quality to which the young player is frequently more sensitive than he is to intonation.

Intonation gradually becomes more and more difficult to control on reeds which have been played on too long, and which are worn out. Student oboists will need to be checked frequently for this condition, as the change in the reed is so gradual that they are frequently not aware that a change has taken place. Insist that a spare reed or two be prepared, broken in and ready to play at all times.

Embouchure and Intonation. The embouchure coupled with the reed is a primary factor in intonation. Even the best of reeds will play out of tune if the embouchure is poorly formed or underdeveloped. An embouchure deficiency can be heard in the tone quality as well as being observed by visual examination. It is for the purpose of good intonation and tone quality that so much emphasis is given to embouchure formation and development. A well formed and developed embouchure is a necessary foundation for good intonation.

The embouchure can correct slight intonation problems through adjusting the pressure with which the reed is held. To make a note higher in pitch contract the embouchure around the reed to increase pressure. To make a note lower in pitch relax the embouchure to reduce pressure. These slight changes in pressure are constant and involuntary in experienced players. Younger players need guidance to develop this facility.

The amount of reed taken into the mouth has considerable effect on pitch and intonation. If too much of the reed is in the mouth in relation to its cut the overall pitch ends to be sharp, especially notes in the second octave. If the half-step between third line B and third space C is too wide it is frequently an indication that there is too much reed in the mouth. Conversely, if too little of the reed is in the mouth in relation to its cut the overall pitch tends to be flat. In both instances the natural tendencies toward sharpness or flatness of certain notes on the instrument will be emphasized.

Dynamics and Intonation. On the oboe, as on most other wind instruments, there is a natural tendency for the pitch to get lower as the tone gets louder, and for the pitch to get sharper as the tone gets softer, with the degree of flatness or sharpness increasing as the level of dynamics approaches the extremes. This must be compensated for by adjusting the embouchure. In order to play louder the student tends to relax the embouchure so that the reed may open up to allow more wind to pass through or to tighten the embouchure as he gets softer to lessen the amount of wind passing through the reed. Since pitch is controlled to a considerable degree by the pressure of the embouchure around the reed there is a corresponding flatting or sharping.

Dynamics are properly controlled by breath support and pressure which controls the velocity of the wind passing through the reed. Students relax their embou-

---

[2]Stauffer, *op. cit.,* p. 111.

chure to play louder rather than increasing breath velocity, and tighten the embouchure rather than decreasing breath velocity. Pitch is maintained through balancing the velocity of the wind through the reed with the pressures of the embouchure around it. When playing fortissimo the slight relaxation of the embouchure is compensated for by an increased velocity of the wind. In a crescendo the wind velocity and embouchure pressure are kept in balance to maintain pitch stability. In playing pianissimo the embouchure pressure may be relaxed slightly if at all, with the pitch maintained through maintaining breath support while decreasing the velocity of the wind through the reed to achieve the proper dynamic level.

Developing the facility for maintaining a constant pitch through long crescendo and diminuendo is one of the ways breath control is developed in students. The tone exercises below are excellent practice in control of pitch through wide dynamic levels. They should be practiced slowly enough that an entire breath is used in each four measures. Maintain constant firm breath support while controlling the dynamics by changing the velocity of the breath through the instrument. Practice exercise "a" in major or minor scale patterns to include the entire range of the instrument in which the student is proficient. Exercise "b" is best practiced chromatically first in the most comfortable range for the student, then extending upward and downward to the extremes of his range. This is also a good exercise for developing the use of the half-hole, and the two octave keys.

Playing Position and Intonation. The angle at which the oboe is held with the body can have considerable influence both on overall pitch and the intonation of individual notes. If the oboe is held at a too great an angle with the body, i.e., greater than forty degrees, the overall pitch is flat with the upper octave even flatter. The same effect results when the head is inclined downward so that the reed enters the mouth on a straight line rather than at the proper angle. The downward position of the head is quite common with beginning players, and must be corrected as soon as it occurs. When

the angle is too great or the head inclined downward good general overall pitch is virtually impossible to obtain, and good intonation completely impossible. Some students attempt to achieve a measure of correction by adjusting a reed to compensate but success with this is rare because complete control of the reed cannot be achieved.

If the instrument is held too close to the body, i.e., at an angle of less than forty degrees, the overall pitch is sharp with the upper octave still sharper in relation to the lower octave. This position also produces a pinched hard sound. The angle of the instrument with the body, whether too great or too small, must be corrected if good intonation is to be achieved. This basic holding position is arrived at very early in the beginning stage of playing the instrument, so it is important that the proper angle be established from the very beginning. Correction of an incorrect angle with an experienced player is a slow and demanding process.

Mechanical Factors and Intonation. The adjustment of the mechanism on the oboe is the most critical of all the woodwind instruments, and keys or plates which do not open wide enough or which open too much will affect the intonation on individual notes. If an individual tone is flat, check to see if the key is opening sufficiently, or if the plate of the first tone hole which is open on that note is raised high enough. If an individual tone is sharp a key or plate may be opening too much. Most brands of oboes have adjusting screws which control the amount of opening on various keys and plates. These adjusting screws should be used to keep the mechanism in the best playing condition. It is well to check all adjusting screws frequently as they move with use and may put the mechanism out of adjustment frequently. If a tone hole or key does not have an adjusting screw, but is open too little or too much, the adjustment should be made by a competent repairman.

Notes in the upper octave which involve the use of the half-hole with the first finger of the left hand may be slightly flat or respond with difficulty if the small vent hole in the plate covered by the first finger

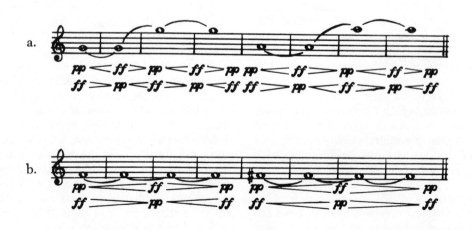

is not clear. Check to see that it is open and clear the hole regularly with a broom straw or a small needle. Avoid increasing the size of this hole through using a needle which is too large since the size of this opening is critical for the best intonation.

The holes covered by the two octave keys are quite small and frequently clogged with foreign matter after a period of use. The keys may be removed from the instrument and the holes cleared with a pipe cleaner.

Summary. An overall sharpness in pitch of the oboe may be caused by one or more of these factors: (1) instrument held to close to the body, (2) too much reed in the mouth, (3) embouchure too tight, (4) a reed which is too sharp for the instrument on which it is being used, (5) a reed which is too stiff. An overall flatness in pitch may be caused by one or more of these factors: (1) instrument held at too great an angle with the body, (2) too little reed in the mouth, (3) embouchure too relaxed, (4) a reed which is too flat for the instrument on which it is being used, and (5) a reed which is too soft.

Intonation difficulties on individual notes may be caused by. (1) a poorly adjusted reed, (2) poorly formed embouchure, (3) improper balance between tightness of the embouchure and breath support, (4) keys or plates too open or too close, (5) a clogged vent hole.

Good intonation is the result of the player's ability to hear intonation accurately and to control it through small variations in breath support and velocity coordinated with increases and decreases in the firmness of the pressure of the embouchure around the reed.

Alternate Fingerings and Intonation. The oboe, as well as other woodwind instruments, has more than one fingering for many notes. Some of these fingerings produce slightly different pitches (as well as tone quality) for the same note, although some produce an identical pitch. The player should be aware that there are alternate fingerings and be able to use them, and should check the pitch relationship between the fingerings for the same note. It is frequently necessary to choose an alternate fingering for the sake of perfect intonation, rather than the fingering which offers the best facility. The player must never hesitate to put intonation before facility. Attention should be paid to the special trill fingerings which are for trilling only, and which must not be used where the note is sufficiently exposed to give an impression of definite pitch. Many trill fingerings are more than a little out of tune but must be used for the sake of facility.

Consult the fingering chart for alternate fingerings and compare their pitches. As the differences between fingerings will vary from instrument to instrument and from player to player, no positive statement as to which alternates are sharp or flat is possible.

TONE

The most valuable asset of any performer is a beautiful tone, and it is to this end that the student must direct his constant attention. The quality of the tone must be the same over the entire range of the instrument and at all dynamic levels. The better the balance of quality over the instrument the better the musical results and the more pleasing the performance to the listener.

The range of the oboe is divided into three registers, designated as the first, second and third octaves (or low, middle, and high register).

First octave   Second octave   Third octave

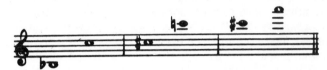

Notes in the lower octave are produced by the fundamental vibration of the air column, those in the upper octave by the column of air vibrating in two segments (the first partial). Notes in the high register are produced by the column of air vibrating in three, four, or five segments—the third, fourth, and fifth partials of the overtone series.

Beginners on the instrument tend to have a discernible different tone quality in each of the three registers. It is true that the quality of tone will be slightly different even in the hands of a professional, but the closer they match the more pleasing the results.

There is no single standard for determining what is a good tone on the oboe or English horn, in fact there are probably greater differences in what is considered the most desirable tone quality on these instruments than any other of the woodwind instruments. The various qualities are described as French, German or American and all three have a place in the United States because so many fine musicians came from France and Germany in the early year of this century to take principal positions in our major symphony orchestras. These men taught the instrument in the way they had learned and the information and style has been passed on from generation to generation of players.

To describe a tone quality accurately in words is impossible and the differences between the French and German sounds on the instrument can be easily heard on the high fidelity recordings made by musicians in these countries. In general the French sound is considered to be a light pure tone with a slight tendency toward reediness to our ears and capable of great variation, while the German sound is dark and heavy, with less potential variation. The American tone quality is a combination of the two combining the dark full sound of the German tone with the flexibility of the French. These various qualities are a product of the type of reed and the embouchure formation being used. There are innumerable variations of both reed and embouchure, most of which are capable of producing what is considered a good oboe tone. No matter what the differences may be if the oboe still sounds like an oboe and if the tone is pleasing it is a good one.

Every teacher and oboist should take advantage of every opportunity to hear live performances of fine instrumentalists. Or if this is not possible, to study the recorded performances of the oboe repertoire on a high quality phonograph. Compare the tone qualities of the various artists. A comparison of the performances of French, German, English and American artists will be quite revealing. All will be quite different, all will be pleasing.

A good tone is the product of all the elements involved in performance: instrument, reed, embouchure and breath support. If any of these is defective then the tone quality suffers accordingly. Problems of tone production and quality are many and varied, but may usually be traced to their source, and must be corrected immediately. Refer also to the sections on reed, embouchure, and breathing.

Following are some of the most prevalent problems or faults in tone:

1. *Small or Pinched Tone.* This is a common fault with beginning oboists, and may be traced to several possible causes. A frequent reason is that the opening in the tip of the reed is too small, a result of the original shaping of the cane or by weakening the sides of the reed during the adjustment process. Consult the section on oboe reeds for possible corrections. If the opening in the tip of the reed is correct, then it is possible that the student is biting the reed through upward pressure with the lower teeth. This can be remedied by asking the student to play flatter by dropping his lower teeth but continuing the lip support around the reed. Unless he also relaxes the breath support, dropping the teeth will not flatten the pitch, but simply free the tone. This fault may also be caused by not having sufficient reed in the mouth, by not having enough lip over the teeth, for the reed cut and embouchure formation being used, or by putting too much pressure on the reed by holding the instrument too close to the body. All of these are physically visible and can be corrected. Instructing the student to check himself in a mirror so that he can actually see what he is doing is advisable.

2. *Squawky Tone.* The squawky tone which can be described as lacking in body and focus, and generally uncontrolled is typical of the beginner although it is sometimes found as well among more advanced students. In the beginner it is caused by a weak, uncontrolled embouchure, but if the basic formation of the embouchure is correct the undesirable tone will gradually disappear. In the more advanced student this tone quality may be caused by a reed which is too stiff for his embouchure causing him to use a large amount of breath to produce a tone. This cause is confirmed if the student is unable to produce a diminuendo into the pianissimo level. Making the proper adjustments on the reed will correct the situation. A squawky tone may also be caused by having too much reed in the mouth, or by having too much lip over the teeth for the type of cut made on the reed.

3. *Hard, Cold Tone.* A tone which is inflexible and which lacks the intangible quality of vitality is described as hard and cold. If embouchure formation is correct this is almost invariably caused by the type of reed being used, usually too stiff for the student. If the usual adjustments on the reed to make it free blowing and responsive in all registers do not remedy the situation, try reeds which are made with a different cut. If the student is making his own reeds have him test with different cuts, or if the reeds he is using are commercial or custom-made reeds try reeds from one or more different makers until a satisfactory tone is achieved. This is a difficult solution for many players since different cuts may require major adjustments in embouchure formation and playing habits. If the student is quite advanced and is playing well in tune with good tone quality except for the coldness of tone introducing the use of a tasteful vibrato would be a solution worth trying. However, the use of the vibrato could be restricted to advanced players.

4. *Weak, Colorless Tone.* A tone which is otherwise smooth in quality, but is lacking in body and carrying power is most often due to lack of proper breathing and breath support. Check the fundamentals of good breath usage with the student, and assign long tone practice with diminuendo and crescendo. The student will need to be told when he is producing the proper sound so that he can associate his physical feeling with the desired sound. It is difficult for many even advanced players to know by listening to themselves when they are producing the proper tone quality and projection.

5. *Control of Soft Tone.* Difficulty in producing and controlling a soft tone is principally due to the inability of the player to project a steady concentrated small stream of air into the instrument. Check breathing and breath support, and have the student practice focusing a steady stream of air into the palm of his hand. Other possible causes may be a reed which is too stiff, or a poorly shaped embouchure.

6. *Dynamics and Tone Quality.* Some students with otherwise good tone quality will lose it when playing at extremes of loudness or softness. This is caused by an undeveloped or poorly formed embouchure, or by lack of proper breath control or a combination of both. In making a crescendo the embouchure must gradually relax to allow the tip of the reed to open while at the same time increasing the velocity of the air. Good control is the product of the proper balance of these two factors, and if they are in the proper balance both tone quality and intonation will remain good. To play a diminuendo the embouchure may tighten slightly around the reed, while decreasing the velocity of air through the instrument, but being very careful to maintain a strong abdominal support of the air stream. With the proper abdominal support, air velocity, and embouchure control tone quality will remain the same at any dynamic level.

TONGUING

Tonguing refers to the manner in which the tongue operates in relation to the reed and breath support in order to articulate the tones. The placement and action of the tongue must be rapid and under complete control at all speeds, and at all dynamic levels. It must, in coordination with breath support, be able to produce on the oboe all varieties of articulation from the hardest staccato to the softest legato.

The manner in which the tongue touches the reed, the place it touches, and how it moves is dependent somewhat upon embouchure formation. There are several points of view on how and where the tongue touches the reed, and each is effective if properly done. In essence the tongue acts as a valve to control the flow of air through the reed, stopping the flow and vibration when it touches the reed, and allowing the vibration to begin again when it is removed. The effectiveness of the tongue is entirely dependent upon proper breath control and support. The interrelation between breath pressure and tongue action allows the production of every conceivable kind of attack from the hardest marcato-staccato to the very smoothest legato within the widest dynamic range. The amount of pressure of the tongue against the reed determines the hardness of the attack, the amount of wind pressure aganist the tongue determines the loudness of the attack.

There are three standard methods of tongue placement used on the oboe, each subject to variations according to the personal desires of the teachers using them. They have several things in common however: (1) the tongue is relaxed. A tongue under tension cannot move rapidly enough, nor can it be controlled; (2) tongue movement is confined to the forward part of the tongue; (3) the tongue acts as a valve for the air and is dependent on good breath support. The three methods may be outlined as follows:

First Method. With the reed in place and the embouchure properly formed, touch the lower blade of the reed at the tip with the top of the tongue just back of the tip. A slight pressure against the reed closes the tip. To start the tone put the tongue in place against the reed and build up air pressure against it. Release the air into the instrument with a tongue action similar to that in pronouncing the syllable "too." The center of the tongue is depressed slightly so that the throat is well open. For a harder attack pronounce the syllable "Tee," and for a softer attack the syllable "Du."

Figures O-41A and O-41B show the front and side view of the tongue in this position.

Second Method. With the reed in place and the embouchure properly formed feel the oval shape of the tip of the reed with the front of the tip of the tongue. This is the placement of the tongue for this style of articulation. The tongue acts physically as a valve to open and close the opening in the tip of the reed. The exact point of contact of the tip of the tongue with the

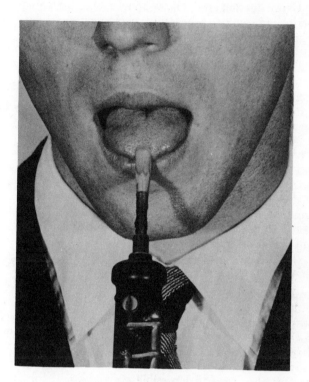

Figure O-41A. Front View.

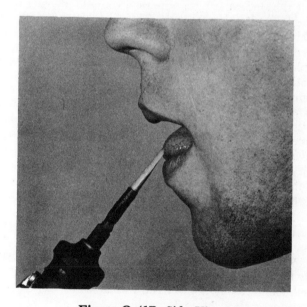

Figure O-41B. Side View.

reed varies from authority to authority and ranges from having the tongue close the tip of the reed by approaching it directly as described, to touching the lower blade as in the previous method but with the very tip of the tongue. To start the tone, put the tongue in place against the tip of the reed, build up air pressure against the tongue and release the air with a tongue action similar to that in pronouncing the syllable "Tu." For a softer attack use the syllable "Du" and for a harder attack the syllable "Tee."

Figure O-42 shows the front view of the tongue in this position.

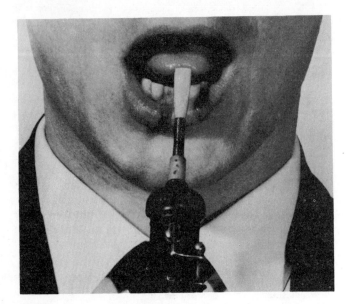

Figure O-42.

Third Method. With the reed in place and the embouchure properly formed, touch the lower lip with the tip of the tongue. Keeping the tip of the tongue in place against the lip the forward part of the tongue moves up to touch the lower blade of the reed. To start the tone, build up air pressure against the tongue and release the air into the instrument with a tongue action similar to that in pronouncing the syllable "Dah." For repeated articulations the tip of the tongue remains in contact with the lower lip with the tongue pivoting against it. Harder attacks are produced by the syllable "Tah" and softer ones by the syllable "Du."

Developing Tongue Action

For the purpose of developing articulation the position of the tongue against the reed is considered the normal position, for it is from this position that it starts the tone. There is no forward or upward movement of the tongue preceding the beginning of the tone since breath support is against the tongue which is in place against the reed. The commonly used word "attack" to describe the articulation of a tone is most unfortunate since it implies both violence and forward movement. The action of the tongue may be gentle or hard depending on the type of articulation desired.

Various types of articulations demand varying lengths of silence between successive notes. The length of this silence is determined by how long the tongue remains in contact with the reed. Hardness of attack is determined by the breath pressure behind the tongue and by how hard the tongue is pressing against the reed. By varying these two factors the entire gamut of bow strokes used by string players can be reproduced on the oboe.

The introduction of tonguing or articulation should be delayed until the student is producing a steady tone of reasonable quality, and has developed facility within the limited range of the begininner. Do not allow the tongue to touch the reed during this preliminary study, but simply start the tone with the breath. This requires that the beginning study be done with music of legato style, and eliminates the rhythmic approach to the beginning study in favor of the melodic approach. The articulation of quarter and eighth notes in the typical beginning method patterns must be done with the tongue and not the breath. Do not allow articulation with the breath alone for once this habit is established it is extremely difficult to break.

Once the tongue is in the correct position against the reed and articulation begun attention must be focused on breath support so that there is a steady stream through the reed upon which the tones rest. The tongue simply interrupts this movement of air through the instrument to detach the notes. A legato style of articulation most successful in the beginning. (See Illustration a.)

After the student is producing the legato articulation reasonably well, he can move to the normal detached sound in which the notes are well separated. There must be a continuing emphasis on a steady stream of air through the reed. The notes are separated simply by leaving the tongue in contact with the reed longer while breath pressure remains constant. This is the most common articulation, used when there is no other articulation indicated, and varied according to the musical demands of the composition. Example b below illustrates a typical exercise for developing this type of articulation.

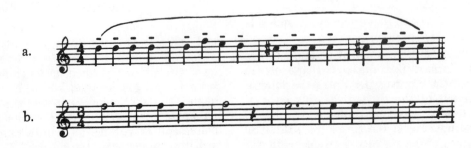

Staccato articulation should not be introduced until both the legato and normal detached articulations are well under control. The same tongue movement and placement and the same steady stream of air is used in staccato articulation. The only difference is that in staccato articulation the tongue returns to the reed to stop the vibration, but the air pressure against the tongue must remain the same during the period of silence as during the production of the tone. Because of the longer period of silence between notes in this type of articulation students are frequently tempted to relax breath support during the silence. If this is done, then the breathing muscles come into operation simultaneously with tongue action, resulting in an accent, and making it virtually impossible to develop a fast staccato. If fairly rapid repetitions of notes are used to introduce the staccato, the concept of an uninterrupted flow of breath is developed and many of the problems involving movement of breathing muscles can be avoided. The following is a typical beginning staccato exercise.

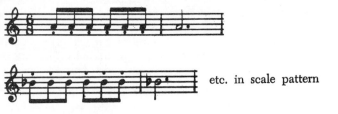

etc. in scale pattern

Common Problems in Tonguing:

1. *Articulation too Heavy.* In this type of sound each note starts with an accent or pop, and is normally caused by too great pressure of the tongue against the reed. The best solution is to have the student practice articulation in the pianissimo level, correcting first the legato type, then the normal detached, and finally the staccato. A reed which is too soft will frequently produce this sound, since the blades do not respond instantly when released by the tongue. If pianissimo practice does not correct this difficulty it is possible that the placement of the tongue against the reed is incorrect for the embouchure and type of reed being used. Vary the tongue placement or experiment with one of the other tongue placements previously described.

2. *Sluggish Tongue.* Inability to tongue rapidly should not be a major concern with beginners, since time and practice is necessary to develop speedy articulation, but in more advanced players where technique has developed past articulation ability, it is a matter of considerable concern. In this condition the reed should be checked first, since a reed which is too stiff for the player makes rapid articulation difficult. If the reed is too stiff there will probably be other symptoms in addition to sluggish articulation.

Some students lack speed in articulation because they are moving the back of their tongue as well as the front. Articulation is confined to the forward portion of the tongue, and the primary motion of the tongue is up and down rather than forward and backward in the mouth. Movement of the back portion of the tongue almost invariably carries with it movements of the throat which can easily be seen. To correct, the entire process of tongue placement and development of articulation must be gone through from the very beginning to form new muscular habits. Some students correct the problem quickly, others are never able to completely overcome the problem.

Sluggish tonguing in many instances is a simple matter of insufficient practice devoted to developing speed and accuracy. Special articulation exercises should be assigned to these students, with specific instructions on how many times each day to practice them, and to use a metronome, and with specific metronomic speeds to use. Any player can develop satisfactory speed and control if he is using his tongue and breath support properly, and if he will spend enough time on the problem. Scales, thirds, and arpeggios as found in most method books practiced with a variety of articulation patterns are the quickest and most efficient way of developing rapid articulation.

3. *Lack of Coordination Between Tongue and Fingers.* This is frequent among the more advanced students who have developed a fair amount of facility on the instrument. It is purely and simply the result of practicing too fast without first working out notes and tonguing carefully. These students must practice slowly, at whatever tempo perfect coordination between fingers and tongue is possible, and gradually increase the speed. Use of a metronome on such exercises is invaluable to maintain a steady tempo and to help in the gradual increase in speed. Major and minor scales and arpeggios making use of various articulation patterns are good media of practice for this purpose.

4. *Slow Staccato.* Some players have difficulty in executing a true staccato rapidly. Other things being correct, this problem can be traced to the lack of breath support and a continuing stream of air through the reed. Such players will be found to be relaxing abdominal support at the end of each note, or cutting off the stream of air in the throat. The concept of the tongue stopping staccato notes as well as starting them with the breath pressure continuing against the tongue during the space of silence will help correct this situation.

5. *Movement of the Jaw in Tonguing.* This is the result of too large or too violent movements of the tongue, frequently accompanied by changes in pitch of the tone. Rather than confining the movement to the front part of the tongue, the student is moving the entire tongue. The solution is to ask the student, no matter what his technical advancement, to practice the basic exercises for developing articulation constantly checking in a mirror on the music stand to eliminate all movement. Jaw movements can occur with all methods of correct tongue placement, as well as with incorrect tongue placement, and present the development of speed in articulation.

Double and Triple Tonguing. Theoretically, double and triple tonguing in the sense of its use on flute and brass instruments is possible on the oboe, but in practice it is very unsatisfactory because it is virtually impossible to match the sounds of the beginnings of the two notes in the double pattern or the three notes in the triple pattern. The double tonguing is done by using the letters "T" and "K" in rapid alternation, the "T" with the tongue in its normal position on the reed and the "K" pronounced with the middle of the tongue against the roof of the mouth which interrupts the flow of air. Triple tonguing uses the letters "T-K-T" or "T-T-K" in rapid succession. Both double and triple tonguing are called for only in the most rapid passages. Most oboists prefer to develop the speed and control of the single tonguing to a degree that it can be used exclusively for both normal and the most rapid articulations. Most authorities agree that students need not be taught double or triple tonguing.

Flutter Tonguing. Flutter tonguing, produced by rolling an "R" so that the tongue flutters against the reed is called for in a few contemporary compositions. Some relaxation of the embouchure with perhaps a little less reed in the mouth will help achieve the best effect.

Accents, Sforzando, Forte-piano. Accents, sforzando, and forte-piano notes must be played in relation to the dynamic level of the musical phrase. A sfzorando is not a note played as loudly as it is possible to play, but simply an isolated note one or two degrees louder than the note which precedes or follows it in the phrase. It demands assistance from the breath so that the breathing mechanism must supply additional support and velocity simultaneously with the release of the reed by the tongue.

The forte-piano requires immediate relaxation of velocity and pressure by the breathing mechanism, coupled with whatever degree of simultaneous support demanded by the musical content of the phrase at the instant the tone starts. Accents indicated above or below the notes must be only one dynamic level above the notes which precede or follow them. Many accents may be accomplished by only increased tongue pressure against the reed, others demand slight movements of the breathing muscles. It must be clearly understood that there are no rapid movements of any breathing muscles in support of tongue action except for accents, sforzando, and forte-piano notes.

TECHNIQUE PROBLEMS

A good technical proficiency on the instrument is one which is accurate, under complete control, and facile. In developing this proficiency the oboist must be aware of certain mechanical or technical problems peculiar to the instrument which must be approached logically. Both the importance of the correct solution and the reasons for a particular solution must be impressed on the student. Unfortunately the literature for the study of the oboe with the possible exception of the Alphonse Leduc edition of the Barret Method does not provide a particularly well organized presentation of these problems, so it is incumbent upon the teacher to make an opportunity to include them in the instruction of the players.

Approached logically, these problems are neither complex to solve, nor complex to use. Many of these technical problems on the instrument demand that the player make a choice between two or more alternatives. Each alternate must be practiced until it becomes an involuntary part of his technique and the use of each alternative made so much a part of his technique that the correct choice becomes involuntary and instantaneous. Players and teachers should not hesitate to mark instructions on the printed music as reminders.

1. *Use of Left and Right Little Fingers.* One or both of the little fingers are involved in the fingering for these notes in the first two octaves:

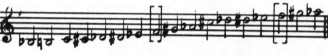

Of these notes only D-sharp—E-flat 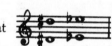 can be played by both the left and right little fingers. (The G-sharp—A-flat has an alternate key operated by the first finger of the right hand which is discussed later.) The problem in playing a passage which has two consecutive little finger notes is to avoid sliding one of the fingers from one key to another if at all possible. Making use of both the left and right D-sharp—E-flat keys and planning ahead to alternate the little fingers will help to avoid excessive sliding. Students should begin using both the left and right D-sharp—E-flat keys very early in their beginning study so that correct use of the little fingers is firmly established as one of the basis for technical advancement.

However, some combinations of notes make it mandatory to slide a finger from one key to another. The proper sliding is done by increasing the curvature of the finger and pressing down so that it slides off the top of one key onto the next one. If the finger does not slide easily an old professional trick is to rub the finger beside the nose where the skin is oily and the finger picks up enough of this oil to slide easily. Rubbing the finger in the hair works equally well. The following example is typical of passages in which sliding the little fingers is mandatory.

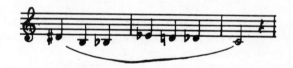

2. *Use of the Two G-Sharp Keys.* There are two fingerings for G-sharp—A-flat: 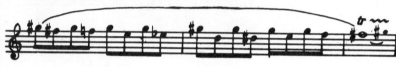 123 G-sharp 000 and 123 4x00, opening the G-sharp key with either the left little finger or with the first finger of the right hand. The normal fingering calls for the use of the left little finger, while the key operated by the first finger of the right hand is primarily a trill key.

3. *Articulated G-Sharp Key.* All standard system oboes have an articulated G-sharp incorporated into the mechanism. This mechanism automatically closes the G-sharp key when the fourth finger is down even though the little finger remains on the key. Use of this key smooths certain technical passages by allowing the little finger to remain stationary on the G-sharp key eliminating the possibility of poor coordination between this finger and others. The example below indicates a typical use of this key. The little finger remains down on the G-sharp key throughout.

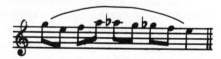

4. *Two Fingerings for F.*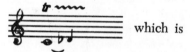

Every oboist from the early beginning stage of development should be familiar with and make constant use of both of the fingerings for F: 123 456x and 123 406(D-sharp). The second of these is called the "fork F." The use of the D-sharp key with either the right or little finger is not necessary if the instrument being used has an F resonance key, but is necessary for those instruments which do not. The fork F fingering is used when the sixth finger is used to cover the sixth hole on the note which precedes or follows the F to avoid sliding this finger from the 6x key to the hole. The first fingering is the normal diatonic or chromatic fingering for F. On most oboes both fingerings produce identical tone qualities and are equally well in tune. It is necessary that both fingerings and directions for their use be introduced very early into the study of the instrument. The following illustrates typical uses of these fingerings.

Diatonic Fingering

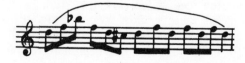

Fork Fingering

5. *Use of Special Plates.* There are two special plates on the standard model oboe which make possible two common trills which without them are impossible. Attention is called to these plates because so few student oboists are aware of their presence on the instrument. Plate 1p on the fingering chart is depressed by extending the first finger to cover it at the same time the finger is closing the tone hole. Its principal use is in the fingering for trilling: 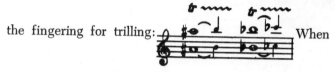 When using this plate the fingering for A-sharp—B-flat is 1 1p20 100 and the fingering for the B-natural—C-flat is 1 1p00 100, with the trill being made by the second finger of the left hand. This plate is also useful in certain trills in the third octave.

Plate 6p on the fingering chart is depressed by extending the sixth finger to depress it at the same time the finger is closing the tone hole. This plate closes the low C key and is a substitute for C key played by the right little finger. When feasible and necessary the plate is used instead of the C key to avoid sliding the right little finger. The most common use of plate 6p is in the trill: which is otherwise impossible to execute. In this trill the fingering for the C is 123 456 6p and the D-flat is obtained by adding the D-flat key with the right little finger to the C fingering. The trill is made by the little finger. Figure 0-43 shows the right hand in position for mking this trill. Note the extension of the sixth finger to close the plate and the little finger on the D-flat key. Note also that the hand position is only slightly changed from the basic guide position.

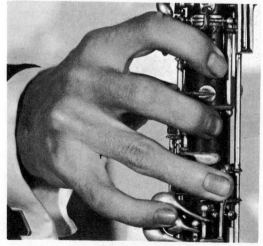

Figure 0-43.

6. *Use of Half-Hole and Two Octave Keys.* Notes in the second octave and the high register are produced by using the half-hole with the first finger, or by one of the two octave keys. Using these correctly on each note as required by the fingering system is most important for the sake of both intonation and tone quality. Insist that students use the correct one from the very beginning of study. These keys are necessary to relieve the pressure in the column of air at a particular place in that column to force it to break into vibrating sections of the right length thus producing the 1st or a higher partial. The notes played with each are indicated below. Notes in the third octave may use any of the three depending on the fingering chosen. Consult the fingering chart for these.

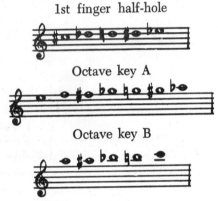

Considerable attention during the process of developing technique on the instrument must be given to developing the proper finger and hand movements used in changing back and forth from one to the other of these. Instruments with a single automatic octave key do not have Octave Key B, the instrument automatically changing vent holes as the notes are fingered. On instruments with the semi-automatic octave key the thumb may be kept in contact with Octave Key A while the first finger opens octave Key B since the mechanism automatically closes Key A when Key B is open. Instruments with no automation require that the thumb be removed from Key A simultaneously with the opening of Key B, and vice versa. The semi-automatic mechanism is the most satisfactory for student use.

7. *Use of Left Little Finger on Two Keys Simultaneously.* For slurring in the lower octave between B-natural and A-flat, or E-flat to A-flat in either the first or second octaves it is frequently advantageous to depress both the keys involved with the left little finger. Distribute the width of the finger between the two keys so that both are fully depressed. The artciulated G-sharp key which is built into the instrument makes this technique possible. Certain fingerings for notes in the high register require two of these keys and depressing them both with the left little finger is advantageous as it frees the little finger of the right hand for other use.

Figure 0-44 shows the placement of the left hand with the little finger in both the G-sharp and D-sharp keys, in the fingering for E-natural in the third octave.

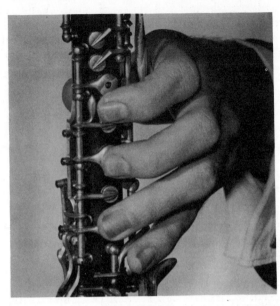

Figure 0-44.

The following excerpt from the slow movement of Dvorak's "New World Symphony" is a notable instance where leaving a finger in place on two keys simplifies the performance immeasurably. The left little finger holds down both the D-sharp and G-sharp keys throughout the entire example, taking advantage of the articulated G-sharp.

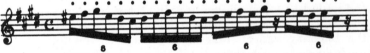

8. *High Register.* Beginners on the oboe should not attempt to play above the top C in the second octave until the embouchure is firmly established and notes in both the first and second octave are played well in tune with good control. Notes in the third octave all have several alternate fingerings. In each instance the first fingering given in the fingering chart is the preferred one. Response of instruments in this register varies and it is well to try the alternate fingerings for each note to see if one of them responds on a particular instrument with better intonation and tone quality than the others. Notes in the third octave require greater embouchure support around the reed than those in the second octave. Avoid biting the reed. Use a firmer breath support. Notes in this register are produced with difficulty if the reed is too soft. It a student has difficulty producing these sounds, try a slightly stiffer reed.

In order for the embouchure to support the reed properly for notes in the third octave more reed is taken into the mouth. The simple process of using more reed in the mouth, even to the point where the upper lip touches the wrapping on the reed, will often make an astounding improvement in students who are having difficulty producing full tones of good quality in the third octave. A comparison of the photographs, Figure O-39 and O-40 will show the extremes in the amount of reed taken into the mouth. Figure O-39 shows the posi-

tion while playing 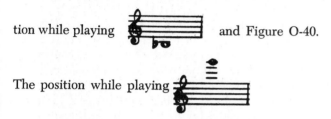 and Figure O-40.

The position while playing

9. *Selection of Alternate Fingerings.* Examination of the oboe fingering chart will reveal that many notes on the instrument have more than one fingering suggested. Some of these have been discussed previously under special headings. Alternate fingerings are provided primarily to facilitate technique, but many on a particular instrument, will also produce a tone of a slightly different pitch, or slightly different tone quality. As the proficiency of the player increases the need for these alternate fingerings increases. Except for the special fingerings for certain notes previously mentioned in this section, there is little need to involve the beginner or intermediate student with numerous alternatives. These alternate fingerings should be given to the student when a special need for that fingering arises in music he is playing. Whenever a particularly difficult or rough fingering problem occurs the student, or teacher, is encouraged to consult the fingering chart to see if an alternate fingering is possible to smooth the sequence or make the fingering easier to master. Alternate fingerings are selected on the basis of facility, intonation, and tone quality according to the demands of the music being played. The wise student and teacher will take full advantage of the many alternatives.

HARMONICS

The use of harmonics for special effects is standard procedure on all string instruments and they are found regularly in musical compositions. The use of harmonics in the same sense on woodwind instruments is rare, but they are used occasionally on the oboe. All the woodwind instruments are capable of producing harmonics on certain notes, but they are never called for on the clarinet and bassoon but appear occasionally in flute and oboe literature.

Harmonics are used on the oboe in piano or pianissimo passages where a light flute-like quality is called for at the discretion of the player. When harmonics are

desired by the composer they are printed with a small circle above them to indicate that they are to be fingered as harmonics in the same way that harmonics are indicated in music for string instruments. Harmonics are produced and controlled with some dififculty, and should be reserved for introduction only to advanced players.

These harmonics are frequently somewhat flatter in pitch than the same notes played normally. If this is the case they may be brought up in pitch by increasing embouchure support around the reed and by increasing breath pressure. Professional players will use harmonics for pianissimo notes which are hard to control with the regular fingering, or which are sharp at this dynamic level.

The example below gives the harmonics used on the oboe and the fingerings used to produce them. Finger the lower notes and overblow a twelfth to produce the harmonics. Oboes with a single automatic octave key cannot play the notes A through C.

Harmonics

Harmonic
Fingering

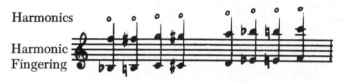

With Octave Key A   With Octave Key B

The following is a melody which can be played entirely in harmonics. If an advanced oboist is available

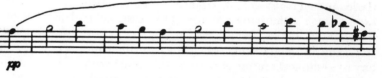

have the example played first with normal full tone and then as harmonics.

TRANSPOSITION FOR THE OBOIST

The oboist is occasionally expected to transpose and play parts written for the English horn on the oboe, and rarely to play oboe parts on the English horn. Advanced players should develop some facility in both transpositions. The ability to transpose and play at sight is acquired only by doing it, slowly at first, and then with increasing speed.

1. *Playing English Horn Parts on the Oboe.* As the English horn is in "F" and the oboe a non-transposing instrument in C, the English horn part is transposed down a perfect fifth when played on the oboe. Since the range of the English horn is lower than that of the oboe, some of the notes in the English horn part cannot be played down a perfect fifth as they actually sound,

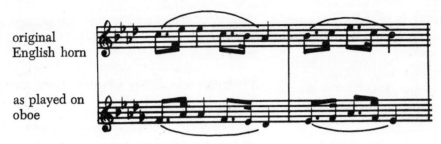

original
English horn

as played on
oboe

but must be played a fourth higher so that they sound an octave above the written notes. To make this transposition add one flat or subtract one sharp from the key signature of the English horn part and transpose down a perfect fifth or up a perfect fourth. The above illustration shows this type of transposition.

2. *Playing Oboe Parts on English Horn.* This transposition involves the reverse of the previous process. To make this transposition add one sharp or subtract one flat from the key signature of the oboe part and transpose up a perfect fifth or down a perfect fourth according to the range of the music being played. The illustration below taken from the Bach "B minor Mass" illustrates the transposition.

SELECTION OF INSTRUMENTS

The system of fingering used on the present day oboes used in the United States developed from principles first applied to the flute by Boehm. This system, called the Conservatory System, was developed by the French firm of Triebert during the mid-nineteenth century, and brought to a high state of development by Loree around 1880. Since that time various improvements have been made on the instrument and its mechanism without, however, changing the basic sytsem.[3] Other systems used in Europe such as the German system, the true Boehm system seem to be gradually losing favor to the Conservatory system, and are never used in this country.

There is perhaps less standardization in mechanism of the oboe than in any other musical instrument, each maker having several models from which to choose, or with extra features which can be added at the option of the buyer. The various options are detailed in the following.

1. *Plateau Keys and Open Tone Holes.* The most fundamental difference in oboe models is found in the option of plateau, or covered tone holes, in contrast to the models with open tone holes as on the clarinet. The plateau system is standard and is used by oboists from beginners to the most polished professional. In it the tone holes are covered by vented plates with pads under them as on the flute rather than directly by the fingers. The open tone hole models require that the tone holes be closed by using the fingers as pads as on the clarinet. Some professionals prefer the open tone holes saying that the tone quality is superior, but these are in the minority. The plateau system is preferable for all school use.

2. *Octave Keys.* The oboe requires two octave keys, and these are available in three different arrangements:

(1) The automatic octave key model in which a single octave key operated by the thumb automatically changes from one vent hole to another according to the fingering being used. This is the arrangement which is standard on the saxophone and on modern alto and bass clarinets. It has the advantage of simplicity for younger students, but the disadvantage of eliminating some excellent fingerings for certain notes in the third octave as well as some of the harmonics. The automatic octave key model is not recommended.

(2) The semi-automatic octave key model incorporates some of the advantages of both the automatic octave key and the double octave key. Two octave keys are provided on the instrument, one operated by the thumb, the other by the first finger of the left hand. The semi-automatic mechanism on this model allows the thumb to be kept on its octave key while the side octave key is being used, the mechanism automatically closing

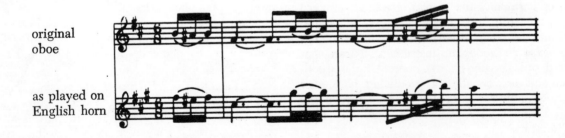

original
oboe

as played on
English horn

---

[3]See Bate, Philip. *The Oboe.* London: Ernest Benn Ltd. 1956 for a fascinating account of the various developments in the construction of the oboe.

the vent hole of the first when the second is opened. This is the preferred arrangement for players on all levels and is the type recommended.

(3) Double octave key instruments have two independent octave keys which must be opened and closed independently by the thumb and first finger of the left hand. This involves complex movements of these fingers and a high degree of coordination which is difficult to develop. This system has no advantages over the semiautomatic arrangement, and is not recommended.

3. *Resonance Keys.* The earlier models of the Conservatory system oboe required the addition of the E-flat key to the fork fingering for F in both the first and second octaves in order to match the resonance of this fingering with the other tones. Many models of oboes now have a resonance key on the side of the instrument which opens automatically when the fork fingering for F is used thus eliminating the necessity of adding the E-flat key with a little finger, and freeing the little finger for use on successive notes. An F resonance key is invaluable and is recommended for use on any level of performance. When examining an oboe the presence of this resonance key can be ascertained by closing the three holes of the right hand, then opening and closing the middle hole while keeping the first and third closed. If there is a key on the side of the body of the instrument which opens and closes simultaneously with the middle hole the instrument has an F resonance key, otherwise there is no F resonance key on the instrument.

The finest oboes of recent manufacture have an additional resonance key on the bell. This key improves the resonance, tone quality and intonation of the low B-flat. If all other considerations are equal when considering the purchase of an instrument the resonance key on the bell is recommended. It is by no means essential, and many manufacturers do not feel that it is essential and do not offer it as an option.

4. *Extra Keys.* Various keys in excess of what has become the standard mechanism are offered on many models. These include a left hand F key operated by the little finger of the left hand; a second G-sharp key operated by the first finger of the right hand which has virtually become standard on the better instruments; a third octave key used only for three notes in the high register; various trill keys, etc. These keys are useful if they are on the instrument, but unless the player is of professional calibre, they are not recommended because of the additional complexity of the mechanism and its accompanying problems.

Recommended Standard Model. The model recommended for use by student musicians on all levels is the Plateau System with the semi-automatic octave key and F resonance key. To this basic complement the better grades of instruments will automatically supply the standard and desirable trill keys, plates, and the extra

G-sharp key. Lower grades of instruments which do not have these extras are satisfactory only for beginning and intermediate students.

STUDENT QUALIFICATIONS AND APTITUDES

The oboe is not a beginning instrument. Before being considered for playing the oboe, a student should have developed something more than basic facility on another woodwind instrument plus the ability to produce a good tone on the instrument, preferably the clarinet. This is the best criteria for advisability of study on the oboe. Most authorities are in agreement that students should not start playing the oboe earlier than the seventh grade because of the stretches required of the fingers and the problems of controlling a small double reed. The benefits of the years of instrumental study prior to the seventh grade, if on another woodwind instrument, can be transferred quickly and easily to the oboe.

A natural aptitude for the oboe may be determined by success in producing a good "crow" on a reed adjusted and prepared for playing by the instructor after some brief instruction on embouchure formation and how to produce the crow. Students who are not immediately successful with some instructive guidance, may soon indicate a good natural aptitude. In the final analysis it is not natural aptitude but desire and persistence which are the greatest of all aptitudes for any instrument.

The English horn should be played only by competent oboists.

CARE OF THE OBOE

Assemble and disassemble with the greatest of care. Review the instructions on assembly of the instrument until they are thoroughly understood and the students are performing the operation easily. Keep the instrument in its case when not in use. Keep the instrument out of direct sunlight and away from all sources of heat. It is mandatory that the instrument be thoroughly dried after each playing, and the habit of doing this thoroughly should be developed from the very first. The process of swabbing does not take much time and will prevent cracks in the wood and help maintain sanitary conditions for playing.

Swabs. Three different types of swabs are available for drying the oboe. Each type has its advantages and disadvantages and its proponents and opponents. The principal problem revolves around the best method of thoroughly drying the very small diameter of the upper joint, and each type of swab gives a solution to this problem as well as for drying the lower joint. The only criteria is that the entire inside of the instrument be thoroughly dried, and the instructor and player are free to choose the type which they feel gets the best results. The three kinds of swabs are:

(1) *Double End Wool Swab.* A stiff wire with a large round wool swab on one end for drying the lower joint and the bell and a small conical shaped wool end for drying the upper joint. The small end of most of these swabs will not go completely through the upper joint but must be inserted and withdrawn from the larger end. This type of swab leaves moisture in the small end of the upper joint which must be cleared by a pipe cleaner, feather, or a special swab for the top joint such as the one made by Artley. The combination of the special top joint swab and the double end wool swab is ideal for younger players.

(2) *Cloth Swabs.* These are small cloths on a drop cord with a weight similar in design to the typical clarinet swab. They usually come in pairs, one for the upper joint and one for the lower joint. Unless the smaller one will pull through the upper joint they are not satisfactory without an additional means of drying the upper part of the top joint as discussed previously. Combined with a top joint swab, however, they are quite satisfactory.

(3) *Turkey Feather.* Using a turkey feather is the traditional way of drying the oboe. These feathers must be long enough to reach through the lower joint. Only feathers with barbs of equal size on either side of the quill should be used. Pheasant tail feathers are equally as useful as the wing tip feathers of the turkey. These feathers may be purchased commercially or prepared by the student. Feathers prepared at home should be washed with lukewarm water and soap to remove the natural oils which prevent the feather from absorbing water. Since the turkey feather is the traditional swab it is used in the illustrations which follow, but wool or cloth swabs may be used with equal success.

The suggested step-by-step process which follows is efficient and should be checked regularly by the instructor until it is easily accomplished by the student.

1. Take the instrument apart in the reverse order of assembly, holding each part exactly as they were held during the process of assembling the instrument. Shake the moisture out of each end of each joint and place the parts carefully in the case before proceeding with drying the inside.

2. Upper joint. Holding the joint in the left hand as shown in Figure O-45, push the feather through from the larger end until the tip extends through the small end. Pull the feather back and forth rotating it at the same time to absorb the moisture. Put the protective cap over the cork and replace joint carefully in case.

3. Lower joint. Hold the lower joint as shown in Figure O-46 (or reverse the left and right hands). Insert the feather from the bottom, rotate and pull back and forth simultaneously. Put the protective cap over the cork and replace joint carefully in the case.

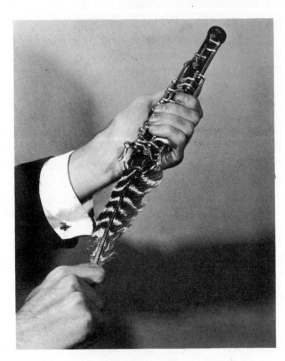

Figure O-45.

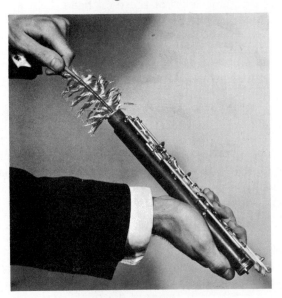

Figure O-46.

4. Hold the bell as shown in Figure O-47. Insert the feather from the bell end, pulling back and forth and rotating simultaneously. Replace bell in case.

5. With a soft cloth or chamois dry the inside of each of the connecting joints.

6. The Reed. Blow the moisture out of the reed and place it carefully in a reed case so that it can dry properly. The inside of the reed should be cleaned once a week or so by drawing a wet pipe cleaner through it carefully (Figure O-48). Insert the pipe cleaner from the

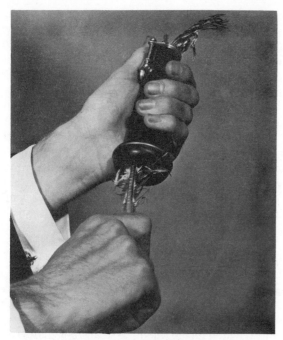

Figure O-47.

cork end pushing then pulling through the tip. Be very careful not to reverse the direction of the cleaner as it will damage the tip of the reed.

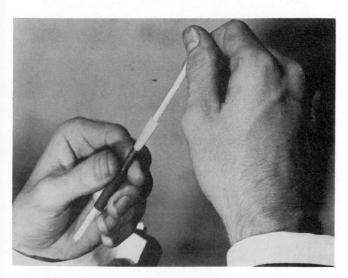

Figure O-48.

Regular Maintenance of the Instrument

1. *Oiling the Bore.* Even though they are made of the hardest wood available—Grenadilla wood—wood instruments are subject to cracking. Careful drying after each playing will help avoid this but authorities recommend that the bore of a wood instrument be oiled with specially prepared bore oil. New instruments should be oiled every two weeks for the first three or four months of use, once a month for the next six months, then four or five times a year. Only the very thinnest coating of oil is desired. The best means of oiling the bore is with a turkey feather kept for this purpose. Let three or four drops of oil run down the bottom of the bore of each joint, then distribute this over the entire inside of the joint by pushing the feather back and forth through the joint rotating it at the same time. Two drops of oil will be sufficient for the bell. Be sure that the upper portion of the top joint is covered well, since this is a critical area for moisture. Be careful that no oil gets into the tone holes or on pads or corks. The outside of the instrument may be oiled very lightly with a few drops of oil distributed by a small, soft cloth, again being very careful that no oil gets onto any pad or cork.

2. *Oiling the Mechanism.* The mechanism, if it is to remain in the best playing condition, must be oiled regularly three or four times a year. Special oil called key oil for this purpose is commercially available. A drop of oil on the end of a needle or toothpick should be put at each pivot screw of each key. Do this carefully so that no oil can get onto the pads. This regular oiling keeps pivot screws from excessive wear and from rusting into place, making repairs and adjustments on the instrument easier.

3. *Adjusting Screws.* These are screws which control the action and clearance of the various keys which act together. These must be perfectly adjusted if the instrument is to respond as it should. Poor adjustment of these makes some notes difficult or impossible to play, and others to play out of tune or with poor quality. There are a number of such screws on the oboe—the better the instrument the more there are. The standard model instrument recommended will have as many as fifteen of these screws including two on the semi-automatic octave keys, one on the articulated G-sharp, two on the F resonance key, etc. Every student past the beginning stage should have a small screwdriver in his case at all times. These screws can be adjusted visually and tested by playing. When a note does not respond, check immediately on the adjusting screws involved in the mechanism for that note. In addition to these adjusting screws, the pivot screws for each key should be tightened regularly to assure the best action of the mechanism.

4. *Dusting the Instrument.* After an instrument has been in use over a period of time, dust collects under the key mechanism. This can and should be removed with a soft water color brush. A cloth should never be used for this purpose as it will snag on the needle springs which will break under pressure.

5. *Shining the Keys.* Keys may be kept in good condition if they are wiped regularly and gently with a soft cloth or chamois to remove perspiration and dirt. This will not only keep the keys from tarnishing, but will prevent corrosion of the plates and keys in the event the player perspires excessively. Silver polish must never be

used on the keys, nor should the keys ever be polished while on the instrument. Using silver polish while the keys are on the instrument will foul pivot screws in the mechanism, and damage pads so that they will leak. Leave polishing up to a competent repairman. Caution students against polishing the keys, but give them careful instructions to keep the instrument clean by wiping the keys.

6. *Bent Keys.* In spite of the best of care, keys sometimes become bent out of line. Bent keys or rods occur with alarming regularity on the instruments of young players, and cause unevenness in technique, or even prevent certain tones from responding at all. No attempt should be made to straighten keys or rods while they are on the instrument. This puts excessive pressure on both the keys and their posts and the instrument may be damaged even more. Keys must be removed from the instrument by a repairman who has the proper tools to stragihten and align them.

7. *Sticking Pads.* If the instrument is not thoroughly dried before it is put into its case, or if the humidity is excessive even temporarily, some pads on the instrument will stick tightly, or will stick momentarily before opening, making technique uneven. Moisture can be removed from sticking pads by placing a cigarette paper between the pad and the tone hole, pressing down on the key firmly. Release the key, move the paper and repeat the process until the key no longer sticks. If this does not relieve the sticking, put the cigarette paper in place, press the key, and pull the paper slowly from under the pad. Repeat the process several times. If the condition reoccurs regularly have the pad replaced. Never use powder on pads to stop sticking.

8. *Water in Tone Holes.* Some instruments tend to collect water in certain tone holes under pads that are normally closed, producing a bubbling sound when these keys are opened. This may be removed by opening the key and blowing into the hole. If time permits take the instrument apart and swab the joint on which this occurs. If a particular hole collects water regularly it may sometimes be corrected by removing the key and coating the inside of the tone hole lightly with vaseline. Avoid a heavy coat of vaseline as it will soak into the pad. Instruments which have the bore oiled regularly tend to collect less water in tone holes than those instruments with a dry bore.

9. *Leaky Pads.* Pads on an instrument wear out with use. Some wear out more rapidly than others and begin to leak, causing the instrument to respond with difficulty on certain notes. To test for leaks take the instrument apart. Plug the lower end of the joint with a cork or with the palm of the hand. Cover the tone holes and close all keys as if playing, avoiding using more pressure against the holes or keys than is used when playing. Blow through the other end with as much pressure as possible. Leaky pads can be identified by leak-

ing air. If a tone hole normally covered by a key and pad held closed by a spring leaks when maximum wind pressure is applied during the test, the spring on that key must be strengthened or replaced by a repairman. A joint in perfect condition will not leak air no matter how much breath pressure is applied.

If the leak cannot be located by the above method, an alternative method which assures positive seating of all pads is to use commercial feeler papers, or strips of cigarette paper about a quarter inch wide. Slide one end of the paper under the pad, put the normal amount of pressure against the pad if the key is not held closed by a spring, and slowly draw the paper out. As long as the pressure against the paper remains constant there is no leak. If the pressure suddenly lessens the pad is not properly seated. Repeat the process completely around the pad so that all edges are tested.

The process of blowing cigarette smoke through the instrument to identify a leak through seeing the cigarette smoke coming out of the leak is not recommended. The nicotine in the smoke coats the pads and if this is done frequently will damage them so that they harden and leak. Repairmen use a small light in the bore of the instrument to find leaks, as the light will shine through the open space of the leak. Teachers responsible for numbers of woodwind instruments might find it advantageous to purchase such a light, as instruments may be tested quickly, accurately, and efficiently with this device.

Pads may leak because they are not seated properly, or because they are worn. A loose membrane on the bottom of the pad indicates that it should be replaced immediately, even though it is not leaking at that time. It soon will be, and if the condition persists it will produce a buzz when that particular key is used to play a note.

10. *Regular Overhaul.* The condition of every instrument must be checked at least once a year by the instructor or by a repairman. Regular maintenance keeps an instrument in good playing condition over a period of years, rather than allowing it to gradually deteriorate becoming increasingly difficult to play. Every instrument must have a complete overhaul every three to five years depending on amount of usage. If fine instruments receive a yearly checkup and regular overhauls they will last in virtually perfect condition for many years. The services of a competent repairman is invaluable and an asset to any program of instrumental instruction.

BIBLIOGRAPHY OF STUDY MATERIALS

The amount of teaching material available for the oboe is not very extensive, although it is adequate if full advantage is taken of what is available. Material on the beginning and lower intermediate levels is particularly limited, with a greater variety of material becoming available as the student's technical facility progresses.

In order that the student will have a well-rounded and interesting course of study which will achieve the most rapid advancement both technically and musically it is recommended that he be studying simultaneously from material in each of these classifications: (1) a method book for continuity and basics, (2) technical studies such as major and minor scales, arpeggios, etc., in various forms and keys; (3) a book of etudes or studies to include various musical styles over a period of time; (4) duets and/or other ensemble experience; and (5) solos with piano acompaniment.

Information about solos, duets and other types of ensembles making use of the oboe is widely available in such places as the Selective Lists of Instrumental Solos and Ensembles published by the National Interscholastic Music Activities Commission and on pages 79-106 of Evelyn Rothwell's "Oboe Technique" published by Oxford University Press. Considerable information about the availability of solos and ensembles as well as other classifications of material for oboe can be obtained from the catalogs of retail stores specializing in woodwind music.[4] A study of these catalogs will reveal far more material than is commonly known, although still not too extensive.

In the sections which follow a cross section of the most widely used material (exclusive of solo and ensemble music) available for oboe is listed. These lists are divided into beginning methods, standard methods, and additional study materials of various kinds. A listing of composers, titles, and publishers such as is given here and in the other sources mentioned is the only starting point for acquiring teaching materials. Only personal acquaintance with the music itself can give the answer to the quality of music, and how and when it could be used. The reader is urged to examine as many of these titles as possible, and to evaluate them whenever possible through actual use.

Beginning Methods

Anzalone, V. *Breeze-Easy Method for Oboe*. Two Volumes. Witmark.

Buck, L. *Elementary Method for Oboe*. Kjos.

Carey, Milburn. *Basic Method for the Oboe*. Carl Fischer.

Gekeler, Kenneth. *Oboe Method*. Three volumes. Belwin, Inc.

Herfurth-Stuart. *A Tune A Day for Oboe*. Boston Music Co.

Hovey, N. W. *Elementary Method for Oboe*. Rubank, Inc.

Skornicka, J. E. and R. Koebner. *Intermediate Method for Oboe*. Rubank, Inc.

Voxman, H. and Wm. Gower. *Advanced Method for Oboe*. Two Volumes. Rubank, Inc.

The methods listed above are the standard type public school beginning methods similar to those written for all woodwind instruments. Younger students who have had little previous experience on another woodwind instrument, or who are having their first woodwind experience on the oboe will need more material than is contained in a single beginning method in order to gain more experience with music of the same technical level. The methods by Carey and Hovey make an excellent combination when used together.

A transfer method. Many fine school oboists are developed by transferring to the oboe a student who has had considerable experience and who has developed good technical facility and musicianship on clarinet or another woodwind. The beginning methods listed above are not suitable for such a student as they progress much too slowly, nor are the Standard Methods suitable for the first few months experience. The following method was designed as a method for the beginner with previous experience and presents technical problems clearly and efficiently and develops facility rapidly. It is highly recommended that it be used when transferring experienced players to the oboe.

Fitch, Wm. D. *The Study of the Oboe*. George Wahr Publishing Co.

Standard Methods

Andraud, Albert. *Practical and Progressive Oboe Method*. Southern Music Co. An extensive collection of exercises, technical studies, and etudes selected from the standard works for oboe. Includes many solos as well. An excellent choice for students who have completed the beginning stage of their development.

Barret, A. *Complete Method for Oboe*. Two editions. Boosey & Hawkes or Alphonse Leduc. Study of this method has become mandatory for all advanced oboists. It contains a wealth of material mostly on an advanced level. The Boosey & Hawkes edition is the original version, while the Leduc edition has been considerably revised and augmented. The material is not progressively arranged.

Langey. *Tutor for Oboe*. Two editions. Carl Fischer or Boosey & Hawkes. An old standard method in the series written by Langey for many instruments. It is primarily in the intermediate level of difficulty.

Niemann. *Method for the Oboe*. Carl Fischer. Another old standard method. The material is mostly on the intermediate level of technical difficulty. Can be used in combination with the Langey to provide more intermediate level material.

---

[4]See appendix IV for a list.

Additional Study Materials

Andraud, Albert. *First Book of Studies for Oboe*. Leduc. *Vade-Mecum of the Oboist*. Southern Music Co. A most important and extensive collection of selected studies from the standard writers for the instrument, and a number of orchestral studies for oboe and English horn.

Bassi. *Twenty-Seven Virtuoso Studies*. Carl Fischer. Transcribed from the original clarinet studies by Iasilli. Fairly difficult.

Bleuzet, Louis. *La Technique du Hautbois* (Oboe Technique). Three volumes. Leduc. English Text. Scales in various forms, chromatic studies, arpeggios, staccato exercises, etc. for advanced student.

Bozza, E. *18 Etudes*. Leduc. Fine studies for advanced student.

Braun, C. A. P. *18 Caprices*. Associated Music Publishers.

Brod. *Etudes et Sonates*. Two volumes. Leduc. Volume one, intermediate, Volume two, more advanced.

Cavallini. *30 Caprices for Oboe*. 2 Volumes. Carl Fischer.

Chopin. *Chopin Studies Transcribed for Oboe*. Gornston Intermediate technical difficulty. Transcribed by Paisner and Gornston

Ferling. *144 Preludes and Studies*. Two volumes. McGinnis & Marx.
18 Studies, Op. 12. Southern Music Co.
The 48 studies are the most famous of all oboe studies, and must be included in the course of study of any student who reaches the upper intermediate level. The opus 12 studies are also in the Vade-Mecum.

Gekeler, K. *Practical Studies for Oboe*. Two volumes. Belwin, Inc.

Labate, Bruno. *Sixteen Daily Exercises for Oboe*. Carl Fischer.

Luft, J. H. *24 Etudes*. Editions Costallat. Early advanced level technically.

Pares, G. *Daily Technical Exercises for Oboe*. Carl Fischer.
Modern Pares Foundation Studies for Oboe. Rubank, Inc. Major and minor scales in various patterns and in keys through four sharps and four flats, these are two editions of the same music.

Salviani. *Studi per Oboe*. Two volumes. Ricordi.

Schiemann. *Seven Characteristic Studies for Oboe*. Edition Musicus.

Singer. *Metodo Teorico-Pratico per Oboe*. Three volumes. Ricordi.

Tustin, Whitney. *Technical Studies*. Peer International Corporation. The most complete book of mechanical technical studies available. Useful on both intermediate and advanced levels. In six sections: scales, intervals, arpeggios, trills, exercises for tonguing, exercises for fingering.

Verroust, S. *24 Melodic Etudes, Op. 65*. Two volumes. Editions Costellat. Excellent intermediate level material. A piano accompaniment to these is also available.

Voxman, H. *Selected Studies for Oboe*. Rubank, Inc. Advanced etudes, scales, and arpeggios in all major and minor keys.

Wiedemann, L. *45 Studies*. Associated Music Publishers.

STUDY AND ACHIEVEMENT QUESTIONS

1. Identify the beginning, intermediate and advanced playing ranges for the oboe.

2. Assemble the instrument, identifying each part, and demonstrating the correct holding position for each operation.

3. Observe beginning, intermediate, and advanced students in the process of assemblying their instruments and fill out the check list for assembly. Describe corrections for any faults.

4. Describe and demonstrate the correct holding position for the oboe including the two rest positions. Demonstrate various common faults in holding positions and describe the effect of each on performance.

5. Demonstrate the correct hand positions for oboe.

6. List the three ways of venting the instrument to produce notes in the second and third octaves, and write on a staff the notes for which each is used.

7. Observe beginning, intermediate, and advanced students and fill out the check list for holding and hand positions. Describe the effect on performance which any faults will have. Prescribe corrections for any faults.

8. Discuss the three basic types of embouchure formation for oboe. Choose one of these and describe and demonstrate the step by step procedure to form it.

9. Observe beginning, intermediate, and advanced students and fill out the check list for embouchure formation. Suggest corrections for any faults.

10. Discuss tuning and intonation for oboe and English horn. What factors will make the instrument flat? What factors will make it sharp? What influence does the mechanism of the instrument have on intonation?

11. Identify the three registers of the instrument with range of each.

12. List the symptoms and corrections for the most commonly found faults in tone quality.

13. Discuss the three methods of tongue placement for articulation and how tongue action is developed.

14. Write on a staff the notes in the first two octaves for which the fingering involves the use of one or both little fingers. Select a passage in which several of these occur and mark the use of the left and right fingers.

15. Identify and describe the use of the two fingerings for F.

16. Write on a staff the harmonics used on the oboe and the fingering for each. Under what circumstances are harmonics used?

17. As considerations for the selection of an instrument for a good high school player discuss the pros and cons of plateau keys vs. open tone holes; whether a single automatic octave key, a semi-automatic octave key, or double octave keys is preferable; and what extra keys should be recommended and why.

18. Discuss the merits of the various kinds of swabs which may be used for drying the oboe.

19. Perform the step by step process of disassembly and cleaning the oboe, having a colleague observe and rate the procedure.

20. Locate the various adjusting screws on an instrument, discover the function of each, and check to see that they are properly set.

21. Discuss the various things involved in the regular maintenance of the oboe.

22. Examine and compare various beginning oboe methods. Select one or two best suited for junior high beginner, one or more suitable for a high school student transferring from clarinet to oboe.

23. Examine available standard methods and additional study materials for oboe and list them with comments. Prepare a suggested list of material to include all five types of material suggested for simultaneous study for an advanced beginner. For an intermediate level student. For an advanced student.

24. Listen to several phonograph records of outstanding oboe soloists. Comment on and compare tone quality, phrasing, articulation and general facility. If the players are other than American describe any nationalistic differences which are discernible.

25. Discuss the use of vibrato on the oboe, and when and how it should be developed.

CHAPTER FOUR

BASSOON

The Bassoon as the bass voice of the double-reed choir has a remarkably large usable range which has been exploited in contemporary music. The contra-bassoon (or double bassoon as it is sometimes called) sounds an octave lower than the bassoon and extends the wood-wind range into that of the string bass, but has not been extensively used. The fingering for the contra-bassoon is identical with that of the bassoon, and it is played, when called for, by a bassoonist just as the English horn is played by an oboist.

The bassoon has defied mechanical development, and the mechanism and technique remain awkward in comparison to the other woodwind instruments. Numerous attempts to adapt the Boehm principles to the bassoon have failed. Today there are two rival fingering systems in use in Europe—the French and German—widely different both mechanically and in tone quality produced. In the United States only the German system, called the Heckel System, is used. The bassoon as we have it today was perfected in the Heckel factory in Germany through several generations since the beginning of the company in 1831. The Heckel mechanical system is made by many manufacturers under their own names. Bassoons made by the Heckel factory are prized possessions of many bassoonists.

The bassoon, written in the bass, tenor, or alto clef is a non-transposing instrument. The beginning, intermediate, and advanced playing ranges are indicated below.

Beginning

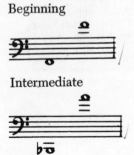

Intermediate

Advanced

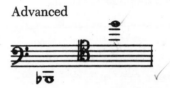

The contra-bassoon, since it is played only by advanced players, makes use of all except the highest portion of the advanced playing range indicated for the bassoon. Some instruments extend the range of the contra-bassoon to the written A one half-step lower than the lowest note on the bassoon. Sounding an octave lower than written, the actual pitch of this note is the same as the lowest note on the piano, making the contra-bassoon capable of producing tones lower than any other instrument of the orchestra or band. The contra-bassoon is written in the bass clef, and sounds an octave lower than written. The example below indicates this transposition.

Written   Sounds

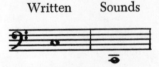

PARTS OF THE BASSOON

Parts of the bassoon are illustrated in Figure B-1. Since much of the literature about the bassoon uses the names, it is well to be able to identify them readily. The parts may be listed as follows:

1. Butt—the end of the bassoon into which are fitted the long joint and the tenor joint.
2. Tenor joint (or Wing joint)—onto which the crook is fitted.
3. Long joint—onto which the bell is fitted.
4. Bell joint.
5. Bocal (or crook) onto which the reed is fitted.

Most bassoons are equipped with two crooks of different lengths.

ASSEMBLING THE INSTRUMENT

Proper assembly and disassembly of the bassoon is of the utmost importance, and must be taught to students from the very first lesson. Probably more damage—bent keys, rods, bent connecting levers, etc.—is done by beginning students to the instrument in putting it together and taking it apart than by all other means combined. Instruments with damaged and out-of-line mechanism do not respond properly, and some of the difficulty that students, especially beginners, have in playing their instruments can be traced to damaged mechanism. The bassoon is, fortunately, somewhat less susceptible to this kind of damage than the oboe or clarinet, so that it is easier to avoid.

The assembly of an instrument must be accomplished wtihout putting pressure on any key or rod which will bend it in any way. An instrument with as many keys as the bassoon is obviously impossible to put together without touching the keys. Before starting the process of assembly, be sure that all cork joints are well greased with prepared cork grease so that undue pressure will not have to be applied to put the parts together. The following step-by-step procedure is given in detail, and every student should practice it carefully until each procedure is correct and automatic. Study the photograph and directions for each step carefully and repeat the operation several times before proceeding to the next.

A. Butt Joint and Long Joint Assembly

1. Figure B-2. With the left hand grasp the long joint with the cluster of keys toward you. The palm of the hand is around the wood, thumb parallel with the long rod. The base of the thumb is near but not touching the rod.

PARTS OF THE BASSOON

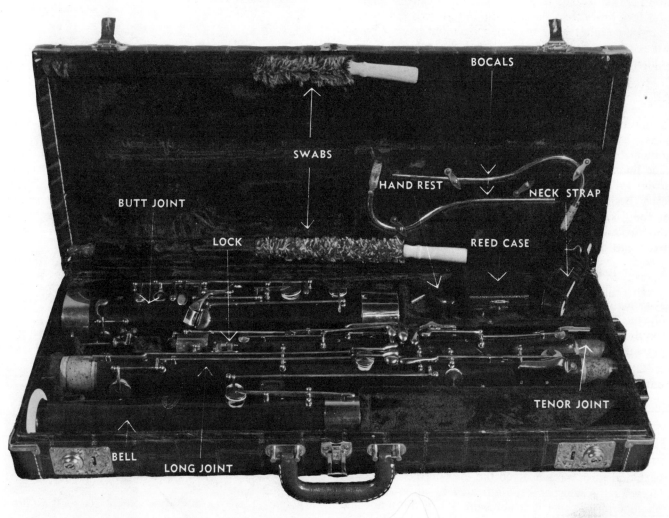

Figure B-1.

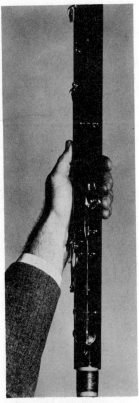

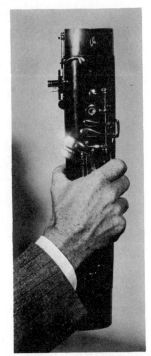

Figure B-2.   Figure B-3.

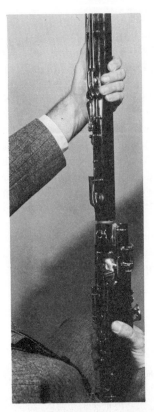

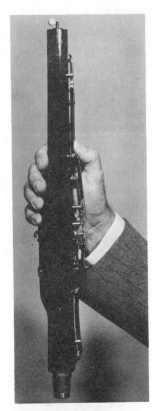

Figure B-4.   Figure B-5.

2. Figure B-3. With the right hand, take the butt joint with the palm over the keys on the tone hole side. The thumb and fingers grasp the wood to hold the joint firmly without pressure of the palm against the keys.

3. Figure B-4. With the end of the butt joint against the leg, and holding the two joints as described, push the two sections together with a slight back and forth twist until the long joint is firmly in place.

B. Butt Joint and Tenor Joint Assembly

1. Figure B-5. Take the tenor joint in the right hand as shown, with the thumb on the pivot screw and pressing the key against the guard. The tips of the fingers are against the wood, and the hand cupped to avoid pressure on the keys.

2. Figure B-6. The left hand holds the assembled butt and long joints against the left leg. Thumb and first finger are on the metal band at the top of the joint, tips of other fingers are on the wood, with second joint of fingers over the holes.

3. Figure B-7. Holding the tenor joint and butt joint as described push the two joints together with a slight back and forth motion. Keep the eyes on the connecting lever for the whisper key (indicated by an arow in the photograph) so that it is not bent. When the tenor and long joints are in place in the butt, check to see that they are properly aligned with each other, and secure the lock which holds them together if the instrument has one.

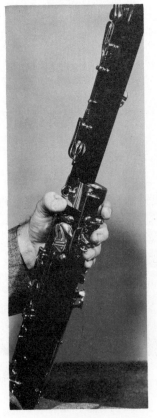

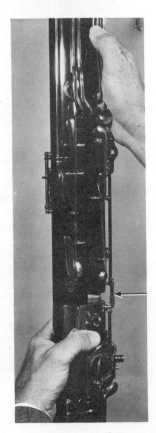

Figure B-6.   Figure B-7.

C. Adding the Bell

1. Figure B-8. The bell is held in the left hand with the fingers on the wood and with the heel of the thumb depressing the single key on the bell to lift the connecting lever.

2. Figure B-9. Rest the heel of the bassoon on the floor and steady the instrument with the right hand. With the left hand holding the bell as indicated push it on and line up the two portions of the connecting lever.

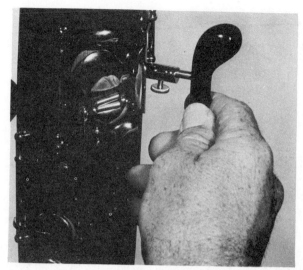

Figure B-10.

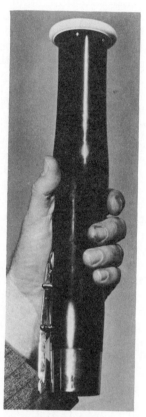 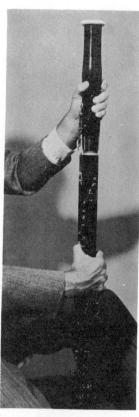

Figure B-8.   Figure B-9.

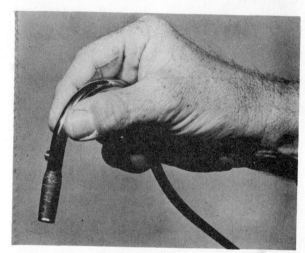

Figure B-11.

D. Completing the Assembly

1. Figure B-10. Insert the thumb rest and line it up vertically with the bassoon, the larger part toward the bell. Adjust the height so the right thumb and fingers will fall into the correct holding position, and tighten the screw.

2. Figure B-11. Hold the bocal with the thumb and forefinger near the vent hold. The remainder of the fingers cup around the part, but control and pressure for adding this piece are in the thumb and forefinger.

3. Figure B-12. With the heel of the bassoon on the floor, push in the bocal with the thumb and forefinger, and line up the vent hole with the pad of the whisper key.

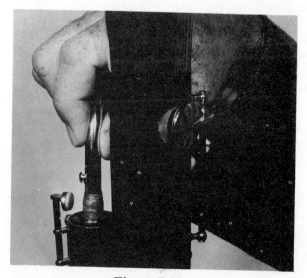

Figure B-12.

4. Figure B-13. Hook the neck strap in the ring and adjust it to the proper length for playing. With the weight on the neck strap and the instrument in playing position balance the instrument with the right hand and add the reed with the left.

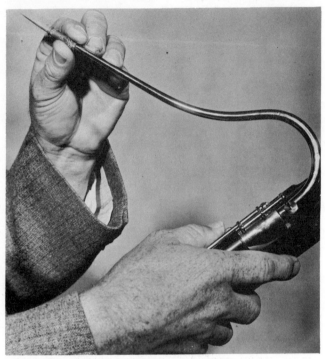

Figure B-13.

Common Faults in Assembly

There are, of course, several possible ways in which the bassoon may be assembled, and various teachers have different methods and procedures. The only criteria for a good procedure is that no pressure is put on rods, plates or keys during the process. The procedure outlined above is a common standard one and may be safely used for beginners. As familiarity with the instrument increases, students may change the procedure to suit themselves. More advanced students will soon take the long joint and the tenor joint from the case together and assemble them with the butt joint at the same time. The following items are the most commonly found faults or inaccuracies in the assembly of the bassoon.

1. *Failure to Grease Cork or Thread Joints.* A container of cork grease is a must for every bassoon. The cork or thread joints of the instrument must be kept well greased so that the connections may be made with ease. If the corks are not greased the instrument is assembled with difficulty and a great deal of pressure is necessary. This excessive pressure can easily cause the hand to grip the instrument too tightly and bend keys or rods. If, after the corks are well greased, a joint is still assembled with difficulty, then the cork is too large. A

cork may be fitted to the correct size by sanding it with fine grain sand paper, being careful not to sand any of the wood of the instrument. If a thread wound joint is too tight, a little of the thread may be unwound to make it the correct size.

If a thread wound joint is so loose that the joint is unsteady in its socket additional linen thread of the same diameter may be wound on to make it the correct size. If a cork joint is too loose wipe off all cork grease and moisten. Some corks will absorb enough water to swell to the correct size. Regrease and replace on the instrument. If the cork joint does not expand sufficiently from the additional moisture apply a little heat entirely around it. This is preferably done with an alcohol lamp, but in an emergency can be applied with a match or cigarette lighter. Hold the match or lighter far enough away that the cork is not burned. If this procedure expands the cork sufficiently, apply cork grease and replace on the instrument. If neither of these procedures expands the cork sufficiently it must be replaced.

2. *Holding Joints Improperly.* Holding the joints improperly puts pressure on keys and rods and soon bends them out of line. It is difficult to hold the various parts of the bassoon so that pressure in the wrong places is avoided, but the method described either avoids pressure on keys, or puts pressure on keys which are ordinarily in a closed position. An instrument which is not in perfect alignment plays with difficulty, has certain notes out of tune, or simply doesn't respond at all. Beginners on the instrument must be taught to hold the parts of the instrument properly during assembly and disassembly and checked frequently to see that they are doing so.

3. *Connecting Levers Out of Line.* With only two connecting levers between the various joints to contend with, the bassoonist is not troubled with this problem as much as the oboist. The connecting lever between the tenor joint and the butt joint closes the whisper key when the right thumb is on the low E key. If this lever is not properly aligned, and the pad on the whisper key is not completely closed, notes in the lowest part of the instrument will be difficult to play and control. The remaining connecting lever, between the long joint and the bell closes the key on the bell to produce the low B-flat. This lever is sometimes bent out of alignment making it impossible to produce this note.

4. *Alignment of Tenor and Long Joints.* The alignment of the tenor and long joints with each other is critical only to the extent that it effects the placement of the left hand and the ability of the fingers and thumb to reach out and operate the various holes and keys involved. In order to assure perfect alignment as well as to stabilize these two joints, many makes of bassoons are provided with a lock to lock the two sections together. Various kinds of locks are found, some in two separate pieces, others in a single piece with the lock operated with a spring. The instructor must examine

the lock in order to instruct the student exactly how to use it. Some students will ignore the lock or be unaware of its use. If there is a lock it must be used. In the absence of a lock correct alignment is made by fitting together the wood projection on the tenor joint and the metal plate under the thumb keys on the long joint. Contact between these two points will help steady these two joints.

5. *The bocal.* The bocal is susceptible to bending if undue pressure is put on it near the reed end. It is common to see in school groups a bassoon bocal with a flat spot where it has been bent. A flat area in the bocal, or any alteration in its shape, changes the tone quality, intonation, and ease of playing. To avoid this kind of damage insist that the crook be held near the cork end as described. Younger students have a tendency to ignore the importance of aligning the vent hole in the crook with the pad which closes it. This should be carefully checked as ease of tone production in the lower register is dependent on its proper operation.

Check List for Assembly

Observe the student in the operation of assemblying the instrument and check the following items. Incorrect items for older students should not be called to their attention until the entire process is completed; younger students should be corrected immediately. If any mistake is made the entire process should be repeated until perfect.

	Yes	No	Comments
1. Were corks examined to see if they were properly greased?			
2. Long joint held properly during assembly with butt?			
3. Butt joint held properly during assembly with long joint?			
4. Tenor joint held properly during assembly with butt?			
5. Butt joint held properly on leg during assembly with tenor joint?			
6. Connecting lever on tenor joint properly aligned?			
7. Long and tenor joints properly aligned and locked?			
8. Bell held properly?			
9. Connecting lever on bell properly aligned?			
10. Crook held properly?			
11. Vent hole aligned with pad?			
12. Reed lined up and secured firmly?			

HOLDING POSITION FOR BASSOON

The way in which the bassoon is held has a direct relationship with the progress of the student, the embouchure formation, tone quality produced, control of intonation, and the development of technical facility. The proper position is one in which the body is in an erect position, with the body balanced comfortably, and in which the arms and hands fall naturally into a position in which there is no muscular tension. This position is one which can be maintained over a period of time without physical exhaustion and which permits freedom and control of the breathing mechanism.

The weight of the bassoon is supported by the neck strap or a seat strap[1] with the instrument balanced by the left and right hands as described in the section on hand position which follows. Adjust the height of the instrument with the strap so that when the head is erect the reed will touch the jaw at the bottom of the lower lip. The reed can be easily taken into the mouth from this position. The butt joint rests against the right hip with the instrument held diagonally across the body so that music can be read with head and eyes straight forward. The bell of the instrument is held forward so that the angle of the crook permits the reed to enter the mouth at a very slight angle. Head erect, chin up, eyes straight ahead, with shoulders up but relaxed. Elbows free from the body. Both feet flat on the floor. Shoulders and back must not touch the back of the chair when playing.

Adjust the music stand so that the music can be easily read from this position. When two students are playing from the same music, angle the chairs slightly toward the center of the stand so that the position of the body and instrument can remain correct.

Seated Position

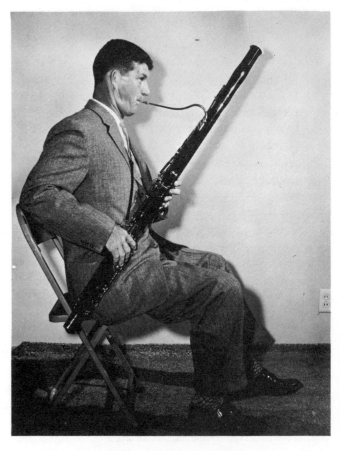

Figure B-15. Side View

Seated Position

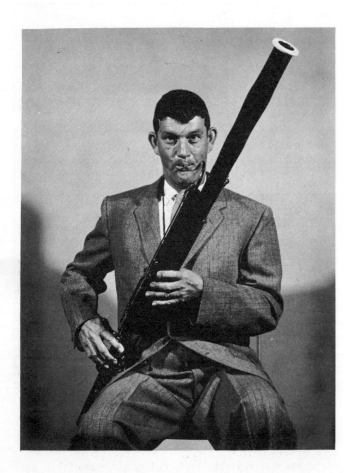

Figure B-14. Front View.

The position of the instrument itself when the player is standing should be identical with that used in the seated position. Only the position of the body itself is changed. Stand erect with feet slightly apart, one foot ahead of the other to help maintain balance. Head remains erect, with chin up and eyes straight ahead. Shoulders up but relaxed, and elbows free from body. Raise the music stand, if one is being used, so that the head does not tilt downward. Every player should regularly spend a portion of his practice time standing to become at ease playing in a standing position.

---

[1]Use of a seat strap is considered later in this chapter.

Standing Position

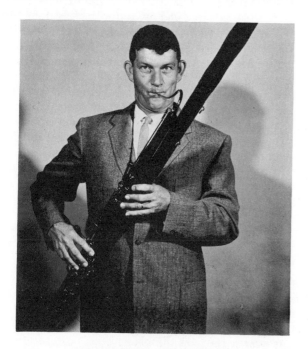

Figure B-16. Front View.

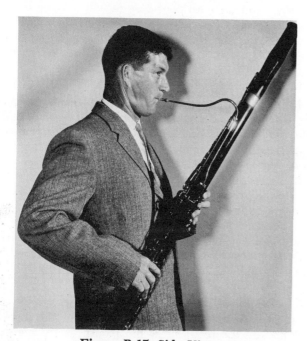

Figure B-17. Side View.

playing position, and the player is free to arrange music and to relax physically.

In the semi-rest position the strap is left hooked and the instrument tilted slightly forward in a relaxed position. This position is used during rests in the music, and when the player must be ready to resume playing immediately. This position, too, permits physical relaxation to avoid fatigue in performing for a period of time.

Rest Position

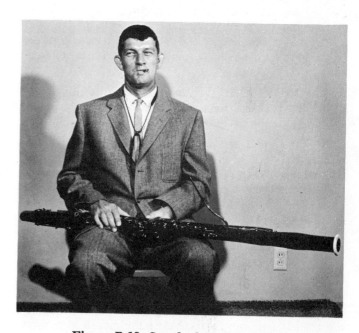

Figure B-18. Standard Rest Position.

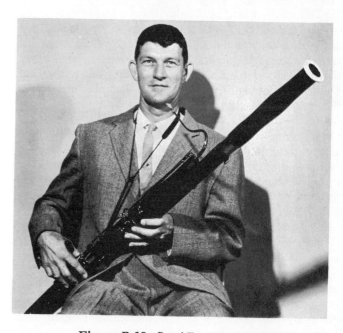

Figure B-19. Semi-Rest Position

In the standard rest position, the neck strap is unhooked and the bassoon is placed diagonally across the legs with the crook up. The reed should be removed from the crook to prevent possible damage. From this position the reed can be returned to the crook and the instrument can be quickly picked up and returned to

Common Faults in Holding Positions

The holding position for an instrument can further rapid musical development, or it can make progress slow and difficult. The exact holding position depends upon and must be adapted to the physical characteristics of the player. Teachers must continually check student positions, especially in the early stages of learning, so that any deviations from the proper position can be immediately corrected before they develop into fixed habits. Once an incorrect position is established, it is extremely difficult to correct. Students themselves must and do learn to feel the right position, and should be encouraged to check their positions daily in front of a mirror both at school and at home. A full-length mirror is an integral part of the well-equipped instrumental room of any school.

The following are the most commonly found faults in holding positions for the bassoon. Check these points specifically and regularly with each student.

1. *Instrument at Wrong Angle with Body.* Because of the two oblique angles, with the front of the body and with the side of the body, which are involved in the playing position there is considerable chance of error. The angle across the front of the body can be checked by looking directly at the student from the front to see that no part of the face is covered by the body of the instrument. If the instrument has a whisper key and most do, the fact that the vent hole in the crook and the pad on the key which closes it must be lined up makes this particular angle easier to arrive at correctly. A final check on this angle is to make sure that the reed is entering the center of the mouth at a right angle rather than entering from one side.

The angle with the side of the body involves more problems, and there is less unanimity of opinion among authorities on exactly what this angle should be. This angle is primarily determined by the angle with which the reed enters the mouth. Most authorities agree that the crook should tilt up slightly so that the reed enters the mouth at a slight angle. Others, and these are by far in the minority, ask that the reed enter the mouth directly, or ask for a greater upward angle. This angle affects tone quality and control and must be subject to constant scrutiny. If the head is erect with the chin up as it should be the reed angle determines how far forward or backward the butt end of the instrument is in relation to the body. If the butt is too far back the left elbow is forced backward too far, putting tension on muscles and ligaments in the right hand. If the butt is too far forward the right hand is pulled out of position, making it difficult for the fingers to operate the holes and keys. The angle of the arm at the elbow should be no less than 90-degrees and preferably greater than this. The physical characteristics of the individual student will help determine the exact angles best for him.

2. *Head Inclined Downward.* This is a most serious deviation from the normal because of the extreme effect it has on tone quality, and is, unfortunately found in students at all stages of development. When the head is inclined downward, unless the butt is drawn correspondingly farther back, the reed enters the embouchure at a downward rather than an upward angle. This puts the primary support for the reed on the upper lip rather than on the lower lip where the best and most accurate control is possible. This downward incline of the head makes the breath enter the reed at an angle and restricts the volume and support by bringing the tip of the reed closer to the tongue. A related undesirable result is the effect this position has on articulation. Because the tip of the reed is close to the tongue, movements of the tongue are restricted, and the reed is contacted by the center of the tongue rather than the forward position. The result is a sluggish tongue and a lack of control and variety on articulation.

3. *Slouched Body.* Varying degrees and kinds of poor posture are almost universal among student players. Common among these are the curved spine with the back against the chair, shoulders curved forward, feet crossed or hung over a rung on the chair. Poor posture affects breathing and breath control to the point that the student finds it impossible to support and control the tone properly. Students with poor posture will become physically tired rather quickly while playing. Poor posture pulls the arms, and consequently the fingers out of position making technique rough. Poor posture in any degree must be corrected immediately. The use of a mirror in correcting is helpful.

4. *Moving the Body While Playing.* Some students have the unfortunate habit of swaying or bouncing their body while playing. Any movement of the body changes the position of the reed in the mouth to a greater or lesser degree, interferes with the coordination of the muscles controlling breath support and in general has undesirable results in performance. Most players who move the body are not aware of the fact that they are doing so. Any movements noted should be called to the attention of the player and corrected immediately and firmly. A correct holding position without any bodily movement is necessary for complete success in performance.

5. *Adjustment of Strap.* The neck or seat strap must be adjusted to support the entire weight of the instrument and so the reed enters the mouth at the correct angle. If the strap is adjusted so that it is too long, the student must duck his head or slouch to get the reed into his mouth. Any attempt to support the weight of the instrument with the hand rest or with the palm of the left hand pulls the hand out of position and tenses the muscles so that the fingers do not move freely. The condition of the strap should be checked when students are found to be having a problem with it to see that it

is not worn to the extent that the lock slides when weight is put on it. The strap must hold the desired length without slipping. Replace worn straps promptly.

HAND POSITIONS

Since the bassoon most desirably is played by a student with previous training on another woodwind instrument—usually clarinet—hand position may not be as much of a problem if the hand position on the previous instrument was good. The size of the student's hand and the length of fingers are more critical on the bassoon than on any other of the woodwind instruments because of the wide stretches necessary to reach and cover the holes and to operate the keys. Students with small hands and/or stubby fingers will have more difficulty achieving the best hand position than students with larger hands and longer fingers. The exact hand position, particularly of the left hand, will of necessity be determined by the size of the player's hands.

The following step-by-step procedure for establishing the hand position on the bassoon should be studied thoroughly with an instrument so that a feel for the position can be developed. Study both the text and the photographs carefully until they are perfectly clear. The "Guide Position" which is given is the fundamental position for hands and fingers and should be maintained at all times except when the fingering for a particular note involves moving a finger temporarily to another location. The guide position puts all fingers into the best position for developing speed and accuracy.

A. Left Hand Position

1. Figure B-20. The bassoon is balanced with the flesh at the base of the forefinger against the wood of the instrument. Position the hand so that the thumb comfortably reaches the whisper key as shown in the photograph. Be sure the hand is not touching the rod which extends up the side of the instrument.

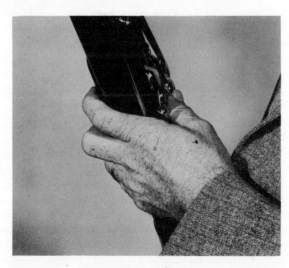

Figure B-20.

2. Figure B-21. The left little finger touches lightly but does not press the D-sharp key. The remaining fingers fall into place covering the three tone holes with the ball of the fingers directly beneath the fingernails.

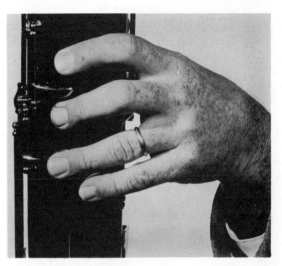

Figure B-21.

B. Right Hand Position

1. Figure B-22. Adjust the height of the hand rest so that the fingers can reach the tone holes and the thumb can close the E key. The crotch of the thumb and forefinger should rest comfortably in the hand rest to help balance the instrument. Wrist should be flat. The thumb may rest on the metal guard plate near the E-key when not in use.

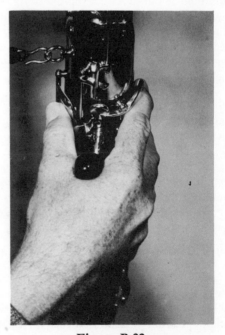

Figure B-22.

2. Figure B-23. The little finger of the right hand touches lightly but does not press the F key. With the little finger in place the remaining fingers fall into place over the two tone holes and G key covering the tone holes with the ball of the finger directly beneath the fingernail.

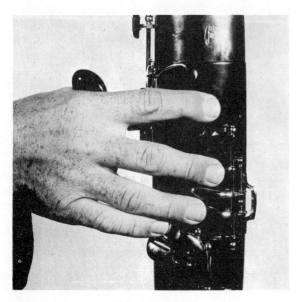

Figure B-23.

C. Guide Position

With the hands in position as described and the balls of the fingers no more than one inch directly above the tone holes a guide position is established which should be maintained constantly. Wrists of both hands should be flat to avoid muscular cramping. In playing, the entire finger moves from the knuckle and closes the tone holes with a snap or click, pressing just hard enough to close the holes. Avoid too much pressure against the plates with the fingers.

D. Special Finger Positions

The bassoon has certain fingerings and keys to operate which tend to pull the hands out of position unless fingers are moved efficiently and with minimum motion. If the correct guide position is established and maintained, these finger movements will come naturally and can be readily developed. A constant check on the use and position of the fingers in these situations is necessary until the movements become habitual.

1. *Half-Hole Position for the First Finger.*

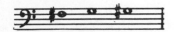

The half-hole position of the first finger functions as a small vent to help secure positively fourth line F-sharp

and fourth space G and G-sharp. To reach the half-hole position the finger is rolled downward by a movement of the second joint of the finger so that half of the tone hole is open and half closed by the finger. The guide

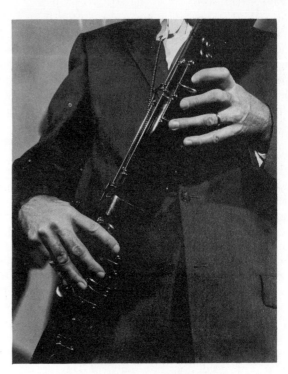

Figure B-24. Guide Position.

position for the remainder of the fingers of the hand must be maintained. Avoid sliding the finger instead of rolling. The motion is that of rolling down to open and rolling up to close. Sliding will slow the movement of the finger so that the notes will not respond.

2. *Right Hand C-sharp.* Key 4x operated by the first finger of the right hand is an alternate fingering for C-sharp used primarily as a trill fingering. Figure B-25 shows the position of the fingers when this key is being used. The first finger stretches slightly to reach the key, but the remainder of the fingers keep the basic guide position. This fingering illustrates the basic principle of moving only the finger or fingers involved in the operation out of position while maintaining the basic guide position so that all the fingers will be in the best position to play notes which follow.

3. *Left Thumb.* With eight (or nine) keys to operate the left thumb requires considerable dexterity in manipulation. The four keys nearest the base of the thumb (D,C,B,B-Flat on the fingering chart) are involved in the four lowest notes on the instrument. To play these

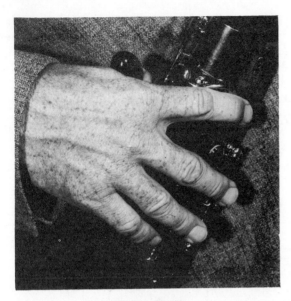

Figure B-25.

notes downward the keys are added one at a time with the D key being depressed by the bottom of the thumb under the first joint, the thumb is slid up to depress the C key, and rolled for the B and B-flat successively. Figure B-26 shows the position of the thumb playing the low B-flat with all four keys depressed. Most modern bassoons have the D, C, and B keys interlocked so that when the C key is depressed the D key is automatically closed, and when the B key is depressed both the D and C keys are automatically depressed. It is not neces-

sary to hold all three keys down with the thumb, although most available fingering charts will so indicate. Taking advantage of this interlocking of the keys simplifies and facilitates technique with these keys.

The three or four keys toward the tip of the thumb are arranged so that the thumb can reach them by moving in a slight arc. These keys are depressed with the portion of the thumb between the ball and the tip, and using a slight arch in the joint of the thumb to clear the other keys. One of the alternate fingerings for fourth space E-flat calls for the use of the whisper key and the C-sharp key, both operated by the tip of the thumb. To do this the width of the thumb is divided between the two keys and both depressed simultaneously.

An alternate fingering for second space C-sharp calls for the use of the low D key with the middle of the thumb and the C-sharp key with the tip. For this the thumb should be flattened so that both keys can be depressed simultaneously. Other notes involve different combinations of right thumb keys. Some experimentation and practice is necessary to perfectly coordinate the operation of these two keys.

Common Faults in Hand and Finger Position

A good hand position is a great asset in the study of the bassoon. Unfortunately the wide stretches necessary to reach keys and holes force students whose hands are not large enough to assume unnatural or strained hand and finger positions. A student whose hand is quite small for the instrument will have difficulty in developing facility since the stretches which he will have to make will tense the muscles and make them slow to respond. However, a physically immature student who is still growing will succeed on the instrument despite small hands, if with the encouragement of his teacher he gradually changes his hand position toward the ideal.

The better the hand position the easier it is to develop facility and control. The first experiences with the instrument must emphasize hand position, and it must be checked continually until the best position for that particular student is established. A beginning player who persists in establishing the proper positions make rapid progress. The use of a mirror of sufficient size so that the student can see the entire length of the instrument is an asset in establishing position.

The following are the most common faults and are those which are instructor should look for. All of these are involved in and help determine the progress of facility and technique.

1. *Hand Rest.* Two common faults are considered in this connection: (1) improper height adjustment and (2) not using the hand rest if the instrument is supported by a neck strap. The height of the hand rest is most important. It must be adjusted so both the thumb and the fingers can reach the various keys and holes easily with the proper amount of curvature and still balance

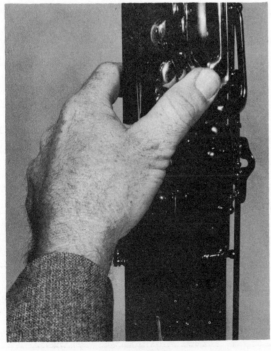

Figure B-26.

Check List for Holding and Hand Positions

The following list of items provides a means of thoroughly checking holding and hand positions while the player is seated. The check must be performed while the student is playing and preferably when he is not aware that the check is being made. Any items which are checked "no" should be corrected with the deviation explained to the student, together with what effect it has on the playing, and why the correct position is important. Students make a more serious effort to correct mistakes if they understand the reason for them.

A. Holding Position

	Yes	No	Comments
1. Angle with front of body correct?			
2. Angle with side of body correct?			
3. Position of head correct?			
4. Neck strap properly adjusted?			
5. Hand rest properly adjusted?			
6. Shoulders up but relaxed?			
7. Elbows free from body?			
8. Body posture good?			
9. Feet in place?			
10. Height of music stand correct?			

B. Hand Positions

	Yes	No	Comments
1. Left hand contacting wood at proper place for supporting the instrument?			
2. Fingers of right hand neither stretched nor cramped because of hand rest adjustment?			
3. Proper part of left thumb contacting keys?			
4. Balls of fingers covering holes?			
5. Left little finger on guide key?			
6. Right little finger on guide key?			
7. Right thumb over E key?			
8. Fingers no more than one inch above open holes?			
9. First finger rolls properly to half-hole position?			
10. Basic guide position maintained?			
11. Wrists flat?			
12. Any signs of muscular tension?			

the instrument securely. The height can be adjusted by the lock screw provided on the instrument. If the student has a small hand, and the hand rest cannot be lowered sufficiently, measure and shorten it by cutting a little off the end. Hand rests are readily available as accessories for the instrument, and the school who has several beginning bassoonists could well have on hand several extra hand rests of varying lengths.

It is mandatory that the hand rest be used if the instrument is being supported by a neck strap. A hand rest is ordinarily not used if the instrument is being supported by a seat strap. Without the hand rest with the neckstrap the student is forced to balance the instrument with the thumb, or by putting a finger against the instrument, limiting technique of the right hand fingers and thumb. Teachers are advised to insist on the use of the hand rest with a neckstrap.

2. *Left Thumb.* The most common problem in the use of the left thumb is that of depressing the D key or the C key with the tip of the thumb rather than beneath the joint. Using the tip of the thumb on these keys makes it impossible to roll the thumb onto the B and B-flat keys or to depress one of the others keys quickly and smoothly. The left thumb is difficult to observe while the student is playing, and it is necessary for the teacher to make a special effort to observe the action.

3. *Muscular Tension.* Symptoms of muscular tension are easily seen, and must not necessarily be attributed to the effort of playing the instrument. Some symptoms are rigid little fingers, uncoordinated finger movements, etc. This tension can be caused by improper positioning of the instrument which puts too much weight on the left hand; not using a hand rest which puts pressure on the right thumb to support the instrument; wrists which are stretched into a curve rather than being virtually flat; a hand rest which is too high or too low; a neck strap adjusted too long or too short; elbows held up rather than relaxed, etc. Any muscular tension should be tracked down to its source and corrected immediately, since the most rapid progress on the instrument is possible only when the body is relaxed.

4. *Little Fingers.* In the suggested guide position the little fingers are touching a key from which it is easy to move rapidly to another key as needed. If the little fingers are not in the guide position, then assurance in this movement is lost. Deviation of the little fingers from the guide position frequently pulls the remainder of the fingers out of position as well. Players with small hands will have difficulty in keeping the little finger of the left hand in position. If keeping the little finger on its guide key causes tension in the hand, then the student must be allowed to relax the little finger into a comfortable position for him. Insist, however, in maintaining the guide position as closely as possible for all students.

EMBOUCHURE FORMATION

An embouchure may be defined as the formation of the performer's lips with supporting muscles, teeth and jaws in relation to the reed which have to do with tone production. The criteria for a good bassoon embouchure may be summarized as follows: a good embouchure is one which over the entire range of the instrument produces (or is capable of producing) a rich, full bodied, clear tone; plays perfectly in tune; allows the full scope of articulations with minimum effort; allows the full range of dynamics to be played with complete control; plays and is controlled with a minimum amount of physical exertion when used with a well adjusted reed. Conversely a poor embouchure is one which violated one or more of these criteria and produces a thin, reedy, nasal tone quality; plays certain notes out of tune; does not allow the full scope of articulations; has a restricted dynamic range; or requires an undue amount of physical exertion. Embouchure is inseparable from the reed and is entirely dependent on having a good, responsive reed. The best embouchure formation cannot play a poor reed, nor will an excellent reed respond properly with a poorly formed embouchure.

The recommendation of various bassoon authorities can be summarized in two basic types of embouchure formation, although the differences between the two are not as great as those found between the two types of clarinet embouchure, and the preponderance of authority lies with one particular formation. As could be expected there are many small variations which are necessary and desirable depending upon the type of reed being used as well as the concept of the desired tone quality. The basic difference between the two approaches to bassoon embouchure is found in whether the cheek muscles and the corners of the mouth are pushed in toward the reed, or whether the cheek muscles are pulled back into a slight "smile" position while the corners of the mouth are pushed in around the reed. For convenience and clarity the first is called a "soft cushion" and the second a "hard cushion," although these terms are relative and not to be taken literally.

The Soft Cushion Embouchure

The soft cushion embouchure has the preponderance of authoritative weight behind it, and is the one most widely recommended. The basic formation of the soft cushion embouchure may be achieved through the following procedure. Check each step with a mirror.

1. Keeping the lips relaxed, drop the lower jaw so that the teeth are about a half inch apart.

2. Pull the lower jaw back to increase the natural overbite. The jaw is kept back while playing.

3. Push the corners of the mouth toward the center as in whistling, forming wrinkles in the lips.

4. Maintaining the contracted position of the lips, roll them over the teeth so that virtually all of the lip

is over the teeth. The exact amount of lip over the teeth varies from student to student depending on whether the lips are average, thin, or thick. Thin lips will need all the lip over the teeth, while those students with thick lips may leave a line of the red of the lip in front of the teeth. Pull the chin muscles down—avoid bunching under the reed.

5. Put the reed between the lips. The reed should be in the mouth far enough that the upper lip is almost touching the first wire. Contract the lips around the reed like a drawstring.

The Hard Cushion Embouchure

The hard cushion embouchure for the bassoon is much less widely recommended than the similar formation on the other woodwind instruments, although some fine performers make use of it. The general experience with this formation has been that school age bassonists develop a good tone quality and control less rapidly than with the soft cushion formation. The hard cushion embouchure may be achieved through the following procedure. Check each step with a mirror.

1. Keeping the lips relaxed, drop the lower jaw so that the teeth are about a half inch apart.

2. Pull the lower jaw back to increase the natural overbite. The jaw is kept back while playing.

3. Pull the corners of the mouth back so that they and the attached cheek muscles are in a slight smiling position.

4. Roll both of the lips over the teeth, keeping the teeth open and the slight smiling position of the corners. The amount of lip over the teeth varies as indicated before according to the thickness of the student's lips. Pull the chin muscles down—avoid bunching under the reed.

5. Insert the reed into the mouth until the upper lip is almost touching the first wire. Tighten the lips around the reed, while maintaining the smile position of the corners.

Setting the Embouchure

Since most begining bassoonists will have had previous experience on another woodwind instrument the same type of embouchure formation used on the previous instrument, either the soft cushion or the hard cushion, will come quite naturally on the bassoon. Before attempting to produce a tone on the instrument, the embouchure must be set with the reed alone. Much time will be saved if this is done.

To find the proper amount of reed in the mouth is a fairly simple process which should be the first order of business. This is done with the reed alone. The well adjusted bassoon reed when blown alone produces a buzz commonly called a "crow," of two distinct pitches —one high and one low pitched. Some good reeds produce more than two pitches but the high and low ones will predominate in the sound. The setting of the em-

bouchure is aimed at finding the exact formation and amount of reed in the mouth which produces this double crow.

Use a reed which has been prepared for playing for either the soft or hard cushion embouchure described, checking in a mirror to see that it is properly formed. Starting with just the tip of the reed between the lips produce a sound using standard abdominal breath support. The sound produced will be a thin reedy buzz. Keeping the sound continuous gradually increase the amount of reed in the mouth until the upper lip touches the wire on the reed. Considerable differences in sound will be readily apparent as the amount of reed in the mouth increases. Try moving it back and forth to note the immediate differences. These differences in sound of the reed alone are magnified many times when the reed is producing a tone on the instrument. This points out the importance of setting the embouchure not only with the proper muscular formation, but with exactly the right amount of reed in the mouth.

Assuming that the reed is properly adjusted, at some point as the amount of reed in the mouth is increased the characteristic "double-crow" of the bassoon reed will be heard with maximum resonance. This is the critical point on the cut of the reed, normally more than half way between the tip and first wire, and determines the amount of reed to be put into the mouth. This point should be approximately centered between the support provided by the upper and lower lips over the teeth. Remember that no matter which embouchure formation is used the lower jaw is pulled back to increase the natural overbite. This means that the position of the upper lip on the reed is slightly forward toward the first wire of the point of maximum vibration while the lower lip and teeth are slightly back toward the tip of the reed in relation to this point. Under normal circumstances this adjustment will have the upper lip almost touching the first wire on the reed.

When this experiment has been completed the student should continue producing a double-crow on the reed until it sounds freely and can be sustained for ten to twenty seconds. Once this is accomplished the reed can be put on the bocal and tones produced on the instrument itself. Continue to emphasize the importance of checking the embouchure formation with the use of a mirror until it is well established—a period of several months.

Checking the Embouchure

The teacher will have to check frequently to make sure the embouchure continues to be correctly formed and is developing properly. Students are not always capable of discovering their own mistakes, or of even knowing when they are right and when they are wrong, since it is just as easy for them to develop the wrong muscular formation as it is the correct one. The embouchure must be established by how it feels in the

Check List for Embouchure Formation

The following check on embouchure formation must be made while the student is playing and preferably when he is not aware that a check is being made. Any errors should be carefully explained to the student, with the correction worked out wtih him while he is observing the embouchure in a mirror. Remedial exercises can be assigned on the basis of this list.

	Yes	No	Comments
1. Sufficient lip over lower teeth?			
2. Sufficient lip over upper teeth?			
3. Lips supporting around entire reed?			
4. Corners of mouth pushed toward center with soft cushion formation?			
5. Corner of mouth pulled back with hard cushion formation?			
6. Reed proper distance in mouth?			
7. Head inclined slightly downward?			
8. Crook at an upward angle toward the mouth?			
9. Cheeks puffed?			
10. Air escaping?			
11. Teeth sufficiently apart?			

mouth and how the tone sounds, as well as how it looks in the mirror. The teacher must tell the student when he is right so he can discover the right feel, hear the right sound, and see the right shape.

Very small variations in embouchure formation are sometimes required to accommodate the physical characteristics of the student. Students with thicker than average lips will not need to put the entire lip over the teeth. Students with a small natural overbite will need to pull the lower jaw back further than students with a large overbite in order to put the points of support in their proper relationship on the reed.

Players with uneven teeth—especially the lower ones—may need to turn the reed slightly to avoid more pressure against one side than the other, since it is necessary that the pressure against the flat of the reed be the same across its width and equal on both the upper and lower blades. If this is necessary the amount that the reed is turned is extremely slight, and care must be taken that the instrument itself is kept in the best playing position.

The amount of pressure or bite against the reed with the lower teeth is frequently difficult to adjust. The

basic concept that the teeth must be kept apart and the reed supported only by the lips must be emphasized. Biting the reed restricts its vibration and prevents good tone production. The lower teeth do control to a degree the amount of support which the lip gives the reed, increasing support for the upper and high registers and decreasing for the lower octave, making small adjustments to control intonation, and assisting in the control of dynamics. If the lower teeth are biting excessive breath pressure is necessary to produce a tone, the tone quality is rough, and the lower notes of the instrument difficult or impossible to produce. Evidence of biting can be seen by examining the inner part of the lip for imprints of the teeth. Asking the player to play flatter will cause him to drop the lower jaw and gives him the feeling of playing flatter although little or no change in pitch will be apparent to the listener. A poorly made or adjusted reed will sometimes force the player to bite in order to control the tone, and for this reason, beginners must be provided with reeds that have been well adjusted and prepared for playing.

Puffing cheeks is sometimes a problem with bassoon players as well as other instrumentalists. This is an inevitable indication of an embouchure problem since it indicates that the cheek muscles involved in the embouchure formation are not supporting properly. Players with puffing cheeks virtually always have an open unfocused tone quality combined with poor intonation. Frequently the player does not realize that his cheeks are puffed, especially if the amount of air between the teeth and cheek is small. The use of a mirror to check is necessary. When the student can actually see that the cheeks are in the right position, and the embouchure correctly formed, he can then feel the muscular support that is necessary to keep the cheeks in position. Playing a note on the instrument with one hand while feeling the cheeks with the other is useful in helping the player feel the right position.

The holding position of the instrument is an important facet of embouchure formation. The bocal must be at a downward angle from the lips to the instrument. It should never be straight nor go upwards from the lips. The height of the instrument must be adjusted by the strap so that when the player's head is erect and straight the reed will touch his lower lip at about the line which divides the lip from the chin. From this position the player tilts his head downward just enough to take the reed into the mouth comfortably. This is the correct playing angle. The instrument must be held so that the reed enters the mouth at a right angle rather than approaching from either side. If the reed enters the mouth at an angle, even a very slight one, the support on the reed becomes slightly diagonal with resulting tone problems.

Air escaping from one corner of the mouth while playing is a clear indication that something, large or small, is wrong with the embouchure formation. With the soft cushion embouchure this means that the lips are not being properly tightened around the reed. The corner of the mouth is either relaxed or is being pulled back enough to release the air. With the hard cushion embouchure, escaping air is the result of too much pulling back of the corner of the mouth. This is corrected by tightening the corner of the mouth and pushing slightly toward the reed. The cause of the escaping air can be seen clearly by examining the embouchure while the student is playing, and corrective measures suggested.

TUNING

The problem of tuning the bassoon is discussed at length in the section on reeds since the basic pitch of the instrument is determined almost entirely by the reed and its relationship with an individual embouchure. Mechanical adjustment of the instrument itself can accomplish only the slightest changes in basic pitch. Refer to the chapter on reeds for information on tuning the reed, and to the section on embouchure for its influence on pitch.

All modern bassoons are made to play to the standard international pitch of A-440, but the construction of the reed and the player's embouchure can make the pitch of the instrument deviate several vibrations in either direction. Tuning is best done with the aid of an electronic tuner where a visual check on the pitch is possible. This is especially important for younger players who have not yet developed an accurate and dependable sense of pitch. Tuning bars, tuning forks or electronic devices which sound a single note are useful comparisons, but are not as useful as a device which provides a visual check of the pitch of all the notes on the instrument.

The piano is probably the poorest source of tuning notes, unless it has been tuned by an expert tuner within the previous few days. Piano pitch is affected by temperature changes which cause the string to stretch or contract, raising and lowering the pitches, and over a period of time the over-all pitch of the instrument gradually sinks lower than the standard A-440. Temperature changes alter the piano and wind instruments in reverse directions. A low temperature raises the pitch of the piano and lowers the pitch of the wind instrument, while a high temperature lowers the pitch of the piano and raises the pitch of the wind instrument. A player who is playing a solo with piano accompaniment must obviously tune and play in tune with it, but other than this the piano is best avoided for tuning purposes.

The bassoon tunes to the standard A for orchestra and either the B-flat or A for band, playing an octave lower than the pitch usually sounded for tuning purposes. The following illustrates this relationship.

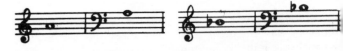

Tuning Note Bassoon Plays   Tuning Note Bassoon Plays

Bocals or Crooks. Once the reed itself is properly tuned, small adjustments on over-all pitch of the instrument can be made by changing the bocal being used. All instruments are provided with two bocals, and an examination will reveal that they are a few millimeters different in length. Following the basic laws of acoustics the longer the bocal the flatter the over-all pitch of the instrument. If a student consistently plays sharp over the instrument he should use a longer bocal, if he consistently plays flat over the instrument he should use a shorter bocal.

Bocals are numbered according to length, normally 1, 2, 3, in order of increasing length. Some manufacturers use the numbers 0, 1, 2, or 0, 1, 2, 3, but always the higher the number the longer the bocal, and the flatter the pitch. If it is necessary to replace a bocal or to purchase one of a different size one made by the manufacturer of the instrument on which it is to be used should be purchased. There are slight differences in length, diameter, and shape from brand to brand, although basically all those used on Heckel system bassoons are copies of those made by the Heckel company. If the length bocal needed is not available in the brand desired, substitute one made by Heckel.

The number is normally stamped on the face of the bocal for easy identification, since differences in length are so small that it is sometimes difficult to make a positive visual comparison of two different bocals. Instruments normally come supplied with number 1 and 2 bocals. If a shorter or longer bocal is needed, they must be purchased separately.

Tuning with Bocal Cork. Very slight adjustments in over-all pitch of the bassoon may be made by adjusting the distance the bocal cork fits into the instrument. The further into the instrument the bocal is the sharper, and conversely farther out the cork is the flatter the instrument. The amount of tuning adjustment that it is possible to make in this manner is limited since the vent hole must be positioned so that it can be covered by its pad.

INTONATION

Even though an instrument is being played with a well tuned reed and the proper bocal has been selected, intonation problems on individual notes still exist. Experienced players adjust to these individual notes automatically, and students must develop a keen sense of discrimination in intonation in order to develop this automatic compensation. The various factors which influence intonation are considered in the following.

Natural Tendencies of the Instrument. The bassoon, because of the combination of acoutical and mechanical factors, probably has more naturally out of tune notes than any other woodwind instrument. These notes may be very slightly or considerably out of tune, and vary somewhat from brand to brand and instrument to instrument. The teacher should be aware of these notes in order to understand the problems of the student and to help him solve them. The following indicates these notes as they are most commonly found.

(a) Notes with a natural tendency to be sharp

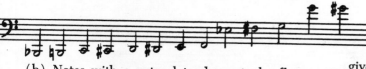

(b) Notes with a natural tendency to be flat

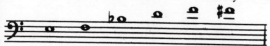

The notes from the lowest B-flat up a perfect fifth to F tend to be sharp on all instruments, and very sharp on some instruments and with some players. These notes pose the most difficult problem in control of in-

tonation on the entire instrument since being sharp in this register is contrary to what the ear expects to hear and no alternate fingerings are available to help in adjusting the pitch. The natural tendencies toward sharping and flatting on the other notes can be compensated for by embouchure, breath support, or through choosing an alternate fingering which is better in tune.

Effect of Reed on Intonation. The nature of the reed being used is of primary importance in intonation. The way it is adjusted, the type of cane used, how it fits the player's embouchure all have an effect on pitch and intonation. The way in which the final adjustments on the reed are made will determine not only whether the instrument is properly tuned to A-440 but how well the instrument will play in tune with itself. Generally a reed which responds well in all registers of the instrument with a good tone quality will also be capable of good intonation over the instrument.

A reed which is too soft will play flat over the range of the instrument and minor adjustments in intonation will be difficult to make. Certain notes, third space E and fourth line F for example, are affected more than others. Notes in the highest register will be quite flat and cannot be brought up to pitch by embouchure adjustments, if indeed they can be played at all.

A reed which is too hard will play generally sharp over the range of the instrument. Here, as well as with the soft reed, certain notes—third space E-flat for example—are affected more than other notes. The lowest notes on the instrument will be difficult to play softly, and will be even sharper than their natural tendencies.

Reeds which have been played too long, and which are worn out gradually become more and more difficult to control in intonation. Student bassoonists will need to be checked frequently for this condition, as the change in the reed is normally so gradual that the student is not aware that a change has taken place. Insist that a spare reed or two be prepared and ready to play at all times.

Effect of Embouchure on Intonation. The embouchure coupled with the reed is a primary factor in intonation. Even the best of reed will play out of tune if the embouchure is poorly formed or undeveloped. An embouchure deficiency can be heard in the tone quality as well as being seen through examination. It is for the dual purposes of good intonation and tone quality that so much emphasis is given to embouchure formation and development. A well formed and developed embouchure is a necessary foundation for good intonation.

The embouchure can make slight corrections in intonation through adjusting the pressure with which the reed is held. This adjusting is made by the lips and their controlling muscles, and not by the lower jaw and teeth. To make a note higher in pitch contract the embouchure around the reed to increase support. To make a note lower in pitch, relax the embouchure to reduce the support. These slight changes in pressure are constant and involuntary in experienced players. Younger players need guidance to develop this facility.

The amount of reed taken into the mouth has considerable effect on intonation—even microscopic changes in the amount frequently can be heard. The skilled bassoonist makes use of the device of using slightly more or less reed in the mouth to help control intonation. For example, the very lowest notes on the instrument have been cited as having a natural tendency to be sharp, and one measure of correction is to take slightly less reed in the mouth when playing these notes. Care must be taken not to use too little reed as this will change tone quality as well as intonation. The highest notes on the instrument are frequently flat in the hands of the student bassoonist. These can be brought up somewhat in pitch through using more reed in the mouth even to the point where the upper lip is actually touching the first wire on the reed.

The lower jaw can help control intonation by moving back and forth slightly under the lower lip. Pulling the lower jaw back slightly flattens the pitch and pushing it forward sharpens the pitch. Used in combination with the amount of reed in the mouth the jaw movement can increase the amount of pitch change possible. If for example, in addition to using less reed in the mouth for the lowest notes on the instrument the lower jaw is also pulled back, a considerably flatter pitch can be achieved than if only one of these changes were made.

Dynamics and Intonation. Like most other wind instruments, the bassoon has a natural tendency to get flat as the tone gets louder and sharper as the tone diminishes in volume, with the degree of flatness or sharpness increasing as dynamics approach the extremes. This must be compensated for by embouchure adjustments. In order to play louder the student tends to relax the embouchure so that the reed tip may open up to allow a great volume of air to pass through, or to tighten the embouchure as he gets softer to lessen the amount of air passing through the reed. Since pitch is controlled to a considerable degree by the pressure for the embou-

chure around the reed there is is a corresponding flattening or sharping.

Dynamics are properly controlled by breath support and pressure which controls the volume or velocity of the air passing through the reed. Students relax their embouchure to play louder rather than increasing breath velocity, and tighten the embouchure to play softer rather than decreasing breath velocity. Pitch is maintained through balancing the velocity of the wind through the reed with the pressure of the embouchure around it. When playing fortissimo the slight relaxation of the embouchure needed to open the tip of the reed more is compensated for by the greatly increased velocity of the air. In a crescendo the wind velocity and embouchure pressure are kept in balance to maintain pitch stability. In playing pianissimo the embouchure may be relaxed slightly, if anything, while the pitch is maintained through a continuing firm breath support while decreasing the velocity of the air through the reed to achieve the desired dynamic level.

Developing the facility for maintaining a constant pitch through long crescendo and diminuendo is one of the best ways to develop breath control. The tone exercises below are excellent practice in control of pitch through wide dynamic levels. They should be practiced slowly enough that an entire breath is used in four measures. Maintain constant firm breath support while controlling the dynamics by changing the velocity of the air through the instrument. Practice exercise "a" in major or minor scale patterns to include the entire range of the instrument in which the student is proficient. Exercise "b" is best practiced chromatically first in the most comfortable range for the student, then extending upward and downward to the extremes of his range. Practicing with the use of a stroboscope which provides a visual check of pitch fluctuations is extremely valuable in connection with developing this facility.

Playing Position and Intonation. Body posture in its relationship with breathing and breath support is an important facet in the control of intonation. Poor posture makes good breath support impossible, and as a result

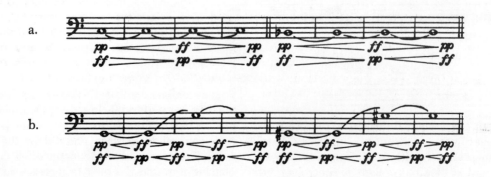

limits its use in the control of intonation. Good posture is so basic **that** it must be given a high priority in teaching.

The position in which the instrument is held in relation to the body has been developed and standardized not only to provide the best playing position to eliminate muscular tension, but so that the embouchure could be formed in the best relationship to the reed and bocal. If the reed is not at a right angle with the lips then pressure is uneven across the reed and intonation problems develop. Similarly if the reed does not enter the mouth at a slightly upward angle control of intonation is difficult or impossible. Playing position is so basic to good performance that unless it is virtually perfect intonation is inevitably poor. Any deviations from standard playing position must be corrected immediately and firmly.

Mechanical Factors and Intonation. Adjustment of the mechanism on the bassoon can control intonation on various notes. Keys or pads which do not open wide enough cause the tone involved to be flat, and conversely if they open too widely these tones will be sharp. If an individual tone is sharp or flat, check first to see that the pads involved are being raised the proper distance from the tone hole. The distance a pad is raised from the tone hole is controlled by the thickness of a buffer cork on the bottom of its key which can be adjusted without too much difficulty. The thickness of the pad itself is frequently involved. The pad may have been too thick when it was put on, or may have swelled through absorbing moisture. These should be replaced by a repairman. Pads which are too thin are rarely found because there is difficulty in seating them and they are replaced in the normal course of putting the instrument in playing condition.

There are several articulated keys on the bassoon where operating a single key opens and/or closes two pads which may be widely separated on the body of the instrument. If the articulation mechanism of these keys is not properly adjusted one of these pads may be too close or too far from a tone hole. The articulations are usually determined by the thickness of a cork beneath one or more of the keys which can be adjusted to give proper clearance.

Keys which are bent up or down or which are bent out of alignment will also cause one or more notes to be out of tune because of the distance of the pad from its tone hole. The instrument should be examined regularly to see that all keys are in the proper alignment. Students become accustomed to out of line keys and are not aware that they should be corrected.

Tone holes covered directly by the fingers frequently become clogged from various causes. A clogged tone hole will change both tone quality and intonation. As a matter of good maintenance all tone holes should be cleaned periodically with a soft cloth or a bent pipe cleaner. It is not always possible to see the foreign material in the holes, so do not depend on a visual examination to determine whether or not they are clean.

The vent hole on the bocal is particularly susceptible to clogging because it is so small. Even a slight bit of foreign material in it will change the intonation of some tones. This hole should be cleared regularly and carefully by running a small broom straw or fine needle through it. Do this carefully to avoid enlarging the size of the hole, which is determined to a close tolerance by the acoustics of the instrument.

Alternate Fingerings and Intonation. An examination of the fingering chart for bassoon given in this book will show that there are alternate fingerings for many notes on the instrument. Some notes have three or four alternate fingerings. Many of these alternate fingerings will produce a tone slightly different in pitch from other fingerings for the same note. This is particularly true in the high register. There is greater pitch variation in the alternate fingerings on the bassoon than on any of the other woodwind instruments. Players must be aware that there are alternate fingerings and be able to use them intelligently. They should, through comparing, be completely aware of the pitch differences between each fingering and choose the fingering which provides the best intonation in a specific musical situation.

Some of these special fingerings tend to be further out of tune than the regular fingerings, and should not be used where the duration of the tone is long enough to give a definite pitch impression. Do not use these special trill fingerings as a substitute for a regular fingering.

If a particular note is out of tune, consult the fingering chart for possible alternate fingerings which could correct the intonation. The intonation differences between fingerings will vary from instrument to instrument and from player to player. No positive statement as to which alternates are sharper and which are flatter is possible. The wise player will take advantage of alternate fingerings, and the more advanced the player the more of these fingerings he should know and use.

TONE

With a range of over three octaves, the bassoon rivals the clarinet in versatility. In spite of this wide usable range the basic quality of the tone produced must be essentially the same throughout. There is however considerable variation in extensity, a feeling of fullness or bigness of tone, between the lowest tones and the highest ones. The lowest tones tend to be large in feeling while the highest ones are smaller in feeling.

There is no particular standardization in the division of the entire bassoon range into registers as there is, for example, on the clarinet. Perhaps the most logical division is based on the acoustical response of the instrument, i.e., those notes produced by the fundamental vibration of the air column, those produced by the first overtone, and those produced by the second or third overtones.[2] Because of the extension of the instrument through the keys operated by the thumbs to extend the range downward an interval of a fifteenth is produced by fundamental vibrations. This is divided into the low register made up of the tones produced by adding thumb keys and the lower middle register made up of the remaining notes produced by six fingers over the holes plus the little fingers. The four registers thus obtained are called: (1) low register, (2) lower middle register, (3) upper middle register, and (4) high register. These are notated as follows:

In the hands of the student bassoonist there is a tendency for each of these registers to have its own individual tone quality. The low register is thick and reedy, the lower middle register the fullest, the upper middle register a little thinner and reedier than the lower, and the high register thin and reedy. An interesting test of the capabilities of the bassoonist to match tone qualities is to make a comparison of the sounds produced on the fourth space F and F-sharp where the tones produced change from the fundamental vibration to the first overtone.

Notes in the high register, because they are products of partial vibrations, have a variety of fingerings available, each being the product of a different harmonic. It will be found that certain instruments produce certain notes with better quality and intonation than other instruments using the same fingering. There are large differences from instrument to instrument in the way in which notes in this register respond.

In the process of developing a good tone the bassoon student must direct his attention not only to producing pleasing sounds, but to matching the basic tone quality over the four registers of the instrument. Beginners have difficulty in producing good quality in both the low and high registers, and should not be forced to play in these sections until their embouchure has developed to the point that control in the middle register is sure and accurate and a good quality has been developed. It is especially important not to force extension of the range upward. A student whose embouchure is not sufficiently developed will make drastic changes in his embouchure, including biting with the lower jaw, in order to play these notes. This changing of his basic embouchure formation slows down its development, and frequently produces a less desirable formation when it is fully developed.

The American concept of good bassoon tone quality as represented by the finest professional musicians in our major symphonies is derived almost entirely from the German school of performance. The French school of bassoon playing has been virtually rejected in this country, primarily because the system of fingering is so different from the Heckel system which we use. The differences in fingering systems are minor when compared to the differences in tone quality produced. The entire bore of the instrument is quite different in the French and Heckel systems and the sounds produced are vastly different in quality. In other chapters it has been suggested that the teacher and student study recorded performances to gain a concept of the best standard quality for the instrument under discussion. This can be done to a certain extent with the bassoon provided the inherent differences between the basic French and German schools of playing are clearly understood. It is virtually impossible to produce the typical good French sound on a Heckel system bassoon, and vice versa. Tone qualities to be desired are those produced by the players in various major orchestras of the United States. Even though the critical listener will hear differences from one player to another, the basic quality is the same—a big, dark tone quality which is capable of great variation and perfect control over the entire range of the instrument.

There are innumerable variations in embouchure formation, which, combined with the various reed cuts and adjustments produce slightly different tone qualities. No matter what combination of reed and embouchure is being used, if the tone produced has the characteristic bassoon sound and if the tone is a pleasing one, then it is a good tone. Teachers and bassoon students alike should take advantage of every opportunity to hear live performances of fine instrumentalists. Take advantage of workshops, demonstrations and clinics sponsored by various educational groups. Every such contact with fine professionals can only be beneficial.

A good tone is the product of all the elements involved in performance: instrument, reed, embouchure and breath control. If any of these is defective the tone quality suffers accordingly. Problems of tone production and quality are many and varied, but may usually be traced to their source, and must be corrected immediately. Refer also to the sections on reed, embouchure, and breathing.

---

[2]See Appendix on Acoustics for details of the overtone series.

Following are some of the most common problems in tone production:

1. *Small or Pinched Tone.* This is a very common problem of student bassoonists. It can be traced to several possible causes, with the reed itself the most likely cause. The tip of the reed may be the wrong shape as a result of poor scraping, or it may not be open sufficiently to vibrate enough to produce a full tone. If the tip is properly shaped but too close together, it may be opened by adjusting the wires on the reed. A reed with a tip which is poorly shaped is best discarded. A reed which is too soft either by scraping too much or which is worn out is difficult to adjust. If after performing the adjustment processes to correct this condition it still doesn't respond, it must be discarded.

If the reed is in good condition and the tone is small or pinched it is possible that the student is biting with the lower jaw, exerting too much pressure against the blades with the teeth. This can be identified by the presence of teeth marks on the inside of the lips which can be felt by the student and frequently seen by the instructor. Corrections for this condition include a review of embouchure information with the student to be sure that he understands that the support for the reed comes from the lips around the reed and not from the teeth pressing against it. Asking the student to play flatter will frequently cause him to drop the lower jaw. If the lips are properly supporting the reed the actual pitch of the tone will not drop, although the student will have the sensation of it doing so. Suggesting that he play a long crescendo will force the student to drop the lower jaw if he is to achieve a fortissimo level. The combination of playing louder and flatter brings the greatest degree of drop of the lower jaw so that the student can actually feel the difference. When the jaw is sufficiently down, the student should be asked to feel the difference and keep the jaw in that position in all his performance. Correction of this pressure with the lower jaw is a slow process which demands persistence by both student and teacher.

If the reed is good and the teeth sufficiently open a small or pinched tone may be caused by having too little reed in the mouth. This is readily recognizable by close examination of the student. The correction is simply to insist that more reed be taken in the mouth. If the reed is a good one the student will immediately hear the difference in the size of the tone he is producing. An additional measure to help find the proper amount of reed in the mouth is to work with the reed alone, moving it back and forth in the mouth to find the place where the best and most characteristic double-crow is heard, as previously explained in the section on embouchure.

2. *Open Squawky Tone.* This tone is described as lacking in body and focus, and generally uncontrolled.

This sound is typical of the very beginner but is, unfortunately, found with more advanced students. In the beginner it is caused by a weak undeveloped embouchure, but if the basic formation of the embouchure is correct and remains correct the undesirable tone will gradually disappear. In the more advanced student this tone quality may be caused by a reed which is too stiff. Ask the student to remove the reed from the instrument for examination, and play to find the double-crow. If an excessive amount of breath is required to blow the reed, or the double-crow is not controllable make the necessary adjustments on the reed as explained in the section on reeds. A further confirmation of the fact that the reed is too stiff can be made by asking the student to play a long crescendo to fortissimo followed by a long decrescendo to pianissimo. If the reed is too stiff he will be unable to play and/or control the tone in the pianissimo range.

If the reed itself is not the cause check for an embouchure formation which does not support the reed sufficiently to control the vibration of the reed. This can be verified by asking the student to play notes in the upper register since these notes are difficult if not impossible to produce without the proper amount of embouchure support around the reed. Appropriate correctional measures include practice of long tones and other exercises for embouchure development.

3. *Hard, Cold Tone.* A tone which is inflexible and which lacks the intangible quality of vitality is described as hard and cold. If embouchure formation is correct this tone quality is almost invariably caused by the type of reed being used, usually one which is too stiff for the student. If the usual adjustments on the reed to make it free blowing and responsive in all registers do not remedy the situation, try reeds which are made with a different cut. If the student is making his own reeds have him test with different cuts, or if the reeds he is using are commercial or custom-made try reeds from one or more different makers until a cut is found with which the student can produce a satisfactory tone. This is a difficult solution for some players since different cuts may require adjustments in embouchure formation and playing habits.

If the student is quite advanced and is playing well in tune with good tone quality except for the coldness of tone introducing the use of a tasteful vibration is a solution worth trying. Vibrato is discussed in another chapter. It is important that the use of the vibrato be restricted to advanced players.

4. *Weak, Colorless Tone.* A tone which is otherwise smooth in quality, but is lacking in body and carrying power is most often due to lack of proper breathing and breath support. Check the fundamentals of good breath usage with the student, and assign long tone practice with diminuendo and crescendo. The student will need to be told when he is producing the proper

sound so that he can associate his physical feeling with the desired sound. It is difficult for many even advanced players to know by listening to themselves when they are producing the proper tone quality and projection.

5. *Control of Soft Tone.* Difficulty in producing and controlling a soft tone is principally due to the inability of the player to project a steady concentrated small stream of air into the instrument. Check breathing and breath support, and have the student practice focusing a steady stream of air into the palm of his hand. Other possible causes may be a reed which is too stiff, or a poorly shaped embouchure.

6. *Dynamics and Tone Quality.* Some students with otherwise good tone quality will loose it when playing at extremes of loudness or softness. This is caused by an undeveloped or poorly formed embouchure, or by lack of proper breath control or a combination of both. In making a crescendo the embouchure must gradually relax to allow the tip of the reed to open while at the same time increasing the velocity of air. Good control is the product of the proper balance of these two factors, and if they are in the proper balance both tone quality and intonation will remain good. To play a diminuendo the embouchure may tighten slightly around the reed, while decreasing the velocity of air through the instrument, but being very careful to maintain a strong abdominal support of the air stream. To play a crescendo the embouchure may relax slightly around the reed while increasing the velocity of air through the instrument, maintaining proper abdominal support. With the best balance of abdominal support, air velocity, and embouchure control tone quality will remain the same at any dynamic level.

TONGUING

Tonguing refers to the manner in which the tongue operates in relation to the reed and breath support in order to articulate the tones. The placement and action of the tongue must be rapid and under complete control at all speeds, and at all dynamic levels. It must, in coordination with breath support, be able to produce on the bassoon all varieties of articulation from the hardest staccato to the softest legato.

The manner in which the tongue touches the reed, the place it touches, and how it moves is dependent somewhat upon embouchure formation. There are several points of view on how and where the tongue touches the reed but the differences are not as great as those on clarinet or oboe, and each is effective if properly done. In essence the tongue acts as a valve to control the flow of air through the reed, stopping the air flow and vibration of the reed when it touches the reed, and allowing the vibration to begin again when it is removed and the air flow is resumed. The effectiveness of the tongue is entirely dependent upon proper breath support and control. The inter-relation between breath

pressure and tongue action allows the production of every conceivable kind of attack from the hardest marcato-staccato to the very smoothest legato within the widest dynamic range. The amount of pressure of the tongue against the reed determines the hardness of the attack, the amount of wind pressure against the tongue determines the loudness of the attack.

There are two standard methods of tongue placement used on bassoon, each subject to small variations according to the personal desires of the teachers using them. Some authorities recommend that different parts of the tongue touch the reed for various types of articulation, a recommendation which makes a great deal of sense on a double-reed instrument. The tongue is simply a means to an end and the way it is used is not as important as the results obtained. No matter what placement and usage of the tongue is recommended certain basic principles are common to all: (1) the tongue is relaxed. A tongue under tension cannot move rapidly enough, nor can it be controlled; (2) tongue movement is confined to the forward part of the tongue; (3) the tongue acts as a valve for the air and is dependent on good breath support. The two most common approaches to tongue placement on the bassoon may be outlined as follows:

First Method. With the reed in place and the embouchure properly formed, touch the tip of the lower blade of the reed with the top of the tongue just back from the tip. A slight pressure against the reed closes the tip. To start the tone put the tongue in place against the reed and build up air pressure against it. Release the air into the instrument with a tongue action similar to that in pronouncing the syllable "too" or "tu." The center of the tongue is depressed slightly so that the throat is open and there is no obstruction to the free flow of air. For a harder attack pronounce the syllable "tee," and for a softer attack the syllable "du."

Second Method. With the reed in place and the embouchure properly formed, touch the tip of the reed with the tip of the tongue. The exact point of contact of the tip of the tongue with the reed varies from authority to authority and ranges from having the tongue close the tip of the reed by approaching it directly, to touching the lower blade as in the previous method but with the tip of the tongue. To start the tone, build up air pressure against the tongue while it is in contact with the reed, and release the air into the instrument with a tongue action similar to that in pronouncing the syllable "Tu." For a softer attack use the syllable "Du," and for a harder attack the syllable "Te."

Developing Tongue Action

For the purpose of developing articulation the position of the tongue against the reed is considered the normal position, for it is from this position that it starts the tone. There is no forward or upward movement of the tongue preceding the beginning of a tone since breath pressure is against the tongue and not the reed. The commonly used word "attack" to describe the articulation of a tone is most unfortunate since it implies both violence and forward movement. The action of the tongue may be gentle or hard depending on the type of articulation desired.

Various types of articulations demand varying lengths of silence between successive notes. The length of this silence is determined by how long the tongue remains in contact with the reed. Hardness of attack is determined by the breath pressure behind the tongue and by how hard the tongue is pressing against the reed. By varying the relationship between breath pressure and tongue pressure articulations which simulate the entire gamut of bow strokes used by string players can be reproduced on the bassoon.

The introduction of tonguing or articulation should be delayed until the student is producing a steady tone of reasonable quality, and has developed facility within the limited range of the beginner. Do not allow the tongue to touch the reed during this preliminary study, but simply start the tone with the breath. This requires that the beginning study be done with music of legato style, and eliminates the rhythmic approach to beginning study in favor of the melodic approach. If the rhythmic approach is used the articulation of quarter and eighth notes in the typical beginning method patterns must be done with the tongue and not the breath. Do not allow articulation with the breath alone for once this habit is established it is extremely difficult to break.

When the tongue is in the correct position against the reed and the study of articulation has begun, attention must be focused on breath support so that there is a steady stream through the reed upon which the tones rest. The tongue simply interrupts this movement of air through the instrument to detach the notes. The following example illustrates the legato style of articulation most successful as the beginning experience with articulation:

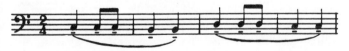

After the student is producing the legato articulation reasonably well, he can move to the normal detached sound in which the notes are well separated. There must be a continuing emphasis on a steady stream of air through the reed. The notes are separated simply by leaving the tongue in contact with the reed longer while breath support remains constant. This is the most common articulation and is used when no other articulation is indicated. It is, of course, varied according to the musical demands of the composition.

The example below illustrates a typical exercise for developing this type of articulation. This exercise may be practiced in scale patterns up and down or adapted to other note sequences in the playing range of the student.

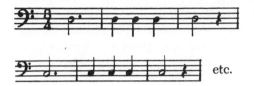

Staccato articulation should not be introduced until both the legato and normal detached articulations are well under control. The same tongue movement and placement and the same steady stream of air is used in staccato articulation. The only difference is that in staccato articulation the tongue returns to the reed to stop the vibration. It is essential that the air pressure against the tongue remain the same during the period of silence as during the production of the tone. Because of the longer period of silence between notes in this type of articulation students are frequently tempted to relax breath support during the silence. If this is done, then the breathing muscles come into operation simultaneously with tongue action, resulting in an accent and making it virtually impossible to develop a fast staccato. For this reason the first introduction to staccato can well utilize as rapidly repeated notes as the student can produce, as well as slower repetition. A typical beginning staccato exercise can be constructed as follows:

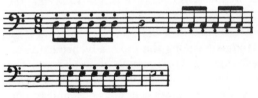

Common Problems in Tonguing

1. *Articulation too Heavy.* In this type of sound each note starts with an accent or pop, and is normally caused by too great pressure of the tongue against the reed. The best solution is to have the student practice articulation at the pianissimo level, correcting first the legato type, then the normal detached, and finally the staccato. A reed which is too soft will frequently produce this sound, since the blades do not respond instantly when released by the tongue. If pianissimo practice does not correct this difficulty it is possible that the placement of the tongue against the reed is incorrect for the embouchure and type of reed being used. Experiment by changing the part of the tongue which contacts the reed to see if a slightly different placement will remedy the situation.

2. *Sluggish Tongue.* Inability to tongue rapidly should not be a major concern with beginners, since time and practice are necessary to develop speedy articulation. In more advanced players where technique has developed past articulation ability, sluggish articulation is a matter of considerable concern. In this condition the reed should be checked first, since a reed which is too stiff for the player makes rapid articulation difficult. If the reed is too stiff there will probably be other symptoms in addition to sluggish response in articulation.

Some students lack speed in articulation because they are moving the back or middle of their tongue as well as the front. Articulation is confined to the forward portion of the tongue, and the primary motion of the tongue is up and down rather than forward and backward in the mouth. Movement of the back portion of the tongue almost invariably carries with it movements of the throat which can be seen. To correct, the entire process of tongue placement and development of articulation must be repeated from the very beginning to form new muscular habits. Some students correct the problem quickly, others are never able to completely overcome the problem.

Sluggish tonguing in most instances is a simple matter of insufficient practice devoted to developing speed and accuracy. Special articulation exercises should be assigned to these students, with specific instructions on how many times each day to practice them, to use a metronome, and with specific metronomic speeds to follow. Any player can develop satisfactory speed and control if he is using his tongue and breath support properly and if he will spend enough time on the problem.

3. *Lack of Coordination Between Tongue and Fingers.* This is frequent among the more advanced players who have developed a fair amount of facility on the instrument. It is purely and simply a product of practicing too fast without first working out notes and tonguing carefully. These students must practice slowly, at whatever tempo perfect coordination between fingers and tongue is possible, and gradually increase the speed. Use of a metronome on such exercises is invaluable to maintain a steady tempo and to help in the gradual increase in speed. Major and minor scales and arpeggios making use of various articulation patterns are good media of practice for this purpose.

4. *Slow Staccato.* Some players have difficulty in executing a true staccato rapidly even though other articulations are executed with sufficient speed. Other things being correct, this problem can be traced to the lack of breath support and a continuing stream of air through the reed. Such players will be found to be relaxing abdominal support at the end of each note, or cutting off the stream of air in the throat. The concept of the tongue stopping staccato notes as well as

starting them with the breath pressure continuing against the tongue during the space of silence will help correct this situation. An improperly adjusted reed will also make rapid staccato impossible, particularly in the low and lower middle registers. Adjust according to directions in the section on reeds.

5. *Movement of the jaw in tonguing.* This is the result of too large or too violent movement of the tongue, frequently accompanied by changes in pitch of the tone. Rather than confine the movement to the front part of the tongue, the student is moving the entire tongue. The solution is to ask the student, no matter what his technical advancement may be, to practice the basic exercises for developing articulation constantly checking in a mirror on the music stand to eliminate all movements. Jaw movements can occur with all methods of correct tongue placement, as well as with incorrect tongue placement, and prevent the development of speed in articulation.

Additional Aspects of Articulation

1. *Double and Triple Tonguing.* Theoretically, double and triple tonguing in the sense of its use on brass instruments is possible on the bassoon, but in practice it is very unsatisfactory because it is virtually impossible to match the sounds of the beginnings of the two notes in the double pattern or the three notes in the triple pattern. The double tonguing is done by using the syllables "Tu-Ku" in rapid alternation, the "Tu" with the tongue in its normal position on the reed and the "Ku" pronounced with the middle of the tongue against the roof of the mouth. Some authorities recommend the syllables "Ti-Ki" because they put more of an arch in the position of the tongue putting it in a better position for the "K" attack. Triple tonguing uses the syllables "Tu-Ku-Tu" or "Tu-Tu-Ku" (Ti-Ki-Ti or Ti-Ti-Ki) in rapid succession. Both double and triple tonguing are useful only in the most rapidly moving passages. Most bassoonists prefer to develop the speed and control of single tonguing to the point where it is used exclusively for both normal and the most rapid articulations. Authorities agree that bassoon students need not be taught double or triple tonguing.

2. *Flutter Tonguing.* Flutter tonguing, produced by rolling an "R" so that the tongue flutters against the reed is called for in a few contemporary compositions. It is an adaptation to woodwinds of the technique which is common and easy on the brass instruments. Among the woodwinds, the flute is the most successful in producing the flutter tongue sound. Some relaxation of the embouchure and complete relaxation of the tongue is necessary to achieve this effect.

3. *Accents, Sforzando, Forte-piano.* Accents, sforzando, and forte-piano notes must be played in relation to the dynamic level of the musical phrase. A sforzando is not a note played as loudly as it is possible to play,

but simply an isolated note one or two degrees louder than the notes which precede or follow it in the phrase. It demands assistance from the breath so that the breathing mechanism supplies additional support and velocity simultaneously with the release of the reed by the tongue.

The forte-piano requires immediately relaxation of velocity and pressure by the breathing mechanism, coupled with whatever degree of simultaneous support at the instant the tone starts demanded by the musical content of the phrase. Accents indicated above or below the notes must be only one dynamic level above the notes which precede or follow them. Many accents may be accomplished by only increased tongue pressure against the reed, others demand slight movements of the breathing muscles. It must be clearly understood that there are no rapid movements of any breathing muscles in support of tongue action except for accents, sforzando, and forte-piano notes.

TECHNIQUE PROBLEMS

A good technical proficiency on the instrument is one which is accurate, under complete control, facile and which permits the performance of all types of musical demands with ease. In developing this proficiency the bassoonist must be aware of certain mechanical or technical problems peculiar to his instrument which must be solved. In teaching, both the importance of the correct solution and the reason for that particular solution must be impressed on the student. Unfortunately the literature for the study of the bassoon does not provide a particularly well organized presentation of these problems, so it is incumbent upon the teacher to take every opportunity to include them in the instruction of his students.

Approached logically, these problems are not difficult to identify, nor complex to solve and put into use. Many of these technical problems demand that the player make a choice between two or more alternatives. Each alternate must be practiced until it becomes an involuntary part of his technical facility and the way and place in which each alternative is used must be made so much a part of his technique that the correct choice becomes automatic. Other technical problems are matters of procedure. Players and teachers should not hesitate to mark instructions on the printed music as reminders.

Following are problems which occur frequently:

1. *Left Thumb.* A good portion of the smoothness of technique which the bassoonist develops is dependent in good measure upon how the left thumb is used. With so many keys to operate considerable dexterity in manipulation is required. The position of the left hand should be checked to see that the wrist is almost flat and that the fingers and thumbs can reach their proper

positions without muscular tension. In playing the notes in the low register of the instrument the forward half or two-thirds of the thumb is used so that each of the four keys involved can be depressed with an absolute minimum of sliding. The D and C keys are depressed by the thumb under the first joint, and the thumb is then rolled to the B and B-flat keys. Avoid sliding the thumb to these keys, although under normal usage the thumb must be slid from the D to the C key. The keys toward the tip of the thumb are depressed with the portion of the thumb near the tip. The thumb moves in a slight arc in order to contact all of these keys most efficiently.

2. *Whisper Key.* The whisper key (sometimes called the pianissimo key) operated by the left thumb which opens and closes the small vent hole in the bocal of the bassoon is a fairly recent addition to the instrument. Some schools and players may have instruments without this valuable aid to playing tones in the upper middle register. It is not an octave key as on the saxophone and oboe, nor a register key as on the clarinet which force a node in the vibrating air column of the instrument. The hole in the bocal of the bassoon is much too small in diameter to do this, but when it is open it does relieve pressure on the air column at this point sufficiently to help the affected notes sound more clearly. Changes in octaves which use the same fingering are controlled primarily by the embouchure and not the whisper key (see use of half-hole below).

The whisper key is closed by the left thumb on all notes in this range:

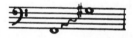

Use of the whisper key is optional on certain notes in the high register which speak better on some instruments when it is closed. Experimentation with an individual player on his instrument is necessary to discover when the key should or should not be used in the high register.

The whisper key is automatically closed when the right thumb depresses the E key, and it is well to develop the habit of removing the left thumb from the whisper key when the right thumb is on this key. This frees the left thumb and makes it instantly available for use on another key.

Many beginners on the instrument neglect to use the whisper key properly since to them the instrument seems to respond just as well without it as with it. Teachers should be alert to this situation because as his facility and tone production develops use of this key becomes absolutely necessary if the best results are to be obtained.

3. *First Finger Half Hole.* The standard fingering for these three notes calls for the first finger to cover only half of its hole:

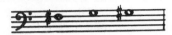

A similar half-hole technique is found as standard procedure on the oboe, and under certain circumstances on the clarinet. Opening the hole half way helps force a node in the vibrating column of air making pitch and intonation more secure. The young bassoonist will soon find that the notes respond when the finger is completely off the hole (as on the flute) as well as when half of the hole is covered. A more advanced bassoonist will know and hear a difference in both tone quality and intonation between a half-hole and a completely open hole. For this reason the teacher must insist on the proper use of the half-hole from the very beginning, for it is difficult to start using it after technique has been developed.

In rapidly moving passages where the tone is not exposed sufficiently to make a firm impression of pitch and quality more advanced students make an exception to this rule. In this circumstance the finger may be taken completely off the hole rather than rolled to the half-hole position in order to facilitate technique. Like the whisper key, use of the half-hole is optional on certain notes in the high register, depending on the player and the instrument being used. Experimentation is necessary to discover when and where it is best used in this register.

4. *Use of Little Fingers.* With only two keys to operate with the left little finger and three with the right, the little fingers have a much simpler operation on bassoon than on the clarinet and oboe. Fingers must be kept in a slight curve to depress the keys rapidly and without muscular tension. Occasionally the little finger will have to be used on different keys on successive notes in spite of the fact that there are alternate fingerings available for some of the notes involved. If there is a satisfactory alternate fingering it is always used in preference to sliding a finger. But if it is necessary to slide the little finger from one key to another make use of the rollers placed on the keys for this purpose. In sliding from one key to the other, keep the finger slightly curved and continue the downward pressure while quickly sliding the finger over the rollers to the next key. The right little finger is never slid from the F to the F-sharp key or vice versa. Rather the regular F-sharp key played with the right thumb is used.

5. *High Register.* Notes in the upper range of the high register are played with difficulty by many students. They should not be attempted nor should students be expected to play these notes until the other registers are well established and they are playing easily with a full tone. A reed which is too soft will make these high notes difficult or impossible to play. An embouchure which is incorrectly formed or immature in development will cause similar difficulties. If the embouchure is well formed and the reed stiff enough, playing these notes can be facilitated by taking more reed into the mouth, even to the extent that the upper lip is actually touching the first wire on the reed. This, combined with a more intense stream of air and firm support around the reed by the lips will help these notes respond with good quality and well in tune. There are many alternate fingerings in this register and the player should try all of them to see which responds with best tone quality and is best in tune for him.

6. *Flick Keys.* Flick keys, or flip keys as they are sometimes known are used to facilitate slurring from notes in the low and lower middle registers to certain notes in the upper middle register. Keys a' and b' operated by the left thumb are used as flick keys. This example shows the notes on which the flick keys may be used for slurring:

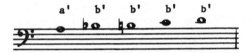

The flick keys function as a momentary vent to help the vibrating column of air break into the proper vibrating segments. The left thumb flicks or flips the key so that it is open for just an instant at the beginning of the note. If the thumb stays on the flick key too long the note doesn't respond at all or responds out of tune. Intermediate students can learn this technique easily, and it is a must for advanced students. Some teachers have been successful in teaching it to students in the beginning level to help them learn a perfect slur to these notes.

A typical use of the flick keys is in octave slurs:

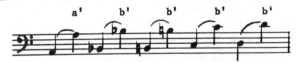

7. *Use of Alternate Fingerings.* Alternate fingerings are provided on an instrument to facilitate technique, and they are selected for use on the basis of ease and smoothness of technical facility as well as tone quality and intonation. There are four notes in the middle registers of the bassoon for which there are two fingerings. Use of both of these fingerings, together with the conditions under which each is used is a desirable part of bassoon instruction on the beginning level. If their introduction and use is delayed the student has developed poor habits of sliding fingers unnecessarily which are difficult to correct.

(a) F-sharp—G-flat: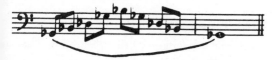

> Regular Fingering: 123 F♯ 456 (Right thumb on F-sharp key)
>
> Alternate Fingering: 123 456 F♯ (Right little finger on F-sharp key)

The regular fingering is used except when the right thumb is needed as part of the fingering of the note which precedes or follows the F-sharp. The most common occurrence of the alternate fingering is when the F-sharp is preceded or followed by an A-sharp, or when G-flat is preceded or followed by a B-flat. A typical use of the alternate fingering on all G-flat's is the following arpeggio. Use of the half-hole for the upper octave, and the whisper key for the lower is necessary

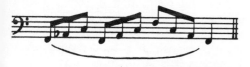

(b) *G-sharp—A-flat:*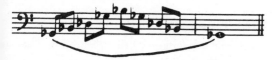

> Regular Fingering: 123 456 G-sharp (Right little finger on G-sharp key)
>
> Alternate Fingering: 123 G-sharp 456 (Right thumb on G-sharp key)

Use of the whisper key on the lower octave and the half-hole on the upper octave is necessary in addition to the fingering indicated. The regular fingering for G-sharp is always used except when the right little finger is needed on another key as part of the fingering for the note which precedes or follows the G-sharp. The most common usage of the alternate fingering is in the lower octave when the G-sharp or A-flat precedes or follows the low F. This passage shows a typical use of the alternate fingering:

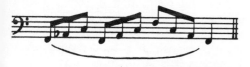

(c) *A-sharp—B-flat:*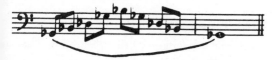

> Regular Fingering: 123 A-sharp 450 (Right thumb on B-flat key)
>
> Alternate Fingering: 123 456x (Sixth finger on B-flat key)

Use of the whisper key on the lower octave is necessary in addition to the fingering indicated. The regular

fingering must always be used when the sixth finger must cover its tone hole as part of the fingering of the note following or preceding. Many students learn the alternate fingering as their standard fingering and treat the thumb B-flat as an alternate. This procedure causes many problems and teachers should be on the lookout for students who are doing this. Situations arise in the music when no matter which fingering is selected either the thumb or sixth finger must slide to the next note. This forces the choice of whether it is better to slide the sixth finger from the B-flat key to the tone hole, or to slide the thumb from the B-flat key to another key. Practices vary in this situation, but most students are able to develop facility in sliding the sixth finger easier than attempting to slide the thumb, although the thumb slides naturally from the B-flat key to the E key. The alternate fingering is used primarily as a chromatic fingering and for trills involving B-flat. The following is a typical passage where the alternate fingering is used:

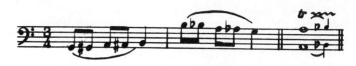

(d) *D-sharp—E-flat:*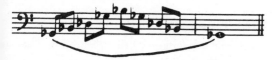

> Regular Fingering: W 103 000
> Alternate Fingering: W 120 000
> c♯

The problems in choosing between these two fingerings are as frequently found in tone quality and intonation as in technical facility. The regular fingering tends to be out of tune and stuffy sounding with beginning bassoonists whose embouchure has not developed and who may be playing on a reed which is not properly adjusted (usually too stiff for them). For this reason, many beginners will use the alternate fingering to get the best quality and intonation rather than for facility. Students should be encouraged to use the regular fingering in spite of how it sounds until they have developed the proper tone quality and intonation. The alternate fingering is used for smoothness in technique, and is mandatory for the trill from D to E-flat.

8. *Tenor Clef.* Because of the extremely wide range of the bassoon a large number of leger lines are necessary when musical passages in the highest portion of the range are rotated in the base clef. To avoid excessive leger lines the tenor clef is used in this range to make note reading easier. All bassoonists past the beginning stage should be able to read tenor clef, and in the course of their progress on the instrument should develop reading facility in this clef equal to that in the bass clef. The teacher should be sure that the tenor clef is introduced as soon as the student is playing in the

upper register. The standard intermediate methods use some tenor clef, and all advanced studies for the instrument make use of it. If additional material is needed to develop facility in reading, useful studies can be found in both the cello and trombone literature.

9. *Alto Clef.* The alto clef is rarely found in bassoon literature, and while the player should have knowledge of it, it is not considered necessary to develop equal facility with the other two clefs. Advanced players will find trombone literature useful in developing facility in both the alto and tenor clefs.

SELECTION OF INSTRUMENTS

Although the bassoon is historically one of the oldest of the woodwind instruments its fingering system is considerably less refined than any of them.[3] The system of fingering used in this country is the Heckel system, developed over a period of years by the Heckel Company in Germany. It is commonly conceded that those instruments made by the Heckel Company are the finest available. Other companies make Heckel system bassoons under their own trade names. While the finest clarinets and oboes available today are made in France, most bassoons are made in Germany. The reason for this is the fact that the French have a different fingering system called the French system which differs greatly both mechanically and tonally with the Heckel system. The French system is not used in this country, and should be avoided when purchasing an instrument.

The standard model bassoon is the Heckel system with twenty-two keys. Some older bassoons which are still in use have only twenty-one keys, lacking the whisper key which is now considered an integral part of the mechanism. Bassoons are made of maple rather than the grenadilla wood used in clarinets and oboes. The wood is sealed inside and out and the outside of the instrument is stained mahogany and finished as are fine pieces of furniture with several coats of lacquer to seal the wood against moisture. An interesting deviation from the standard mahogany color is a fine American made instrument which is available in an ebony color finish. The interior of the instrument is specially treated to seal it against moisture. Virtually all instruments now have the tenor joint lined with rubber or a plastic substance to further seal it against moisture, and the small side of the butt joint is lined either with metal or rubber. These inner linings protect the instrument against moisture in the places where moisture tends to collect, and as a result cracks in the wood of a bassoon are considerably less frequent than in the wood of an oboe or clarinet. All instruments purchased for school use should have these inner linings.

The variety of models of bassoons available, unlike the oboe for example, is practically nil. If an instrument other than the standard twenty-two key Heckel system is desired, extra keys can be added on order from the factory, or added to the instrument after it is received by an expert repairman. The most useful of these additional keys is the high D key which is added to the tenor joint above the b′ key operated by the left thumb, and used for slurring to D second space above the bass clef. This key is a widely used addition to the instrument and is recommended for advanced players.

Other refinements of the mechanism which are found but rarely include a locking mechanism for the whisper key which locks the key in place leaving the left thumb free to operate other keys, an A-flat to B-flat trill key added to the cluster of keys played by the right thumb, etc. None of these and many others available are recommended for school use since the need for them is so limited, and they add complexity to the already complex key system of the instrument.

STUDENT QUALIFICATIONS AND APTITUDES

The bassoon is not a beginning instrument. The best criteria for advisability of study of the bassoon is the demonstration of fine tone production and basic technique on another woodwind instrument. The clarinet is an excellent pre-bassoon instrument. Physical size of the potential student is of primary importance because of the long reaches and stretches demanded of the fingers in playing the instrument. Most students younger than seventh grade are not physically large enough to play the instrument, and are best started on another woodwind and then transferred to the bassoon. In addition to size physical qualifications which will prove to be of advantage include fairly even teeth, an upper lip which is not too short to cover the teeth comfortably, a natural or greater than natural overbite (students with an underbite or protruding lower jaw have difficulty with the instrument), and fingers of normal or longer length.

A natural aptitude for the bassoon may be determined by his success in producing a good double crow on a reed adjusted and prepared for playing by the instructor after some brief instruction on embouchure formation and how to produce the crow. Students who are not immediately successful in producing the crow may, with instruction, soon exhibit a good natural aptitude. In the final analysis it is not natural aptitude but desire and persistence which are the greatest of all aptitudes for any instrument.

CARE OF THE BASSOON

The instrument must be assembled and disassembled with the greatest of care. Review the instructions on assembly of the instrument until they are thoroughly understood and the students are performing the operation

---

[3]For an interesting history of the development of the instrument see Langwill, Lyndesay. *The Bassoon and Double Bassoon.* London: Hinrichen, Ltd. n.d.

easily. Keep the instrument in its case when not in use. The instrument is damaged by excess heat. Keep the instrument either in or out of the case out of the direct sun and away from all sources of heat. It is basic to good care of the instrument that it be thoroughly dried after each playing, and the habit of doing this thoroughly should be developed from the very first. The process of swabbing does not take much time, and will keep the instrument in good condition and maintain sanitary conditions for playing.

Swabs

The type of swab used and the way in which it is used determines the thoroughness with which the instrument is dried inside. Various kinds of swabs are used in cleaning the instrument, and the player chooses the type he likes best. These are described below.

1. *Wool Swabs.* Figure B-27 shows the pair of wool swabs which are the traditional type used for bassoon. The two sizes are to fit the large and small sections of the instrument. These have the advantage of maximum convenience in use, but must be used with care. The wire on which the wool is mounted can and does scratch the bore of the instrument unless handled carefully.

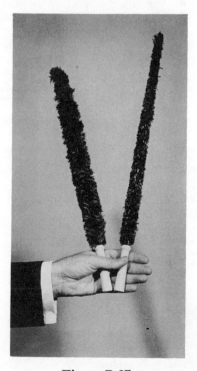

Figure B-27.

2. *Cleaning Rod.* Use of an aluminum cleaning rod similar to the rod used in cleaning the flute is an excellent method of cleaning the bassoon. A piece of silk or soft lint-free cotton cloth of the dimensions shown in

Figure B-28 is used. The small end of the cloth is pulled through the opening in the rod. To clean the tenor joint the rod is used as a weight to carry the cloth through the joint. To clean the butt joint the cloth is wrapped around the rod.

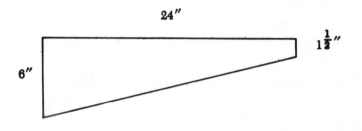

Figure B-28.

First put a corner of the large end through as in Figure B-29. Pull the cloth up and over the end as in Figure B-30 and wrap the cloth loosely around the rod as shown in Figure B-31. Continue winding until all the cloth is around the rod, and hold the end against the rod with the forefinger while cleaning the butt joint.

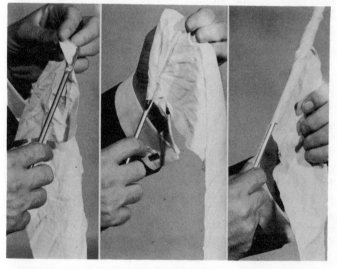

Figure B-29.   **Figure B-30.**   **Figure B-31.**

3. *Cloth and Drop Cord.* A small piece of soft lint-free cloth, or a small triangle of chamois tied to a weighted drop cord similar to the typical clarinet swab is sometimes used for cleaning the tenor joint. The cord must be long enough to drop completely through the tenor joint. The cord and cloth must *not* be pulled through the butt joint because of the small rods which go through the instrument to articulate keys on either side of the joint. The cloth can be pushed down into the butt joint with the end of a wool swab to the end

and pulled out by the string simultaneously with the wool swab.

To summarize the pair of wool swabs traditionally used for cleaning the inside of the bassoon while the most convenient may damage the bore by scratching it and as they wear will drop lint into the bore and tone holes. The cleaning rod is recommended by a majority of bassoon teachers as it gives maximum flexibility to clean all parts equally well and the cloth used can be kept clean and lint-free. The cloth and drop cord are frequently combined with the cleaning rod and is used instead of the rod for drying the tenor joint.

4. *Bocal Brush.* A small brush about a half-inch in diameter mounted on a long flexible wire designed specifically to clean the inside of the bassoon bocal. Because of its shape, small diameter, and location next to the reed the bocal is much more susceptible to the accumulation of sediment than other parts of the instrument. If allowed to accumulate this sediment soon changes the size and shape of the bore and makes playing more difficult and uncertain. Regular use of the bocal brush and an occasional washing out with lukewarm water will keep the bocal clean and free blowing.

Cleaning the Bassoon

The following step-by-step process in cleaning the instrument is an efficient one which should be taught the student from the very beginning. As he gains experience he can adapt the process to his personal liking.

1. Take the instrument apart in reverse order of assembly, holding each part exactly as it was held during the process of assembling the instrument. As each joint is removed shake any moisture out of the ends. Place the parts carefully in the case before beginning the swabbing process.

2. Shake the moisture out of the bocal from both ends. Blow through it from the large end to force water out. Clean thoroughly with the bocal brush. The small end may be cleaned with a pipe cleaner (Figure B-32) on which the end has been bent to keep it from falling through. In addition to regular use of the bocal brush once each week or so the bocal should be thoroughly cleaned by running a stream of lukewarm water through it.

3. Using the type of swab selected, dry the tenor joint. If a cloth and drop cord are being used drop the weight from the small end (Figure B-33). Pull the cloth through a couple of times being very careful that it does not snag the key which protrudes from the top. (Figure B-34.) If a cleaning rod and cloth are being used the rod is dropped into the joint from the top and the cloth pulled through a couple of times. If wool swabs are used the smaller wool swab is inserted from the large end of the joint (Figure B-35) and pushed back and forth to clean.

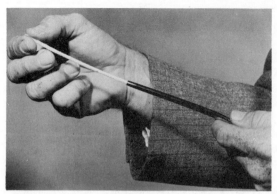

Figure B-32.

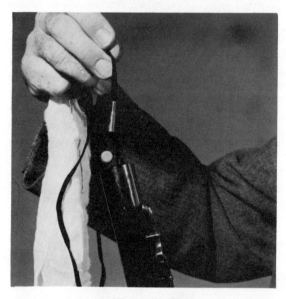

Figure B-33.

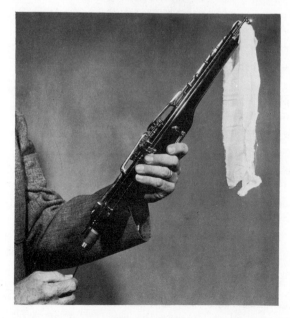

Figure B-34.

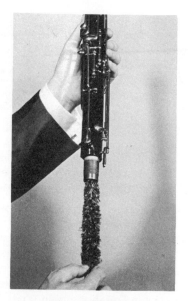

Figure B-35.

4. Shake excess water from the small side of the butt joint. The small side of the joint is cleaned first with the smaller of the wool swabs, or with the cleaning rod on which the cloth has been wound as described. (Figure B-36.) Be sure to hold the end of the cloth with the fingers so that it will not unwind on the rod.

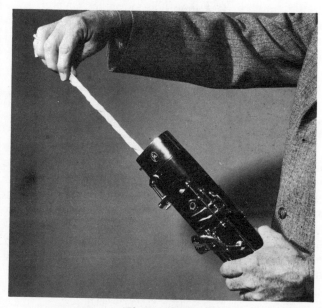

Figure B-36.

5. The larger side of the butt joint is cleaned with the larger of the two wool swabs (Figure B-37) or with the cleaning rod and cloth. Even though very little water collects in this side of the joint it should be cleaned as a matter of precaution.

6. The long joint and the bell rarely collect moisture but should be cleaned occasionally. They are cleaned with the larger of the two wool swabs (Figure B-38) or by the cloth and drop cord or the cleaning rod used as they were on the tenor joint.

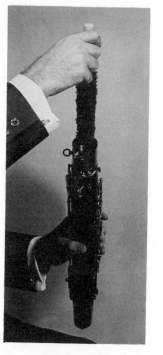

Figure B-37.   **Figure B-38.**

7. Because of the way in which the tone holes for the fingers are bored into the body of the instrument water sometimes collects in them. The first tone hole on the tenor joint is especially susceptible. During rehearsal or performance this water must be blown out. If there is sufficient time the hole affected can be dried with a pipe cleaner and the joint thoroughly swabbed as described.

8. With a soft cloth or chamois wipe the outside of the wood and keys to remove moisture and fingerprints. Place the instrument carefully in the case checking to see that each joint is properly positioned with the right side up.

9. Blow the moisture out of the reed and place it carefully in a reed case so that it can dry properly. The inside of the reed should be cleaned once a week by drawing a wet pipe cleaner through it carefully. Insert the cleaner from the bottom of the reed and pull it carefully out of the tip. Move cleaner from side to side as it is being pulled through to clean the entire surface of the blades. Repeat the process several times. Be very careful not to reverse the direction of the cleaner as it will damage the tip of the reed. A quick way to clean the reed is to run lukewarm or cold water through

it from a tap. The pressure of the stream of water will force out accumulation although this is not a good substitute for the pipe cleaner.

Regular Maintenance of the Instrument

1. *Oiling the Mechanism.* The mechanism, if it is to remain in the best playing condition, must be oiled regularly three or four times a year. Special oil, called key oil, is available for this purpose. A drop of oil on the end of a needle or toothpick should be put at each pivot screw of each key. Do this carefully so that no oil gets on the pads. This regular oiling keeps pivot screws from excessive wear and from rusting into place, making repairs and adjustments on the instrument easier.

2. *Dusting the Instrument.* After the instrument has been in use over a period of time, dust collects under the key mechanism. This can and should be removed with a soft water-color brush. A cloth should never be used for this purpose.

3. *Shining the Keys.* Keys will be kept in good condition if they are wiped regularly and gently with a soft cloth or chamois to remove perspiration and dirt as directed in the previous section. This will not only keep the keys from tarnishing, but will prevent corrosion of the plating in the event the player perspires excessively. Silver polish must never be used on the keys, nor should the keys ever be polished while on the instrument. Using silver polish while the keys are on the instrument will clog pivot screws in the mechanism and damage pads so that they will leak. Leave polishing up to a competent repairman. Caution student against polishing the keys, but give them careful instructions to keep the instrument clean by wiping the keys.

4. *Bent Keys.* In spite of the best of care, keys sometimes become bent out of line causing unevenness in technique, or even preventing certain tones from responding at all. No attempt should be made to straighten keys or rods while they are on the instrument. This puts excessive pressure on both keys and their posts and the instrument may be damaged even more. Keys must be adjusted by a repairman who has the proper tools to straighten and align them.

5. *Sticking Pads.* If the instrument is not thoroughly dried before it is put into the case, or if the humidity is excessive even temporarily some pads on the instrument may stick tightly, or will stick momentarily before opening. This sticking can frequently be eliminated by placing a cigarette paper between the pad and the tone hole and pressing the key down firmly. Release the key, move the paper, and repeat the process until the key no longer sticks. If this does not relieve the sticking, put the cigarette paper in place, press the key, and pull the paper slowly from under the pad. Repeat the process several times.

If the cigarette paper does not relieve the sticking dip the end of a pipe cleaner into a cleaning fluid such as carbon tetrachloride, benzine or denatured alcohol. Wipe the pad with this fluid, and dry thoroughly with another pipe cleaner. Since this removes the natural oil from the pad, replace the oil by putting a very light coat of key oil over the pad with a pipe cleaner. Wipe off excess key oil with a dry pipe cleaner.

If none of these processes relieves the sticking, the pad should be replaced. Never use powder on pads in an attempt to stop sticking. It is rarely successful and damages the pad so that it begins to deteriorate rapidly.

6. *Leaky Pads.* Pads on instruments wear out with use. Some wear out more rapidly than others and begin to leak, causing the instrument to respond with difficulty on certain notes. Other pads which are in good condition may leak because they are improperly seated over the tone holes. If some notes respond with difficulty, with a change in tone quality and intonation in comparison with surrounding notes, there is a strong possibility of a leak in the instrument. Finding the exact source of the leak on a bassoon is somewhat more awkward than a similar operation on clarinet or flute.

To test for leaks take the instrument apart. Close one end of the joint to be tested with a cork or the palm of the hand, cover tone holes and close all keys as if playing and blow through the other end with as much pressure as possible. Leaky pads can be identified by the air leaking through. If a tone hole normally covered by a pad held closed by a spring leaks when maximum pressure is applied during the test, the spring on that key must be strengthened or replaced by a repairman. A joint in perfect condition will not leak no matter how much breath pressure is applied.

If the leak is located an examination of the pad will determine whether it should be replaced or simply reseated. Accuracy in seating pads is determined best by the use of commercial feeler papers or strips of cigarette papers about a quarter inch wide. Slide one end of the paper under the pad, put the normal amount of pressure against the pad if the key is not held closed by a spring, and slowly draw the paper out. As long as the pressure against the paper remains constant there is no leak. If the pressure suddenly lessens the pad is not properly seated. Repeat the process completely around the pad so that all edges are tested.

The process of blowing cigarette smoke through the instrument to identify a leak by seeing the smoke come out of the leak is not recommended. The nicotine in the smoke coats the pads and if this is done frequently will damage them so that they harden and leak. Repairmen use a small light in the bore of the instrument to find leaks as the light will shine through the open space of the leak.

7. *Regular Overhaul.* The condition of every instrument must be checked at least once each year by the instructor or by a repairman. Regular maintenance keeps an instrument in good playing condition over a period of years, rather than allowing it to gradually deteriorate and become increasingly difficult to play. Every instrument must have a complete overhaul every three to five years depending on amount of usage. If fine instruments receive a yearly checkup and regular overhaul they will last in virtually perfect condition for many years. The services of a competent repairman are invaluable and an asset to any program of instrumental instruction.

ACCESSORIES

There are certain accessories for the bassoon which are designed to make performance easier or more convenient for the player, or to protect the instrument against damage. The most common of these are discussed in the following.

Neck Strap. The traditional suspension of the instrument is by a neck strap which supports the instrument and which makes use of the right hand in the hand rest. Use of the hand rest is mandatory when a neck strap is used. Neck straps may be thick cords, or may have a wide leather neck piece which is more comfortable for the student as the cord around the neck frequently becomes uncomfortable when playing for long periods of time. The strap must be adjustable so that the instrument may be easily adjusted to the proper playing position, and the adjusting mechanism such that it will not gradually slip when the weight of the instrument is put on it. The instructor will need to check the condition of neck straps occasionally as they wear and do not stay in adjustment. This wear is so gradual that the students are frequently not aware of the problem and their playing suffers.

Seat Strap. A seat strap rather than a neck strap is becoming more and more widely used to support the weight of the instrument. This type of suspension of the instrument is advantageous in that it removes the weight of the instrument from the neck, and relieves the right hand of the necessity of assisting in the support of the instrument. A seat strap is simply a belt with a snap on the end which snaps into a ring holder on the cap at the bottom of the butt joint. The belt is placed over the chair, the amount of strap over the edge of the chair adjusted to hold the bassoon at the right height, and the player sits on the belt to keep it from slipping.

Bassoons do not come from the factory equipped for the use of a seat strap—they must be altered for this type of suspension. The most simple alteration is the addition of a metal band with a ring over the cap of the butt joint. This can be easily added by the student or the instructor, and the seat strap snaps into the ring

to support the instrument. These add-on metal ring holders are commercially available and are not expensive.

Some bassoonists prefer to alter the cap on the butt end of the instrument by drilling a hole in the rib at the bottom and attaching a ring holder through the hole. This must be done by a professional repairman since special drilling tools are necessary.

The right hand rest is not used with the seat strap, freeing the right hand from its restrictive influence. It is desirable that a plate similar to the right-hand thumb plate be added to the instrument on which the first finger of the right hand can rest. On some bassoons the thumb rest can be shifted to serve this function, although it is advisable that it be left in place since the neck strap and the normal hand-rest for the right hand will be needed for playing the instrument in a standing position. A competent repairman can add the first finger rest plate. A protective plate over the A-sharp and F-sharp keys on the bottom of the butt joint is also a desirable addition when the instrument is adapted to the seat strap.

Floor Stand. Two types of floor stands may be used with the bassoon. The first type is used to hold the instrument safely when it is not being played. The bassoon is held in a fairly upright position so that water does not run into the holes, and the stand protects the instrument from possible damage through being knocked off of a chair, or stepped on if it is placed on the floor. This type of stand is highly recommended for safety of the instrument and is not expensive. Models are available which fold up compactly for convenience in carrying, although they will not fit inside the normal bassoon case.

The second type of floor stand holds the instrument in playing position so that neither a neck or seat strap is necessary. It functions similarly to the stand whcih holds the baritone saxophone in playing position. Regular use of this type of stand is not recommended for school use as it tends to put the student into an awkward and somewhat unnatural playing position. Use of this type of stand is normally used only by players in studio-type orchestras who are doubling on several instruments and must have them in position for rapid changes from one to another.

BIBLIOGRAPHY OF STUDY MATERIALS

In comparison to that available for the other woodwind instruments study material written especially for bassoon is meager. And unless it is carefully selected tends to lack stylistic variety and is frequently downright uninteresting. For this reason the wise instructor will make generous use of appropriate materials written for cello and trombone which frequently is ideal for bassoon when appropriate phrasing is added to put it into the woodwind idiom.

So that the student will have a well-rounded and interesting course of study which will achieve the most rapid advancement both technically and musically it is recommended that he be studying simultaneously from material in each of these classifications: (1) a method book for continuity and basics; (2) technical studies such as major and minor scales, arpeggios, etc., in various forms and keys; (3) a book of etudes or studies to include various musical styles over a period of time; (4) duets and/or other ensemble experience; and (5) solos with piano accompaniment.

Information about solos, duets and other types of ensembles making use of the bassoon is widely available in such places as the Selective Lists of Instrumental Solos and Ensembles published by the National Inter-scholastic Music Activities Commission. Considerable information about the availability of solos and ensembles as well as other classifications of material for bassoon can be obtained from the catalogs of retail stores specializing in woodwind music.[4] A study of these catalogs will reveal far more material than is commonly known, although still not too extensive.

In the sections which follow a cross-section of the most widely available material (exclusive of solo and ensemble music) for bassoon is listed. These lists are divided into beginning methods, standard methods, and additional study materials of various kinds. A listing of composers, titles, and publishers such as is given here and in the other sources mentioned is only the starting point for acquiring teaching materials. Only personal acquaintance with the music itself can give the answer to the quality of music, and how and when it could be used. The reader is urged to examine as many of these titles as possible, and to evaluate them whenever possible through actual use.

Beginning Methods

Anzalone, V. *Breeze-Easy Method for Bassoon.* Two Volumes. Witmark.

Buck, Lawrence. *Elementary Method for Bassoon.* Neil A. Kjos.

Herfurth-Stuart. *A Tune A Day for Bassoon.* Boston Music Co.

Lentz, Don. *Method for Bassoon.* Two Volumes. Belwin, Inc.

Skornicka, J. E. *Elementary Method for Bassoon.* Rubank, Inc.

Voxman, H. *Intermediate Method for Bassoon.* Rubank, Inc.

Voxman, H. & W. Gower. *Advanced Method for Bassoon.* Two Volumes. Rubank, Inc.

Standard Methods

Bourdeau, E. *Grande Methode Complete de Bassoon.* Leduc. Text in English and French. For use by more advanced students. Scales, interval studies, scales in thirds in a wide range and making use of tenor clef. Concludes with a series of etudes on an advanced level and in all major and minor keys. Fingerings indicated in early portion of the method are for the French system bassoon. Fingerings for the Heckel system are not indicated.

Langey. *Tutor for Bassoon.* Carl Fischer. An old standard which contains much useful material in the traditional nineteenth century style. Useful on upper intermediate level. Some duets and a couple of trios.

Weissenborn, J. *Practical Method for the Bassoon.* Carl Fischer. The standard method for bassoon which all bassoonists use. Basic to the study of the instrument. Useful for early intermediate level.

Additional Study Materials

Bitsch. *20 Studies for Bassoon.* Leduc. Contemporary style, quite advanced.

Dherin, G. & P. Pierne. *Nouvelle Technique du Bassoon.* Two Volumes. Henry Lemoine & Co. Paris. Volume One by Dherin is quite advanced technical exercises in all keys. Volume Two by Pierne is advanced etudes.

Flament. *Technical Exercises.* Seven Volumes. Leduc. The volumes are classified as follows: 1. long tones, 2. staccato exercises, 3. exercises in accentuation, 4. miscellaneous studies, 5. cello studies of Duport, 6. daily studies, 7. study of reed adjustment.

Gambaro, J. B. *18 Studies.* International.

Haultier, J. *Le Debutant Bassooniste.* A. Leduc. For early intermediate level. Ranges to G in upper register. Basic technical exercises in all keys. Uses tenor and bass clef.

Jacobi, C. *Six Caprices.* International.

Jancourt, E. *26 Melodic Studies.* International. *Method for Bassoon, op. 15.* Two Volumes. Costallat. *32 Progressive Exercises.* Costallat.
Bassoon Studies. Belwin. Selected from the method by Collins. These are slightly more advanced studies than Volume Two of the Weissenborn studies.

Kopprasch. *60 Studies for Bassoon.* Two Volumes. International, Cundy-Bettoney. The standard studies used for many instruments adapted for bassoon by Kovar. Upper intermediate level.

Kreutzer. *Studies Op. 6.* Leduc. The famous violin studies transcribed for bassoon.

4See Appendix IV for a list.

McDowell, P. *First Book of Practical Studies for Bassoon.* Belwin.
  Second Book of Practical Studies for Bassoon. Belwin.

Milde, L. *25 Studies in Scales and Chords, Op. 24.* International, Cundy-Bettoney.
  Concert Studies, Op. 26. Two Volumes. International, Cundy-Bettoney.

Oubradous, F. *Gammes et Exercises Journaliers.* (Scales and Daily Exercises). Three Volumes. A. Leduc. Tone studies, scales, thirds, fourths, arpeggios, articulation exercises in three octave ranges and in all major and minor keys. Excellent for lower advanced level.

Pares, C. *Scales and Daily Exercises for Bassoon.* Carl Fischer.
  Modern Foundation Studies for Bassoon. Rubank, Inc. Two versions of the same material. The Carl Fischer is the original. The Rubank edition revised by Harvey Whistler keeps the exercises in an easier range.

Petrov, I. A. *Scale Studies.* International.

Piard, Marius. *Enseignement Du Contrebassoon.* A. Leduc. A volume designed to orient the bassoonist to the contrabassoon quickly and efficiently, using exercises, etudes, and presenting a large number of excerpts from orchestral works using the contrabassoon.
  16 Characteristic Studies for Bassoon. International.
  Quatre-vignt-dix Etudes pour le Bassoon. Three Volumes. Costallat. The 16 studies are on the lower advanced level, and the 90 studies are quite advanced.

Satzenhofer, J. *24 Studies for Bassoon.* International.

Slama. *66 Studies in All Keys.* International.

Vaulet, A. *20 Studies for Bassoon.* Rubank.

Vobaron. *Thirty-Four Etudes for Bassoon.* Cundy-Bettoney.
  Four Lessons and Seventeen Studies. Cundy-Bettoney.

Weissenborn, J. *Bassoon Studies, Op. 8.* Two Volumes. Carl Fischer. International, Cundy-Bettoney. Volume One "for beginners" is useful on the intermediate level and has short technical studies in seven sections: essential kinds of expression, tenor clef, brief scale exercises in all keys, arpeggios and chord exercises, chromatic scales, progressions in thirds, fourths, sixths, octaves and tenths, and embellishments. These are basic studies which all students should cover. Volume Two is slightly more advanced. It is reprinted in the Fischer edition of the Weissenborn method and also available separately.

STUDY AND ACHIEVEMENT QUESTIONS

1. Identify and write on a staff the beginning, intermediate, and advanced playing ranges for bassoon.
2. Assemble the bassoon identifying each part as it is taken from the case and demonstrating the correct holding position for each operation.
3. Observe beginning, intermediate, and advanced students (when available) in the process of assembling their instruments and fill out the check list for assembly. Describe corrections for any faults.
4. Demonstrate the correct holding positions for the bassoon. Demonstrate commonly found faults and describe their effect on performance.
5. Demonstrate the guide positions for the hands. Instruct a student who is unfamiliar with the instrument in how to arrive at this guide position.
6. Observe various students during performance and fill out check lists for holding and hand positions. Suggest appropriate corrections for any faults.
7. Discuss the two general types of embouchure formation for bassoon. Select one and demonstrate the step by step formation. Describe and demonstrate the process of how the proper amount of reed in the mouth is arrived at.
8. Observe various students during performance and fill out check lists for embouchure formation. If any faults are observed describe their effect on performance, and suggest corrections.
9. How is the basic tuning of the bassoon done? How is the bocal involved in tuning?
10. What factors will make the overall pitch of the bassoon flat? Sharp? What factors influence the pitch of individual notes?
11. Identify the four registers of the bassoon range by writing the notes in each on a staff.
12. List the most common problems in tone production on the bassoon together with their causes and corrections.
13. Describe the two most common approaches to tongue placement on the bassoon. What basic principles do they have in common?
14. Describe and demonstrate the use and action of the left thumb. The right thumb.
15. What is the function of the whisper key? On what notes must it be closed by the thumb? On what notes does it close automatically.
16. On what notes is the first finger half-hole position used? What is the purpose of the half-hole?
17. What are flick keys? On what notes are they used? When and why are they used?
18. List the notes on the bassoon for which there are standard alternate fingerings. Give the fingering for each alternate and an example of how and when it is used.
19. Discuss student qualifications and aptitudes for study of the bassoon.

20. Discuss the advantages, disadvantages and uses of the various kinds of swabs available for use with the bassoon.

21. Perform the step by step process of disassembly and cleaning the bassoon, having a colleague observe and rate the procedure.

22. List the items to be considered in the regular maintenance of the instrument.

23. Discuss the pros and cons of the neck strap, the seat strap, and the floor stand to hold the bassoon.

24. Examine and compare various beginning bassoon methods. Select one or two best suited for a junior high beginner, and one or two best suited for a high school student transferring from clarinet.

25. Examine available standard methods and additional study materials for bassoon and list them with comments. Prepare a suggested list of material to include all five types of material suggested for simultaneous study for an advanced beginner. For an intermediate level student. For an advanced student.

26. Listen to several phonograph records of outstanding bassoonists. Compare and comment on tone quality, phrasing, articulation. If the players are other than American describe any nationalistic differences which are discernible.

27. Discuss the use of vibrato on the bassoon, together with when and how it should be developed.

CHAPTER FIVE

SAXOPHONE

Since its invention in 1846 by Adolph Sax of Paris the saxophone has received an acceptance in the musical world which is remarkable for the divergence of usages to which it has been put. Excepting only the flute among the woodwind instruments the saxophone is the most perfect instrument from the standpoint of both acoustics and mechanism. Only very minor alterations and additions have been made to its basic mechanism since its introduction. As a newcomer historically speaking, the saxophone lacks musical literature in various musical styles available for the other woodwinds, and clearly defined schools or performance styles have not become as apparent as those for the other woodwinds. The development of performance styles and pedagogical approaches to the teaching of an instrument have always centered around fine performers in major symphony orchestras over the world or in various conservatories or schools of music. The saxophone has not had this treatment since it is not a regular part of the symphony orchestra, and it is only comparatively recently that students have been allowed to "major" on the saxophone at schools of music in the United States. Certain European music schools have considered the saxophone an instrument suitable for major study for some time, but the influence of these schools has not been widely felt in the United States.

As a result of this situation, the saxophone in the United States generally speaking, has the lowest performance standards of any woodwind instrument. Educators who act as adjudicators for public school festivals will affirm the fact that more often than not the saxophone section of a band is the weakest by far of all sections in the group. An analysis of the problem reveals that while the technical facility of the players in this section is adequate, the concept of tone quality is woefully lacking. This is due primarily to two factors. First, there is a lack of professional saxophone players in the field of legitimate music to set the same high standard that is found on the other woodwinds. Second, the traditional association and use of the saxophone in the field of popular music where the concept of tone quality changes from year to year depending on the style of musical entertainment in vogue, and where many of the star performers who have not had a legitimate musical training and succeed on the basis of raw talent alone, develop highly individual tone qualities. This is not necessarily to be condemned as the entertainment business demands individuality of the kind no other personality can duplicate.

The fact remains, unhappy as it may be, that the saxophone as a medium of musical expression has not been developed in the United States to anywhere the extent found on other wind instruments. This situation can and must be remedied by intelligent and diligent teaching. It is no more difficult to produce beautiful sounds, fine phrasing, and all the other aspects of artistic performance on the saxophone than on any other woodwind instrument. Indeed, some teachers hold the view that progress toward this goal can be more rapid on the saxophone than on some of the other woodwind instruments. Be this as it may the saxophone is an instrument deserving of serious study, of serious teaching, and sufficient literature exists to make this possible. A fine saxophone section is one of the most valuable assets a band can have. The sounds produced as a section and in the ensemble of the group will pay handsome rewards to the teacher who develops them. As a solo instrument or in ensembles the saxophone is a flexible and musically pleasing medium of expression.

THE SAXOPHONE FAMILY

While only the Alto, Tenor and Baritone saxophones are widely used, the addition of the Soprano and Bass instruments to the choir produces a pitch range almost as great as that of the clarinet family. While the Soprano saxophone is provided for in many band scores, the Bass instrument, unfortunately, has virtually disappeared from the secondary school instrumentation.

Fingerings for all instruments in the saxophone family are identical, and a player may transfer from one to another easily with only embouchure adjustments to contend with. The basic embouchure is the same for all the instruments with adjustments made according to the size of the mouthpiece of the instrument. Since the Alto saxophone is the most widely used, discussions in this chapter will center around it, with special problems and differences between it and the other instruments in the family noted in the course of the discussion.

Except for some models of the Soprano and Bass which do not have the two lowest notes, all the instruments in the family have the same theoretical *written* range:

but all are transposing instruments and *sound* in different ranges.

The transpositions and ranges in which each instrument sounds is as follows:

1. *B-flat Soprano*: Sounds a whole step lower than written.

Written   Sounds   Range of Actual Sounds

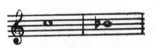
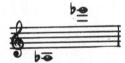

2. *E-flat Alto*: Sounds a major sixth lower than written.

Written   Sounds   Range of Actual Sounds

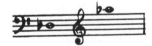

3. *B-flat Tenor*: Sounds a major ninth lower than written.

Written   Sounds   Range of Actual Sounds

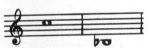
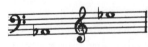

4. *E-flat Baritone*: Sounds an octave plus a major sixth lower than written.

Written   Sounds   Range of Actual Sounds

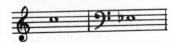
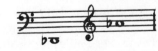

5. *B-flat Bass* (rarely found): Sounds two octaves plus a whole step lower than written.

Written   Sounds   Range of Actual Sounds

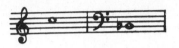
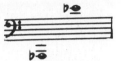

In addition to the preceding instruments a Soprano saxophone in C, sounding the pitch as written is occasionally found. The C-melody saxophone is a Tenor saxophone in C. Although it is obsolete an occasional beginning student will bring such an instrument from home since it is identical in appearance with the B-flat Tenor and considerable diplomacy is necessary on the part of the teacher to explain why it can't be used. The reason it can't be used is simply that there is no music written for it to play in a band or in a beginning class.

PLAYING RANGES

Because of the acoustics of the saxophone, the beginner on this instrument can extend his playing range more rapidly than on the other woodwinds. In actual practice, however, the highest notes are not utilized on the Tenor and Baritone instruments as much as they are on the Alto. A very advanced player on the Alto, through use of additional harmonics, can extend the playing range of his instrument above the normal high F. This is discussed later in this chapter, and fingerings for these notes given in an additional section of the fingering chart. The two playing ranges on the instrument are described as the easy range and the complete range as follows:

Easy Range   Complete Range

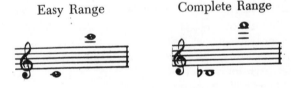

PARTS OF THE SAXOPHONE

Parts of all members of the saxophone family are the same: body, neck, mouthpiece, ligature, mouthpiece cap, reed, and neck strap, and differ only in size.[1] The instrument pictured is an Alto. The type of case illustrated provides a place for a fitted B-flat clarinet case on the shelf where the mouthpiece and neck are shown, and a flute case in the brackets on the lid as a convenience for those players who double these instruments.

---

[1]The Soprano is normally straight and with body and neck as a single unit.

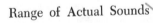

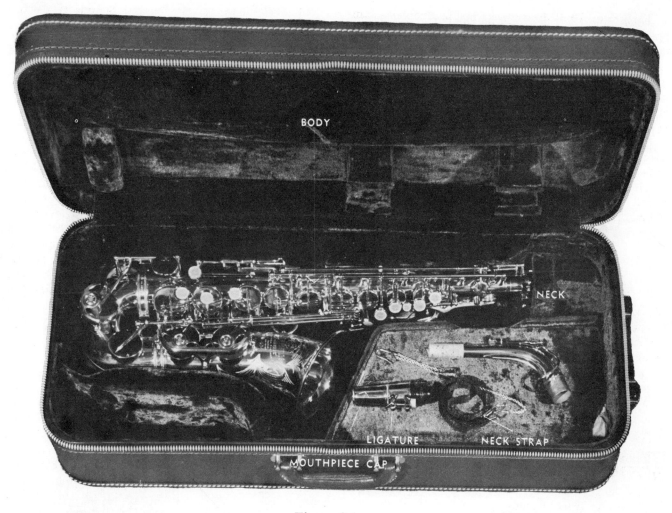

Figure S-1.

ASSEMBLING THE INSTRUMENT

All members of the saxophone family are assembled in the same fashion, and the Alto saxophone is used in the photographs. Proper assembly and disassembly of the instrument is of the utmost importance, and must be taught to students from the very first lesson. Probably more damage—bent keys, rods, bent connecting levers, etc.—is done to instruments in putting them together and taking them apart than by all other means combined. The mechanism of the saxophone is rugged, but the long rods, the large cups for the pads, the connecting levers as well as the side keys are easily bent out of line. Instruments with damaged mechanism do not respond properly. A great deal of the difficulty students, especially beginners, have in playing their instruments can be traced to damaged mechanism which causes leaky pads. For this reason, as well as for the simple necessity of keeping the instrument in perfect mechanical condition, proper habits of assembly must be firmly established.

The assembly of an instrument must be accomplished without putting pressure on any key or rod which will bend it in any way. It is obviously impossible to put together the saxophone without touching the mechanism, so in selecting the way in which the parts are held the hands and fingers must be in a position against parts of the mechanism which are not affected by the slight pressure put on them. The following step-by-step procedure is given in detail, and every student should practice it carefully until each procedure is correct and automatic. After some experience with the instrument, the student will adjust this procedure to his personal tastes.

Before starting the process make sure that the cork end of the neck is well greased with prepared cork grease. Study the photograph and directions for each step carefully and repeat the operation several times before proceeding to the next.

1. Take the neck strap out of the case and put it into position around the neck. Examine the device on

it which adjusts its length, and operate it to become familiar with its adjustment. The exact length will be determined later.

2. Figure S-2. Grasp the instrument by the bell away from the keys and lift it from the case. Holding it by the bell, hook the neck strap on to the circle on the body of the instrument. Continuing to hold the bell, remove the end plug which protects the connective lever for the octave key.

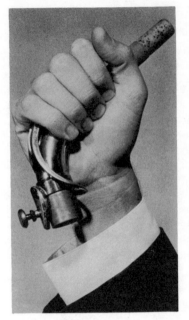
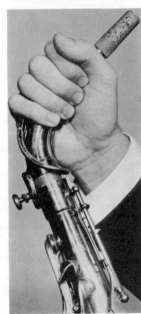

Figure S-3.   Figure S-4.

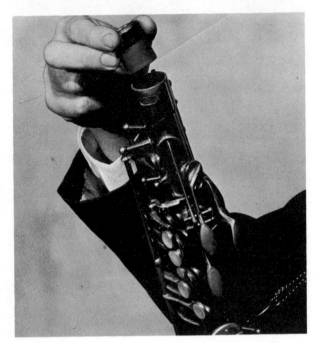

Figure S-2.

3. Figure S-3. Remove the neck from the case and hold it in the palm of the right hand so that the octave key is held down firmly. Check the tension screw which holds the neck in place on the instrument to see that it is loose. This screw appears either on the neck as in the photograph, or at the top sleeve of the body. Check to see that the sleeve which fits into the body is clean and polished. If it is clean but does not slide into place easily lubricate it with cork grease or vaseline.

4. Figure S-4. Holding the body of the instrument with the left hand, push the neck on, keeping the eyes on the connecting lever to avoid turning the neck in such a way that this lever will be bent. Bending this lever during this process is a very common problem with beginners. Push neck fully on the body.

5. Figure S-5. Line up the brace on the bottom of the neck so that it is centered on the connecting lever on the body of the instrument. The exact adjustment varies with the brand of instrument and with the playing position used by the student. Tighten the tension screw to hold the neck firmly in place.

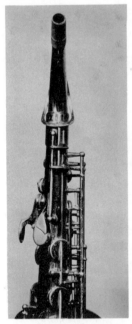
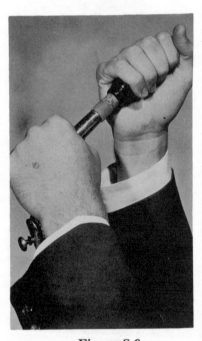

Figure S-5.   Figure S-6.

6. Figure S-6. Hold the mouthpiece in the palm of the right hand, with the left hand on the neck, palm holding down the octave key. The weight of the instrument is on the neck strap. Push on the mouthpiece so that at least half of the cork is covered. The exact distance of the mouthpiece is determined by

the tuning process. If the instrument has a tuning screw on the neck in addition to a cork, the mouthpiece must be pushed on to cover the entire cork.

Placing the Reed on the Mouthpiece

Placement of the reed on the mouthpiece is highly critical since the way in which it is fitted to the mouthpiece affects its response and tone quality to a considerable degree. Placement and procedure is the same for all instruments in the saxophone family. If the reed is put on the mouthpiece and the ligature slipped over it there is danger that the ligature will chip or split the reed if it touches it. Many reeds are damaged this way by students, and even advanced players have been known to ruin a good reed by inadvertently hitting it with the ligature. To avoid the slightest chance of damage, and as a matter of efficient procedure it is recommended that the ligature be put on first and the reed slipped under it. The following step-by-step outline should be carefully followed by all saxophonists from the very beginning stage to the most advanced.

1. Figure S-7. Put ligature with loosened screws on the mouthpiece with screws on the flat side of the mouthpiece. With the weight of the instrument on the neck strap, hold the ligature forward on the mouthpiece with the left thumb and slide the reed underneath the ligature.

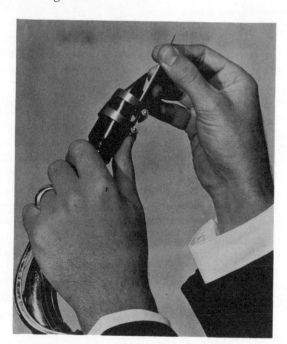

Figure S-7.

2. Figure S-8. With the thumbs in the position shown in the photograph, line up the reed on the mouthpiece so that there is equal space from side to side and centered on the flat portion of the mouthpiece.

About a sixty-fourth of an inch of the black of the tip should be seen when looking directly at the tip.

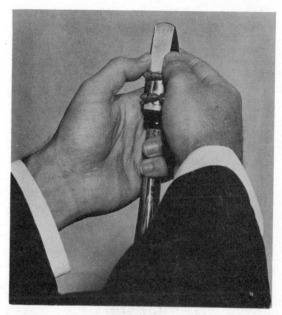

Figure S-8.

3. Figure S-9. Hold the reed in place firmly with the left thumb and tighten first the upper screw and then the lower screw snugly. Avoid tightening them too much as this will pull the reed out of position and restrict its vibration.

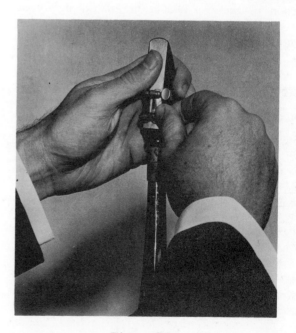

Figure S-9.

4. Figure S-10. Turn the mouthpiece so that the reed is flat on the lower lip when the instrument is in playing position. The flat portion of the mouthpiece will be off center with the brace on the neck of the instrument.

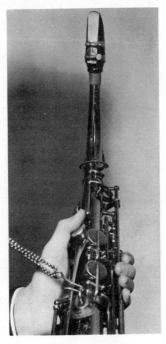

Figure S-10.

5. Figure S-11. When the instrument is not in use the mouthpiece cap should be in place. In order to avoid chipping the end of the reed with the cap, the upper portion of the cap should be placed lightly against the curved portion of the mouthpiece and slid into position keeping contact with the mouthpiece.

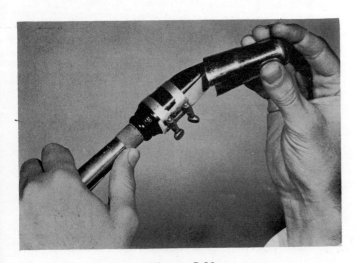

Figure S-11.

Common Faults in Assembly

There are various incorrect procedures in assembling a saxophone which are commonly seen among students. The younger the student and the less experienced he is the more often he violates the best procedures. Advanced players have learned through experience the value of careful assembly, and rarely, if ever, deviate from an accepted method of preparing his instrument for playing, although he won't always follow exactly the procedures previously outlined. If the opportunity arises, observe carefully how a professional saxophone player takes his instrument from the case and puts it together, the care and detail with which the reed is put on the mouthpiece, and the way in which the instrument is tested to assure that everything is operating properly.

The following items are the most frequent faults:

1. *Holding the Parts Incorrectly.* This puts undue pressure on keys and rods which eventually forces them out of adjustment. Bent keys rub against each other and move sluggishly or stick; bent rods cause the key to stick against its pivot screw; pad cups bent out of line even very slightly will cause the pad to leak.

2. *Failure to Grease Cork on Neck.* Since there is only one cork which connects parts of the saxophone, unlike the clarinet, oboe, and bassoon, the young saxophone student does not feel the necessity of having a container of cork grease in his case to the extent that players on the other instruments feel the need, and is apt to ignore this important procedure. Teachers should make sure that every student has cork grease in his case. Assuming that the cork is the proper diameter to fit the mouthpiece a small amount of grease applied once a week or oftener if necessary and spread evenly over the cork will make the mouthpiece slide into place easily. Excess grease must be wiped off with a soft cloth. Corks which are too large for the mouthpiece, or which are not greased make it difficult to put the mouthpiece in place and cause excess pressure against the mechanism of the instrument with the result of possible damage. If a cork is excessively tight after being greased it may be rubbed down with very fine sandpaper to the proper size. Corks which are not the proper size or which are not greased are easily damaged by forcing the mouthpiece on and will crack or tear making the mouthpiece even more difficult to put in place, and will eventually break off entirely.

3. *Bent or Out of Line Connecting Lever.* The connecting lever which projects from the top of the body of the saxophone, fitting under a metal circle on the neck to operate the upper octave key, is the most vulnerable key on the instrument because of its exposed position. It is frequently bent in the case because the student neglects to use the protective plug provided with the instrument. The instrument will fit solidly

Check List for Assembly

Observe the student in the operation of assembling the saxophone and check the following items. Incorrect items for older students should not be called to their attention until the entire process is completed; younger students should be corrected immediately. If any mistake is made the entire process should be repeated until perfect.

	Yes	No	Comments
1. Protective plug in place in the end of the body?			
2. Cork on the neck examined to see that it was well greased?			
3. Neck strap put around neck before assembly started?			
4. Body of instrument picked up by bell away from any keys?			
5. Body of instrument immediately attached to neck strap?			
6. Connecting sleeve on neck examined and/or wiped clean?			
7. Neck held properly during placement on body?			
8. Neck properly aligned with body of instrument?			
9. Mouthpiece held properly during placement on cork?			
10. Ligature placed on mouthpiece before reed.			
11. Reed correctly placed on mouthpiece.			
12. Ligature tightened to proper degree.			

in the case only if this plug is in place. When the plug is missing the body of the instrument is free in the case and this connecting lever is bent. A second cause of a bent connecting lever is the failure of the student to hold the neck properly during the process of assembly, allowing the ring under which the lever fits to hit the lever, or by twisting the neck too far from side to side which, on some instruments, will cause the ring to press against the lever. Remind the student to hold the neck properly, and to keep the eyes on this lever while the neck is being put in place. A bent lever will stick and cause difficulties in the operation of the octave key, or will cause the automatic second octave key to function improperly.

An out of line connecting lever, that is one which while it is not bent is not properly aligned with the neck through improper alignment of the neck and body of the instrument, will not allow proper operation of the octave key. Usually the result is that the pad on the octave key on the neck will not close firmly and it is impossible or difficult to play any notes on the instrument in the lower octave. Somewhat less frequently the result is that the connecting lever will not open the pad on the neck, and tones in the second octave are difficult or impossible to produce. The problem of an out of line connecting lever is usually a product of a poor holding and playing position for the instrument. Check the holding position, body position, and hand position and correct as needed.

4. Bent Keys or Rods. Bent keys or rods are most frequently the result of improper assembly of the instrument. The clusters of keys played by the left and right forefingers are the most vulnerable to damage because of their exposed location on the instrument. Other keys, especially the cups and pads covering the holes on the top of the instrument may also be bent out of line during the process of assembly or disassembly. Even if the keys or rods are not bent to the point of causing leaks they should be realigned by an expert repairman as soon as they are discovered. They must be removed from the instrument for straightening—never attempt to straighten a key while it is on the instrument. This puts tremendous pressure on the posts and pivot screws and can easily break them, making a major repair job out of a minor one. It is best to leave these adjustments to an expert who has the proper knowledge and tools.

5. *Reed Improperly Placed on the Mouthpiece.* The way in which the reed is placed on the mouthpiece determines to a large degree how the instrument will respond. Inexperienced players do not understand the importance of perfect reed placement, and teachers must check constantly to see that it is done properly. Check first to see that it is properly centered both at the tip and at the butt. A reed which is crooked is hard to blow, squeaks, and does not respond properly. If the reed is centered properly in relation to the sides of the mouthpiece, check the distance of its tip from the tip of the mouthpiece. When looking directly across the tip of the reed toward the mouthpiece just a hairline of black of the mouthpiece should be seen. Reeds which are too far down from the tip or which extend past the tip of the mouthpiece require greater wind

pressure to produce a tone than when they are properly placed. There are minor deviations from this rule of placement which can be used in emergencies which are discussed elsewhere.

HOLDING POSITIONS FOR THE SAXOPHONE

The manner and position in which the saxophone is held affect both directly and indirectly such important musical items as tone quality, intonation and technical facility. The proper position is one in which the body is in a comfortable erect .position, in which the hands and arms fall naturally into position, and which permits the formation and development of the best embouchure, breath control, and technical facility. Authorities are in virtually unanimous agreement on what the proper playing positions are for all the instruments in the saxophone family, and the ones given here follow this standard. Basic seated, standing and rest positions are given here, with details of hand and finger positions in the next section.

The saxophone is held to the right of the body with the instrument resting against the side of the leg. The body of the instrument is slightly out of the vertical position with the bottom slightly further back. The right arm is relaxed with the elbow pushed back very slightly to put the right hand into the best playing position. This angle is critical as it puts the mouth-

Alto Saxophone

Seated Position

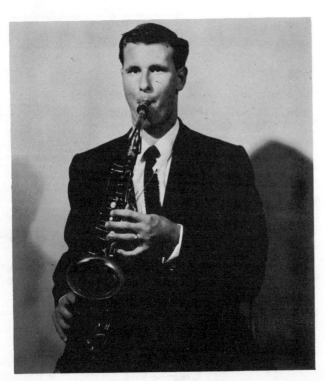

Figure S-12. Front View

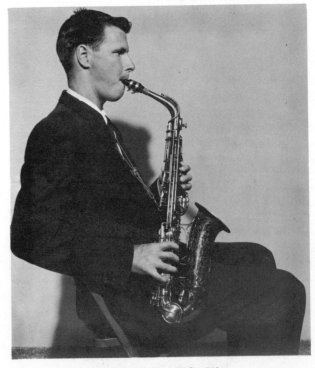

Figure S-13. Side View

piece into the mouth at the slight upward angle to permit the best embouchure formation. The mouthpiece is adjusted on the neck cork so that the reed is absolutely flat with the lower lip and teeth. The weight of the instrument is on the neck strap, and the instrument is balanced by the right and left thumbs and the mouth. Adjust the length of the neck strap so that the end of the mouthpiece touches the center of the lower lip. Head erect, chin up, eyes straight ahead, with shoulders up but relaxed. Elbows hang free from the body. Both feet flat on the floor. Shoulders and back must not touch the back of the chair when playing. Adjust the height of the music stand so that music can be easily read in this position. When two students are playing from the same music, angle the chairs slightly toward the center of the stand so that the position of the body and instrument can remain correct.

The position of the instrument when the player is standing should be identical with the seated position; only the position of the body itself is changed. Since the instrument doesn't rest against the body in the standing position, it is held in position by the right thumb. Stand erect with feet slightly apart, one foot ahead of the other to help maintain balance. Head remains erect, with chin up and eyes straight ahead. Shoulders up but relaxed, and elbows free from the body. Raise the music stand, if one is being used, so that the head does not tilt downward. Every player should regularly spend a portion of his practice time standing to become at ease playing in a standing position.

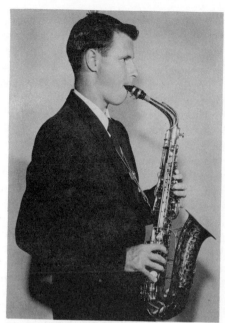

Figure S-15. Side View

The Alto saxophone falls quite naturally into a rest position across the body with the curve of the bell resting on the right leg. The neck strap must be left in position on the instrument. In this position the player is relaxed, is free to arrange music, and the instrument can be returned to playing position quickly and efficiently.

Standing Position

Rest Position

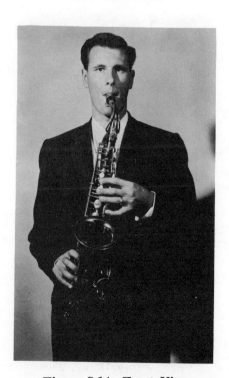

Figure S-14. Front View

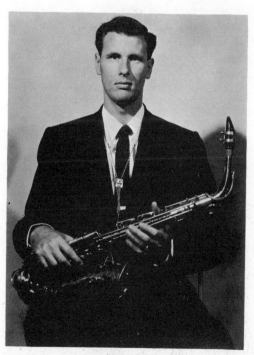

Figure S-16.

Tenor Saxophone

The Tenor saxophone is held to the right of the body with the instrument resting against the side of the leg, the weight of the instrument on the neck strap. Adjust the length of the neck strap so that the end of the mouthpiece touches the center of the lower lip. No weight should be supported by the right thumb. The Tenor saxophone is further out of a vertical line—the bottom being further back—than the Alto. The neck of the instrument is a different shape than that of the Alto so that the mouthpiece will enter the mouth at the same angle as that of the Alto instrument. Adjust the neck of the instrument so that it is at right angles with the mouth when the head is turned very slightly to the right. Adjust the mouthpiece so that the reed is absolutely flat on the lower lip and teeth. The instrument is balanced on the neck strap by the left and right thumbs and by the mouth. Head erect, chin up, eyes straight ahead, with shoulders up but relaxed. Elbows hang free from the body. Both feet flat on the floor. Turn the chair slightly to the right so that the right arm is not against the back. Shoulders and back do not contact the back of the chair while playing. Adjust the height of the music stand for easy reading so that the head is tilted neither up nor down.

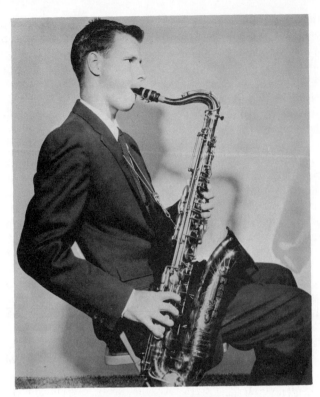

Figure S-18. Side View

The position of the instrument when the player is standing is identical with that in the seated position; only the position of the body itself is changed. Since the instrument doesn't rest against the body in the

Seated Position

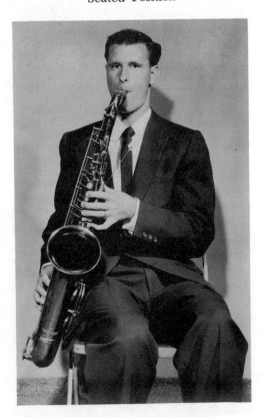

Figure S-17. Front View

Standing Position

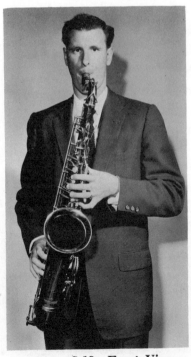

Figure S-19. Front View

standing position, it is held in position by a forward pressure of the right thumb. Stand erect with feet slightly apart, one foot ahead of the other to help maintain balance. Head remains erect, with chin up and eyes straight ahead. Shoulders up but relaxed, and elbows free from the body. Adjust the music stand so that the head does not tilt downward. Practice in the standing position regularly.

The Tenor saxophone falls quite naturally into a rest position across the body with the curve of the ball resting on the right leg. The neck strap must be left in position on the instrument. From this position the instrument can be quickly returned to playing position.

Baritone Saxophone

Seated Position

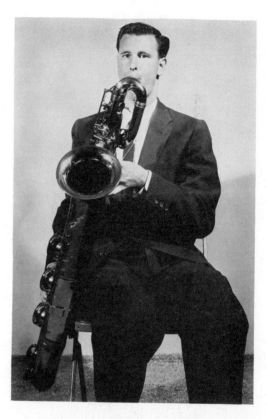

Figure S-22. Front View.[2]

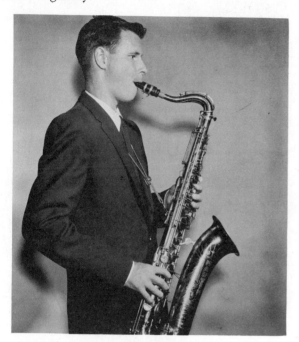

Figure S-20. Side View

Rest Position

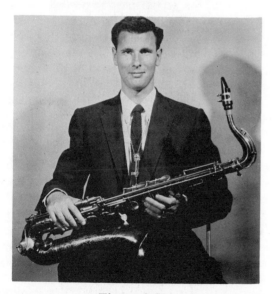

Figure S-21.

The Baritone saxophone may be supported by a neck strap or by a stand. These photographs show the instrument in position held by a neck strap, and the following series with a stand. The bulk of this instrument causes it to be considerably out of the vertical position in order to place the hands in a comfortable playing position. The exact angle is determined by the angle at which the mouthpiece enters the mouth. The instrument rests against the player's right leg or against the chair and is balanced by the right and left thumbs and the mouth. The right thumb must support no weight. Adjust the length of the neck strap so that the tip of the mouthpiece touches the center of the lower lip.

---

[2]The bell of the instrument photographed is longer than standard to provide for the optional low "A."

Adjust the neck of the instrument so that it is at right angles with the mouth when the head is turned very slightly to the right. Adjust the mouthpiece so that the reed is absolutely flat on the lower lip and teeth. Head erect, chin up, eyes straight ahead, with shoulders up but relaxed. Elbows hang free from the body. Both feet flat on the floor. Turn the chair slightly to the right so that the right arm is not against the back. Shoulders and back of the body do not contact the back of the chair while playing. Adjust the height of the music stand for easy reading so that the head is tilted neither up nor down.

The Baritone saxophone, because of its weight and bulk, is not comfortable to play in a standing position although some dance band players do so. If it is played in the standing position the position of the instrument must be identical with that in the seated position so that the same embouchure, breath support, and hand position can be used.

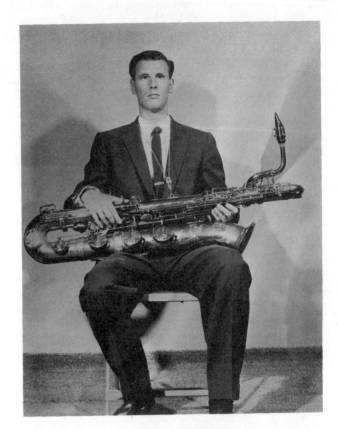

Figure S-24.

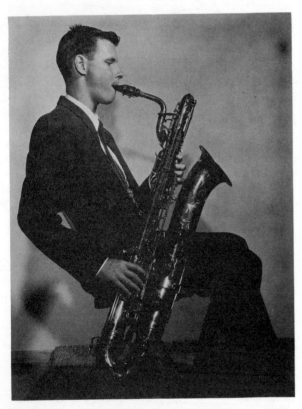

Figure S-23. Side View.[3]

The Baritone saxophone must be lifted into its rest position across the legs, but once in this position it is comfortably balanced and held securely by the neck strap. The player must allow several seconds to put the instrument back into playing position.

[3]*Ibid*

The use of a stand to support the Baritone saxophone and to hold it in the proper playing position is common with professional players and is highly recommended for school musicians. These stands are readily available, and are provided with rollers so that they can be easily moved into position. A metal band with a plate and a slot which fits onto the stand is put around the bell of the instrument. This remains on the instrument permanently and permits it to be taken from the stand and put into its case. The height, the front to back angle with the player, and the side to side angle with the player must be adjustable so that the instrument can be adjusted to be in the same perfect playing position when on the stand as when it is held with the neck strap. These adjustments are critical and are different for each player, but once they are made they are locked into position. Young players are especially appreciative of the stand for the instrument as it removes the strain of the weight of the instrument and gives them complete freedom of movement. Since the stand holds the instrument securely, and moves easily on rollers no rest position is necessary.

Positions with Instrument in Stand

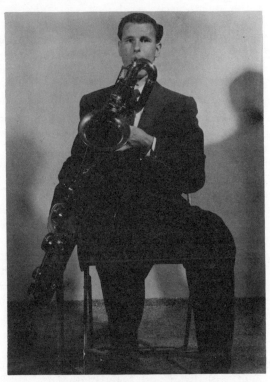

Figure S-25. Front View.

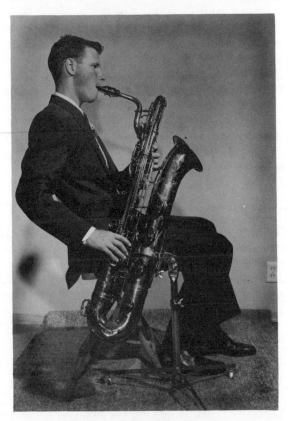

Figure S-26. Side View.

Soprano Saxophone

The Soprano saxophone being small enough is constructed in a straight line like the oboe and clarinet. Some Soprano saxophones made in the same shape as the Alto with the up-turned bell are still in use, although this shape is no longer available in new instruments. If the curved bell instrument is used, the directions given for the Alto saxophone apply to it. If the straight Soprano is being used it is held directly in front of the center of the body, with the instrument at an angle of thirty-five to forty-five degrees with the body. This makes a more acute angle at which the mouthpiece enters the embouchure, similar to that for the clarinet, but Soprano saxophone mouthpieces are constructed for this angle. Students transferring to the Soprano from another instrument in the saxophone family have a tendency to hold the instrument too far out from the body so that the mouthpiece feels the same in the mouth as it did on the previous instrument. This should be discouraged and corrected as an angle which is too great will produce an open uncontrolled sound. The Soprano saxophone properly played produces a clear, bell-like tone of great power and beauty.

Bass Saxophone

If the Bass saxophone is used, and it makes a valuable addition to any concert band, it must be held in a stand. The instrument is simply too heavy for anyone to play comfortably for long if the weight is supported by a neck strap. The stand for this instrument must be carefully adjusted in the same fashion described for the Baritone saxophone in order to get the proper angle of the reed with the embouchure. The size of the mouthpiece and reed permit little deviation from this angle if the proper tonal response is to be achieved.

Common Faults in Holding Positions

The holding position for an instrument can further rapid musical development, or it can make real progress difficult. Teachers must continually check student positions for it is important that any deviations from a normal position be corrected immediately before the incorrect position becomes habitual. Once an incorrect position is established, it is extremely difficult to correct. Students themselves must learn to feel the right position, and should be encouraged to check their positions daily in front of a mirror both at school and at home. A full-length mirror is an integral part of the well-equipped instrumental room of every school.

The following are the most commonly found faults in holding positions on the saxophones:

1. *Bottom of Instrument Too Far Back.* Perhaps the most common fault in the holding position, and one which causes problems both in embouchure and technique, is that of holding the bottom of the instrument too far back so that the side of the instrument is resting

against the hip rather than the leg. An instrument in this position pulls the right elbow so far back that it must be held up which develops muscular tension in the arm and shoulders which in turn causes problems in finger technique in the right hand as well as adversely affecting breathing. With the instrument too far back, unless the head is tilted downward which is highly undesirable, the angle at which the mouthpiece enters the embouchure is incorrect and results in a thin reedy tone quality in most instances. If the head is tilted downward to keep the angle of the mouthpiece in the proper relationship with the embouchure, breathing and breath control suffer because of the cramped position of the throat.

The correct angle of the saxophone in its front-to-back relationship with the body is determined by the angle at which the mouthpiece enters the embouchure with the chin up in the normal position. No other consideration is pertinent. The exact angle is somewhat dependent on the physical size of the player and adjustments may need to be made to achieve the proper angle of the mouthpiece. If the mouthpiece angle is correct then the instrument will fall into the correct position where both the right and left arms and hands will be in a comfortable relaxed position on the instrument, and the body held in an equally comfortable erect position.

This problem may be caused by having the neck strap adjusted so that it is too short which pulls the instrument back to release the pressure on the player's neck. Put the instrument in the correct playing position—then adjust the neck strap to the proper length. Check photographs to note the difference in the front to back relationship between the Alto, Tenor, and Baritone instruments.

The Soprano saxophone which is straight like an oboe or clarinet, must be held at an angle of approximately forty degrees with the body just as the clarinet is held. The mouthpiece of this instrument is designed for the clarinet angle in the embouchure rather than the angle called for on the other instruments of the family. The Baritone and Bass instruments on stands require that the stand be carefully adjusted for the angle under consideration, and the assistance of the teacher in making this adjustment, as well as the adjustment for height, is virtually mandatory for all but the most experienced players.

2. *Head Inclined Downward.* This problem is encountered in students on all stages of development, and may or may not be associated with the problem just discussed. When the head is inclined downward, the neck is constricted which restricts the flow of air through the instrument, and support of the embouchure around the mouthpiece is difficult to achieve. If the instrument itself is in the proper position and head is inclined downward the support of the lower teeth is moved to a point

forward of that provided by the upper teeth on the top of the mouthpiece, producing an underbite with which it is virtually impossible to develop an acceptable tone quality. The correction for this condition is to insist that the instrument be in the proper playing position and that the head be erect with the chin up, and the eyes straight ahead. The use of a large mirror is a necessity so that the student can check his position frequently.

3. *Slouched Body.* Varying degrees of poor posture occur almost universally—shoulders slumped or curved forward, leaning against the back of the chair with spine curved, bending forward so that the shoulders sag downward, feet crossed or hung over a rung on the chair or various combinations of these. Poor posture affects breathing and breath control to the point that students may find it impossible to support the tone adequately. It pulls the arms, and consequently the fingers out of position making technique rough. The importance of good posture cannot be overemphasized. It is basic to musical development, and the wise instructor will maintain a continual vigilance to be sure that it is established and maintained by every student.

4. *Adjustment of Neck Strap.* The adjustment of the neck strap on the saxophone of any size allows little deviation from the correct length if it is to support the intsrument with head and body in the best positions. The standard adjustment of the neck strap is one, with the instrument in playing position, which allows the mouthpiece to fall naturally into the embouchure without tilting the head up or down. An adjustment which is too long or too short forces the student to raise or lower his head which is not only a muscular strain if continued over a period of time, but also forces the embouchure into an unnatural formation. It is important that the neck strap be one which will maintain the desired length without slipping when the weight of the instrument is put on it. The same comments made concerning the adjustment of the neck strap apply to the height of the stand used for the Baritone or Bass instrument.

HAND POSITIONS

The same basic hand position is used on all instruments in the saxophone family, the only difference being the slightly wider spread of the fingers as the size of the instrument gets larger. This position may be defined as one in which the fingers fall naturally into place and are completely relaxed without any muscular tension in the fingers, wrists, arms or shoulders. It is only in this perfectly relaxed condition that it is possible to develop rapid, accurate and dependable facility.

Proper position and shape of the hands on the instrument must be stressed from the very beginning of saxophone study, and checked in detail regularly until it is habitual. If the student is transferring to the saxophone from the clarinet or another woodwind instrument and has achieved correct hand positions on the preivous instrument, achieving the proper positions on the saxophone will come quite naturally with some instruction.

Even the youngest students can achieve this correct position, and indeed, progress much faster with the correct placement than with one which deviates slightly. Many of the difficulties beginners have in playing from one octave range to the other, in crossing the break between C-sharp and D, in playing the lowest notes, etc., can be traced to faulty hand and finger positions. Poor hand position becomes even more of a handicap when the student attempts to extend the range into the third octave. It is very easy for beginners who have not acquired a feel for the instrument to deviate to a position which temporarily feels better or gives them a greater sense of security. It is a truism that the proper placement of hands develops a faster sense of security and better technical facility sooner than an incorrect one. Perhaps the greatest service a teacher can give the student is to insist that he establish and maintain this correct position.

The following step-by-step procedure for establishing the hand position should be studied thoroughly, preferably with an instrument with which to experiment. Study both the text and the photographs carefully until they are perfectly clear. The "Guide Position" which is given is the fundamental position for hands and fingers and should be maintained at all times except when the fingering for a note involves moving a finger temporarily to another location. This position on the instrument may be compared to the position on the typewriter which makes it possible to develop speed and accuracy so quickly on that machine. It is used on the saxophone for exactly the same reason.

A. Right Hand Position

1. Figure S-27. The right thumb contacts the thumb rest on the flesh to the side of and at the base of the nail. The ball of the thumb is against the body or a plate

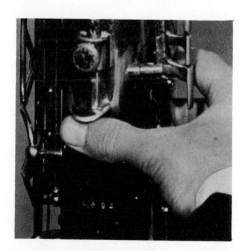

Figure S-27.

on the instrument. Notice the "U" shape formation of the thumb and forefinger which put the fingers into position on the top of the instrument. Notice also that the thumb rest on this particular instrument can be adjusted up and down for the best and most comfortable position for the player's hand. Not all instruments have this feature.

2. Figure S-28. The right little finger touches lightly the C key, and the remaining fingers fall in a natural curve without tension and contact the pearl buttons of their tone holes with the bottom of the finger beneath the forward portion of the nail.

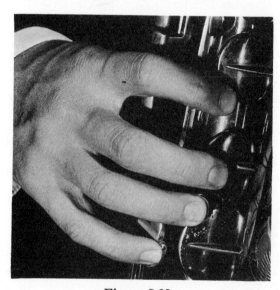

Figure S-28.

B. Left Hand Position

1. Figure S-29 and Figure S-30. The left thumb has the function of operating the octave key. It is placed at

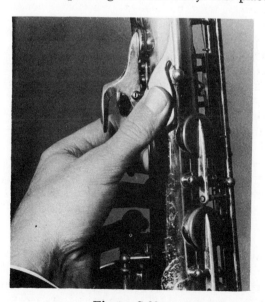

Figure S-29.

a diagonal angle across the instrument so that the fleshy part of the ball is on the plate provided for it, and the tip of the finger is touching but not pressing the octave key.

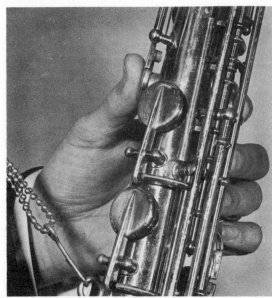

Figure S-30.

2. Figure S-31. The octave key is controlled by vertical movements of the first joint of the thumb. The placement of the octave key on some instruments requires that the thumb be lifted off the plate on which it rests as in the photograph, while others permit the octave to be depressed by a smaller vertical movement of the first joint so that the ball of the thumb remains in contact with the plate. The latter mechanical arrangement is somewhat more efficient from the standpoint of technique.

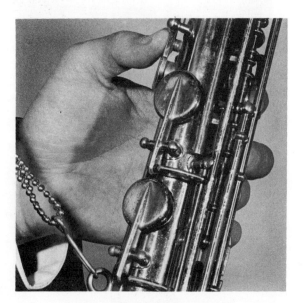

Figure S-31.

3. Figure S-32. The left little finger touches lightly the G-sharp key, and the remaining fingers fall into a natural curve without tension to contact the pearl buttons of their tone holes with the bottom of the finger beneath the forward portion of the nail.

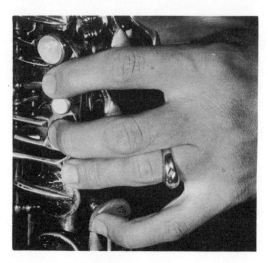

Figure S-32.

C. Guide Position

1. Figure S-33. With the thumbs and fingers in the proper positions, the wrists are almost flat, and the thumbs and forefingers of both hands form a "U." If this shape is a "V" the wrists are out of place and the student will have difficulty reaching the little finger keys.

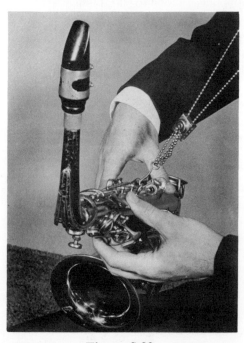

Figure S-33.

2. Figure S-34. With the thumbs and little fingers in place as described above, and the remaining fingers touching their respective buttons, a guide position is established which should be maintained constantly. Note that the fingers are at approximately a ninety degree angle to the instrument. Avoid more than the slightest deviation from this right angle relationship. The entire finger moves from the knuckle and closes the tone holes with a snap or click, pressing just hard enough to close the tone holes. Avoid using too much pressure with the fingers. The fingers preferably should be in contact with their key or pearl button at all times. Avoid lifting the fingers high above the keys and closing them by pounding.

most commonly used movements in this respect. Study both the text and the photograph, and try the movement on an instrument if possible, until they are clearly understood.

1. Figures S-35 and S-36. First finger right hand playing B-flat: This key, called the side B-flat, is contacted and depressed by the first joint of the right forefinger. The finger is straightened and moved directly down from the knuckle to press the key. The second, third, and little fingers of the hand must remain in the basic guide position. Avoid pressing the key by rotating the wrist which pulls the remaining fingers out of position.

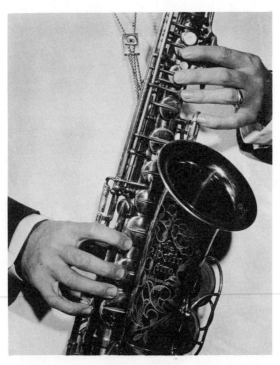

Figure S-34.

Movement of Fingers from Guide Position

Fingerings for certain notes on the instrument tend to pull the hands out of position unless fingers are moved efficiently and with minimum motion of both the finger involved and the entire hand. Some keys on the saxophone require that the hand be pulled out of position in order to reach them, and when this occurs the hand should be returned immediately to the perfect guide position. These movements do not seem to come naturally to all students, but can be readily developed if they are understood and the teacher provides music to practice which isolates the problem. A constant check on finger positions for these keys is necessary until the movements become habitual. The following are the

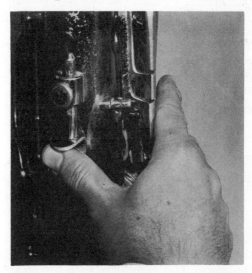

Figure S-35.

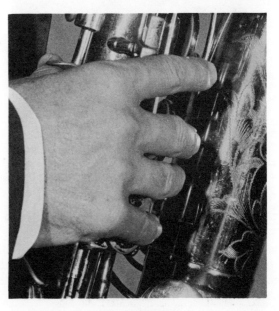

Figure S-36.

2. The center key of this group of three operated by the side of the right forefinger is one of the two regular fingerings for C: 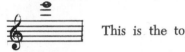. On most instruments it can be conveniently operated in the same way as the B-flat key, by extending only the forefinger slightly upwards. Keep the second, third, and little fingers in the guide position. Players with small hands and/or short fingers may have to use a movement similar to that described below for F. In any event, use a minimum of hand motion.

3. Figure S-37. First finger right hand playing E: This is the top key played by the right forefinger and its distance from the finger requires that the wrist be rotated very slightly to the left in order that it can be reached. It is contacted by the left side of the finger between the knuckle and first joint. The little finger will be pulled off its guide key, but the movement of the wrist and hand must be as small as possible. Avoid large movements of the forearm, and elevating the elbow to reach this key.

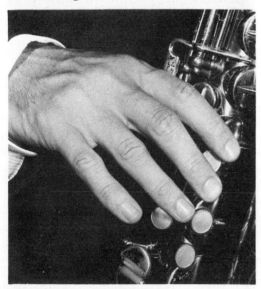

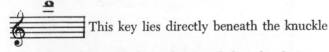
Figure S-37.

4. Figure S-38. First finger left hand playing D. This key lies directly beneath the knuckle of the first finger and is depressed by the bottom of the knuckle with a slight downward movement of the knuckles of the hand. The second, third, and little fingers of the hand must be kept in the guide position. Avoid straightening and lifting all the fingers of the

hand while depressing this key. Avoid also depressing the key by rotating the wrist. Both of these are common faults with students.

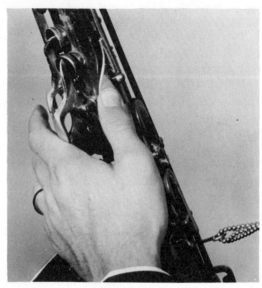
Figure S-38.

5. Figure S-39. First finger left hand playing E-flat: Two keys operated by the first finger are involved in this fingering, and both lie conveniently beneath the finger when the hand is in the guide position. The D key, as explained above, is depressed by the bottom of the knuckle. The E-flat key is depressed by the finger beneath the first joint. Keep the second, third and little fingers in the guide position. Avoid both straightening all the fingers of the hand and a rotating of the wrist when playing this note.

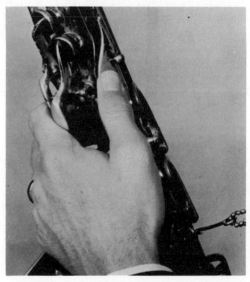
Figure S-39.

6. The third side key of the cluster of three on the upper left side of the instrument lies directly beneath and is operated by the bottom of the *second* finger at the first joint. It is added to the D and E-flat keys played by the first finger of the left hand, and the E key operated by the first finger of the right hand to produce the

high F: To open this key the second finger is straightened slightly and moved downward. The third and little fingers will have to be moved slightly from the guide position in order for this finger to operate the key, but this movement should be kept at a minimum. Avoid straightening all the fingers, rolling the wrist, and pulling the hand too far away from the guide position.

7. Figure S-40. First finger left hand on key 1x—the pearl button above the normal position for the first finger. This key is involved in a standard alternate fingering for the high F, and opens the same tone hole as the side F key. It is operated by moving the first finger from its normal position to this key, making a wider spacing between the first and second fingers. Use of this key is a valuable asset to good technique.

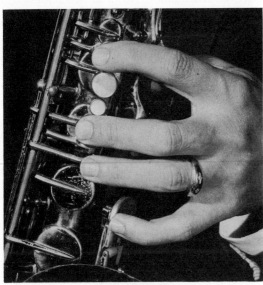

Figure S-40.

8. Figure S-41. Little finger left hand on low B-flat key: The cluster of keys played by the left little finger play, in addition to the G-sharp, low B-flat, B-natural and C-sharp. The shape of these keys varies considerably in different brands as a result of the effort to make them more accessible and easy to use. They are depressed by the bottom of the tip of the little finger which must be kept in a curved

position. Students with small hands will have difficulty in reaching the low B-flat key which requires considerable extension of the finger. Avoid, if at all possible, rolling the wrist and hand down to put the little finger closer to these keys. Keep the hand as close to the guide position as possible. These keys are provided with rollers so that the finger may slide more easily from one to another in playing legato passages. Considerable practice is necessary to gain facility with these keys.

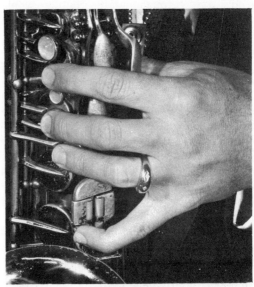

Figure S-41.

Common Faults in Hand and Finger Position

Because of the nature of the mechanics of the instrument and the fact that the saxophone was invented rather than being the result of decades of devolpment by trial and error the hand and finger positions are worked out to best fit the human hand and the saxophone student has a considerable advantage over students of the other woodwinds in this respect. This relative perfection in the mechanical arrangement is disadvantageous in a way in that sounds can be produced and a small amount of technique developed with hand and finger positions deviating greatly from the proper positions to the degree which if applied to the clarinet or bassoon no sequence of sounds could be produced. The saxophone does not demand correct holding, hand or finger positions as a prerequisite to a minimum of success, and for this reason the teacher's attention is not called aurally to a poor position on the instrument. A conscious effort should be made to check position on the saxophone as regularly and with the same degree of exactitude as for other woodwind instruments.

A player whose hand and finger positions are poor develops facility slowly and seldom if ever progresses to the point where he would be considered a good performer. A beginning student who persists in quickly establishing the proper positions makes rapid progress in acquiring technical facility. There is a direct relationship between how the instrument is held, hand and finger positions and success on the instrument. Many potentially fine players are discouraged in the beginning stages because their teacher does not insist on the best position.

It is, therefore, of the utmost importance that proper positions be established from the very beginning of saxophone study, through careful continuous checking by the teacher and by the student himself who must check his positions in a mirror daily until they are established. Some teachers take the attitude that positions are not important for elementary school beginners, and that poor positions can be corrected when the student becomes more advanced. Nothing could be more unfortunate than this attitude, since many students are discouraged from continuing, and even those who do continue with the instrument have great difficulty in correcting non-standard positions once the muscular pattern has been established incorrectly. It is so easy and simple to do it correctly in the beginning and so difficult to correct that every teacher who is truly interested in his pupil's progress will do everything possible to establish the proper habits from the very beginning.

The common faults which are listed here occur over and over again in students. Some of them are directly related to the holding position of the instrument itself which must be correct before hand and finger positions can be established. All of these faults have an adverse affect on facility and technique—making some progressions rough, some difficult and others impossible.

1. *Left Thumb.* The left thumb must be held in the diagonal angle described in the holding position, with the pad of thumb on the button, and with the corner of the finger operating the octave key. The thumb must never lose contact with the instrument while playing. There are several common deviations from this standard position:

(a) The thumb is held almost parallel with the body of the instrument rather than diagonal. While it is possible to operate the octave key from this position, the fingers are pulled out of position on top of the instrument frequently to the point that the student cannot reach the keys operated by the little finger. Remedial measures include changing the direction of the thumb to the diagonal so that the thumb and forefinger form the "U" as pictured above, and insisting that the left little finger remain in contact with its guide key.

(b) The thumb slides back and forth over the button to open and close the octave key rather than operating it with a vertical movement of the joint. This results in sluggish and inaccurate operation of the octave key with resultant technical difficulties. The best reme-

dial measure is to position the thumb properly and then have the student play octave intervals up from the first to the second octaves in which the only difference in fingering is the opening of the octave key. Scales in octaves provide readily accessible material. It should be noted that slurring the octave interval down from the second to the first octave on notes where the fingering is the same except for the octave key is difficult on the saxophone so the slurs should be only up. The following is typical of other material which can be used for this purpose:

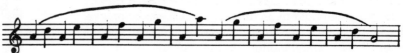

(c) The thumb is removed entirely from the button and held free from the instrument when playing in the first octave. Beginners especially are susceptible to this difficulty, and frequently have trouble replacing the thumb in the proper position when it is needed for the octave key. Insist that the left thumb be in contact with its button at all times, for if it isn't the basic holding position of the instrument is difficult to maintain.

2. *Right Thumb.* The position of the right thumb is critical for both balancing the instrument in the proper playing position, and for putting the fingers of the right hand into the best guide position for developing facility. The position of the right thumb on the saxophone is easier to achieve and maintain than on the oboe and clarinet where the thumb actually supports the weight of the instrument. There are two common faults with the position of the right thumb on the saxophone:

(a) Pushing the thumb too far under the instrument so that it contacts the rest too far from the end of the finger. Some students contact the support at the first joint of the thumb and some even higher. The thumb support should contact the side of the finger at the base of the nail as shown in the photograph illustrating the right hand position. This condition of contacting the support too far up on the thumb can frequently be detected by merely looking at the student's thumb since an incorrect position will cause a callous on any player who spends enough time playing the instrument to be considered an average performer. No callous will develop if the thumb is in the proper position. When the thumb is too far under the instrument the fingers on top are forced into an unnaturally acute angle so that the fingers contact the key buttons with the tip rather than the natural pad on the finger beneath the nail. Younger players especially have difficulty in contacting the buttons with the natural pad since their fingers are short, so it is even more important for them to have the thumb properly positioned. Further, when the fingers are at an acute angle which approaches the instrument directly, there is considerable muscular tension which makes rapid and accurate coordination of the fingers difficult.

When this condition is corrected with intermediate or advanced students there is a noticeable improvement in facility and smoothness of technique in the space of a few days.

(b) A second, and less frequent fault, is that of contacting the thumb rest with the nail itself so that the side of the finger rather than the ball is against the body of the instrument. This puts the pressure of the forward support of the instrument in such a way that a great deal of muscular tension is needed to steady the instrument and the student tires quickly. It also turns the hand slightly downward making it dificult for the fingers to contact their keys in the correct way. Fortunately this faulty position is easy to correct if discovered before it becomes habitual. Students are grateful for the correction since they are immediately more comfortable playing the instrument.

3. *Little Fingers.* The guide position calls for each little finger to be in contact with a key so that they will be in a position to move rapidly and easily to other keys which they operate. If they are not on the guide keys, then there is a slight delay in putting the finger in place, making for rough technique. Beginners whose little finger positions have not been established frequently go so far as to take their instrument out of the mouth to look at the keys to see exactly where the little finger should go. If the fingers are on the proper guide key then they soon move naturally to the desired location. The most frequently found fault in the placement of the little fingers is to find them sticking straight up in the air—a tense position which also tenses up the other fingers. The left little finger is frequently placed underneath the keys, apparently to help keep the instrument in playing position. The best, and perhaps the only, remedial measure is to insist that the fingers remain in the guide position actually touching their respective keys.

4. *Finger Positions.* If the thumbs and little fingers are properly located, the remaining six fingers should fall naturally into place on their respective buttons. The best procedure for keeping these fingers in position is to insist that they remain in contact at all times with the buttons during the beginning stage of development. It is permissible for more advanced students to lift the fingers no more than one-half inch directly above the buttons. There are three commonly found faults in the positions of these fingers, each having an adverse effect on technical development.

(a) The fingers are not curved into the most natural relaxed position, where there is a complete absence of tension so they move quickly and accurately from the knuckle. The correct curve is established by the "U" shape formed by the thumb and forefinger, with the other fingers following the curve of the forefinger. An incorrect position of these fingers is caused by an in-correct position of the thumb or by the wrist being either too low (usually) or too high. Check and correct as necessary although some persistence will be needed to correct a long established habit.

(b) Lifting the fingers too high—more than one-half inch above the buttons—is rather common, even among advanced players, and causes unevenness in rapidly moving passages. Since the fingers usually are unequal distances above the buttons it takes a slightly longer space of time for the finger highest above to close the key than it does for the finger which is closest. This space of time is microscopic, but it is enough that unevenness can be heard, and in less advanced players actually produces the unwanted grace note. It is signicant to note that this fault is never found among the finest players.

(c) Contacting the buttons with the tips of the fingers is most frequently encountered with inexperienced players, but is occasionally found with more advanced students. It happens when the fingers do not fall in the natural curve described above, and may occur even though the remainder of the hand position is correct. It is frequently the result of a faulty position of the right thumb (see above), and if this is the case is easily corrected. Using the tips of the fingers to contact the buttons causes the fingers to be in an unnatural position creating muscular tension and stiff movements. The remedial action for this problem is to insist that the front portion of the pad of the finger directly beneath the nail be centered on the button. On most instruments these pearl buttons are slightly concave which assists in finding the best position. It should be noted at this point that procedure of centering the ball of the finger tip over the pearl button in the same manner in which the finger is centered over a tone hole of the clarinet and bassoon is not necessary on the saxophone, although players with small hands will find it convenient to do so. Mature players should contact the buttons somewhat forward on the finger in relationship to the center of the natural pad of the finger.

5. *Angle of Hands.* The standard placement of the hands on the saxophone places the fingers of both hands at an almost perfect right angle to the instrument. The mechanism of the instrument is constructed in such a way that this approach is easily achieved. With the hands in this position the keys, with the exceptions previously discussed, lie well under the fingers and hand so that all can be reached with a minimum of displacement of the hand. Insist on the correct angle from the very beginning of study, having the student check this in a mirror if he is having a problem.

6. *Side Keys.* The side keys played by the first finger of the right hand and the first and second fingers of the left hand are normally not introduced until the students has established his basic hand positions and has acquired some technical facility on the intstrument.

Check List for Holding and Hand Positions

The following list of items provides a thorough check of holding positions and hand positions, and is limited to the seated positions for the instruments. The check should be performed while the student is playing and preferably when he is not aware that the check is being made. Any items which are checked "No" should be corrected with the deviation explained to the student, what effect it has on his playing, and why the correct position is important. Students make a more serious effort to correct mistakes if they thoroughly understand the reasons for them.

A. Holding Position

	Yes	No	Comments
1. Angle with front of body correct?			
2. Angle with side of body correct?			
3. Position of head correct?			
4. Neck strap properly adjusted?			
5. Shoulders up but relaxed?			
6. Elbows free from body?			
7. Body posture good?			
8. Feet in place?			
9. Height of music stand correct?			

B. Hand Positions

1. Right thumb contacting thumb rest properly?			
2. Left thumb at diagonal across instrument?			
3. Tip of left thumb above or touching octave key?			
4. Fingers curved?			
5. Right little finger touching guide key?			
6. Left little finger touching guide key?			
7. Thumbs and forefingers form a "U"?			
8. Fingers across instrument at right angle?			
9. Wrists virtually flat?			
10. Octave key operated by vertical movements of the first joint?			
11. Fingers contacting buttons at right place?			
12. Left side keys properly operated?			
13. Right side keys properly operated?			
14. Guide position consistently maintained?			

If he has established his position properly, introduction and operation of these keys will pose no problem provided he is given careful instruction on how they are used along with study material with which to develop facility. Unless this is done, there is a tendency for students to pull the entire hand out of position to operate one of these keys which has an adverse effect on the entire basic hand position. The key to success with the left hand keys is to depress the key with the right part of the finger—the D key with the bottom of the knuckle of the first finger, the E-flat key with the first finger at the first joint, the F key by the second finger at the first joint, while keeping the other fingers in or as close to the guide position as possible. When this is done properly students can acquire just as much facility with these keys as with any other keys on the instrument, and failure to do so is a product of improper operation. The three side keys operated by the first finger of the right hand—B-flat, C, and high E require a minimum of movement with the hand, keeping as close to guide position as possible. The most common fault in their operation is found where the player removes his entire hand from the instrument and depresses these keys with the side of the finger with the rest of the hand helping to push. This makes slow, rough, and uncertain technique because of the time it takes to replace the hand in the guide position. To correct, first establish correct use of the B-flat key with the second, third, and little fingers in the guide position, and finally the F key pulling the hand as little from the guide position as necessary to reach the key.

EMBOUCHURE FORMATION

An embouchure may be defined as the formation of the performer's lips with supporting muscles, teeth and jaws in relation to the mouthpiece and reed which have to do with tone production. The criteria for a good embouchure may be summarized as follows. A good embouchure is one which over the entire range of the intsrument: (1) produces (or has the potential of producing) a rich, full bodied, clear tone; (2) plays perfectly in tune; (3) allows the player to use the full scope of articulations from the hard short staccato to the smoothest legato at all dynamic levels and without adverse effect on the tone quality; (4) allows the player to use the full range of dynamics from the very softest to the very loudest under complete control and without affecting either pitch or tone quality; (5) and is controlled with a minimum amount of physical exertion; (6) once developed can be maintained with a reasonable amount of practice.

Conversely a poorly formed embouchure is one with which: (1) the tone quality is reedy, thin, nasal, or which changes quality from register to register on the instrument; (2) plays the upper register or lower register out of tune consistently, or with which it is difficult or impossible to adjust the pitch of individual tones; (3) produces staccato notes which are hard, with mechanical noises, or which have poor tone quality; (4) has a restricted dynamic range in which tonal body is lost at soft levels, and very loud levels impossible to produce or control; (5) requires an undue amount of physical exertion; (6) deteriorates rapidly without persistent practice.

There are considerable differences in the kinds of embouchure formations used on the saxophone, primarily because of the lack of any great number of artist-teachers to develop and set a standard. Investigation reveals, however, that there are only two basic saxophone embouchures in use by the better players, each subject to minor variations depending primarily on the concept of the desired tone quality. The major difference between the two is found in the shape of the lower lip, one embouchure bunches the lower lip to a greater or lesser degree, the other stretches it to a lesser or greater degree. For convenience and clarity the bunched lower lip formation is called a "Soft Cushion" and the stretched lower lip a "Hard Cushion," although the words soft and hard must not be taken literally.

The Soft Cushion Embouchure

The basic formation of the soft cushion embouchure can be achieved through the following step-by-step procedure: Check each step with a small mirror on the music stand.

1. Keeping the lips lightly together drop the lower jaw so that the teeth are about three-eighths of an inch apart.

2. Shape the lips as if saying the letter "O." The corners of the mouth are slightly compressed and there are wrinkles in the lips, especially the lower one.

3. With the teeth open and the lips in the "O" position the rim of the lower lip which divides it from the chin should be directly in front of the top edge of the front teeth. Feel this with a finger and raise or lower the jaw until this relationship is correct.

4. Maintaining this position insert the mouthpiece of the saxophone into the mouth allowing the reed to push the lower lip over the teeth. If the winkles on the lower lip are maintained, the line dividing the lip from the chin is directly over the front edge of the lower teeth. Students with thicker than average lips will probably adjust so that less lip is over the teeth. Contract the lips and especially the corners of the mouth inward and around the mouthpiece so that no air can escape.

5. In order to vibrate freely the end of the reed must be clear of any contact with the lip for three-eighths to a half-inch on the Alto saxophone, more on the Tenor, and still more on the Baritone instrument. The amount of mouthpiece in the mouth is determined by the mouthpiece itself. As a rule of the thumb, the support of the lower teeth against the lip should be at the

point on the reed where the lay of the mouthpiece starts breaking away from the reed. Some deviations from this are possible, but examine the mouthpiece to find this point, and apply the principle to all instruments in the saxophone family. This distance varies from one-half to three-fourths of an inch on the Alto saxophone.

6. The upper teeth rest, but do not press, on the top of the mouthpiece somewhat forward of the position of the lower teeth.

7. The lower teeth remain in the open position established in step three above, and must not bite or exert pressure against the lower lip. The reed and mouthpiece is supported and controlled by inward pressure toward the center of the mouthpiece by the upper and lower lips and by the corners of the mouth.

8. The first efforts at tone production should be with the mouthpiece alone. Check the embouchure formation in the mirror, and using standard breath support produce a tone by blowing without using the tongue. Continuing practicing with the mouthpiece alone until a steady natural tone of the highest pitch can be sustained for at least ten seconds. Check constantly in the mirror to be certain that the effort of blowing and producing a tone does not change the shape of the embouchure. When this is accomplished the student is ready to proceed with tone production on the entire instrument.

Any experienced teacher will verify the fact that while it is fairly simple to explain and form the embouchure in the manner given above, maintaining it in perfect condition over a period of weeks and months while the student is struggling with tone production and fingering problems is an entirely different matter. For this reason it is suggested that every student who is working on embouchure formation, whether he is at the beginning, intermediate, or advanced level, have a small mirror on the music stand for constant reference. The embouchure must be established by how it feels in the mouth and how the tone sounds, as well as how it looks in the mirror, and this is done only with the careful assistance of the teacher.

Common Faults in Soft Cushion Embouchure Formation

Analyzing the problem a student is having with his embouchure must be done both visually and aurally since some faults are not apparent to the eye but must be heard. It is frequently difficult to analyze and isolate an embouchure problem since the tonal symptoms indicating a difficulty in embouchure formation may indicate as well a problem with breath support or with the reed or mouthpiece being used which must also be discovered and corrected. These factors are virtually inseparable in performance. Following are some of the most frequent mistakes in embouchure.

1. Perhaps the most frequent mistake in the formation of the soft cushion embouchure is indicated by the presence of a dimple in one or both cheeks. These are caused when one muscle is pulling back the corner of the mouth to stretch the lip, while at the same time another muscle is attempting the proper contraction of the lips. This is a serious problem since the pulling back of the corner or corners of the mouth lessens the support of the lip against the reed with a consequent loss of tone quality. Students with this condition tire easily because of the muscular tension resulting from muscles pulling against each other rather than working together. Unfortunately this condition is difficult to correct, and the only solution is to practice long sustained tones while the student watches himself in a mirror to see that the dimple doesn't return. Because it is so difficult to correct, it is of the utmost importance to avoid the problem from the beginning rather than letting it develop.

2. The amount of lower lip over the teeth depends on the size of the lips of the student, although all should start as directed in the embouchure formation with the line separating lip from chin directly over the front edge of the teeth, as this will be correct for the normal lip. The student will make an adjustment himself, or can be directed to do so if his progress on the instrument indicates that such an adjustment should be made. If there is too much lip over the teeth the tone is open and squawky, but too much mouthpiece in the mouth produces the same symptoms so a visual check is necessary. Too little lip over the teeth produces a cushion which is too small to control the vibrations of the reed and a very nasal reedy tone quality is produced which is quite flat in pitch, especially in the upper register. Too little mouthpiece in the mouth produces much the same sound so a visual check is necessary.

3. Biting the reed with the lower teeth is another fault which is frequently found in students on all stages of advancement. This excess pressure against the reed restricts the amount of vibration possible, and produces a thin stuffy tone with little body, and requires considerable more breath pressure to produce a tone than the correct procedure. Reducing this pressure by dropping the lower jaw back into the open position immediately frees the tone and improves both body and quality. The strength of reed being used may need to be changed at the same time.

4. The amount of mouthpiece to put in the mouth is dependent on several variables—facial characteristics, mouthpiece, and reed—and the final determination is made by ear, moving the mouthpiece back and forth slightly to secure the best tone quality. The length and amount of the curvature of the lay, the size of the opening at the tip, and the strength of the reed being used help determine the exact location of the mouthpiece. Regardless of the size of the mouthpiece, whether for

the Soprano saxophone or for the Baritone saxophone, the lower teeth must be slightly back of the point at which the lay starts breaking from the reed in order that the cushion of the lip may control its vibration. A mouthpiece with a slight curvature and small opening at the tip requires that the lower teeth be fairly close to the break-away point, while a mouthpiece with a larger curvature and wide opening at the tip requires that the lower teeth support the cushion closer to the tip of the mouthpiece and farther away from the break-away point.

5. Puffing cheeks is a problem with many beginners as well as with some more advanced students. They indicate a lack of support by the cheek muscles which may or may not affect the amount of support the corners of the mouth are giving the mouthpiece and reed. Puffed cheeks are always an indication that breath support necessary to produce a good tone is not properly focused and directed into the mouthpiece. Frequently the student does not realize that the cheeks are puffed, and the use of a mirror to check is invaluable. When the student can see that the cheeks are not puffed he can then feel the muscular support which is necessary to keep them in place and make the correction.

6. Escaping air from one corner of the mouth while playing is another clear indication that something is wrong with the embouchure formation. Normally it means that the lips are not being kept in a circle with pressure against the mouthpiece from all directions, but are being relaxed at that corner. The imagery of suggesting that the lips act as a draw-string closing around the mouthpiece is frequently helpful.

The Hard Cushion Embouchure

The hard cushion embouchure is formed in virtually diametric opposition to the soft cushion, and like the soft cushion is subject to many variations. The basic formation of this embouchure can be achieved through the following step-by-step procedure. Use a mirror on the music stand to check each step.

1. Drop the lower jaw so that the teeth are about three-eighths of an inch apart, allowing the lips to open also.

2. Draw the lower lip over the teeth so that approximately one-half of the red of the lips is covering the teeth. Test by putting a finger against the lip to see that the front edge of the upper teeth is in the center of the lip.

3. Using the "smile" muscles pull the corners of the mouth back in a smiling position.

4. The chin is held firm in a flat and pointed position pulling the lower lip against the teeth, forming a hard cushion upon which the reed rests.

5. Put the mouthpiece in the mouth so that the upper teeth are resting approximately three-fourths of

an inch from the tip for the Alto saxophone, more for lower pitched instruments. This distance is determined and adjusted by following the previous discussion on how much mouthpiece to use in the mouth.

6. The corners of the mouth are pushed together to prevent air from escaping while maintaining the smiling position.

7. A slight downward pressure of the upper lip and a slight upward pressure of the lower lip provide the support for the mouthpiece and reed.

8. First efforts at tone production should be made with the mouthpiece alone as previously described.

Common Faults in Hard Cushion Embouchure Formation

Problems encountered in forming the proper hard cushion embouchure may be summarized as follows:

1. The amount of lip over the lower teeth is dependent on the size and thickness of the lips of the individual student. Students with very thin lips may need to put the entire lip over the lower teeth, while students with thick lips may need to use as little as one-third of the lower lip. The correct distance can be determined by a visual check and by the tone quality produced.

2. The amount of mouthpiece in the mouthpiece is determined by the nature of the teeth of the student as well as factors previously discussed in connection with the soft cushion formation, and is equally important to the success of the hard cushion formation.

3. The chin must be kept pointed at all times as it is this muscular tension in a downward direction which maintains the hard cushion over the lower teeth. If the chin is relaxed or pushed up the cushion is lost and there is too much pressure against the reed which restricts its vibration and results in poor tone quality. A stretched soft cushion produces the poorest imaginable tone quality on the instrument.

4. The corners of the mouth should maintain the smile position and the most frequently encountered problem in this connection is that they are pulled back too far into a position similar to the make-up on a happy clown. This exaggerated position makes control difficult and often causes air leakage around the mouthpiece. This condition can be corrected by pushing the corners of the mouth slightly toward the mouthpiece, while relaxing the tension on the smile muscles.

5. Biting or excess pressure of the lower teeth against the reed is quite frequent. Excess pressure restricts the reed vibration, demands excess breath pressure to produce a tone, makes high tones difficult to play in tune, and inhibits the development of a good tone quality.

Insist that the teeth remain apart as described. If there is too much pressure the student can feel well defined indentations on the inside of his lower lip with his tongue and will complain of a "sore lip."

The problems involving the mouthpiece, the reed, and puffing cheeks are similar with those encountered with soft cushion formation and need not be repeated here.

Check List for Embouchure Formation

The following check on embouchure formation must be made while the student is playing and preferably when he is not aware that a check is being made. Any errors should be carefully explained to the student, the correction worked out with him while he is observing the embouchure in a mirror. Remedial exercises can be assigned on the basis of this list.

A. *Soft Cushion Embouchure*

	Yes	No	Comments
1. Lips rounded with wrinkles?			
2. Mouthpiece proper distance in mouth?			
3. Corners of lips pushed inward?			
4. Sufficient lip over lower teeth?			
5. Are lower teeth biting?			
6. Cheeks puffed?			
7. Dimples in cheek?			
8. Air escaping?			

B. *Hard Cushion Embouchure*

1. Mouthpiece proper distance in mouth?			
2. Proper amount of lip over lower teeth?			
3. Chin firm and pointed?			
4. Cheeks in proper smiling position?			
5. Lower lip smooth and firm?			
6. Corners pushed in slightly?			
7. Are lower teeth biting?			
8. Cheeks puffed?			
9. Air escaping?			

TUNING

All saxophones must be carefully and regularly tuned to the standard international pitch of A-440. The instruments are made to be in tune with themselves at this pitch, and playing sharper or flatter than this standard will cause intonation problems on the instrument. Tuning for saxophones as for all wind instruments is best when done with an electronic aid which provides a visual check on the pitch. Tuning bars and tuning forks are useful for checking single notes through the use of "beats" or direct comparisons but are not as useful as an instrument which can check the pitch of all the notes on the instrument, nor are they as useful for beginning players who have not developed a sense of pitch discrimination on their instrument.

The saxophone is tuned with the mouthpiece. If the instrument is flat when tuning push the mouthpiece further on the cork, if the instrument is sharp when tuning pull the mouthpiece out so less cork is covered. The amount of cork covered by the mouthpiece is to some extent determined by the nature of its construction, but in general saxophones are made to sound A-440 when approximately half the cork is covered by the mouthpiece. Some brands of saxophones are provided with an adjustable tuning screw on the neck of the instrument in place of a long cork. On these instruments the mouthpiece must be placed completely over the cork and against the tuning screw. Such instruments may be sharpened by turning the screw to the left, and flattened by turning the screw to the right. This type of construction has the advantage of being able to return the mouthpiece to the neck and play at the same pitch previously determined.

Following are the standard band B-flat tuning notes and the note which each instrument plays for tuning purposes.

1. *Soprano Saxophone*

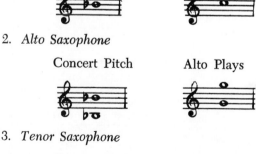

2. *Alto Saxophone*

3. *Tenor Saxophone*

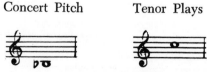

4. *Baritone Saxophone*

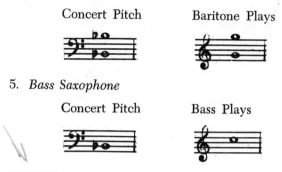

5. *Bass Saxophone*

INTONATION

Accoustically the saxophone, in its normal range, uses only pitches which are products of the fundamental vibration of the air column or of the first harmonic (an octave higher). Since the octave harmonic is double the frequency rate of the fundamental in both the tempered scale and the natural scale, from a theoretical point of view every note on the instrument should be perfectly in tune. Instrument manufacturers have gone to great lengths to produce such an instrument, and it is probable that almost all intonation problems experienced on the saxophone are due to factors other than the physical acoustics of the instrument. Among the woodwind instruments only the flute approaches these ideal conditions. Following are some factors which bear on the problems of intonation:

Natural Tendencies of the Instrument. Generally speaking because of the effect of the embouchure, reed and mouthpiece on the pitch the saxophones have a tendency to be sharp on both the lowest and highest notes in their range and flat in the upper portion of the second octave. Not all players will play all notes in these ranges sharp or flat, but these are areas to watch. These tendencies are the same on all instruments in the saxophone family.

Tendency to be sharp

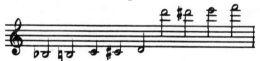

Tendency to be flat

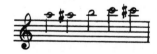

Effect of Reed on Intonation. A reed which is too hard tends to make the instrument sharp while a reed which is too soft tends to make the instrument flat. A soft reed emphasizes the natural tendencies of the notes and does not respond well to embouchure adjustments, so in addition to a general pitch flatness the instrument is out of tune with itself. A student who consistently plays flat, but whose embouchure formation is correct, is playing on a reed which is too soft. If he is given a harder reed the overall flatness disappears rather quickly, although he will probably protest that it is too hard to blow, but most students will make the adjustment to a slightly stiffer reed quite readily. The student who has been using a reed which is too hard compensates for the overall sharpness by pulling out the mouthpiece. This in turn makes the instrument out of tune with itself making multiple intonation problems which are impossible to solve. Providing the embouchure formation is correct, a student who has to pull the mouthpiece out an excessive amount to play at the standard pitch is playing on a reed which is too stiff. This tuning habit is frequently the best clue to an overly stiff reed. If he is given a softer reed the pitch will be lowered although he will complain about the tone quality he is producing, even though no change will be apparent to the listener.

Effect of Embouchure on Intonation. The embouchure is the primary controlling factor in intonation on any woodwind instrument. The pitch of most tones on the saxophones can be considerably altered either up or down by the embouchure. A properly formed and developed embouchure playing on a reed of the correct strength for the mouthpiece can control the pitch of individual notes on the instrument within the normal deviations easily and with facility to achieve perfect intonation.

The amount of mouthpiece in the mouth is critical to good intonation. If there is too little mouthpiece in the mouth restricting the amount of reed which is vibrating the upper octave in the range will be flat in spite of the natural tendencies of the highest tones to be sharp. It is virtually impossible to play in tune in this range without sufficient mouthpiece in the mouth no matter how hard the student bites with his lower jaw. This biting in an attempt to play in tune needless to say causes other serious complications. Too much mouthpiece in the mouth tends to make the general pitch of the instrument flat, but even more important makes pitch control of individual notes difficult because the support of the reed by the lower lip is placed so far forward on the reed that embouchure adjustments have little or no effect on the vibration of the reed.

The angle at which the saxophone is held determines the way in which the embouchure can control it. If the instrument is held too far forward so that the mouthpiece enters the mouth almost straight rather than at the recommended upward direction, the embouchure does not support the reed sufficiently and there is an overall flatness in pitch. If the bell of the instrument is held too far back the mouthpiece enters the mouth at too much of an upward angle and the resulting unequal support of the mouthpiece by the embouchure

causes the overall pitch to be sharp. Both of these positions affect certain notes on the instrument to a greater extent than others and the embouchure can not make the necessary adjustments for correct intonation. The importance of the angle at which the instrument is held can be verified by experimenting with the student sustaining an open C-sharp while moving the instrument back and forth. There will be a marked change in both pitch and tone quality, and the best position can be discovered.

Effect of Mouthpiece on Intonation. Mouthpieces with a close lay tend to be sharper than mouthpieces with an open lay, although the player through proper reed selection and embouchure formation can compensate for these natural tendencies of the mouthpiece. A close lay restricts the amount of compensation the embouchure can make in pitch, while an open lay although allowing sufficient compensation to be made is difficult to control because of the kind of reed it is necessary to use. This is only one of the reasons why it is necessary to select a mouthpiece with a medium length lay with medium tip opening.

All mouthpieces do not have the same internal dimension—i.e., throat and bore size and shape—and all brands mouthpieces do not fit all brands of instruments. They will, of course, physically fit over the cork on the neck, but may be acoustically unsuited for the instrument. This problem is especially acute on the saxophone where there are so many different brands of mouthpieces available, some designed to produce the type of tone quality currently in vogue in the popular field professional circles. If a student is having serious intonation problems and other possible causes have been checked, have him try other mouthpieces of different brands. If the mouthpiece construction is the problem some quite serious intonation difficulties can be solved by changing mouthpieces, although the student will not suddenly cease playing out of tune and start playing in tune because of the automatic adjustments his embouchure has been making to accommodate the out-of-tune mouthpiece. These automatic embouchure adjustments can be changed in a short space of time if the student concentrates on intonation. However, the mouthpiece has its greatest influence on tone quality, and is not to be blamed for poor intonation until all other causes have been checked and corrected.

Dynamics and Intonation. There is a universal tendency for the saxophonist to play flatter as he gets louder and sharper as he gets softer, the degree of flatness or sharpness increasing as the degree of dynamics approaches the extremes. This must be compensated for by embouchure adjustments. The student has the tendency to increase the pressure of the lower lip against the reed when playing softly and to decrease the support of the lip as he gets louder. This tendency is especially apparent in students who do not use the proper abdominal breath support.

To overcome sharpness when playing softly relax the embouchure slightly, decrease the velocity of the air through the instrument but maintain the same firm support of the breath with the diaphragm and abdominal muscles that is used when playing with full tone. To prevent becoming progressively flatter and flatter as the loudness of a tone increases, drop the lower teeth slightly to allow a greater width of vibration of the reed, but slightly increase the pressure of the lips around the mouthpiece to retain control of this greater amplitude of reed movement. Relaxing the embouchure when playing softly allows a great length of the reed to vibrate which lowers the natural pitch of the reed itself and hence the pitch of the tone being played and overcomes the sharpness. Dropping the lower jaw and increasing the pressure around the mouthpiece when playing loudly allows the maximum length of the reed to vibrate in order to produce a loud tone while the increased pressure of the lower lip against it raises its natural rate of vibration to maintain the proper pitch. The dynamic levels between a normal mezzo-piano and a mezzo-forte usually require little or no adjustment for intonation.

The tone exercises below are excellent practice in control of pitch through wide dynamic levels. Practice them slowly enough to use an entire breath on each slur. Maintain constant firm breath support while controlling dynamics by changing velocity of the breath through the instrument at the same time embouchure compensations are made.

Practice exercise "a" in major and minor scale patterns to include the entire range of the instrument in which the student is proficient. Exercise "b" is best practiced chromatically using a restricted range which the student is capable of controlling well, and gradually extending the range upward and downward to cover his entire proficient range. This is also a good exercise for developing change of octaves. Check to see that the student is operating the octave key by vertical movements of the joint of the thumb.

Intonation in Ensemble. The ability to tune the saxophone to the standard pitch and to play the instrument in tune with itself is essential. However very few saxophonists do much playing alone, but rather with other instruments in ensemble. For this reason, playing the instrument itself in tune is only the starting point for good intonation. The player must listen to other instruments and make slight adjustments so that he is exactly in tune with the other players. Other woodwind instruments have natural tendencies toward out of tuneness which are different from those on the saxophone; brass instruments have different problems, and the piano still others. The musically intelligent player will recognize these different problems, and will compromise his intonation for the sake of perfect ensemble intonation. Training in listening and hearing intonation is the most valuable contribution an instrumental teacher can make to his students. But it must be emphasized that the basis for good ensemble intonation must be the ability to play the instrument in tune with itself at the standard pitch.

TONE

There is no single standard by which to measure tone quality on the saxophone. The lack of acceptance of the instrument as a legitimate subject of study on the collegiate level has made it impossible to develop and mold a standard of achievement toward which the student can aspire. The prevalence of the saxophone in the dance band field tends to obscure its use in other fields of music, and to in effect, set in the minds of the student performers a bewildering multitude of constantly changing concepts of tone quality. Where in serious music tone quality is constant and unvarying in its development with use, concepts and standards widely known and accepted, the tone quality of the saxophone in the dance band fluctuates from year to year, from style to style, and from individual to individual. The saxophonist must apply the same standards of tone quality expected on the other wind instruments: body, brilliance, control, smoothness, consistency, etc. to his instrument, and reject highly individualized and transient concepts of quality used by entertainers.

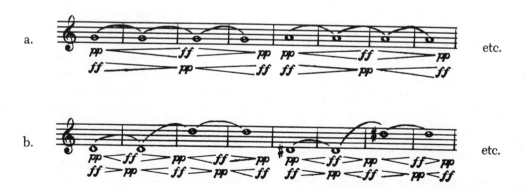

The eminent saxophone virtuoso Sigurd Rascher points out in one of his books for the instrument[4] that Adolphe Sax, the inventor of the saxophone, had in mind an instrument that should be as flexible as a string instrument, as powerful as one of the brasses, and possess an expressive power equal to that of the cello. This ideal can be attained provided serious study and effort is applied to the study of the instrument.

In order to identify the exact notes intended when discussing the saxophone, the range of the instrument is divided into three segments which are understood and remembered if called simply the first octave, the second octave, and the third octave. The notes in the first octave are produced by fundamental vibrations of the air column, those in the second octave by the first harmonic (the air column vibrating in two equal segments), and those in the third octave—actually only a part of an octave—by side keys operated by the first and second fingers of the left hand and by the first finger of the right hand. These three segments of the saxophone's playing ranges are sometimes called low register, middle register, and high register and should be understood to have the same meaning as first, second, and third octaves. These three octaves are identified as follows:

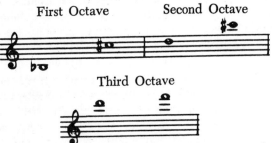

The playing range of the Alto saxophone can be extended a full octave or more above the high F indicated as the top limit of the range through the use of harmonics other than the first, or octave harmonic. It is possible, although difficult, to produce a series of seven or eight harmonic or overtones with each fingering in the first octave just as a brass player produces the series by using valves. (Refer to the section on acoustics for the harmonic series if necessary). Not all of these harmonics will be in tune with the tempered scale and the practical fingerings for notes in this extended range must be determined by experimentation and vary from individual to individual. The practice of extending the range is limited to the Alto saxophone, and is not practical on other instruments in the choir. Only the most experienced and advanced students should attempt to develop this extended range for it is demanding of concentrated effort over a period of time. Notes in this range are called for rarely in difficult solo compositions for the Alto, and never in the normal band or orchestra

literature. In the field of popular music, however, these notes are being more and more widely used with good effect in styles where the player is called upon to improvise. Players wishing to develop facility in the extended range are advised to study the book "Top Tones for the Saxophone" by Sigurd Rascher previously mentioned, or "Modern Fingering System for Saxophone" by Jay Arnold published by Shapiro, Bernstein & Co. A chart of fingerings for notes in the extended range is included with the fingering chart for the saxophone which are successful for many players, although it is quite possible that they will not work for all. Each individual must, in the end, determine the exact fingering for each note for himself through careful experimentation as his control and facility in the extended range develops. An electronic tuning aid should be used in this connection.

A good tone is the product of all the elements involved in performance: the instrument, mouthpiece, reed, embouchure, and breath support. If any of these is defective than the tone quality suffers accordingly. Problems of tone production and quality are many and varied, but may usually be traced to their source and steps taken to correct the problem immediately. Following are some of the most prevalent problems or faults in tone:

1. *Small, Pinched, or Muffled Tone.* Assuming a good mouthpiece and reed, a small, pinched, or muffled tone may be caused by too much pressure on the reed with the lower jaw, or by having too little mouthpiece in the mouth. Adjust the distance in the mouth by experimentation to the point of optimum quality and fullness, yet avoiding the tendency of the tone to break into a higher partial which is caused by too much mouthpiece in the mouth. Too much pressure against the reed can be remedied by asking the student to play flatter. This will cause him to relax the pressure of the lower jaw and free the vibration of the reed. Unless he also relaxed the support of the lip against the reed, he will not actually play flatter in pitch, the effect will simply be a freer tone quality.

2. *Squawky Tone.* The squawky tone which can be described as lacking in body and focus, generally uncontrolled, and commonly flat in pitch is caused by or a combination of three things. Not enough pressure on the reed with the lower lip; poor embouchure formation evidenced by not enough support around the mouthpiece with the upper lip, and the corners of the mouth, as well as the lower lip, or by a poor reed. Corrections for these have been discussed previously.

3. *Hard, Cold Tone.* A tone which is inflexible and which lacks the intangible quality of vitality is described as hard and cold. This is caused by a mouthpiece which

---

[4]Rascher, Sigurd M. *Top Tones for the Saxophone.* New York: Carl Fischer. 1941.

has a lay which is too open and too long, or by a reed which is too hard.

4. *Squeaking.* Squeaking on the saxophone is not a common problem with most students as it is on the clarinet, but when it occurs it is caused by a leaky pad which must be identified and replaced; by a reed which has a built-in squeak; or by an incorrect embouchure which is putting unequal pressure across the reed because of irregular length lower teeth or because the mouthpiece is not adjusted to be parallel with the teeth.

5. *Weak, Colorless Tone.* A tone which is otherwise smooth in quality but is lacking in body, quality and carrying power is most often due to lack of proper breathing and breath support. If all other conditions are good, the breath support can be corrected with diligent effort.

6. *Loud, Raucous Tone.* This quality is always the result of too much breath support, combined frequently with a very open mouthpiece and stiff reed, which overblows the instrument and presses it beyond the controllable dynamic range of the player. Insisting on a full dynamic range extending well into the pianissimo level, and limiting the volume the student is allowed to produce will correct this problem. In making this correction it is important to see to it that the student continues to use the proper breath support, and achieves the lower dynamic levels by reducing the velocity of air through the instrument rather than the support for the air.

7. *Control of Soft Tone.* Difficulty in producing and controlling a soft tone is principally due to the inability of the player to project a steady concentrated small stream of air into the instrument. Check breathing and breath support, and have the student practice focusing a steady stream of air into the palm of his hand. Other possible causes may be a reed which is too stiff, a mouthpiece which is too open, or a poorly shaped embouchure. Check all three if breath support is not the solution.

8. *Dynamics and Tone Quality.* Some students will lose their tone quality when playing at extremes of loudness and softness. This is normally due to an undeveloped embouchure. Keep the volume of tone within the ability of the embouchure to retain control, and concentrate on embouchure development through the use of the proper exercises.

TONGUING

Tonguing refers to the manner in which the tongue operates in relation to the reed and breath support in order to articulate the tones. This placement and action must be rapid and under complete control at all speeds. It must, in coordination with breath support, be able to produce on the saxophone all varieties of articulation from the hardest staccato to the softest legato. In short, at least the Alto saxophone must be able to match sound for sound the effects of the entire gamut of bow strokes used on the violin. As the instruments in the saxophone family get physically large the complete variety of articulations available for the Alto become more and more difficult to produce. The large mouthpiece and reed of the Baritone instrument responds somewhat more slowly and with a less variety of attacks than are available on the Alto instrument, although few school musicians take full advantage of its potential in this respect.

The manner in which the tongue touches the reed, the place it touches, and how it moves is dependent somewhat upon the embouchure formation, on the lay of the mouthpiece, and the stiffness of the reed being used. There are several ways in which the tongue touches the reed and in the way in which it moves, each with backing from fine woodwind instructors, and each effective within the style of performance being taught. There seems to be one point upon which all authorities are agreed in this respect however, and that is that *the tongue never touches the tip of the reed.* No matter which style of tonguing is used the tongue must contact the reed away from the tip. Indeed, if there is a sufficient amount of mouthpiece in the mouth, touching the tip of the reed with the tip of the tongue is virtually impossible, and if it is accomplished the tongue is forced into an unnatural and inflexible position.

The function of the tongue is simply to act as a valve to control the flow of breath through the mouthpiece, stopping the breath and vibration when it touches the reed, and allowing the vibration to begin again when it is removed and the air flow begins again. Effective tonguing and articulation is entirely dependent upon the flow of air, and hence upon proper breath support and control. The inter-relationship between breath pressure and tongue pressure against the reed allows the production of a broad range of attacks from the hardest marcato-staccato to the very smoothest legato within the widest dynamic range. The amount of pressure of the tongue against the reed determines the hardness of the attack, the amount of wind pressure against the tongue determines the loudness of the attack.

There are three basic methods of tongue placement used on the saxophone, each subject to many variations according to the personal desires of the teachers using them. All are effective, although perhaps not equally so, if properly executed. All standard methods have at least three things in common: (1) the tongue is relaxed. A tongue under tension cannot move rapidly enough, nor can it be controlled; (2) tongue movement is confined to the forward part of the tongue. The base or root of the tongue is down to permit an open throat and does not move; (3) the tongue acts as a valve for the air and is dependent on good breath support.

The three basic methods may be outlined as follows:

1. *First Method.* This method is used with the soft cushion embouchure previously described and is the method taught by many fine saxophone teachers. When properly developed and used it produces maximum flexibility and facility, and is adaptable to solo, ensembles, band and orchestra performance. This method in combinaiton with the soft cushion embouchure is recommended by the author. This method of tonguing is discussed in some detail in Lucien Calliet's "Method for Saxophone, Book One" published by Belwin, Inc. where material for its development is presented.

With the mouthpiece in playing position, and the embouchure corectly formed, feel with the tip of the tongue the junction of the reed and lower lip. The reed and lip form a small "V" shaped pocket. The tongue should be in this pocket with the top of the tip of the tongue curved up and touching the reed lightly about a half-inch from the tip on the Alto.

To start the tone, build up wind pressure against the tongue. Release the air into the instrument with tongue action similar to that in pronouncing the syllable "too." The center of the tongue is depressed slightly so that the tongue will not lie flat on the reed. Figure S-42 below shows this tongue position.

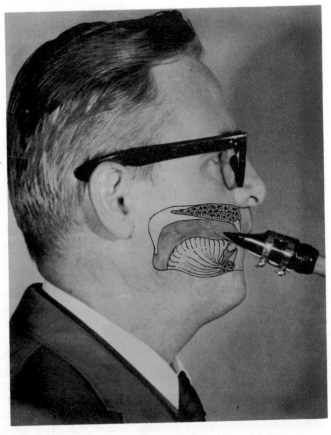

Figure S-42.

2. *Second Method.* This method is used with the hard cushion embouchure previously described, and is recommended by the many fine teachers who use the hard cushion. It is less successful when used with the soft cushion embouchure. It produces considerable flexibility and is adapted to all types of performance.

With the mouthpiece in place and the embouchure properly formed, the tongue is drawn up and back with the tip pointed. The center of the tongue is arched and the throat kept open. Action of the tongue is forward contacting the reed about a quarter of an inch from its tip with the top of the tongue about an eighth of an inch from its tip. Pressure of the tongue against the reed may be light or heavy depending on the type of articulation desired. To start the tone place the tongue against the reed, build up air pressure against it, and release the air with a tongue action similar to that in pronouncing "du."

3. *Third Method.* This method is used with either the soft cushion or the hard cushion embouchure. With the mouthpiece in place and the embouchure properly formed, the tip of the tongue is anchored against the base of the lower teeth. Keeping the tip anchored against the teeth the tongue moves up and forward to contact the reed between a quarter and a half-inch from its tip. The point on the tongue which contacts the reed is found naturally and is determined by its natural placement. Experience with advanced students who use this method has indicated that this technique of using the tongue does not have the potential of as great a variety of articulations as either of the previous methods, nor is speed and control developed as rapidly or to as great an extent. Unless there is a strong personal preference for this method, it should be used with caution.

Soprano, Tenor, Baritone, and Bass Saxophone. Any of the three methods of tongue placement and action described above for the Alto saxophone can be successfully used on the Soprano, Tenor, Baritone and Bass instruments. Normally the Soprano, Baritone or Bass saxophone are played after some experience on either the Alto or Tenor instrument, and the same method of tongue placement and action should be used on them that the student has already developed. The difference between the various sizes of saxophone will be found in the point at which the tongue contacts the reed. As the reeds and mouthpieces get larger there is more reed in the mouthpiece and the point of contact of tongue and reed is further away from the tip of the reed. The placement of the tongue in relation to the lower lip and teeth remains essentially the same regardless of size of the mouthpiece. Because of the larger reed and the fact that its response is slower it becomes increasingly difficult to produce a short staccato or to articulate as rapidly as we go from the Soprano to the Bass instrument.

Variety in Articulation. Once correct tongue action is established according to the method selected, variety in articulation can be developed. The exact sounds desired are determined by musical taste and style. A great variety of articulations is possible on the saxophone through the use of varying degrees of pressure of the tongue against the reed combined with varying amounts of breath support and velocity of wind through the instrument. This can be illustrated by a student playing in the following ways:

1. Sustain a second line G at a good solid *forte* level. While maintaining this dynamic level and keeping the length of the notes the same start with maximum tongue pressure against the reed and play a series of notes with gradually diminishing pressure of the tongue.

2. Do the same maintaining a *piano* level for the second line G, but starting with minimum pressure against the reed and play a series of notes with gradually increasing pressure of the tongue. It will be found that tongue pressure beyond a certain point will introduce an objectionable amount of mechanical noise.

3. Using the second line G softly play a series of staccato notes simultaneously increasing both loudness of the tone and pressure of the tongue against the reed. Be sure to eliminate any movement of the breathing muscles. Experimentation will show that the louder the staccato note the greater the tongue pressure needed to control it, and if the result is to be musically pleasing, the louder the staccato the longer duration it must have.

The success of these experiments depends on the degree of advancement of the player performing them. An advanced player will be able to carry the illustrations much farther and show a greater variety of articulated sounds.

Common Articulation Problems

There are several common problems in connection with articulation on the saxophone some of them occurring in combination. Articulation is so basic to satisfactory performance that it must be accomplished well if the player is to have any measure of success with the instrument. The following are the most commonly found problems:

1. *Hard Attack.* This is the result of either too much tongue pressure against the reed in relation to the amount of breath support, or too much tongue in contact with the reed. The inter-relationship between tongue pressure and breath support is rather easy to correct. The problem of too much tongue in contact with the reed—sometimes to the point of laying flat against considerable portion of the reed—is much more of a problem to correct. A special effect on the instrument, the slap tongue, is produced with the tongue in the flat position on the reed, but in normal articulation only a very small area of the tongue must contact the reed. The correction involves a return to the basic procedures and concepts of tongue placement, and a gradual re-training of

the muscles of the tongue to the correct position. The hard, percussive attack is frequently associated with movements of the lower jaw which must also be eliminated.

2. *Sluggish Tongue.* A sluggish tongue which does not permit rapid articulations may be the result of incorrect placement and movement of the tongue, moving the breathing muscles simultaneously with the tongue, or simply a matter of insufficient practice to gain speed. If a variety of articulations can be controlled and successfully produced at slow speeds, it is probable that the placement and movement of the tongue is correct. If this is the case speed may be gained by diligent practice making use of various articulation patterns with major and minor scales, thirds, and arpeggios. Use of a metronome for maintaining a constant tempo and to increase speed gradually is essential. An incorrect placement and movement of the tongue usually produces a sluggish response because the tongue is tense or is making too large motions with the entire tongue rather than only the front portion moving. If this is the case, then a return to the basic position of the tongue and a gradual development of articulation from the beginning is required. Moving the breathing muscles simultaneously with the movement of the tongue from the reed is relatively easy to detect since there will be visible body movements. This may occur with either correct or incorrect breathing. The habit of moving breathing muscles with the tongue can be corrected by reviewing correct breathing to get support and by emphasizing the concept that the pressure of the air against the tongue must be constant throughout a series of articulated notes with the function of the tongue that of a valve.

3. *Poor Staccato.* A poor staccato or no staccato at all, if tongue placement is otherwise correct, is caused by lack of sustained, continuous breath support to the tip of the mouthpiece. The support is being relaxed between staccato notes and then tightened simultaneously with the beginning of the note by the tongue. Check breathing carefully, since if this is the cause the air is most frequently being inhaled with a chest movement rather than by the diaphragm and abdominal muscles. A good dependable staccato is rarely possible with incorrect breath placement.

If a check reveals that placement of breath is correct and the support continuous, then a poor staccato is the result of incorrect tongue placement or movement. Frequently the cause is simply that the student is not returning the tongue quickly enough to its place on the reed to stop the vibration. This can be developed by practicing slow repeated notes at a very soft dynamic level, increasing the dynamic level as proficiency is attained. Many students are simply afraid to stop a note with their tongue and need encouragement to do so in the case of the staccato.

4. *Lack of Coordination Between Tongue and Fingers.* This is the result of practicing and playing too fast without the essential slow working out process. Slow down the tempo until the tongue and fingers are perfectly coordinated, and increase speed gradually. Do not allow the student to exceed the maximum tempo at which there is perfect coordination between tongue and fingers. Use of a metronome to maintain a constant tempo is mandatory.

5. *Movement of the Jaw in Tonguing.* This is the result of too large or too violent movements of the tongue. Rather than confining the movement to the front portion of the tongue the student is moving the entire tongue. The solution is to require the student, no matter what his technical advancement, to practice basic exercises for developing articulation constantly checking in a mirror on the music stand to eliminate all movement. Jaw movements can occur with all methods of correct tongue placement, as well as with incorrect tongue placement.

Flutter Tonguing. Technically speaking flutter tonguing is not an articulation but a special tonal effect which has come into use in twentieth century music. The flutter tongue is produced by rolling the tongue rapidly against the reed as in rolling the letter "R" in "b-r-r-r," producing a very rapid tremolo. There is no set speed for the roll, but the more rapid the tongue movement the more effective the sound. There is no standard notation to indicate flutter tonguing, and notes or passages to be flutter tongued usually contain the verbal directions to do so.

Double and Triple Tonguing. The standard technique of double or triple tonguing used for very rapid articulations on the flute and on all brass instruments is not practical on the saxophone, although some professional players profess to make use of them. The double tongue is done on the flute by tongue movements used in pronouncing the syllables "tu-ku" in rapid sequence. It is not practical on the saxophone since the second syllable, the "ku" stops the flow of air when the center of the tongue strikes the roof of the mouth. The alternation of the tongue against the reed and the tongue against the roof of the mouth produces two entirely different sounds which are impossible to match. Triple tongue, produced on the flute by the use of the syllables "tu-ku-tu" is impractical for the same reason. Saxophone players must develop the speed and control of the single tonguing to the point where it can be used at all speeds. Composers and arrangers who are familiar with the instrument will not write passages which cannot be played with the single tongue movement.

TECHNIQUE PROBLEMS

A good technical proficiency on the saxophone is one which is accurate, under complete control, and facile. In developing this proficiency the saxophonist must be aware of certain mechanical or technical problems peculiar to the instrument which must be understood and approached in a logical fashion. While in the training of the saxophone student some of the problems or technical procedures which will be discussed are not introduced until the student is quite advanced, many of them will be quite valuable to students who are still in the intermediate stage of their development, while still others are suitable for introduction even earlier. For this reason every instructor must be fully aware of the various possibilities of solving certain technical problems, and introduce them whenever the problem arises in the day to day work of the student. Among the most important things in developing a fine technical proficiency is to have a command of all the fingerings possible for every note together with the knowledge of how and when to use each. The book by Jay Arnold "Modern Fingering System for the Saxophone" published by Shapiro, Bernstein & Co. has the most complete listing of fingerings available together with musical examples illustrating the use of each, although the book does not provide enough musical material to fully develop their use. Any teacher responsible for saxophone students past the beginning stage should be familiar with the book and have it available for ready reference.

Approached logically and with full information on available choices technical problems on the saxophone are neither complex to solve, nor complex to use. Intelligent selection and use of alternate fingerings and other devices will simplify technical problems to an extent undreamed of by the uninformed. Both the importance of the correct solution and the reasons for a particular solution must be impressed on the student. Each alternative must be practiced until it becomes an involuntary part of the player's technique and how each alternative is used must be made so much a part of his technique that the correct choice becomes involuntary and instantaneous. Both players and teachers should not hesitate to mark instructions on the printed pages as reminders.

1. *Use of Little Fingers.* Two problems arise in connection with the use of the little fingers in achieving technical facility. The first of these is that of having them in the proper position to reach and depress any key involved with a minimum of motion. The guide position is established for this purpose, but care should be taken to see that the fingers remain in the natural curved position in so far as possible. This curved position gives them maximum strength since on some instruments the number and strength of the springs involved in playing low B-flat for example, requires considerable pressure to close the key. Avoid too much curve which makes the finger contact the key with its tip. There is little strength in this motion. The right little finger with only two keys to operate poses little problem, but the four keys operated by the left little finger require accuracy, dexterity, and strength to operate properly. Many players

never gain much facility in using the lowest notes on the instrument because of faulty use of the little fingers.

The second problem in the use of the little fingers is that of sliding from one to another when successive notes require the same finger to be in two different locations, especially when the notes are slurred. Almost all brands of instruments provide rollers on these keys to facilitate this process. To slide from one key to another, keep the little finger curved and without relaxing the downward pressure on the key, slide the finger with a sideways motion to the new location. Do not roll the hand to move the finger, do not flatten the hand or the little finger to contact the second key with the middle or side of the little finger. Considerable practice is necessary to perfect the technique of sliding, and most teachers find it necessary to assign particular exercises for this purpose.

2. *Left Thumb*. The position and movements of the left thumb previously described are those which, if carefully observed, will eliminate any problems with this finger. However, many beginners find it difficult to establish this and fall into a variety of bad habits which are a detriment to their technical advancement. A constant check of this finger is advisable throughout the beginning stages of study. Emphasize to the student that the thumb must remain in contact with its button at all times, and that the octave key is operated by vertical movements of the first joint. Assigning exercises which cross back and forth between the first and second octaves so that the student's attention is focused on the operation of the octave key will help correct a poor habit, although if the habit is firmly established its correction will take a period of time.

3. *Leaving Down One or More Fingers Throughout a Passage*. Rapidly moving passages involving certain combinations of notes can frequently be made smoother if some of the fingers and/or keys can be kept down throughout even though they are not involved in the basic fingerings for all the notes. This basic principle can be applied to all woodwind instruments. Advanced players make use of this technique without being conscious of it, but it is frequently a great aid to less experienced players if they can be directed to make use of it. Some combinations will affect the pitch of other notes in the passage, while others will have no effect. Use of this technique is limited to those instances where there is no appreciable change in intonation of any of the notes, but is always usable where the notes are moving so rapidly that none of the notes are sufficiently exposed for the ear to detect incorrect intonation. Following are some examples illustrating this technique.

(a) leave first two fingers of right hand down throughout.

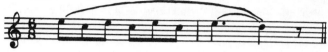

(b) leave three fingers of right hand down throughout.

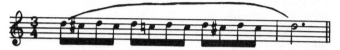

(c) leave three fingers and little finger of right hand down throughout.

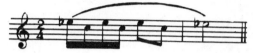

(d) leave right little finger on c key and left little finger on d-flat key down throughout.

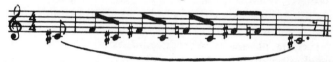

4. *Articulated G-sharp Key*. The G-sharp key played by the left little finger is articulated in two ways on the saxophone: (1) If the G-sharp key is depressed by the little finger, the pad which opens a tone hole to produce the note will automatically close when any of the tone holes operated by the three fingers of the right hand are closed. Thus in a sequence of notes containing several G-sharp's (or A-flat's) and notes fingered by the right hand the left little finger depresses the G-sharp key throughout, making the progression smoother and easier technically than if the little finger released and depressed the key each time a G-sharp appeared. Keeping the little finger down has no effect on the pitch of the other notes in the right hand and this technique may be used at any speed. The following example illustrates a typical use of this procedure:

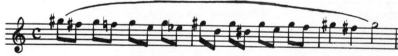

(2) When the B-flat, B-natural or C-sharp keys are depressed by the left little finger the G-sharp key is automatically depressed.[5] With this type of articulated mechanism the G-sharp can be played with the three fingers of the left hand down plus any of the four keys operated by the left little finger. This eliminates the necessity of sliding the little finger back and forth in sequences of notes which involve the left little finger and permits

---

[5]Not all instruments have this interlocking mechanism.

a smooth legato technique in situations where a legato would otherwise be impossible. Fingering the G-sharp with any one of the other keys of the left little finger has no appreciable effect on intonation and this device may be used regardless of the speed of the notes. Following is a typical example. Finger the G-sharp with the left little finger key used on the note which precedes it if that finger is involved in the fingering of that note, or if the left litle finger is not involved in the note preceding the G-sharp, prepare for the note which follows it by using that key for the G-sharp. Left little finger keys to be used for each G-sharp (or A-flat) are indicated above the note in the example.

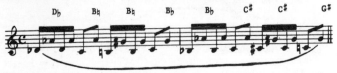

Without the use of this articulation of the G-sharp this example would be impossible to play legato, but using the fingerings indicated a perfect legato is possible and the rapid movement of notes no problem at all. This procedure should be introduced to students when the need arises in music which they are playing and referred to until it becomes an automatic part of their technique.

5. *Selection and Use of Alternate Fingerings.* There are alternate fingerings for some notes in each of the three octave range of the saxophone which match the standard basic fingerings perfectly in tone quality and intonation. If the smoothest and most useful technique is to be developed it is necessary that these alternates be learned, when and how they are to be used, and the best choice made each time there is a choice. This choice should be the one which gives the smoothest progression and the best facility and intonation. Notes in the example following have standard alternate fingerings. Each quarter note indicates a fingering for that pitch. Special trill fingerings which sacrifice intonation for facility are not included in this list.

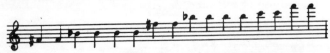

These are all fingerings which should be learned and facility developed by the student before or during the intermediate stage of development. Unless full advantage is taken of the potentials of the instrument, technical development is slowed, or smooth facility never achieved. Following is a consideration of each fingering and its uses:

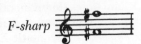

Two fingerings: (1) 123 050 Diatonic Fingering
　　　　　　　 (2) 123 406x Chromatic Fingering

Use of the chromatic fingering is mandatory where F and F-sharp (or G-flat) follow each other if perfect smoothness is to be achieved. The only exception to this rule is found when the fingering of the note preceding or following the F-sharp involves the sixth finger on the button of the tone hole. Following are typical passages using these fingerings:

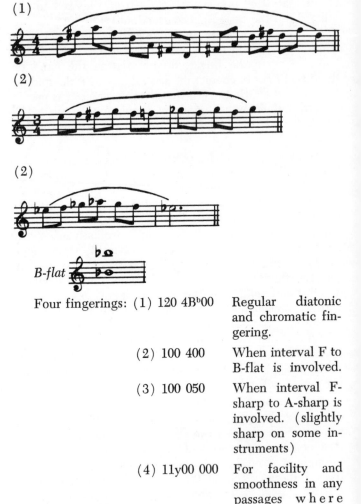

Four fingerings: (1) 120 4B♭00 　Regular diatonic and chromatic fingering.

(2) 100 400 　When interval F to B-flat is involved.

(3) 100 050 　When interval F-sharp to A-sharp is involved. (slightly sharp on some instruments)

(4) 11y00 000 　For facility and smoothness in any passages where there is no B-natural.

The first fingering, the regular diatonic and chromatic fingering, is the most frequently used of all the fingerings. It is the preferred fingering in chromatic passages, in sharp keys, and in any passage where B-natural occurs. The second fingering produces a perfectly in tune B-flat and is useful when the interval of F to B-flat or B-flat to F occurs, as well as certain passages in which notes fingered with the right hand skip to the B-flat. The third fingering, a cross fingering, is slightly sharp on some instruments but may be used on these when the B-flat is not an exposed note. It is useful in passages involving the interval of F-sharp to A-sharp or A-sharp to F-sharp. Both the second and third fingerings should be introduced rather early in saxophone study as they permit students with limited facility to play these intervals more smoothly and accurately than when the regular diatonic fingering is used. The fourth fingering in which the first finger of the left hand closes both the first tone hole and key ly is one of the most useful, but at the same time one of the most neglected fingerings on the instrument. It provides a fingering for B-flat which utilizes only one finger on the instrument and makes this note as convenient to play as B-natural with the resultant smoothness and rapid facility not possible with the use of the regular diatonic fingering. The only limitation on its use is that the passage not contain B-natural since to produce B-natural the finger would have to slide off of key ly. In this respect its use is analogous to the use of the thumb B-flat lever on the flute. This fourth fingering is considered as a useful alternate, perhaps even the standard, fingering for flat keys. Use of this fingering should be delayed until the regular diatonic fingering is established, but then introduced and established in the student's technique. Following are typical passages in which each of the four fingerings are used:

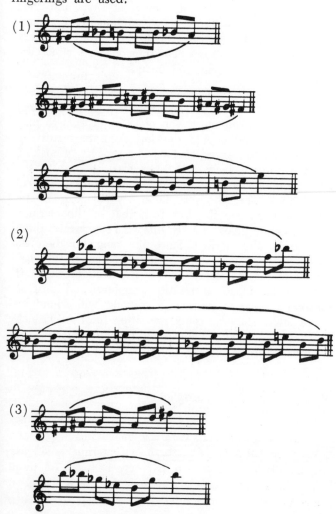

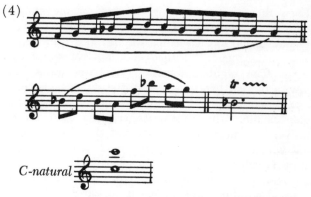

C-natural

Two fingerings: (1) 020 000 diatonic fingering
(2) 100 4C00 chromatic fingering

The first fingering is the standard fingering for C, while the second is for chromatic passages and where the C follows or precedes B-natural if the right hand is not involved in the fingering of the note immediately preceding or following the C. It is difficult to release key 4C and depress a tone hole simultaneously with the right hand. Use the second fingering, when possible to overcome the inherent roughness which results in the rapid changes from B-natural to the diatonic fingering for C. Following are typical usages of these two fingerings:

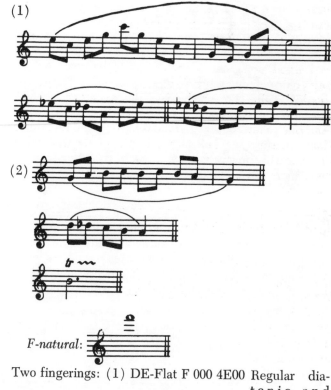

F-natural:

Two fingerings: (1) DE-Flat F 000 4E00 Regular diatonic and chromatic fingering.

(2) 1x20 000 Alternate fingering.

Even though it is the highest note in the normal range of the saxophone this F occurs with considerable frequency in the music written for the Alto instrument, with some frequency for the Tenor but rarely for the Baritone. The regular fingering, involving three side keys with the left hand and one in the right is awkward and considerable practice and experience is necessary to gain facility. The regular fingering is used almost exclusively by most saxophonists, but the alternate fingering which provides a tone of equal quality and intonation is valuable in situations where it can be used. This fingering calls for the first finger to be moved from its normal location and stretched upward to key 1x. Virtually every brand of saxophone has this key located in such a way that it is impossible to slide the finger to it—the finger must be picked up from the first tone hole and replaced in its new location. If this key could be moved so that the finger could conveniently roll or slide, it would be of far greater use. It was added to the instrument as an auxiliary key many years after the invention of the instrument by Sax primarily for the interval of C to F in the major arpeggio and for instances where the high F is isolated. This fingering cannot be used conveniently when the first finger is in place on its tone hole on the preceding note, or must be on the tone hole on the note following. This example illustrates typical uses of both fingerings:

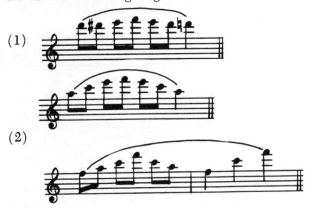

6. *Trill Fingerings.* Although most trills on the saxophone may be done with the basic and alternate fingerings previously discussed, some notes require special fingerings in order to provide smoothness and speed. Many of these special trill fingerings sacrifice either tone quality or intonation for the sake of facility and must not be used on notes which are sufficiently exposed to give a true impression of pitch and quality. In addition to their use in trilling these special fingerings are valuable in playing grace notes, mordents, or turns which would otherwise be difficult or impossible to execute. In a trill the lower note is played with a regular fingering and the upper note with the trill fingering. A special chart of trill fingerings is provided following the fingering chart.

TRANSPOSITIONS FOR THE SAXOPHONE

While the saxophonist in the normal band or orchestra routine is rarely called upon to transpose and play a part written for another instrument, the situation does occasionally arise. In those schools which include a dance band in the curriculum the need for facility in transposition frequently becomes a matter of importance, and in the professional dance band field various transpositions are so common as to be considered an essential part of the performer's skill. Certainly the advanced school player should develop facility in the more common transpositions for his instrument. This facility is acquired only by doing it, slowly at first, and then with increasing speed. Regular assignments in transposition of study material should be a part of every advanced student's lessons. The transpositions which are most commonly encountered include:

1. *Playing B-flat Clarinet Parts on the Alto Saxophone.* The need for this transposition is so frequent that the Alto saxophonist who plays or expects to play in a dance band should develop accurate facility in sight-reading this transposition. The process of making the transposition from the B-flat clarinet part to the Alto saxophone is to play the clarinet notes a perfect fifth higher. The Alto saxophone key signature is one sharp more or one flat less than that of the clarinet. This interval gives exactly the same concert pitch sounded by the clarinet. Since the range of the Alto saxophone does not extend as high as that of the clarinet, notes for the clarinet above B-flat above the staff cannot be produced on the Alto saxophone and must be transposed down a perfect fourth and will sound an octave lower than the pitches written for the clarinet. The following example illustrates the interval and key signature transpositions.

Clarinet Key: C	Saxophone Key: G	Clarinet Key: G	Saxophone Key: D	Clarinet Key: E-flat	Saxophone Key: B-flat

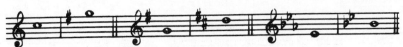

2. *Playing Bass Clarinet Parts on the Baritone Saxophone.* In large studio bands the Baritone saxophone player frequently doubles on Bass clarinet. If in the school band this player does not have a Bass clarinet, the parts written for it may be transposed and played on the Baritone saxophone with exactly the same transposition as that used for the B-flat clarinet to Alto saxophone. As both the Bass clarinet and Baritone saxophone sound an octave lower than written this transposition will have the Baritone playing exactly the same pitches as those written for the Bass clarinet. The same limitation in the upper range applies as for the Alto saxophone transposition.

3. *Playing Alto Saxophone from Piano Music.* Playing from a piano part or scales, tuning chords, etc., from a given concert key or from parts written for a non-transposing instrument such as flute is a useful facility to acquire. Flute and oboe are frequent doubles for the Alto saxophone in the studio band, and playing from piano music is frequently recreational in nature which helps encourage development. To sound the same note as the concert key the Alto saxophone plays a major sixth higher than written. The key signature is obtained by adding three sharps or subtracting three flats from the signature of the piano. Example No. 1 illustrates the interval and key signature transpositions. The same transposition is used for playing Baritone saxophone from piano music, but the saxophone sounds an octave lower than the piano note.

4. *Playing Tenor Saxophone from Piano Music.* The need for transposing from a concert key for the Tenor saxophone is as great as that for the Alto saxophone both in the normal school band routine and for recreation, and for those players in the school dance band. The problem with this transposition is that the range in which the Tenor saxophone sounds is an octave lower than those of the oboe, flute, or voice lines on piano sheet music. With this transposition the Tenor saxophone will sound an octave lower than the written pitches for the original part. This transposition is a major second higher than the written note, sounding an octave lower. The

key signature for the Tenor saxophone is obtained by adding two sharps or subtracting two flats from the original signature. Example No. 2 illustrates the interval and key signature transpositions.

5. *Playing Oboe Parts on B-flat Soprano Saxophone.* Since the oboe cannot be played satisfactorily in a marching band, many directors ask the oboe players to play a Soprano saxophone when marching. As the playing range of the Soprano saxophone is almost identical with that of the oboe, it is a most satisfactory substitute for this purpose and the student transposes the oboe part. The same transposition can be used when playing from a piano, violin, or flute part. This transposition is accomplished in the same way as that described above for playing Tenor saxophone from piano music. The Soprano saxophone will sound the same pitch as the original part.

6. *Playing B-flat Clarinet Parts on Tenor Saxophone.* As both instruments are B-flat instruments the clarinet part may be read as written but will sound an octave lower when played on the Tenor saxophone. Not all parts are satisfactory in the musical texture when sounding an octave lower than written, and the Tenor saxophone should play the notes an octave higher where possible if he is to blend with other B-flat clarinets. In dance band the Tenor saxophone player is expected to double on B-flat clarinet, and playing clarinet parts on the saxophone is not a desirable substitute.

7. *Playing Alto Saxophone Parts on the Tenor Saxophone.* This procedure will be necessary very infrequently in the school dance band, although advanced players who play professionally should have this facility. The need for this transposition arises most frequently in the "Tenor band" style which uses no Alto saxophones but which may play some arrangements in which parts are written for the Alto. In this case the original Alto saxophone part is transposed and played on the Tenor. The problem of the differences in range of actual sounds of the two instruments can be solved only by having the Tenor saxophone play those notes which are out of range an octave lower. To sound the same pitch as the Alto,

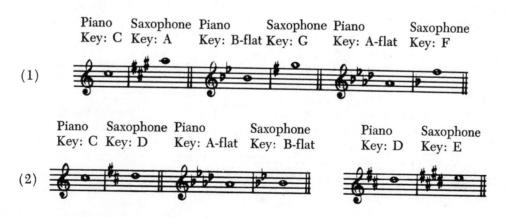

Piano Saxophone Piano Saxophone Piano Saxophone
Key: C Key: A Key: B-flat Key: G Key: A-flat Key: F

(1)

Piano Saxophone Piano Saxophone Piano Saxophone
Key: C Key: D Key: A-flat Key: B-flat Key: D Key: E

(2)

the Tenor saxophone transposes the note written for the Alto a perfect fourth higher, or a perfect fifth lower to sound an octave below the Alto pitch. The transposed key signature is obtained by adding one flat or subtracting one sharp from the Alto saxophone signature. Example No. 3 illustrates the interval and key signature transposition.

8. *Playing Tenor Saxophone Parts on the Alto Saxophone.* There is very little need for this transposition as the difference in the pitch range of the two instruments does not lend itself to good musical results in most circumstances. The transposition for playing Tenor saxophone parts on the Alto saxophone is the same as that described for transposing from B-flat clarinet parts. With the transposition up a perfect fifth, the Alto saxophone will sound an octave higher than the Tenor saxophone pitch, and the Alto saxophone should play his transposed note an octave lower whenever the range of the instrument permits.

9. *Playing Bassoon Parts on Baritone Saxophone.* With the chronic shortage of bassoon players in many school systems, some directors who have good Baritone saxophone players available ask them to transpose and play the bassoon parts in band or orchestra. This must be considered a temporary expediency as the tone quality of the Baritone saxophone is quite different from that of the bassoon, but it does cover the part and get the job done. Transposing from the bassoon part, or any other part written in bass clef, is the simplest of all transpositions. To accomplish this change the bass clef to a treble clef and add three sharps or subtract three flats from the bass clef signature. Other than this purely mechanical process the player must adjust for accidentals in the original part by raising or lowering the pitch of his note in the same way and to the same degree that the written accidental altered the original. With some instruction and experience the average school musician is able to do this accurately. Example No. 4 illustrates the interval and key signature transposition.

SELECTION OF INSTRUMENTS

The saxophone was invented by the great artisan of wind instruments Adolphe Sax who patented the instrument in 1846. It was the result of his experiments with applying a single reed mouthpiece to the ophicleide, a now obsolete brass instrument played with a cup mouthpiece but having tone holes and pads rather than valves. He was fascinated with mixture of woodwind and brass tone qualities which resulted and gradually evolved the shape and mechanism of the saxophone which he patented. In general appearance the modern saxophone is little different from the original, but many refinements in the mechanism have been made to expand its technical potentials. The original Sax instruments' range was from low B-natural to the high D. A low B-flat has been added as well as the high notes from D to F. Other changes include the articulations for the G-sharp key, the alternate F-sharp key, and a single automatic octave key replacing the two separate octave keys of the original.

Today the mechanism of the saxophone is so standardized that there is a single model available from all manufacturers, differing mechanically only in shape and placement of keys and finger buttons. The teacher and student is not forced to make a decision between various models having different numbers of keys as he is when selecting a clarinet or oboe.

The same three different grades of instruments, determined by musical standards, are found in the saxophone just as in the other woodwinds. These grades are determined by tone quality produced by the instrument, by the accuracy of its intonation, by the mechanism which must be rugged and capable of easy and long lasting adjustment, by beauty and permanence of its finish, and by the general standards and control of production reflected in the amount and skill of the hand work involved. The grade of instrument must be selected to fit the use to which the student will put it. An instrument suitable for the elementary school begin-

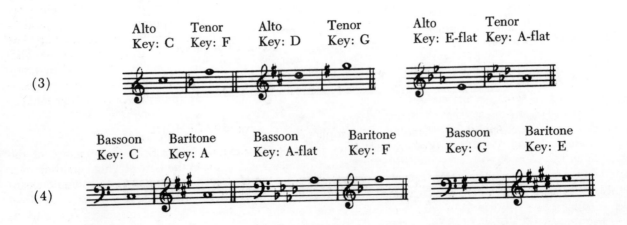

Alto   Tenor   Alto   Tenor   Alto   Tenor
Key: C Key: F   Key: D Key: G   Key: E-flat Key: A-flat

(3)

Bassoon Baritone   Bassoon   Baritone   Bassoon Baritone
Key: C   Key: A   Key: A-flat Key: F   Key: G   Key: E

(4)

ner is not necessarily suited to the advanced high school or college player. There are considerable differences in the quality of instruments produced by various manufacturers as well as in the various lines of instruments produced by the same manufacturer. Price is not always, even though it is frequently an indication of quality. The higher the standard of tone quality and other musical values expected of the student, the more carefully the instrument must be selected. Select a saxophone with the same high standards and care used in selecting the best oboe or clarinet.

The standard finish for all the saxophones is a brass lacquer, which although giving virtually the same appearance on every brand, is subject to great fluctuation in lasting quality. Until recent years a gold lacquer, giving the instrument a gold rather than a brass color, was an optional choice in finish. This gold lacquer is still available from some manufacturers. Until the development of the gold and brass lacquer, the instruments were silver plated. The silver plate gave a permanent finish to the instrument, while lacquer deteriorates and wears and must be replaced periodically, but was dropped apparently because of the higher cost. The type of exterior finish on the body and keys of the instruments has no effect at all on the tone quality, and is selected for other reasons. The heavy brass lacquer is recommended for all student instruments.

An optional extra key to extend the range down a half-step to A is available in some brands of Baritone saxophones. The Baritone instrument used for illustrations in this chapter has this extension to low A. This extra key requires lengthening the bell of the instrument, and some redistribution of tone holes on the lower part of the instrument. It has no effect on the tone quality of the instrument, nor upon its intonation. This extra key is useful in symphonic bands and in dance bands playing special arrangements where it is called for. It is recommended only for advanced students. This extra key is available only on the Baritone instrument.

STUDENT QUALIFICATIONS AND APTITUDES

The Alto and Tenor saxophones are good beginning instruments, and the comments in this section refer only to them. The Soprano, Baritone, and Bass saxophones should be played only by competent performers on either the Alto or Tenor saxophone. It should be noted that because of the great differences in the cost of a saxophone and a clarinet suitable for young beginners, many teachers prefer to place elementary school age beginners on the clarinet rather than the saxophone. Students who have demonstrated good tone production and basic technique on the clarinet will make rapid progress on the saxophone.

Standards of physical aptitudes for the saxophone are not always reliable. Any student with normal teeth, lip, and chin formation can play the saxophone successfully.

Thick lips and thin lips, crooked teeth and straight teeth, and to some extent overbite and underbite can all be accommodated within the normal embouchure formation without any adverse results on future development.

It is obvious that the student must be physically large enough so that he may hold the instrument with the proper hand position before he begins to study the saxophone. Students who are too small to play the instrument develop poor hand positions which are extremely difficult to correct, make slow progress and tend to become discouraged because of the physical handicap. Whether the student is large enough to play the instrument can be easily determined by asking him to hold the assembled instrument with the assistance of a properly adjusted neck strap. Place his right hand in position. If the thumb is in the right place, can he reach the three tone hole buttons with the fingers curved and contact the buttons properly. If he can do this, see if he can reach the C key with the little finger without pulling the hand out of position. If he is successful in all of this, test the left hand with the thumb in position; will his fingers reach over the side keys to reach the tone buttons and retain their curved shape? Students who can do this can easily reach the G-sharp and C-sharp keys with the little finger. Small hands will have trouble extending the little finger to the B-natural and B-flat keys, but this should be of little concern as these notes do not normally appear very early in the study of the instrument.

Having been checked for physical size, a natural aptitude for the instrument may be determined by the success of the prospective student in producing a steady natural tone of the highest pitch with the mouthpiece and reed alone after some instruction on embouchure. Students who are immediately successful and who are able to produce and sustain a strong clear tone for five to ten seconds may be said to have a natural aptitude for the instrument, and are ready to begin study. Other students may fail this test for some time, but with instruction and guidance may develop an aptitude. Such students should not be denied the opportunity to study saxophone on this basis alone, since the difference between those who quickly accomplish this tone production and those who must work to develop it disappears soon after formal study of the instrument begins. Success or failure on the instrument is determined by many other factors. In the final analysis desire and persistence are the greatest of all aptitudes for any instrument.

CARE OF THE SAXOPHONE

Simple but regular and careful maintenance of the saxophone will keep it in the best playing condition over a long period of time. Careless handling, sporadic cleaning, and lack of attention soon begins to have an effect on how the instrument plays and responds. It is important that the basic procedures for care of the instrument be emphasized from the very beginning of saxophone study so that they are correctly done and become habitual. Care of the instrument starts with the assembly and disassembly of the instrument. Review the instructions on assembly of the instrument until they are thoroughly understood and the students are performing the operation easily. Disassembly is done in the same manner, but in the exact reverse order of assembly. Keep the instrument in its case when not in use for maximum protection. Heat is the greatest enemy of the instrument. Keep it, in or out of its case, out of direct sunlight and away from radiators and other sources of heat.

Cleaning the Instrument

It is mandatory that the inside of the saxophone—body, neck, and mouthpiece be thoroughly dried after each playing. Establish this routine from the very beginning of study. Many saxophone players have the unfortunate habit of entirely neglecting this process. Swabbing the instrument does not take much time, and will prevent the accumulation of dirt and grime inside the instrument, as well as helping to maintain sanitary conditions for playing. To dry the instrument properly each case should be equipped with the following:

1. *A Swab.* To clean the inside of the body of the instrument. The best and most efficient is a chamois with a center brush attached to a cord with a weight to pull the cord through the instrument. The cord must be long enough to drop entirely through the body of the instrument. This type of swab comes in two sizes, one for Alto and one for Tenor. The Tenor swab can be adapted for use on the Baritone by replacing the cord with one of sufficient length. The Soprano saxophone can be cleaned with the Alto swab, or with a clarinet chamois swab provided the cord is long enough.

2. *A Neck Cleaner.* A flexible metal wire with a soft wool swab on one end and a stiff brush on the other. The wool swab end is pushed through the neck to dry moisture, while the brush end is used to clean out any accumulated deposits. The neck is the most critical poriton of the swabbing process; using a neck cleaner is the only way it can be kept clean. These come in only one size, and can be used on all saxophones.

3. *A Chamois or Soft Cloth.* To clean the inside and outside of the mouthpiece. Because of the danger of chipping the mouthpiece neither the swab or the neck cleaner can be used on the mouthpiece. This chamois or cloth, but preferably another, is used to wipe the upper part of the bell and the outside of the instrument.

The following routine for cleaning the saxophone is a standard one which should be followed carefully until the player is sufficiently advanced to make satisfactory changes to suit himself. The instrument pictured is the Alto saxophone, but the same process is followed on all instruments in the family.

1. *Mouthpiece.* Remove the mouthpiece from the instrument. Loosen the ligature and slide the reed from under it; then remove the ligature. Wipe off the reed with the chamois and put it in a reed case or aside to be returned to the mouthpiece. Roll the chamois to fit the inside of the mouthpiece. Push the smaller end through the mouthpiece, and pull through carefully as in Figure S-43, or push back and forth until the mouthpiece is completely dry. Return the ligature to the mouthpiece and slide under the reed if it is not kept in a reed case. If the reed is returned to the mouthpiece, put it in playing position, and tighten the ligature screws just enough to hold the reed. If the ligature screws are too tight there is danger of damaging the facing of the mouth piece if the instrument is exposed to heat. Put the mouthpiece cap in place as shown in the directions for assembly, and return the mouthpiece to its place in the case.

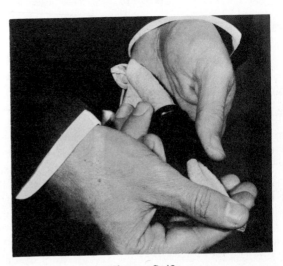

Figure S-43.

2. *Neck.* Loosen the tension screw and remove the neck from the body of the instrument. Carefully shake the moisture out of each end. Then holding the neck as shown in Figure S-44 push the wool swab of the neck cleaner into the neck from the large end and back and forth through the neck to thoroughly dry it. Once each week this should be followed by a thorough brushing with the brush end of the neck cleaner. Return neck to its place in the case.

3. *Body.* Holding the body of the saxophone by the bell away from the keys unhook the neck strap. Tilt and shake the body to remove excess moisture from small end. Drop the weight on the end of the swab cord into the bell and rotate the instrument so that it falls out the other end. Pull the swab through the body as in Figure S-45. Repeat this process several times if necessary to remove all moisture.

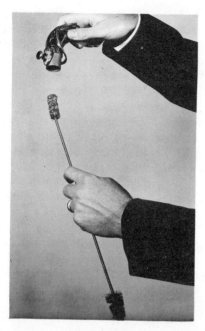

Figure S-44.

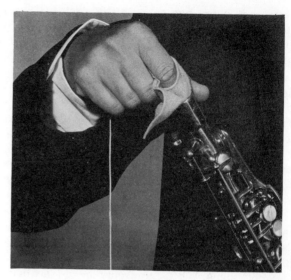

Figure S-46.

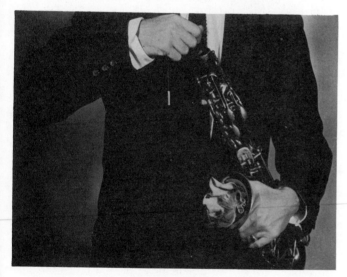

Figure S-45.

Regular Maintenance of the Instrument

If the saxophone received good care and a regular schedule of maintenance is followed it will remain in the best playing condition over a long period of time. Instruments which are in poor condition are difficult to play and result in poor players. Observing the following suggestions will help keep the saxophone in the perfect mechanical condition so necessary for success on the instrument.

1. *Oiling the Mechanism*. The mechanism must be oiled regularly three or four times each year. A special oil, called key oil, is available under various brand names for this purpose. A drop of oil on the end of a needle or toothpick should be at each pivot screw of each key. Do this carefully so that no oil can get onto the pads. This regular oiling keeps pivot screws from excessive wear and from rusting in place, making any repairs and adjustments on the instrument easier to accomplish.

2. *Corks and Felts*. A casual examination of the saxophone will reveal a number of bumper corks or felts against which keys rest either in an open or a closed position. These not only keep the mechanism silent in operation but determine the height to which the pads rise above the holes. This height is critical as it has a considerable adverse effect on intonation if it is incorrect. Two very critical adjusting corks appear on the cup of the tone hole just above the first finger of the right hand. One of these closes a tone hole on the articulated G-sharp, the other a tone hole higher on the instrument when the first or second finger of the right hand is used for a fork B-flat fingering. If either of these are worn or damaged the tone holes do not close and that fingering will not respond. If either of the fingerings does not operate properly suspect these corks first. Some of the better instruments have adjusting screws in con-

4. *Connecting Joint*. Using a portion of the chamois around the index finger clean the inside of the connecting joint on the top of the body as in Figure S-46. Insert the end plug for storage in case.

5. *Outside of Instrument*. Using the chamois or soft cloth wipe the inside portion of the bell that can be reached with the hand, then the outside of the bell to remove finger prints. Continue to wipe the body of the instrument on which no keys are attached. Once a week the entire key mechanism should be wiped free of fingerprints and dust. If this is done regularly and thoroughly the instrument's finish will remain in good condition.

nection with these two corks so that they may be kept in perfect adjustment by the player. If any of the corks or felt bumpers are lost or badly worn they should be replaced by a repairman.

3. *Dusting the Instrument.* If the instrument is wiped carefully after each use as suggested above, very little dust will accumulate. However, over a period of time some dust will be found beneath the key mechanism where the regular wiping does not reach. This dust can be removed with a soft watercolor brush. If a cloth is used, it must be handled very carefully so it will not snag on the needle springs which break under pressure.

4. *Polishing the Instrument.* The body and key mechanism of the saxophone will remain in good condition if wiped regularly as directed. After a long period of use the lacquer is worn away in places where the hands contact the keys and body, and the lacquer begins to loose its sheen. When this occurs the old lacquer must be removed and the entire instrument relacquered—a job for an expert. Students must be cautioned against attempting to polish a lacquered instrument with silver polish or a polishing cloth as such a procedure damages or removes the lacquer entirely, calling for an expensive relacquer job.

5. *Bent Rods or Keys.* In spite of the best of care, keys or rods sometimes become bent out of line. This occurs with alarming regularity on the instruments of young players, and cause unevenness in technique, or even prevent some tones from responding at all. The long rods on the right side of the instrument are especially susceptible to damage. No attempt should be made to straighten keys or rods while they are on the instrument. This puts excessive pressure on both the keys and their posts and the instrument may be damaged even more. This adjustment must be made by a repairman who has the proper knowledge and tools to straighten and align them. Caution students against trying to do it themselves.

6. *Sticking Pads.* The saxophone is not especially susceptible to sticking pads because of the large size of most of the pads and the fact that they have rather strong springs. If a student is having a problem with sticking pads, it is probably because he has failed to dry the instrument thoroughly before returning it to the case. Excessively high humidity might also be the cause. The pad most likely to stick is that of the G-sharp key as it is both opened and closed with a spring because of its articulation with other keys. This is discovered when the student fingers G-sharp, but the instrument plays G-natural. It can be unstuck by depressing the G-sharp key and lifting the pad from the hole with the forefinger of the right hand.

The moisture which causes pads to stick can be removed by placing a cigarette paper between the pad and the tone hole, and pressing down firmly on the key. Release the key, move the paper and repeat the pro-

cess until the key no longer sticks. If this does not relieve the sticking, put the cigarette paper in place, press the key, and pull the paper slowly from under the pad. Repeat the process several times. If the pad persists in sticking, it should be replaced. Never use powder on pads in attempt to stop sticking as it damages the pad so it deteriorates.

7. *Leaky Pads.* Pads on an instrument wear out with use. Some wear out more rapidly than others and begin to leak, causing the instrument to respond with difficulty on certain notes. Pads deteriorate so slowly that the player is frequently not aware that the condition exists. For this reason a close inspection of the condition of the pads on every instrument should be made every three or four months.

There are two methods of determining whether a pad is seated properly or whether it is leaking. The first is by the use of commercial feeler or papers or strips of cigarette paper about a quarter inch wide. Slide one end of the paper under the pad, put the normal amount of pressure against the pad if the key is not held closed by a spring, and slowly draw the paper out. As long as the pressure against the paper remains constant there is no leak. If the pressure suddenly lessens the pad is not properly seated. Repeat the process completely around the pad so that all edges are tested. The second method is that used most frequently by professional repairmen. This is through the use of a small electric light on the end of a rod which is dropped into the bore of the instrument. When the light is held close to a leaky pad, it will shine through the pad and the exact source of the leak can be determined. Teachers responsible for the condition of numbers of woodwind instruments will find it advantageous to purchase such a light.

Regular Overhaul. The condition of every instrument must be checked at least once each year by the instructor or by a repairman. Regular maintenance keeps an instrument in playing condition over a period of years, rather than allowing it to gradually deteriorate becoming increasingly difficult to play and more expensive to repair. Every instrument must have a complete overhaul every three to five years depending on the amount of usage. If instruments receive a yearly checkup, a regular overhaul, and proper daily maintenance they will last in virtually perfect condition for many years.

BIBLIOGRAPHY OF STUDY MATERIALS

Except for beginning methods very little study material for saxophone is of recent vintage. Much of it is arrangements of standard material written originally for another instrument. However, a careful appraisal of available materials will indicate sufficient music to carry the saxophonist to the same technical and musical proficiency expected of the other woodwind instruments. The saxophone student should, and must, take advantage of the instructional material published for oboe. It is in the same playing range demanded of the saxophone and will greatly expand the possibilities for variety in musical styles and content.

For the most rapid technical and musical advancement it is recommended that the student study simultaneously from material in each of these classifications: (1) a method book; (2) technical studies in various keys; (3) a book of etudes or studies to include various musical styles over a period of time; (4) duets and/or other ensemble experience; and (5) solos with piano accompaniment.

Information about solos, duets and other types of ensembles making use of the saxophone is widely available from such sources as the Selective Lists of Instrumental Solos and Ensembles published by the National Interscholastic Music Activities Commission. Considerable information about the availibility of solos and ensembles as well as other classifications of material for saxophone can be obtained from the catalogs of retail stores specializing in woodwind music.[6]

In the sections which follow a cross-section of the most widely used material (exclusive of solo and ensemble music) available for saxophone is listed. These lists are divided into beginning methods, standard methods, and additional study materials of various kinds. A listing of composers, titles, and publishers such as is given here and the other sources mentioned is only the starting point for acquiring teaching materials. Only personal acquaintance with the music itself can give the answer to the quality of the music, and how and when it could be used. The reader is urged to examine as many of these titles as possible, and to evaluate them whenever possible through actual use.

Beginning Methods

Bodegraven, Paul van. *Adventures in Saxophone Playing.* Two volumes. Staff Music Publishing Co. An excellent, if not the best beginning method for the young student.

Calliet, Lucien. *Method for Saxophone.* Two volumes. Belwin, Inc. An excellent method. Has more material and progresses slightly faster than the Bodegraven. Combines well with the Bodegraven to give more material on various levels. Develops articulation especially well.

Colin-Lindeman. *Saxophone Made Easy.* Two Volumes. Charles Colin.

Gornston, David. *Very First Saxophone Method.* Edward Schuberth & Co.

Herfurth, C. Paul. *A Tune A Day For Saxophone.* Boston Music Co.

Hovey, N. W. *Elementary Method for Saxophone.* Rubank, Inc.

Pease, D. J. *Saxophone Method.* Pro Art.

Skornicka. *Intermediate Method for Saxophone,* Rubank, Inc.

Voxman-Gower. *Advanced Method for Saxophone.* Rubank, Inc.

Vereecken, Ben. *Junior Saxophone Method.* Rubank, Inc. A good source for supplementary melodic material.

Standard Methods

Henton, H. B. *Beginners Method for Saxophone.* Theodore Presser.

Klose-Gay. *Methode Complete pour Saxophone.* Leduc. English and French text. Modeled after and making use of much of the material in the Klose clarinet method with considerable additional material this is by far the best method for the serious student who has recahed the upper intermediate stage of development. Material is too difficult to follow directly after an "advanced" beginning method.

Iasilli, G. *Modern Conservatory Method for Saxophone.* Two Volumes. Carl Fischer.

Mayeur, A. *Method for Saxophone.* Carl Fischer or Leduc.

Vereecken, B. *Foundation to Saxophone Playing.* Carl Fischer.

The Saxophone Virtuoso. Carl Fischer. The first of these, while described as an elementary method on the title page, is not a beginning method in the present-day understanding of the word. It is suitable to follow a beginning method. The second has more advanced material in the form of twenty-four advanced studies. The first portion of this book is concerned with transpositions (including for C-melody saxophone!), and the second section with transposing for any saxophone through the use of the seven c clefs.

Ville, Paul de. *Universal Method for the Saxophone.* Carl Fischer. The best and most complete of the American publications, but is not arranged in progressive order of difficulty.

Wiedoeft, R. *Modern Method for Saxophone.* Two Volumes. Robins. With a copyright date of 1950 the Klose is the only one of these methods which presents a modern viewpoint and material. The deVille was copyrighted in 1908, the Vereecken in 1917 and 1919, the Mayeur in 1911, the Iasilli in 1927, the Wiedoeft in 1927, and the Henton in 1928. These dates reflect the tremendous popularity of the saxophone in the United States during the first part of this century, but unfortunately are woefully out of date for contemporary teaching techniques and interests.

---

[6] See Appendix IV for a list.

Additional Study Material

Arnold, Jay. *Fingered Scales for Saxophones.* Shapiro, Bernstein & Co.

Modern Fingering System for Saxophone. Shapiro, Bernstein & Co.

The second of these presents a most extensive series of fingerings with examples of when and how each is used, and carries the range above the high F. The fingered scales applies this fingering to scales in various forms with the option of extending them above the high F.

Bassi, L. *27 Virtuoso Studies.* Carl Fischer. Transcribed. by Iasilli from the original clarinet method. Advanced level.

Blemant. *20 Melodic Studies.* Two Volumes. Leduc.

Capelle. *20 Grand Studies for Saxophone.* Leduc.

Cragun. *Thirty Melodic Caprices.* Rubank, Inc.

Twenty Etudes. Rubank, Inc.

Chopin. *Chopin Studies Transcribed for Saxophone.* David Gornston. Intermediate level Chopin melodies transcribed by Paisner and Gornston.

Endresen. *Supplementary Studies for Saxophone.* Rubank, Inc.

Ferling. *48 Studies.* Southern Music Co., Leduc. The Southern Music company edition is the original oboe version. The Leduc edition is edited by Mule for saxophone and includes additional original studies in various keys. The other Ferling studies listed in the oboe chapter are also excellent for saxophone.

Gatti. *35 Melodious Technical Exercises.* Carl Fischer. *Studies on Major and Minor Scales.* Carl Fischer.

Hovey, Nilo. *First Book of Practical Exercises for Saxophone.* Belwin. Excellent begining level supplementary material.

Daily Exercises for Saxophone. Belwin. Fine work of Albert and Pares.

Klose, H. *25 Exercises for Saxophone.* Carl Fischer.

Labanchi. *33 Concert Etudes.* Three Volumes. Carl Fischer.

Lazarus. *Grand Virtuoso Saxophone Studies.* Belwin, Inc.

Luft, J. H. *24 Etudes.* Editions Costallat. Lower advanced level.

Mule, M. *24 Easy Studies after Samie.* Leduc.

Scales and Arpeggios. Three Volumes. Leduc.

18 Studies after Berbiguier. Leduc.

Daily Exercises after Terschak. Leduc.

30 Grand Studies after Soussmann. Two Volumes. Leduc.

52 Studies After Boehm, Terschak and Furstenau. Three Volumes. Leduc.

Miscellaneous Studies in All Keys. Leduc.

These studies, arranged by the famous French Virtuoso from standard works for other instruments, are some of the most musical and useful material available for saxophone. They are listed roughly in progressive order of difficulty.

Pantaleo. *Six Virtuoso Caprices.* Carl Fischer. Lower advanced level of difficulty.

Pares, C. *Scales and Daily Exercises for Saxophone.* Carl Fischer.

Modern Foundation Studies for Saxophone. Rubank, Inc. Two versions of the same material.

Rascher, S. *Top-Tones for the Saxophone.* Carl Fischer. In a brief book of twenty-four pages Mr. Rascher clearly presents a technique for developing the playing range above high F through the use of harmonics. Indispensible for the alto saxophonist who wishes to extend his range.

158 Saxophone Exercises. Wilhelm Hansen. Quite advanced technical exercises built around various chord structures. Does not use the range above high F. Excellent material for the advanced student.

Salviani. *Exercises for Saxophone.* Carl Fischer.

Teal, Larry. *The Saxophonist's Workbook.* University Music Press.

Tustin, Whitney. *Technical Studies.* Peer International Corporation. The most complete book of mechanical technical studies available. Useful on both intermediate and advanced levels. In six sections: scales, intervals, arpeggios, trills, exercises for tonguing, exercises for fingering.

Voxman, H. *Selected Studies for Saxophone.* Rubank, Inc.

STUDY AND ACHIEVEMENT QUESTIONS

1. Discuss the possible reasons for the lack of performance standards for the saxophone.

2. What is the theoretical written range for the saxophone?

3. Select a band arrangement scored for a full complement of saxophones. Transpose the saxophone parts to the pitches they actually sound and make a two-line piano score of these parts.

4. Identify the easy and complete range for the instrument.

5. Assemble a saxophone identifying each part as it is taken from the case and demonstrating the correct holding positions for each operation. Show how the neck strap is correctly adjusted.

6. Demonstrate the correct procedure for placing a reed on the saxophone mouthpiece. Add the protective cap.

7. Observe one or more beginning, intermediate and advanced saxophone students and fill out the check list for assembly. Suggest corrections for any faults.

8. Describe and demonstrate the correct holding and hand positions for the saxophone. Instruct a student

unfamiliar with the instrument in how to achieve the correct positions.

9. Observe one or more beginning, intermediate and advanced saxophone students and fill out the check list for holding and hand positions. Describe the effect any faults will have on performance and suggest appropriate corrections.

10. Discuss and demonstrate correct and incorrect placement and use of the left thumb. The correct placement of the right thumb. Demonstrate hand positions for correct use of the side keys.

11. Describe and discuss the two basic embouchure formations for saxophone. Select one and demonstrate the step by step procedure in its formation. Do the same with a student who is unfamiliar with the instrument.

12. List the most commonly found faults in the type embouchure selected and describe the effect of each on performance.

13. Observe various students during performance and fill out check lists for embouchure formation. If any faults are observed identify their effect on performance, and suggest corrections.

14. What are the factors which will make the pitch of a saxophone flat? Sharp? Instruct an advanced player on how to demonstrate some of them.

15. Identify by writing on the staff the three registers in the saxophone's range.

16. What is meant by an "extended range" for the saxophone? How is this achieved?

17. List the most common problems in tone production on the saxophone together with their causes and corrections.

18. Describe the three basic methods for tongue placement for articulation. How does this placement differ on the Alto, Tenor and Baritone instruments?

19. What is an articulated G-sharp key? How does it function?

20. List all the notes which have alternate fingerings, demonstrate each, and illustrate how each is used.

21. Identify the various transpositions which may be required of a saxophonist and describe how each is made.

22. What three items are needed for the regular cleaning of the instrument?

23. Perform the process of disassembly and cleaning. Discuss the regular maintenance of the instrument.

24. How may sticking pads be corrected? How may leaky pads be identified?

25. Make a comparative analysis of as many beginning saxophone methods as you have available. Select and rank them in order of preference.

26. Examine available standard methods and additional study materials for saxophone and list them with comments. Examine and list oboe study material which you consider suitable for saxophone.

27. Prepare a suggested list of study material to include all five types of material suggested for simultaneous study for an upper beginning level student. For an intermediate level student. For an advanced student.

28. Attend a music festival event which includes saxophone solos and ensembles. Observe the players and make a detailed critique of as many as possible on details of holding positions, hand positions, embouchure formation, tuning, intonation, tone quality, articulation and technique. Describe any faults found in any of these, the symptoms, possible causes, and corrections for each.

CHAPTER SIX

MOUTHPIECES AND REEDS

The quality, intonation, and control of the tone of the clarinet and saxophone is influenced by and, to a great extent, determined by the mouthpiece together with the reed and the embouchure. Of these basic factors involved in the production of the tone, only the mouthpiece remains constant. Further it can be measured and produced so that under careful quality control in production any number can be made which will respond exactly alike. Embouchures vary considerably from player to player, and even from day to day with the same player. The quality of response in reeds cannot be predicted. They wear out and must be replaced. Because of the variation in embouchure and reed it is most important that the one stable item—the mouthpieces—be carefully selected and cared for.

A tone is produced on the clarinet and saxophone by the vibration of the reed which acts as a flap beating against the mouthpiece alternately opening and closing the tip opening. When the tip opening is closed, the stream of air is interrupted, and when the reed breaks free from its contact with the mouthpiece the air stream flows into the instrument. This rapid pulsation of air into the instrument sets the column of air into vibration and produces a tone. The length of the column of air is determined by the fingering being used for a particular note, and forces the reed to vibrate in the natural frequency of the note being fingered.

The mouthpiece must be constructed so that the vibration of the reed can be controlled by the embouchure in such a way as to produce the desired pitch and tone quality. The length of the table (or lay) and the amount of curvature determine how much of the reed moves and how far it must move. The opening at the tip determines how far the flexible tip of the reed must move to stop the flow of air. The size and shape of these parts of the mouthpiece in relation to the vibration of the reed becomes of the utmost importance when it is realized that the reed strikes the mouthpiece 146 times each second for the Chalameau F and 1395 times

each second for the G in the high register on the clarinet. For this to occur such a large number of times each second in such a way as to produce the best sounds demands a fine mouthpiece.

Achieving the proper number of vibrations per second to produce the desired pitch is the most simple of the problems. A poor mouthpiece, even combined with a poor reed and embouchure formation will produce a pitch. A pitch is not enough. The tone must be of a pleasing characteristic quality for the instrument. The quality of a tone is determined by the form of the sound wave produced. The best wave form will produce a good quality, another shape wave will produce a poor quality. The basic forms of the sound waves which can be produced are determined by both the internal and external shape and dimensions of the mouthpiece. This basic form determines the limits within which the reed and embouchure can operate to produce and control the type of sound produced. If the physical characteristics of a mouthpiece do not produce a basic wave form which is capable of being controlled and shaped to produce the desired tone quality even with the best embouchure and the finest reed it will not be possible to develop a good tone.

The loudness of the tone produced on a single reed mouthpiece is determined primarily by the amplitude of the vibration of the reed. The greatest amplitude, hence the loudest tone possible, is determined by the length and amount of curve on the facing and by the amount of tip opening. From this maximum amount of vibration the embouchure tightens and controls the amplitude for less volume of tone. If the greatest amplitude is not large enough the student cannot play with a full tone no matter how much the embouchure is relaxed. If the facing is long and the tip quite open an embouchure which is quite strong is required to play a soft tone with good quality and control. Selecting a reed to fit the mouthpiece will sometimes aleviate this situation, although usually at the expense of tone quality.

PARTS OF THE MOUTHPIECE

The construction of mouthpieces for all clarinets and saxophones is basically the same. The size is changed to fit the instrument on which it is being used, but the identification of parts and the influence of these parts is the same on all. Figure R-1 which is a drawing of a B-flat clarinet mouthpiece identifies in standard nomenclature the parts of the mouthpiece.[1]

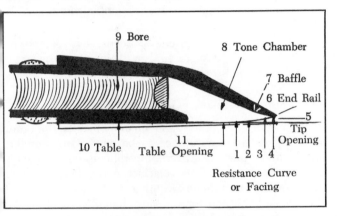

CLARINET MOUTHPIECE—CROSS SECTION

Figure R-1.

The manner in which the mouthpiece is constructed, i.e., the shape of the tone chamber, the size of the bore, the length and shape of the table opening, and the size of the tip opening determine the kind and quality of tone the mouthpiece is capable of producing. Upon this potential the reed and embouchure are selected and developed to produce the desired tone quality. There is no scientific evidence that a mouthpiece needs to be fitted to a particular individual or to a particular embouchure formation in order to achieve a desired tone quality. A mouthpiece with a medium facing and a medium tip opening, provided it is constructed accurately with all specifications correct, will be the best choice for every student.

The parts of the mouthpiece identified in the drawing may be described as follows:

1, 2, 3, 4. *The Facing*, resistance curve, or lay is the portion on the flat side which slants away from the reed. The facing varies greatly both in length and in the amount of curvature. A short lay requires less mouthpiece in the mouth, and frequently produces a stuffy tone quality with little volume or projection. An excessively long lay requires more than the normal amount of mouthpiece in the mouth. Because of the greater length of reed which is vibrating it is more difficult to control, demands more than normal breath pressure, frequently produces a rough tone and is tiring to play. A long facing usually requires a soft reed, while a short facing calls for a stiff reed.

5. *Tip Opening*. This is the distance between the mouthpiece and the reed at the tip. The tip opening is described as close, medium, or wide, each with some variation depending on the length of the facing. The amount of tip opening is determined by the amount of curvature on the facing as well as its length. It is this opening which provides the resistance to the flow of breath into the instrument. A close opening offers great resistance, requires a stiff reed, and produces a small stuffy tone quality. A wide opening offers little resistance, requiring a soft reed, a strong embouchure and is difficult to control. A medium opening is recommended for all students at all levels of advancement. It provides optimum resistance, uses a medium stiff reed, and normal embouchure support. The medium opening produces the tone quality commonly accepted as typical of the instrument regardless of the type of embouchure formation used.

6. *End Rail*. The end rail is the edge of the mouthpiece tip against which the tip of the reed beats. This is a critical portion of the mouthpiece, which must be perfectly smooth, not too wide, and the same width from side to side. The width varies with the instrument for which the mouthpiece is made. On the B-flat clarinet it should be no wider than one thirty-second of an inch. If the end rail is too wide the reed responds slower because it has a tendency to stick on the surface, and it is difficult to articulate properly. The shape of the end rail must correspond exactly with the shape of the reed for that instrument. The mark of a well made mouthpiece is in the finishing of this end rail which must be carefully done by hand.

7. *Baffle*. The baffle is produced when the end rail is completed and the inside of the mouthpiece is leveled off to fit the tone chamber. The height of this baffle is critical in tone production. If it is too high the mouthpiece squeaks. If it is too low it is difficult to produce and control notes in the upper register of the instrument. Some mouthpieces which are otherwise well made, will be unusable because of the height of the baffle.

8. *Tone Chamber*. The tone chamber is the interior of the mouthpiece under the facing, extending from the tip to the beginning of the bore. The proportions of the tone chamber determine to a degree the type of response the mouthpiece will give and the quality of tone it will produce. Most brands of mouthpieces use the same shape tone chamber for all models for a particular instrument, varying only the facing and tip opening. A few will have a choice of tone chambers, and if they are available will make this fact known. The size and

[1]Reproduced by permission of Mr. Arlie Richardson, Supervisor of Instrumental Music in the Oakland, California Public Schools.

shape of the tone chamber varies considerably from brand to brand, and is one aspect of the mouthpiece which may be seen easily with a visual examination. It is wise to stay with a medium bore and to avoid radical variations from the standard.

9. *Bore*. The bore is the cylindrical, or mostly cylindrical, portion which fits on the barrel joint. The size and shape of the bore must be a continuation of the bore of the instrument upon which it is used. All instruments of the same type do not use exactly the same bore, nor is the size of the mouthpiece bore identical in all cases. If the tone of the instrument is uneven, or if there are serious intonation problems which cannot otherwise be identified the student should try another mouthpiece preferably of another brand which has a different bore.

10. *Table*. The table is the flat portion of the mouthpiece on which the reed is held by the ligature. If the reed is to respond properly it is important that the table be perfectly flat. A well finished mouthpiece will have a perfectly symetrical shaped table on which the reed can be centered.

11. *Table Opening*. The table opening is the space over the tone chamber on which the reed vibrates. Its size is the result of the basic side of the tone chamber and the length of the table. On mouthpieces for a particular instrument the width is determined by the standard reed size for that instrument and by the width of the side rails. The width may vary slightly without influencing the tone. If the opening is too wide or too narrow reeds will not fit properly, and such a mouthpiece should be promptly discarded.

12. *Side Rails*. The side rails are not shown in the illustration. They are the edges of the table opening which are shaped to make the facing of the mouthpiece. These rails must be perfectly smooth if the reed is to vibrate properly. A slight bump in a side rail will cause air to leak through the edge of the reed. The facing on the side rails must be absolutely identical on either side of the opening. If they are not, more of one side of the reed vibrates because it is damped by contact with the rail further back than the other side. This irregular vibration causes many problems in tone production and control which must be compensated for by the embouchure.

CRITERIA FOR A GOOD MOUTHPIECE

While the physical specifications of a mouthpiece determine how it will respond, the criteria by which a mouthpiece may be judged are musical ones. As such they are subjective rather than objective in nature, and may be summarized as follows.

A good mouthpiece is one which:

1. Produces a tone which has good body, typical of the best produced on the instrument, and matching in quality in all registers.

2. Plays perfectly in tune in all registers with no more than normal embouchure adjustments.

3. Allows the easy production of all types of articulations from hard short staccato to broad legato at all dynamic ranges.

4. Has a wide dynamic range over which the tone quality remains constant.

5. Does not require too much or too little mouthpiece in the mouth so that a standard embouchure may be formed.

6. Is not highly critical of reeds, but is one for which it is fairly easy to find and adjust a satisfactory reed of medium strength.

RECOMMENDATION FOR A MOUTHPIECE

Authorities do not all agree unanimously on the brand or facing of the mouthpiece to be used. One standard brand offers thirteen different combinations of facings and tip openings for the clarinet and seven combinations for the saxophone. Another offers eleven for the clarinet and thirteen for the saxophone. It is interesting to note that while all brands offer a wide selection, most brands indicate which are their most popular facings. Regardless of the brand, three out of four of the facings indicated as being the most popular fall within the recommendation of a medium length with a medium tip opening.

This confirms the most general consensus of authorities that all students on any level of advancement should play on a mouthpiece with a medium facing and medium tip opening. Mr. Arlie Richardson who has done intensive research in the field of single reed mouthpieces makes the statement in connection with clarinet mouthpieces: "In recording and observing many national and regional bands composed of students selected from all over the United States, I have found that the chairs held after auditions to be in direct ratio to the type of mouthpiece played, and that as few as two of forty-eight players played anything but a medium facing."

Even more important than the maker's designation of medium facing and medium tip is how closely the individual mouthpiece meets the maker's specifications for that particular model of mouthpiece. The facing is put on by hand following pre-set dies, rather than being put on automatically by machine. The various measurements on a mouthpiece must be accurate within a thousandth of an inch, and the necessary handwork allows for considerable error. Quality control in the matter of facings seems to vary from day to day. Measurements made of twenty-eight B-flat clarinet mouthpieces made by a famous company and having the same model number revealed that no two were exactly alike in all their dimension. Measurements made of a number of clarinet and saxophone mouthpieces made by another well known company failed to turn up a single one which was not defective in some critical part or another. This explains the experience of most teachers that no two mouthpieces play exactly alike even though they have the same model number.

In selecting a mouthpiece the more advanced students should thoroughly test a number of mouthpieces by playing on them. In this test various reeds must be used for not all reeds fit all mouthpieces. This testing must be done over a period of several days since the embouchure compensates for variations in both reed and mouthpiece. When the choice is narrowed down to two or three, the player should try many reeds on each, for one of the best criteria for a good mouthpiece is its quality for responding to various kinds of reeds rather than being highly critical of the type of reed with which it will respond.

In addition to the playing test, it is well to actually measure the physical characteristics of the mouthpiece. Until recently this has been possible only with home made or laboratory instruments. The LeBlanc company has available a mouthpiece gauge kit for B-flat clarinet mouthpieces at the present time, and it is anticipated that similar kits for the other clarinets as well as for the saxophones will become available in the future. This kit consists of a tip gauge, and three metal shims of different thicknesses to measure the curvature of the facing. The mouthpiece is measured by holding it table down on a piece of plate glass marked off with sixteenths of an inch. A B-flat clarinet medium tip will measure .0431 inches in height with the gauge in the center. A medium curve facing will measure .0015 inches at 10/16 inch, .010 inches at 7/16 inch, .024 inches at 4/16 inch, and .034 inches at 2/16 inch. These measurements are average and slight deviations in either direction would also indicate medium measurements. Use of the metal shims are especially useful to indicate whether or not the lay is warped. Teachers responsible for a number of clarinet students, or responsible for purchasing mouthpieces for schools will find the kit most useful in securing mouthpieces which are not defective. Checking student mouthpieces will often reveal that the mouthpiece is defective and changing mouthpieces will result in a rapid and startling improvement.

There are many brands of mouthpieces available today, and some of them are excellent musical tools. Generally speaking the best mouthpieces are made of machined rod-rubber or of crystal glass. Inferior mouthpieces are made of poorer quality rod-rubber or molded plastic. However, with the proper manufacturing methods and quality control it is theoretically possible to make mouthpieces of molded rubber or plastic which are equal in quality to the best rod-rubber and crystal. The buyer has no way of knowing the playing qualities of any mouthpiece without a trial and measuring. The rod-rubber and crystal mouthpieces are considered better because of the amount of handwork and the quality con-

trol which goes into the production of first-line mouthpieces. No clarinet or mouthpiece is possible without handwork and the amount of handwork is reflected in the price, although a high price does not necessarily indicate a mouthpiece of high quality. There is no evidence that the material of which a mouthpiece is made has any effect at all on the type of tone quality it produces. Rod-rubber, crystal, or molded rubber or plastic will all produce equally good tone quality if the dimensions of the mouthpiece—the bore, tone chamber, resistance curve and tip opening—are identical.

MOUTHPIECE DEFICIENCIES

Many difficulties students have in performance could be remedied if they would change to a good mouthpiece. Even the youngest beginner must have a good mouthpiece since he will progress much faster and be more satisfied with the results if he does have one. It is recommended that the mouthpieces which the makers supply with the inexpensive school instruments be replaced with a good quality mouthpiece, or that the instruments be purchased with the brand and model mouthpiece specified. It is obvious that the further advanced the student is in his performance the more important it is that he have the best possible mouthpiece with which to work.

It must be pointed out, however, that many problems which are attributed to mouthpieces are actually caused by embouchure formation, tongue placement, or reeds. If all these are correct, or if it is virtually impossible to find a reed which responds satisfactorily then it is the mouthpiece which should be suspected. Some common problems in connection with mouthpieces are the following:

1. *Warped Lay.* A lay is warped when the rail on one side touches the bottom of the reed at a different distance from the tip than the rail on the other side. Some mouthpieces come from the maker with the facing warped. A mouthpiece may be tested for a warped lay by running a thin paper such as a cigarette paper between the mouthpiece and the reed. When the paper has reached as far as it will go it should be straight across the reed. If not the facing is warped at this point. The lay may be warped at any point on the facing as well as the end tested at the paper. Other locations may be tested for warping by using metal shims similar to those mentioned in the clarinet mouthpiece gauge kit with the mouthpiece held against the plate glass.

A warped lay may be caused during the process of making it, by a ligature which is consistently too tight, by subjecting the mouthpiece to excessive head, or by washing the mouthpiece in hot water. A mouthpiece with a warped lay requires that the embouchure adjust to it, needs specially adjusted reed, and may squeak. A warped mouthpiece can be avoided by keeping it away from heat, removing the reed and storing it in a reed case after playing, tightening the ligature just enough to hold the reed firmly in place rather than as tight as it will go, and making sure by testing and measuring that it is in perfect condition before it is purchased.

2. *Refacing the Lay.* A warped mouthpiece may be corrected by having it refaced. There are many specialists over the country who have the knowledge and tools to not only correct warping but to put an entire facing on the mouthpiece. They can duplicate in a mouthpiece the exact dimensions of another. Many teachers have worked out formulae for the facing which works best for their students, and recommend that the students use this facing put on by a specialist. If a mouthpiece is otherwise a good one, then it is worth having refaced.

3. *Blows Too Hard.* This is caused by a mouthpiece with a lay that is too long or by a tip that is too close. The length and tip opening may be determined by measurements. The condition of blowing too hard may also be caused by a reed that is too stiff. The first remedy is to attempt to find a reed which fits the mouthpiece and responds according to the criteria for a good reed. If this does not correct the difficulty, other mouthpieces should be tried or the mouthpiece refaced.

4. *To Little Resistance.* When a mouthpiece has too little resistance measuring the tip opening and the length of the facing will indicate a tip which is too open, or a reed which is too soft on a long lay, or both. Attempt first to correct the condition with a reed. If this fails try other mouthpieces, or have the mouthpiece refaced to a medium length lay and medium open tip.

5. *Stuffy Tone.* This is the product of a short lay or a close tip, or a combination of both. A stiffer reed may remedy the situation, however the tone and intonation will be controlled with difficulty. A mouthpiece which produces a stuffy tone is best discarded.

6. *Intonation.* A properly proportioned mouthpiece will play with good intonation, assuming a good embouchure and reed. A mouthpiece with a tone chamber which is too large will cause the instrument to play sharp. This condition is most often found in "novelty" mouthpieces rather than in standard brands. If the size and taper of the bore of the mouthpiece does not properly match the bore of the instrument there will be intonation problems. This again is found frequently in novelty brands rather than in standard brands. Most of the serious intonation problems attributed to a standard mouthpiece of the medium dimensions will, upon careful investigation, be found to be embouchure problems. Or if only the throat tones are sharp or flat in relation to the rest of the instrument the barrel joint is too short or too long. Defective barrel joints are the result of using a joint which the manufacturer did not provide for that instrument, or because it has been shortened by being cut off in the repair shop. The various registers of the instrument cannot be played in tune if the barrel joint is too short or too long.

Single Reeds

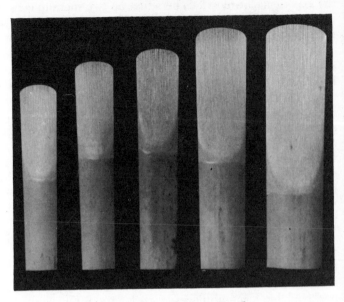

Figure R-2. Clarinet Reeds

Left to right: E-flat clarinet, B-flat (or A) clarinet, Alto clarinet, Bass clarinet, and Contra-bass clarinet

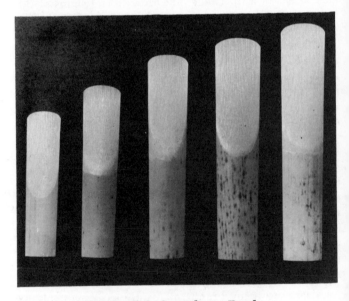

Figure R-3. Saxophone Reeds.

Left to right: Soprano saxophone, Alto saxophone, Tenor saxophone, Baritone saxophone, and Bass saxophone.

CLARINET AND SAXOPHONE REEDS

The reed has been described as the "soul" of the instrument, perhaps by a player who had just found a good one, as a "nightmare" by another, as well as in various other shades of purple prose. But the fact remains that the reed poses a problem for every player from the rank beginner to the most seasoned professional. Excellent instruments and mouthpieces can be purchased and kept in perfect condition, a good embouchure formed and developed, smooth and facile technique acquired—all of these remain more or less permanent acquisitions of the performer. But even the best of reeds last only a few days or a few weeks at the most, and the player is faced with the necessity of finding another one on which to play, and then another, and another, and another endlessly. No wonder some players have the chronic disease known as "reeditis," which can and should be avoided at all costs.

While oboe and bassoon students learn the art of reed making and adjustment as a regular normal part of the study of their instrument, and soon gain enough experience to make their own reeds from a blank piece of cane, clarinet and saxophone students are rarely if ever given instruction on how to select a reed, much less how to adjust them. Teachers of these instruments would be wise to include regular instruction on adjustment of single reeds. The information is well known, standardized, and easily accessible. There are no secrets of the trade, and the selection and adjustment of single reeds is not particularly time consuming.

It is not the purpose of this book to go into great detail or into an involved discussion of reeds. Rather it is the intent to present the basic facts in organized fashion—those facts which the teacher needs to know and use in his everyday activities. Those who are interested in great detail may consult the fine books by Opperman and Jaffrey.[2]

SELECTING THE REED

All clarinet and saxophone reeds are machine made, and as a result are not tested and adjusted as are oboe and bassoon reeds which are mostly hand made. As a result the cost of single reeds is considerably less than the double reeds, which makes it possible for the clarinet and saxophone player to exercise greater selectivity as to the reeds he actually uses. The best procedure for selecting single reeds is to buy them by the box of twenty-five in order to have enough from which to select. A good player will find four or five reeds in a box which he can use with very little adjustment. Another four or five can be used, but require more adjustment. The remaining reeds he will discard as being unusable. If it is impossible for students to buy reeds by the box, they should purchase them a half dozen at a time, and expect to discard three of them.

The selection of a reed is a highly personal matter, since only the person who is to play it can make the selection. The reasons for this are numerous, and per-

haps help explain why reeds are such a problem for some players and no problem at all for others. How a reed responds is determined by the player's embouchure and mouthpiece as well as the inherent characteristics of the reed itself. A reed which does not respond at all for one individual on his instrument plays beautifully for another. A mouthpiece which is defective in any of several respects will make it difficult if not impossible to find a satisfactory reed. Thus the first prerequisite for a good reed is a good mouthpiece.

The individual embouchure formation has a tremendous effect on reed response, although the nearer to a standard formation the embouchure is the less difficulties there are in finding a satisfactory reed to produce the desired tone quality. A good embouchure, then, is the second prerequisite for finding a good reed. This, unfortunately, eliminates the beginner who has only a start toward developing an embouchure, but even he can make study on the instrument infinitely easier by having a reed which best fits his needs. The instructor must assume responsibility for seeing that he has a suitable reed, for a reed which is to hard or too soft or poorly proportioned can have disastrous results on a beginning embouchure.

Before discussing the points to be considered in selecting a reed a vocabulary for identification of the various parts of the reed should be established. The illustration shown on page 236 identifies parts of the reed which will be referred to throughout this discussion.

CRITERIA FOR A GOOD REED

Whether a reed is a good one for an individual player or isn't a good reed for him is a subjective judgment. Players themselves can judge how a reed responds when they play on it, but frequently can't judge exactly how it sounds to others because vibrations which are not heard by another person are transmitted from the mouthpiece through the upper teeth to the ear. The teacher can be of great assistance to the student through listening and commenting on how various reeds sound. The student will soon learn how the best reeds feel to him when he is playing and will be in a better position to judge final tone quality for himself.

The following criteria for a good reed can act as guide-lines in the selection of a reed:

A good reed is one which:

1. Responds freely and easily over the entire range of the instrument.
2. Plays all registers of the instrument well in tune without adjustments in embouchure formation or lip pressure.

[2]Opperman, Kalman. *Handbook for Making and Adjusting Single Reeds.* New York: Chappell & Co., 1956, and Jaffrey, K. S. *Reed Mastery.* Summer Hill: Australia The Author, 1956, which is available from woodwind supply houses in the U. S.

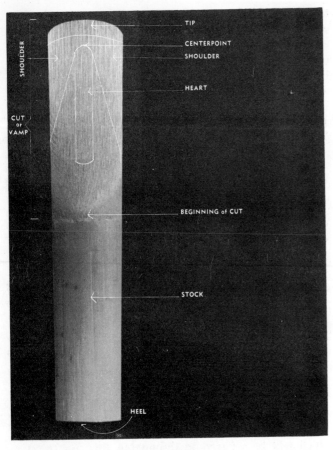

Figure R-4.

3. May be controlled throughout the full dynamic range.
4. Produces a rich, clear bodied tone of the same quality over the entire range of the instrument.
5. Can be played without a too great wind pressure and without tiring the embouchure.
6. Allows the complete scope of articulations from hard staccato to legato detached to be played in all registers of the instrument.

Reed Strength. The first thing to consider in the selection of a reed is its strength. Most brands of reeds are classified by strength: 1, 1½, 2, 2½, 3, 3½, 4, 4½, 5 according to the resistance of the tip to bending as measured on a standard reed gauge, with number 1 being the softest and number 5 the hardest. In addition some brands use the designations "soft," medium-soft," "medium," "medium-hard," and "hard," either with or without the number designation. These classifications are extremely unreliable since they represent only a general indication of the resistance of the tip and not the general shape of the vamp, do not consider the inherent characteristic of the cane itself, and are made when the reed is dry and unplayed although it is common knowledge that a reed moist as it is in playing responds quite differently than a dry one. Testing the twenty-five reeds

in a box marked no. 2 or medium strength will easily show that every range of strength from very soft to very hard is included among them. It must be clearly understood that selecting a reed simply by number or classification is no guarantee of getting the exact strength desired, however since they are merchandised in this fashion this must be the starting point. For the average student, beginning, intermediate, or advanced, playing with a standard embouchure on a good mouthpiece of medium facing and medium opening the medium or medium-soft classification should be used. There is a widespread old wives tale that beginners must start with very soft reeds and gradually increase the strength of the reed used as they gain proficiency until they are playing on a very hard reed. This fallacy should be dispensed with once and for all. Beginners are frequently deliberately given a reed which is too soft until breath support and embouchure are set, and this is to be commended but they do not progress from strength no. 1 to 2, 3, 4, 5 in the way they must increase their shoe size as their bodies grow.

The hardness or softness of a reed in relation to a particular mouthpiece is determined by the nature of the lay on that particular mouthpiece, as well as the type and formation of embouchure being used by the player. In general an open lay calls for a softer reed and a close lay for a harder reed. Only by a careful experimentation with many reeds can the clarinetist determine the type of reed best suited to his mouthpiece and embouchure.

A reed is too stiff for a player when it is hard to blow, offering too much resistance, and requiring more than normal breath pressure to produce a tone. A second symptom of a reed which is too hard is that it produces a heavy, hard and coarse quality of tone in the low register.

A reed which is too soft produces a thin, reedy tone quality, and frequently won't play the higher notes at all. The clarion register is difficult to play in tune, generally being flat in pitch, and the lower notes in the chalameau register buzz. It requires less than normal breath pressure to produce a tone. Some soft reeds may be adjusted to play well, and this type of adjustment is discussed later.

Both hard and soft reeds frequently squeak. Squeaks are caused by faulty cutting of the vamp during the manufacturing process which makes it vibrate out of balance. The cane is thicker on one side of the center point than on the other, one side of the tip is thicker than the other, or the cane is inherently faulty in the heart section. A reed which is either too hard or too soft and squeaks as well poses a difficult problem in adjustment which cannot always be carried out. On the other hand a reed which is of the right strength and which possess the other attributes of a good reed but squeaks can frequently be adjusted so that it plays well.

The Cane. The color of the cane from which the reed is made can offer some criteria of quality. The bark on the stock of well seasoned cane from which the best reeds come is a deep golden yellow color, and irregular brown or dark colored marks in the bark do not affect its quality. Indeed, some players feel that these indicate the best quality cane. Reeds on which the bark on the stock is light yellow or has a greenish look are usually improperly seasoned, or simply poor cane. Immature can is also indicated by extreme roughness in the grain of the vamp which can be both seen and felt.

An even better indication of the quality of cane is the way in which the grains run. This can be seen by holding the reed up to the light or using a shadow box with a ground glass. The best cane has the grain running absolutely straight, with the hard grains (the darker streaks) evenly distributed across the vamp and with part of them running entirely to the tip of the reed. Reeds in which the grains run at an angle across the vamp play unevenly and frequently squeak. Reeds which have no hard grains extending to the tip tend to be too soft, or if playable, to wear out rapidly.

Shape of the Vamp. The way in which the vamp is cut or shaped determines how the reed will play, regardless of the quality of the cane from which it is made. The Vandoren reed has been the standard against which all single reeds have been measured for many years, and the style of vamp used on these reeds is generally accepted as being the best. The way in which the reed is cut can be determined by holding it up to a light and observing the light and dark areas. The darker the area the thicker the cane. If an imaginary line is drawn from the heel to the tip down the center of the reed the shadows should be exactly the same on either side. If they are not, one side is thicker than the other, and adjustments are made until both sides are identical. The more nearly symetrical the reed the better the cut. The difference between soft and hard reeds can clearly be seen by comparing the amount and shape of the light and dark areas.

The basic cut of the reed is as follows. The tip is a very thin area extending back about an eighth of an inch from the end which must be the same thickness for the entire width of the reed. When held to the light it is a very pale color.

The flexibility of the tip of the reed is all-important in the selection of a reed. It is determined not only by the thickness of the tip, but by the general proportion of the entire vamp—the shape and thickness of the heart, the location and thickness of the center point, the thickness of the shoulders and how they are graduated. If there is a single test of the hardness or softness of a reed it is in the response of the tip. The most accurate way of testing this flexibility, aside from playing the reed, is to gently move the tip across the thumb nail to

ascertain how much pressure is necessary to flex it back. The more pressure needed the harder the reed. It should flex evenly across the entire width, and if it does not, should be adjusted until it does.

The tip area is identified in Figure R-6.

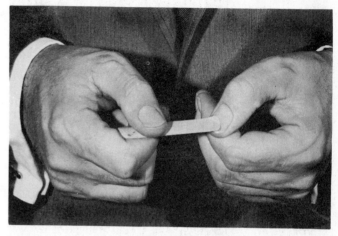

Figure R-5.

Figure R-7 shows the heart of the reed which extends from the stock to the center point and which gradually becomes thinner as it approaches the center point. It is graduated toward the edge with the edges considerable thinner than the center line. The shape is roughly that of an inverted "V" which shows clearly as a shadow when the reed is held toward the light.

The shoulders, Figure R-8 extend from the heart toward the edges and toward the tip, gradually growing thinner (lighter in color when held toward the light) as they approach the points on either side at which the edges and the back line of the tip meet. The shadows shown by the shoulders should be identical and symetrical. Much of the control of the vibration, and much of the adjusting of the reed is done in the shoulder area.

In summary the selection of a reed is made by (1) the color; (2) the way the grains run; (3) an examination of the cut by holding it toward the light; and (4) testing the resistance of the tip by running it across the thumb nail and (5) testing it on the instrument. Considerable experience is needed both in judging a reed from its physical characteristics and hearing various kinds of reeds played on the instrument. How it plays on the instrument is the final determining factor. Regardless of how it looks, if it plays well it is a good reed, and players must, as part of the selection of a reed, give it a playing test on the instrument to make a final judgment, and to ascertain what adjustments, if any, need to be made, or if adjustments are possible at all if it is a poor reed.

Tip of single   Heart area of   Shoulder area of a
      reed.   single reed.   single reed.

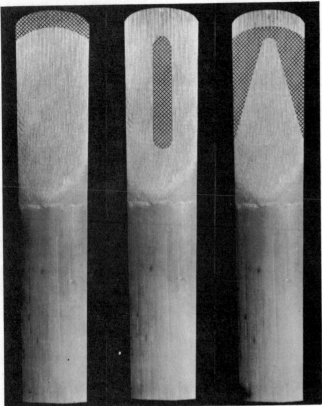

Figure R-6.   Figure R-7.   Figure R-8.

ADJUSTING THE SINGLE REED

Proficiency in making adjustments on the reed is virtually mandatory for every teacher involved in teaching single reed instruments, because the students must be taught how to do it for themselves, and they must learn by example. This technique can only be learned by experience, and every teacher should experiment and work with reeds at great length. A great many reeds will be ruined but the knowledge and technique acquired are well worth the cost in time and money.

Tools and materials used in adjusting single reeds are simple to acquire and the following must be available:

1. *Scraping Knife.* A reed knife such as those sold for making oboe and bassoon reeds; or a pocket knife; or a single-edged razor blade. The knives must be kept honed to a sharp edge, and the razor blades discarded when they become dull. Many players carry a razor blade in their cases so that it will always be available.

2. *Plate Glass.* A piece of plate glass at least two by four inches, or some other hard material which can be kept absolutely flat.

3. *Sandpaper.* Fine grained sandpaper No. 8/0.

4. *Dutch Rush.* Also known as Swamp Grass which grows wild around rivers, lakes and swampy areas in many sections of the United States. It is commercially processed and is available in music stores. It is normally used wet, and must be soaked in water for several minutes so that one end can be pressed flat in order to obtain sufficient working surface. It may be used dry although the small working surface on the rounded material makes slow progress. Dutch rush is used for smoothing and polishing the vamp, and for making smaller adjustments to the shoulder or tip area of the reed than are possible with a knife.

5. A *Reed Clipper.* This is used for trimming the tip of soft reeds. The type and model should be selected carefully so that the shape of the cut it makes matches exactly the shape of the tip of the mouthpiece and/or the original shape of the reed. In addition it must have a screw adjustment for small adjustments in the amount of reed to be clipped off. Take along several useless reeds for testing shape, adjustment, **and** sharpness of the cutting blade when the clipper is **being** selected.

The Cordier brand reed trimmer is recommended. This company makes reed trimmers for B-flat clarinet, Alto clarinet, Bass clarinet, Alto saxophone, Tenor saxophone, and Baritone saxophone reeds. Players on these instruments should have their own reed trimmer, and the well-equipped teacher will have a full set available for his students.

The purpose of adjusting a reed is to make corrections in the proportions of the vamp which are imperfect. The adjustments are made by scraping or sanding parts of the shoulders, adjusting and relocating the center point of the cut, re-proportioning the heart, and, rarely, evening the thickness across the tip. All scraping or sanding movements are made in one direction with the grain of the wood and only toward the tip of the reed. All adjustments are made with the reed moist in playing condition.

The reed selected for adjustment should be the most nearly perfect reed selected from a group of six or more. Many players prefer to select the best three or four reeds from a box of twenty-five for final adjusting. Not all reeds can be adjusted for satisfactory playing and the better the response at the time the adjusting process is started, the better the final success will be in adjusting the reed. Only a very few reeds will be found that respond perfectly without some adjusting being necessary. The chances are practically a hundred per cent that if a student is handed or purchases two or three reeds at a time all of them will require adjustment to a greater or lesser degree. It should be emphasized again that proficiency in reed adjustment can only be learned by experience. Each single operation must be small and the reed tested on the instrument before making another adjustment. The process is one of continual testing by playing. It is easy to ruin a reed with even the slightest too much scraping, or rubbing or clipping. Proceed cautiously!

Soft Reeds. Soft reeds are identified by a thin reedy sound which requires little breath pressure for tone production, and which usually play out of tune. They are reeds on which the tip is too flexible. This can be seen when tested against the thumb nail, and when the reed is held to the light the tip section is almost transparent and extends farther than normal from the end putting the center point of the cut too far from the tip. This condition is corrected by clipipng the tip with the reed clipper.

Put the reed in the clipper carefully being sure that both the heel and tip are exactly centered. Adjust the reed so that only a hair line of cane is cut off. The biggest danger in using the reed clipper is in cutting off too much of the reed. Very small amounts of cane removed make enormous differences in how the reed responds. It is better to clip twice to get the desired response than it is to risk taking off too much at once. When this is done test the reed again. If it is still too soft repeat the process. Once the reed is clipped to the desired strength it may play properly, or it may show need for further adjustment of any of the kinds discussed in the following paragraphs. Clipping a soft reed doesn't automatically make it a good reed.

Slightly Hard Reeds. These are the reeds which meet the general criteria for good reeds except that they blow a little hard, or on which the chalameau register tone quality is rough while the clarion register is good. Fortunately a good many reeds fall into this category. Many players deliberately choose this type of reed since it may soften to the desired strength after a few hours of playing, and if not, have suffecient reserve strength to allow the necessary minor adjustments. Reeds of this kind will generally have a perfectly formed tip section, but be slightly too thick in one or both shoulder areas. If the reed doesn't play in, then the shoulder areas should be scraped gently with the knife to lighten the shadow when held to the light. The two shoulders should match perfectly. Polish the entire vamp with the Dutch Rush.

Medium Hard Reeds. These reeds required a greater breath pressure to produce a tone than do the slightly hard class and are somewhat rough not only in the chalameau register but also in the clarion register. The degree of hardness is such that they are uncomfortable to play on, and as a consequence cannot be brought into playing condition through use. This type of reed will have shoulders and tips which are thicker than the slightly hard group, and the center point of the cut may be closer to the end of the reed than is necessary for the best response. Corrections on this kind of reed should be made in the following order: (1) Using the knife, scrape the shoulder areas so that both have identical shadows but not as light in color as the finished reed will be. The reed should respond a little freer when tried on the instrument. (2) With the Dutch Rush thin the tip area uniformly across the width of the reed until its color is almost that desired for the finished reed. It should be tested several times during this process to avoid taking off too much. (3) With the knife scrape the front portion of the heart section if the center point is closer than one-eighth inch to the tip, or if the general area of the center point is dark. Make this adjustment very gradually and test frequently. (4) Hold the reed to the light and check the color and shape of the shoulders and tip. Remove uneven dark spots with the knife, making sure that both sides of the center line are identical. (5) When these operations are completed the reed should respond as a slightly hard reed and treatment continued as suggested for that classification of reed. Conclude the adjustment by polishing the entire vamp with Dutch Rush.

Very Hard Reeds. These are reeds which require an extraordinary amount of wind pressure to produce a tone, and with a hard, rough and squawky tone quality. These reeds have an overall thickness which is much greater than normal, some to the extent that this additional thickness is readily noticeable at the heel. Some have the overall vamp too thick—the tip area is dark, the shoulders dark and the heart section much wider and longer than normal. Some few simply have a tip section which is little or no thinner than the shoulders. The adjustments on this type of reed should be done in this sequence, testing frequently: (1) Using very light strokes of the knife and following the line of the grain remove the excess cane from the tip section. Test on the instrument frequently, and continue until the reed responds well, which it will if the only trouble was the tip section, or until the thickness of the tip is almost that of the normal reed. (2) If this process does not complete the adjustment of the reed, thin the shoulder sections with the knife, keeping the graduation from the center line to the edge correct and balancing each side. Test frequently. If when the graduation and thickness is near normal and the reed doesn't respond proceed to the next step. (3) With light strokes of the knife thin the heart section, paying particular attention to the area near the center point so that it blends into the shoulders and tip. Test frequently. (4) Perform steps two and three alternately, testing frequently, until the reed responds as a slightly hard reed. (5) Make final adjustments on shoulders and tip area with the knife and then Dutch Rush. (6) Polish entire vamp with Dutch Rush.

Squeaky Reeds. Reeds which are otherwise perfect may squeak. Soft reeds squeak and reeds of varying degrees of hardness may squeak. The process of bringing soft or hard reeds to the proper playing condition frequently removes the squeak. If when the proper degree of stiffness is reached and they still squeak, the same remedial measures as for a good reed can be applied to them.

Squeaks may also be caused by leaky pads, faulty position of fingers over the tone holes, or by fingers touching keys so not all squeaks can be attributed to a faulty reed. If a student doesn't squeak on several reeds, but does with one, then it is safe to assume that the squeak is built into the reed. Reeds normally squeak when slurring across the break, especially open G to third line B-natural, and rapid slurring back and forth between these two notes will identify most, but not all, squeaky reeds.

Squeaks are the result of uneven vibrations by the reed. These may be caused by a heavy or thick spot on one of the shoulders, by a thick spot in the tip area, or by a thick spot in the heart near the center point. These thick places in the tip and in the shoulders show up as dark spots when the reed is held to the light. When they are located rub them down to the proper thickness with the Dutch Rush, or if they are especially thick begin the process with the knife and finish with the Dutch Rush. Only the Dutch Rush should be used on the tip area. Test frequently during the process. If when any heavy areas in tip or shoulders are removed and blended into the surrounding areas the squeak still remains the squeak is in the heart of the reed. Rub the heart with Dutch Rush over its entire length. Test frequently, since small changes in the heart area make large differences in reed response. If after all these operations are performed the squeak persists throw the reed away! Reeds are inexpensive and the apprehension of playing on a reed that may squeak at any time puts a severe strain on the performer.

CARE OF THE REED

A good reed is worth preserving, and a few simple measures will lengthen its useful life. Some students persist in using a reed long past its useful life, and a regular weekly reed inspection should be part of the regular routine of the instrumental class, band, and orchestra. A simple inspection will reveal reeds with chips out of the tips, splits, dirty reeds, reeds on instruments played by girls coated with lipstick, reeds with jagged tips, etc. etc., ad infinitum. Any one of these conditions has an affect not only on how the instrument sounds, but on the ease with which it plays. Many students do not realize the importance of having a good reed to play on and it is the responsibility of the teacher to see that they do have good reeds until this importance becomes apparent to the player. Any reeds with any of the conditions mentioned above should be replaced immediately.

Much damage to reed of younger players occurs while on the instrument. The tip is brushed against the clothing, hit against a chair or music stand or any one of a number of other contacts any one of which will damage it beyond reasonable use. Reeds are frequently split or chipped by the ligature if it is put on the mouth-piece after the reed is in place. It is for this reason that the ligature should be put over the mouthpiece and the reed slipped under it as standard practice. Putting the cap over the mouthpiece, if carelessly done often chips or splits the reed. The importance of avoiding this type of accident through reasonable care must be emphasized continuously, but especially with beginning students.

When the instrument is taken apart reeds should always be removed from the mouthpiece and stored in a reed case or reed holder. Cane is susceptible to warpage when drying out after use, and the reed is preserved best if it is held firmly in place on a flat surface after being wiped dry of excess moisture. Several commercial reed containers which do this efficiently are available and hold two to four reeds thus providing ready accessible storage for reeds which are ready to use. Keeping the reed in a reed case rather than on the mouthpiece will also protect the mouthpiece from possible damage if it is exposed to heat while the ligature is tightly in place. Some teachers recommend a piece of plate glass of the size to fit into the instrument case on which the reeds are held by wide rubber bands. This is more usable with the Chesterfield model case than with the fitted cases which do not have much excess storage in them. Plate glass or commercial reed cases are inexpensive and well worth the slight investment to preserve the reeds. Figure R-9 shows an excellent commercial reed case.

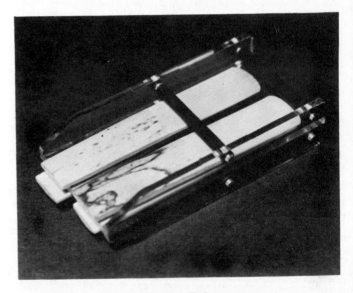

Figure R-9.

After a reed has been used several times the underside, or flat side, may warp. Or you may be able to see the shape of the tone chamber of the mouthpiece on the underside of the reed, since it tends to sink into the hollow space in the mouthpiece. This latter condition may be caused by having the ligature too tight which puts too much pressure against the reed. But whatever the cause the warp or unevenness should be removed if the reed is to continue to play well. This may be done by scraping the bottom of the reed with a knife or razor blade, or rubbing it gently over the sandpaper. If the sandpaper is used, protect the tip of the reed by sliding a piece of paper between it and the sandpaper.

The reed must be kept clean of accumulated dirt and saliva deposits or the pores of the cane become clogged and the reed loses response. These deposits may be washed off with warm water, or scraped off with a knife or Dutch Rush. If the scraping method is used care must be taken not to take off any of the wood which would weaken the reed.

In recent years many experiments have been made with plastic reeds, and there are several brands on the market. Plastic reeds are still in the developmental stage and do not give as good results as cane reeds. The plastic reeds have the higher overtones present in great intensity which gives them a rather thin and brittle tone. They lack the flexibility and depth of tone of a good reed of French cane. Because of their many shortcomings, plastic reeds cannot be recommended for use on any of the woodwind instruments.

OBOE AND ENGLISH HORN REEDS

Comparison of an oboe reed (left) with an English horn reed.

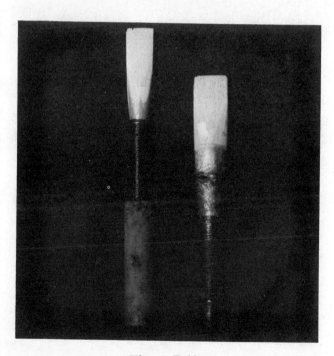

Figure R-10.

The selection, adjustment and care of the reed for the oboe or English horn is a subject which should be thoroughly understood by every player on these instru-

ments, and by every teacher who is responsible for students on these instruments. The double reed functions both as a mouthpiece and as the tone generator for the instrument, and as such its response is highly critical. The type of reed being used determines tone quality, influences embouchure formation, and all aspects of performance. For these reasons the reed should be carefully selected and adjusted to fit both the student and the instrument he is using.

Every oboist past the beginning stage should be able to adjust commercial reeds, and if he is a serious student of the instrument should learn how to make his own reeds from the blank cane. Most oboists learn the art of reed making and adjustment as a regular normal part of the study of their instrument. Many teachers consider this as important a part of their learning as developing technique, tone quality or phrasing. No oboist's training is considered complete until he is proficient in making and adjusting reeds. Beginners on the instrument will first develop the facility for adjustment and then progress into the complete production of reeds.

The present discussion is limited to selection, adjustment and care of the oboe reed. The problems involved in making reeds are beyond the scope of this book, and are best learned through personal instruction from one who is skilled in the art. The considerations here will be limited to those aspects of the problem which the teacher needs to know and use in his everyday activities.

Before discussing the oboe reed it is necessary to establish a vocabulary for identification of the various parts of the reed. The designations are the standard ones widely found in published literature. Figure R-11 identi-

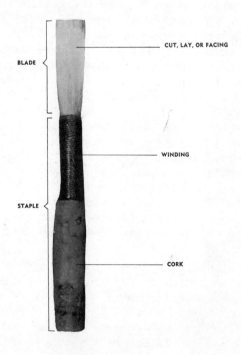

Figure R-11.

fies the parts. The staple is the metal tube on which the cane is fitted, and has a cork on the end to fit into the socket on the oboe. The blades are the two pieces of cane which make the reed. The winding is the thread which holds the blades onto the staple. The portion of the blades from which the bark has been cut is known as the cut, scrape, lay or facing.

HOW AN OBOE REED IS MADE

In order to adjust and care for oboe reeds it is desirable to understand the complete process of how they are made, even though skill in performing these operations is expected only of advanced oboists. Understanding the procedures will provide a basis upon which adjustments can be made. The following sequence of photographs illustrates a standard procedure in making an oboe reed as performed by a professional oboist and highly skilled reed maker.

1. Figure R-12. Cured, uncut cane from which oboe reeds are made is available in various diameters. The diameter of the cane determines to some extent the shape of the oval tip of the finished reed. The diameters of the pieces of cane illustrated are 14 mm, 12 mm, and 10 mm. The 12 mm is considered the standard size.

2. Figure R-13. The cane is split into three equal sections with a three blade knife called a splitting arrow.

3. Figure R-14. Three pieces of cane produced when the cane is split.

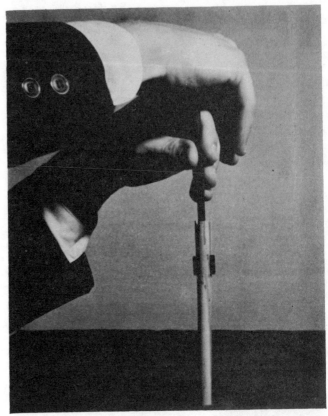

Figure R-13.

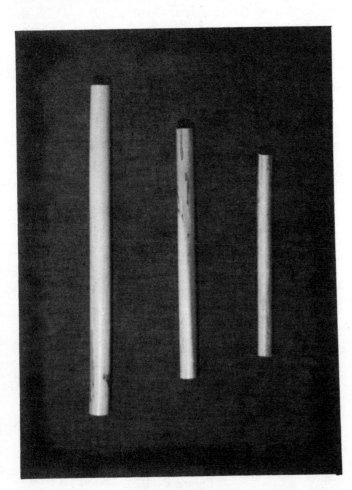

Figure R-12.

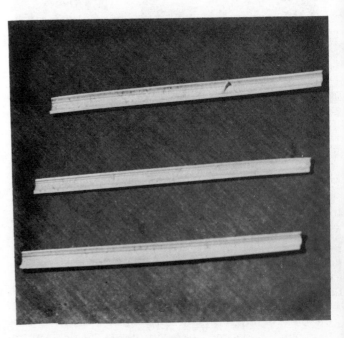

Figure R-14.

4. Figure R-15. Each piece of cane is cut to size by pushing it through a plane-like instrument called the filiere. Beginning with this procedure, all subsequent operations are done with the cane thoroughly soaked so that it is pliable.

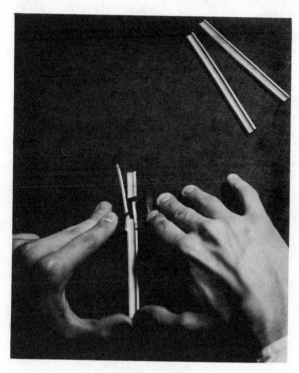

Figure R-15.

5. Figure R-16. The cane is then cut to the correct length on a machine known as a guillotine.

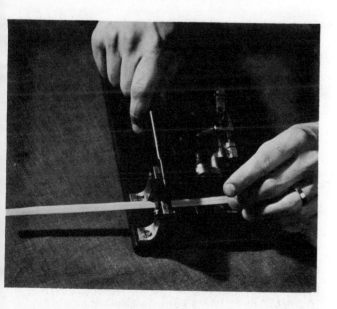

Figure R-16.

6. Figure R-17. When the cane is the correct length it is placed in the gouger and the inside is planed to the correct shape and thickness.

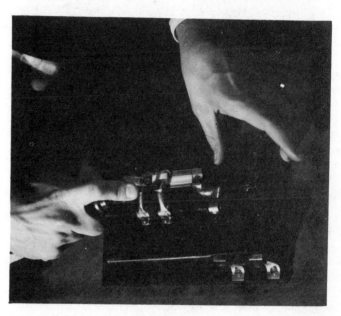

Figure R-17.

7. Figure R-18. The gouged cane is placed on the cane easel which has an etched line marking the exact center of the length. With the cutting knife a notch is made through the bark at this point which will become the tip of the finished reed. Some players buy cane which has been finished to this point from which to make their own reeds. It is described as "gouged cane."

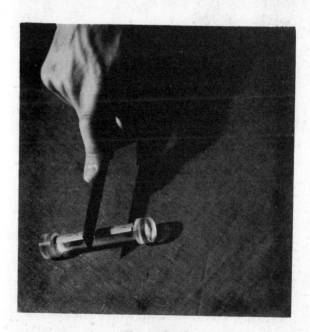

Figure R-18.

8. Figure R-19. The cane is folded over the knife blade at the point where the notch was made.

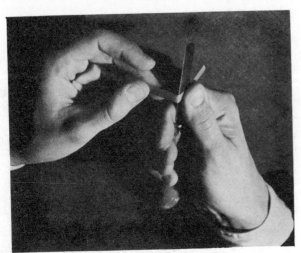

Figure R-19.

9. Figure R-20. The folded cane is placed on an instrument called a shaper and the edges are cut with a knife or single edge razor blade to the exact shape of the finished reed. When this process has been completed the cane is described as "gouged, shaped and folded" and it is this type of prepared cane that most oboists purchase to make their own reeds.

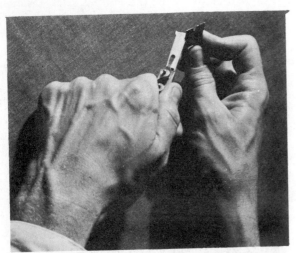

Figure R-20.

10. Figure R-21. This photograph compares the cane in three stages. From bottom to top: filiered and cut to size, gouged, and shaped.

11. Figure R-22. The shaped cane is returned to the easel and the narrow ends of the cane which will be bound on the tube are thinned with a knife so that they will be flexible enough to fit tightly on the tube.

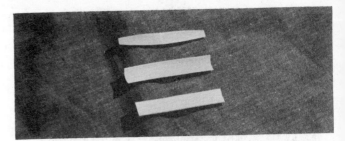

Figure R-21.

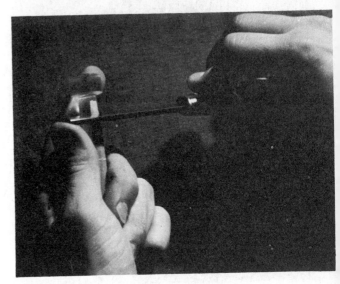

Figure R-22.

12. Figure R-23. The cane is folded over the tube which is oval rather than perfectly round in shape. The cane is fitted to the flat sides.

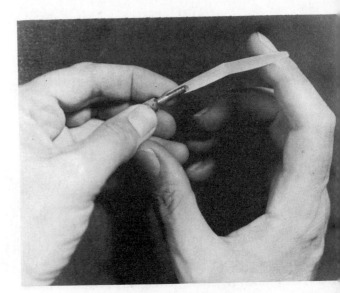

Figure R-23.

13. Figure R-24. With the end of the binding thread attached to something which will hold it securely the thread is wrapped once around the reed at the edge of the tube. With the thread in place the cane is straightened and positioned on the tube and the thread secured.

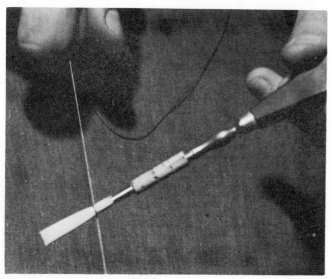

Figure R24.

14. Figure R-25. The thread is wound tightly around the reed and stapled down to the cork where it is tied securely. At this point the blank cane is ready for scraping.

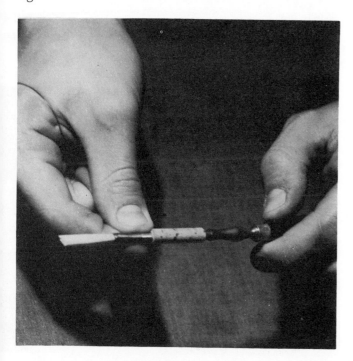

Figure R-25.

15. Figure R-26. The back of the cut is scraped on either side of the spine of the red to form the general outline of the final cut. Both blades are scraped in identical fashion. This reed will be made in what will be described later as a long "W" cut. In the photographs the reed is being held with the fingers during the scraping process. Some professionals and most students feel more secure when the reed is held on a mandrel during all scraping, and this is the general recommendation.

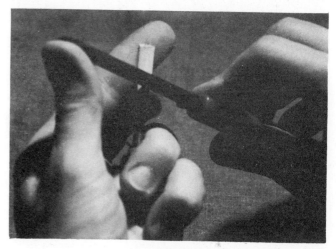

Figure R-26.

16. Figure R-27. The tip of each blade is thinned and shaped.

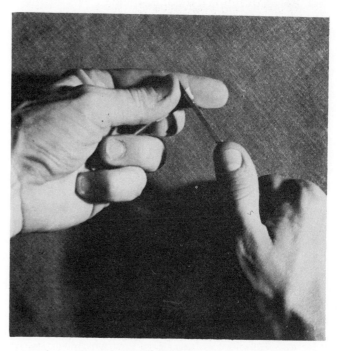

Figure R-27.

17. Figure R-28. The end of the reed is split with the plaque, and we now have the basic double reed. At this point the reed is classified as "semi-finished" and will produce a tone.

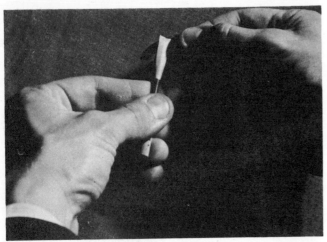

Figure R-28.

The steps which are necessary to finish the reed and put it into perfect playing condition are similar to those described later in the adjusting process and are not shown here. Those who are interested in the detailed process of making oboe reeds may consult the excellent books by Mayer and Rohner[3], or Artley[4] and others.

TYPES OF OBOE REEDS AVAILABLE

Although the advanced oboist is expected to make his own reeds, the great majority of student oboists will purchase reeds which are ready made. Many schools purchase oboe reeds by the dozens for their oboists. Since the success of these students is dependent upon how the reed responds it is most important that they be purchased wisely and with full knowledge of the choices available. There are three general types of ready made reeds available which can be described as follows:

1. *Semifinished Commercial Reeds.* These are mass produced for general retail distribution in much the same way that single reeds are produced and distributed. On some brands the lay is cut by machine rather than by hand. The designation "semi-finished' 'indicates that the purchaser must put the finishing touches on the reed himself, as the reed is in the same state of adjustment as the reed in step fifteen in the preceding outline of how an oboe reed is made. These finishing touches include tuning the reed to fit his embouchure and instrument, finishing the cut on both blades, smoothing the surfaces. Reeds of this type vary greatly in the

amount of finishing necessary. Unless the teacher or the student has developed some skill in adjusting reed this type of reed is seldom satisfactory. Unfortunately some semi-finished reeds which have very little work remaining to be done are not designated as such when they are sold and many players attempt to play them without making the finishing touches. Many of the difficulties student oboists have can be traced to this situation. If the brand of reeds being used responds poorly, and requires considerable adjustment to achieve a good response they are most certainly of the semi-finished class.

2. *Finished Commercial Reeds.* Other types of commercial reeds generally available in music stores are classified as "finished" reeds. That is, the scrape has been finished and the reed tuned either by measurement or by actually playing it on an instrument. Some brands of these finished commercial reeds are graded according to strength in the same way single reeds are graded in strengths 1, 2, 3, 4, 5 with the number one the softest and the number five the hardest. The grading of oboe reeds in this fashion is a more reliable indication of their actual strength than is the grading of single reeds. The oboe reed probably will have been tested by a player and sterilized before shipment. This is not always the case however, since other and less accurate means of determining strengths are available.

It is not always possible to judge by merely looking at the reed whether it is finished or semi-finished. It must be tried on the instrument. Even the finished reeds frequently need adjustment to suit the individual player. If a teacher or player finds a brand of commercial reeds which are consistently satisfactory without adjustment he is indeed fortunate. The way in which commercial reeds are adjusted is the same as that for all oboe reeds and these processes are discussed later in this chapter.

3. *Custom Made Reeds.* These are reeds made by professional players to individual order. Professional players in all sections of the country cater to school musicians and will make reeds for beginning, intermediate or advanced students which are fitted and tuned to a particular brand and model of oboe (or English horn). These reeds are usually made in the same way and with the same care the professional makes reeds for himself and are finished and ready to play when received.

It is highly recommended that this type of reed be secured for all school oboists until they learn to make their own, or at least have arrived at the place where they are competent to make adjustments on their reeds. If there is not a near-by professional oboist to supply reeds the names and addresses of professional players who specialize in making reeds for school use can be

---

[3]Mayer, Robert and Traugott Rohner. *Oboe Reeds: How to Make and Adjust Them.* Glen Ellyn, Illinois: The Instrumental Company. 1953.
[4]Artley, Joe. *How To Make Double Reeds.* Old Greenwich, Conn.: Jack Spratt Woodwind Shop. Second Edition, 1953.

found in the classified advertisements in such magazines as the *Instrumentalist* and *School Musician*. Try reeds from several makers until those best suited for the student and instrument are found.

Figure R-29 shows three typical oboe reeds. Number 1 is a custom made reed with a long "W' cut which is ready to play without further adjustment. Number 2 is an imported finished commercial reed with a medium long "U" cut. The lay of this reed was cut by machine and completed with a minimum of handwork. Note that the blades are not aligned. This reed would need considerable adjusting before responding properly. Number 3 is a domestic finished commercial reed using a long "U" cut. The lay is cut by hand even though the reeds are made on an assembly-line basis. This reed would require some adjusting in order to respond properly.

Variations in cuts are found in the length of the blade from which the bark has been removed, in the shape of the bark remaining where the cut begins, as well as the proportions of the thickness of the cane at various places on the cut. The cut gets its name from the shape of the bark at the beginning of the cut. This bark takes on the general shape of a "U," a "V," or a "W," and the reeds are described as having a "U," "V" or "W" cut. In addition the length of the cut as well as its shape varies considerably and is described as short, medium or long. The length is added to the designation of shape and we find the designations of short "U" cut, medium "U" cut, long "U" cut, and similar designations for the "W" and "V" shapes. This gives the designations for the nine basic types of cuts for oboe reeds. Figure R-30 illustrates some of the various cuts.

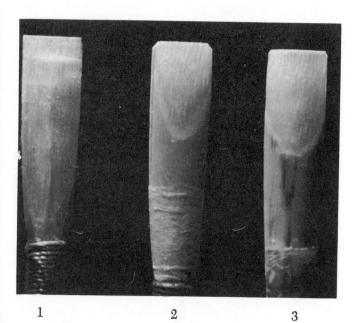

Figure R-29.

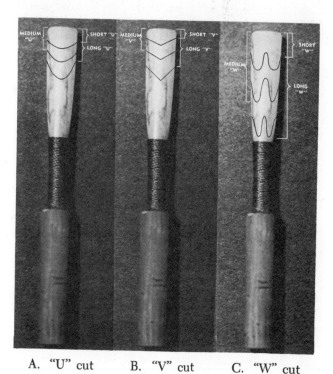

A. "U" cut   B. "V" cut   C. "W" cut

Figure R-30.

TYPES OF CUT

The term *cut* (scrape or facing) refers to the portion of the blades from which the bark of the cane has been removed, and specifically to the shape and proportion of the tip, shoulders, back and spine. There are various standard and basic cuts for the oboe reed, each subject to considerable variation in the hands of the individual maker. These variations are made to achieve the response, control and tone quality desired by the individual player. Each professional oboist, and eventually each student oboist who makes his own reeds, will arrive after much experimentation at a cut which best suits his individual needs. Students should experiment with various types of cuts in order to select the type which best meets his requirements.

When the innumerable variations in the proportions of the thickness of the cane at various points on the cut is added to the nine basic types a bewildering multitude of different cuts becomes available. Each type of cut responds somewhat differently for an individual player and will produce a slightly different tone quality. The type of cut which is best for a specific player is a highly personal decision and is primarily dependent upon the tone quality desired, and the shape and development of the embouchure. Any player can learn to play successfully on any type of cut so long as the reed is well-made and adjusted for optimum response.

It must be emphasized that the type of cut is a primary factor in determining the ultimate tone quality which the player will produce. Experience with listening to advanced players who use various types of cuts will soon clearly indicate the tone quality each cut produces, and the teacher can make a choice on this basis.

Both the semi-finished and finished commercial reeds as well as custom made reeds are available in a variety of cuts. In the commercial brands each brand will feature a particular cut, although the semi-finished reeds tend to be mostly short or medium "U" cuts. The professional who makes custom made reeds will make only that cut which he has found most successful for his purposes. One of the reasons why it is recommended that custom made reeds from several makers be given a trial is to provide experience on several types of cuts. Teachers are urged to try a variety of makers in order to discover one or two types of reeds which are consistently good and which respond easily and produce the best quality of tone for their students.

CRITERIA FOR A GOOD REED

Whether the student makes his own reeds or buys them already made, no matter what type of cut is used, the criteria for a good reed are the same. These criteria are applied to the musical results obtained by a specific student. Therefore, a good reed is one that for the individual using it:

1. Responds freely and easily over the entire range of the instrument.
2. Plays all octaves of the instrument well in tune without undue adjustments in embouchure or lip pressure.
3. May be controlled throughout the full dynamic range in all octaves of the instrument.
4. Produces a rich, clear bodied tone of the same quality over the entire range of the instrument.
5. Provides the correct resistance to wind pressure.
6. Allows the complete scope of articulations from hard staccato to soft legato to be played in all octaves.

Reeds must be suited to the individual who is going to use them—to his embouchure, his instrument and, for more advanced players, to fit the demands of the type of music he is playing. The reed must be made to play in tune at A-440 on the instrument on which it is being used. Different makes of oboes require reeds and/or staples of different lengths to play at the standard pitch. The oboe itself is not tuned, the reed is tuned so that the instrument is at the correct pitch.

Some embouchures require certain types of reeds so that the high notes or the low notes can be played in tune. Since it is not possible for an oboist to try many reeds to find one which is satisfactory, he must be able to adjust a particular reed in order to make it respond correctly. He must know how to care for it so that its useful life will be prolonged.

Every player should have three or more reeds adjusted, broken in and ready to play at all times. While it is not generally recommended that the oboist rotate reeds from day to day as is sometimes recommended for a clarinetist, it is dangerous to play on the same reed until it completely deteriorates. As the reed deteriorates the embouchure makes adjustments to compensate for the reed deficiencies, and when a new reed is selected to play the embouchure must be readjusted to it. For this reason the oboist should practice occasionally on a reed which he is not using in performance in order to break it in as well as to help maintain an embouchure which is not set inflexibly to a particular reed.

TOOLS AND MATERIALS FOR ADJUSTING OBOE REEDS

In order to perform the operations necessary to adjust the response of an oboe reed certain tools and materials are necessary. Additional tools and materials are necessary to produce a finished reed from blank cane. The compliment of tools and materials for making adjustments should be a part of the equipment of every teacher responsible for oboe instruction. As soon as the student has progressed to the place where he is mature enough and his oboe playing has been stabilized he too should acquire these tools and begin to adjust reeds for himself. Figure R-31 shows the basic tools and materials for oboe reed adjusting. From left to right these are: file, cutting knife, scraping knife, mandrel, billot (above), plaque (below), and fishskin (or goldbeater's skin).

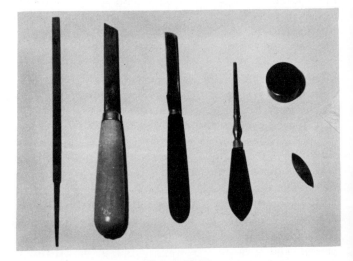

Figure R-31.

A description of these and additional items is summarized as follows. Details of their use in adjusting appears in the section on adjustment.

1. *File.* A fine file or emery boards are used for taking cane off the sides of the reed, or for making major adjustments to the cut.

2. *Cutting Knife.* One of the two knives needed for reed adjustment, the cutting knife is used for cutting off the tip of the reed. The edge of the cutting knife is honed to a razor sharp straight edge. The scraping knife has a rolled edge and must not be used as a cutting knife.

3. *Scraping Knife.* The scraping knife or reed knife as it is also designated is used only for scraping the cane. The scraping knife must have a rigid blade and be of steel which will hold a sharp edge. Hollow ground blades are not satisfactory, and a special reed knife is an investment which will last indefinitely. A folding reed knife which folds like a pocket knife is available and is preferred by some players because the cutting edge is protected when it is closed. The edge of the scraping knife is rolled into a slight "J" shape as the final operation in the sharpening process in order that it will catch the wood evenly. Because of this rolled edge and the fact that it is designed to scrape only in one direction models for right handed and left handed use are available.

4. *Mandrel.* The mandrel fits into the tube of the reed and is used to hold the reed while working on it. The mandrel must fit the inside of the staple perfectly, and may be used to straighten bent staples as well as for holding the reed. The use of a mandrel when working on oboe reeds is optional, although many players prefer to use one. A different mandrel of the proper size to fit the tube is necessary for the English horn reed.

5. *Billot.* The billot, or cutting block, is a round block about an inch in diameter with a slightly convex upper surface. It may be made of grenadilla wood or plastic, and is used to provide a firm shaped surface for trimming the tip of the reed.

6. *Plaque.* The plaque is inserted between the blades of the reed whenever any scraping is being done in order to prevent damage to the tip section. The same plaque may be used for oboe and English horn reeds. It is pushed gently between the blades about a half-inch or until it extends an eighth to a quarter inch on either side of the reed. The correct placement of the plaque is shown in photographs later in this section.

7. *Fishskin.* Fishskin or goldbeater's skin is a tough clear material wrapped around the reed away from the cut to prevent air leaks. This wrapping is not a standard part of the finished reed, but is added only if testing of the reed indicates air leaks. Addition of fishskin to a finished reed is quite frequently a necessary part of its final adjustment.

8. *Clear Fingernail Polish.* Clear fingernail polish or lacquer or a special reed cement is applied over the goldbeater's skin and the thread wrapping to seal it and to keep the skin in place. A half and half mixture of clear fingernail polish and fingernail polish remover is as effective as fingernail polish alone and dries much more rapidly.

9. *Soft Brass Wire.* Soft brass wire is sometimes applied to the oboe reed to hold the tip of the blades open. The application of a wire to an oboe reed is a last resort measure and is not recommended as a common practice. The English horn reed is normally supported by the wire which is a permanent part of the standard reed construction.

10. *Small Pliers with Wire Cutter.* For applying wire to oboe and English horn reeds. The special bassoon reed making pliers may be used for this purpose.

11. *Dutch Rush.* Dutch rush is sometimes recommended for making fine adjustments to the cut of the reed and for the final polishing of the entire scrape. It is used wet and removes extremely small amounts of cane. For this reason it can be more safely used by inexperienced players than a reed knife.

12. *Knife Sharpening Materials.* The cutting knife and especially the scraping knife must be kept razor sharp at all times. A dull cutting knife will not cut the tip of the reed cleanly, and may even split one of the blades. A dull scraping knife cannot be controlled when scraping the reed, and may do more damage than good. A fine oil stone is necessary for keeping the knives sharp. Some reed makers use a leather strop in conjunction with the oil stone.

The sharpening of the scraping knife is an especially important process. The first step in this process is to polish the flat side by rubbing the entire side flat against the stone as shown in Figure R-32. This removes the rolled edge or "J" hook which is necessary for the scraping process. When this is accomplished the bevel edge is polished so that there is a fine, razor sharp straight edge on it. When the bevel edge is sharp, slowly straighten the knife to the vertical position as shown in Figure R-33 for about six light strokes to roll the edge slightly into the "J" hook.

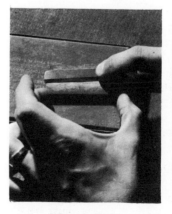 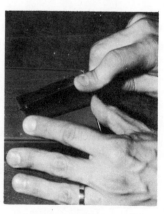

Figure R-32.   **Figure R-33.**

AREAS OF REED TO BE SCRAPED FOR ADJUSTMENT

The areas of the reed which may need adjustment are well defined no matter which type of cut is being used. The exact size and shape of each area will vary with the type of cut and with the individual reed maker. Examine the reed carefully to locate the size, shape and proportions of each area before attempting to make an adjustment. Figures R-34 and R-35 show the various areas for adjustment. Each area influences a particular aspect of the reed's response. Figure R-34 identifies the areas as they appear on a "W" cut reed and Figure R-35 as they appear on a "U" cut reed. The areas of the "V" cut are similar to those on the "U" cut.

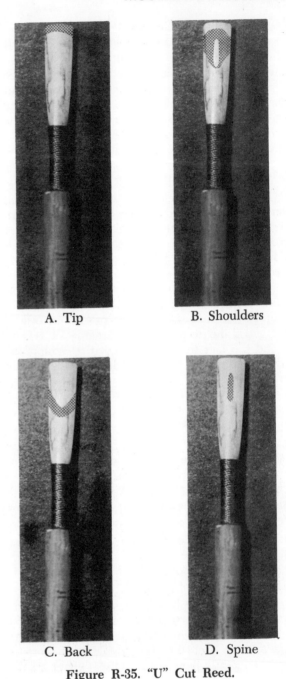

A. Tip   B. Shoulders

C. Back   D. Spine

Figure R-35. "U" Cut Reed.

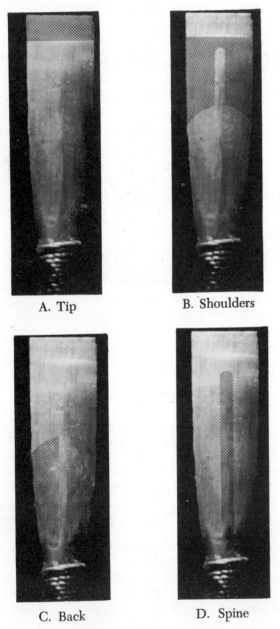

A. Tip   B. Shoulders

C. Back   D. Spine

Figure R-34. "W" Cut Reed.

The areas and their function are as follows:

1. *Tip.* The tip must be uniformly thin across the entire width of the reed, except for the short "U" cut which uses a half moon shape tip. Scrape toward the tip with the knife parallel with the tip, very little at a time, and testing frequently. The thinner the tip the easier the reed will blow and the more reedy the sound will be. The adjustment of the thickness must be determined by balancing tone quality and easy for blowing with the other areas of adjustment as described in the testing routine.

In scraping the tip, the scraping knife is held in the tips of the fingers as shown in Figure R-36. Figure R-37 illustrates how the reed is held securely against the forefinger by the thumb. Note the placement of the plaque in the reed. The knife rests against the thumb and in this illustration is in position for scraping the center section of the tip. The scraping is done by rotating the cutting edge toward the tip with the fingers and wrist, with the knife pivoting against the thumb.

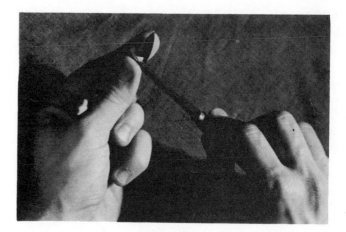

Figure R-38.

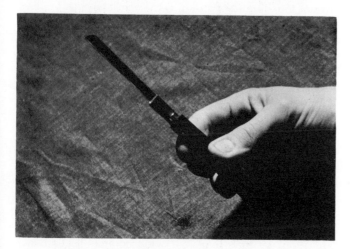

Figure R-36.

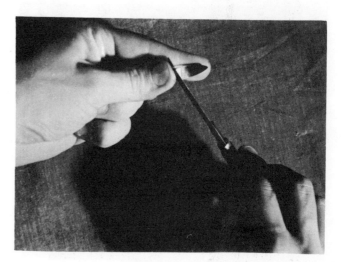

Figure R-39.

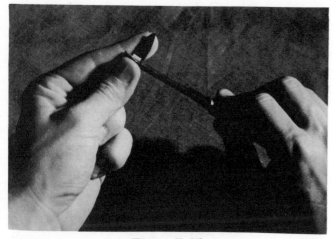

Figure R-37.

The corners of the tip are scraped with the reed held in the same position as for the center scrape. The angle of the knife is changed to move diagonally toward the corner of the tip being scraped. The direction of the scrape is toward the corner with the cutting edge of the knife rotated by the tip of the fingers and the wrist and pivoting against the thumb. Figure R-38 shows the position of the knife for scraping the right corner of the tip, and Figure R-39 the position for scraping the left corner. The tips of both blades must be scraped to identical proportions.

2. *Shoulders.* The shoulders determine to a great extent the basic flexibility or strength of the reed. The two shoulders are thicker at the spine and at the base of the cut getting progressively thinner toward the sides and tip. Figure R-40 shows the way in which the scraping knife is held for scraping the shoulders. It is held firmly in the fingers with the thumb braced on the top. Figure R-41 shows the reed in place for scraping the left shoulder area. Notice that the end of the knife is against the thumb and is in position for beginning the scrape. This scrape is done toward the corner of the tip rather than straight forward with a forward motion of the forearm with the knife pivoting on the thumb.

3. *Back.* The back supports the vibration of the shoulders and is slightly thicker. The length of the scrape of the back helps control the basic pitch of the reed. The further back it is extended within the basic cut the flatter the reed. The thinner the back is, the thinner the shoulders will be and the softer the reed's strength which will make the tone quality more reedy. The back

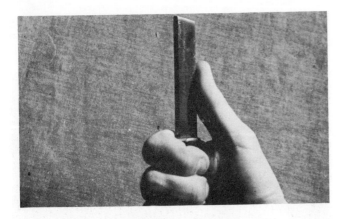

Figure R-40.

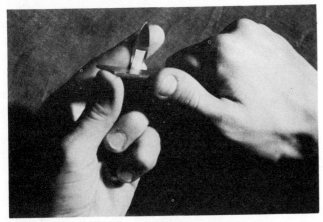

Figure R-41.

also affects the response of the low notes on the instrument. The back is scraped with the knife and reed held as for the shoulder scrape. The knife is held parallel with the tip and the scraping is done toward the tip while moving the knife from the center to the side of the reed with a movement of the thumb.

4. *Spine.* The spine is the center or heart of the reed which tapers in thickness toward the tip. Some types of cuts for oboe reeds do not have a clearly defined spine section, but if there is one it should be scraped only as a last resort. If in spite of other adjustments, the reed continues to be too stiff, the thickness and taper of the spine must be brought into the proper relationship with the remainder of the cut. It is scraped with the knife held as for the shoulder cut parallel to the tip, and very lightly. A very little cane removed from this section will have a great effect on the response of the reed.

TESTING AND CORRECTING REED RESPONSE

An oboe reed may be tested in several ways to see what adjustments, if any, need to be made to make it suitable for a particular player. All of the following tests

can be performed in sequence, and if the reed does not respond properly on any one of them, adjustments should be made to correct the response before proceeding to the next test. The reed must be moistened to the proper playing condition before starting the testing. No adjustments are ever made on a dry reed.

The reed is soaked in a small amount of fresh water to put it in playing condition. A small glass vial deep enough to hold enough water to immerse the reed up to, but not touching the fishskin if the skin has been applied, or up to the end of the cut. The winding must never under any circumstances be soaked. The length of time needed to soak a reed into playing condition varies with the reed and type of cane. Soak until the sides close, but avoid soaking too long. The longer the reed has been played the longer it will take to soak it.

1. *Air Leakage*

Test: Testing for leakage of air through the sides of the reed is done by stopping the end of the tube with a finger and blowing into the reed with some pressure. If air escapes from between the blades this should be corrected before proceeding to the next test.

Correction: Wrap goldbeater's skin around the reed in the area shown in Figure R-42. Cut a piece of the skin about an inch long and wide enough (a half inch is usually sufficient) to cover the affected area. Moisten with saliva the area of the reed where the skin is to be wound. Locate one end of the strip of skin carefully in place in the center of one of the blades and wrap tightly around the reed. A slight spiral downward so that the skin covers at least a quarter inch of the thread wrapping will help keep it in place. When the skin is wound in place moisten the entire surface of the skin with saliva. When this is dry apply a coat of clear fingernail polish over the skin and the wrapping to seal the skin permanently in place. Keep the polish off of the cane.

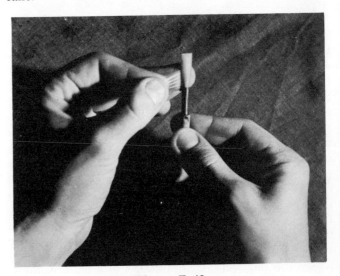

Figure R-42.

2. Basic Strength of Reed.

Test: Stop the end of the tube with a finger and suck the air out of the reed. When taken from the mouth the blades of a properly adjusted reed will stay closed for a second and then open with a slight pop. If the end remains closed the reed is too soft, if the end does not close at all to form the vacuum the reed is too stiff, or a leak has not been sealed.

Corrections: (1) If the tip does not close test the thickness of the tip. First moisten the inside with saliva, then insert the plaque. The thickness of the tip can be seen when the plaque is pressed gently against each blade as shown in Figure R-43. The tip should be sufficiently transparent so that the plaque can be seen through it, and should be the same thickness entirely across the reed. Scrape the tip section of both blades until they are equally transparent. Retest the reed and if this procedure has not corrected the condition proceed with the next correction.

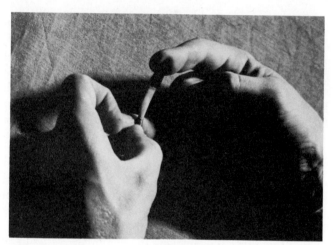

Figure R-43.

(2) If, after the tip has been tested and adjusted as directed the reed will not form a vacuum, test, then the flexibility of the cut by pressing the blades together with the thumb and forefinger about a half-inch from the tip as shown in Figure R-44. If the blades require considerable pressure to close the tip they are too thick and must be scraped. Experience will quickly indicate the proper pressure needed to close the tip. While this test is performed the tip should close from the edges toward the center, with the exact center being the last place to close. If the tip does not close last in the exact center a diminuendo is difficult to play. This condition is corrected by cutting the back of the lay to relieve the side which closes last. This procedure will sometimes be the only adjustment needed to correct the strength of the reed. If this does not make the correction scrape the shoulders of both blades to a uniform thickness and blend them into the tip area to maintain balance.

Be sure that the reed remains moist. Test the reed frequently during the scraping both with the vacuum test and the crow of the reed as outlined later.

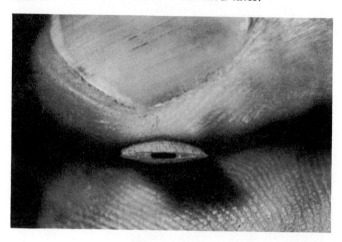

Figure R-44.

(3) A tip which remains closed when the vacuum test is made may be much too soft, or the curvature of the blades may be so slight that there is not enough spring in them to open the tip. A tip which remains closed in the vacuum test will more often than not close easily when it is played so that no sound can be produced. A reed which is in this condition for either cause can seldom be adjusted for excellent response, although adjustments can be made so that it can be played. If the curvature of the blades is satisfactory a tip which is too soft can be identified when the plaque is inserted as directed in number one above. A tip which is too soft will be almost completely transparent. The correction is to cut off a portion of the tip and if necessary rescrape the reed to the proper pitch and response.

If the reed which is otherwise satisfactory closes because of the slight curvature of the blades and generally weak shoulder areas, the tip may be held open by adding a wire as far back on the reed as possible. Figure R-45 shows a typical location. Use two turns of wire around the reed and twist the ends together. The twist controls the pressure against the reed and the amount the tip is held open. Adjust to achieve the desired opening. A wire is seldom necessary with a medium or long "W" cut, but is more frequently used with a medium or short "U" cut. Many oboists prefer to discard a reed rather than using a wire to hold the tip open, while others will use a wire as part of the normal process of making a reed. English horn reeds may have a wire as part of its regular construction. The objection to wiring a reed is due to the fact that basic dynamic changes are made by opening and closing the tip. If the tip is naturally open it can be easily closed by the embouchure, but if it is held open by a wire it is difficult to control with the embouchure. Usually only quite soft reeds need a wire and the tone quality is not good, and is not improved by the wiring.

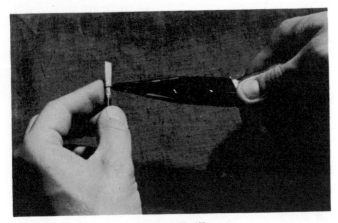

Figure R-45.

3. *Crow or Cackle of the Reed.*

Test: Testing the crow or cackle is done by placing the reed a little further into the mouth than it is placed for playing. Blow with a steady, but unfocused stream of air. When a sound is produced in this way a good reed will have a characteristic even and well-defined double crow. The correct crow must have both the high sound and the low sound present in about equal balance. Experience will enable a player to determine a great many things about a reed from the way in which it crows. Many reed makers will not even put the reed on the oboe until the crow is satisfactorily adjusted.

Corrections: (1) A high pitched squeak is produced by a reed that is too stiff. This may be accounted for by a tip which is too thick, a tip which is too short, or by shoulders or back being too thick. Test and adjust the tip area as previously described to the proper length and thickness, testing the sound of the crow frequently. If the high pitched sound persists after the tip is adjusted scrape the shoulders and back section a very little at a time, testing the crow frequently. Unless the reed is an exceptionally stiff one this should produce the proper crow. If the reed is very stiff it may be necessary to take a little cane off the spine section. This must be done extremely carefully, very little cane at a time, and the reed tested frequently. Keep the length, shape, and proportions of both blades the same. Do not touch the tip section of the reed if it has been previously adjusted.

(2) If only a low pitch is present the tip is too long, too soft, or both. If the tip section is properly cut then the facing is too long. In both instances the pitch of the reed will probably be flat. The correction for a too long or too soft tip is to trim the tip back very very little at a time until the correction is made. Once the tip is responding correctly, the basic strength and pitch of the

reed may be adjusted if necessary. If the tip area is not the cause a facing which is too long is corrected by cutting off a little of the tip and reshaping the forward portion of the cut and tip. This process may make the reed play sharp and must be carefully done.

The tip may be trimmed with the cutting knife and billot. With the reed in place on the billot prepare for the cut with the knife flat on the blade of the reed. With the knife in this position the cutting edge may be lined up exactly parallel with the tip and the amount to be removed determined accurately. When the edge is in position roll the knife up to the vertical position for the cutting as shown in Figure R-46. The cutting is done with pressure of both hands on the blade.

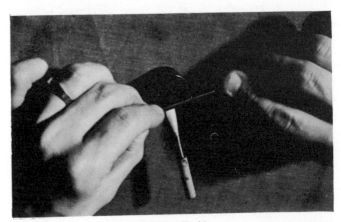

Figure R-46.

Some oboists prefer to trim the tip with a pair of ordinary sewing scissors. When the scissors are used the two blades are pressed firmly together with the thumb and forefinger of the left hand. The reed is placed against the lower scissor blade, lined up parallel with it and the amount to be clipped determined as in Figure R-47. The trimming is done by holding the reed firmly against the lower scissor blade and cutting with a single movement of the scissors.

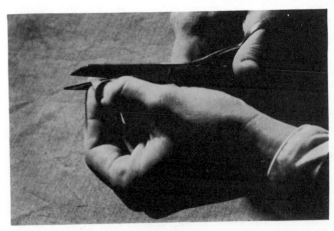

Figure R-47.

4. *Matching the Blades.*

Test: Test the reed in correct playing position in the normally formed embouchure without the instrument. (Note the difference between this position and the crow position.) It should produce a clear tone. Turn the reed over so that the position of the blades is reversed in the mouth. The tone produced in this position should be identical with the previous sound.

Correction: If the tones produced with the reed in both positions are not identical then the blades are scraped unevenly and do not match. A careful visual examination will usually show the difference between the blades so that they can be scraped to match. Not all oboe reeds match exactly or respond identically when the blades are reversed. If, in spite of careful adjustments the response is still slightly different—one position responding better than the other—mark the upper blade of the better position so that the player can always play wtih this blade up.

5. *Checking Pitch.*

Test: Put the reed on the instrument, warm up the instrument, and test the pitch to see that the reed plays exactly at A-440 when the tube is pushed into the instrument as far as it will go. All oboists should have a tuning fork for this purpose. A stroboscopic tuner where a visual check of the pitch can be made is more convenient and may be used when available.

Corrections: (1) If the reed is very slightly sharp, the tube can be pulled no more than a sixteenth of an inch from the instrument without adverse effect on the way in which the instrument will respond. If the tube is pulled more than a sixteenth of an inch, the instrument will be out of tune with itself, some notes will respond poorly, and tone quality on some notes will suffer.

(2) If the reed is too sharp to be corrected by pulling the tube, then the pitch can be flattened by slightly lengthening the cut. Scrape lightly the back area an equal amount on both blades. Test frequently and continue until the reed is brought to the correct pitch.

(3) If the reed is flat, the pitch may be raised by trimming a small amount off the tip, as previously described. Cut off only the smallest amount of the tip at one time Test carefully, and repeat the process if necessary. Be very careful not to cut off too much so that the reed is sharp. If the trimming process to bring the reed up to pitch makes it stiff and difficult to blow, first scrape to reform the proper tip area. If reforming the tip does not correct the stiffness the entire cut may require scraping and adjusting.

6. *Intonation of Upper Octave.*

Test: If the A-440 is in tune, test to see if the octave above can be played perfectly in tune with normal adjustment in embouchure pressure. If the upper A is flat in relation to the lower one, then all the upper notes

will be flat and the reed must be adjusted to compensate for this.

Correction: Assuming that the player's embouchure is properly formed and developed, there are several possible corrections for flatness in the upper notes. Perform the following operations in sequence until the situation is corrected:

(1) The tip of the reed may be too open, i.e., too round. If this is the case, correct as described under correction two of the basic strength tests previously described.

(2) Narrow the reed by filing both sides lightly with a file or emery board. Place the reed solidly on a table top. Holding it firmly file parallel with the table, moving the file back and forth gently as shown in Figure R-48. Test the reed frequently to avoid taking too much off. Watch the tip opening during this process to see that it does not become too close.

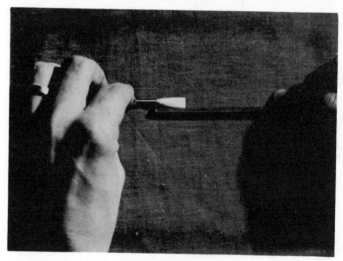

Figure R-48.

(3) Slide one blade sideways so that they are very slightly out of parallel. If this does not help the intonation, shift them in the other direction and retest.

(4) Cut a sixty-fourth of an inch off the tip of the reed. This will solve the out-of-tune upper octave which is caused by a tip which is too thin and/or too long without changing the over-all pitch of the reed.

If the reed otherwise responds well with satisfactory tone quality and none of these procedures solves the problem of flatness in the upper octave, then it is caused by the student's embouchure being undeveloped and/or poorly formed and the solution lies in the embouchure rather than the reed.

The upper A will almost never be sharp, this sharpness can be corrected by the appropiate adjustment in the embouchure. If this sharpness occurs regularly on several different well adjusted reeds, check the embouchure formation of the student. It is likely that he is biting the reed with his lower teeth or wedging it between the upper and lower teeth.

7. *Response of Lowest Notes.*

Test: Test the response of the reed on the lowest four or five notes of the instrument. They should speak readily at a piano level and should not have a reedy quality.

Correction: If the low notes do not speak at a piano level or respond with difficulty thin the blade by scraping lightly the portions of the shoulder near the spine. Test frequently during this process since if too much is taken off response of other notes of the instrument will change. Be sure that both blades are scraped equally.

ENGLISH HORN REEDS

English horn reeds have the same basic cuts and adjustments as those described for oboe reeds. It normally has a shorter tip proportionately than an oboe reed to respond better on the higher notes and for better intonation. It will, as well, have a more pronounced spine. The English horn reed is made on a staple which fits directly on the crook of the instrument, and usually has a wire in place to adjust the tip opening.

All the tools except the mandrel used in adjusting oboe reeds can be used for adjusting English horn reeds. A special English horn mandrel to fit the staple is necessary to hold the reed while working on it. The tests and corrections used for the oboe reed apply also to the English horn reed with adjustments for its slightly different proportioned cut. Students who are skilled in adjusting oboe reeds can easily adapt this skill to the English horn reed with some experience.

CARE OF THE OBOE AND ENGLISH HORN REED

A good, well responding oboe or English horn reed is a valuable possession and should have meticulous care if it is to have a long useful life. The rules for caring for reeds are simple and if followed will prolong their useful life:

1. Keep the fingers off of the tip of the reed.

2. Keep reeds in a reed case so that they will dry out slowly and completely. Plastic tubes seal too tightly for this purpose. If such a tube is used punch a small hole in the cap. Figure R-49 shows a typical oboe reed case.

3. Always soak the reed as directed before playing. Never play on a dry or partially moist reed. Clear water is better than saliva for this purpose. Most oboists carry a small water-tight bottle in their case for this purpose.

4. Clean the inside of the reed every week or two with a wet pipe cleaner when the reed is well soaked. Insert the wet pipe cleaner through the tube from the cork and and force it gently through the tip of the reed. Then pull it through the reed slowly moving it from side to side so that all inside surfaces are cleaned. Re-

peat the process two or three times. Figures R-50 and R-51 illustrates this procedure.

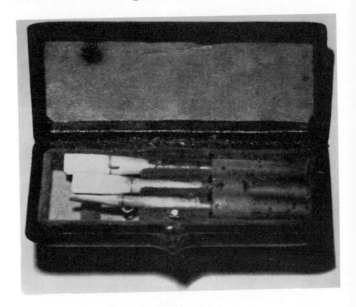

Figure R-49.

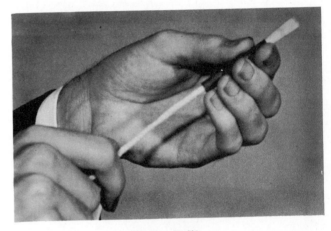

Figure R-50.

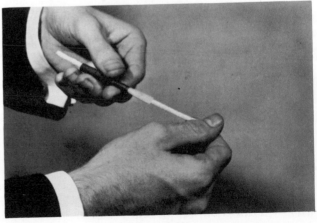

Figure R-51.

BASSOON REEDS

The reed is perhaps the most important part of the bassoon, since in combination with the embouchure and the instrument itself it is the determining factor in how the instrument will sound. Even the best embouchure cannot make a poor reed sound well, while a good reed is a valuable assistant for an undeveloped embouchure. The response of a good reed is limited by a poor instrument or an instrument in poor condition. The finest instrument cannot make a poor reed sound or respond correctly. In order to isolate the influence, response, and control of the reed it is necessary to have the instrument in good playing condition, and a properly formed embouchure which has been developed past the beginning stages. If the embouchure is poorly formed or undeveloped it is impossible to isolate and identify many incorrect factors as being caused specifically by the reed. Many of the symptoms of a poorly responding reed may be caused by the embouchure.

The selection, adjustment and care of the bassoon reed is a subject which should be thoroughly understood by every player and by every teacher who is responsible for these students. This is a widely neglected and misunderstood subject possibly because the information is not readily available. There is no mystery to the bassoon reed. Its selection and adjustment is no more complicated than for the oboe and single reeds, and is readily understood and performed after some experience by anyone familiar with the instrument. One writer on the subject is of the opinion that anyone, after making a dozen reeds from blank cane will be able to turn out a reed which will be very playable. Not everyone will agree with this statement, but certainly the subject of bassoon reeds is not one which should be considered difficult or impossible to understand.

Every bassoonist past the beginning stage should be able to adjust ready made reeds. If he is a serious student of the instrument he should learn how to make his own reeds from the blank cane. Most bassoonists who are fortunate enough to study with a teacher skilled in reed making learn the art of reed making and adjustment as a regular normal part of the study of their instrument. Many teachers consider this as important as any other aspect of study. Certainly no bassoonist's training can be considered complete until he is proficient in making and adjusting reeds. Beginners on the instrument will first develop the facility for adjustment and then progress into the complete production of reeds.

The present discussion is limited to the selection, adjustment and care of the bassoon reed. The problems involved in making reeds are beyond the scope of this book, and are best learned through personal instruction from one who is skilled in the art. The considerations here will be limited to those aspects of the problem which the teacher needs to know and use in his everyday activities.

PARTS OF THE BASSOON REED

Before discussing the bassoon reed it is necessary to establish a vocabulary for identification of the various parts of the reed. The designations here are the standard ones which are in almost universal use. Figure R-52 identifies these parts.

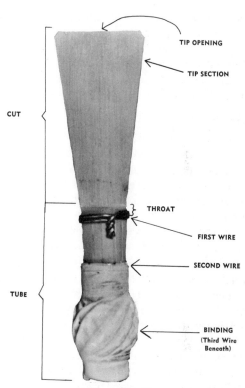

Figure R-52.

The *tip* section is an inverted "U" similar to that found in single reeds and will be illustrated later. The *tip opening* refers to the space between blades. The *cut* (also called the facing, lay or scrape) is that portion of the reed from which the bark has been cut. Its length, contours and thickness control the vibration of the blades and must be carefully controlled. The *shoulder* is the point at which the cut begins. The *throat* is the interior of the reed from the first wire to the shoulder. Its shape may be perfectly round or slightly elliptical when observed from the back of the reed. The function of the throat section is to blend the tube into the cut blades and it determines to some extent the amount of arch in the blades. Its shape may be adjusted by the first wire. The *tube* extends from the first wire to the bottom of the reed. Regardless of the shape of the throat the tube section, both inside and out, must be perfectly round. The two halves of the reed are held together by three wires. The *first wire* is near the shoulder, the *second wire* about a half inch down the tube from it, and the *third wire*, beneath the binding, is about a quarter of an inch from the end. The first and second wires influence the response of the reed and are used in making certain adjustments. The function of the *binding* is to help hold the two pieces of cane together, to seal possible leaks in this area, and to provide a place for the fingers to grip the reed securely. The binding is nylon or cotton thread wound in a ball over the third wire, with a single layer extending to the second wire. It is covered with a coat of reed cement, or collodion to seal the reed and binding against air leaks. The wrapping is traditionally red in color, but some makers use other colors. The neatness and skill with which the binding is applied to the reed is one obvious way to judge the quality of workmanship in a reed.

HOW A BASSOON REED IS MADE

The process of making a bassoon reed from cane tubes is quite similar to that described in making an oboe reed. The diameter of the cane used is about nine-eighth inches—somewhat larger than that used for oboe reeds. A few more steps are necessary because the bassoon reed is not mounted on a staple. The steps in producing the bassoon reed are performed in this order: splitting, gouging, sanding the inside, scoring on the easel, removing the bark from the center inch of cane on the easel, filing this portion which will become the tip of the reed, notching either side of the cane at the center, folding over shaper, shaping, beveling the edges, cutting the tube section to the correct length, applying the three wires, with the reed on the mandrel finishing the blades with knife and file, wrapping the thread, reaming the tube to fit the bocal and final tuning and adjustments. This process is described and illustrated in detail in the book "How to Make Double-Reeds."[5]

Cane for making bassoon reeds is available in five different forms in decreasing order of the amount of work remaining to complete the reed: (1) bulk, (2) straight gouged, (3) gouged and shaped, (4) gouged, shaped and folded, (5) gouged, shaped, folded and profiled. The profiled cane has the basic cut of both blades completed, usually by machine, and requires only wiring, wrapping and completing the cut to produce a finished reed. The profiling is often referred to as "roughing out the tip" and should be understood as having the same meaning. The more proficient and particular the bassoonist is in making reeds the more work he wants to do himself on the reeds. Professionals will start with bulk cane. An excellent way for a student bassoonist to learn the art of reed making is to start with the fifth class of cane listed above and work his way back through the list as his proficiency develops. The fourth type—gouged, shaped and folded—is that most frequently used by experienced student bassoonists as it saves a great deal of time while

giving them complete control over the shape and contours of the lay. There are considerable differences in brands of cane available in all five forms. Several brands should be tried until the one best suited is found.

TYPES OF BASSOON REEDS AVAILABLE

Although the advanced bassoonist is expected and wants to make his own reeds, the great majority of students will purchase reeds which are ready-made. Many schools purchase them by the dozens for their bassoonists. Since the success of these students is dependent upon how the reed responds it is most important that they be purchased wisely and with full knowledge of the choices available. There are three general types of ready-made reeds available which can be described as follows:

1. *Semi-finished Commercial Reeds.* These are mass produced for general retail distribution in the same way that single reeds are produced and distributed. Several machines have been perfected which produce a semi-finished bassoon reed virtually without handwork. The value of these machines lies in the consistency of the cut and in producing reeds at a lower cost. The description "semi-finished" indicates that the purchaser must perform the final adjustments for the best response. This includes tuning the reed to fit his embouchure and instrument, finishing the cut on both blades, and smoothing the surfaces. Unless the teacher or student has developed some skill in adjusting reeds, this type of reed is seldom satisfactory. Many semi-finished reeds are not designated as such when they are sold and many students attempt to play them without making the final adjustments, with the consequent multitude of problems a poorly adjusted reed brings.

2. *Finished Commercial Reeds.* Other types of commercial reeds generally available in music stores are classified as "finished" reeds. That is, the cut has been finished and the reed is in playing condition. Some brands of these finished commercial reeds are graded according to strength in the same way single reeds are graded. Strengths, 1, 2, 3, 4, 5, etc., are available. The lower the number the softer the strength. Even though the reed is classified as finished it must be tried on the instrument and adjustments made to suit the individual player. If this kind of reed is used several brands must be tried to find the one which is most consistently satisfactory and needs the least adjusting.

3. *Custom Made Reeds.* This class of reeds is made by professional players to individual order. There are many professional players in all sections of the country who will make reeds for students, and who will adapt the reed to the level of advancement of the student. These reeds are normally made in the same way and with

---

[5]Artley, Joe. *How To Make Double Reeds.* Old Greenwich, Conn.: Jack Spratt. Second Edition, 1953.

the same care the professional makes reeds for himself. Since they are not mass produced the quality is consistently high.

It is highly recommended that this type of reed be secured for all school bassoonists at least until their embouchure and facility has developed to the point that they have enough assurance to learn how to adjust their own reeds. If there is not a nearby professional bassoonist to supply reeds the names and addresses of professional players who specialize in making reeds for school use can be found in the classified advertisements in such magazines as the *Instrumentalist* and *School Musician*. Try reeds from several makers until those best suited for the student and instrument are found.

TYPES OF CUT

There are two basic types of bassoon reeds, the French and the German. In the chapter on the bassoon vast differences are pointed out between the French system instruments and the Heckel system or German instruments both in mechanics of the key work and in the type of tone quality produced. Only the German or Heckel system bassoon is used in this country. Since the German type reed is designed for the Heckel bassoon it is the only type which should be used. The French cut reed will not respond or produce the desired tone quality when it is used on a Heckel bassoon. Unless the finished reeds are imported from a French maker it is highly improbable that the French cut will be found on the market. Avoid using any bassoon reed described as having a French cut.

Within the basic German cut which is universally used in this country, there are probably as many variations in length, width, shape and over-all size as there are people making bassoon reeds. Reeds for no other instrument vary so greatly. In spite of this the general shape of the cut remains the same, with only the proportions of the various areas changed. For this reason the areas described for adjustment, and the way the adjustments are made can be applied to any standard reed.

CRITERIA FOR A GOOD REED

Whether the student makes his own reeds or buys them already made the criteria for a good reed are the same. A good reed is one that for the individual using it:

1. Responds freely and easily over the entire range of the instrument.

2. Plays all registers of the instrument in tune without undue embouchure adjustments.

3. May be controlled throughout the full dynamic range in all registers.

4. Produces a rich, clear bodied tone of the same quality over the entire range of the instrument.

5. Provides the correct resistance to wind pressure.

6. Allows the complete scope of articulations to be played in all registers.

Reeds must be suited to the individual who is going to use them—to his embouchure and his instrument. The reed must be made to play in tune on his instrument since the pitch of the instrument itself can be changed very little with other adjustments. Unlike the clarinetist, the bassoonist cannot try a dozen or more reeds to find one that responds well, but must learn to adjust a particular reed to make it fit his needs. He must know how to care for it so that its useful life will be prolonged.

Every player should have at least three reeds adjusted and broken in and ready to play at any time. He should break in the reeds and adjust them over a period of several days since the reed changes as it is played on for the first few hours. After this it will not change except to gradually deteriorate with use. The embouchure will adjust to a particular reed, so it is important that the bassoonist not use one reed exclusively, but occasionally play on others to keep the embouchure flexible.

TOOLS AND MATERIALS FOR ADJUSTING BASSOON REEDS

In order to perform the operations necessary to adjust the response of a bassoon reed certain tools and materials are necessary. This complement should be a part of the equipment of every teacher responsible for bassoon students. When the student has progressed far enough he should acquire these tools and learn to adjust his reeds. Figure R-53 shows the basic equipment for adjusting bassoon reeds. From left to right the items are: file, cutting knife, scraping knife, reamer, mandrel, shaped plaque, billot (above), pliers (top).

A description of these and additional items is summarized as follows. Details of their use in adjusting appears in the section on adjustment.

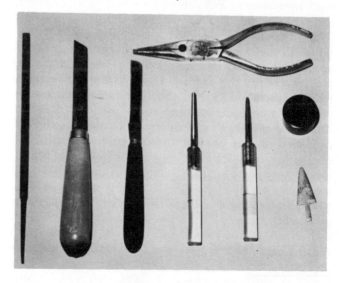

Figure R-53.

1. *File*. For finishing the cut, rather than using the scraping knife. A "piller" file which has the serrations completely to the end is preferred.

2. *Cutting Knife*. Used for cutting off tip of reed. Must not be used for scraping.

3. *Scraping Knife*. The scraping or reed knife is used only for scraping the cane. It is identical with the oboe scraping knife. Refer to the section on oboe reeds for details of its shape and how it is kept sharp.

4. *Mandrel*. Fits into the tube of the reed, and is used to hold the reed while working on it. One with a short handle is preferable for the adjusting process. It must be the same size as the small end of the bocal being used.

5. *Reamer*. For enlarging the end of the tube so that the reed will fit the bocal properly. Like the mandrel, the reamer should match the size of the bocal.

6. *Plaque*. The plaque is inserted between the blades of the reed whenever any scraping is being done in order to prevent damage to the tip section. There are two shapes of plaques available, an oval shape similar to the standard oboe plaque and a shaped plaque as illustrated in the photograph. The shaped plaque is identical with the shape of the reed and is advantageous in that it supports the blades more firmly than the flat oval shape, and its smaller size has a minimum protrusion around the blades so that the knife or file can be worked to the edge of the reed. Both are useful in the adjusting process.

7. *Billot*. The billot, or cutting block, is a round block about an inch and a half in diameter made of wood or plastic, and with a slightly convex upper surface. It is used to provide a firm shaped surface for trimming the tip of the reed.

8. *Pliers*. For adjusting the wires on the reed. A small, narrow end pair with a cutting edge is desirable. The special pliers made for use with bassoon reeds have a hole in them for shaping the cane over the mandrel, but are not necessary for simple adjustments.

9. *Dutch Rush*. Used for making fine adjustment in the cut and for the final polishing of the entire lay. It may be used wet or dry and is recommended for beginners learning the art of adjustment because it removes cane very slowly. Fine grain sandpaper or a fine grain emery board may be used instead of the Dutch Rush.

10. *Soft Brass Wire*. For replacing the wire bindings on the reed in the event this becomes necessary.

AREAS OF REED TO BE SCRAPED FOR ADJUSTMENT

The areas of the reed which may need adjustment are well defined no matter what the size and shape of the reed. The exact size and shape of each area will vary slightly with each type of reed. Examine the reed carefully to locate the size, shape and proportions of each area before attempting to make an adjustment. Figure R-54 shows the various areas for adjustment. Each area influences a particular aspect of the reed's response.

A. Spine   B. Sides   C. Tip

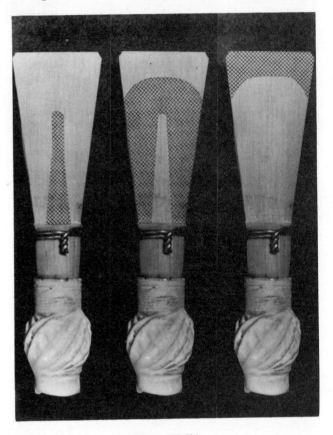

Figure R-54.

The areas and their function are as follows:

1. *Spine*. The spine is the center or heart of the reed which tapers in thickness toward the tip. It controls the vibrations of the sides and influences the strength of the reed. If the reed is too stiff this portion of the reed should be scraped only after the tip and sides have been properly proportioned. Scrape very little at a time and test frequently. This portion of the reed has its greatest influence on the low register of the instrument.

In scraping the spine and the back portion of the sides, the knife is held between the fingers and thumb. It is held parallel with the tip of the reed. The scrape is made straight forward toward the tip and keeping the blade parallel with the tip. Figure R-55 shows the starting position for this scrape.

2. *Sides*. These areas are tapered in thickness from the spine to the edge of the reed and toward the tip area. The sides along with the tip determine the stiffness of the reed. If the tip is properly proportioned and

the reed is too stiff scrape the sides to make it softer. The sides must be blended smoothly into both the heart and tip sections.

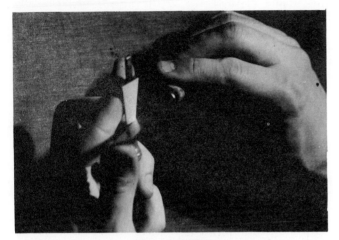

Figure R-55.

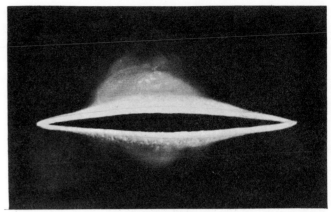

Figure R-57.

In scraping the forward portion of the sides the knife is held as shown in Figure R-56 and braced against the thumb. The direction of the scrape is diagonally toward the edge of the reed.

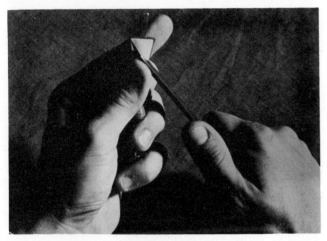

Figure R-56.

3. *Tip.* The tip area is in the shape of an inverted "U" and tapers in thickness toward the corners. When looking at the tip opening the blades should curve evenly, and must match exactly. The blade is thickest in the center and gradually tapers to a very thin line at the corners. Both sides of the center of the blade should be identical, and both blades should match. Figure R-57 shows the shape of the tip opening. The two blades should be approximately one-sixteenth of an inch apart in the center of the tip opening.

In scraping the tip, the scraping knife is held as shown in Figure R-58 in the cupped fingers with the thumb on top. Notice how the knife rests against the thumb. The knife rotates against thumb and the direction of the knife is toward the corner of the reed.

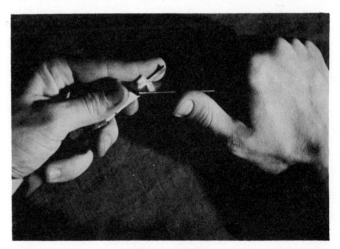

Figure R-58.

ADJUSTING BASSOON REED WITH WIRES

The two visable wires on the bassoon reed bind the two sections of the reeds together as their primary function. In doing so they exert pressure against the top and bottom as well as the sides of the blades. These pressures control the amount of curvature in the blades and thereby the size and to some extent the shape of the tip opening. The two wires are adjusted to control both the tip opening and curvature of the blades.

The wires are squeezed from either the top and bottom or from the sides with the pliers. Do not tighten the wires by twisting the ends. If the wires are too tight either by twisting the ends or by squeezing, the reed may crack. The first wire is especially susceptible to cracking the reed, even to the point of extending the crack into the cut. When tightening the second wire the circular shape of the tube must not be disturbed. If this wire is tightened very much it may be necessary to ream the end of the reed so that it will fit on the bocal.

Changing the tip opening affects both tone quality and pitch, so adjusting with the wires must be done gradually and cautiously. A tip which is more open will produce a fuller and darker tone, be slightly higher in pitch, and have more resistance. A tip which is more closed will produce a thinner, reedier sound, be slightly flatter in pitch and have less resistance.

The first wire when squeezed on the sides will open the tip. When squeezed on the top and bottom the first wire will close the tip. The second wire when squeezed on the sides will close the tip. When squeezed on the top and bottom the second wire will open the tip. Notice that the two wires have an opposite effect on the tip when squeezed on the top and bottoms and on the sides. To open the tip squeeze the sides of the first wire or the top and bottom of the second wire. To close the tip squeeze the top and bottom of the first wire or the sides of the second wire.

The reed may be opened or closed an even greater amount by using both of the wires. The decision on whether to make the adjustment with the first or second wires or both of them depends on the nature of the reed itself. The first wire makes a greater change in the curvature of the blade and tip than does the second while opening and closing it. Therefore if the tip opening is too round or too flat in shape begin by adjusting the first wire. If the curvature of the blades is correct and the tip is too open or too close begin by adjusting the second wire. If the adjustment of one wire does not correct the problem, both should be used. Experience will quickly indicate whether or not adjustment of the wires is called for and how this adjustment should be done.

TESTING AND CORRECTING REED RESPONSE

A bassoon reed is tested in several ways to see what adjustments, if any, need to be made to make it suitable for a particular player. The testing and adjustments must be done slowly and carefully, testing the reed after each adjustment. Students have a tendency to over adjust in the learning stage. While some over adjusting can be corrected, cane which is scraped away cannot be put back. Emphasize the process of small adjustments between each testing of the reed.

All adjustments, including those made with the wires, must be made with the reed soaked to the proper playing condition. The reed is soaked in a small amount of fresh water. A small glass vial deep enough to hold sufficient water to immerse the reed up to the first wire is sufficient, and all bassoonists should have one in their case. The length of time needed to soak a reed varies with the reed type of cane, anywhere from three to twenty minutes. The reed is sufficiently moist when the sides

close. This is the only dependable criteria for the length of time needed. Avoid soaking the reed too long. Do not wet the circular tube section, for if it becomes soaked and expands the binding tends to come loose after it dries.

After the reed has been soaked make the following tests. The tests for leaks should be first, followed by the "crow" test. The remainder may be performed in any sequence.

1. *Air Leakage in Reed.*

Test: Stop the end of the reed with a finger and blow air into the tip with considerable pressure. If air leaks out the seams make one or both corrections.

Correction: (1) Soak the reed longer—as much as twenty minutes—to see if the sides will close firmly. Many leaks will be stopped by this simple process.

(2) If soaking the reed does not stop the leak, the wires must be tightened. With the pliers twist the end of each wire, one-half turn and test the reed. If it still leaks twist each another half-turn and test. Continue until the leak stops, but avoid tightening the wires so much that the shape of the throat or tube is changed or the vibration of the blades is damped.

2. *Air Leakage at Bocal Connection.*

Test: Using the bocal alone, put the reed in place with a slight twisting motion. Close the cork end of the bocal and the whisper key vent hole with the fingers and blow firmly through the reed. If the air leaks at the juncture of reed and bocal correct as follows.

Correction: Ream the end of the reed very carefully (Figure R-59) so that it is perfectly round and will fit further on the bocal. It should fit at least a quarter of an inch over the bocal.

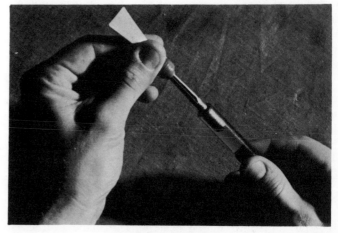

Figure R-59.

3. *Crow of the Reed.*

Test: Testing the crow of the reed is done by putting the reed between the lips with just enough pressure around it to keep the air from escaping, and with the lips almost touching the first wire. Blow with a steady, unfocused stream of air. When a sound is produced in this way on a good reed it will produce the characteristic double crow. This sound must have both high and low pitch sounds in it with the low pitch somewhat more prominent.

With some experience the bassoonist can judge the quality of the reed quite accurately from how it crows. No further tests should be made on the reed until attempts have been made to produce a satisfactory crow. If the high pitch predominates and the sound takes more than normal breath pressure to produce, the tip is too open and/or the reed is too stiff. If little or no high pitch is present and the sound takes less than normal breath pressure to produce, the tip is too close and/or the reed is too soft.

Correction: (1) If the reed is well soaked alter the tip opening by squeezing it with the thumb and forefinger. Squeeze the top and bottom of the tip for less opening. Squeeze the corners of the tip for a greater opening. This must be done with a gentle pressure in order not to crack the reed. If the reed is basically a good one the tip opening can be adjusted with this procedure. Make the adjustment and test the crow. Repeat two or three times if necessary. If the tip opening is still incorrect adjust with the wires.

(2) If adjusting the tip as directed in the first correction does not produce the correct crow, proceed with the test of the basic strength of the reed.

4. Basic Strength of Reed.

Test: The test will help verify the crow test. Stop the end of the tube with a finger and suck the air out of the reed. When taken from the mouth the blades of a properly adjusted reed will stay closed for a second or two and then open with a slight pop. If the end remains closed the reed is too soft or the tip opening too close. If the end does not close at all to form the vacuum the reed is too stiff, or a leak has not been sealed.

Correction: Repeat the test for air leakage to eliminate this as a cause. Check the tip opening to see that it is correct. If there is no air leakage and the tip opening is correct this test should confirm the conclusion made in the crow test, that the reed is too stiff or too soft. Proceed with the appropriate test and adjustment given for a stiff reed or soft reed.

5. Stiff Reed.

Test: The crow test reveals a stiff reed when the high pitch predominates and it is hard to blow. The basic strength test indicates a stiff reed when the vacuum fails to form. For an additional test, put the reed in place on the instrument and play third space E-flat with the 103 000 fingering. Compare this pitch with the octave below. If the third space note is sharp the reed is too

stiff. Play the notes in the low register—B-flat to F below the staff. If the reed is too stiff it responds slowly and these notes will have a rough quality and be impossible to play softly.

Correction: (1) Most commercial reeds are deliberately left stiff so that the purchaser can adjust them to his needs. If the tip opening is correct and the reed is stiff, the entire facing must be scraped or filed to make the blades thinner. This must be done evenly over both blades so they are in perfect balance. Remember, it is easy to take off too much cane. Make the crow and basic strength test frequently during this process until the reed successfully passes them. When it does, test the E-flat and the low register. If the E-flat responds properly but the low register does not, proceed with the next correction.

(2) The response of the lower octave on a reed which is otherwise correct is adjusted by additional scraping on the side areas of the reed. Scrape both sides of both blades evenly, a very little amount at a time. Test frequently so that too much cane is not removed. Continue until the proper response is achieved.

6. Soft Reed.

Test: The crow test indicates a soft reed when there is little or no high pitch present and the sound takes less than normal breath pressure to produce. The basic strength test identifies a soft reed when the end remained closed. For an additional test, put the reed in place on the instrument and play third space E-natural starting softly and making a gradual crescendo. If the tone cracks before the fortissimo is reached the reed is too soft. Notes in the low register will have a very reedy quality on a soft reed, and notes in the high register will be difficult or impossible to play in tune. The basic pitch of the reed will be flat, and difficult to control. A reed is too soft because the tip area alone is too thin, the sides and tip area both are too thin, or because the spine alone or in combination with the sides and tip is too thin. Adjustment is difficult or impossbile and it is for this reason that testing the reed after each minute adjustment has been emphasized. In some areas, the spine, for example, a very little cane removed has a great effect on the strength of the reed. Since most commercial reeds are deliberately left too stiff and the usual problem is to bring them down to the desired strength, almost all reeds which are too soft are that way because of over adjustment on the part of the player.

Correction: (1) If the reed is only slightly soft work with the wire adjustments to see if it can be brought to the proper strength by increasing the curvature of the blades and the tip opening.

(2) Put the reed on the billot and with the cutting knife cut off a sixteenth of an inch from the tip. Starting

with the crow test repeat the adjusting process. Pay careful attention to the basic pitch of the reed as cutting off the tip may make it too sharp.

(3) If the reed has been used for a period of time and has become too soft because the blades have lost some of their elasticity clean the inside of the reed with a pipe cleaner as directed in the section on care of the reed and put it aside to dry out for a week or more. If the reed is still too soft, try the first two corrections.

(4) If none of these corrections brings the reed to the proper strength discard it. Nothing is more useless and discouraging for a player than a soft reed which produces a poor tone quality, and cannot be controlled or played in tune.

7. *Pitch of Reed.*

Test: Generally, but not always the pitch of a stiff reed is sharp, the pitch of a soft reed is flat. During the process of adjusting the reed the pitch must be checked frequently. If the response of the reed is good and needs no further adjustment, but the pitch is sharp or flat make the appropriate correction. If a particular brand of reed is consistently sharp or flat for the instrument on which it is being used it is too long or too short for that instrument. Try other brands.

Correction: (1) If the reed is slightly flat ream the tube so that it fits further on the bocal. Increase the depth very little at a time and test frequently. This distance is critical for if it goes on too far the response of the instrument is altered. The reed under no circumstances must be reamed to the extent that the end of the bocal is any further into the reed than the first wire, and even this is risky.

(2) If reaming does not bring the reed up to pitch change to a shorter bocal. Bocals are discussed in the bassoon chapter. If this doesn't bring it up to pitch the reed should be discarded, for the student will begin biting in order to play in tune.

(3) If the reed responds well in all ways, but is sharp use a longer bocal if a longer one is available. If this does not bring it to the correct pitch continue with the following corrections which will change the response of the reed somewhat so that attention must be given to the response as well as the pitch.

(4) If the reed is slightly sharp check the thickness of the tip area and remove a very little cane. Check the response of the reed in articulation so that the tip is not made too thin. Readjust wires as needed.

(5) If the reed is still sharp check the thickness of the side areas and remove a little cane, but keep the sides and both blades in balance.

(6) If this does not correct the sharpness remove a very little cane from the forward portion of the spine section of each blade, and blend into the side sections.

Do this very slowly and carefully and test frequently for the pitch and strength of the reed changes rapidly with this adjustment.

8. *Matching the Blades.*

Test: During this discussion of adjusting the reed the point has been repeatedly made that both blades must be identical in shape and thickness at all points. The greater the deviation in the perfect symetry of the two blades the poorer the reed. This matching of the blades should be a consideration in each step of the adjusting process. Two tests can be applied. First, with the reed wet and saliva inside the reed insert a flat plaque. Press the plaque against the entire tip area to observe the thickness at the tip and to feel the resistance to the pressure at various points in the area. Test the corners of the tip area. Alternate the process between the two blades. The more transparent the cane the thinner it is. Adjust by scraping to balance as necessary. Second, the side areas and the forward portion of the spine is tested by pressing these areas against the plaque with the thumb and forefinger. Alternate blades to compare. A little experience will soon enable the player to feel the relative resistance to the pressure at various points. Third, polish the entire cut of the reed by rubbing it with dry Dutch Rush. An observation of the polished cane will reveal any irregularities, unevenness or bumps in the cut. This polishing has an additional advantage of sealing the pores of the cane.

Correction: Adjust as necessary to balance the blades. Major adjustments can be made with the scraping knife. Minor adjustments and adjustments to small areas are best done with wet Dutch Rush with the end pinched to make a flat surface. Fine grain sandpaper or a fine grain emery board may be used instead of the Dutch Rush if handled carefully.

9. *Intonation of Reed.*

Test: A reed on which the response has been adjusted according to the previous tests and which is responding well will normally play with good intonation. If the reed is a good one but plays out of tune, the fault almost always lies in the embouchure or in the instrument itself. The relationships of embouchure and the instrument to intonation are discussed in the chapter on bassoon.

Correction: Repeat various tests, especially the crow and basic strength tests, to see if further adjustments need to be made in the response of the reed. If response checks out and the student has intonation problems on several reeds the correction lies elsewhere than the reed. If a student who has been playing well in tune has intonation problems with a new reed which has been adjusted for response the construction of that particular reed is faulty and it should be discarded or have major alterations made.

10. *Articulation and the Reed.*

Test: Play major scales and arpeggios through all registers of the instrument with legato and staccato articulations. If the reed does not respond as desired make corrections.

Correction: Articulation response is controlled almost entirely by the tip area of the reed. If the reed does not articulate properly, assuming of course that the student's tongue placement and action is correct, adjust the tip area for balance over the various registers of the instrument. Check tip opening in the center which should be one sixteenth to three thirty-seconds. If the tip opening is too small articulation in the low register is difficult, if the tip opening is too wide articulation in the high register is difficult. Adjust the opening to balance these. The thickness of the blades at the very tip is critical. They must be thicker in the center of the blade and thin toward the edges, with both blades identical. Using wet Dutch Rush thin the forward quarter inch of the blade as necessary, testing frequently. Good response in articulation is the result of the best balance and relationship between the size of the tip opening and the thickness of the forward portion of the blades. If articulation response is satisfactory except for excess reed noises, cut off a small portion of both corners of the reed.

11. *Response of Lowest Notes.*

Test: Test the low register—B-flat to F below the staff—in scale and arpeggio passages both slurred and legato. If the notes respond with difficulty the reed is too stiff or the tip opening too close.

Correction: (1) Check first the tip opening. Notes in this register articulate sluggishly when the tip is too close. Adjust the tip opening with the wires if necessary.

(2) If tip opening is correct and the reed responds well in other registers of the instrument but not in the low register the spine of the reed is too thick. Thin the entire spine section of both blades very gradually and testing frequently until correct response is achieved.

CARE OF THE BASSOON REED

Once the reed is adjusted and responding well it can be kept in good condition with care. The rules for caring for the reeds are simple and if followed will prolong their useful life.

1. Always soak the reed as directed before playing or adjusting. Clear water is better than saliva for this purpose. A small water tight glass should be kept in the case for this purpose.

2. Keep the reeds in a reed case so that they will dry out slowly and completely to retain their form. Some reed cases have a mandrel on which they are stored. The plastic tubes in which commercial reeds are merchandised are not a suitable substitute for reed storage unless a hole is punched in the cap. Otherwise they seal too tightly for the proper drying of the reed. Figure R-60 shows a typical bassoon reed case.

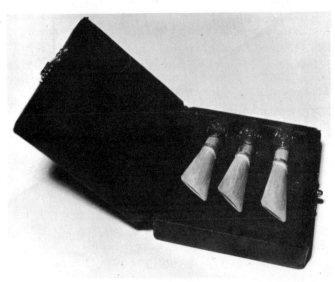

Figure R-60.

3. Clean the inside of the reed every week or ten days with a wet pipe cleaner when the reed is well soaked. Insert the pipe cleaner from the round end and force it gently through the tip of the reed. Then pull it through the reed slowly moving it from side to side so that all inside surfaces are cleaned. Repeat the process two or three times.

4. Keep the outside of the blades clean so that the vibration of the blades is not restricted. A light polishing with Dutch Rush will clean the surface. Girls who play bassoon should remove their lipstick before playing, and remove any accumulation with the Dutch Rush or with the edge of an emery board. The discoloration of the blades which remains after the lipstick is removed will not harm the reed.

5. Protect the reed when it is in place on the bocal. When the instrument is to be in the rest position for a few minutes remove the reed from the bocal and put it in the mouth or behind an ear for protection.

STUDY AND ACHIEVEMENT QUESTIONS

Mouthpieces

1. Define and identify on a single reed mouthpiece: facing, tip opening, end rail, baffle, tone chamber, bore, table, table opening, side rails. Describe effect of each on response.

2. Obtain several B-flat clarinet or Alto saxophone mouthpieces of different brands. Compare the shape and size of the various parts. Determine whether or not the end rail and side rails meet specifications. Have a member of the class who is proficient on

the instrument play on each of the mouthpieces to compare tone quality and general response.

3. Using a gauge kit for B-flat clarinet mouthpieces measure the tip opening and facing of as many as you can. Number each mouthpiece and prepare a chart of these measurements. Indicate any which have a warped lay. Indicate on the chart whether the tip opening is close, medium, or open and whether the lay is short, medium, or long. Have a member of the class who is proficient on the instrument play each of these to compare measurements with tone quality and general response.

Single Reeds

4. Identify parts of a single reed: tip, shoulder, heart, center point, cut, stock, heel.

5. Select at random six B-flat clarinet or Alto saxophone reeds from a box of medium strength, and number them on the back. Describe each in terms of color, grain, cut, and tip resistance. Estimate their probable quality and arrange them in progressive order from best to poorest.

6. Using the same reeds have a competent player on the instrument test them. On the basis of the playing test and the previous visual examination describe any adjustments which need to be made on each to bring them to the best playing condition, after indicating the degree of hardness of each.

7. Secure the minimum tools and equipment for adjusting single reeds. Practice the following operations: (1) scraping and balancing the shoulders; (2) scraping and balancing the tip; (3) adjusting the heart section to put the centerpoint in the proper place and of the right thickness; (4) trimming the tip.

8. Select a reed which is too soft. Deliberately cut off too much of the tip. Reshape the entire lay to bring tip, shoulders and heart section into the proper balance.

9. Adjust a reed for someone who is proficient on the instrument having him play on the reed after each adjustment. Experience will enable you to hear as well as see the adjustments which are necessary.

10. From a mixed collection of reeds for various sizes of clarinets identify the instrument for which each is intended. Do the same for a mixed collection of saxophone reeds. Mix the clarinet and saxophone reeds together and identify the instrument for which each is intended.

11. Describe in detail the care of a single reed.

Oboe Reeds

12. Define and identify on an oboe reed: staple, blades, winding, cut.

13. Outline the shape of the blade of an oboe reed, draw and label the various types of cuts available.

14. Examine a collection of oboe reeds from various sources and describe the shape and length of cut on each.

15. Secure the minimum tools and equipment for adjusting an oboe reed. Identify each and practice holding it or putting it in place without adjusting a reed.

16. Practice the following scrapes: center and sides of the tip, shoulders, back (if clearly defined on the type of cut selected), and spine.

17. Perform the following, which can be done even though you are not an oboist, on one or more oboe reeds: (1) test for air leakage, (2) practice applying goldbeaters skin, (3) test for basic strength of reed and make necessary corrections, (4) test the crow and make necessary corrections. Use commercial reeds for this as custom made reeds will need little or no adjustment.

18. Adjust a reed for someone who is proficient on the instrument having him test after each adjustment. Perform the step by step test and correction procedure until the reed is responding properly.

19. Discuss how an oboe reed may be kept in good playing condition over a period of time.

Bassoon Reeds

20. Define and identify on a bassoon reed: tip, tip opening, cut, shoulder, throat, tube, first wire, second wire, binding. On the cut identify: spine, side areas, tip area.

21. Practice adjusting the bassoon reed with the first and second wires. Observe and describe how each adjustment effects the reed.

22. Secure the minimum tools and equipment for adjusting a bassoon reed. Identify each and practice holding it or putting it in place without adjusting a reed.

23. Practice the following scrapes on a reed: center and sides of the tip area, front and back portion of each of the sides, front portion of the spine. Be sure reed and knife are properly held for each operation.

24. Perform the following, which can be done even though you are not a bassoonist on one or more reeds: (1) test reed for air leakage, (2) test for air leakage at bocal connection, (3) the crow test, (4) and the test of basic strength. Make the necessary corrections after each test.

25. Adjust a reed for someone who is proficient on the instrument having him test after each adjustment. Perform the step by step test and correction procedure until reed response is correct.

26. Discuss care of the bassoon reed.

CHAPTER SEVEN

CONCLUSION

Teaching the woodwind instruments with good results becomes a fairly simple process when the instruments themselves are fully understood and when appropriate techniques, procedures and materials are used in an abundant variety. The instruments in the woodwind family have a great many things in common and when these are understood and advantage taken of them understanding the instructional process becomes more efficient. Rather than five distinct and separate instruments they become a unified whole.

Careful selection of the students who will study a woodwind instrument as well as helping the prospective student select the specific instrument he wishes to study is basic to success. This must be a cooperative decision between the teacher and student. The student's responsibility is to have a real interest in the instrument and to consider it worth learning so that he will conscientiously apply himself to the study. The teacher's responsibility is to see that the student has the intellectual capacity to comprehend and utilize instruction and musical information, that he has sufficient innate musical talent to succeed, and preferably that he has a natural aptitude for the instrument selected.

The natural progress of success or failure during the first year or so of study of the instrument eliminates those with insufficient interest, little musical talent and lacking the intellectual capacity for the instruction. Those who continue with an instrument will succeed or fail, will make rapid, slow or no progress depending partly upon themselves but to a great extent upon the skill of the teacher in motivating them through instruction which is carefully planned to proceed in small increments of learning and which build to a goal that the student can recognize and accomplish.

MUSICAL LEARNING

The things which must be taught are surprisingly few in number but of unlimited depth so that they must be developed over a period of years. These may be classified generally as notation, tone production, ear training, technical facility, and sight reading. Each is independent of the others yet a deficiency in one area will handicap development in others. They are separate but at the same time closely inter-related.

Notation, the written language of music, is of itself not difficult to learn provided the information is well organized and presented. It is best learned independently of an instrument and then applied to it. By learning notation independently the student can focus his attention upon it without distraction. The teacher can make use of drills, memory devices, workbook sheets, regular reviews and tests until the subject is thoroughly learned. In this way both pitch and rhythmic notation can be quickly assimilated to provide a basis for instrumental study, rather than being slowly acquired as a part of and to the detriment of the instrumental instruction.

Tone production, that is the development of a beautiful sound on the instrument, is the goal of every musician. Without a beautiful sound musical expression is limited. Tone production is dependent upon several things, each of which can be isolated, described, and understood by the student. These include the instrument; the mouthpiece and/or reed or embouchure hole; embouchure formation, development and control; and inhalation, exhalation and support of breath. Each of these factors is considered in detail in the chapters on each instrument. Tone is the object of all performance, its quality the result of all performance and practice.

Ear training is an aspect of woodwind instruction which is frequently considered only incidentally or indirectly if at all, yet is one of the important determining factors in the musical development of the student. The ear is concerned with hearing, identifying, comparing and controlling the four basic aspects of a musical tone: pitch, loudness, rhythm and tone quality. If the student clearly recognizes that he is responsible for hearing only four different kinds of things the process of learning to hear and control them becomes much easier for him.

The ability to hear and discriminate these four aspects of a musical sound is an innate capacity which every student has to a greater or lesser degree. Some students are born with a high capacity for this type of discrimination and it is easy for them to develop, others are born with less capacity and have more difficulty in developing a proficiency. These differences in innate capacities must be recognized and students handled accordingly.

In hearing pitch the student is involved hearing the exact pitch of the note and any intonation faults it might have. He is involved in hearing a series of melodic intervals. He hears the note he is playing as one of the notes in a harmonic structure. He is involved in hearing and correctly performing melodic ornaments such as grace notes, trills, turns, etc. All of these can be isolated or combined but can and must be developed to the student's level of musical understanding and technical proficiency on the instrument.

In hearing loudness the student is involved in hearing the exact degree of loudness of any particular note. He is hearing changes in dynamics as in crescendo, diminuendo, attacks, and releases. He is hearing volume of sound of both himself and the other players and the interrelation between the two. He can detect inbalance in loudness or erratic and incorrect changes.

Rhythm is the most basic of all musical elements. Everyone can feel the beat of heavily accented music such as marches. The student in hearing rhythm or time is involved in much more than simply hearing the beat. He is concerned with the actual duration of each individual tone he produces and of each individual rest. He is concerned with tempo and tempo changes. He is concerned with the precision of attack and release both in relation to what he is playing and in relation to any other performers. He is concerned with the length of notes in various articulations: staccato, marcato, half-staccato, legato, etc. He is concerned with changes in tempo—accelerando, ritards, fermatas, etc. He hears and is sensitive to small degrees of erratic and incorrect tempo and in the duration of notes and rests.

The ability to discriminate good, bad, or indifferent tone quality either in himself or in others is one of the most difficult aspects of ear training to develop. This ability is dependent to a great extent upon having a mental image of what the ideal tone quality should be so that a comparison between what he hears and the mental image can be made. It is for this reason that it is so important for every student on any level of achievement to hear live and record performances of music, especially that featuring their own instrument, as often and as consistently as possible. Innumerable other benefits occur from this experience in addition to acquiring a concept of tone quality. Appendix III lists recordings which may be used for this purpose, and teachers should encourage, or even require, attendance at public concerts. In hearing tone quality the student will develop an exact and objective concept of tone quality. He will become sensitive to variations in tone quality from one instrument to another, from one player to another on the same instrument, and in variations in tone quality on an instrument which are the result of the register in which it is played, in loudness or softness of the tone, and in how the breath supports the tone.

The goals of ear training as a portion of woodwind instruction are not achieved quickly. They are a portion of the student's work as long as he continues to play the instrument. As he gains experience on the instrument and in listening to music his powers of discrimination increase. The degree of acuity of discrimination which the teacher expects of him and he demands of himself must increase simultaneously. As he gains facility in hearing, the accumulated knowledge is transferred to his own playing which improves accordingly.

Technical facility is the product of neuro-muscular patterns which are established through repetition. It is not an isolated factor in performance, but must be based on ear training so that technique is developed and controlled to achieve the highest musical results. Technical facility is the result of intelligent conscientious practice of appropriate musical materials. Suitable materials for this are listed in the chapter on each instrument. These materials must be at the level of the student, neither too easy nor too difficult. They must be varied and interesting. In practicing the student should recognize what he is learning. He should repeat each new pattern or sequence until its use becomes habitual. He should review regularly and in cycles so that he loses nothing that he has acquired. Most teachers will assign specific music to review rather than depending on the student to do it for himself. If these suggestions are followed a sound technical facility will be acquired.

The ability to read at sight is one of the most valuable assets any performer can have. It is the culmination of musical learning as it combines the student's knowledge of notation, tone production, ear training and technical facility. Musicians gain facility in sight reading only by reading at sight as much as possible. A portion of every lesson, every band or orchestra rehearsal should be spent in sight reading in order to develop this facility. Students should be provided with material and encouraged to sight read regularly outside of lessons and rehearsals. Once this ability is developed other aspects of musical performance become easier to control.

The process of learning to play a woodwind instrument is one in which the various segments of learning are clearly defined, in which the objectives in each segment are clear, and in which the teacher can offer guidance and assistance. The teacher must not lose sight of the objectives of each facet of learning: notation, tone production, ear training, technical facility and sight reading. Concentrate attention on the portion of each which is appropriate to the student or class, rather than simply on "playing" the instrument.

ORGANIZATION OF INSTRUCTION

The typical beginner on a woodwind instrument is started in one of three types of instruction: (1) A heterogeneous grouping of instruments such as a beginning band, (2) a homogeneous grouping of instruments such as a beginning clarinet class, or (3) individual instuction. Each of these types of instruction is dictated by the particular circumstances of the school or personal situation and each has its advantages.

A heterogeneous grouping of instruments is advantageous in that the situation provides maximum motivation for the young student, but has certain disadvantages as well. Beginning band books which provide instructional material for all woodwind, brass and percussion instruments must of necessity comprise the amount and sequence of material to accommodate the various instruments. Material which is naturally adapted to the woodwinds is difficult for brasses. Material which is naturally adapted to the beginning brass student has little or no functional value for the woodwind student. For this reason progress is at a snail's pace for every instrument and the actual accomplishment of the individual student is not at all commensurate with the amount of time consumed in the effort.

If the heterogeneous grouping is used the method selected for class use must be supplemented with additional material designed specifically for each instrument. Instruction from the supplementary material can be distributed through the lesson period alternating the use of specific instruments and the entire group. Additional material from other sources must be given to those students who are high achievers so that even within the basic class organization each student is constantly working at his own maximum level. This is admittedly a difficult problem in class management. It requires that the teacher have a great knowledge of available materials and the ability to organize their use. This information is part of the tools of the trade and is most certainly not too much to expect, nor is it difficult to acquire if direct attention is paid to it. A wealth of suitable materials for all the woodwind instruments which can be used as a starting point for this information is listed in the chapter on that instrument.

The homogeneous grouping for instruction—like instrument classes—may be used on beginning, intermediate or advanced levels of instruction. It provides incentive for the student while at the same time permitting the selection of music suitable for that instrument which is uncompromised by being adjusted to problems of other instruments. Even on the beginning level like instrument classes are preferable. Once past the elementary stage student ability and accomplishments become so diverse that like instrument classes or individual insturction are the only way in which real progress can be accomplished.

Individual instruction, or private lessons, is by far the most successful way of teaching and learning a woodwind instrument. Some will make the point that class instruction gives better motivation for the very beginner than individual instruction. There is no doubt that competition with other players is a great incentive to many students, and many instructors wisely take full advantage of this. On the other hand the larger the class the less individual attention each student receives. This may lead to the establishment of incorrect habits in embouchure, hand position, fingering, breath support, articulation and other facets of performance. Habits established at the beginning level are extremely difficult to change and require considerable effort on the part of the student and considerable skill and patience on the part of the instructor to correct. It would be a more efficient use of student and instructor time to use the individual attention necessary to correct bad habits earlier in the instructional process to keep them from developing.

Private lessons in addition to the beginning class instruction are ideal to combine the advantages of each and should be encouraged. Any student who is seriously interested in learning to play his instrument should be strongly encouraged to take private lessons no matter what his level of advancement. It is safe to say, and all authorities will agree, that no real advanced level of technical or musical accomplishment is possible without individual instruction.

INSTRUCTIONAL MATERIALS

The best organization of instructional materials on any technical level involves a five classification program. Material in each of these classifications is used simultaneously to provide a well rounded musical experience, provide stimulation to the study of the instrument, and to maintain interest through a variety of materials, to to assure a continual advancement in technical and musical proficiency. At least one assignment in each of the five classifications must be given for each lesson. The amount of material available for each instrument is sufficient to introduce this type of instruction early in the beginning stage and to carry it through to a high artistic level. Except for information about solo and ensemble literature which is readily available elsewhere, a broad cross section of materials available in the other classifications is given in the chapter on each instrument.

The five classifications of materials and musical experiences may be listed as follows:

1. A *Method Book*. These are basic to the study of the instrument and provide continuity. Methods books for every instrument are available which are suitable

for students from the very beginning stages to the most advanced. American publishers have been very active in providing methods books for the elementary levels of study, and they exist in large numbers for virtually every instrument. Theoretically they are organized to progress in easy stages and to provide sufficient material for the establishment of the factors being learned. In practice the various beginning methods vary tremendously in the success with which they do this.

In general it is best to use two or three beginning methods simultaneously and to coordinate assignments in them in order to provide sufficient material on the same problem for the beginner to firmly establish the technical facility being learned. Teachers of students on the elementary level have a general tendency to expect too little of their students and to give them too little to do. Instructors of woodwind instruments would be wise to model their instructional procedures on the successful private piano teacher of young beginners who normally has each student working out of three or four books of similar material at the same time. For example, in the beginning study of clarinet Paul van Bodegraven's "Adventures in Clarinet Playing" and James Collis' "Modern Course for the Clarinet" make an excellent pair. Oother combinations are possible for the clarinet and effective combinations for the other instruments can be easily selected. Material in the other four classifications must be introduced as soon as the student progresses to the point where suitable material is available.

Methods books for other levels of advancement are available for each instrument. These are listed in the chapter for each instrument in sections called "Beginning Methods" which includes series made up of two or three volumes sometimes under the same title and sometimes called beginning, intermediate, and advanced even though they are in reality different levels of beginning books.

The second group of method books is described as "Standard Methods." These are the traditional methods such as Klose for clarinet, Altes for flute, Barret for oboe, Weissenborn for bassoon, and Mayeur for saxophone. For the most part these are more than fifty years old, are not arranged progressively, and do not take advantage of contemporary teaching techniques. They must be used, however, since the material they contain is basic to the study of the instrument. It is incumbent upon the teacher to assign the material in the correct order for a particular student. None of these is suitable for a beginning student, but most contain material from the intermediate to the most advanced level. Most students will use one or more of these over a period of a year or two or more in combination with other materials. The total number of standard method books for all the woodwind instruments is not large and a skilled teacher will become familiar with all of them.

2. *Technical Studies.* By technical studies is meant the mechanical note patterns which are common to all musical styles and in which the student develops a basic technical facility which can be applied to all his playing. These involve major and minor scales; major, minor, diminished and augmented triads; dominant, diminished, and other forms of seventh chords all in various patterns, various ranges, and in every key. To these is added mechanical exercises to establish finger patterns which are difficult on that particular instrument and which will enable the student to gain facility in using all possible alternate fingerings.

Such studies are available which are suitable for students on any level of advancement past the beginning stage. Many of these are incorporated in the standard methods, others are published separately. The Pares studies which are available for all woodwind instruments are almost exclusively scale studies suitable for the lower intermediate level. For clarinet the Albert "Twenty-four Varied Scales and Exercises," books I, II and III of the Kroepsch "416 Progressive Daily Studies," and Part III of the Baermann "Method for Clarinet" are typical of this material. The three volume "Scales and Daily Exercises" for bassoon by Oubradous; the "Scales and Arpeggios—480 Exercises" of Moyse for flute; sections of the Andraud "Vade Mecum" for oboe; and Arnold's "Fingered Scales" or Rascher's "158 Exercises" for saxophone are representative of this kind of material on a more advanced level. Other material of this nature on every technical level is listed in the "additional study materials" section of each chapter.

The skilled teacher will take full advantage of this common core of technique which has universal application and keep his students working with it at their maximum level. Consistent use of this type of study is a shortcut to technical proficiency on any instrument.

3. *Etudes or Studies.* These are books of studies of varying lengths each of which is concerned with developing a facility in a particular segment of study. Such studies concern themselves with tone control, phrasing, staccato, articulation patterns, a particular key, etc., and differ from technical studies in that they are musical rather than mechanical. The student practices them primarily for musical results with technical facility a subordinate objective. Material of this kind is available for every level of technical advancement past the early beginning stage.

Much of the study material available for each instrument is of this nature, since it is possible to include all musical styles from Baroque through Contemporary so that the student becomes familiar with various styles as they apply to his instrument. So much of the available material of this nature is in the nineteenth century style that it is necessary to make a real effort to find suitable materials in other styles. Even so, much of the study of style must be relegated to the solo and ensemble classifications.

Typical of the books of etudes available are the Lo Presti "20 Melodic Studies for Clarinet" which are of lower intermediate level of difficulty. The "40 Studies" and "32 Studies" for clarinet by Rose; the Ferling "48 Studies" for oboe or saxophone; the studies by Berbiguier and Anderson for flute; the Weissenborn "Studies, Op. 8" and the Jancourt studies for bassoon. Much material in this classification is listed in the "Additional Study Materials" section in the chapter for each instrument. The teacher must become familiar with as many of these as possible.

4. *Duets or Other Ensemble Music.* The opportunity to play with another instrument or instruments is an integral part of the study of any instrument on any level. Ensemble experience is an important aspect of ear training in that the student must relate his pitch, loudness, rhythm and tone quality to other players. Duets for like instruments are especially valuable since the clear texture gives an opportunity for hearing and comparing. If the student is taking private lessons playing duets with the teacher gives him an auditory model to follow in the matters of tone quality, phrasing, intonation and style. Much musical learning is accomplished by the process of imitation and this experience is invaluable.

Playing duets, trios, quartets, etc. with other student players provides a different kind of valuable experience for all. Learning to play together, to become sensitive to the playing of others, and to become an integral part o fa musical group is a part of becoming a good player. Such experiences can be encouraged and provided on a regular organized basis, on a volunteer basis or as a recreational activity which the student does on his own. The more of this type of activity the better for the student.

Duets are frequently included in the standard methods books. Volumes of duets by a single composer are available as well as compilation of selected duets of various composers. These are available on virtually every level of technical advancement. NIMAC publishes Selective Music Lists of graded ensembles and catalogs of retail stores specializing in woodwind music have considerable additional listings.

5. *Solos.* Every woodwind instrument is a solo instrument. Opportunities for performing a solo with piano accompaniment must be provided for every student. Such performances provide an incentive for practice and develop self confidence to a degree no other activity can provide. Solos on every level from the most elementary to the most advanced are available for every instrument. So many are available in fact that the problem is not finding a solo but in finding the best solo for a particular student at a particular time.

Solo experience can be provided for students in any type of class instructions as well as those taking individual instruction. Every student should have several solos of various kinds ready to play at any time and should be preparing others at the same time. They should be encouraged to play all of them from memory and over a period of time develop complete confidence in their ability to do so. The NIMAC lists give graded solos for all instruments although this list is highly selective and does not include a very high percentage of the available solo material for any instrument. This list is a useful starting point but must be considerably expanded in most categories to acquire sufficient teaching materials. In this area also the catalogs of retail companies are most useful.

BEGINNING METHODS

There are numerous beginning methods for each instrument, some of them very excellent both from the standpoint of pedagogy and musical content, others strong on pedagogy and weak on musical content, and still others weak on both points. Since the excitement in starting the study of a new and strange instrument wears off rapidly once the student realizes that a real effort is necessary, his initiative and interest must be sustained by the material he is studying. Dreary mechanical exercises, endless repetition of the same thing, difficult technical problems introduced without sufficient preparation or material to accomplish them, and the lack of musically satisfying melodies soon turn what could be pleasant into a dissatisfying experience. Students lose interest and either fail to make satisfactory progress or drop the study of the instrument entirely. Probably the most important decision a teacher will ever make for a student is what book or books to use for his very beginning experience.

Examine and evaluate all beginning methods for each instrument. Do they progress in small increments of learning, are the problems presented in logical order, is sufficient material included to establish habits for each problem, is the musical content varied and interesting or is it trite and mechanical? What books can be combined to give the student sufficient material on the same level of difficulty? At what point in the book, if at all, can solos with piano accompaniment be introduced? Does the book contain duets or trios, and if not at what point can this experience be introduced? Beginners need a variety of approaches to the same problem. The young beginners, especially, do not realize the value of many repetitions of the same music but will practice different music containing the same problems and achieve the same result. Take full advantage of this fact.

New beginning methods for each instrument appear regularly. Examine these carefully and compare them with those previously selected. There is a tendency among music teachers to consider a new publication superior to all others simply because it is new. This is not necessarily true. The new publication may well be inferior to older publications. Excellent new material is being published and should be used, but not simply because it is new, but because a careful evaluation points out its usefulness.

PRACTICE

All teachers assign music for the students to practice, but few tell them how to practice. Practice is a habit with students and the sooner this habit is established the more successful he will be. He must understand that a certain amount of daily practice is required, and that daily means seven days a week. He should have a specific time to practice each day, rather than changing times from day to day according to his other activities. Schedule a specific hour of the day, with the cooperation of the parents of younger children, which is set aside for practice. If this is done, other activities do not interfere and a habit of regular practice is established. It is effective to have the student keep a record of the time practiced each day and report regularly to his teacher.

Daily practice on all five classifications of materials is required. In addition regular reviews of previously learned material must be scheduled so that the player does not lose command of that particular facility. The review makes excellent material with which to begin the practice session, or the practice session can begin with typical warm-up material such as long tones, slow scales, etc. The student should learn to devote his full mental powers to his practicing, rather than letting his mind wander. Suggestions by the teacher of specific items in each portion of the assignment to which he must pay attention will help the student. The student should alternate periods of complete concentration with periods of rest and relaxation. Many students, especially the younger ones, will profit more from two shorter practice periods during the day rather than one long one.

Many students both experienced and inexperienced practice too fast. One of the most dificult problems of the teacher is to make the student realize the value of slow practice, and to teach him restraint in the matter of tempo. Use of a metronome is helpful provided the student is instructed on when and how to use it, and does not let it become a crutch. Practicing too fast makes rough technique, poor musicianship in the matter of musical values and phrasing, establishes uncontrolled articulation, and eliminates much of the value of the practice period in the important areas of ear training. Showing the student frequently in class or lesson how to practice will help impress upon him the old axiom that haste makes waste.

A carefully planned assignment plus the efficient use of practice time can help the student overcome any weaknesses he might have in tone, technique, intonation and phrasing. During the practice session he can listen to his tone quality carefully, correct or develop his embouchure with the use of a mirror, select and experiment with reeds if he is playing a reed instrument, spending as much time as necessary to accomplish his assignment.

New material is best practiced first slowly and completely through. This first impression is the most important so the student must go slowly enough that every note is correct and that correct fingering choices are made. Fingerings can be marked on the music if desirable. This is followed by several slow repetitions to establish notes and fingerings. By this time the difficult sections of a few notes or a measure or so can be identified. Practice is continued by isolating and practicing only these difficult sections until the sequence is established. If the sequence is particularly difficult practice two or three notes, add another note and continue to repeat, then add other notes one by one until the entire sequence can be played easily. Finally practice the phrase in which this sequence occurs. When this is done with each section the entire study can be practiced slowly at first and then with gradually increasing speed until the proper tempo is reached. Practicing the entire study, especially if it is a page or two in length, without working out the difficult sections is a poor use of time and will not achieve the desired results.

Individual practice sessions where the player can hear himself are invaluable in developing intonation on the instrument. Students must be taught to hear correct intonation by using an electronic device or by playing with an experienced player. They become accustomed to the temperament of their own instrument and accept it as being correct even though it might not be. Hearing correct intonation does not come naturally, it must be acquired. A study of intonation and how to correct deficiencies must be a continual part of instruction if the students is to become able to help himself acquire perfection.

Phrasing is worked out in practice, and is the final objective of all the other aspects of performance. Instruction in phrasing is frequently neglected in favor of instruction in technique. Technique without good phrasing is valueless. Students must be taught to recognize phrases, periods and sections of a composition, together with repetitions and contrasting sections which make up good musical form. An understanding of the simple structures of music is easy to acquire and gives the student a concrete basis upon which to build his phrasing. Developing good phrasing is a slow process in which the student needs considerable help. Ends of phrases, places to breathe, slight nuances in dynamics should be marked in the music by the teacher so the student can practice intelligently. As the student gains musical experience and technical facility various musical styles must be introduced together with details of how each style is phrased and how they differ from each other.

BREATHING AND BREATH CONTROL

Correct inhalation, exhalation and breath support forms the foundation for woodwind performance without which only limited success is possible. The only correct breathing is that described as diaphragmatic. This is exactly the same breathing process that is taught in playing brass instruments, singing and public speaking. Details of diaphragmatic breathing are so widely known and taught that they need not be repeated here. Those who are interested in the physiology of the breathing process should consult the article on inhalation in one of the large standard encyclopedias where it is thoroughly and simply explained. Once this is understood teaching it becomes simpler.

Every teacher has his or her own set of words to describe correct breathing as well as procedures used in teaching it. The reader is encouraged to observe as many skilled teachers as possible in their teaching procedures and techniques which they feel will be successful. A variety of ways of explaining and doing the same thing is valuable. In teaching the woodwinds correct breathing and breath support must be taught from the very beginning of study, review regularly, checked regularly and corrected if necessary until it becomes habitual with the student. Many many problems which woodwind players have can be traced to incorrect breathing and breath support. The importance of doing it properly cannot be emphasized enough.

ACOUSTICS AND WOODWIND INSTRUMENTS

A knowledge of *why* a woodwind instrument sounds and responds as it does is as important as knowing *how* it sounds and responds to adjustments. This *why* is the product of the study of acoustics of music and forms an essential basis for completely understanding how the instruments operate. The finest woodwind teaching is based on a thorough knowledge of what to do and how to do it as well as why it is being done. A complete course in the acoustics of music should be a part of every instrumental teacher's training. Such a complete consideration of acoustics is beyond the scope of this book, but the basic aspects of the subject as they concern the woodwind instruments are presented.

PERCEPTION OF SOUND

In order that a sound may be heard three things are necessary: (1) a vibrating object, (2) a medium of transmission, and (3) a receiver. The vibrating object in the woodwind instruments may be a single reed as on the clarinets and saxophones; a double reed as on the oboe, English horn and bassoon; or an edge tone which produces the tone on the flute. In each instance the vibrating object is reinforced by the enclosed column of air inside the instrument to amplify the tone so that it can be heard.

The medium of transmission is normally the air, but sound travels through any substance which has elasticity. Through the walls from one room to another, for example. Sound vibrations travel at the rate of 1,132 feet per second (almost 800 miles per hour) through the air when it is at 70 degrees Fahrenheit, faster when the air is warmer and slower when the air is cooler.

The receiver is normally the ear which can hear vibrations as slow as twenty per second and as fast as twenty thousand per second. The receiver may also be a microphone which changes the vibrations into electrical energy and makes it possible to record the sounds for future study.

PITCH

The fundamental pitch of a note is determined by the frequency of the vibration stated in terms of the number of vibrations per second. The faster the vibration the higher the pitch; the slower the vibration the flatter the pitch. The standard pitch to which all instruments is tuned is A-440, meaning that there are four hundred and forty vibrations per second for this note. The A an octave above has 880 vibrations per second, and the A an octave lower 220 vibrations per second. In woodwind instruments the frequency of the vibration is determined primarily by the length of the enclosed air column. The longer the column the lower the pitch. Thus if we start with all the holes on the instrument closed and open them one by one the pitch is raised as each hole is opened. This is the physical basis for the fingering of a woodwind instrument. In addition to the fundamental pitches of the air column, woodwind instruments make use of harmonics of this fundamental which will be considered in the following section.

The fundamental pitch of a note on any woodwind instrument is the product of the *ratio* of the distance from the tip of the mouthpiece or flute embouchure hole to the first open hole on the instrument. For this reason the distance between the tone holes becomes less and less as they become closer to the mouth, and their diameter decreases. A brief examination of any of the woodwinds but especially the B-flat clarinet will indicate the extent of these differences.

The importance of understanding the effect of this ratio and how it affects both pitch and intonation can be illustrated on the B-flat clarinet. If the tuning barrel is pulled out one-eighth of an inch the third-line B-flat will be lowered one-fourth of a half-step while the third-line B-natural will be lowered only one-twelfth of a half-step. This adjustment has three times as much effect on the shortest length of pipe as it does on the longest. The more the barrel joint is pulled the greater the differences between the amount of change in these two notes. So that the ratios could be kept constant the three note three-place tuning procedure which is presented in the clarinet chapter is important, and must be used for the best intonation.

Double reed instruments are tuned to the basic pitch primarily through reed adjustments rather than adjusting the connections between the various joints and the ratios in the air column maintained. This is also the reason why the importance of the placement of the end plug on the flute was stressed in the flute chapter. If it is out of place the ratios are wrong and the instrument out of tune with itself.

A further relationship between the length of the enclosed air column is illustrated by the differences in sizes of the instruments in the clarinet family as we go down in pitch from E-flat, to B-flat, to A, to Alto, to Bass, to Contra-Bass. The importance of the ratio between the mouth and the first open hole on pitch can be seen by comparing the size of the Alto and Baritone saxophones. The Baritone saxophone sounds an octave lower than the Alto saxophone, but is more than twice the size.

Other factors which influence pitch to a slight degree are:

1. *Temperature.* It has been previously indicated that the speed at which a sound vibration travels is determined by the temperature of the air. The colder the air the slower the vibration travels. The warmer the air the faster the vibration travels. The slower it travels inside an instrument the fewer vibrations per second and the flatter the pitch and conversely for warmer temperatures. An instrument which is tuned to A-440 at a temperature of 70 degrees Fahrenheit with the same adjustment will sound approximately A-435 at 60 degrees Fahrenheit. The implications of this effect of temperature on woodwind instruments are most significant, and point out the importance of having the instrument properly warmed up before tuning. Instruments which are tuned at the beginning of a rehearsal before they are warmed up, will play considerably sharp when they have been warmed up by playing. Playing in rooms which are overheated, or playing outside at cold or hot temperatures not only influences the basic pitch of the instruments, but makes playing them in tune virtually impossible.

2. *Humidity.* Humidity affects the fundamental frequency of a wood instrument in that a high humidity will cause the wood to swell and low humidity will cause it to shrink. Fortunately, the wood used in woodwind instruments is treated to minimize this condition. A further precaution is found in the suggestion that the bores of wood instruments be oiled regularly. The same condition of high humidity in the instrument pre-

vails when it is not thoroughly swabbed before it is put in its case, and this is one of the reasons why this process is so important. Rapid changes from low to high humidity will cause the wood to expand and shrink and eventually crack. All cracks are the result of this expansion and contraction. The result on pitch of the expansion of an instrument under conditions of high humidity when the wood expands is to make it flatter. Conversely, when low humidity shrinks the instrument the pitch becomes sharper. The consequences of playing a wood instrument in the sun on a hot dry day in summer combines high temperature and low humidity to the point that no amount of adjusting could possibly bring the fundamental pitch down to A-440.

3. *Wind Pressure.* An increase in the amount of wind pressure into the instrument will sharpen the fundamental pitch of a woodwind instrument slightly. This does not occur with most players as the natural sharpening is counteracted by embouchure adjustments. If, however, the wind pressure is increased too much the instrument will break into a harmonic which in the case of the single reed instruments is called a squeak. The flute makes use of this breaknig into a harmonic by using increased wind pressure as one of the means of playing in the second and third octaves.

TONE QUALITY

The tone quality or timbre of an instrument is determined by what harmonics are present in the tone and their relative intensities. Harmonics are the result of partial vibrations of the air column. At the same time it is vibrating in two, three, four, five, six or more parts. The vibration as a whole produces the fundamental and is the pitch we hear. When it vibrates in two equal parts a tone one octave above the fundamental is produced, when vibrating in three equal parts a tone a twelfth above the fundamental is produced, when vibrating in four equal parts a tone two octaves above the fundamental is produced, etc. All these and more may be produced simultaneously in various strengths and, combined, determine the tone quality. When all the overtones are combined with the fundamental and graphed the curved line is called the wave form. The potential overtone series which is identical for every fundamental tone on every musical instrument is shown on page 276.[1]

The series is given on C. A similar series may be constructed for every fundamental on the instrument. The portion of the range of each instrument which is produced by the fundamental vibration is indicated in the section on Tone in the chapter for that instrument.

In addition to the fundamental vibration, each woodwind instrument makes use of partial vibrations of the

---

[1]The black notes indicate harmonic frequencies which only approximate these pitches.

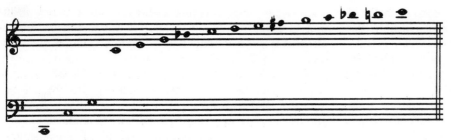

air column to increase its playing range. When a partial is used in the playing range the air column is forced to vibrate in its frequency and the vibration frequency of the fundamental itself is eliminated. The partial is produced as the predominant sound through the use of vent holes which force the column of air to vibrate in segments rather than as a whole. These vent holes are called the register key on the clarinet, the octave key on the oboe and saxophone. In addition the first finger halfhole position on the oboe, and bassoon and the first finger entirely open on the flute function as vent holes, and are a part of the regular fingering for certain notes.

The complicated fingerings for notes in the highest registers of each instrument are the result of selecting the harmonic from one of the fundamentals to produce the pitch, opening a key to vent the air column so that it will vibrate at the correct speed, and finally opening or closing other tone holes which will make the note exactly in tune without altering the fundamental fingering. The multiplicity of fingerings for a particular high note is the product of using various fundamentals to produce it.

Special harmonic fingerings for a few notes are presented in the chapters on oboe and flute where they are used for limited functions. The extension of the range of the Alto saxophone above the normal high F is done through the utilization of additional harmonics which are not normally used on the instrument. Additional fingerings for many notes on any woodwind instrument can be discovered by applying the principle of harmonics.

The nature of the construction of the clarinets causes them to produce only every other harmonic. The first harmonic above the fundamental which can be produced on the clarinet is the twelfth. The octave is missing. For this reason the clarinet is described as overblowing a twelfth, while all the other woodwinds can produce all the notes in the harmonics, and overblow an octave. Thus on the clarinet the fundamental fingering is duplicated on notes a twelfth above, while on the flute, oboe, saxophone and bassoon the fundamental fingering is duplicated an octave above.

Each instrument in the woodwind group characteristically produces tones with a particular complex of harmonics. Since this basic complex is a product of the instrument itself rather than the player a saxophone

tone is clearly recognizable as saxophone tone even though it ma be also described as an excellen average, or poor tone quality. Th same can be applied to the othe woodwinds.

With the general nature of th harmonics a product of the instru ment itself, the relative intensitie and the inter-relationships between them are controllec by the individual player. It is the inter-relationship whicl determines whether a tone is a striking beautiful one o a sound which is downright bad. The nature of the number and format of harmonics present is a produc of the size and shape of the mouthpiece or flute em bouchure hole, the shape, proportions and response o the reed, the control of the wind pressure, and the formation and control of the embouchure. Each of these is considered elsewhere in its relationship to tone quality

LOUDNESS

Loudness is the product of the amplitude of vibra tion, and/or the force of vibration in the air column The wider the vibration the greater the force in the ai column and the louder the tone is. In the case of the reed instruments the amplitude of vibration is deter mined by the distance the reed moves in vibrating. A mouthpiece with a close lay does not permit the reec to vibrate as far as a mouthpiece with an open lay and thus in general does not permit the production of a full volume of tone. This is only one of the reasons why the lay of a mouthpiece is so important. The tip opening of the double reeds will determine how far the blades can vibrate. If the tip opening is too small there is suf ficient amplitude to produce only a weak tone. This is one reason why tip opening is stressed.

The extent of the amplitude of vibration of a reed, and the force of the vibration of the air column on both the reeds and flute is primarily a product of wind pressure. Hence the player blows harder to play louder, and less hard to play softer. The infinite variety in loud ness of various tones which is so essential to good musi cal phrasing is dependent upon subtle changes in wind pressure. In order that these can be controlled it is neces sary that breathing, breath support and breath control be developed if artistic performance is to be achieved.

DURATION

The duration of a tone, or how long it sounds, is determined by how long the vibratory source continues to vibrate. Or to put it more simply how long the wind pressure is continued. Since rhythm in music is deter mined by duration of tones, and by the infinite subtle variations which are inherent in good musical style duration becomes a matter of importance. Duration of tones in addition to the continuing wind pressure is determined by the articulation process on woodwinds. Various articulations are used for notes of different lengths, and the tongue functions as a valve to start and stop the flow of air into the instrument and thereby the duration of the notes.

SUMMARY

The various aspects of musical sounds exist as physical phenomenon of the sound wave produced by the instrument and are heard by the ear which produces a psychological reaction. The corresponding physical and psychological attributes of a sound can be summarized as follows:

Physical	*Psychological*
Frequency	Pitch
Harmonic content (wave form)	Tone quality
Amplitude	Loudness
Duration	Duration

The following films provide a useful explanation and demonstration of the various aspects of sound. The first one gives a short overview and demonstration, while the three part series provides more detail and gives more elaborate demonstrations.

1. *Nature of Sound.* Coronet Instructional Films. 10 minutes. Black and White or Color. Demonstration of frequency, transmission, amplitude, and timbre.

2. *Science in the Orchestra.* British Information Service, Distributed by McGraw-Hill Text Films. Black and White prints only.

   Part   I. "Hearing the Orchestra." 13 minutes. Frequency, amplitude, timbre and transmission.
   Physiology of hearing.

   Part II. "Exploring the Instruments." 12 minutes.
   Vibrations, playing ranges of instruments, experiments in harmonics.

   Part III. "Looking at Sounds." 10 minutes.
   The harmonic structure of the tones of several instruments is shown and compared. An oboe tone is made to sound like a flute by electronically altering its harmonic structure.

An excellent source of more detailed information written clearly and in non-technical language is the paper-back book *Horns, Strings, and Harmony* by Arthur H. Benade published in 1960 by the Anchor Book division of Doubleday & Company.

VIBRATO

In the instruction of woodwind instruments the subject of vibrato arises with many students on the intermediate level, and with virtually every student on an advanced level. The subject of vibrato is especially important to the student who is playing or who is interested in playing in a dance band. While this desire is frequently the motivating factor for a consideration of vibrato, it is of equal or greater importance for the player to understand its use in serious music as well.

The vibrato is an integral part of all vocal tones, in fact one authority states that there can be no true vocal tone without it. Its use is universally accepted as being good vocal technique. The use of vibrato is equally universal on string instruments, and the development of a satisfactory vibrato is a mandatory part of string instruction. Brass instruments virtually all make use of a tasteful vibrato, but restrict its use primarily to solo passages.

The use of the vibrato on all woodwind instruments except the clarinet is virtually mandatory in solo passages if the performance is to be judged a fine one. Development of a tasteful well controlled vibrato is necessary for complete success in flute, oboe, bassoon and saxophone performance. In the field of serious music vibrato is rarely used in the clarinet, although at least two of the finest performer-teachers of the last decade consider vibrato essential to the clarinet tone under certain circumstances for the most expressive interpretation. It is quite possible, indeed probable, that vibrato on the clarinet will become as widely used as on any of the other woodwind instruments.

Vibrato is used only on notes that are of sufficient duration to sustain a vibrato. It is never used in fast moving passages. No matter on what instrument the vibrato is being used it must be under perfect control consciously used and never involuntary. It must not always be used, but only when good musical taste demands it. In orchestra and band use of the vibrato must be reserved for solo passages. Intonation suffers when it is used in the ensemble portions of the performance.

DEFINITION

A good vibrato in music is a regular pulsation, generally involving changes in pitch, intensity and timbre which produces a pleasing mellowness and richness of tone.

TYPES OF VIBRATO

There are four general types of vibrato used in music. These involve three of the elements which go to make up musical sounds: pitch, intensity and timbre. These types of vibrato may be described as follows:

1. Parallel vibrato which involves increasing and decreasing intensity and raising and lowering the pitch at the same time and at the same rate of speed.

2. Opposite relationship vibrato in which pitch is raised and lowered at the same rate of speed that intensity is increased and decreased but in opposite directions.

3. Pitch vibrato in which the pitch alone changes.

4. Intensity vibrato in which the intensity alone changes.

All four types are in common use on woodwind instruments, some instrumentalists using more than one of them according to the demands of the music.

CONFUSIONS ABOUT VIBRATO

Among musicians there is more disagreement and confusion about vibrato and its uses than any other single factor in performance. Most of the confusion results because the ear, even of a trained musician, does not hear vibrato as it actually exists in the tone. Many people cannot hear vibrato as a separate entity, but hear it only as part of tone quality in general. Because of the intangibles of the musical tone the ear does not hear the speed of the vibrato as it actually exists, nor the amount of pitch fluctuation as being as large as it actually is.

The vibrato is also frequently confused with tremolo. Many of the objections to the use of vibrato should be aimed at the tremolo. The tremolo is a rapid and wide dynamic variation of the tone without any pitch deviation. It must not be confused with the intensity vibrato which has a much slower rate of speed and a small and carefully controlled amount of dynamic variation. Needless to say the tremolo should never under any circumstances be used on a woodwind instrument.

WHAT IS GOOD VIBRATO

What one person might consider a good vibrato would not be considered good by another. Many persons, even musicians, cannot hear it at all, and to others even a slight vibrato can be irritating. Because of this great difference in hearing there is a question of what rate of vibrato is artistic. The rate of speed of the vibrato gives it life. If the rate is too slow, the tone gives an effect of laboriousness, heaviness and sluggishness. If the rate is too fast, its effect is lost and frequently approaches the tremolo in sound.

A scientific analysis of the vibrato of outstanding artists reveals that a rate of speed between five and eight pulsations per second can be accepted as standard. Slower than five or faster than eight pulsations per second are extremely rare in artistic performances.

The amount of pitch fluctuation in these analysis has been established at about one-half step—one quarter tone below and one quarter tone above the actual pitch. Small deviations on either side of the half-step interval are common, but too great a deviation is considered poor taste.

The amount of pitch variation must be equally divided above and below the correct pitch of the tone without vibrato. The ear hears the tone at its average pitch. If most of the pitch change of the vibrato is above the actual true pitch of the tone the effect will be that of sharpening the pitch. If most of the pitch change in the vibrato is below the actual true pitch of the tone, the effect will be that of flatting the tone.

Although the actual amount of pitch fluctuation in the vibrato has been found to be approximately a half-step the ear hears it as being one-half or even less of this amount. A pitch fluctuation that is much smaller than a half-step will not be heard in such a way as to be effective. The actual amount of pitch fluctuation may be heard only by greatly reducing the rate of speed.

TYPES OF VIBRATO FOR WOODWINDS

There are three methods of producing a vibrato on woodwind instruments. There are many variations and combinations of these three methods. In fact, the same player may use each method at various times, depending on the effect he wishes to produce. However, most players will prefer to develop one type which will be flexible enough to cover any situation which might arise. The standard ways of producing the vibrato may be described as follows:

1. *Diaphramatic Vibrato.* This type of vibrato is produced by increasing and decreasing the wind pressure against the embouchure by controlled motions of the diaphragm and abdominal muscles in exactly the same way the vocal vibrato is produced. As we have seen in the study of acoustics an increase in wind pressure raises the pitch of a tone and at the same time makes it louder, while decreasing the wind pressure lowers the pitch of the tone while making it softer. When this method is used on a woodwind instrument it produces the most effective type of vibrato—the parallel described above—in that there are simultaneous fluctuations in both pitch and intensity. This is the ideal and most widely taught method of producing a vibrato on any of the woodwinds. It is the ideal method because no change in embouchure is necessary, it can be freely used and controlled thoroughut the entire pitch and dynamic ranges of the instrument and is capable of great variation.

2. *Jaw Motion.* This type of vibrato is produced by slight up and down motions of the lower jaw producing changes in the pressure of the lips against the reed. When the pressure increases the pitch is raised when the pressure decreases the pitch is lowered. This method is rarely used on the flute, but can achieve a vibrato through slight changes in direction of the wind across the embouchure hole. Producing a vibrato in this fashion comes quite naturally to all except flute students, and is probably the method which they will use if they are not given instruction in the diaphragmatic vibrato. Some teachers recommend this vibrato because it is relatively simple and easy to learn. The advantages of the jaw motion are that it may be employed with equal freedom on any note in the pitch range of the particular instrument, and is subject to ease of control within a wide dynamic range. Its disadvantages are that the movement of the jaw usually results in too wide fluctuations in pitch, the amount of pitch variation changes in the various registers of the instrument, and the constant movement of the lower jaw impairs embouchure development especially in students who have not reached a quite advanced level. It is almost always true that when a student who has not fully developed his embouchure begins using this type of vibrato there is a marked deterioration in his tone quality both with and without the vibrato.

3. *Throat Motion.* In this method the vibrato is produced by successive contraction and expansion of the throat muscles. When singers use this type of vibrato the motion is quite visible. A very dramatic vibrato is produced in this manner but it is the least desirable of the methods because it impairs the breathing, the player using it tires quickly, the vibrato produced in this

fashion is difficult to control and is capable of but little variation. Unless this type of vibrato is perfectly controlled the result will be an objectionable tremolo rather than a vibrato. This type of vibrato is not recommended.

DEVELOPING A VIBRATO

A good vibrato will add an effective richness and mellowness to the tone of any instrument. On any woodwind instrument the vibrato should be the last of all technical problems to be studied. No attempt should be made to develop a vibrato until the player has not only developed a good technique, but has also developed a strong embouchure and is producing a tone of good quality without a vibrato. And most important of all, not until the player has developed sufficient musicianship to know exactly when and how the vibrato should be used.

The diaphragmatic vibrato is recommended as the ideal method for all woodwind instruments. Developing it requires thorough and careful study, but once developed it can be varied in many ways for use in all kinds of musical expression. A successful method of developing this vibrato may be outlined as follows:

1. Playing a strong clear tone in the middle register of the instrument increase and decrease the pressure of the air against the embouchure with the diaphragm and abdominal muscles. Move slowly until there are definite changes in the pitch as well as the loudness of the tone. Be sure that the embouchure formation itself does not move or change.

2. Set a metronome to sixty beats per minute. Practice until there is one movement up and down of the tone to each beat.

3. After the fluctuations come easily at this speed, increase the metronome speed little by little to 120 beats per minute, keeping one complete movement of the tone per beat.

4. After the one fluctuation per beat comes easily at these speeds, move the metronome back to sixty beats per minute. Practice successive vibratos of one, two, three and four fluctuations per beat. Do the same thing, gradually increasing the metronome tempo to 100 beats per minute.

The speed of the ideal vibrato ranges from four pulsations per beat at a speed of 72 up to four pulsations per beat at a speed of 120. The speed to be used depends on the musical content. Expect some fluctuation in the intensity as well as the pitch of the tone.

5. After the vibrato is under perfect control practice slow melodies—folk tunes, chorale melodies, or hymn melodies—using vibrato only on the half notes and whole notes.

Remember that use of the vibrato is the exception rather than the rule on woodwind instruments. It is not used continually, but only in solo passages, and only on notes of sufficient duration to establish an effective vibrato. A good vibrato cannot be developed overnight. Rather it must be slowly and carefully developed over a period of weeks and months until it is under perfect control. Do not attempt to rush the process.

PHONOGRAPH RECORDINGS

The general availability of phonograph recordings of excellent quality and the high quality reproduction units which are widely available make possible an important adjunct to woodwind teaching. The opportunity to hear fine artists in performance is essential to the learning process of any instrument. This helps the student arrive at a concept of tone quality and phrasing which he would not be possible to acquire in any other way. Students should be encouraged to listen carefully and often to recorded performances. If a copy of the musical score is available at the same time it should be used.

In the sections which follow a few recordings of special interest are identified by company and number. However, recordings are introduced and disappear from the market sometimes quite rapidly. For this reason compositions which have been recorded and have been available on long playing records are listed without further identification. Whether or not they are currently available can be checked quickly by referring to the Schwann catalog or to the "Phonolog" an all-inclusive and classified catalog which most record shops have available.

In selecting recordings the differences in concept of the best tone quality and performance style between artists in various countries should be kept in mind. French, German, Italian, Dutch, Scandinavian, and to some extent English artists have quite different concepts from each other and from the American concept. For this reason it is generally best to select recordings by American artists for study purposes, although the comparison in sounds from nation to nation is in itself an interesting study.

FLUTE

Recordings of Special Interest

1. *Eighteenth Century Flute Duets.* Washington Records WR 419. Music of Schultze, Quantz, Telemann, and Stamitz played by Julius Baker and Jean Pierre Rampal.

2. *Flute Contest Music.* Two records. Lanier Records. Volume One record No. 5238, Volume Two record No. 6129. Available from H. & A. Selmer, Inc., Elkhart, Indiana. Played by Charles DeLaney. Compositions selected from NIMAC Festival lists. Volume One includes music by Handel, J. S. Bach, Pessard, Kohler, Godard, Anderson, Lewallen, Enesco, Mozart, Busser, Martin and Honneger. Volume Two music of Teleman, Handel, Anderson, Quantz, Bournonville, Hue, Ganne, Widor, Ibert, and Gaubert.

3. *William Kincaid.* Performances by the solo flutist of the Philadelphia orchestra are ideal for study purposes. Three solo recordings are available:

   A. "Music for the Flute" Columbia ML 4339. Music by Marcello, Hindemith, Saint-Saens, Caplet, Debussy.

   B. William Kincaid Plays the Flute, Vol. I. Intermediate Award Artists Series AAS 705. Ten compositions.

   C. William Kincaid Plays the Flute, Vol. II. Advanced. Award Artists Series AAS 706. Five compositions.

4. *Marcel Moyse.* The great French flutist, flute teacher at the Paris Conservatory, and editor of a large number of flute books has three recordings available. They are available from McGinnis & Marx, or from Mr. Moyse at 183 Western Avenue, Brattleboro, Vermont.

   A. "The French School at Home" Record No. 99. Recordings of typical flute studies by Moyse, Soussmann, Furstenau, Andersen.

   B. "Flute Excerpts" Record No. M-101. Solos and two trio sonatas.

   C. "A Marcel Moyse Flute Recital" Record No. M-102. Solos by Debussy, Taffanel, Wetzger, Tchaikovsky, Genin, Couperin, Doppler, Ferroud, Dvorak, Roussel.

5. *John Wummer*. Flutist of the New York Philharmonic. Sonatas by Frederick the Great and Quantz played by John Wummer, flute; and Fernado Valenti, harpsichord.

Westminster SWN 18070. Handel—Ten Flute Sonatas. Westminster WAL 218.

Recorded Repertoire

Bach, C. P. E. Concerto in G for Flute and Orchestra

Bach, J. S. Suite No. 2 in B Minor for Flute and Strings

Bach, J. S. Suite for Flute and Figured Bass in C minor

Bach, W. F. Sonata in F for 2 flutes

Boccherini. Concerto in D Major for flute and strings

Boismortier, J. D. Concerto in A Minor for five flutes

Chedeville, N. Sonata No. 3 in C Minor, op. 8 for two flutes

Cimarosa, D. Concerto for 2 flutes and orchestra

Debussy. Sonata No. 2 for flute, viola and harp

Foote, Arthur. A Night Piece for flute and strings

Gluck. Concerto in G Major for flute and orchestra

Gluck. Dance of the Spirits

Gordeli. Concerto in D for flute and orchestra, op. 8

Gretchaninoff, A. Fantasy on Bashkir Themes for flute and harp, op. 125

Griffes, Charles. Poem for Flute and Orchestra

Handel. Sonatas for Flute and Harpsichord, op. 1

Haydn. Flute Concerto in D

Hindemith, Paul. Sonata for Flute and Piano

Hindemith, Paul. Sonatine for two flutes

Ibert, Jacques. Concerto for Flute and Orchestra

Ibert, Jacques. Entracte for Flute and Guitar

Mozart. Andante in C Major for flute and string orchestra

Mozart. Concerto for Flute and Harp in C major, K. 299

Mozart. Flute Quartets (flute, violin, viola, cello) D major, K. 285; C major, K. 285b; A major, K. 298

Quantz. Concerto in G major for flute and string orchestra

Pergolesi. Flute Concerto No. 1 in G major

Tartini. Concerto in G major for Flute

Varese, Edgard. Density 21.5

Vivaldi. Antonio. Concerto in C Major for picolo, strings and cembalo

Vivaldi, Antonio. Concerto for flute, oboe, bassoon and figured bass in G minor

Vivaldi, Antonio. Sonata for flute and figured bass in D minor

Vivaldi, Antonio. Six Concertos, op. 10 for flute, strings, and continuo

OBOE

Recorded Repertoire

Albinoni. Concerto in B-flat for Oboe and Strings, op. 7, No. 3

Bach, J. C. Andante for oboe and orchestra

Bach, J. S. Adagio-Arioso

Bach, J. S. Concerto in C minor for oboe and violin

Bach, J. S. Concerto in A major for oboe d'amore, strings and continue

Bach, J. S. Sinfonia from Easter Oratorio

Bach. J. S. Sinfonias: Cantatas 12, 21, and 156

Beethoven. Trio, Op. 87 for two oboes and English horn

Beethoven. Variations on Mozart's "Reich Mir" for two oboes and English horn

Beethoven. Rondino in E-flat major for two oboes and English horn

Britten, Benjamin. Fantasy for Oboe and Strings, op. 2

Cimarosa. Concerto for Oboe and Strings

Donovan, Richard. Suite for oboe and string orchestra

Fiocco. Adagio for oboe and strings

Handel. Concerto in G minor for oboe and strings

Haydn. Concerto in C for oboe and orchestra

Hindemith. Sonata for Oboe and Piano

Loeffler. Two Rhapsodies for Oboe, Viola and Piano

Marcello. Concerto in C minor for Oboe and Strings

Mozart. Concerto in C major for oboe and orchestra, K. 314

Mozart. Quartet in F for oboe, violin, viola, cello, K. 370

Strauss, Richard. Concerto for Oboe and Small Orchestra

Teleman. Partita No. 5 in E minor for Oboe and Harpsichord

Teleman. Sonata in C minor for Oboe and Harpsichord

Teleman. Concerto in F minor for oboe, strings, and continuo

Vaughan-Williams. Concerto for Oboe and Strings

Vivaldi, Antonio. Concerto in D minor for oboe, strings and cembalo

CLARINET

Recordings of Special Interest

1. *In Tribute to Simeon Bellison*. Classic Editions CE 1001. Four compositions played by the late Simeon Bellison who was solo clarinetist of the New York Philharmonic for many years.

2. *Reginald Kell-Clarinet Encores*. Decca DL 9926. Pieces by Handel, Corelli, Beethoven, Ravel, Debussy, Richardson, Godard, and Benjamin played with piano accompaniment.

Decca DL 9941. Reginald Kell with Brooks Smith, piano in performances of the Saint-Saens Sonata, Alec Templeton Pocket Size Sonata, Szalowski Sonatina, and the Vaughan Williams Six Studies in English Folk Song.

3. *Robert McGinnis Plays the Clarinet.* Award Artists Series AAS 33-702. The solo clarinetist of the New York Philharmonic in performances of music by Mozart, Schumann, Bassi, Pierne, Brahms, Avon, Bergson, and Thiere all of which appear on various recommended lists of solos for Festivals.

Recorded Repertoire

Bartok. Contrasts for Piano, Violin and Clarinet

Berg, Alban. Four Pieces for Clarinet and Piano, op. 5

Brahms. Sonata, Op. 120, No. 1 for Clarinet and Piano

Brahms. Sonata, Op. 120, No. 2 for Clarinet and Piano

Brahms. Quintet in B minor, op. 115 for Clarinet and Strings

Brahms. Trio in A minor, op. 114 for clarinet, cello, and piano

Copland. Concerto for clarinet and orchestra

Debussy. Premiere Rhapsodie for Clarinet and orchestra

Hindemith. Concerto for clarinet and orchestra

Hindemith. Sonata for clarinet and piano

Khachaturian, Aram. Trio for Clarinet, violin, and piano (1932)

Manevich, A. Concerto for clarinet and orchestra

Mozart. Concerto for clarinet and orchestra

Mozart. Quintet in A major, K. 581, for clarinet and strings

Mozart. Trio in E-flat major, K. 498 for clarinet, viola and piano

Milhaud. Suite for clarinet, violin and piano

Spohr. Clarinet Concerto in F minor

Stamitz, Johann. Concerto for clarinet, strings, and continuo in B-flat major

Stravinsky. Three pieces for clarinet solo

Weber. Concertino for clarinet and orchestra, op. 26

Weber. Concerto No. 1 in F minor, op. 73 for clarinet and orchestra

Weber. Concerto No. 2 in E-flat major, op. 74 for clarinet & orchestra

Weber. Grand Duo Concertante for clarinet and piano, op. 48

Weber. Variations on an air from Silvania, op. 33 for clarinet and piano

BASSOON
Recorded Repertoire

Hindemith. Sonata for Bassoon and piano

Mozart. Concerto in B-flat major for bassoon and orchestra, K. 191

Rosetti, Antonio. Concertino in E-flat for bassoon and orchestra

Weber. Concerto in F major for bassoon and orchestra, op. 75

Vivaldi, Antonio. Concerto for bassoon in e minor

SAXOPHONE
Recordings of Special Interest

1. *Sigurd Rascher—A Classical Recital on the Saxophone.* Concert Hall CHS 1156. The greatest saxophone soloist of the present day in performances of nine compositions by various composers with piano accompaniment. This record dramatically illustrates the extended range above high F for which Mr. Rascher is unique.

   Sigurd Rascher Plays the Saxophone. Volume 1, Volume 2. Award Artist Series. AAS 703 and AAS 708. Volume 1 has nineteen compositions by various composers all of which are grades 2, 3, or 4 on the New York State School Music Association Manual. Volume 2 is advanced music and includes the sonatas for Alto saxophone and piano by Eccles, Creston, and Heiden; the Galliard sonata for Tenor saxophone and piano; and short pieces by Handel, Fiocco, and Bozza for Alto and piano.

Recorded Repertoire

Creston, Paul. Sonata for Saxophone and piano, op. 19

Debussy. Rhapsody for Saxophone and orchestra

Glazounov. Concerto for Saxophone and string orchestra

Ibert. Concertino da Camera for Alto saxophone and chamber orchestra

WOODWIND QUINTET

The only standard woodwind ensemble, and one which has a large repertoire available, is the "French Quintet" consisting of flute, oboe, clarinet, bassoon, and French horn. This medium gives an opportunity to compare and study woodwind style and performance techniques.

Records of Special Interest

1. *Philadelphia Woodwind Qunintet.* This group, made up of the first chair players of the Philadelphia Symphony, has several records available. Among them is Columbia ML 5093 which has compositions by Hindemith, Ibert, Bozza, Haydn, and Beethoven; and Columbia ML 5217 which is a performance of the Schoenberg Quintet. op. 26.

Recorded Repertoire

Barber, Samuel. Summer Music for a Woodwind Quintet

Berezowsky. Suite for wind quintet, op. 11

Bozza. Scherzo for wind quintet, op. 48

Bozza. Variations sur un theme libre, op. 40

Dahl, Ingolf. Allegro and arioso for five wind instruments (1942)

Etler, Alvin. Quintet for winds (1955)

Fine, Irvine. Partita for woodwind quintet

Francaix. Quintet

Goeb, Roger. Prairie songs for woodwind quintet

Ibert. Trois Pieces Breves

Janacek. Concertino for woodwind quintet and piano

Janacek. Mladi (Youth Suite, 1924) woodwind quintet and bass clarinet

Milhaud. La Cheminee du Roi Rene (1942)

Milhaud. Two Sketches: Madrigal, Pastoral

Nielsen, Carl. Quintet for wind instruments, op. 43

Schoenberg. Woodwind Quintet, op. 26

Taffanel, Paul. Quintet

Villa-Lobos. Quintette in forme de choros

Wilder, Alec. Quintet for woodwinds

OTHER COMBINATIONS

Beethoven. Rondino in E-flat Major (2 ob., 2 cl., 2 bsn., 2 bsn., 2 hns.)

Beethoven. Quintet. Op. 16 (ob., cl., bsn., hn., pf.)

Beethoven. Rondino in E-flat major (2 bo., 2 cl., 2 bsn., 2 hns.)

Beethoven. Septeti n E-flat. Op. 20 (cl., bsn., hn., strings)

Berger, Arthur. Quartet in c major (1941) (fl., ob., cl., bsn.)

Glanville-Hicks. Concertino da Camera (fl., cl., bsn., pf.)

Glinka, Michael. Trio Pathetique (cl., bsn., pf.)

Gounod. Little Symphone in B-flat (2 fl., 2 ob., 2 cl., 2 hn., 2 bsn.)

Haydn. Divertimento in C major (fl., ob., 2 cl., 2 hns., strings)

Haydn. Sinfonia Concertante, op. 84 (ob., bsn., vln., clo., orch.)

Hill. E. B. Sextet, op. 39 (fl., ob., cl., hn., bsn., pf.)

Honneger. Concerto da camera for flute, English horn, and string orchestra

Honneger. Rhapsodie for flute, oboe, clarinet and piano

Jongen, Joseph. Concerto, op. 124 (fl., ob., cl., bsn., hn.)

Milhaud. Pastorale for oboe, clarinet and bassoon (1936)

Milhaud. Sonata for flute, oboe, clarinet and piano (1918)

Milhaud. Suite (d'apre Corrette) for oboe, clarinet, bassoon

Mozart. Divertimenti: K. 166, K. 186, K. 213, K. 240, K. 252, K. 253, K. 270, K. 289. (2 ob., 2 bsn., 2 hns.)

Mozart. Quintet in E-flat Major, K. 425 (ob., cl., bsn., hn., pf.)

Mozart. Sinfonia Concertant in E-flat, K. 297b. Solo oboe, clarinet, bassoon and horn with orchestra

Piston, Walter. Three Pieces for flute, clarinet, bassoon

Poulenc. Sextet (woodwind quintet and piano)

Poulene. Trio for oboe, bassoon and piano

Prokofieff. Overture on Hebrew Themes, op. 35 (cl., str. quartet, piano)

Prokofieff. Quintet, op. 39 for oboe, clarinet, violin, viola, bass

Quantz. Trio Sonata for flute, oboe, piano

Ravel. Introduction and Allegro for harp, flute, clarinet, and string quartet

Rieti, V. Sonata for flute, oboe, bassoon, piano

Rimsky-Korsakoff. Quintet in B-flat (fl., cl., bsn., hn., pf.)

Roland. Suite dans le Gout Espagnol (ob., bsn., trpt., harpsichord)

Saint-Saens. Caprice sur des airs danois et russes (fl., ob., cl., pf.)

Schonberg. Suite, op. 29 (E-flat clarinet, B-flat clarinet, bass clarinet, violin, viola, cello and piano)

Schubert. Eine Kleine Trauermusik (2 ob., 2 cl., 2 hn., 2 bsn.)

Schubert. Octet, op. 166 (cl., bsn., hn., and strings)

Spohr. Nonette in F, op. 31. Woodwind quintet and string quartet

Stamitz, Karl. Concerto for clarinet, bassoon and orchestra

Strauss, R. Duet-Concertino for clarinet and bassoon with string orchestra and harp.

Strauss, R. Serenade for wind instruments in E-flat major, op. 7

Stravinsky. Octet for wind instruments (fl., cl., 2 bsn., 2trpt., 2 tromb.)

Stravinsky. The Soldier's Tale (cl., bsn., tromb., trpt., violin, bass, perc.)

Teleman, G. F. Trio sonata in c minor for flute, oboe, and piano

Thompson, R. Suite for oboe, clarinet, viola

Villa-Lobos. Bachiana Brasilieras No. 6 for flute and bassoon

Villa-Lobos. Choros No. 2 for flute and clarinet

Villa-Lobos. Quartet for flute, oboe, clarinet and bassoon

Villa-Lobos. Quintet enforme de choros (fl., ob., cl., bsn., English horn)

Villa-Lobos. Trio for oboe, clarinet and bassoon

Vivaldi, A. Concerto for flute, oboe, bassoon & figured bass in G minor

Weber, Ben. Concertino for flute, oboe, clarinet & str. quartet, op. 45.

Weiss, A. Trio for clarinet, viola, cello

OF GENERAL INTEREST

1. *Spotlight on Winds.* Vox DL 312. Two long playing records of demonstrations of woodwind instruments of today and their predecessors.

2. *The Complete Orchestra.* Music Education Record Corporation, Box 445, Englewood, N. J. Woodwinds demonstrated include flute, piccolo, clarinet, E-flat clarinet, bass clarinet, oboe, English horn, bassoon, contra-bassoon. Performances are excellent. Conducted by Wheeler Beckett.

3. *First Chair.* Columia ML 4629. Features first chair players of the Philadelphia Orchestra in performances with the orchestra under the direction of Eugene Ormandy. Woodwind compositions include: Griffes "Poem for Flute"; Handel—"Concerto in g minor for Oboe"; Burrill Phillips—"Concert Piece for bassoon and string orchestra"; Weber—"Concertino for clarinet and orchestra."

4. *American Music for Solo Winds and String Orchestra.* Mercury MG 50076. Eastman Rochestra Orchestra directed by Howard Hanson. Compositions include Wayne Barlow "The Winter's Past for oboe"; Bernard Rogers "Soliloquy for flute"; Kent Kennan "Night Soliloquy for flute"; Homer Keller "Serenade for Clarinet"; Howard Hanson "Serenade for flute, strings and harp"; Howard Honson "Pastorale for oboe, strings, and harp."

5. *Eastman Wind Ensemble.* Mercury Records. Excellent source for study of woodwinds in band. A number of recordings by this group under the direction of Frederick Fennell are available. Especially recommended are MG 50176 "Mozart—Serenade in B-flat major, K. 361"; MG 50173 "Winds in Hi-Fi" including Grainger "Lincolnshire Posey"; Rogers "Three Japanese Dances"; Milhaud "Suite Francaise" and Strauss "Serenade in E-flat major"; and MG 50143 which includes Hindemith "Symphony in B-flat"; Schoenberg "Theme and Variations, op. 43a"; and Stravinsky "Symphonies of Wind Instruments."

6. *Selmer Demonstration Records.* London Records. Although these are older records the quality of woodwind performances by the French artists is astounding. The series includes: (1) The Flute played by Fernad Marseau, LS 1096; (2) The Clarinet, two records of solos played by Ulysse Delacluse, LS 987 and LS 1097; (3) Two records of a clarinet sextet "Sextuor de Clarinettes de Paris" made up of E-flat, B-flat, A, Alto, Bass, and Contra-bass instruments. LS 1077 and LS 1096; (4) The Saxophone, two records of solos played by Marcel Mule, LS 986 and LS 1187; and (5) A record of a saxophone quartet "Quatuor de Saxophones" made up of soprano, alto, tenor and baritone instruments. LS 1188.

7. *Music Minus One.* Performances of chamber music and concerti with one part omitted. Gives advanced players an opportunity to perform with original instrumentation. A record player with a variable speed adjustment is desirable so that the pitch can be adjusted. Printed music for the missing part is provided with the record. Records available include: MMO 106 Mozart: 3 flute quartets; MMO 107 Handel: 3 Flute sonatas and Telemann: 3 flute sonatas; MMO 301 Oboe concerti by Handel, Telemann and Vivaldi; MMO 61 Brahms: Clarinet Quintet, op. 115; MMO 71 Mozart: Clarinet Quintet K. 581; MMO 103 Piano and wind Quintets by Beehoven and Mozart with the clarinet part omitted; and MMO 104 Piano and wind Quintets by Beethoven and Mozart with the bassoon part omitted. The series is being enlarged.

8. *Kjos Solo Records.* A series of seven inch long playing records of solos from the Kjos catalog. Each record has six solos in the easy to medium difficulty range. Recording artists are not identified. The series to date includes: Two records for flute, IM 11 and IM 12; three records for clarinet, IM 13, IM 14, 15, and two records for Alto saxophone IM 16 and IM 17.

SOURCES OF MUSIC FOR WOODWINDS

I. Your regular music dealer is the best sources of supply. He can obtain music of any publisher through his usual channels. A request for music should identify composer, exact title, opus number if available, publisher, and the instrument or instrumental combination for which it is written.

II. The following retail stores maintain a large stock of woodwind music and process mail orders promptly. They publish catalogs which include music of both domestic and foreign publishers, and will send lists of materials when they are available. In requesting these lists identify the instrument or instruments in which you are interested.

McGinnis & Marx
408 Second Avenue
New York 10, New York

M. Baron and Company
8 West 45th. Street
New York 19, New York

Jack Sprat Woodwind Shop
21-23 West End Avenue
Old Greenwich, Conecticut

Southern Music Company
1100 Broadway
San Antonio 6, Texas

III. The catalogs of the following publishers (among many) contain music of interest in the woodwind field:

Associated Music Publishers, Inc. 1 West 47th Street, New York 36, N.Y.
(American source for music of a number of foreign publishers, their catalogs are composites of all of them)

Belwin, Inc. 250 Maple Avenue, Rockeville Center, New York

Boosey and Hawkes, Inc. P.O. Box 418, Lynbrook, New York

Broude Bros. 56 W. 45th Street, New York, 19, N. Y.

Cundy-Bettoney Co. Hyde Park, Boston 36, Mass.

Carl Fischer, Inc. 62 Cooper Square, New York 3, N. Y.

International Music Co. 509 Fifth Avenue, New York 17, N. Y.

Kjos Music Co., 525 Busse, Park Ridge, Ill.

Mills Music, Inc. 1619 Broadway, New York 19, N. Y.

Music Publishers Holding Corp. 619 West 54th Street, New York 19, N. Y.

Oxford University Press, 114 Fifth Avenue, New York, N. Y.

C. F. Peters Corp. 373 Fourth Avenue, New York 16, N. Y.

Pro Art Publications, 469 Union Avenue, Westbury, N. Y.

Ricordi & Co. 16 W. 61st Street, New York, N. Y.

Rubank, Inc. 5544 W. Armstrong Avenue, Chicago 30, Ill.

G. Schirmer, Inc. 609 Fifth Avenue, New York 17, N. Y.

IV. Special listings which include music for woodwinds:

1. Cobbett, Walter W. *Cyclopedic Survey of Chamber Music.* Two volumes, London: Oxford University Press. 1929-30. The standard reference work in this field. Out of print but available in most libraries.

2. Helm, Sanford M. *Catalog of Chamber Music for Wind Instruments.* Ann Arbor, Michigan: The Author. 1952.

3. Hauser, Roy. *Compendium of Chamber Music for Woodwinds.* Bloomington, Indiana: University of Indiana Press, 1959.

4. National Association of Schools of Music. *Solo Literature for the Wind Instruments.* Bulletin

No. 31 of the Association. 1951. These lists are intended primarily for the college level and are representative of the best music available for the various instruments.

5. NIMAC. *Selective Music Lists. Instrumental and Vocal Solos, Instrumentala nd Vocal Ensembles.* Washington, D. C.: National Interscholastic Music Activities Commission. 1961. Available from Music Educators National Conference, 1201 Sixteenth St., N.W., Washington 6, D. C. Lists are selective and graded. Intended for public school use.

BIBLIOGRAPHY

GENERAL

Baines, Anthony. *Woodwind Instruments and Their History*. New York: W. W. Norton & Co. 1957. 382 pp.

Brand, Erick D. *Band Instrument Repair Manual*. Elkhart, Indiana: Erick D. Brand. 4th edition, 1946.

Cahn, M. M. *The Instrumentalist's Handbook and Dictionary*. San Francisco, Calif.: Forman Publishing Co. 1958. 106 pp.

Galpin, Francis W. *A Textbook of European Musical Instruments*: Their origin, history, and character. New York: J. DeGraff, 1956. 256 pp.

Geiringer, Karl. *Musical Instruments, Their History in Western Culture*. New York: Oxford University Press. 1945. 278 pp.

Palmer, Harold G. *Teaching Techniques of the Woodwinds*. Rockville Center, N. Y.: Belwin, Inc. 1952. 70 pp.

Sachs, Cur. *The History of Musical Instruments*. New York: W. W. Norton. 1940. 505 pp.

————. *Woodwind Anthology*. New York: Woodwind Magazine, 1952. Reprinted by McGinnis and Marx.

FLUTE

Boehm, Theolbald. *The Flute and Flute Playing*. New York: McGinnis & Marx, 1960. 198 pp. A facsimile reprint of the revised edition of 1922 translated by Dayton C. Miller. Boehm's original version in German was published in 1871. An extremely important book on the development of the Boehm system as well as Boehm's views on flute playing.

Chapman, F. B. *Flute Technique*. London: Oxford University Press, 1958. 84 pp. Chapters on breath control, finger control, tongue control, practice, care of the flute, and an extensive list of flute music.

DeLorenzo, Leonardo. *My Complete Story of the Flute*. New York: Citadel Press. 1951. 493 pp. Personal reminiscences about flute, flutists, and flute music.

Fitzgibbon, H. Macaulay. *The Story of the Flute*. New York: Charles Scribner's Sons. 1914. 292 pp.

Miller, Dayton C. *Catalog of Books and Literature Relating to the Flute*. Cleveland, Ohio: The Author. 1935. 120 pp.

Putnik, Edwin. *Flute Pedagogy and Performance*. Part I: Basic Esentials. Chicago: Estes Music Co. 1955. 59 pp.

Rockstro, Richard S. *The Flute*. London: Rudall, Carte & Co. Revised Edition 1920. (Originally published in 1890). 64 pp. Complete title page reads: "A treatise on the construction, the history, and the practice of the flute, including a sketch of the elements of acoustics and critical notices of sixty celebrated flute players." One of the important standard books on the flute.

Welch, Christopher. *History of the Boehm Flute*. London: Rudall, Carte & Co. New York: G. Schirmer. 1896. 504 pp. Facsimile reprint: McGinnis & Marx.

Wilkins, Frederick. *The Flutist's Guide*. Elkhart, Indiana: The author. 1957. Available from the Conn Corporation, Elkhart, Indiana. A book of 84 pages with accompanying illustrative long playing record.

OBOE

Bate, Philip. *The Oboe: An Outline of its History, Development and Construction*. London: Ernest Been, Ltd. 1956. 195 pp.

McAninch, Daniel A. *Technical Problems of the Oboe in the Woodwind Quintet*. Rochester, New York: University of Rochester Press, 1957 microprint copy of original thesis.

Rothwell, Evelyn. *Oboe Technique*. London: Oxford University Press. 1953. 106 pp. Chapters on producing a sound, brath control, embouchure control, tongue control, finger control, care of the instrument, reeds and their care, practice, and an extensive list of music for oboe and English horn.

Russell, Myron E. *The Oboe: A Comparison Study of Specifications With Musical Effectiveness.* Ann Arbor, Michigan: University Microfilms. L. 953. Publication No. 5723.

Sprenkle, Robert & David Ledet. *The Art of Oboe Playing.* Evanston, Illinois: Summy-Birchard. 1961. 96 pp.

CLARINET

Cummings, Frank & Carl Gutmann. *Band Instrument Repair Manual Series I: Clarinet.* Berkeley, California: Don Kelelr Music Co. 1953. 27 pp.

Eby, W. M. *The Clarinet And Its Care.* New York: Walter Jacobs Co. 1927. 13 pp.

Eby, W. M. *The Clarinet Embouchure.* New York: Walter Jacobs Co. 1927. 18 pp.

McCathrey, Don. *Playing and Teaching the Clarinet Family.* San Antonio, Texas: Southern Music Company. 1959.

Miller, Jean R. *A Spectrum Analysis of Clarinet Tones.* Ann Arbor, Michigan: Unversity Microfilms. 1956. Publication No. 19, 120.

Opperman, Kalmen. *Repertory of the Clarinet.* New York: G. Ricordi & Co. 1960. 140 pp.

Seltzer, George A. *A Study of Some Technical Problems for the Clarinet Family in Orchestral Literature.* Rochester, New York: University of Rochester Press, 1959 microprint copy of original typescript.

Stein, Keith. *The Art of Clarinet Playing.* Evanston, Illinois: Summy-Bichard. 1958. 80 pp.

Rendall, Francis G. *The Clarinet, Some Notes Upon Its History and Construction.* New York: Philosophical Library. 1954. 182 pp.

Thurston, Frederick. *Clarinet Technique.* London: Oxford University Press. 1956. 98 pp.

Willaman, Robert. *The Clarinet and Clarinet Playing.* New York: Carl Fischer, Inc. 1949. 316 pp.

BASSOON

Heckel, Wilhelm H. *The Bassoon.* Old Greenwich, Conn. Jack Spratt. Revised edition 1940. Translated from the German by Langwill and Waples.

Langwill, Lyndesay. *The Bassoon and Double Bassoon.* London: Hinrichen Edition, Ltd. n.d. 40 pp.

Spencer, William. *The Art of Bassoon Playing.* Evanston, Illinois: Summy-Birchard. 1958. 77 pp.

REEDS

Artley, Joe. *How to Make Double-Reeds.* Old Greenwich, Conn.: Jack Spratt. Second Edition 1953. 35 pp.

Eby, W. M. *Reed Knowledge.* New York: Walter Jacobs, Inc. 1925. 16 pages. Considers clarinet and saxophone reeds.

Larson, Glen & Harry Baxter. *Oboe Reed Technique.* Los Angeles, California: Baxter-Northup Co. 1933. 16 pp.

Jaffrey, K. S. *Reed Mastery.* Summer Hill, Australia. The Author. 1956. 50 pp. Considers clarinet and saxophone reeds.

Mayer, Robert & Traugott Rohner. *Oboe Reeds: How To Make and Adjust Them.* Glen Ellyn, Illinois: The Instrumentalist Co. 1953. 54 pp.

Opperman, Kalmen. *Handbook for Making and Adjusting Single Reeds.* New York: Chappell & Co. 1956. 40 pp.

Spratt, Jack. *How to Make Your Own Clarinet Reds.* Stamford, Conn.: Jack Spratt. 1956. 24 pp.

ACOUSTICS

Benade, Arthur H. *Horns, Strings & Harmony—The Science of Enjoyable Sounds.* Science Study Series. 1960. Garden City, N. Y.: Anchor Books, Doubleday & Co., Inc. (Paperback)

Bartholomew, W. T. *Acoustics of Music.* New York: Prentice-Hall, Inc. 1942. 238 pp.

Culver, Charles A. *Musical Acoustics.* 4th edition N.Y.: McGraw-Hill. 1956. 305 pp.

Jeans, James. *Science and Music.* New York: Macmillan Co., 1939.

Olson, Harry F. *Elements of Acoustical Engineering.* New York: D. Van Nostrand Co. 1947. 539 pp.

Richardson, G. W. *Acoustics of Orchestral Instruments and the Organ.* London: Edward Arnold & Co. 1929. 158 pp.

Stauffer, Donald W. *Intonation Deficiencies of Wind Instruments in Ensemble.* Washington, D. C.: Catholic University of America Press. 1954. 191 pp. Photo offset of a doctorate dissertation.

Journal of the Acoustical Society of America

Benade, A. H. "On Woodwind Bores." Vol. XXXI, Feb. 1949, p. 137.

Benade, A. H. "On the Mathematical Theory of Woodwind Finger Holes." Vol. XXXII, Dec. 1960, p. 1591.

Backus, John. "Vibrations of the Reed and the Air Column i nthe Clarinet." Vol. XXXIII, June 1961, p. 806.

Ghosh, R. N. "Theory of the Clarinet." Vol. IX, January 1938.

McGinnis, C. S. & R. Pepper. "Intonation of the Boehm Clarinet." Vol. XVI, 1945, p. 188.

McGinnis, C. S. & H. Hawkins. "Experimental Study of the Tone Quality of the Boehm Clarinet." Vol. XIV, 1943, p. 228.

McGinnis & Gallagher. "Mode of Vibration of a Clarinet Reed." Vol. XXII, 1941, p. 529.

Parker, S. E. "Analyses of the Tones of Wooden and Metal Clarinets." Vol. XIX, 1947, p. 415.

Young, R. W. "Dependence of Tuning of Wind Instruments on Temperature." Vol. XVII, 1946, p. 187.

MAGAZINES

The following magazines have articles of interest to woodwind teachers and players. Consult the Music Guide for specific articles.

> *The Instrumentalist*
> *Journal of Research in Music Education*
> *Journal of the Music Educators National Conference*
> *School Musician*
> *Woodwind World*

The following magazines are no longer published but if back files are available in libraries they have considerable material of interest in the woodwind field.

> *Clarinetist Magazine*
> *Etude Music Magazine*
> *Woodwind Magazine*

FINGERING CHARTS FOR

FLUTE
OBOE
CLARINET
BASSOON
SAXOPHONE

Flute Fingering Chart

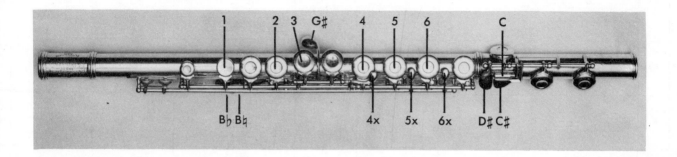

X—indicate keys operated by fingers normally covering holes. When these keys are used the hole operated by that finger remains open.

T—Left thumb on either lever except where indicated otherwise. Normal position is on the B-natural lever.

The D-sharp key is down on all notes except Low C, C-sharp, the two D-naturals, and the highest B-flat, B natural, and C.

( )—Parenthesis indicate that the use of that key or hole is optional in that fingering, depending on intonation and resonance on a particular instrument.

			Left Hand	Right Hand				Left Hand	Right Hand
C		1.	T 123	456 C	A		10.	T 120	000
C♯		2.	T 123	456 C♯	A♯		11. 12. 13.	T 100 TB♭ 100 T 100	400 000 4x00
D		3.	T 123	456	B		14.	TB 100	000
D♯		4.	T 123	456 D♯	C		15.	100	000
E		5.	T 123	450	C♯		16.	000	000
F		6.	T 123	400	D		17.	T 023	456
F♯		7.	T 123	006	D♯		18.	T 023	456 D♯
G		8.	T 123	000	E		19.	T 123	450
G♯		9.	T 123 G♯	000	F		20.	T 123	400

			Left Hand	Right Hand
F♯		21.	T 123	006
G		22.	T 123	000
G♯		23.	T 123 G♯	000
A		24.	T 12 0	000
A♯		25.	T 100	400
		26.	TB♭ 100	000
		27.	T 100	4x00
B		28.	TB 100	000
C		29.	100	000
C♯		30.	000	000
D		31.	T 023	000 D♯
D♯		32.	T 123 G♯	456 D♯
E		33.	T 120	450

			Left Hand	Right Hand
F		34.	T 103	400
F♯		35.	TB 103	006
G		36.	123	000
G♯		37.	023 G♯	000
A		38.	T 020	400
A♯		39.	T 000	4 5x0 (D♯)
		40.	T 000	4 06x (D♯)
B		41.	TB 103	006x (D♯)
C		42.	123 G♯	400 D♯ or C♯
C♯		43.	020 G♯	400 C♯
		44.	020 G♯	406 C
D		45.	T 003	450 C
D♯		46.	T 003	400 C
		47.	T 003	45x0 C

Flute Harmonic Fingerings

			Left Hand	Right Hand
G#		1.	T 123 G#	456 C#
A		2.	T 120	456 (no D#)
A#		3.	T 103	456 D#
B		4.	T 103	450 D#
C		5.	123	400 D#
C#		6.	T 023	456 C#

			Left Hand	Right Hand
D		7.	T 023	05x0 D#
D#		8.	T 023 G#	006x D#
E		9.	T 120	456x D#
F		10.	T 103	400 C#
F#		11.	TB 103	050 C#

Flute Trill Fingerings

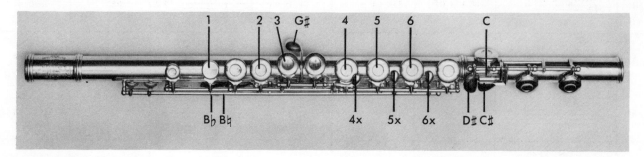

A composite fingering is given for the notes in a trill. The trill is made with the fingers and/or keys circled. Only special trill fingerings are included. Trills which are executed with regular fingerings are not included.

			Left Hand	Right Hand
E / F♯		1.	T 123	④ 50
F / G♭		2.	T 123	④ 06
F♯ / G♯		3.	T 123 G♯	006
A / B♭		4.	T 1 ② 0	100
		5.	T 1 ② 0	4x00
		6.	TB♭ 1 ② 0	000
A♯ / B		7.	TB♮ 100	④ 00
		8.	TB♮ 100	(4x) 00
B♭ / C		9.	Ⓣ 100	400
		10.	(TB♭) 100	000
		11.	Ⓣ 100	4x00
B / C♯		12.	Ⓣ ① 00	000
C / D		13.	100	0 (5x) 0
C / D♭		14.	① 00	000
C♯ / D		15.	000	0 (5x) 0
C♯ / D♯		16.	000	00 (6x)

			Left Hand	Right Hand
E / F♯		17.	T 123	④ 50
F / G♭		18.	T 123	④ 06
F♯ / G♯		19.	T 123 (G♯)	006
A / B♭		20.	T 1 ② 0	400
		21.	T 1 ② 0	4x00
		22.	TB♭ 1 ② 0	000
A♯ / B		23.	TB♮ 100	④ 00
		24.	TB♮ 100	(4x) 00
B♭ / C		25.	Ⓣ 100	400
		26.	(TB) 100	000
		27.	Ⓣ 100	4x00
B / C♯		28.	TB 100	0 (5x) 0
		29.	TB ① 00	000
C / D♭		30.	① 00	000
		31.	123	④ 50
C / D		32.	100	00 (6x)
		33.	100	0 (5x) 0
C♯ / D		34.	000	0 (5x) 0
C♯ / D♯		35.	000	0 (5x) (6x)

FLUTE FINGERING CHART

			Left Hand	Right Hand
D Eb		36. 37.	T 023 G♯ T 023	000 00 (6x)
D E		38.	T 02 ③	000
D♯ E		39. 40. 41.	T 12 ③ G♯ T 12 ③ (G♯) T 123 G♯	456 456 45 ⑥
Eb F		42. 43.	T 1 ② 3 G♯ T 1 ② ③ G♯	456 456
E F		44.	T 1 ② 0	450
E F♯		45.	Ⓣ 120	450
F Gb		46.	T 103	④ 06
F G		47.	Ⓣ 103	400

			Left Hand	Right Hand
F♯ G		48.	Ⓣ 103	006
F♯ G♯		49.	Ⓣ ① 03	006
G Ab		50. 51.	123 ① 23	0 (5x) 0 000
G A		52. 53.	T 12 ③ T 02 ③	000 056
G♯ A		54. 55.	023 G♯ T 02 ③ G♯	0 (5x) 0 000
Ab Bb		56.	023 G♯	0 (5x) (6x)
A Bb		57. 58.	TB 0 ② 0 T 020	400 40 (6x)
B C		59.	ⓉⒷ 103	00 (6x)

Oboe Fingering Chart

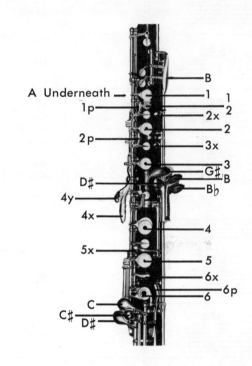

A Underneath

B
1 — 1
1p
2x — 2
2
2p
3x
3
G#
B
D#
Bb
4y
4x
4
5x
5
6x
6p
6
C
C#
D#

( )–Keys or fingers in parenthesis indicate its use in that fingering is optional, depending on intonation and resonance on a particular instrument.

x, y–indicate keys operated by fingers normally covering holes. When these keys are used the hole operated by that finger remains open unless specifically indicated that they are to be closed.

			Left Hand	Right Hand
Bb		1.	123 Bb	456 C
		2.	123 Bb	4566p
B		3.	123 B	456 C
		4.	123 B	4566p
C		5.	123	456 C
		6.	123	4566p
C#		7.	123	456 C#
		8.	123	4566p C#
D		9.	123	456
D#		10.	123 D#	456
		11.	123	456 D#
E		12.	123	450
F		13.	123	456x
		14.	123	406 (D#)

			Left Hand	Right Hand
F#		15.	123	400
G		16.	123	000
G#		17.	123 G#	000
		18.	123	4x00
		19.	*123	4y00
A		20.	120	000
A#		21.	120	400
		22.	*103 G#	000
B		23.	100	000
		24.	11p00	400
		25.	103 Bb	456 C
		26.	120 B	456 C
C		27.	100	400
		28.	020	000
		29.	103	456 C
		30.	½23	456 C
C#		31.	½23	456 C#
		32.	000	400

*Plateau model only.

Note		#	Left Hand	Right Hand
D		33.	½23	456
D♯		34.	½23 D♯	456
		35.	½23	456 D♯
E		36.	A 123	450
F		37.	A 123	456x
		38.	A 123	406 (D♯)
F♯		39.	A 123	400
G		40.	A 123	000
G♯ **		41.	A 123 G♯	000
		42.	A 123	4x00
		43.	*A 123	4y00
A		44.	B 120	000
A♯		45.	B 120	400
		46.	B 103	000
B		47.	B 100	000
		48.	B 11p20	400
		49.	B 103	456 (D♯)

Note		#	Left Hand	Right Hand
C		50.	B 100	400
		51.	023	450
C♯		52.	023	400 C
		53.	B 000	400
		54.	½23	400
D		55.	½23	000 (C)
		56.	023	000 (C)
D♯		57.	½23 B	056
		58.	½23 G♯	000 C
		59.	½23	4x00 (C)
		60.	A ½23	000
E		61.	A ½23 G♯ D♯	056
		62.	A ½23 (B)	4x56 D♯
		63.	A ½23 G♯	056 D♯
F		64.	A ½20 G♯ D♯	056
		65.	A ½20 (B)	4x56 D♯
		66.	A ½20 G♯	056 D♯
F♯		67.	A 120	456x C
		68.	A ½20	400 C
		69.	A 120	400 C
		70.	A 120	406
G		71.	A 103	400
		72.	A 11p00 (G♯)	400 C
		73.	A ½00 G♯ D♯	400 C
		74.	A ½20	406x
G♯		75.	A 103 B	056
		76.	A 100	400 (C)
		77.	A 103	006 C
A		78.	A 003 (B)	056 (D♯)
		79.	A 000	400
		80.	A ½03 G♯	006 D♯
		81.	A ½03 B	4x06
		82.	A 023	050

*Plateau model only.

**English Horn use octave key B.

Oboe Harmonic Fingerings

Note		#	Left Hand	Right Hand
F		1.	A 123 B♭	456 C
F♯		2.	A 123 B	456 C
G		3.	A 123	456 C
G♯		4.	B 123	456 C♯

Note		#	Left Hand	Right Hand
A		5.	B 123	456
A♯		6.	B 123	456 D♯
B		7.	B 123	450
		8.	B 103 B♭	456 C
C		9.	B 123	456x

Oboe Trill Fingerings

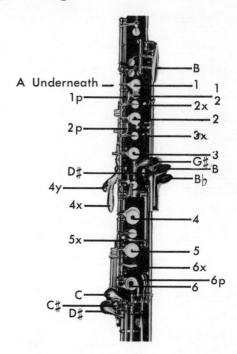

A composite fingering is given for the notes in a trill. The trill is made with the fingers and/or keys circled. Only special trill fingerings are included. Trills which are executed with regular fingerings are not included.

			Left Hand	Right Hand
B / C♯		1.	123 ⒷВ	456 C♯
C / D♭		2.	123	4566p Ⓒ♯
C♯ / D♯		3.	123 D♯	456 Ⓒ♯
E♭		4.	123	4 ⑤ 6 D♯
F		5.	123 D♯	4 ⑤ 6
F		6.	123	④ 56x
G		7.	123	④ 06
F♯ / G♯		8.	123 G♯	④ 00
G / A♭		9.	123	④x 00
G♯ / A		10.	*12 ③	4y00

			Left Hand	Right Hand
A♭		11.	1 ② 3 G♯	000
B♭		12.	1 ② 3	4x00
		13.	**123 G♯	④y 00
A♯		14.	1 ② 0 G♯	400
B		15.	11p ② 0	400
B / C♯		16.	10 ③x	000
C		17.	① 00	400
D♭		18.	10 ③x	400
C		19.	1 ②x 0	400
D		20.	100	4 ⑤x 0
C♯ / D♯		21.	½23 D♯	456 C♯
D♯ / E		22.	½23 D♯	45 ⑥
E♭		23.	½23	4 ⑤ 6 D♯
F		24.	½23 D♯	4 ⑤ 6

*Plateau model only.

**Open hole model only.

300

OBOE FINGERING CHART

Note	No.	Left Hand	Right Hand
F / G	25. / 26.	A 123	④ 56x / ④ 06
F# / G#	27.	A 123 G#	④ 00
G / Ab	28.	A 123	④x 00
G# / A	29.	*A 12 ③	4y00
Ab / Bb	30. / 31.	A 1 ② 3 G# / A 1 ② 3	000 / 4x00
A# / B	32. / 33.	B 1 ② 0 G# / B 11p ② 0	400 / 400
B / C#	34.	B 10 ③x	000
C / Db	35. / 36.	B 10 ③x / B ① 00	400 / 400
C / D	37. / 38.	B 1 ②x 0 / B 100	400 / 4 ⑤x 0
C# / D	39.	023	④ 00 C
C# / D#	40.	023 G#	④ 00 C
D / Eb	41. / 42.	½23 / ½23 Ⓖ#	④x 00 C / 000

Note	No.	Left Hand	Right Hand
D / E	43. / 44.	½2 ③ / A 023 G#	000 / ④ 06x
D# / E	45. / 46.	½2 ③ G# / ½2 ③	056 / 4y00 C
Eb / F	47. / 48.	½ 2 ③ G# / ½ 2 ③	000 C / 4x00 C
E / F	49. / 50.	A ½2 ③ B / A ½2 ③ G# D#	4x56 D# / 056
E / F#	51. / 52.	A ½ ② ③ G# D# / A ½ ② ③ B	056 / 4x56 D#
F / Gb	53. / 54.	A ½ ② 0 B / A ½ ② 0 G# D#	4x56 D# / 056
F / G	55. / 56. / 57.	A ① ② 0 G# D# / A ① ② 0 B / A 11p ② ③	056 / 4x56 D# / 400 C
F# / G	58. / 59.	A 11p ② 0 / **A 11p ② 0	400 C / 406x
F# / G#	60. / 61.	A 1 ② 0 / A 1 ② 0	400 C / 456x
G / Ab	62.	A 10 ③	400
G / A	63.	A ① 0 ③	400

*Plateau model only.

**Open hole model only.

Clarinet Fingering Chart

x, y, z, zz—indicate keys operated by one of the fingers normally covering a hole. When they are used the hole is left open.

A, G-sharp operated by 1st finger; T-thumb hole and R—Register key by left thumb; E, F, F-sharp and G-sharp by little fingers.

( )—Parenthesis indicate that the use of that key or hole is optional in that fingering, depending on intonation and resonance on a particular instrument.

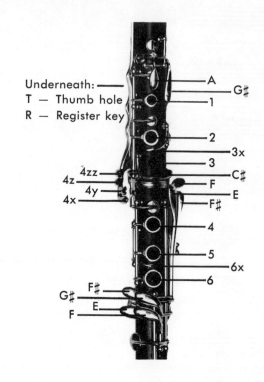

Underneath: ——
T — Thumb hole
R — Register key

			Left Hand	Right Hand
E		1.	T 123 E	456
F		2.	T 123	456 F
		3.	T 123 F	456
F♯		4.	T 123 F♯	456
		5.	T 123	456 F♯
G		6.	T 123	456
G♯		7.	T 123	456 G♯
A		8.	T 123	450
A♯		9.	T 123	400
B		10.	T 123	050
		11.	T 123	406x

			Left Hand	Right Hand
C		12.	T 123	000
C♯		13.	T 123 C♯	000
D		14.	T 120	000
D♯		15.	T 120	4x00
		16.	T 123x	000
		17.	T 100	400
		18.	T 100	050
		19.	*T 103	000
E		20.	T 100	000
F		21.	T 000	000
F♯		22.	100	000
		23.	T 000	4xy 00
G		24.	000	000

*7 ring model only.

302

Note		No.	Left Hand	Right Hand
G#		25.	G# 00	000
A		26.	A 00	000
A#		27.	R A00	000
		28.	A00	4z00
B		29.	TR 123 E	456
		30.	TR 123	456 E
		31.	A00	4zz00
		32.	R A00	4z00
C		33.	TR 123	456 F
		34.	TR 123 F	456
		35.	R A00	4zz00
C#		36.	TR 123 F#	456
		37.	TR 123	456 F#
D		38.	TR 123	456
D#		39.	TR 123	456 G#
E		40.	TR 123	450
F		41.	TR 123	400
F#		42.	TR 123	050
		43.	TR 123	406x
G		44.	TR 123	000
G#		45.	TR 123 G#	000
		46.	TR 120	450
A		47.	TR 120	000
A# Bb		48.	TR 120	4x00
		49.	TR 123x	000
		50.	TR 100	400
		51.	TR 100	050
		52.	TR 023 C#	000
		53.	*TR 103	000

Note		No.	Left Hand	Right Hand
B		54.	TR 100	000
C		55.	TR 000	000
C#		56.	TR 023	450
		57.	TR 000	4xy00
D		58.	TR 023	400 G#
D#		59.	TR 023	406x G#
		60.	TR 023	006 G#
		61.	TR 023	050 G#
E		62.	TR 023	000 G#
F		63.	TR 023 C#	000 G#
		64.	TR 123 C#	456
F#		65.	TR 020	000 G#
		66.	TR 120	456 G#
G		67.	TR 020	450 G#
		68.	TR 100	400 G#
		69.	TR 023	450 G#
		70.	TR 023x	000 G#
		71.	TR 020	4x00 G#
		72.	TR 003 C#	000 G#
		73.	TR 100	450 G#
G#		74.	TR 023	400 F#
		75.	TR 023	400 G#
		76.	TR 003	400 G#
		77.	TR 023	006 F
A		78.	TR 023	000 F#
		79.	TR 023	000 G#
		80.	TR 023 F	4x00 G#
A#		81.	TR G#23 (C#)	4xy00
		82.	TR 123 (C#)	456 F
		83.	TR 023 (C#)	456 F
		84.	R 123	456 F
B		85.	TR 120	450 F#
		86.	TR 120	450 G#
		87.	TR G#120 C#	450 G#
		88.	TR 020 F#	450 (G#)
C		89.	TR G#00	400 G#
		90.	TR 103x	406x G#
		91.	TR A00	450 G#
		92.	TR 100	400 G#

*7 ring model only.

Clarinet Trill Fingerings

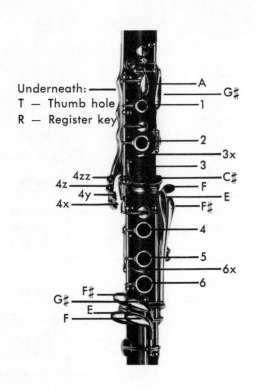

Underneath:
T — Thumb hole
R — Register key

			Left Hand	Right Hand
B C♯		9. 10. 11.	T 123 Ⓒ♯ T 123 Ⓒ♯ **T 123 C♯	050 406x 0 ⑤ 0
C♯ D		12. 13.	T 12 ③ C♯ T 12 ③ Ⓒ♯	000 000
C♯ D♯		14. 15.	T 123 C♯ *T 1 ② 3 C♯	④x00 000
D♯ E		16. 17. 18.	T 1 ② 0 T 100 *T 10③	4x00 ④00 000
E♭ F		19.	T ①②0	4x00
E F♯		20. 21.	Ⓣ 100 T 100	000 ④xy 00
F G♭		22.	T 000	④xy 00
F G		23.	T Ⓖ♯00	000
F♯ G♯		24.	T Ⓖ♯00	4xy00
G♯ A		25.	G♯00	④z 00
A♭ B♭		26.	G♯00	④zz 00
A B♭		27.	A00	④z 00
A B		28.	A00	④zz 00
A♯ B		29.	R A00	④z 00
B♭ C		30.	R A00	④zz 00

A composite fingering is given for the notes in a trill. The trill is made with the fingers and/or keys circled. Only special trill fingerings are included. Trills which are executed with regular fingerings are not included.

			Left Hand	Right Hand
E F		1. 2.	T 123 Ⓔ T 123 F	456 F 456 Ⓔ
E F♯		3. 4.	T 123 Ⓕ♯ T 123 E	456 E 456 Ⓕ♯
F G♭		5. 6.	T 123 Ⓕ♯ T 123 F	456 F 456 Ⓕ♯
F♯ G♯		7.	T 123 F♯	456 Ⓖ♯
A♯ B		8.	T 123	40 ⑥x

*7 ring model only.

**Model with articulated C#-G# key only

304

CLARINET FINGERING CHART

			Left Hand	Right Hand
B / C		31. / 32.	TR 123Ⓔ / TR 123 F	456 F / 456Ⓔ
B / C#		33. / 34.	TR 123 Ⓕ# / TR 123 E	456 E / 456 Ⓕ#
C / Db		35. / 36.	TR 123 Ⓕ# / TR 123 F	456 F / 456 Ⓕ#
C# / D#		37.	TR 123 F#	456 Ⓖ#
F / Gb		38.	TR 123	40Ⓖ#
F# / G#		39. / 40. / 41.	TR 123 Ⓒ# / TR 123 Ⓒ# / **TR 123 C#	050 / 406x / 0Ⓢ0
G# / A		42. / 43. / 44.	TR 12③ Ⓒ# / TR 123 C# / TR 120	000 / ④x00 / ④Ⓢ0
Ab / Bb		45. / 46.	TR ①23 C# / *TR 1②3 C#	000 / 000
A# / B		47. / 48.	TR 1②0 / TR 100	4x00 / ④00
Bb / C		49. / 50.	TR ①②0 / TR 123x	4x00 / ④xy00
B / C#		51. / 52. / 53.	Ⓣ®100 / TR 103 / TR 100	000 / 45Ⓢ / ④xy00
C / Db		54.	TR 000	④xy00
C / D		55. / 56.	TR Ⓖ#00 / TR 000	000 / ④z00

			Left Hand	Right Hand
C# / D#		57. / 58.	TR 023 / TRⒶ23	④50 / 450
Eb / F		59. / 60. / 61.	TR 02③ / TR 02③ / TR 02③	406x G# / 050 G# / 006 G#
E / F		62. / 63.	TR 023 Ⓒ# / TR 023	000 G# / ④x00 G#
F / Gb		64. / 65.	TR 02③ Ⓒ# / TR 023 C#	000 G# / ④x00 G#
F / G		66.	TR 0②3 C#	000 G#
F# / G		67. / 68.	TR 020 / TR 1②0	④x00 G# / 456 G#
F# / G#		69. / 70.	TR 023 / TR 020	4Ⓢ⑥ G# / ④xy00 G#
G / Ab		71.	TR 023	④50 G#
G / A		72.	TR 023	④Ⓢ0 G#
G# / A		73.	TR 023	0Ⓢ0 G#
Ab / Bb		74.	TR Ⓐ②③	4xy00 G#
A / Bb		75.	TRⒶ23	000 G#

*7 ring model only.

**Model with articulated C#-G# key only

Bassoon Fingering Chart

x—indicates key operated by one of the fingers normally covering a hole. When they are used the hole is left open.

( )—Parenthesis indicate that the use of that key or hole is optional in that fingering, depending on intonation and resonance on a particular instrument.

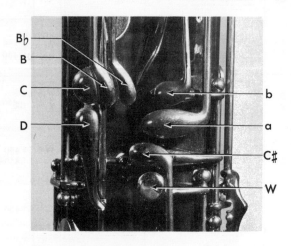

Left Thumb

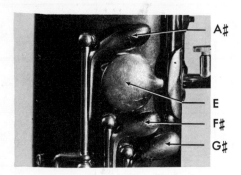

Right Thumb

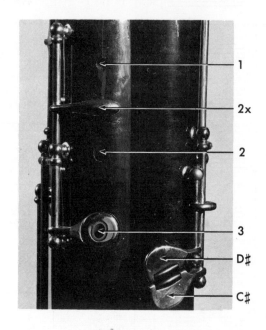

Left Hand

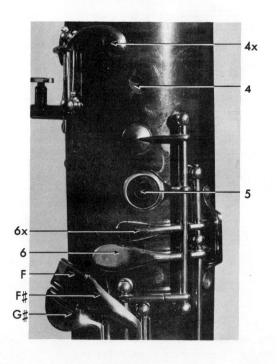

Right Hand

			Left Thumb	Left Hand	Right Thumb	Right Hand
B♭		1.	BB♭	123	E	456 F
B		2.	B	123	E	456 F
C		3.	C	123	E	456 F
C		4.	C	123 C♯	E	456 F
D		5.	D	123	E	456 F

Note		No.	Left Thumb	Left Hand	Right Thumb	Right Hand
D#		6.	D	123 D#	E	456 F
E		7.		123	E	456 F
F		8.	W	123		456 F
F#		9.	W	123	F#	456
		10.	W	123	F#	456 F#
		11.	(W)	123	E-F#	456 F#
G		12.	W	123		456
G#		13.	W	123		456 G#
		14.	W	123	G#	456
A		15.	W	123		450
A#		16.	W	123	A#	450
		17.	W	123		456x
B		18.	W	123		400
C		19.	W	123		000
C#		20.	Dc# / W	123		000
		21.	(W)	123	E	4x00 F
D		22.	W	120		000
D#		23.	W	103		000
		24.	Wc#	120		000
		25.	W	103 D#	A#	050
E		26.	W	100		000
F		27.	W	000		000
F#		28.	(W)	½23	F#	456
		29.	(W)	½23		456 F#
		30.	(W)	½23	E F#	456 F#

Note		No.	Left Thumb	Left Hand	Right Thumb	Right Hand
G		31.	(W)	½23		456
G#		32.	(W)	½23		456 G#
		33.	(W)	½23	G#	456
A		34.		123		450
A#		35.		123	A#	450
		36.		123		456x
B		37.		123		400
C		38.		123		000
C#		39.	C#	123		056 F
D		40.		120		000
		41.		120		056 F
D#		42.		120		(4)56
		43.	C#	120		000
		44.		120		006
E		45.	.	103 D#		(4)56
		46.		100		000
F		47.		103 (D#)		450
		48.		023 (D#)		450
		49.		100		450
F#		50.	W	½23 (D#)	A#	400
		51.		023 D#	A#	450
		52.		103 (D#)		450
		53.		020 D#		450 F
		54.		020		400
		55.		000 D#	G#	050
G		56.	W	½23 (D#)		400 F
		57.	W	½23 D#		000 G#
		58.	W	½23 (D#)		000
G#		59.	W	½23 (D#)		006
		60.	W	½23 (D#)	A#	000 F
A		61.	a c#	123 (D#)		006
		62.	a c#	123 (D#)		000 F
A#		63.	a c#	123 (D#)		450 F

			Left Thumb	Left Hand	Right Thumb	Right Hand
B		64.	b	120 (D♯)	A♯	450 F
C		65. 66.	b b	100 (D♯) 100 (D♯)	A♯	450 F 000
C♯		67. 68.	b b	103 (D♯) 103 (D♯)		406 (G♯) 406 (F)

			Left Thumb	Left Hand	Right Thumb	Right Hand
D		69. 70.	*b *b	003 (D♯) 003 (D♯)		006 F 006 G♯
D♯		71. 72.	*b c♯	02x3 (D♯) ½23	G♯	(4x)06 G♯ 4x00
E		73. 74.	c♯ ac♯	½23 ½2(3) D♯	G♯	056 456x

*Use key d on instruments which have this extra key.

Bassoon Trill Fingerings

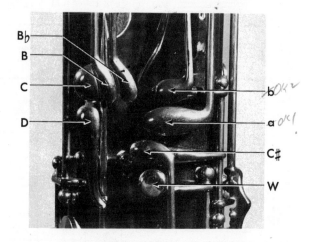

Left Thumb

A composite fingering is given for the notes in a trill. The trill is made with the fingers and/or keys circled. Only special trill fingerings are included. Trills which are executed with regular fingerings are not included.

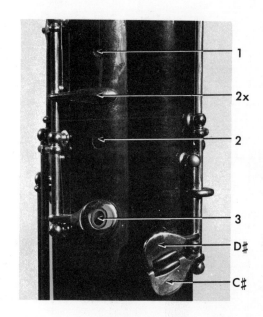

Left Hand

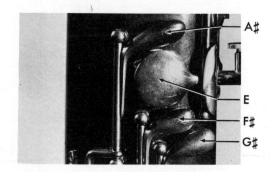

Right Thumb

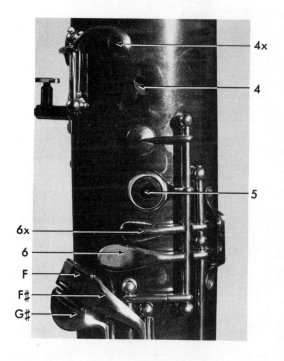

Right Hand

			Left Thumb	Left Hand	Right Thumb	Right Hand
D♯ E		1.	Ⓓ	123 D♯	E	456 F
E♭ F		2.	Dw	123 D♯	Ⓔ	456 F
F G♭		3.	W	123	Ⓕ♯	456 F
F♯ G♯		4.	W	123	F♯	456 Ⓖ♯
		5.	W	123	Ⓖ♯	456 F♯
G♯ A		6.	W	123	G♯	45 ⑥

BASSOON FINGERING CHART

Note		#	Left Thumb	Left Hand	Right Thumb	Right Hand
A#/B		7.	W	123	A#	4⑤0
Bb/C		8.	W	123	A#	④⑤0
B/C#		9.	W	12③	A#/E	050
C/Db		10.	W	123		④x 00
		11.	W	123	(A#)	④x 00
C#/D		12.	(W)	12③	E	4x00 (F)
C#/D#		13.	Dc#/W	12③		000
D/Eb		14.	(c#)	120		000
		15.	W	12③x		000
Eb/F		16.	Wc#	①②0		000
		17.	W	103		④⑤⑥Ⓕ
E/F#		18.	W	1②x 0		000
F/Gb		19.	W	0②x 0		000
F/G		20.	W	0②③		456
F#/G#		21.		½123	F#	456 Ⓖ#
		22.		½123	G#	456 F#
G/A		23.		123		45⑥
G#/A		24.	W	½2③		456 G#
Ab/Bb		25.		123	A#	45⑥
		26.		123		④⑤6 G#
A#/B		27.		123	A#	4⑤0

Note		#	Left Thumb	Left Hand	Right Thumb	Right Hand
Bb/C		28.		12③	A#	450
		29.		123	A#	④⑤0
B/C#		30.		12③		400
C/Db		31.		123	(C#)	000
		32.		123		④x 00
C#/D		33.		12③		056 F#
C#/D#		34.	C#	12③		056 F
D/Eb		35.		120		00⑥
D/E		36.		1②0 (D#)		000
D#/E		37.		120		(4)56 Ⓖ#
		38.		① 20		(4)56
Eb/F		39.		①②0		(4)56
E/F#		40.		103 (D#)		4⑤6
F/Gb		41.	(W)	(½)23 D#		4⑤0
F/G		42.	(W)	(½)23 D#		④⑤0
F#/G#		43.	W	½23 D#	A#	④⑤0 (G#)
		44.	W	020 D#	A#	④⑤0 G#
G/Ab		45.	W	½23 D#	(A#)	④x 00 G#
G/A		46.	W	½23 (D#)		④x 0 ⑥ G#
		47.	W	½23 (D#)		00⑥ G#
		48.	ⓐc#	½23		400 F
		49.	ⓑⓐ	½23		400 F
G#/A		50.	C#/ⓐ	½23 (D#)		006

			Left Thumb	Left Hand	Right Thumb	Right Hand	
Ab Bb		51.	Ⓒ# ⓐ	♭123 (D#)		④⑤0 F	✓
A Bb		52.	a c#	123 (D#)		④⑤0 F	✓
A B		53.	a	123 (D#)	A#	④⑤0 F	✓

			Left Thumb	Left Hand	Right Thumb	Right Hand	
A# B		54.	a c#	12③		450 F	
Bb C		55. 56.	b ac#	1②③ 1②③		450 F ④⑤0 F	
B C		57.	b	1②0 (D#)	A#	450 F	

Saxophone Fingering Chart

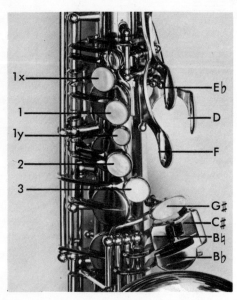

Left Hand

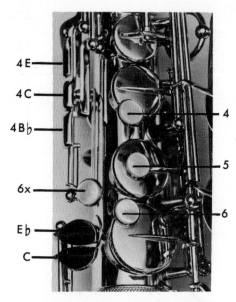

Right Hand

x, y—indicate keys operated by one of the fingers normally covering a hole. When they are used the hole is left open.

( )—Parenthesis indicate that use of that key is optional in that fingering, depending on intonation and resonance on a particular instrument.

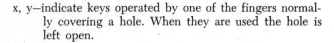

			Left Hand	Right Hand
Bb		1.	123 Bb	456 C
B		2.	123 B	456 C
C		3.	123	456 C
C♯		4.	123 C♯	456 C
D		5.	123	456
D♯		6.	123	456 Eb
E		7.	123	450
F		8.	123	400

			Left Hand	Right Hand
F♯		9.	123	050
		10.	123	406x
G		11.	123	000
G♯		12.	123 G♯	000
A		13.	120	000
A♯		14.	120	4Bb00
		15.	100	400
		16.	100	050
		17.	11y00	000
B		18.	100	000
C		19.	020	000
		20.	100	4C00
C♯		21.	000	000

Left table (upper)

Note		No.	Left Hand	Right Hand
D		22.	T 123	456
D#		23.	T 123	456 Eb
E		24.	T 123	450
F		25.	T 123	400
F#		26.	T 123	050
		27.	T 123	406x
G		28.	T 123	000
G#		29.	T 123 G#	000
A		30.	T 120	000

Right table (upper)

Note		No.	Left Hand	Right Hand
A#		31.	T 120	4Bb00
		32.	T 100	400
		33.	T 100	050
		34.	T 11y00	000
B		35.	T 100	000
C		36.	T 020	000
		37.	T 100	4C00
C#		38.	T 000	000
D		39.	T D000	000
D#		40.	T DEb000	000
E		41.	T DEb000	4E 000
F		42.	T DEbF 000	4E 000
		43.	T 1x20	000

Saxophone Extended Range

Left table (lower)

Note		No.	Left Hand	Right Hand
F#		44.	T 103	400 (Eb)
		45.	T 100	450 (Eb)
G		46.	T 103	006 (Eb)
		47.	T 020	450 (Eb)
G#		48.	T 103	000 (Eb)
		49.	T 020	050 (Eb)
A		50.	T 023	456 (Eb)
		51.	T 023	000 (Eb)
A#		52.	T 003	450 (Eb)
B		53.	T DEb 000	000 (Eb)
		54.	T Eb 100	450 (Eb)

Right table (lower)

Note		No.	Left Hand	Right Hand
C		55.	T DEb000	000 (Eb)
		56.	T 100	450 (Eb)
C#		57.	T DEb000	4E00 (Eb)
		58.	T Eb100	450 (Eb)
D		59.	T 1x00	000 (Eb)
		60.	T Eb100	000 (Eb)
D#		61.	T 1x20	400 (Eb)
		62.	T 020	050 (Eb)
E		63.	T 020	450 (Eb)
F		64.	T 103	400 (Eb)
		65.	T DEb020	450 (Eb)

Saxophone Trill Fingerings

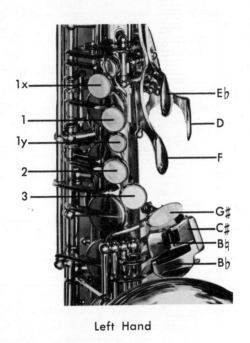

Left Hand

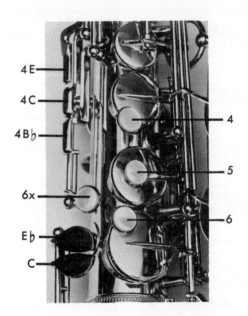

Right Hand

A composite fingering is given for the notes in a trill. The trill is made with the fingers and/or keys circled. Only special trill fingerings are included. Trills which are executed with regular fingerings are not included.

			Left Hand	Right Hand
C♯ / D		1.	123 C♯	456 Ⓒ
D♯ / E		2.	123	45 ⑥ Eb
Eb / F		3.	123	4 ⑤ ⑥ Eb
F / Gb		4.	123	40 ⑥ₓ
F♯ / G♯		5.	123 G♯	0 ⑤ 0
Ab / Bb		6.	123 G♯	④Bb 000
		7.	11y ② ③ G♯	000
A♯ / B		8.	1 ② 0	4Bb000

			Left Hand	Right Hand
Bb / C		9.	① 20	4Bb000
B / C		10.	100	④C 000
C / D		11.	Ⓔb 020	000
C♯ / D		12.	Ⓔb 000	000
C♯ / D♯		13.	000	④E 000
D♯ / E		14.	T 123	45 ⑥ Eb
Eb / F		15.	T 123	4 ⑤ ⑥ Eb

SAXOPHONE FINGERING CHART

			Left Hand	Right Hand	
F Gb		16.	T 123	40 (6x)	✓
F♯ G♯		17.	T 123 G♯	0 ⑤ 0	✓
Ab Bb		18. 19.	T 123 G♯ T 11y ② ③ G♯	(4Bb) 000 000	✓
A♯ B		20.	T 1 ② 0	4Bb000	✓
Bb C		21.	T ① 20	4Bb000	✓

			Left Hand	Right Hand	
B C		22.	T 100	(4C) 000	✓
C D		23.	T (Eb) 020	000	✓
C♯ D♯		24.	T 000	(4E) 000	✓
D E		25.	T D (F) 000	000	✓
E F		26. 27.	T DEb (F) 000 T 1x2 ③	4E 000 000	✓

315

THE SYNTHESIS OF YOGA

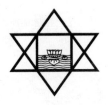

Sri Aurobindo

The Synthesis of Yoga

LOTUS PRESS
Box 325, Twin Lakes, WI 53181 USA
email: lotuspress@lotuspress.com
website: www.lotuspress.com

This edition is published and distributed in the United States
by Lotus Press, Box 325, Twin Lakes, WI 53181 USA by
arrangement with Sri Aurobindo Ashram Trust, Copyright
Department, Pondicherry 605 002 India.

ISBN: 0-941524-65-5 paperbound
0-941524-66-3 hardbound
Library of Congress Catalogue Card No. 91-76706
Second Impression: 1996
Third Impression: 2001
Printed at Sri Aurobindo Ashram Press
Pondicherry, India

Printed in India

Publisher's Note

The Synthesis of Yoga first appeared serially in the monthly review *Arya* between August 1914 and January 1921. Each instalment was written immediately before its publication. The work was left incomplete when the *Arya* was discontinued. Sri Aurobindo never attempted to complete the *Synthesis*; he did, however, lightly revise the Introduction, thoroughly revise all of Part I, "The Yoga of Divine Works", and significantly revise several chapters of Part II, "The Yoga of Integral Knowledge". More than thirty years elapsed between the first appearance of the *Synthesis* in the *Arya* and the final stages of its incomplete revision. As a result, there are some differences of terminology between the revised and unrevised portions of the book.

In 1948 the chapters making up "The Yoga of Divine Works" were published as a book by the Sri Aurobindo Library, Madras. No other part of *The Synthesis of Yoga* appeared in book-form during Sri Aurobindo's lifetime. In 1955 an edition comprising the Introduction and four Parts was brought out by the Sri Aurobindo International University Centre. The present edition, which has been checked against all manuscripts and printed texts, includes for the first time the author's revisions to the Introduction and Chapters XV–XVII of Part II, and an incomplete continuation of Part IV entitled "The Supramental Time Consciousness".

Contents

CONTENTS

PART II

THE YOGA OF INTEGRAL KNOWLEDGE

CONTENTS

CONTENTS

PART III

THE YOGA OF DIVINE LOVE

CONTENTS

CONTENTS

The Synthesis of Yoga

"All life is Yoga."

Introduction

The Conditions of the Synthesis

Chapter I

Life and Yoga

THERE are two necessities of Nature's workings which seem always to intervene in the greater forms of human activity, whether these belong to our ordinary fields of movement or seek those exceptional spheres and fulfilments which appear to us high and divine. Every such form tends towards a harmonised complexity and totality which again breaks apart into various channels of special effort and tendency, only to unite once more in a larger and more puissant synthesis. Secondly, development into forms is an imperative rule of effective manifestation; yet all truth and practice too strictly formulated becomes old and loses much, if not all, of its virtue; it must be constantly renovated by fresh streams of the spirit revivifying the dead or dying vehicle and changing it, if it is to acquire a new life. To be perpetually reborn is the condition of a material immortality. We are in an age, full of the throes of travail, when all forms of thought and activity that have in themselves any strong power of utility or any secret virtue of persistence are being subjected to a supreme test and given their opportunity of rebirth. The world today presents the aspect of a huge cauldron of Medea in which all things are being cast, shredded into pieces, experimented on, combined and recombined either to perish and provide the scattered material of new forms or to emerge rejuvenated and changed for a fresh term of existence. Indian Yoga, in its essence a special action or formulation of certain great powers of Nature, itself specialised, divided and variously formulated, is potentially one of these dynamic elements of the future life of humanity. The child of immemorial ages, preserved by its vitality and truth into our modern times, it is now emerging from the secret schools and ascetic retreats in which it had taken refuge and is seeking its place in the future sum of living human powers and utilities. But it has first to rediscover itself, bring to the surface the profoundest reason of its being in that general truth and that unceasing aim of Nature which it represents, and find by virtue of this new self-knowledge and self-appreciation its own recovered and larger synthesis. Reorganising itself, it will enter more easily and powerfully into the reorganised life of the race which its processes claim to lead within into the most secret penetralia and upward to the highest altitudes of existence and personality.

In the right view both of life and of Yoga all life is either consciously or subconsciously a Yoga. For we mean by this term a methodised effort towards self-perfection by the expression of the secret potentialities latent in the being and — highest condition of victory in that effort — a union of the human individual with the universal and transcendent Existence we see partially expressed in man and in the Cosmos. But all life, when we look behind its appearances, is a vast Yoga of Nature who attempts in the conscious and the subconscious to realise her perfection in an ever-increasing expression of her yet unrealised potentialities and to unite herself with her own divine reality. In man, her thinker, she for the first time upon this Earth devises self-conscious means and willed arrangements of activity by which this great purpose may be more swiftly and puissantly attained. Yoga, as Swami Vivekananda has said, may be regarded as a means of compressing one's evolution into a single life or a few years or even a few months of bodily existence. A given system of Yoga, then, can be no more than a selection or a compression, into narrower but more energetic forms of intensity, of the general methods which are already being used loosely, largely, in a leisurely movement, with a profuser apparent waste of material and energy but with a more complete combination by the great Mother in her vast upward labour. It is this view of Yoga that can alone form the basis for a sound and rational synthesis of Yogic methods. For then Yoga ceases to appear something mystic and abnormal which has no relation to the ordinary processes of the World-Energy or the purpose she keeps in view in her two great movements of subjective and objective self-fulfilment; it reveals itself rather as an intense and exceptional use of powers that she has already manifested or is progressively organising in her less exalted but more general operations.

Yogic methods have something of the same relation to the customary psychological workings of man as has the scientific handling of the force of electricity or of steam to their normal operations in Nature. And they, too, like the operations of Science, are formed upon a knowledge developed and confirmed by regular experiment, practical analysis and constant result. All Rajayoga, for instance, depends on this perception and experience that our inner elements, combinations, functions, forces, can be separated or dissolved, can be new-combined and set to novel and formerly impossible workings or can be transformed and resolved into a new general synthesis by fixed internal processes. Hathayoga similarly depends on this perception and experience that the vital forces and functions to which our life is normally subjected and whose ordinary operations seem set and indispensable, can be mastered and the operations changed or suspended with results that would otherwise be impossible and that seem miraculous to those who have not seized the rationale of their process. And if in some other of its forms this character of Yoga is less apparent, because they are more intuitive and less mechanical, nearer, like the Yoga of Devotion, to a supernal ecstasy or, like the Yoga of Knowledge, to a supernal infinity of consciousness and being, yet they too start from the use of some principal faculty in us by ways and for ends not contemplated in its everyday spontaneous workings. All methods grouped under the common name of Yoga are special psychological processes founded on a fixed truth of Nature and developing, out of normal functions, powers and results which were always latent but which her ordinary movements do not easily or do not often manifest.

But as in physical knowledge the multiplication of scientific processes has its disadvantages, as that tends, for instance, to develop a victorious artificiality which overwhelms our natural human life under a load of machinery and to purchase certain forms of freedom and mastery at the price of an increased servitude, so the preoccupation with Yogic processes and their exceptional results may have its disadvantages and losses. The

Yogin tends to draw away from the common existence and lose his hold upon it; he tends to purchase wealth of spirit by an impoverishment of his human activities, the inner freedom by an outer death. If he gains God, he loses life, or if he turns his efforts outward to conquer life, he is in danger of losing God. Therefore we see in India that a sharp incompatibility has been created between life in the world and spiritual growth and perfection, and although the tradition and ideal of a victorious harmony between the inner attraction and the outer demand remains, it is little or else very imperfectly exemplified. In fact, when a man turns his vision and energy inward and enters on the path of Yoga, he is popularly supposed to be lost inevitably to the great stream of our collective existence and the secular effort of humanity. So strongly has the idea prevailed, so much has it been emphasised by prevalent philosophies and religions that to escape from life is now commonly considered as not only the necessary condition, but the general object of Yoga. No synthesis of Yoga can be satisfying which does not, in its aim, reunite God and Nature in a liberated and perfected human life or, in its method, not only permit but favour the harmony of our inner and outer activities and experiences in the divine consummation of both. For man is precisely that term and symbol of a higher Existence descended into the material world in which it is possible for the lower to transfigure itself and put on the nature of the higher and the higher to reveal itself in the forms of the lower. To avoid the life which is given him for the realisation of that possibility, can never be either the indispensable condition or the whole and ultimate object of his supreme endeavour or of his most powerful means of self-fulfilment. It can only be a temporary necessity under certain conditions or a specialised extreme effort imposed on the individual so as to prepare a greater general possibility for the race. The true and full object and utility of Yoga can only be accomplished when the conscious Yoga in man becomes, like the subconscious Yoga in Nature, outwardly conterminous with life itself and we can once more, looking out both on the path and the achievement, say in a more perfect and luminous sense: "All life is Yoga."

Chapter II

The Three Steps of Nature

WE RECOGNISE then, in the past developments of Yoga, a specialising and separative tendency which, like all things in Nature, had its justifying and even imperative utility and we seek a synthesis of the specialised aims and methods which have, in consequence, come into being. But in order that we may be wisely guided in our effort, we must know, first, the general principle and purpose underlying this separative impulse and, next, the particular utilities upon which the method of each school of Yoga is founded. For the general principle we must interrogate the universal workings of Nature herself, recognising in her no merely specious and illusive activity of a distorting Maya, but the cosmic energy and working of God Himself in His universal being formulating and inspired by a vast, an infinite and yet a minutely selective Wisdom, *prajñā prasṛtā purāṇī* of the Upanishad, Wisdom that went forth from the Eternal since the beginning. For the particular utilities we must cast a penetrative eye on the different methods of Yoga and distinguish among the mass of their details the governing idea which they serve and the radical force which gives birth and energy to their processes of effectuation. Afterwards we may more easily find the one common principle and the one common power from which all derive their being and tendency, towards which all subconsciously move and in which, therefore, it is possible for all consciously to unite.

The progressive self-manifestation of Nature in man, termed in modern language his evolution, must necessarily depend upon three successive elements. There is that which is already evolved; there is that which, still imperfect, still partly fluid, is persistently in the stage of conscious evolution; and there is that which is to be evolved and may perhaps be already displayed, if not constantly, then occasionally or with some regularity of recurrence, in primary formations or in others more developed and, it may well be, even in some, however rare, that are near to the highest possible realisation of our present humanity. For the march of Nature is not drilled to a regular and mechanical forward stepping. She reaches constantly beyond herself even at the cost of subsequent deplorable retreats. She has rushes; she has splendid and mighty outbursts; she has immense realisations. She storms sometimes passionately forward hoping to take the kingdom of heaven by violence. And these self-exceedings are the revelation of that in her which is most divine or else most diabolical, but in either case the most puissant to bring her rapidly forward towards her goal.

That which Nature has evolved for us and has firmly founded is the bodily life. She has effected a certain combination and harmony of the two inferior but most fundamentally necessary elements of our action and progress upon earth, — Matter, which, however the too ethereally spiritual may despise it, is our foundation and the first condition of all our energies and realisations, and the Life-Energy which is our means of existence in a material body and the basis there even of our mental and spiritual activities. She has successfully achieved a certain stability of her constant material movement which is at once sufficiently steady and durable and sufficiently pliable and mutable to provide a fit dwelling-place and instrument for the progressively manifesting god in humanity. This is what is meant by the fable in the Aitareya Upanishad which tells us that the gods rejected the animal forms successively offered to them by the Divine Self and only when man was produced, cried out, "This indeed is perfectly made," and consented to enter in. She has effected also a working compromise between the inertia of matter and the active Life that lives in and feeds on it, by which not only is vital existence sustained, but the fullest developments of mentality are rendered possible. This equilibrium constitutes the basic status of Nature in man and is termed in the language of Yoga his gross body composed of the material or food sheath and the nervous system or vital vehicle.[1]

If, then, this inferior equilibrium is the basis and first means of the higher movements which the universal Power contemplates and if it constitutes the vehicle in which the Divine here seeks to reveal Itself, if the Indian saying is true that the body is the instrument provided for the fulfilment of the right law of our nature, then any final recoil from the physical life must be a turning away from the completeness of the divine Wisdom and a renunciation of its aim in earthly manifestation. Such a refusal may be, owing to some secret law of their development, the right attitude for certain individuals, but never the aim intended for mankind. It can be, therefore, no integral Yoga which ignores the body or makes its annulment or its rejection indispensable to a perfect spirituality. Rather, the perfecting of the body also should be the last triumph of the Spirit and to make the bodily life also divine must be God's final seal upon His work in the universe. The obstacle which the physical presents to the spiritual is no argument for the rejection of the physical; for in the unseen providence of things our greatest difficulties are our best opportunities. A supreme difficulty is Nature's indication to us of a supreme conquest to be won and an ultimate problem to be solved; it is not a warning of an inextricable snare to be shunned or of an enemy too strong for us from whom we must flee.

Equally, the vital and nervous energies in us are there for a great utility; they too demand the divine realisation of their possibilities in our ultimate fulfilment. The great part assigned to this element in the universal scheme is powerfully emphasised by the catholic wisdom of the Upanishads. "As the spokes of a wheel in its nave, so in the Life-Energy is all established, the triple knowledge and the Sacrifice and the power of the strong and the purity of the wise. Under the control of the Life-Energy is all this that is established in the triple heaven."[2] It is therefore no integral Yoga that kills these vital energies, forces them into a nerveless quiescence or roots them out as the source

---

[1] *annakoṣa* and *prāṇakoṣa*.   [2] Prasna Upanishad II. 6 and 13.

of noxious activities. Their purification, not their destruction, — their transformation, control and utilisation is the aim in view with which they have been created and developed in us.

If the bodily life is what Nature has firmly evolved for us as her base and first instrument, it is our mental life that she is evolving as her immediate next aim and superior instrument. This in her ordinary exaltations is the lofty preoccupying thought in her; this, except in her periods of exhaustion and recoil into a reposeful and recuperating obscurity, is her constant pursuit wherever she can get free from the trammels of her first vital and physical realisations. For here in man we have a distinction which is of the utmost importance. He has in him not a single mentality, but a double and a triple, the mind material and nervous, the pure intellectual mind which liberates itself from the illusions of the body and the senses, and a divine mind above intellect which in its turn liberates itself from the imperfect modes of the logically discriminative and imaginative reason. Mind in man is first emmeshed in the life of the body, where in the plant it is entirely involved and in animals always imprisoned. It accepts this life as not only the first but the whole condition of its activities and serves its needs as if they were the entire aim of existence. But the bodily life in man is a base, not the aim, his first condition and not his last determinant. In the just idea of the ancients man is essentially the thinker, the Manu, the mental being who leads the life and the body,[3] not the animal who is led by them. The true human existence, therefore, only begins when the intellectual mentality emerges out of the material and we begin more and more to live in the mind independent of the nervous and physical obsession and in the measure of that liberty are able to accept rightly and rightly to use the life of the body. For freedom and not a skilful subjection is the true means of mastery. A free, not a compulsory acceptance of the conditions, the enlarged and sublimated conditions of our physical being, is the high human ideal. But beyond this intellectual mentality is the divine.

The mental life thus evolving in man is not, indeed, a

---

[3] *manomayaḥ prāṇaśarīranetā.* Mundaka Upanishad II. 2. 8.

common possession. In actual appearance it would seem as if it were only developed to the fullest in individuals and as if there were great numbers and even the majority in whom it is either a small and ill-organised part of their normal nature or not evolved at all or latent and not easily made active. Certainly, the mental life is not a finished evolution of Nature; it is not yet firmly founded in the human animal. The sign is that the fine and full equilibrium of vitality and matter, the sane, robust, long-lived human body is ordinarily found only in races or classes of men who reject the effort of thought, its disturbances, its tensions, or think only with the material mind. Civilised man has yet to establish an equilibrium between the fully active mind and the body; he does not normally possess it. Indeed, the increasing effort towards a more intense mental life seems to create, frequently, an increasing disequilibrium of the human elements, so that it is possible for eminent scientists to describe genius as a form of insanity, a result of degeneration, a pathological morbidity of Nature. The phenomena which are used to justify this exaggeration, when taken not separately, but in connection with all other relevant data, point to a different truth. Genius is one attempt of the universal Energy to so quicken and intensify our intellectual powers that they shall be prepared for those more puissant, direct and rapid faculties which constitute the play of the supra-intellectual or divine mind. It is not, then, a freak, an inexplicable phenomenon, but a perfectly natural next step in the right line of her evolution. She has harmonised the bodily life with the material mind, she is harmonising it with the play of the intellectual mentality; for that, although it tends to a depression of the full animal and vital vigour, need not produce active disturbances. And she is shooting yet beyond in the attempt to reach a still higher level. Nor are the disturbances created by her process as great as is often represented. Some of them are the crude beginnings of new manifestations; others are an easily corrected movement of disintegration, often fruitful of fresh activities and always a small price to pay for the far-reaching results that she has in view.

We may perhaps, if we consider all the circumstances, come

to this conclusion that mental life, far from being a recent appearance in man, is the swift repetition in him of a previous achievement from which the Energy in the race had undergone one of her deplorable recoils. The savage is perhaps not so much the first forefather of civilised man as the degenerate descendant of a previous civilisation. For if the actuality of intellectual achievement is unevenly distributed, the capacity is spread everywhere. It has been seen that in individual cases even the racial type considered by us the lowest, the negro fresh from the perennial barbarism of Central Africa, is capable, without admixture of blood, without waiting for future generations, of the intellectual culture, if not yet of the intellectual accomplishment of the dominant European. Even in the mass men seem to need, in favourable circumstances, only a few generations to cover ground that ought apparently to be measured in the terms of millenniums. Either, then, man by his privilege as a mental being is exempt from the full burden of the tardy laws of evolution or else he already represents and with helpful conditions and in the right stimulating atmosphere can always display a high level of material capacity for the activities of the intellectual life. It is not mental incapacity, but the long rejection or seclusion from opportunity and withdrawal of the awakening impulse that creates the savage. Barbarism is an intermediate sleep, not an original darkness.

Moreover the whole trend of modern thought and modern endeavour reveals itself to the observant eye as a large conscious effort of Nature in man to effect a general level of intellectual equipment, capacity and farther possibility by universalising the opportunities which modern civilisation affords for the mental life. Even the preoccupation of the European intellect, the protagonist of this tendency, with material Nature and the externalities of existence is a necessary part of the effort. It seeks to prepare a sufficient basis in man's physical being and vital energies and in his material environment for his full mental possibilities. By the spread of education, by the advance of the backward races, by the elevation of depressed classes, by the multiplication of labour-saving appliances, by the movement towards ideal social and economic conditions, by the labour of Science towards an improved health, longevity and sound physique in civilised humanity, the sense and drift of this vast movement translates itself in easily intelligible signs. The right or at least the ultimate means may not always be employed, but their aim is the right preliminary aim, — a sound individual and social body and the satisfaction of the legitimate needs and demands of the material mind, sufficient ease, leisure, equal opportunity, so that the whole of mankind and no longer only the favoured race, class or individual may be free to develop the emotional and intellectual being to its full capacity. At present the material and economic aim may predominate, but always, behind, there works or there waits in reserve the higher and major impulse.

And when the preliminary conditions are satisfied, when the great endeavour has found its base, what will be the nature of that farther possibility which the activities of the intellectual life must serve? If Mind is indeed Nature's highest term, then the entire development of the rational and imaginative intellect and the harmonious satisfaction of the emotions and sensibilities must be to themselves sufficient. But if, on the contrary, man is more than a reasoning and emotional animal, if beyond that which is being evolved, there is something that has to be evolved, then it may well be that the fullness of the mental life, the suppleness, flexibility and wide capacity of the intellect, the ordered richness of emotion and sensibility may be only a passage towards the development of a higher life and of more powerful faculties which are yet to manifest and to take possession of the lower instrument, just as mind itself has so taken possession of the body that the physical being no longer lives only for its own satisfaction but provides the foundation and the materials for a superior activity.

The assertion of a higher than the mental life is the whole foundation of Indian philosophy and its acquisition and organisation is the veritable object served by the methods of Yoga. Mind is not the last term of evolution, not an ultimate aim, but, like body, an instrument. It is even so termed in the language of

Yoga, the inner instrument.[4] And Indian tradition asserts that this which is to be manifested is not a new term in human experience, but has been developed before and has even governed humanity in certain periods of its development. In any case, in order to be known it must at one time have been partly developed. And if since then Nature has sunk back from her achievement, the reason must always be found in some unrealised harmony, some insufficiency of the intellectual and material basis to which she has now returned, some over-specialisation of the higher to the detriment of the lower existence.

But what then constitutes this higher or highest existence to which our evolution is tending? In order to answer the question we have to deal with a class of supreme experiences, a class of unusual conceptions which it is difficult to represent accurately in any other language than the ancient Sanskrit tongue in which alone they have been to some extent systematised. The only approximate terms in the English language have other associations and their use may lead to many and even serious inaccuracies. The terminology of Yoga recognises besides the status of our physical and vital being, termed the gross body and doubly composed of the food sheath and the vital vehicle, besides the status of our mental being, termed the subtle body and singly composed of the mind sheath or mental vehicle,[5] a third, supreme and divine status of supra-mental being, termed the causal body and composed of a fourth and a fifth vehicle[6] which are described as those of knowledge and bliss. But this knowledge is not a systematised result of mental questionings and reasonings, not a temporary arrangement of conclusions and opinions in the terms of the highest probability, but rather a pure self-existent and self-luminous Truth. And this bliss is not a supreme pleasure of the heart and sensations with the experience of pain and sorrow as its background, but a delight also self-existent and independent of objects and particular experiences, a self-delight which is the very nature, the very stuff, as it were, of a transcendent and infinite existence.

---

[4] *antaḥkaraṇa.*   [5] *manaḥ-koṣa.*   [6] *vijñānakoṣa* and *ānandakoṣa.*

Do such psychological conceptions correspond to anything real and possible? All Yoga asserts them as its ultimate experience and supreme aim. They form the governing principles of our highest possible state of consciousness, our widest possible range of existence. There is, we say, a harmony of supreme faculties, corresponding roughly to the psychological faculties of revelation, inspiration and intuition, yet acting not in the intuitive reason or the divine mind, but on a still higher plane, which see Truth directly face to face, or rather live in the truth of things both universal and transcendent and are its formulation and luminous activity. And these faculties are the light of a conscious existence superseding the egoistic and itself both cosmic and transcendent, the nature of which is Bliss. These are obviously divine and, as man is at present apparently constituted, superhuman states of consciousness and activity. A trinity of transcendent existence, self-awareness and self-delight[7] is, indeed, the metaphysical description of the supreme Atman, the self-formulation, to our awakened knowledge, of the Unknowable whether conceived as a pure Impersonality or as a cosmic Personality manifesting the universe. But in Yoga they are regarded also in their psychological aspects as states of subjective existence to which our waking consciousness is now alien, but which dwell in us in a superconscious plane and to which, therefore, we may always ascend.

For, as is indicated by the name, causal body (*kāraṇa*), as opposed to the two others which are instruments (*karaṇa*), this crowning manifestation is also the source and effective power of all that in the actual evolution has preceded it. Our mental activities are, indeed, a derivation, selection and, so long as they are divided from the truth that is secretly their source, a deformation of the divine knowledge. Our sensations and emotions have the same relation to the Bliss, our vital forces and actions to the aspect of Will or Force assumed by the divine consciousness, our physical being to the pure essence of that Bliss and Consciousness. The evolution which we observe and of which

---

[7] *saccidānanda.*

we are the terrestrial summit may be considered, in a sense, as an inverse manifestation, by which these supreme Powers in their unity and their diversity use, develop and perfect the imperfect substance and activities of Matter, of Life and of Mind so that they, the inferior modes, may express in mutable relativity an increasing harmony of the divine and eternal states from which they are born. If this be the truth of the universe, then the goal of evolution is also its cause, it is that which is immanent in its elements and out of them is liberated. But the liberation is surely imperfect if it is only an escape and there is no return upon the containing substance and activities to exalt and transform them. The immanence itself would have no credible reason for being if it did not end in such a transfiguration. But if human mind can become capable of the glories of the divine Light, human emotion and sensibility can be transformed into the mould and assume the measure and movement of the supreme Bliss, human action not only represent but feel itself to be the motion of a divine and non-egoistic Force and the physical substance of our being sufficiently partake of the purity of the supernal essence, sufficiently unify plasticity and durable constancy to support and prolong these highest experiences and agencies, then all the long labour of Nature will end in a crowning justification and her evolutions reveal their profound significance.

So dazzling is even a glimpse of this supreme existence and so absorbing its attraction that, once seen, we feel readily justified in neglecting all else for its pursuit. Even, by an opposite exaggeration to that which sees all things in Mind and the mental life as an exclusive ideal, Mind comes to be regarded as an unworthy deformation and a supreme obstacle, the source of an illusory universe, a negation of the Truth and itself to be denied and all its works and results annulled if we desire the final liberation. But this is a half-truth which errs by regarding only the actual limitations of Mind and ignores its divine intention. The ultimate knowledge is that which perceives and accepts God in the universe as well as beyond the universe; the integral Yoga is that which, having found the Transcendent, can return upon the universe and possess it, retaining the power freely to descend as well as ascend the great stair of existence. For if the eternal Wisdom exists at all, the faculty of Mind also must have some high use and destiny. That use must depend on its place in the ascent and in the return and that destiny must be a fulfilment and transfiguration, not a rooting out or an annulling.

We perceive, then, these three steps in Nature, a bodily life which is the basis of our existence here in the material world, a mental life into which we emerge and by which we raise the bodily to higher uses and enlarge it into a greater completeness, and a divine existence which is at once the goal of the other two and returns upon them to liberate them into their highest possibilities. Regarding none of them as either beyond our reach or below our nature and the destruction of none of them as essential to the ultimate attainment, we accept this liberation and fulfilment as part at least and a large and important part of the aim of Yoga.

The Threefold Life

NATURE, then, is an evolution or progressive self-manifestation of an eternal and secret existence, with three successive forms as her three steps of ascent. And we have consequently as the condition of all our activities these three mutually interdependent possibilities, the bodily life, the mental existence and the veiled spiritual being which is in the involution the cause of the others and in the evolution their result. Preserving and perfecting the physical, fulfilling the mental, it is Nature's aim and it should be ours to unveil in the perfected body and mind the transcendent activities of the Spirit. As the mental life does not abrogate but works for the elevation and better utilisation of the bodily existence, so too the spiritual should not abrogate but transfigure our intellectual, emotional, aesthetic and vital activities.

For man, the head of terrestrial Nature, the sole earthly frame in which her full evolution is possible, is a triple birth. He has been given a living frame in which the body is the vessel and life the dynamic means of a divine manifestation. His activity is centred in a progressive mind which aims at perfecting itself as well as the house in which it dwells and the means of life that it uses, and is capable of awaking by a progressive self-realisation to its own true nature as a form of the Spirit. He culminates in what he always really was, the illumined and beatific spirit which is intended at last to irradiate life and mind with its now concealed splendours.

Since this is the plan of the divine Energy in humanity, the whole method and aim of our existence must work by the interaction of these three elements in the being. As a result of their separate formulation in Nature, man has open to him a choice between three kinds of life, the ordinary material existence, a life of mental activity and progress and the unchanging spiritual beatitude. But he can, as he progresses, combine these three forms, resolve their discords into a harmonious rhythm and so create in himself the whole godhead, the perfect Man.

In ordinary Nature they have each their own characteristic and governing impulse.

The characteristic energy of bodily Life is not so much in progress as in persistence, not so much in individual self-enlargement as in self-repetition. There is, indeed, in physical Nature a progression from type to type, from the vegetable to the animal, from the animal to man; for even in inanimate Matter Mind is at work. But once a type is marked off physically, the chief immediate preoccupation of the terrestrial Mother seems to be to keep it in being by a constant reproduction. For Life always seeks immortality; but since individual form is impermanent and only the idea of a form is permanent in the consciousness that creates the universe, — for there it does not perish, — such constant reproduction is the only possible material immortality. Self-preservation, self-repetition, self-multiplication are necessarily, then, the predominant instincts of all material existence. Material life seems ever to move in a fixed cycle.

The characteristic energy of pure Mind is change, and the more our mentality acquires elevation and organisation, the more this law of Mind assumes the aspect of a continual enlargement, improvement and better arrangement of its gains and so of a continual passage from a smaller and simpler to a larger and more complex perfection. For Mind, unlike bodily life, is infinite in its field, elastic in its expansion, easily variable in its formations. Change, then, self-enlargement and self-improvement are its proper instincts. Mind too moves in cycles, but these are ever-enlarging spirals. Its faith is perfectibility, its watchword is progress.

The characteristic law of Spirit is self-existent perfection and immutable infinity. It possesses always and in its own right the immortality which is the aim of Life and the perfection which is the goal of Mind. The attainment of the eternal and the realisation of that which is the same in all things and beyond all things, equally blissful in universe and outside it, untouched by the imperfections and limitations of the forms and activities in which it dwells, are the glory of the spiritual life.

In each of these forms Nature acts both individually and collectively; for the Eternal affirms Himself equally in the single form and in the group-existence, whether family, clan and nation or groupings dependent on less physical principles or the supreme group of all, our collective humanity. Man also may seek his own individual good from any or all of these spheres of activity, or identify himself in them with the collectivity and live for it, or, rising to a truer perception of this complex universe, harmonise the individual realisation with the collective aim. For as it is the right relation of the soul with the Supreme, while it is in the universe, neither to assert egoistically its separate being nor to blot itself out in the Indefinable, but to realise its unity with the Divine and the world and unite them in the individual, so the right relation of the individual with the collectivity is neither to pursue egoistically his own material or mental progress or spiritual salvation without regard to his fellows, nor for the sake of the community to suppress or maim his proper development, but to sum up in himself all its best and completest possibilities and pour them out by thought, action and all other means on his surroundings so that the whole race may approach nearer to the attainment of its supreme personalities.

It follows that the object of the material life must be to fulfil, above all things, the vital aim of Nature. The whole aim of the material man is to live, to pass from birth to death with as much comfort or enjoyment as may be on the way, but anyhow to live. He can subordinate this aim, but only to physical Nature's other instincts, the reproduction of the individual and the conservation of the type in the family, class or community. Self, domesticity, the accustomed order of the society and of the nation are the constituents of the material existence. Its immense importance in the economy of Nature is self-evident, and commensurate is the importance of the human type which represents it. He assures her of the safety of the framework she has made and of the orderly continuance and conservation of her past gains.

But by that very utility such men and the life they lead are condemned to be limited, irrationally conservative and earth-bound. The customary routine, the customary institutions, the inherited or habitual forms of thought, — these things are the life-breath of their nostrils. They admit and jealously defend the changes compelled by the progressive mind in the past, but combat with equal zeal the changes that are being made by it in the present. For to the material man the living progressive thinker is an ideologue, dreamer or madman. The old Semites who stoned the living prophets and adored their memories when dead, were the very incarnation of this instinctive and unintelligent principle in Nature. In the ancient Indian distinction between the once born and the twice born, it is to this material man that the former description can be applied. He does Nature's inferior works; he assures the basis for her higher activities; but not to him easily are opened the glories of her second birth.

Yet he admits so much of spirituality as has been enforced on his customary ideas by the great religious outbursts of the past and he makes in his scheme of society a place, venerable though not often effective, for the priest or the learned theologian who can be trusted to provide him with a safe and ordinary spiritual pabulum. But to the man who would assert for himself the liberty of spiritual experience and the spiritual life, he assigns, if he admits him at all, not the vestment of the priest but the robe of the Sannyasin. Outside society let him exercise his dangerous freedom. So he may even serve as a human lightning-rod receiving the electricity of the Spirit and turning it away from the social edifice.

Nevertheless it is possible to make the material man and his life moderately progressive by imprinting on the material mind the custom of progress, the habit of conscious change, the fixed idea of progression as a law of life. The creation by this means of progressive societies in Europe is one of the greatest triumphs of Mind over Matter. But the physical nature has its revenge; for the progress made tends to be of the grosser and more outward kind and its attempts at a higher or a more rapid movement bring about great wearinesses, swift exhaustions, startling recoils.

It is possible also to give the material man and his life a moderate spirituality by accustoming him to regard in a religious spirit all the institutions of life and its customary activities. The creation of such spiritualised communities in the East has been one of the greatest triumphs of Spirit over Matter. Yet here, too, there is a defect; for this often tends only to the creation of a religious temperament, the most outward form of spirituality. Its higher manifestations, even the most splendid and puissant, either merely increase the number of souls drawn out of social life and so impoverish it or disturb the society for a while by a momentary elevation. The truth is that neither the mental effort nor the spiritual impulse can suffice, divorced from each other, to overcome the immense resistance of material Nature. She demands their alliance in a complete effort before she will suffer a complete change in humanity. But, usually, these two great agents are unwilling to make to each other the necessary concessions.

The mental life concentrates on the aesthetic, the ethical and the intellectual activities. Essential mentality is idealistic and a seeker after perfection. The subtle self, the brilliant Atman,[1] is ever a dreamer. A dream of perfect beauty, perfect conduct, perfect Truth, whether seeking new forms of the Eternal or revitalising the old, is the very soul of pure mentality. But it knows not how to deal with the resistance of Matter. There it is hampered and inefficient, works by bungling experiments and has either to withdraw from the struggle or submit to the grey actuality. Or else, by studying the material life and accepting the conditions of the contest, it may succeed, but only in imposing temporarily some artificial system which infinite Nature either rends and casts aside or disfigures out of recognition or by withdrawing her assent leaves as the corpse of a dead ideal. Few and far between have been those realisations of the dreamer in Man which the world has gladly accepted, looks back to with a fond memory and seeks, in its elements, to cherish.

---

[1] Who dwells in Dream, the inly conscious, the enjoyer of abstractions, the Brilliant. Mandukya Upanishad 4.

When the gulf between actual life and the temperament of the thinker is too great, we see as the result a sort of withdrawing of the Mind from life in order to act with a greater freedom in its own sphere. The poet living among his brilliant visions, the artist absorbed in his art, the philosopher thinking out the problems of the intellect in his solitary chamber, the scientist, the scholar caring only for their studies and their experiments, were often in former days, are even now not unoften the Sannyasins of the intellect. To the work they have done for humanity, all its past bears record.

But such seclusion is justified only by some special activity. Mind finds fully its force and action only when it casts itself upon life and accepts equally its possibilities and its resistances as the means of a greater self-perfection. In the struggle with the difficulties of the material world the ethical development of the individual is firmly shaped and the great schools of conduct are formed; by contact with the facts of life Art attains to vitality, Thought assures its abstractions, the generalisations of the philosopher base themselves on a stable foundation of science and experience.

This mixing with life may, however, be pursued for the sake of the individual mind and with an entire indifference to the forms of the material existence or the uplifting of the race. This indifference is seen at its highest in the Epicurean discipline and is not entirely absent from the Stoic; and even altruism does the works of compassion more often for its own sake than for the sake of the world it helps. But this too is a limited fulfilment. The progressive mind is seen at its noblest when it strives to elevate the whole race to its own level whether by sowing broadcast the image of its own thought and fulfilment or by changing the material life of the race into fresh forms, religious, intellectual, social or political, intended to represent more nearly that ideal of truth, beauty, justice, righteousness with which the man's own soul is illumined. Failure in such a field matters little; for the mere attempt is dynamic and creative. The struggle of Mind to elevate life is the promise and condition of the conquest of life by that which is higher even than Mind.

That highest thing, the spiritual existence, is concerned with what is eternal but not therefore entirely aloof from the transient. For the spiritual man the mind's dream of perfect beauty is realised in an eternal love, beauty and delight that has no dependence and is equal behind all objective appearances; its dream of perfect Truth in the supreme, self-existent, self-apparent and eternal Verity which never varies, but explains and is the secret of all variations and the goal of all progress; its dream of perfect action in the omnipotent and self-guiding Law that is inherent for ever in all things and translates itself here in the rhythm of the worlds. What is fugitive vision or constant effort of creation in the brilliant Self is an eternally existing Reality in the Self that knows[2] and is the Lord.

But if it is often difficult for the mental life to accommodate itself to the dully resistant material activity, how much more difficult must it seem for the spiritual existence to live on in a world that appears full not of the Truth but of every lie and illusion, not of Love and Beauty but of an encompassing discord and ugliness, not of the Law of Truth but of victorious selfishness and sin? Therefore the spiritual life tends easily in the saint and Sannyasin to withdraw from the material existence and reject it either wholly and physically or in the spirit. It sees this world as the kingdom of evil or of ignorance and the eternal and divine either in a far-off heaven or beyond where there is no world and no life. It separates itself inwardly, if not also physically, from the world's impurities; it asserts the spiritual reality in a spotless isolation. This withdrawal renders an invaluable service to the material life itself by forcing it to regard and even to bow down to something that is the direct negation of its own petty ideals, sordid cares and egoistic self-content.

But the work in the world of so supreme a power as spiritual force cannot be thus limited. The spiritual life also can return upon the material and use it as a means of its own greater

---

[2] The Unified, in whom conscious thought is concentrated, who is all delight and enjoyer of delight, the Wise. . . . He is the Lord of all, the Omniscient, the inner Guide. Mandukya Upanishad 5, 6.

fullness. Refusing to be blinded by the dualities, the appearances, it can seek in all appearances whatsoever the vision of the same Lord, the same eternal Truth, Beauty, Love, Delight. The Vedantic formula of the Self in all things, all things in the Self and all things as becomings of the Self is the key to this richer and all-embracing Yoga.

But the spiritual life, like the mental, may thus make use of this outward existence for the benefit of the individual with a perfect indifference to any collective uplifting of the merely symbolic world which it uses. Since the Eternal is for ever the same in all things and all things the same to the Eternal, since the exact mode of action and the result are of no importance compared with the working out in oneself of the one great realisation, this spiritual indifference accepts no matter what environment, no matter what action, dispassionately, prepared to retire as soon as its own supreme end is realised. It is so that many have understood the ideal of the Gita. Or else the inner love and bliss may pour itself out on the world in good deeds, in service, in compassion, the inner Truth in the giving of knowledge, without therefore attempting the transformation of a world which must by its inalienable nature remain a battlefield of the dualities, of sin and virtue, of truth and error, of joy and suffering.

But if Progress also is one of the chief terms of world-existence and a progressive manifestation of the Divine the true sense of Nature, this limitation also is invalid. It is possible for the spiritual life in the world, and it is its real mission, to change the material life into its own image, the image of the Divine. Therefore, besides the great solitaries who have sought and attained their self-liberation, we have the great spiritual teachers who have also liberated others and, supreme of all, the great dynamic souls who, feeling themselves stronger in the might of the Spirit than all the forces of the material life banded together, have thrown themselves upon the world, grappled with it in a loving wrestle and striven to compel its consent to its own transfiguration. Ordinarily, the effort is concentrated on a mental and moral change in humanity, but it may extend itself also to the alteration of the forms of our life and its institutions so that they too may be a better mould for the inpourings of the Spirit. These attempts have been the supreme landmarks in the progressive development of human ideals and the divine preparation of the race. Every one of them, whatever its outward results, has left Earth more capable of Heaven and quickened in its tardy movements the evolutionary Yoga of Nature.

In India, for the last thousand years and more, the spiritual life and the material have existed side by side to the exclusion of the progressive mind. Spirituality has made terms for itself with Matter by renouncing the attempt at general progress. It has obtained from society the right of free spiritual development for all who assume some distinctive symbol, such as the garb of the Sannyasin, the recognition of that life as man's goal and those who live it as worthy of an absolute reverence, and the casting of society itself into such a religious mould that its most customary acts should be accompanied by a formal reminder of the spiritual symbolism of life and its ultimate destination. On the other hand, there was conceded to society the right of inertia and immobile self-conservation. The concession destroyed much of the value of the terms. The religious mould being fixed, the formal reminder tended to become a routine and to lose its living sense. The constant attempts to change the mould by new sects and religions ended only in a new routine or a modification of the old; for the saving element of the free and active mind had been exiled. The material life, handed over to the Ignorance, the purposeless and endless duality, became a leaden and dolorous yoke from which flight was the only escape.

The schools of Indian Yoga lent themselves to the compromise. Individual perfection or liberation was made the aim, seclusion of some kind from the ordinary activities the condition, the renunciation of life the culmination. The teacher gave his knowledge only to a small circle of disciples. Or if a wider movement was attempted, it was still the release of the individual soul that remained the aim. The pact with an immobile society was, for the most part, observed.

The utility of the compromise in the then actual state of the world cannot be doubted. It secured in India a society which lent itself to the preservation and the worship of spirituality, a country apart in which as in a fortress the highest spiritual ideal could maintain itself in its most absolute purity unoverpowered by the siege of the forces around it. But it was a compromise, not an absolute victory. The material life lost the divine impulse to growth, the spiritual preserved by isolation its height and purity, but sacrificed its full power and serviceableness to the world. Therefore, in the divine Providence the country of the Yogins and the Sannyasins has been forced into a strict and imperative contact with the very element it had rejected, the element of the progressive Mind, so that it might recover what was now wanting to it.

We have to recognise once more that the individual exists not in himself alone but in the collectivity and that individual perfection and liberation are not the whole sense of God's intention in the world. The free use of our liberty includes also the liberation of others and of mankind; the perfect utility of our perfection is, having realised in ourselves the divine symbol, to reproduce, multiply and ultimately universalise it in others.

Therefore from a concrete view of human life in its threefold potentialities we come to the same conclusion that we had drawn from an observation of Nature in her general workings and the three steps of her evolution. And we begin to perceive a complete aim for our synthesis of Yoga.

Spirit is the crown of universal existence; Matter is its basis; Mind is the link between the two. Spirit is that which is eternal; Mind and Matter are its workings. Spirit is that which is concealed and has to be revealed; mind and body are the means by which it seeks to reveal itself. Spirit is the image of the Lord of the Yoga; mind and body are the means He has provided for reproducing that image in phenomenal existence. All Nature is an attempt at a progressive revelation of the concealed Truth, a more and more successful reproduction of the divine image.

But what Nature aims at for the mass in a slow evolution, Yoga effects for the individual by a rapid revolution. It works by a quickening of all her energies, a sublimation of all her faculties. While she develops the spiritual life with difficulty and has constantly to fall back from it for the sake of her lower realisations, the sublimated force, the concentrated method of Yoga can attain directly and carry with it the perfection of the mind and even, if she will, the perfection of the body. Nature seeks the Divine in her own symbols: Yoga goes beyond Nature to the Lord of Nature, beyond universe to the Transcendent and can return with the transcendent light and power, with the fiat of the Omnipotent.

But their aim is one in the end. The generalisation of Yoga in humanity must be the last victory of Nature over her own delays and concealments. Even as now by the progressive mind in Science she seeks to make all mankind fit for the full development of the mental life, so by Yoga must she inevitably seek to make all mankind fit for the higher evolution, the second birth, the spiritual existence. And as the mental life uses and perfects the material, so will the spiritual use and perfect the material and the mental existence as the instruments of a divine self-expression. The ages when that is accomplished, are the legendary Satya or Krita[3] Yugas, the ages of the Truth manifested in the symbol, of the great work done when Nature in mankind, illumined, satisfied and blissful, rests in the culmination of her endeavour.

It is for man to know her meaning, no longer misunderstanding, vilifying or misusing the universal Mother, and to aspire always by her mightiest means to her highest ideal.

---

[3] Satya means Truth; Krita, effected or completed.

Chapter IV

The Systems of Yoga

THESE relations between the different psychological divisions of the human being and these various utilities and objects of effort founded on them, such as we have seen them in our brief survey of the natural evolution, we shall find repeated in the fundamental principles and methods of the different schools of Yoga. And if we seek to combine and harmonise their central practices and their predominant aims, we shall find that the basis provided by Nature is still our natural basis and the condition of their synthesis.

In one respect Yoga exceeds the normal operation of cosmic Nature and climbs beyond her. For the aim of the Universal Mother is to embrace the Divine in her own play and creations and there to realise It. But in the highest flights of Yoga she reaches beyond herself and realises the Divine in Itself exceeding the universe and even standing apart from the cosmic play. Therefore by some it is supposed that this is not only the highest but also the one true or exclusively preferable object of Yoga.

Yet it is always through something which she has formed in her evolution that Nature thus overpasses her evolution. It is the individual heart that by sublimating its highest and purest emotions attains to the transcendent Bliss or the ineffable Nirvana, the individual mind that by converting its ordinary functionings into a knowledge beyond mentality knows its oneness with the Ineffable and merges its separate existence in that transcendent unity. And always it is the individual, the Self conditioned in its experience by Nature and working through her formations, that attains to the Self unconditioned, free and transcendent.

In practice three conceptions are necessary before there can be any possibility of Yoga; there must be, as it were, three consenting parties to the effort, — God, Nature and the human soul or, in more abstract language, the Transcendental, the Universal and the Individual. If the individual and Nature are left to themselves, the one is bound to the other and unable to exceed appreciably her lingering march. Something transcendent is needed, free from her and greater, which will act upon us and her, attracting us upward to Itself and securing from her by good grace or by force her consent to the individual ascension.

It is this truth which makes necessary to every philosophy of Yoga the conception of the Ishwara, Lord, supreme Soul or supreme Self, towards whom the effort is directed and who gives the illuminating touch and the strength to attain. Equally true is the complementary idea so often enforced by the Yoga of devotion that as the Transcendent is necessary to the individual and sought after by him, so also the individual is necessary in a sense to the Transcendent and sought after by It. If the Bhakta seeks and yearns after Bhagavan, Bhagavan also seeks and yearns after the Bhakta.[1] There can be no Yoga of knowledge without a human seeker of the knowledge, the supreme subject of knowledge and the divine use by the individual of the universal faculties of knowledge; no Yoga of devotion without the human God-lover, the supreme object of love and delight and the divine use by the individual of the universal faculties of spiritual, emotional and aesthetic enjoyment; no Yoga of works without the human worker, the supreme Will, Master of all works and sacrifices, and the divine use by the individual of the universal faculties of power and action. However Monistic may be our intellectual conception of the highest truth of things, in practice we are compelled to accept this omnipresent Trinity.

For the contact of the human and individual consciousness with the divine is the very essence of Yoga. Yoga is the union of that which has become separated in the play of the universe with its own true self, origin and universality. The contact may take place at any point of the complex and intricately organised consciousness which we call our personality. It may be effected in the physical through the body; in the vital through the action of

---

[1] Bhakta, the devotee or lover of God; Bhagavan, God, the Lord of Love and Delight. The third term of the trinity is Bhagavat, the divine revelation of Love.

those functionings which determine the state and the experiences of our nervous being; through the mentality, whether by means of the emotional heart, the active will or the understanding mind, or more largely by a general conversion of the mental consciousness in all its activities. It may equally be accomplished through a direct awakening to the universal or transcendent Truth and Bliss by the conversion of the central ego in the mind. And according to the point of contact that we choose will be the type of the Yoga that we practise.

For if, leaving aside the complexities of their particular processes, we fix our regard on the central principle of the chief schools of Yoga still prevalent in India, we find that they arrange themselves in an ascending order which starts from the lowest rung of the ladder, the body, and ascends to the direct contact between the individual soul and the transcendent and universal Self. Hathayoga selects the body and the vital functionings as its instruments of perfection and realisation; its concern is with the gross body. Rajayoga selects the mental being in its different parts as its lever-power; it concentrates on the subtle body. The triple Path of Works, of Love and of Knowledge uses some part of the mental being, will, heart or intellect as a starting-point and seeks by its conversion to arrive at the liberating Truth, Beatitude and Infinity which are the nature of the spiritual life. Its method is a direct commerce between the human Purusha in the individual body and the divine Purusha who dwells in every body and yet transcends all form and name.

Hathayoga aims at the conquest of the life and the body whose combination in the food sheath and the vital vehicle constitutes, as we have seen, the gross body and whose equilibrium is the foundation of all Nature's workings in the human being. The equilibrium established by Nature is sufficient for the normal egoistic life; it is insufficient for the purpose of the Hathayogin. For it is calculated on the amount of vital or dynamic force necessary to drive the physical engine during the normal span of human life and to perform more or less adequately the various workings demanded of it by the individual life inhabiting this frame and the world-environment by which it is conditioned.

Hathayoga therefore seeks to rectify Nature and establish another equilibrium by which the physical frame will be able to sustain the inrush of an increasing vital or dynamic force of Prana indefinite, almost infinite in its quantity or intensity. In Nature the equilibrium is based upon the individualisation of a limited quantity and force of the Prana; more than that the individual is by personal and hereditary habit unable to bear, use or control. In Hathayoga, the equilibrium opens a door to the universalisation of the individual vitality by admitting into the body, containing, using and controlling a much less fixed and limited action of the universal energy.

The chief processes of Hathayoga are *āsana* and *prāṇāyāma*. By its numerous *āsanas* or fixed postures it first cures the body of that restlessness which is a sign of its inability to contain without working them off in action and movement the vital forces poured into it from the universal Life-Ocean, gives to it an extraordinary health, force and suppleness and seeks to liberate it from the habits by which it is subjected to ordinary physical Nature and kept within the narrow bounds of her normal operations. In the ancient tradition of Hathayoga it has always been supposed that this conquest could be pushed so far even as to conquer to a great extent the force of gravitation. By various subsidiary but elaborate processes the Hathayogin next contrives to keep the body free from all impurities and the nervous system unclogged for those exercises of respiration which are his most important instruments. These are called *prāṇāyāma*, the control of the breath or vital power; for breathing is the chief physical functioning of the vital forces. Pranayama, for the Hathayogin, serves a double purpose. First, it completes the perfection of the body. The vitality is liberated from many of the ordinary necessities of physical Nature; robust health, prolonged youth, often an extraordinary longevity are attained. On the other hand, Pranayama awakens the coiled-up serpent of the Pranic dynamism in the vital sheath and opens to the Yogin fields of consciousness, ranges of experience, abnormal faculties denied to the ordinary human life while it puissantly intensifies such normal powers and faculties as he already possesses.

These advantages can be farther secured and emphasised by other subsidiary processes open to the Hathayogin.

The results of Hathayoga are thus striking to the eye and impose easily on the vulgar or physical mind. And yet at the end we may ask what we have gained at the end of all this stupendous labour. The object of physical Nature, the preservation of the mere physical life, its highest perfection, even in a certain sense the capacity of a greater enjoyment of physical living have been carried out on an abnormal scale. But the weakness of Hathayoga is that its laborious and difficult processes make so great a demand on the time and energy and impose so complete a severance from the ordinary life of men that the utilisation of its results for the life of the world becomes either impracticable or is extraordinarily restricted. If in return for this loss we gain another life in another world within, the mental, the dynamic, these results could have been acquired through other systems, through Rajayoga, through Tantra, by much less laborious methods and held on much less exacting terms. On the other hand the physical results, increased vitality, prolonged youth, health, longevity are of small avail if they must be held by us as misers of ourselves, apart from the common life, for their own sake, not utilised, not thrown into the common sum of the world's activities. Hathayoga attains large results, but at an exorbitant price and to very little purpose.

Rajayoga takes a higher flight. It aims at the liberation and perfection not of the bodily, but of the mental being, the control of the emotional and sensational life, the mastery of the whole apparatus of thought and consciousness. It fixes its eyes on the *citta*, that stuff of mental consciousness in which all these activities arise, and it seeks, even as Hathayoga with its physical material, first to purify and to tranquillise. The normal state of man is a condition of trouble and disorder, a kingdom either at war with itself or badly governed; for the lord, the Purusha, is subjected to his ministers, the faculties, subjected even to his subjects, the instruments of sensation, emotion, action, enjoyment. Swarajya, self-rule, must be substituted for this subjection. First, therefore, the powers of order must be helped to overcome the powers of disorder. The preliminary movement of Rajayoga is a careful self-discipline by which good habits of mind are substituted for the lawless movements that indulge the lower nervous being. By the practice of truth, by renunciation of all forms of egoistic seeking, by abstention from injury to others, by purity, by constant meditation and inclination to the divine Purusha who is the true lord of the mental kingdom, a pure, glad, clear state of mind and heart is established.

This is the first step only. Afterwards, the ordinary activities of the mind and sense must be entirely quieted in order that the soul may be free to ascend to higher states of consciousness and acquire the foundation for a perfect freedom and self-mastery. But Rajayoga does not forget that the disabilities of the ordinary mind proceed largely from its subjection to the reactions of the nervous system and the body. It adopts therefore from the Hathayogic system its devices of *āsana* and *prāṇāyāma*, but reduces their multiple and elaborate forms in each case to one simplest and most directly effective process sufficient for its own immediate object. Thus it gets rid of the Hathayogic complexity and cumbrousness while it utilises the swift and powerful efficacy of its methods for the control of the body and the vital functions and for the awakening of that internal dynamism, full of a latent supernormal faculty, typified in Yogic terminology by the *kuṇḍalinī*, the coiled and sleeping serpent of Energy within. This done, the system proceeds to the perfect quieting of the restless mind and its elevation to a higher plane through concentration of mental force by the successive stages which lead to the utmost inner concentration or ingathered state of the consciousness which is called Samadhi.

By Samadhi, in which the mind acquires the capacity of withdrawing from its limited waking activities into freer and higher states of consciousness, Rajayoga serves a double purpose. It compasses a pure mental action liberated from the confusions of the outer consciousness and passes thence to the higher supra-mental planes on which the individual soul enters into its true spiritual existence. But also it acquires the capacity of that free and concentrated energising of consciousness on its object which our philosophy asserts as the primary cosmic energy and the method of divine action upon the world. By this capacity the Yogin, already possessed of the highest supra-cosmic knowledge and experience in the state of trance, is able in the waking state to acquire directly whatever knowledge and exercise whatever mastery may be useful or necessary to his activities in the objective world. For the ancient system of Rajayoga aimed not only at Swarajya, self-rule or subjective empire, the entire control by the subjective consciousness of all the states and activities proper to its own domain, but included Samrajya as well, outward empire, the control by the subjective consciousness of its outer activities and environment.

We perceive that as Hathayoga, dealing with the life and body, aims at the supernormal perfection of the physical life and its capacities and goes beyond it into the domain of the mental life, so Rajayoga, operating with the mind, aims at a supernor-mal perfection and enlargement of the capacities of the mental life and goes beyond it into the domain of the spiritual existence. But the weakness of the system lies in its excessive reliance on abnormal states of trance. This limitation leads first to a certain aloofness from the physical life which is our foundation and the sphere into which we have to bring our mental and spiritual gains. Especially is the spiritual life, in this system, too much associated with the state of Samadhi. Our object is to make the spiritual life and its experiences fully active and fully utilisable in the waking state and even in the normal use of the functions. But in Rajayoga it tends to withdraw into a subliminal plane at the back of our normal experiences instead of descending and possessing our whole existence.

The triple Path of devotion, knowledge and works attempts the province which Rajayoga leaves unoccupied. It differs from Rajayoga in that it does not occupy itself with the elaborate training of the whole mental system as the condition of perfec-tion, but seizes on certain central principles, the intellect, the heart, the will, and seeks to convert their normal operations by turning them away from their ordinary and external preoccu-pations and activities and concentrating them on the Divine. It differs also in this, — and here from the point of view of an integral Yoga there seems to be a defect, — that it is indifferent to mental and bodily perfection and aims only at purity as a condition of the divine realisation. A second defect is that as actually practised it chooses one of the three parallel paths exclusively and almost in antagonism to the others instead of effecting a synthetic harmony of the intellect, the heart and the will in an integral divine realisation.

The Path of Knowledge aims at the realisation of the unique and supreme Self. It proceeds by the method of intellectual reflection, *vicāra*, to right discrimination, *viveka*. It observes and distinguishes the different elements of our apparent or phenomenal being and rejecting identification with each of them arrives at their exclusion and separation in one common term as constituents of Prakriti, of phenomenal Nature, creations of Maya, the phenomenal consciousness. So it is able to arrive at its right identification with the pure and unique Self which is not mutable or perishable, not determinable by any phenomenon or combination of phenomena. From this point the path, as ordinarily followed, leads to the rejection of the phenomenal worlds from the consciousness as an illusion and the final immergence without return of the individual soul in the Supreme.

But this exclusive consummation is not the sole or inevitable result of the Path of Knowledge. For, followed more largely and with a less individual aim, the method of Knowledge may lead to an active conquest of the cosmic existence for the Divine no less than to a transcendence. The point of this departure is the realisation of the supreme Self not only in one's own being but in all beings and, finally, the realisation of even the phenomenal aspects of the world as a play of the divine consciousness and not something entirely alien to its true nature. And on the basis of this realisation a yet further enlargement is possible, the conversion of all forms of knowledge, however mundane, into activities of the divine consciousness utilisable for the perception of the one and unique Object of knowledge both in itself and through the play of its forms and symbols. Such a method might well lead to the elevation of the whole range of human intellect and perception to the divine level, to its spiritualisation and to the justification of the cosmic travail of knowledge in humanity.

The Path of Devotion aims at the enjoyment of the supreme Love and Bliss and utilises normally the conception of the supreme Lord in His personality as the divine Lover and enjoyer of the universe. The world is then realised as a play of the Lord, with our human life as its final stage, pursued through the different phases of self-concealment and self-revelation. The principle of Bhakti Yoga is to utilise all the normal relations of human life into which emotion enters and apply them no longer to transient worldly relations, but to the joy of the All-Loving, the All-Beautiful and the All-Blissful. Worship and meditation are used only for the preparation and increase of intensity of the divine relationship. And this Yoga is catholic in its use of all emotional relations, so that even enmity and opposition to God, considered as an intense, impatient and perverse form of Love, is conceived as a possible means of realisation and salvation. This path, too, as ordinarily practised, leads away from world-existence to an absorption, of another kind than the Monist's, in the Transcendent and Supra-cosmic.

But, here too, the exclusive result is not inevitable. The Yoga itself provides a first corrective by not confining the play of divine love to the relation between the supreme Soul and the individual, but extending it to a common feeling and mutual worship between the devotees themselves united in the same realisation of the supreme Love and Bliss. It provides a yet more general corrective in the realisation of the divine object of Love in all beings not only human but animal, easily extended to all forms whatsoever. We can see how this larger application of the Yoga of Devotion may be so used as to lead to the elevation of the whole range of human emotion, sensation and aesthetic perception to the divine level, its spiritualisation and the justification of the cosmic labour towards love and joy in our humanity.

The Path of Works aims at the dedication of every human activity to the supreme Will. It begins by the renunciation of all egoistic aim for our works, all pursuit of action for an interested aim or for the sake of a worldly result. By this renunciation it so purifies the mind and the will that we become easily conscious of the great universal Energy as the true doer of all our actions and the Lord of that Energy as their ruler and director with the individual as only a mask, an excuse, an instrument or, more positively, a conscious centre of action and phenomenal relation. The choice and direction of the act is more and more consciously left to this supreme Will and this universal Energy. To That our works as well as the results of our works are finally abandoned. The object is the release of the soul from its bondage to appearances and to the reaction of phenomenal activities. Karmayoga is used, like the other paths, to lead to liberation from phenomenal existence and a departure into the Supreme. But here too the exclusive result is not inevitable. The end of the path may be, equally, a perception of the Divine in all energies, in all happenings, in all activities, and a free and unegoistic participation of the soul in the cosmic action. So followed it will lead to the elevation of all human will and activity to the divine level, its spiritualisation and the justification of the cosmic labour towards freedom, power and perfection in the human being.

We can see also that in the integral view of things these three paths are one. Divine Love should normally lead to the perfect knowledge of the Beloved by perfect intimacy, thus becoming a path of Knowledge, and to divine service, thus becoming a path of Works. So also should perfect Knowledge lead to perfect Love and Joy and a full acceptance of the works of That which is known; dedicated Works to the entire love of the Master of the Sacrifice and the deepest knowledge of His ways and His being. It is in this triple path that we come most readily to the absolute knowledge, love and service of the One in all beings and in the entire cosmic manifestation.

Chapter V

The Synthesis of the Systems

BY THE very nature of the principal Yogic schools, each covering in its operations a part of the complex human integer and attempting to bring out its highest possibilities, it will appear that a synthesis of all of them largely conceived and applied might well result in an integral Yoga. But they are so disparate in their tendencies, so highly specialised and elaborated in their forms, so long confirmed in the mutual opposition of their ideas and methods that we do not easily find how we can arrive at their right union.

An undiscriminating combination in block would not be a synthesis, but a confusion. Nor would a successive practice of each of them in turn be easy in the short span of our human life and with our limited energies, to say nothing of the waste of labour implied in so cumbrous a process. Sometimes, indeed, Hathayoga and Rajayoga are thus successively practised. And in a recent unique example, in the life of Ramakrishna Paramhansa, we see a colossal spiritual capacity first driving straight to the divine realisation, taking, as it were, the kingdom of heaven by violence, and then seizing upon one Yogic method after another and extracting the substance out of it with an incredible rapidity, always to return to the heart of the whole matter, the realisation and possession of God by the power of love, by the extension of inborn spirituality into various experience and by the spontaneous play of an intuitive knowledge. Such an example cannot be generalised. Its object also was special and temporal, to exemplify in the great and decisive experience of a master-soul the truth, now most necessary to humanity, towards which a world long divided into jarring sects and schools is with difficulty labouring, that all sects are forms and fragments of a single integral truth and all disciplines labour in their different ways towards one supreme experience. To know, be and possess the Divine is the one thing needful and it includes or leads up to all the rest; towards this sole good we have to drive and this attained, all the rest that the divine Will chooses for us, all necessary form and manifestation, will be added. The synthesis we propose cannot, then, be arrived at either by combination in mass or by successive practice. It must therefore be effected by neglecting the forms and outsides of the Yogic disciplines and seizing rather on some central principle common to all which will include and utilise in the right place and proportion their particular principles, and on some central dynamic force which is the common secret of their divergent methods and capable therefore of organising a natural selection and combination of their varied energies and different utilities. This was the aim which we set before ourselves at first when we entered upon our comparative examination of the methods of Nature and the methods of Yoga and we now return to it with the possibility of hazarding some definite solution.

We observe, first, that there still exists in India a remarkable Yogic system which is in its nature synthetical and starts from a great central principle of Nature, a great dynamic force of Nature; but it is a Yoga apart, not a synthesis of other schools. This system is the way of the Tantra. Owing to certain of its developments Tantra has fallen into discredit with those who are not Tantrics; and especially owing to the developments of its left-hand path, the Vama Marga, which not content with exceeding the duality of virtue and sin and instead of replacing them by spontaneous rightness of action seemed, sometimes, to make a method of self-indulgence, a method of unrestrained social immorality. Nevertheless, in its origin, Tantra was a great and puissant system founded upon ideas which were at least partially true. Even its twofold division into the right-hand and left-hand paths, Dakshina Marga and Vama Marga, started from a certain profound perception. In the ancient symbolic sense of the words Dakshina and Vama, it was the distinction between the way of Knowledge and the way of Ananda, — Nature in man liberating itself by right discrimination in power and practice of its own energies, elements and potentialities and Nature in man liberating itself by joyous acceptance in power and practice of its own energies, elements and potentialities. But in both paths there was in the end an obscuration of principles, a deformation of symbols and a fall.

If, however, we leave aside, here also, the actual methods and practices and seek for the central principle, we find, first, that Tantra expressly differentiates itself from the Vedic methods of Yoga. In a sense, all the schools we have hitherto examined are Vedantic in their principle; their force is in knowledge, their method is knowledge, though it is not always discernment by the intellect, but may be, instead, the knowledge of the heart expressed in love and faith or a knowledge in the will working out through action. In all of them the lord of the Yoga is the Purusha, the Conscious Soul that knows, observes, attracts, governs. But in Tantra it is rather Prakriti, the Nature-Soul, the Energy, the Will-in-Power executive in the universe. It was by learning and applying the intimate secrets of this Will-in-Power, its method, its Tantra, that the Tantric Yogin pursued the aims of his discipline, — mastery, perfection, liberation, beatitude. Instead of drawing back from manifested Nature and its difficulties, he confronted them, seized and conquered. But in the end, as is the general tendency of Prakriti, Tantric Yoga largely lost its principle in its machinery and became a thing of formulae and occult mechanism still powerful when rightly used but fallen from the clarity of their original intention.

We have in this central Tantric conception one side of the truth, the worship of the Energy, the Shakti, as the sole effective force for all attainment. We get the other extreme in the Vedantic conception of the Shakti as a power of Illusion and in the search after the silent inactive Purusha as the means of liberation from the deceptions created by the active Energy. But in the integral conception the Conscious Soul is the Lord, the Nature-Soul is his executive Energy. Purusha is of the nature of Sat, the being of conscious self-existence pure and infinite; Shakti or Prakriti is of the nature of Chit, — it is power of the Purusha's self-conscious existence, pure and infinite. The relation of the two exists between the poles of rest and action. When the Energy is absorbed in the bliss of conscious self-existence, there is rest; when the Purusha pours itself out in the action of its Energy, there is action, creation and the enjoyment or Ananda of becoming. But if Ananda is the creator and begetter of all becoming, its method is Tapas or force of the Purusha's consciousness dwelling upon its own infinite potentiality in existence and producing from it truths of conception or real Ideas, *vijñāna*, which, proceeding from an omniscient and omnipotent Self-existence, have the surety of their own fulfilment and contain in themselves the nature and law of their own becoming in the terms of mind, life and matter. The eventual omnipotence of Tapas and the infallible fulfilment of the Idea are the very foundation of all Yoga. In man we render these terms by Will and Faith, — a will that is eventually self-effective because it is of the substance of Knowledge and a faith that is the reflex in the lower consciousness of a Truth or real Idea yet unrealised in the manifestation. It is this self-certainty of the Idea which is meant by the Gita when it says, *yo yac-chraddhaḥ sa eva saḥ*, "whatever is a man's faith or the sure Idea in him, that he becomes."

We see, then, what from the psychological point of view, — and Yoga is nothing but practical psychology, — is the conception of Nature from which we have to start. It is the self-fulfilment of the Purusha through his Energy. But the movement of Nature is twofold, higher and lower, or, as we may choose to term it, divine and undivine. The distinction exists indeed for practical purposes only; for there is nothing that is not divine, and in a larger view it is as meaningless, verbally, as the distinction between natural and supernatural, for all things that are are natural. All things are in Nature and all things are in God. But, for practical purposes, there is a real distinction. The lower Nature, that which we know and are and must remain so long as the faith in us is not changed, acts through limitation and division, is of the nature of Ignorance and culminates in the life of the ego; but the higher Nature, that to which we aspire, acts by unification and transcendence of limitation, is of the nature of Knowledge and culminates in the life divine. The passage from the lower to the higher is the aim of Yoga; and this passage may effect itself by the rejection of the lower and escape into the higher, — the ordinary view-point, — or by the transformation of the lower and its elevation to the higher Nature. It is this, rather, that must be the aim of an integral Yoga.

But in either case it is always through something in the lower that we must rise into the higher existence, and the schools of Yoga each select their own point of departure or their own gate of escape. They specialise certain activities of the lower Prakriti and turn them towards the Divine. But the normal action of Nature in us is an integral movement in which the full complexity of all our elements is affected by and affects all our environments. The whole of life is the Yoga of Nature. The Yoga that we seek must also be an integral action of Nature, and the whole difference between the Yogin and the natural man will be this, that the Yogin seeks to substitute in himself for the integral action of the lower Nature working in and by ego and division the integral action of the higher Nature working in and by God and unity. If indeed our aim be only an escape from the world to God, synthesis is unnecessary and a waste of time; for then our sole practical aim must be to find out one path out of the thousand that lead to God, one shortest possible of short cuts, and not to linger exploring different paths that end in the same goal. But if our aim be a transformation of our integral being into the terms of God-existence, it is then that a synthesis becomes necessary.

The method we have to pursue, then, is to put our whole conscious being into relation and contact with the Divine and to call Him in to transform our entire being into His. Thus in a sense God Himself, the real Person in us, becomes the sadhaka of the sadhana[1] as well as the Master of the Yoga by whom the lower personality is used as the centre of a divine transfiguration and the instrument of its own perfection. In effect, the pressure of the Tapas, the force of consciousness in us dwelling in the Idea of the divine Nature upon that which we are in our entirety, produces

---

[1] *Sādhana*, the practice by which perfection, *siddhi*, is attained; *sādhaka*, the Yogin who seeks by that practice the *siddhi*.

its own realisation. The divine and all-knowing and all-effecting descends upon the limited and obscure, progressively illumines and energises the whole lower nature and substitutes its own action for all the terms of the inferior human light and mortal activity.

In psychological fact this method translates itself into the progressive surrender of the ego with its whole field and all its apparatus to the Beyond-ego with its vast and incalculable but always inevitable workings. Certainly, this is no short cut or easy sadhana. It requires a colossal faith, an absolute courage and above all an unflinching patience. For it implies three stages of which only the last can be wholly blissful or rapid, — the attempt of the ego to enter into contact with the Divine, the wide, full and therefore laborious preparation of the whole lower Nature by the divine working to receive and become the higher Nature, and the eventual transformation. In fact, however, the divine Strength, often unobserved and behind the veil, substitutes itself for our weakness and supports us through all our failings of faith, courage and patience. It "makes the blind to see and the lame to stride over the hills." The intellect becomes aware of a Law that beneficently insists and a succour that upholds; the heart speaks of a Master of all things and Friend of man or a universal Mother who upholds through all stumblings. Therefore this path is at once the most difficult imaginable and yet, in comparison with the magnitude of its effort and object, the most easy and sure of all.

There are three outstanding features of this action of the higher when it works integrally on the lower nature. In the first place it does not act according to a fixed system and succession as in the specialised methods of Yoga, but with a sort of free, scattered and yet gradually intensive and purposeful working determined by the temperament of the individual in whom it operates, the helpful materials which his nature offers and the obstacles which it presents to purification and perfection. In a sense, therefore, each man in this path has his own method of Yoga. Yet are there certain broad lines of working common to all which enable us to construct not indeed a routine system, but yet some kind of Shastra or scientific method of the synthetic Yoga.

Secondly, the process, being integral, accepts our nature such as it stands organised by our past evolution and without rejecting anything essential compels all to undergo a divine change. Everything in us is seized by the hands of a mighty Artificer and transformed into a clear image of that which it now seeks confusedly to present. In that ever-progressive experience we begin to perceive how this lower manifestation is constituted and that everything in it, however seemingly deformed or petty or vile, is the more or less distorted or imperfect figure of some element or action in the harmony of the divine Nature. We begin to understand what the Vedic Rishis meant when they spoke of the human forefathers fashioning the gods as a smith forges the crude material in his smithy.

Thirdly, the divine Power in us uses all life as the means of this integral Yoga. Every experience and outer contact with our world-environment, however trifling or however disastrous, is used for the work, and every inner experience, even to the most repellent suffering or the most humiliating fall, becomes a step on the path to perfection. And we recognise in ourselves with opened eyes the method of God in the world, His purpose of light in the obscure, of might in the weak and fallen, of delight in what is grievous and miserable. We see the divine method to be the same in the lower and in the higher working; only in the one it is pursued tardily and obscurely through the subconscious in Nature, in the other it becomes swift and self-conscious and the instrument confesses the hand of the Master. All life is a Yoga of Nature seeking to manifest God within itself. Yoga marks the stage at which this effort becomes capable of self-awareness and therefore of right completion in the individual. It is a gathering up and concentration of the movements dispersed and loosely combined in the lower evolution.

An integral method and an integral result. First, an integral realisation of Divine Being; not only a realisation of the One in its indistinguishable unity, but also in its multitude of aspects which are also necessary to the complete knowledge of it by the relative consciousness; not only realisation of unity in the Self, but of unity in the infinite diversity of activities, worlds and creatures.

Therefore, also, an integral liberation. Not only the freedom born of unbroken contact and identification of the individual being in all its parts with the Divine, *sāyujya-mukti*, by which it can become free[2] even in its separation, even in the duality; not only the *sālokya-mukti* by which the whole conscious existence dwells in the same status of being as the Divine, in the state of Sachchidananda; but also the acquisition of the divine nature by the transformation of this lower being into the human image of the Divine, *sādharmya-mukti*, and the complete and final release of all, the liberation of the consciousness from the transitory mould of the ego and its unification with the One Being, universal both in the world and the individual and transcendentally one both in the world and beyond all universe.

By this integral realisation and liberation, the perfect harmony of the results of Knowledge, Love and Works. For there is attained the complete release from ego and identification in being with the One in all and beyond all. But since the attaining consciousness is not limited by its attainment, we win also the unity in Beatitude and the harmonised diversity in Love, so that all relations of the play remain possible to us even while we retain on the heights of our being the eternal oneness with the Beloved. And by a similar wideness, being capable of a freedom in spirit that embraces life and does not depend upon withdrawal from life, we are able to become without egoism, bondage or reaction the channel in our mind and body for a divine action poured out freely upon the world.

The divine existence is of the nature not only of freedom, but of purity, beatitude and perfection. An integral purity which shall enable on the one hand the perfect reflection of the divine Being in ourselves and on the other the perfect outpouring of its Truth and Law in us in the terms of life and through the right

---

[2] As the Jivanmukta, who is entirely free even without dissolution of the bodily life in a final Samadhi.

functioning of the complex instrument we are in our outer parts, is the condition of an integral liberty. Its result is an integral beatitude, in which there becomes possible at once the Ananda of all that is in the world seen as symbols of the Divine and the Ananda of that which is not-world. And it prepares the integral perfection of our humanity as a type of the Divine in the conditions of the human manifestation, a perfection founded on a certain free universality of being, of love and joy, of play of knowledge and of play of will in power and will in unegoistic action. This integrality also can be attained by the integral Yoga.

Perfection includes perfection of mind and body, so that the highest results of Rajayoga and Hathayoga should be contained in the widest formula of the synthesis finally to be effected by mankind. At any rate a full development of the general mental and physical faculties and experiences attainable by humanity through Yoga must be included in the scope of the integral method. Nor would these have any *raison d'être* unless employed for an integral mental and physical life. Such a mental and physical life would be in its nature a translation of the spiritual existence into its right mental and physical values. Thus we would arrive at a synthesis of the three degrees of Nature and of the three modes of human existence which she has evolved or is evolving. We would include in the scope of our liberated being and perfected modes of activity the material life, our base, and the mental life, our intermediate instrument.

Nor would the integrality to which we aspire be real or even possible, if it were confined to the individual. Since our divine perfection embraces the realisation of ourselves in being, in life and in love through others as well as through ourselves, the extension of our liberty and of its results in others would be the inevitable outcome as well as the broadest utility of our liberation and perfection. And the constant and inherent attempt of such an extension would be towards its increasing and ultimately complete generalisation in mankind.

The divinising of the normal material life of man and of his great secular attempt of mental and moral self-culture in the individual and the race by this integralisation of a widely perfect spiritual existence would thus be the crown alike of our individual and of our common effort. Such a consummation being no other than the kingdom of heaven within reproduced in the kingdom of heaven without, would be also the true fulfilment of the great dream cherished in different terms by the world's religions.

The widest synthesis of perfection possible to thought is the sole effort entirely worthy of those whose dedicated vision perceives that God dwells concealed in humanity.

Part I

The Yoga of Divine Works

Chapter I

The Four Aids

YOGA-SIDDHI, the perfection that comes from the practice of Yoga, can be best attained by the combined working of four great instruments. There is, first, the knowledge of the truths, principles, powers and processes that govern the realisation — *śāstra*. Next comes a patient and persistent action on the lines laid down by this knowledge, the force of our personal effort — *utsāha*. There intervenes, third, uplifting our knowledge and effort into the domain of spiritual experience, the direct suggestion, example and influence of the Teacher — *guru*. Last comes the instrumentality of Time — *kāla*; for in all things there is a cycle of their action and a period of the divine movement.

*
* *

The supreme Shastra of the integral Yoga is the eternal Veda secret in the heart of every thinking and living being. The lotus of the eternal knowledge and the eternal perfection is a bud closed and folded up within us. It opens swiftly or gradually, petal by petal, through successive realisations, once the mind of man begins to turn towards the Eternal, once his heart, no longer compressed and confined by attachment to finite appearances, becomes enamoured, in whatever degree, of the Infinite. All life, all thought, all energising of the faculties, all experiences passive or active, become thenceforward so many shocks which disintegrate the teguments of the soul and remove the obstacles to the inevitable efflorescence. He who chooses the Infinite has been chosen by the Infinite. He has received the divine touch without which there is no awakening, no opening of the spirit; but once it is received, attainment is sure, whether conquered swiftly in the course of one human life or pursued patiently through many stadia of the cycle of existence in the manifested universe.

Nothing can be taught to the mind which is not already concealed as potential knowledge in the unfolding soul of the creature. So also all perfection of which the outer man is capable, is only a realising of the eternal perfection of the Spirit within him. We know the Divine and become the Divine, because we are That already in our secret nature. All teaching is a revealing, all becoming is an unfolding. Self-attainment is the secret; self-knowledge and an increasing consciousness are the means and the process.

The usual agency of this revealing is the Word, the thing heard (*śruta*). The Word may come to us from within; it may come to us from without. But in either case, it is only an agency for setting the hidden knowledge to work. The word within may be the utterance of the inmost soul in us which is always open to the Divine; or it may be the word of the secret and universal Teacher who is seated in the hearts of all. There are rare cases in which none other is needed, for all the rest of the Yoga is an unfolding under that constant touch and guidance; the lotus of the knowledge discloses itself from within by the power of irradiating effulgence which proceeds from the Dweller in the lotus of the heart. Great indeed, but few are those to whom self-knowledge from within is thus sufficient and who do not need to pass under the dominant influence of a written book or a living teacher.

Ordinarily, the Word from without, representative of the Divine, is needed as an aid in the work of self-unfolding; and it may be either a word from the past or the more powerful word of the living Guru. In some cases this representative word is only taken as a sort of excuse for the inner power to awaken and manifest; it is, as it were, a concession of the omnipotent and omniscient Divine to the generality of a law that governs Nature. Thus it is said in the Upanishads of Krishna, son of Devaki, that he received a word of the Rishi Ghora and had the knowledge. So Ramakrishna, having attained by his own internal effort the central illumination, accepted several teachers in the different paths of Yoga, but always showed in the manner and swiftness of his realisation that this acceptance was a concession to the general rule by which effective knowledge must be received as by a disciple from a Guru.

But usually the representative influence occupies a much larger place in the life of the sadhaka. If the Yoga is guided by a received written Shastra, — some Word from the past which embodies the experience of former Yogins, — it may be practised either by personal effort alone or with the aid of a Guru. The spiritual knowledge is then gained through meditation on the truths that are taught and it is made living and conscious by their realisation in the personal experience; the Yoga proceeds by the results of prescribed methods taught in a Scripture or a tradition and reinforced and illumined by the instructions of the Master. This is a narrower practice, but safe and effective within its limits, because it follows a well-beaten track to a long familiar goal.

For the sadhaka of the integral Yoga it is necessary to remember that no written Shastra, however great its authority or however large its spirit, can be more than a partial expression of the eternal Knowledge. He will use, but never bind himself even by the greatest Scripture. Where the Scripture is profound, wide, catholic, it may exercise upon him an influence for the highest good and of incalculable importance. It may be associated in his experience with his awakening to crowning verities and his realisation of the highest experiences. His Yoga may be governed for a long time by one Scripture or by several successively, — if it is in the line of the great Hindu tradition, by the Gita, for example, the Upanishads, the Veda. Or it may be a good part of his development to include in its material a richly varied experience of the truths of many Scriptures and make the future opulent with all that is best in the past. But in the end he must take his station, or better still, if he can, always and from the beginning he must live in his own soul beyond the limitations of the word that he uses. The Gita itself thus declares that the Yogin in his progress must pass beyond the written Truth, — *śabdabrahmātivartate* — beyond all that he has heard and all that he has yet to hear, — *śrotavyasya śrutasya ca.* For he is not the sadhaka of a book or of many books; he is a sadhaka of the Infinite.

Another kind of Shastra is not Scripture, but a statement of the science and methods, the effective principles and way of working of the path of Yoga which the sadhaka elects to follow. Each path has its Shastra, either written or traditional, passing from mouth to mouth through a long line of Teachers. In India a great authority, a high reverence even is ordinarily attached to the written or traditional teaching. All the lines of the Yoga are supposed to be fixed and the Teacher who has received the Shastra by tradition and realised it in practice guides the disciple along the immemorial tracks. One often even hears the objection urged against a new practice, a new Yogic teaching, the adoption of a new formula, "It is not according to the Shastra." But neither in fact nor in the actual practice of the Yogins is there really any such entire rigidity of an iron door shut against new truth, fresh revelation, widened experience. The written or traditional teaching expresses the knowledge and experiences of many centuries systematised, organised, made attainable to the beginner. Its importance and utility are therefore immense. But a great freedom of variation and development is always practicable. Even so highly scientific a system as Rajayoga can be practised on other lines than the organised method of Patanjali. Each of the three paths of the *trimārga*[1] breaks into many bypaths which meet again at the goal. The general knowledge on which the Yoga depends is fixed, but the order, the succession, the devices, the forms must be allowed to vary; for the needs and particular impulsions of the individual nature have to be satisfied even while the general truths remain firm and constant.

An integral and synthetic Yoga needs especially not to be bound by any written or traditional Shastra; for while it embraces the knowledge received from the past, it seeks to organise it anew for the present and the future. An absolute liberty of experience and of the restatement of knowledge in new terms and new combinations is the condition of its self-formation.

---

[1] The triple path of Knowledge, Devotion and Works.

Seeking to embrace all life in itself, it is in the position not of a pilgrim following the highroad to his destination, but, to that extent at least, of a path-finder hewing his way through a virgin forest. For Yoga has long diverged from life and the ancient systems which sought to embrace it, such as those of our Vedic forefathers, are far away from us, expressed in terms which are no longer accessible, thrown into forms which are no longer applicable. Since then mankind has moved forward on the current of eternal Time and the same problem has to be approached from a new starting-point.

By this Yoga we not only seek the Infinite, but we call upon the Infinite to unfold himself in human life. Therefore the Shastra of our Yoga must provide for an infinite liberty in the receptive human soul. A free adaptability in the manner and the type of the individual's acceptance of the Universal and Transcendent into himself is the right condition for the full spiritual life in man. Vivekananda, pointing out that the unity of all religions must necessarily express itself by an increasing richness of variety in its forms, said once that the perfect state of that essential unity would come when each man had his own religion, when not bound by sect or traditional form he followed the free self-adaptation of his nature in its relations with the Supreme. So also one may say that the perfection of the integral Yoga will come when each man is able to follow his own path of Yoga, pursuing the development of his own nature in its upsurging towards that which transcends the nature. For freedom is the final law and the last consummation.

Meanwhile certain general lines have to be formed which may help to guide the thought and practice of the sadhaka. But these must take as much as possible the form of general truths, general statements of principle, the most powerful broad directions of effort and development rather than a fixed system which has to be followed as a routine. All Shastra is the outcome of past experience and a help to future experience. It is an aid and a partial guide. It puts up signposts, gives the names of the main roads and the already explored directions, so that the traveller may know whither and by what paths he is proceeding.

The rest depends on personal effort and experience and upon the power of the Guide.

*
* *

The development of the experience in its rapidity, its amplitude, the intensity and power of its results, depends primarily, in the beginning of the path and long after, on the aspiration and personal effort of the sadhaka. The process of Yoga is a turning of the human soul from the egoistic state of consciousness absorbed in the outward appearances and attractions of things to a higher state in which the Transcendent and Universal can pour itself into the individual mould and transform it. The first determining element of the siddhi is, therefore, the intensity of the turning, the force which directs the soul inward. The power of aspiration of the heart, the force of the will, the concentration of the mind, the perseverance and determination of the applied energy are the measure of that intensity. The ideal sadhaka should be able to say in the Biblical phrase, "My zeal for the Lord has eaten me up." It is this zeal for the Lord, — *utsāha*, the zeal of the whole nature for its divine results, *vyākulatā*, the heart's eagerness for the attainment of the Divine, — that devours the ego and breaks up the limitations of its petty and narrow mould for the full and wide reception of that which it seeks, that which, being universal, exceeds and, being transcendent, surpasses even the largest and highest individual self and nature.

But this is only one side of the force that works for perfection. The process of the integral Yoga has three stages, not indeed sharply distinguished or separate, but in a certain measure successive. There must be, first, the effort towards at least an initial and enabling self-transcendence and contact with the Divine; next, the reception of that which transcends, that with which we have gained communion, into ourselves for the transformation of our whole conscious being; last, the utilisation of our transformed humanity as a divine centre in the world. So long as the contact with the Divine is not in some considerable degree established, so long as there is not some measure of sustained identity, *sāyujya*, the element of personal effort must normally predominate. But in proportion as this contact establishes itself, the sadhaka must become conscious that a force other than his own, a force transcending his egoistic endeavour and capacity, is at work in him and to this Power he learns progressively to submit himself and delivers up to it the charge of his Yoga. In the end his own will and force become one with the higher Power; he merges them in the divine Will and its transcendent and universal Force. He finds it thenceforward presiding over the necessary transformation of his mental, vital and physical being with an impartial wisdom and provident effectivity of which the eager and interested ego is not capable. It is when this identification and this self-merging are complete that the divine centre in the world is ready. Purified, liberated, plastic, illumined, it can begin to serve as a means for the direct action of a supreme Power in the larger Yoga of humanity or superhumanity, of the earth's spiritual progression or its transformation.

Always indeed it is the higher Power that acts. Our sense of personal effort and aspiration comes from the attempt of the egoistic mind to identify itself in a wrong and imperfect way with the workings of the divine Force. It persists in applying to experience on a supernormal plane the ordinary terms of mentality which it applies to its normal experiences in the world. In the world we act with the sense of egoism; we claim the universal forces that work in us as our own; we claim as the effect of our personal will, wisdom, force, virtue the selective, formative, progressive action of the Transcendent in this frame of mind, life and body. Enlightenment brings to us the knowledge that the ego is only an instrument; we begin to perceive and feel that these things are our own in the sense that they belong to our supreme and integral Self, one with the Transcendent, not to the instrumental ego. Our limitations and distortions are our contribution to the working; the true power in it is the Divine's. When the human ego realises that its will is a tool, its wisdom ignorance and childishness, its power an infant's groping, its virtue a pretentious impurity, and learns to trust itself to that which transcends it, that is its salvation. The apparent freedom and self-assertion of our personal being to which we are so profoundly attached, conceal a most pitiable subjection to a thousand suggestions, impulsions, forces which we have made extraneous to our little person. Our ego, boasting of freedom, is at every moment the slave, toy and puppet of countless beings, powers, forces, influences in universal Nature. The self-abnegation of the ego in the Divine is its self-fulfilment; its surrender to that which transcends it is its liberation from bonds and limits and its perfect freedom.

But still, in the practical development, each of the three stages has its necessity and utility and must be given its time or its place. It will not do, it cannot be safe or effective to begin with the last and highest alone. It would not be the right course, either, to leap prematurely from one to another. For even if from the beginning we recognise in mind and heart the Supreme, there are elements of the nature which long prevent the recognition from becoming realisation. But without realisation our mental belief cannot become a dynamic reality; it is still only a figure of knowledge, not a living truth, an idea, not yet a power. And even if realisation has begun, it may be dangerous to imagine or to assume too soon that we are altogether in the hands of the Supreme or are acting as his instrument. That assumption may introduce a calamitous falsity; it may produce a helpless inertia or, magnifying the movements of the ego with the Divine Name, it may disastrously distort and ruin the whole course of the Yoga. There is a period, more or less prolonged, of internal effort and struggle in which the individual will has to reject the darkness and distortions of the lower nature and to put itself resolutely or vehemently on the side of the divine Light. The mental energies, the heart's emotions, the vital desires, the very physical being have to be compelled into the right attitude or trained to admit and answer to the right influences. It is only then, only when this has been truly done, that the surrender of the lower to the higher can be effected, because the sacrifice has become acceptable.

The personal will of the sadhaka has first to seize on the egoistic energies and turn them towards the light and the right;

once turned, he has still to train them to recognise that always, always to accept, always to follow that. Progressing, he learns, still using the personal will, personal effort, personal energies, to employ them as representatives of the higher Power and in conscious obedience to the higher Influence. Progressing yet farther, his will, effort, energy become no longer personal and separate, but activities of that higher Power and Influence at work in the individual. But there is still a sort of gulf or distance which necessitates an obscure process of transit, not always accurate, sometimes even very distorting, between the divine Origin and the emerging human current. At the end of the process, with the progressive disappearance of egoism and impurity and ignorance, this last separation is removed; all in the individual becomes the divine working.

*
* *

As the supreme Shastra of the integral Yoga is the eternal Veda secret in the heart of every man, so its supreme Guide and Teacher is the inner Guide, the World-Teacher, *jagad-guru*, secret within us. It is he who destroys our darkness by the resplendent light of his knowledge; that light becomes within us the increasing glory of his own self-revelation. He discloses progressively in us his own nature of freedom, bliss, love, power, immortal being. He sets above us his divine example as our ideal and transforms the lower existence into a reflection of that which it contemplates. By the inpouring of his own influence and presence into us he enables the individual being to attain to identity with the universal and transcendent.

What is his method and his system? He has no method and every method. His system is a natural organisation of the highest processes and movements of which the nature is capable. Applying themselves even to the pettiest details and to the actions the most insignificant in their appearance with as much care and thoroughness as to the greatest, they in the end lift all into the Light and transform all. For in his Yoga there is nothing too small to be used and nothing too great to be attempted. As the servant and disciple of the Master has no business with pride or egoism because all is done for him from above, so also he has no right to despond because of his personal deficiencies or the stumblings of his nature. For the Force that works in him is impersonal — or superpersonal — and infinite.

The full recognition of this inner Guide, Master of the Yoga, lord, light, enjoyer and goal of all sacrifice and effort, is of the utmost importance in the path of integral perfection. It is immaterial whether he is first seen as an impersonal Wisdom, Love and Power behind all things, as an Absolute manifesting in the relative and attracting it, as one's highest Self and the highest Self of all, as a Divine Person within us and in the world, in one of his — or her — numerous forms and names or as the ideal which the mind conceives. In the end we perceive that he is all and more than all these things together. The mind's door of entry to the conception of him must necessarily vary according to the past evolution and the present nature.

This inner Guide is often veiled at first by the very intensity of our personal effort and by the ego's preoccupation with itself and its aims. As we gain in clarity and the turmoil of egoistic effort gives place to a calmer self-knowledge, we recognise the source of the growing light within us. We recognise it retrospectively as we realise how all our obscure and conflicting movements have been determined towards an end that we only now begin to perceive, how even before our entrance into the path of the Yoga the evolution of our life has been designedly led towards its turning-point. For now we begin to understand the sense of our struggles and efforts, successes and failures. At last we are able to seize the meaning of our ordeals and sufferings and can appreciate the help that was given us by all that hurt and resisted and the utility of our very falls and stumblings. We recognise this divine leading afterwards, not retrospectively but immediately, in the moulding of our thoughts by a transcendent Seer, of our will and actions by an all-embracing Power, of our emotional life by an all-attracting and all-assimilating Bliss and Love. We recognise it too in a more personal relation that from the first touched or at the last seizes us; we feel the eternal presence of a supreme Master, Friend, Lover, Teacher. We recognise it in the essence of our being as that develops into likeness and oneness with a greater and wider existence; for we perceive that this miraculous development is not the result of our own efforts: an eternal Perfection is moulding us into its own image. One who is the Lord or Ishwara of the Yogic philosophies, the Guide in the conscious being (*caitya guru* or *antaryāmin*), the Absolute of the thinker, the Unknowable of the Agnostic, the universal Force of the materialist, the supreme Soul and the supreme Shakti, the One who is differently named and imaged by the religions, is the Master of our Yoga.

To see, know, become and fulfil this One in our inner selves and in all our outer nature, was always the secret goal and becomes now the conscious purpose of our embodied existence. To be conscious of him in all parts of our being and equally in all that the dividing mind sees as outside our being, is the consummation of the individual consciousness. To be possessed by him and possess him in ourselves and in all things is the term of all empire and mastery. To enjoy him in all experience of passivity and activity, of peace and of power, of unity and of difference is the happiness which the Jiva, the individual soul manifested in the world, is obscurely seeking. This is the entire definition of the aim of integral Yoga; it is the rendering in personal experience of the truth which universal Nature has hidden in herself and which she travails to discover. It is the conversion of the human soul into the divine soul and of natural life into divine living.

*
* *

The surest way towards this integral fulfilment is to find the Master of the secret who dwells within us, open ourselves constantly to the divine Power which is also the divine Wisdom and Love and trust to it to effect the conversion. But it is difficult for the egoistic consciousness to do this at all at the beginning. And, if done at all, it is still difficult to do it perfectly and in every strand of our nature. It is difficult at first because our egoistic habits of thought, of sensation, of feeling block up the avenues by which we can arrive at the perception that is needed. It is difficult afterwards because the faith, the surrender, the courage requisite in this path are not easy to the ego-clouded soul. The divine working is not the working which the egoistic mind desires or approves; for it uses error in order to arrive at truth, suffering in order to arrive at bliss, imperfection in order to arrive at perfection. The ego cannot see where it is being led; it revolts against the leading, loses confidence, loses courage. These failings would not matter; for the divine Guide within is not offended by our revolt, not discouraged by our want of faith or repelled by our weakness; he has the entire love of the mother and the entire patience of the teacher. But by withdrawing our assent from the guidance we lose the consciousness, though not all the actuality — not, in any case, the eventuality — of its benefit. And we withdraw our assent because we fail to distinguish our higher Self from the lower through which he is preparing his self-revelation. As in the world, so in ourselves, we cannot see God because of his workings and, especially, because he works in us through our nature and not by a succession of arbitrary miracles. Man demands miracles that he may have faith; he wishes to be dazzled in order that he may see. And this impatience, this ignorance may turn into a great danger and disaster if, in our revolt against the divine leading, we call in another distorting Force more satisfying to our impulses and desires and ask it to guide us and give it the Divine Name.

But while it is difficult for man to believe in something unseen within himself, it is easy for him to believe in something which he can image as extraneous to himself. The spiritual progress of most human beings demands an extraneous support, an object of faith outside us. It needs an external image of God; or it needs a human representative, — Incarnation, Prophet or Guru; or it demands both and receives them. For according to the need of the human soul the Divine manifests himself as deity, as human divine or in simple humanity — using that thick disguise, which so successfully conceals the Godhead, for a means of transmission of his guidance.

The Hindu discipline of spirituality provides for this need of the soul by the conceptions of the Ishta Devata, the Avatar and the Guru. By the Ishta Devata, the chosen deity, is meant, — not some inferior Power, but a name and form of the transcendent and universal Godhead. Almost all religions either have as their base or make use of some such name and form of the Divine. Its necessity for the human soul is evident. God is the All and more than the All. But that which is more than the All, how shall man conceive? And even the All is at first too hard for him; for he himself in his active consciousness is a limited and selective formation and can open himself only to that which is in harmony with his limited nature. There are things in the All which are too hard for his comprehension or seem too terrible to his sensitive emotions and cowering sensations. Or, simply, he cannot conceive as the Divine, cannot approach or cannot recognise something that is too much out of the circle of his ignorant or partial conceptions. It is necessary for him to conceive God in his own image or in some form that is beyond himself but consonant with his highest tendencies and seizable by his feelings or his intelligence. Otherwise it would be difficult for him to come into contact and communion with the Divine.

Even then his nature calls for a human intermediary so that he may feel the Divine in something entirely close to his own humanity and sensible in a human influence and example. This call is satisfied by the Divine manifest in a human appearance, the Incarnation, the Avatar — Krishna, Christ, Buddha. Or if this is too hard for him to conceive, the Divine represents himself through a less marvellous intermediary, — Prophet or Teacher. For many who cannot conceive or are unwilling to accept the Divine Man, are ready to open themselves to the supreme man, terming him not incarnation but world-teacher or divine representative.

This also is not enough; a living influence, a living example, a present instruction is needed. For it is only the few who can make the past Teacher and his teaching, the past Incarnation and his example and influence a living force in their lives. For this need also the Hindu discipline provides in the relation of the Guru and the disciple. The Guru may sometimes be the Incarnation or World-Teacher; but it is sufficient that he should represent to the disciple the divine wisdom, convey to him something of the divine ideal or make him feel the realised relation of the human soul with the Eternal.

The sadhaka of the integral Yoga will make use of all these aids according to his nature; but it is necessary that he should shun their limitations and cast from himself that exclusive tendency of egoistic mind which cries, "My God, my Incarnation, my Prophet, my Guru," and opposes it to all other realisation in a sectarian or a fanatical spirit. All sectarianism, all fanaticism must be shunned; for it is inconsistent with the integrity of the divine realisation.

On the contrary, the sadhaka of the integral Yoga will not be satisfied until he has included all other names and forms of Deity in his own conception, seen his own Ishta Devata in all others, unified all Avatars in the unity of Him who descends in the Avatar, welded the truth in all teachings into the harmony of the Eternal Wisdom.

Nor should he forget the aim of these external aids which is to awaken his soul to the Divine within him. Nothing has been finally accomplished if that has not been accomplished. It is not sufficient to worship Krishna, Christ or Buddha without, if there is not the revealing and the formation of the Buddha, the Christ or Krishna in ourselves. And all other aids equally have no other purpose; each is a bridge between man's unconverted state and the revelation of the Divine within him.

*
* *

The Teacher of the integral Yoga will follow as far as he may the method of the Teacher within us. He will lead the disciple through the nature of the disciple. Teaching, example, influence, — these are the three instruments of the Guru. But the wise Teacher will not seek to impose himself or his opinions on the passive acceptance of the receptive mind; he will throw in only what is productive and sure as a seed which will grow under the divine fostering within. He will seek to awaken much more than to instruct; he will aim at the growth of the faculties and the experiences by a natural process and free expansion. He will give a method as an aid, as a utilisable device, not as an imperative formula or a fixed routine. And he will be on his guard against any turning of the means into a limitation, against the mechanising of process. His whole business is to awaken the divine light and set working the divine force of which he himself is only a means and an aid, a body or a channel.

The example is more powerful than the instruction; but it is not the example of the outward acts nor that of the personal character which is of most importance. These have their place and their utility; but what will most stimulate aspiration in others is the central fact of the divine realisation within him governing his whole life and inner state and all his activities. This is the universal and essential element; the rest belongs to individual person and circumstance. It is this dynamic realisation that the sadhaka must feel and reproduce in himself according to his own nature; he need not strive after an imitation from outside which may well be sterilising rather than productive of right and natural fruits.

Influence is more important than example. Influence is not the outward authority of the Teacher over his disciple, but the power of his contact, of his presence, of the nearness of his soul to the soul of another, infusing into it, even though in silence, that which he himself is and possesses. This is the supreme sign of the Master. For the greatest Master is much less a Teacher than a Presence pouring the divine consciousness and its constituting light and power and purity and bliss into all who are receptive around him.

And it shall also be a sign of the teacher of the integral Yoga that he does not arrogate to himself Guruhood in a humanly vain and self-exalting spirit. His work, if he has one, is a trust from above, he himself a channel, a vessel or a representative. He is a man helping his brothers, a child leading children, a Light kindling other lights, an awakened Soul awakening souls, at highest a Power or Presence of the Divine calling to him other powers of the Divine.

*
* *

The sadhaka who has all these aids is sure of his goal. Even a fall will be for him only a means of rising and death a passage towards fulfilment. For once on this path, birth and death become only processes in the development of his being and the stages of his journey.

Time is the remaining aid needed for the effectivity of the process. Time presents itself to human effort as an enemy or a friend, as a resistance, a medium or an instrument. But always it is really the instrument of the soul.

Time is a field of circumstances and forces meeting and working out a resultant progression whose course it measures. To the ego it is a tyrant or a resistance, to the Divine an instrument. Therefore, while our effort is personal, Time appears as a resistance, for it presents to us all the obstruction of the forces that conflict with our own. When the divine working and the personal are combined in our consciousness, it appears as a medium and a condition. When the two become one, it appears as a servant and instrument.

The ideal attitude of the sadhaka towards Time is to have an endless patience as if he had all eternity for his fulfilment and yet to develop the energy that shall realise now and with an ever-increasing mastery and pressure of rapidity till it reaches the miraculous instantaneousness of the supreme divine Transformation.

Chapter II

Self-Consecration

ALL YOGA is in its nature a new birth; it is a birth out of the ordinary, the mentalised material life of man into a higher spiritual consciousness and a greater and diviner being. No Yoga can be successfully undertaken and followed unless there is a strong awakening to the necessity of that larger spiritual existence. The soul that is called to this deep and vast inward change, may arrive in different ways to the initial departure. It may come to it by its own natural development which has been leading it unconsciously towards the awakening; it may reach it through the influence of a religion or the attraction of a philosophy; it may approach it by a slow illumination or leap to it by a sudden touch or shock; it may be pushed or led to it by the pressure of outward circumstances or by an inward necessity, by a single word that breaks the seals of the mind or by long reflection, by the distant example of one who has trod the path or by contact and daily influence. According to the nature and the circumstances the call will come.

But in whatever way it comes, there must be a decision of the mind and the will and, as its result, a complete and effective self-consecration. The acceptance of a new spiritual idea-force and upward orientation in the being, an illumination, a turning or conversion seized on by the will and the heart's aspiration, — this is the momentous act which contains as in a seed all the results that the Yoga has to give. The mere idea or intellectual seeking of something higher beyond, however strongly grasped by the mind's interest, is ineffective unless it is seized on by the heart as the one thing desirable and by the will as the one thing to be done. For truth of the Spirit has not to be merely thought but to be lived, and to live it demands a unified single-mindedness of the being; so great a change as is contemplated by the Yoga is not to be effected by a divided will or by a small portion of the energy or by a hesitating mind. He who seeks the Divine must consecrate himself to God and to God only.

If the change comes suddenly and decisively by an overpowering influence, there is no further essential or lasting difficulty. The choice follows upon the thought, or is simultaneous with it, and the self-consecration follows upon the choice. The feet are already set upon the path, even if they seem at first to wander uncertainly and even though the path itself may be only obscurely seen and the knowledge of the goal may be imperfect. The secret Teacher, the inner Guide is already at work, though he may not yet manifest himself or may not yet appear in the person of his human representative. Whatever difficulties and hesitations may ensue, they cannot eventually prevail against the power of the experience that has turned the current of the life. The call, once decisive, stands; the thing that has been born cannot eventually be stifled. Even if the force of circumstances prevents a regular pursuit or a full practical self-consecration from the first, still the mind has taken its bent and persists and returns with an ever-increasing effect upon its leading preoccupation. There is an ineluctable persistence of the inner being, and against it circumstances are in the end powerless, and no weakness in the nature can for long be an obstacle.

But this is not always the manner of the commencement. The sadhaka is often led gradually and there is a long space between the first turning of the mind and the full assent of the nature to the thing towards which it turns. There may at first be only a vivid intellectual interest, a forcible attraction towards the idea and some imperfect form of practice. Or perhaps there is an effort not favoured by the whole nature, a decision or a turn imposed by an intellectual influence or dictated by personal affection and admiration for someone who is himself consecrated and devoted to the Highest. In such cases, a long period of preparation may be necessary before there comes the irrevocable consecration; and in some instances it may not come. There may be some advance, there may be a strong effort, even much purification and many experiences other than those that are central or supreme; but the life will either be spent in preparation or, a certain stage having been reached, the mind pushed by an insufficient driving-force may rest content at the limit of the effort possible to it. Or there may even be a recoil to the lower life, — what is called in the ordinary parlance of Yoga a fall from the path. This lapse happens because there is a defect at the very centre. The intellect has been interested, the heart attracted, the will has strung itself to the effort, but the whole nature has not been taken captive by the Divine. It has only acquiesced in the interest, the attraction or the endeavour. There has been an experiment, perhaps even an eager experiment, but not a total self-giving to an imperative need of the soul or to an unforsakable ideal. Even such imperfect Yoga has not been wasted; for no upward effort is made in vain. Even if it fails in the present or arrives only at some preparatory stage or preliminary realisation, it has yet determined the soul's future.

But if we desire to make the most of the opportunity that this life gives us, if we wish to respond adequately to the call we have received and to attain to the goal we have glimpsed, not merely advance a little towards it, it is essential that there should be an entire self-giving. The secret of success in Yoga is to regard it not as one of the aims to be pursued in life, but as the one and only aim, not as an important part of life, but as the whole of life.

*
* *

And since Yoga is in its essence a turning away from the ordinary material and animal life led by most men or from the more mental but still limited way of living followed by the few to a greater spiritual life, to the way divine, every part of our energies that is given to the lower existence in the spirit of that existence is a contradiction of our aim and our self-dedication. On the other hand, every energy or activity that we can convert from its allegiance to the lower and dedicate to the service of the higher is so much gained on our road, so much taken from the powers that oppose our progress. It is the difficulty of this wholesale conversion that is the source of all the stumblings in the path of Yoga. For our entire nature and its environment, all our personal and all our universal self, are full of habits and of influences that are opposed to our spiritual rebirth and work against the whole-heartedness of our endeavour. In a certain sense we are nothing but a complex mass of mental, nervous and physical habits held together by a few ruling ideas, desires and associations, — an amalgam of many small self-repeating forces with a few major vibrations. What we propose in our Yoga is nothing less than to break up the whole formation of our past and present which makes up the ordinary material and mental man and to create a new centre of vision and a new universe of activities in ourselves which shall constitute a divine humanity or a superhuman nature.

The first necessity is to dissolve that central faith and vision in the mind which concentrate it on its development and satis-faction and interests in the old externalised order of things. It is imperative to exchange this surface orientation for the deeper faith and vision which see only the Divine and seek only after the Divine. The next need is to compel all our lower being to pay homage to this new faith and greater vision. All our nature must make an integral surrender; it must offer itself in every part and every movement to that which seems to the unregenerated sense-mind so much less real than the material world and its objects. Our whole being — soul, mind, sense, heart, will, life, body — must consecrate all its energies so entirely and in such a way that it shall become a fit vehicle for the Divine. This is no easy task; for everything in the world follows the fixed habit which is to it a law and resists a radical change. And no change can be more radical than the revolution attempted in the integral Yoga. Everything in us has constantly to be called back to the central faith and will and vision. Every thought and impulse has to be reminded in the language of the Upanishad that "That is the divine Brahman and not this which men here adore." Every vital fibre has to be persuaded to accept an entire renunciation of all that hitherto represented to it its own existence. Mind has to cease to be mind and become brilliant with something beyond it. Life has to change into a thing vast and calm and intense and powerful that can no longer recognise its old blind eager narrow self of petty impulse and desire. Even the body has to submit to a mutation and be no longer the clamorous animal or the impeding clod it now is, but become instead a conscious servant and radiant instrument and living form of the spirit.

The difficulty of the task has led naturally to the pursuit of easy and trenchant solutions; it has generated and fixed deeply the tendency of religions and of schools of Yoga to separate the life of the world from the inner life. The powers of this world and their actual activities, it is felt, either do not belong to God at all or are for some obscure and puzzling cause, Maya or another, a dark contradiction of the divine Truth. And on their own opposite side the powers of the Truth and their ideal activities are seen to belong to quite another plane of consciousness than that, obscure, ignorant and perverse in its impulses and forces, on which the life of the earth is founded. There appears at once the antinomy of a bright and pure kingdom of God and a dark and impure kingdom of the devil; we feel the opposition of our crawling earthly birth and life to an exalted spiritual God-consciousness; we become readily convinced of the incompatibility of life's subjection to Maya with the soul's concentration in pure Brahman existence. The easiest way is to turn away from all that belongs to the one and to retreat by a naked and precipitous ascent into the other. Thus arises the attraction and, it would seem, the necessity of the principle of exclusive concentration which plays so prominent a part in the specialised schools of Yoga; for by that concentration we can arrive through an uncompromising renunciation of the world at an entire self-consecration to the One on whom we concentrate. It is no longer incumbent on us to compel all the lower activities to the difficult recognition of a new and higher spiritualised life and train them to be its agents or executive powers. It is enough to kill or quiet them and keep at most the few energies necessary, on one side, for the maintenance of the body and, on the other, for communion with the Divine.

The very aim and conception of an integral Yoga debar us from adopting this simple and strenuous high-pitched process.

The hope of an integral transformation forbids us to take a short cut or to make ourselves light for the race by throwing away our impedimenta. For we have set out to conquer all ourselves and the world for God; we are determined to give him our becoming as well as our being and not merely to bring the pure and naked spirit as a bare offering to a remote and secret Divinity in a distant heaven or abolish all we are in a holocaust to an immobile Absolute. The Divine that we adore is not only a remote extra-cosmic Reality, but a half-veiled Manifestation present and near to us here in the universe. Life is the field of a divine manifestation not yet complete: here, in life, on earth, in the body, — *ihaiva*, as the Upanishads insist, — we have to unveil the Godhead; here we must make its transcendent greatness, light and sweetness real to our consciousness, here possess and, as far as may be, express it. Life then we must accept in our Yoga in order utterly to transmute it; we are forbidden to shrink from the difficulties that this acceptance may add to our struggle. Our compensation is that even if the path is more rugged, the effort more complex and bafflingly arduous, yet after a certain point we gain an immense advantage. For once our minds are reasonably fixed in the central vision and our wills are on the whole converted to the single pursuit, Life becomes our helper. Intent, vigilant, integrally conscious, we can take every detail of its forms and every incident of its movements as food for the sacrificial Fire within us. Victorious in the struggle, we can compel Earth herself to be an aid towards our perfection and can enrich our realisation with the booty torn from the Powers that oppose us.

*
* *

There is another direction in which the ordinary practice of Yoga arrives at a helpful but narrowing simplification which is denied to the sadhaka of the integral aim. The practice of Yoga brings us face to face with the extraordinary complexity of our own being, the stimulating but also embarrassing multiplicity of our personality, the rich endless confusion of Nature. To the ordinary man who lives upon his own waking surface, ignorant of the self's depths and vastnesses behind the veil, his psychological existence is fairly simple. A small but clamorous company of desires, some imperative intellectual and aesthetic cravings, some tastes, a few ruling or prominent ideas amid a great current of unconnected or ill-connected and mostly trivial thoughts, a number of more or less imperative vital needs, alternations of physical health and disease, a scattered and inconsequent succession of joys and griefs, frequent minor disturbances and vicissitudes and rarer strong searchings and upheavals of mind or body, and through it all Nature, partly with the aid of his thought and will, partly without or in spite of it, arranging these things in some rough practical fashion, some tolerable disorderly order, — this is the material of his existence. The average human being even now is in his inward existence as crude and undeveloped as was the bygone primitive man in his outward life. But as soon as we go deep within ourselves, — and Yoga means a plunge into all the multiple profundities of the soul, — we find ourselves subjectively, as man in his growth has found himself objectively, surrounded by a whole complex world which we have to know and to conquer.

The most disconcerting discovery is to find that every part of us — intellect, will, sense-mind, nervous or desire self, the heart, the body — has each, as it were, its own complex individuality and natural formation independent of the rest; it neither agrees with itself nor with the others nor with the representative ego which is the shadow cast by some central and centralising self on our superficial ignorance. We find that we are composed not of one but many personalities and each has its own demands and differing nature. Our being is a roughly constituted chaos into which we have to introduce the principle of a divine order. Moreover, we find that inwardly too, no less than outwardly, we are not alone in the world; the sharp separateness of our ego was no more than a strong imposition and delusion; we do not exist in ourselves, we do not really live apart in an inner privacy or solitude. Our mind is a receiving, developing and modifying machine into which there is being constantly passed from moment to moment a ceaseless foreign flux, a streaming mass of disparate materials from above, from below, from outside. Much more than half our thoughts and feelings are not our own in the sense that they take form out of ourselves; of hardly anything can it be said that it is truly original to our nature. A large part comes to us from others or from the environment, whether as raw material or as manufactured imports; but still more largely they come from universal Nature here or from other worlds and planes and their beings and powers and influences; for we are overtopped and environed by other planes of consciousness, mind planes, life planes, subtle matter planes, from which our life and action here are fed, or fed on, pressed, dominated, made use of for the manifestation of their forms and forces. The difficulty of our separate salvation is immensely increased by this complexity and manifold openness and subjection to the in-streaming energies of the universe. Of all this we have to take account, to deal with it, to know what is the secret stuff of our nature and its constituent and resultant motions and to create in it all a divine centre and a true harmony and luminous order.

In the ordinary paths of Yoga the method used for dealing with these conflicting materials is direct and simple. One or another of the principal psychological forces in us is selected as our single means for attaining to the Divine; the rest is quieted into inertia or left to starve in its smallness. The Bhakta, seizing on the emotional forces of the being, the intense activities of the heart, abides concentrated in the love of God, gathered up as into a single one-pointed tongue of fire; he is indifferent to the activities of thought, throws behind him the importunities of the reason, cares nothing for the mind's thirst for knowledge. All the knowledge he needs is his faith and the inspirations that well up from a heart in communion with the Divine. He has no use for any will to works that is not turned to the direct worship of the Beloved or the service of the temple. The man of Knowledge, self-confined by a deliberate choice to the force and activities of discriminative thought, finds release in the mind's hushed inward-drawn endeavour. He concentrates on the idea of the self, succeeds by a subtle inner discernment in distinguishing its silent presence amid the veiling activities of Nature, and through the perceptive idea arrives at the concrete spiritual experience. He is indifferent to the play of the emotions, deaf to the hunger-call of passion, closed to the activities of Life, — the more blessed he, the sooner they fall away from him and leave him free, still and mute, the eternal non-doer. The body is his stumbling-block, the vital functions are his enemies; if their demands can be reduced to a minimum, that is his great good fortune. The endless difficulties that arise from the environing world are dismissed by erecting firmly against them a defence of outer physical and inner spiritual solitude; safe behind a wall of inner silence, he remains impassive and untouched by the world and by others. To be alone with oneself or alone with the Divine, to walk apart with God and his devotees, to entrench oneself in the single self-ward endeavour of the mind or Godward passion of the heart is the trend of these Yogas. The problem is solved by the excision of all but the one central difficulty which pursues the one chosen motive-force; into the midst of the dividing calls of our nature the principle of an exclusive concentration comes sovereignly to our rescue.

But for the sadhaka of the integral Yoga this inner or this outer solitude can only be incidents or periods in his spiritual progress. Accepting life, he has to bear not only his own burden, but a great part of the world's burden too along with it, as a continuation of his own sufficiently heavy load. Therefore his Yoga has much more of the nature of a battle than others; but this is not only an individual battle, it is a collective war waged over a considerable country. He has not only to conquer in himself the forces of egoistic falsehood and disorder, but to conquer them as representatives of the same adverse and inexhaustible forces in the world. Their representative character gives them a much more obstinate capacity of resistance, an almost endless right to recurrence. Often he finds that even after he has won persistently his own personal battle, he has still to win it over and over again in a seemingly interminable war, because his inner existence has already been so much enlarged that not only it contains his own being with its well-defined needs and experiences, but is in solidarity with the being of others, because in himself he contains the universe.

Nor is the seeker of the integral fulfilment permitted to solve too arbitrarily even the conflict of his own inner members. He has to harmonise deliberate knowledge with unquestioning faith; he must conciliate the gentle soul of love with the formidable need of power; the passivity of the soul that lives content in transcendent calm has to be fused with the activity of the divine helper and the divine warrior. To him as to all seekers of the spirit there are offered for solution the oppositions of the reason, the clinging hold of the senses, the perturbations of the heart, the ambush of the desires, the clog of the physical body; but he has to deal in another fashion with their mutual and internal conflicts and their hindrance to his aim, for he must arrive at an infinitely more difficult perfection in the handling of all this rebel matter. Accepting them as instruments for the divine realisation and manifestation, he has to convert their jangling discords, to enlighten their thick darknesses, to transfigure them separately and all together, harmonising them in themselves and with each other, — integrally, omitting no grain or strand or vibration, leaving no iota of imperfection anywhere. An exclusive concentration, or even a succession of concentrations of that kind, can be in his complex work only a temporary convenience; it has to be abandoned as soon as its utility is over. An all-inclusive concentration is the difficult achievement towards which he must labour.

*
* *

Concentration is indeed the first condition of any Yoga, but it is an all-receiving concentration that is the very nature of the integral Yoga. A separate strong fixing of the thought, of the emotions or of the will on a single idea, object, state, inner movement or principle is no doubt a frequent need here also; but this is only a subsidiary helpful process. A wide massive opening, a harmonised concentration of the whole being in all its parts and through all its powers upon the One who is the All is the larger action of this Yoga without which it cannot achieve its purpose. For it is the consciousness that rests in the One and that acts in the All to which we aspire; it is this that we seek to impose on every element of our being and on every movement of our nature. This wide and concentrated totality is the essential character of the Sadhana and its character must determine its practice.

But even though the concentration of all the being on the Divine is the character of the Yoga, yet is our being too complex a thing to be taken up easily and at once, as if we were taking up the world in a pair of hands, and set in its entirety to a single task. Man in his effort at self-transcendence has usually to seize on some one spring or some powerful leverage in the complicated machine that his nature is; this spring or lever he touches in preference to others and uses it to set the machine in motion towards the end that he has in view. In his choice it is always Nature itself that should be his guide. But here it must be Nature at her highest and widest in him, not at her lowest or in some limiting movement. In her lower vital activities it is desire that Nature takes as her most powerful leverage; but the distinct character of man is that he is a mental being, not a merely vital creature. As he can use his thinking mind and will to restrain and correct his life impulses, so too he can bring in the action of a still higher luminous mentality aided by the deeper soul in him, the psychic being, and supersede by these greater and purer motive-powers the domination of the vital and sensational force that we call desire. He can entirely master or persuade it and offer it up for transformation to its divine Master. This higher mentality and this deeper soul, the psychic element in man, are the two grappling hooks by which the Divine can lay hold upon his nature.

The higher mind in man is something other, loftier, purer, vaster, more powerful than the reason or logical intelligence. The animal is a vital and sensational being; man, it is said, is distinguished from the animal by the possession of reason. But that is a very summary, a very imperfect and misleading account of the matter. For reason is only a particular and limited utilitarian and instrumental activity that proceeds from something much greater than itself, from a power that dwells in an ether more luminous, wider, illimitable. The true and ultimate, as distinguished from the immediate or intermediate importance of our observing, reasoning, inquiring, judging intelligence is that it prepares the human being for the right reception and right action of a Light from above which must progressively replace in him the obscure light from below that guides the animal. The latter also has a rudimentary reason, a kind of thought, a soul, a will and keen emotions; even though less developed, its psychology is yet the same in kind as man's. But all these capacities in the animal are automatically moved and strictly limited, almost even constituted by the lower nervous being. All animal perceptions, sensibilities, activities are ruled by nervous and vital instincts, cravings, needs, satisfactions, of which the nexus is the life-impulse and vital desire. Man too is bound, but less bound, to this automatism of the vital nature. Man can bring an enlightened will, an enlightened thought and enlightened emotions to the difficult work of his self-development; he can more and more subject to these more conscious and reflecting guides the inferior function of desire. In proportion as he can thus master and enlighten his lower self, he is man and no longer an animal. When he can begin to replace desire altogether by a still greater enlightened thought and sight and will in touch with the Infinite, consciously subject to a diviner will than his own, linked to a more universal and transcendent knowledge, he has commenced the ascent towards the superman; he is on his upward march towards the Divine.

It is, then, in the highest mind of thought and light and will or it is in the inner heart of deepest feeling and emotion that we must first centre our consciousness, — in either of them or, if we are capable, in both together, — and use that as our leverage to lift the nature wholly towards the Divine. The concentration of an enlightened thought, will and heart turned in unison towards one vast goal of our knowledge, one luminous and infinite source of our action, one imperishable object of our emotion is the starting-point of the Yoga. And the object of our seeking must be the very fount of the Light which is growing in us, the very origin of the Force which we are calling to move our members. Our one objective must be the Divine himself to whom, knowingly or unknowingly, something always aspires in our secret nature. There must be a large, many-sided yet single concentration of the thought on the idea, the perception, the vision, the awakening touch, the soul's realisation of the one Divine. There must be a flaming concentration of the heart on the seeking of the All and Eternal and, when once we have found him, a deep plunging and immersion in the possession and ecstasy of the All-Beautiful. There must be a strong and immovable concentration of the will on the attainment and fulfilment of all that the Divine is and a free and plastic opening of it to all that he intends to manifest in us. This is the triple way of the Yoga.

*
* *

But on that which as yet we know not how shall we concentrate? And yet we cannot know the Divine unless we have achieved this concentration of our being upon him. A concentration which culminates in a living realisation and the constant sense of the presence of the One in ourselves and in all of which we are aware, is what we mean in Yoga by knowledge and the effort after knowledge. It is not enough to devote ourselves by the reading of Scriptures or by the stress of philosophic reasoning to an intellectual understanding of the Divine; for at the end of our long mental labour we might know all that has been said of the Eternal, possess all that can be thought about the Infinite and yet we might not know him at all. This intellectual preparation can indeed be the first stage in a powerful Yoga, but it is not indispensable: it is not a step which all need or can be called upon to take. Yoga would be impossible, except for a very few, if the intellectual figure of knowledge arrived at by the speculative or meditative Reason were its indispensable condition or a binding preliminary. All that the Light from above asks of us that it may begin its work is a call from the soul and a sufficient point of support in the mind. This support can be reached through an

insistent idea of the Divine in the thought, a corresponding will
in the dynamic parts, an aspiration, a faith, a need in the heart.
Any one of these may lead or predominate, if all cannot move
in unison or in an equal rhythm. The idea may be and must
in the beginning be inadequate; the aspiration may be narrow
and imperfect, the faith poorly illumined or even, as not surely
founded on the rock of knowledge, fluctuating, uncertain, easily
diminished; often even it may be extinguished and need to be
lit again with difficulty like a torch in a windy pass. But if once
there is a resolute self-consecration from deep within, if there is
an awakening to the soul's call, these inadequate things can be a
sufficient instrument for the divine purpose. Therefore the wise
have always been unwilling to limit man's avenues towards God;
they would not shut against his entry even the narrowest portal,
the lowest and darkest postern, the humblest wicket-gate. Any
name, any form, any symbol, any offering has been held to be
sufficient if there is the consecration along with it; for the Divine
knows himself in the heart of the seeker and accepts the sacrifice.

But still the greater and wider the moving idea-force behind the consecration, the better for the seeker; his attainment
is likely to be fuller and more ample. If we are to attempt an
integral Yoga, it will be as well to start with an idea of the Divine
that is itself integral. There should be an aspiration in the heart
wide enough for a realisation without any narrow limits. Not
only should we avoid a sectarian religious outlook, but also all
one-sided philosophical conceptions which try to shut up the Ineffable in a restricting mental formula. The dynamic conception
or impelling sense with which our Yoga can best set out would be
naturally the idea, the sense of a conscious all-embracing but all-
exceeding Infinite. Our uplook must be to a free, all-powerful,
perfect and blissful One and Oneness in which all beings move
and live and through which all can meet and become one. This
Eternal will be at once personal and impersonal in his self-
revelation and touch upon the soul. He is personal because he is
the conscious Divine, the infinite Person who casts some broken
reflection of himself in the myriad divine and undivine personalities of the universe. He is impersonal because he appears to us

as an infinite Existence, Consciousness and Ananda and because he is the fount, base and constituent of all existences and all energies, the very material of our being and mind and life and body, our spirit and our matter. The thought, concentrating on him, must not merely understand in an intellectual form that he exists, or conceive of him as an abstraction, a logical necessity; it must become a seeing thought able to meet him here as the Inhabitant in all, realise him in ourselves, watch and take hold on the movement of his forces. He is the one Existence: he is the original and universal Delight that constitutes all things and exceeds them: he is the one infinite Consciousness that composes all consciousnesses and informs all their movements: he is the one illimitable Being who sustains all action and experience: his will guides the evolution of things towards their yet unrealised but inevitable aim and plenitude. To him the heart can consecrate itself, approach him as the supreme Beloved, beat and move in him as in a universal sweetness of Love and a living sea of Delight. For his is the secret Joy that supports the soul in all its experiences and maintains even the errant ego in its ordeals and struggles till all sorrow and suffering shall cease. His is the Love and the Bliss of the infinite divine Lover who is drawing all things by their own path towards his happy oneness. On him the Will can unalterably fix as the invisible Power that guides and fulfils it and as the source of its strength. In the impersonality this actuating Power is a self-illumined Force that contains all results and calmly works until it accomplishes, in the personality an all-wise and omnipotent Master of the Yoga whom nothing can prevent from leading it to its goal. This is the faith with which the seeker has to begin his seeking and endeavour; for in all his effort here, but most of all in his effort towards the Unseen, mental man must perforce proceed by faith. When the realisation comes, the faith divinely fulfilled and completed will be transformed into an eternal flame of knowledge.

*
* *

Into all our endeavour upward the lower element of desire will

at first naturally enter. For what the enlightened will sees as the
thing to be done and pursues as the crown to be conquered,
what the heart embraces as the one thing delightful, that in us
which feels itself limited and opposed and, because it is limited,
craves and struggles, will seek with the troubled passion of an
egoistic desire. This craving life-force or desire-soul in us has to
be accepted at first, but only in order that it may be transformed.
Even from the very beginning it has to be taught to renounce all
other desires and concentrate itself on the passion for the Divine.
This capital point gained, it has to be taught to desire, not for
its own separate sake, but for God in the world and for the
Divine in ourselves; it has to fix itself upon no personal spiritual
gain, though of all possible spiritual gains we are sure, but on
the great work to be done in us and others, on the high coming
manifestation which is to be the glorious fulfilment of the Divine
in the world, on the Truth that has to be sought and lived and
enthroned for ever. But last, most difficult for it, more difficult
than to seek with the right object, it has to be taught to seek in the
right manner; for it must learn to desire, not in its own egoistic
way, but in the way of the Divine. It must insist no longer, as
the strong separative will always insists, on its own manner of
fulfilment, its own dream of possession, its own idea of the right
and the desirable; it must yearn to fulfil a larger and greater Will
and consent to wait upon a less interested and ignorant guidance.
Thus trained, Desire, that great unquiet harasser and troubler of
man and cause of every kind of stumbling, will become fit to be
transformed into its divine counterpart. For desire and passion
too have their divine forms; there is a pure ecstasy of the soul's
seeking beyond all craving and grief, there is a Will of Ananda
that sits glorified in the possession of the supreme beatitudes.

When once the object of concentration has possessed and
is possessed by the three master instruments, the thought, the
heart and the will, — a consummation fully possible only when
the desire-soul in us has submitted to the Divine Law, — the
perfection of mind and life and body can be effectively fulfilled
in our transmuted nature. This will be done, not for the personal
satisfaction of the ego, but that the whole may constitute a fit

temple for the Divine Presence, a faultless instrument for the divine work. For that work can be truly performed only when the instrument, consecrated and perfected, has grown fit for a selfless action, — and that will be when personal desire and egoism are abolished, but not the liberated individual. Even when the little ego has been abolished, the true spiritual Person can still remain and God's will and work and delight in him and the spiritual use of his perfection and fulfilment. Our works will then be divine and done divinely; our mind and life and will, devoted to the Divine, will be used to help fulfil in others and in the world that which has been first realised in ourselves, — all that we can manifest of the embodied Unity, Love, Freedom, Strength, Power, Splendour, immortal Joy which is the goal of the Spirit's terrestrial adventure.

The Yoga must start with an effort or at least a settled turn towards this total concentration. A constant and unfailing will of consecration of all ourselves to the Supreme is demanded of us, an offering of our whole being and our many-chambered nature to the Eternal who is the All. The effective fullness of our concentration on the one thing needful to the exclusion of all else will be the measure of our self-consecration to the One who is alone desirable. But this exclusiveness will in the end exclude nothing except the falsehood of our way of seeing the world and our will's ignorance. For our concentration on the Eternal will be consummated by the mind when we see constantly the Divine in itself and the Divine in ourselves, but also the Divine in all things and beings and happenings. It will be consummated by the heart when all emotion is summed up in the love of the Divine, — of the Divine in itself and for itself, but love too of the Divine in all its beings and powers and personalities and forms in the Universe. It will be consummated by the will when we feel and receive always the divine impulsion and accept that alone as our sole motive force; but this will mean that, having slain to the last rebellious straggler the wandering impulses of the egoistic nature, we have universalised ourselves and can accept with a constant happy acceptance the one divine working in all things. This is the first fundamental siddhi of the integral Yoga.

It is nothing less that is meant in the end when we speak of the absolute consecration of the individual to the Divine. But this total fullness of consecration can only come by a constant progression when the long and difficult process of transforming desire out of existence is completed in an ungrudging measure. Perfect self-consecration implies perfect self-surrender.

*
* *

For here, there are two movements with a transitional stage between them, two periods of this Yoga, — one of the process of surrender, the other of its crown and consequence. In the first the individual prepares himself for the reception of the Divine into his members. For all this first period he has to work by means of the instruments of the lower Nature, but aided more and more from above. But in the later transitional stage of this movement our personal and necessarily ignorant effort more and more dwindles and a higher Nature acts; the eternal Shakti descends into this limited form of mortality and progressively possesses and transmutes it. In the second period the greater movement wholly replaces the lesser, formerly indispensable first action; but this can be done only when our self-surrender is complete. The ego person in us cannot transform itself by its own force or will or knowledge or by any virtue of its own into the nature of the Divine; all it can do is to fit itself for the transformation and make more and more its surrender to that which it seeks to become. As long as the ego is at work in us, our personal action is and must always be in its nature a part of the lower grades of existence; it is obscure or half-enlightened, limited in its field, very partially effective in its power. If a spiritual transformation, not a mere illumining modification of our nature, is to be done at all, we must call in the Divine Shakti to effect that miraculous work in the individual; for she alone has the needed force, decisive, all-wise and illimitable. But the entire substitution of the divine for the human personal action is not at once entirely possible. All interference from below that would falsify the truth of the superior action must first be inhibited or rendered impotent, and it must be done by our own free choice. A continual and always repeated refusal of the impulsions and falsehoods of the lower nature is asked from us and an insistent support to the Truth as it grows in our parts; for the progressive settling into our nature and final perfection of the incoming informing Light, Purity and Power needs for its development and sustenance our free acceptance of it and our stubborn rejection of all that is contrary to it, inferior or incompatible.

In the first movement of self-preparation, the period of personal effort, the method we have to use is this concentration of the whole being on the Divine that it seeks and, as its corollary, this constant rejection, throwing out, *katharsis*, of all that is not the true Truth of the Divine. An entire consecration of all that we are, think, feel and do will be the result of this persistence. This consecration in its turn must culminate in an integral self-giving to the Highest; for its crown and sign of completion is the whole nature's all-comprehending absolute surrender. In the second stage of the Yoga, transitional between the human and the divine working, there will supervene an increasing purified and vigilant passivity, a more and more luminous divine response to the Divine Force, but not to any other; and there will be as a result the growing inrush of a great and conscious miraculous working from above. In the last period there is no effort at all, no set method, no fixed sadhana; the place of endeavour and tapasya will be taken by a natural, simple, powerful and happy disclosing of the flower of the Divine out of the bud of a purified and perfected terrestrial nature. These are the natural successions of the action of the Yoga.

These movements are indeed not always or absolutely arranged in a strict succession to each other. The second stage begins in part before the first is completed; the first continues in part until the second is perfected; the last divine working can manifest from time to time as a promise before it is finally settled and normal to the nature. Always too there is something higher and greater than the individual which leads him even in his personal labour and endeavour. Often he may become, and remain for a time, wholly conscious, even in parts of his being permanently conscious, of this greater leading behind the veil, and that may happen long before his whole nature has been purified in all its parts from the lower indirect control. Even, he may be thus conscious from the beginning; his mind and heart, if not his other members, may respond to that seizing and penetrating guidance with a certain initial completeness from the very first steps of the Yoga. But it is the constant and complete and uniform action of the great direct control that more and more distinguishes the transitional stage as it proceeds and draws to its close. This predominance of a greater diviner leading, not personal to ourselves, indicates the nature's increasing ripeness for a total spiritual transformation. It is the unmistakable sign that the self-consecration has not only been accepted in principle but is fulfilled in act and power. The Supreme has laid his luminous hand upon a chosen human vessel of his miraculous Light and Power and Ananda.

Self-Surrender in Works —
The Way of the Gita

LIFE, NOT a remote silent or high-uplifted ecstatic Beyond-Life alone, is the field of our Yoga. The transformation of our superficial, narrow and fragmentary human way of thinking, seeing, feeling and being into a deep and wide spiritual consciousness and an integrated inner and outer existence and of our ordinary human living into the divine way of life must be its central purpose. The means towards this supreme end is a self-giving of all our nature to the Divine. Everything must be given to the Divine within us, to the universal All and to the transcendent Supreme. An absolute concentration of our will, our heart and our thought on that one and manifold Divine, an unreserved self-consecration of our whole being to the Divine alone — this is the decisive movement, the turning of the ego to That which is infinitely greater than itself, its self-giving and indispensable surrender.

The life of the human creature, as it is ordinarily lived, is composed of a half-fixed, half-fluid mass of very imperfectly ruled thoughts, perceptions, sensations, emotions, desires, enjoyments, acts, mostly customary and self-repeating, in part only dynamic and self-developing, but all centred around a superficial ego. The sum of movement of these activities eventuates in an internal growth which is partly visible and operative in this life, partly a seed of progress in lives hereafter. This growth of the conscious being, an expansion, an increasing self-expression, a more and more harmonised development of his constituent members is the whole meaning and all the pith of human existence. It is for this meaningful development of consciousness by thought, will, emotion, desire, action and experience, leading in the end to a supreme divine self-discovery, that Man, the mental being, has entered into the material body. All the rest is either auxiliary and subordinate or accidental and otiose; that only matters which sustains and helps the evolution of his nature and the growth or rather the progressive unfolding and discovery of his self and spirit.

The aim set before our Yoga is nothing less than to hasten this supreme object of our existence here. Its process leaves behind the ordinary tardy method of slow and confused growth through the evolution of Nature. For the natural evolution is at its best an uncertain growth under cover, partly by the pressure of the environment, partly by a groping education and an ill-lighted purposeful effort, an only partially illumined and half-automatic use of opportunities with many blunders and lapses and relapses; a great portion of it is made up of apparent accidents and circumstances and vicissitudes, — though veiling a secret divine intervention and guidance. In Yoga we replace this confused crooked crab-motion by a rapid, conscious and self-directed evolution which is planned to carry us, as far as can be, in a straight line towards the goal set before us. In a certain sense it may be an error to speak of a goal anywhere in a progression which may well be infinite. Still we can conceive of an immediate goal, an ulterior objective beyond our present achievement towards which the soul in man can aspire. There lies before him the possibility of a new birth; there can be an ascent into a higher and wider plane of being and its descent to transform his members. An enlarged and illumined consciousness is possible that shall make of him a liberated spirit and a perfected force — and, if spread beyond the individual, it might even constitute a divine humanity or else a new, a supramental and therefore a superhuman race. It is this new birth that we make our aim: a growth into a divine consciousness is the whole meaning of our Yoga, an integral conversion to divinity not only of the soul but of all the parts of our nature.

*
* *

Our purpose in Yoga is to exile the limited outward-looking

ego and to enthrone God in its place as the ruling Inhabitant of the nature. And this means, first, to disinherit desire and no longer accept the enjoyment of desire as the ruling human motive. The spiritual life will draw its sustenance not from desire but from a pure and selfless spiritual delight of essential existence. And not only the vital nature in us whose stamp is desire, but the mental being too must undergo a new birth and a transfiguring change. Our divided, egoistic, limited and ignorant thought and intelligence must disappear; in its place there must stream in the catholic and faultless play of a shadowless divine illumination which shall culminate in the end in a natural self-existent Truth-consciousness free from groping half-truth and stumbling error. Our confused and embarrassed ego-centred small-motived will and action must cease and make room for the total working of a swiftly powerful, lucidly automatic, divinely moved and guided unfallen Force. There must be implanted and activised in all our doings a supreme, impersonal, unfaltering and unstumbling will in spontaneous and untroubled unison with the will of the Divine. The unsatisfying surface play of our feeble egoistic emotions must be ousted and there must be revealed instead a secret deep and vast psychic heart within that waits behind them for its hour; all our feelings, impelled by this inner heart in which dwells the Divine, will be transmuted into calm and intense movements of a twin passion of divine Love and manifold Ananda. This is the definition of a divine humanity or a supramental race. This, not an exaggerated or even a sublimated energy of human intellect and action, is the type of the superman whom we are called to evolve by our Yoga.

In the ordinary human existence an outgoing action is obviously three-fourths or even more of our life. It is only the exceptions, the saint and the seer, the rare thinker, poet and artist who can live more within themselves; these indeed, at least in the most intimate parts of their nature, shape themselves more in inner thought and feeling than in the surface act. But it is not either of these sides separated from the other, but rather a harmony of the inner and the outer life made one in fullness and transfigured into a play of something that is beyond them which will create the form of a perfect living. A Yoga of works, a union with the Divine in our will and acts — and not only in knowledge and feeling — is then an indispensable, an inexpressibly important element of an integral Yoga. The conversion of our thought and feeling without a corresponding conversion of the spirit and body of our works would be a maimed achievement.

But if this total conversion is to be done, there must be a consecration of our actions and outer movements as much as of our mind and heart to the Divine. There must be accepted and progressively accomplished a surrender of our capacities of working into the hands of a greater Power behind us and our sense of being the doer and worker must disappear. All must be given for a more direct use into the hands of the divine Will which is hidden by these frontal appearances; for by that permitting Will alone is our action possible. A hidden Power is the true Lord and overruling Observer of our acts and only he knows through all the ignorance and perversion and deformation brought in by the ego their entire sense and ultimate purpose. There must be effected a complete transformation of our limited and distorted egoistic life and works into the large and direct outpouring of a greater divine Life, Will and Energy that now secretly supports us. This greater Will and Energy must be made conscious in us and master; no longer must it remain, as now, only a superconscious, upholding and permitting Force. There must be achieved an undistorted transmission through us of the all-wise purpose and process of a now hidden omniscient Power and omnipotent Knowledge which will turn into its pure, unobstructed, happily consenting and participating channel all our transmuted nature. This total consecration and surrender and this resultant entire transformation and free transmission make up the whole fundamental means and the ultimate aim of an integral Karmayoga.

Even for those whose first natural movement is a consecration, a surrender and a resultant entire transformation of the thinking mind and its knowledge, or a total consecration, surrender and transformation of the heart and its emotions, the consecration of works is a needed element in that change. Otherwise, although they may find God in other-life, they will not be able to fulfil the Divine in life; life for them will be a meaningless undivine inconsequence. Not for them the true victory that shall be the key to the riddle of our terrestrial existence; their love will not be the absolute love triumphant over self, their knowledge will not be the total consciousness and the all-embracing knowledge. It is possible, indeed, to begin with knowledge or Godward emotion solely or with both together and to leave works for the final movement of the Yoga. But there is then this disadvantage that we may tend to live too exclusively within, subtilised in subjective experience, shut off in our isolated inner parts; there we may get incrusted in our spiritual seclusion and find it difficult later on to pour ourselves triumphantly outwards and apply to life our gains in the higher Nature. When we turn to add this external kingdom also to our inner conquests, we shall find ourselves too much accustomed to an activity purely subjective and ineffective on the material plane. There will be an immense difficulty in transforming the outer life and the body. Or we shall find that our action does not correspond with the inner light: it still follows the old accustomed mistaken paths, still obeys the old normal imperfect influences; the Truth within us continues to be separated by a painful gulf from the ignorant mechanism of our external nature. This is a frequent experience because in such a process the Light and Power come to be self-contained and unwilling to express themselves in life or to use the physical means prescribed for the Earth and her processes. It is as if we were living in another, a larger and subtler world and had no divine hold, perhaps little hold of any kind, upon the material and terrestrial existence.

But still each must follow his nature, and there are always difficulties that have to be accepted for some time if we are to pursue our natural path of Yoga. Yoga is after all primarily a change of the inner consciousness and nature, and if the balance of our parts is such that this must be done first with an initial exclusiveness and the rest left for later handling, we must accept the apparent imperfection of the process. Yet would the ideal working of an integral Yoga be a movement, even from the beginning, integral in its process and whole and many-sided in its progress. In any case our present preoccupation is with a Yoga, integral in its aim and complete movement, but starting from works and proceeding by works although at each step more and more moved by a vivifying divine love and more and more illumined by a helping divine knowledge.

* * *

The greatest gospel of spiritual works ever yet given to the race, the most perfect system of Karmayoga known to man in the past, is to be found in the Bhagavad Gita. In that famous episode of the Mahabharata the great basic lines of Karmayoga are laid down for all time with an incomparable mastery and the infallible eye of an assured experience. It is true that the path alone, as the ancients saw it, is worked out fully: the perfect fulfilment, the highest secret[1] is hinted rather than developed; it is kept back as an unexpressed part of a supreme mystery. There are obvious reasons for this reticence; for the fulfilment is in any case a matter for experience and no teaching can express it. It cannot be described in a way that can really be understood by a mind that has not the effulgent transmuting experience. And for the soul that has passed the shining portals and stands in the blaze of the inner light, all mental and verbal description is as poor as it is superfluous, inadequate and an impertinence. All divine consummations have perforce to be figured by us in the inapt and deceptive terms of a language which was made to fit the normal experience of mental man; so expressed, they can be rightly understood only by those who already know, and, knowing, are able to give these poor external terms a changed, inner and transfigured sense. As the Vedic Rishis insisted in the beginning, the words of the supreme wisdom are expressive only to those who are already of the wise. The Gita at its cryptic close may seem by its silence to stop short of that solution for which we are seeking; it pauses at the borders of the highest spiritual mind and does not cross them into the splendours of the supramental

---

[1] *rahasyam uttamam.*

Light. And yet its secret of dynamic, and not only static, identity with the inner Presence, its highest mystery of absolute surrender to the Divine Guide, Lord and Inhabitant of our nature, is the central secret. This surrender is the indispensable means of the supramental change and, again, it is through the supramental change that the dynamic identity becomes possible.

What then are the lines of Karmayoga laid down by the Gita? Its key principle, its spiritual method, can be summed up as the union of two largest and highest states or powers of consciousness, equality and oneness. The kernel of its method is an unreserved acceptance of the Divine in our life as in our inner self and spirit. An inner renunciation of personal desire leads to equality, accomplishes our total surrender to the Divine, supports a delivery from dividing ego which brings us oneness. But this must be a oneness in dynamic force and not only in static peace or inactive beatitude. The Gita promises us freedom for the spirit even in the midst of works and the full energies of Nature, if we accept subjection of our whole being to that which is higher than the separating and limiting ego. It proposes an integral dynamic activity founded on a still passivity; a largest possible action irrevocably based on an immobile calm is its secret, — free expression out of a supreme inward silence.

All things here are the one and indivisible eternal transcendent and cosmic Brahman that is in its seeming divided in things and creatures; in seeming only, for in truth it is always one and equal in all things and creatures and the division is only a phenomenon of the surface. As long as we live in the ignorant seeming, we are the ego and are subject to the modes of Nature. Enslaved to appearances, bound to the dualities, tossed between good and evil, sin and virtue, grief and joy, pain and pleasure, good fortune and ill fortune, success and failure, we follow helplessly the iron or gilt and iron round of the wheel of Maya. At best we have only the poor relative freedom which by us is ignorantly called free-will. But that is at bottom illusory, since it is the modes of Nature that express themselves through our personal will; it is force of Nature, grasping us, ungrasped by us that determines what we shall will and how we shall will it. Nature, not an independent ego, chooses what object we shall seek, whether by reasoned will or unreflecting impulse, at any moment of our existence. If, on the contrary, we live in the unifying reality of the Brahman, then we go beyond the ego and overstep Nature. For then we get back to our true self and become the spirit; in the spirit we are above the impulsion of Nature, superior to her modes and forces. Attaining to a perfect equality in the soul, mind and heart, we realise our true self of oneness, one with all beings, one too with That which expresses itself in them and in all that we see and experience. This equality and this oneness are the indispensable twin foundation we must lay down for a divine being, a divine consciousness, a divine action. Not one with all, we are not spiritual, not divine. Not equal-souled to all things, happenings and creatures, we cannot see spiritually, cannot know divinely, cannot feel divinely towards others. The Supreme Power, the one Eternal and Infinite is equal to all things and to all beings; and because it is equal, it can act with an absolute wisdom according to the truth of its works and its force and according to the truth of each thing and of every creature.

This is also the only true freedom possible to man, — a freedom which he cannot have unless he outgrows his mental separativeness and becomes the conscious soul in Nature. The only free will in the world is the one divine Will of which Nature is the executrix; for she is the master and creator of all other wills. Human free-will can be real in a sense, but, like all things that belong to the modes of Nature, it is only relatively real. The mind rides on a swirl of natural forces, balances on a poise between several possibilities, inclines to one side or another, settles and has the sense of choosing: but it does not see, it is not even dimly aware of the Force behind that has determined its choice. It cannot see it, because that Force is something total and to our eyes indeterminate. At most mind can only distinguish with an approach to clarity and precision some out of the complex variety of particular determinations by which this Force works out her incalculable purposes. Partial itself, the mind rides on a part of the machine, unaware of nine-tenths of its motor agencies in Time and environment, unaware of its past preparation and future drift; but because it rides, it thinks that it is directing the machine. In a sense it counts: for that clear inclination of the mind which we call our will, that firm settling of the inclination which presents itself to us as a deliberate choice, is one of Nature's most powerful determinants; but it is never independent and sole. Behind this petty instrumental action of the human will there is something vast and powerful and eternal that oversees the trend of the inclination and presses on the turn of the will. There is a total Truth in Nature greater than our individual choice. And in this total Truth, or even beyond and behind it, there is something that determines all results; its presence and secret knowledge keep up steadily in the process of Nature a dynamic, almost automatic perception of the right relations, the varying or persistent necessities, the inevitable steps of the movement. There is a secret divine Will, eternal and infinite, omniscient and omnipotent, that expresses itself in the universality and in each particular of all these apparently temporal and finite inconscient or half-conscient things. This is the Power or Presence meant by the Gita when it speaks of the Lord within the heart of all existences who turns all creatures as if mounted on a machine by the illusion of Nature.

This divine Will is not an alien Power or Presence; it is intimate to us and we ourselves are part of it: for it is our own highest Self that possesses and supports it. Only, it is not our conscious mental will; it rejects often enough what our conscious will accepts and accepts what our conscious will rejects. For while this secret One knows all and every whole and each detail, our surface mind knows only a little part of things. Our will is conscious in the mind, and what it knows, it knows by the thought only; the divine Will is superconscious to us because it is in its essence supra-mental, and it knows all because it is all. Our highest Self which possesses and supports this universal Power is not our ego-self, not our personal nature; it is something transcendent and universal of which these smaller things are only foam and flowing surface. If we surrender our conscious will and allow it to be made one with the will of the Eternal, then, and then only, shall we attain to a true freedom; living in the divine liberty, we shall no longer cling to this shackled so-called free-will, a puppet freedom ignorant, illusory, relative, bound to the error of its own inadequate vital motives and mental figures.

*
 * *

A distinction has to be firmly seized in our consciousness, the capital distinction between mechanical Nature and the free Lord of Nature, between the Ishwara or single luminous divine Will and the many executive modes and forces of the universe.

Nature, — not as she is in her divine Truth, the conscious Power of the Eternal, but as she appears to us in the Ignorance, — is executive Force, mechanical in her steps, not consciously intelligent to our experience of her, although all her works are instinct with an absolute intelligence. Not in herself master, she is full of a self-aware Power[2] which has an infinite mastery and, because of this Power driving her, she rules all and exactly fulfils the work intended in her by the Ishwara. Not enjoying but enjoyed, she bears in herself the burden of all enjoyments. Nature as Prakriti is an inertly active Force, — for she works out a movement imposed upon her; but within her is One that knows, — some Entity sits there that is aware of all her motion and process. Prakriti works containing the knowledge, the mastery, the delight of the Purusha, the Being associated with her or seated within her; but she can participate in them only by subjection and reflection of that which fills her. Purusha knows and is still and inactive; he contains the action of Prakriti within his consciousness and knowledge and enjoys it. He gives the sanction to Prakriti's works and she works out what is sanctioned by him for his pleasure. Purusha himself does not execute; he maintains Prakriti in her action and allows her to express in energy and process and formed result what he perceives in his knowledge. This is the distinction made by the Sankhyas; and although it is not all the true truth, not in any way the highest truth either

---

[2] This Power is the conscious divine Shakti of the Ishwara, the transcendent and universal Mother.

of Purusha or of Prakriti, still it is a valid and indispensable practical knowledge in the lower hemisphere of existence.

The individual soul or the conscious being in a form may identify itself with this experiencing Purusha or with this active Prakriti. If it identifies itself with Prakriti, it is not master, enjoyer and knower, but reflects the modes and workings of Prakriti. It enters by its identification into that subjection and mechanical working which is characteristic of her. And even, by an entire immersion in Prakriti, this soul becomes inconscient or subconscient, asleep in her forms as in the earth and the metal or almost asleep as in plant life. There, in that inconscience, it is subject to the domination of tamas, the principle, the power, the qualitative mode of obscurity and inertia: sattwa and rajas are there, but they are concealed in the thick coating of tamas. Emerging into its own proper nature of consciousness but not yet truly conscious, because there is still too great a domination of tamas in the nature, the embodied being becomes more and more subject to rajas, the principle, the power, the qualitative mode of action and passion impelled by desire and instinct. There is then formed and developed the animal nature, narrow in consciousness, rudimentary in intelligence, rajaso-tamasic in vital habit and impulse. Emerging yet farther from the great Inconscience towards a spiritual status the embodied being liberates sattwa, the mode of light, and acquires a relative freedom and mastery and knowledge and with it a qualified and conditioned sense of inner satisfaction and happiness. Man, the mental being in a physical body, should be but is not, except in a few among this multitude of ensouled bodies, of this nature. Ordinarily he has too much in him of the obscure earth-inertia and a troubled ignorant animal life-force to be a soul of light and bliss or even a mind of harmonious will and knowledge. There is here in man an incomplete and still hampered and baffled ascension towards the true character of the Purusha, free, master, knower and enjoyer. For these are in human and earthly experience relative modes, none giving its single and absolute fruit; all are intermixed with each other and there is not the pure action of any one of them anywhere. It is their confused and inconstant interaction that determines the experiences of the egoistic human consciousness swinging in Nature's uncertain balance.

The sign of the immersion of the embodied soul in Prakriti is the limitation of consciousness to the ego. The vivid stamp of this limited consciousness can be seen in a constant inequality of the mind and heart and a confused conflict and disharmony in their varied reactions to the touches of experience. The human reactions sway perpetually between the dualities created by the soul's subjection to Nature and by its often intense but narrow struggle for mastery and enjoyment, a struggle for the most part ineffective. The soul circles in an unending round of Nature's alluring and distressing opposites, success and failure, good fortune and ill fortune, good and evil, sin and virtue, joy and grief, pain and pleasure. It is only when, awaking from its immersion in Prakriti, it perceives its oneness with the One and its oneness with all existences that it can become free from these things and found its right relation to this executive world-Nature. Then it becomes indifferent to her inferior modes, equal-minded to her dualities, capable of mastery and freedom; it is seated above her as the high-throned knower and witness filled with the calm intense unalloyed delight of his own eternal existence. The embodied spirit continues to express its powers in action, but it is no longer involved in ignorance, no longer bound by its works; its actions have no longer a consequence within it, but only a consequence outside in Prakriti. The whole movement of Nature becomes to its experience a rising and falling of waves on the surface that make no difference to its own unfathomable peace, its wide delight, its vast universal equality or its boundless God-existence.[3]

* * *

[3] It is not indispensable for the Karmayoga to accept implicitly all the philosophy of the Gita. We may regard it, if we like, as a statement of psychological experience useful as a practical basis for the Yoga; here it is perfectly valid and in entire consonance with a high and wide experience. For this reason I have thought it well to state it here, as far as possible in the language of modern thought, omitting all that belongs to metaphysics rather than to psychology.

These are the conditions of our effort and they point to an ideal which can be expressed in these or in equivalent formulae.

To live in God and not in the ego; to move, vastly founded, not in the little egoistic consciousness, but in the consciousness of the All-Soul and the Transcendent.

To be perfectly equal in all happenings and to all beings, and to see and feel them as one with oneself and one with the Divine; to feel all in oneself and all in God; to feel God in all, oneself in all.

To act in God and not in the ego. And here, first, not to choose action by reference to personal needs and standards, but in obedience to the dictates of the living highest Truth above us. Next, as soon as we are sufficiently founded in the spiritual consciousness, not to act any longer by our separate will or movement, but more and more to allow action to happen and develop under the impulsion and guidance of a divine Will that surpasses us. And last, the supreme result, to be exalted into an identity in knowledge, force, consciousness, act, joy of existence with the Divine Shakti; to feel a dynamic movement not dominated by mortal desire and vital instinct and impulse and illusive mental free-will, but luminously conceived and evolved in an immortal self-delight and an infinite self-knowledge. For this is the action that comes by a conscious subjection and merging of the natural man into the divine Self and eternal Spirit; it is the Spirit that for ever transcends and guides this world-Nature.

*
* *

But by what practical steps of self-discipline can we arrive at this consummation?

The elimination of all egoistic activity and of its foundation, the egoistic consciousness, is clearly the key to the consummation we desire. And since in the path of works action is the knot we have first to loosen, we must endeavour to loosen it where it is centrally tied, in desire and in ego; for otherwise we shall cut only stray strands and not the heart of our bondage. These are the two knots of our subjection to this ignorant and divided Nature, desire and ego-sense. And of these two desire has its native home in the emotions and sensations and instincts and from there affects thought and volition; ego-sense lives indeed in these movements, but it casts its deep roots also in the thinking mind and its will and it is there that it becomes fully self-conscious. These are the twin obscure powers of the obsessing world-wide Ignorance that we have to enlighten and eliminate.

In the field of action desire takes many forms, but the most powerful of all is the vital self's craving or seeking after the fruit of our works. The fruit we covet may be a reward of internal pleasure; it may be the accomplishment of some preferred idea or some cherished will or the satisfaction of the egoistic emotions, or else the pride of success of our highest hopes and ambitions. Or it may be an external reward, a recompense entirely material, — wealth, position, honour, victory, good fortune or any other fulfilment of vital or physical desire. But all alike are lures by which egoism holds us. Always these satisfactions delude us with the sense of mastery and the idea of freedom, while really we are harnessed and guided or ridden and whipped by some gross or subtle, some noble or ignoble, figure of the blind Desire that drives the world. Therefore the first rule of action laid down by the Gita is to do the work that should be done without any desire for the fruit, *niṣkāma karma*.

A simple rule in appearance, and yet how difficult to carry out with anything like an absolute sincerity and liberating entireness! In the greater part of our action we use the principle very little if at all, and then even mostly as a sort of counterpoise to the normal principle of desire and to mitigate the extreme action of that tyrant impulse. At best, we are satisfied if we arrive at a modified and disciplined egoism not too shocking to our moral sense, not too brutally offensive to others. And to our partial self-discipline we give various names and forms; we habituate ourselves by practice to the sense of duty, to a firm fidelity to principle, a stoical fortitude or a religious resignation, a quiet or an ecstatic submission to God's will. But it is not these things that the Gita intends, useful though they are in their place; it aims at something absolute, unmitigated, uncompromising, a turn, an attitude that will change the whole poise of the soul. Not the mind's control of vital impulse is its rule, but the strong immobility of an immortal spirit.

The test it lays down is an absolute equality of the mind and the heart to all results, to all reactions, to all happenings. If good fortune and ill fortune, if respect and insult, if reputation and obloquy, if victory and defeat, if pleasant event and sorrowful event leave us not only unshaken but untouched, free in the emotions, free in the nervous reactions, free in the mental view, not responding with the least disturbance or vibration in any spot of the nature, then we have the absolute liberation to which the Gita points us, but not otherwise. The tiniest reaction is a proof that the discipline is imperfect and that some part of us accepts ignorance and bondage as its law and clings still to the old nature. Our self-conquest is only partially accomplished; it is still imperfect or unreal in some stretch or part or smallest spot of the ground of our nature. And that little pebble of imperfection may throw down the whole achievement of the Yoga!

There are certain semblances of an equal spirit which must not be mistaken for the profound and vast spiritual equality which the Gita teaches. There is an equality of disappointed resignation, an equality of pride, an equality of hardness and indifference: all these are egoistic in their nature. Inevitably they come in the course of the sadhana, but they must be rejected or transformed into the true quietude. There is too, on a higher level, the equality of the stoic, the equality of a devout resignation or a sage detachment, the equality of a soul aloof from the world and indifferent to its doings. These too are insufficient; first approaches they can be, but they are at most early soul-phases only or imperfect mental preparations for our entry into the true and absolute self-existent wide evenness of the spirit.

For it is certain that so great a result cannot be arrived at immediately and without any previous stages. At first we have to learn to bear the shocks of the world with the central part of our being untouched and silent, even when the surface mind, heart, life are strongly shaken; unmoved there on the bedrock of our life, we must separate the soul watching behind or immune deep within from these outer workings of our nature. Afterwards, extending this calm and steadfastness of the detached soul to its instruments, it will become slowly possible to radiate peace from the luminous centre to the darker peripheries. In this process we may take the passing help of many minor phases; a certain stoicism, a certain calm philosophy, a certain religious exaltation may help us towards some nearness to our aim, or we may call in even less strong and exalted but still useful powers of our mental nature. In the end we must either discard or transform them and arrive instead at an entire equality, a perfect self-existent peace within and even, if we can, a total unassailable, self-poised and spontaneous delight in all our members.

But how then shall we continue to act at all? For ordinarily the human being acts because he has a desire or feels a mental, vital or physical want or need; he is driven by the necessities of the body, by the lust of riches, honours or fame, or by a craving for the personal satisfactions of the mind or the heart or a craving for power or pleasure. Or he is seized and pushed about by a moral need or, at least, the need or the desire of making his ideas or his ideals or his will or his party or his country or his gods prevail in the world. If none of these desires nor any other must be the spring of our action, it would seem as if all incentive or motive power had been removed and action itself must necessarily cease. The Gita replies with its third great secret of the divine life. All action must be done in a more and more Godward and finally a God-possessed consciousness; our works must be a sacrifice to the Divine and in the end a surrender of all our being, mind, will, heart, sense, life and body to the One must make God-love and God-service our only motive. This transformation of the motive force and very character of works is indeed its master idea; it is the foundation of its unique synthesis of works, love and knowledge. In the end not desire, but the consciously felt will of the Eternal remains as the sole driver of our action and the sole originator of its initiative.

Equality, renunciation of all desire for the fruit of our works, action done as a sacrifice to the supreme Lord of our nature and of all nature, — these are the three first Godward approaches in the Gita's way of Karmayoga.

Chapter IV

The Sacrifice, the Triune Path and the Lord of the Sacrifice

THE LAW of sacrifice is the common divine action that was thrown out into the world in its beginning as a symbol of the solidarity of the universe. It is by the attraction of this law that a divinising principle, a saving power descends to limit and correct and gradually to eliminate the errors of an egoistic and self-divided creation. This descent, this sacrifice of the Purusha, the Divine Soul submitting itself to Force and Matter so that it may inform and illuminate them, is the seed of redemption of this world of Inconscience and Ignorance. "For with sacrifice as their companion," says the Gita, "the All-Father created these peoples." The acceptance of the law of sacrifice is a practical recognition by the ego that it is neither alone in the world nor chief in the world. It is its admission that, even in this much fragmented existence, there is beyond itself and behind that which is not its own egoistic person, something greater and completer, a diviner All which demands from it subordination and service. Indeed, sacrifice is imposed and, where need be, compelled by the universal World-Force; it takes it even from those who do not consciously recognise the law, — inevitably, because this is the intrinsic nature of things. Our ignorance or our false egoistic view of life can make no difference to this eternal bedrock truth of Nature. For this is the truth in Nature, that this ego which thinks itself a separate independent being and claims to live for itself, is not and cannot be independent nor separate, nor can it live to itself even if it would, but rather all are linked together by a secret Oneness. Each existence is continually giving out perforce from its stock; out of its mental receipts from Nature or its vital and physical assets and acquisitions and belongings a stream goes to all that is around it. And always again it receives something from its environment gratis or in return for its voluntary or involuntary tribute. For it is only by this giving and receiving that it can effect its own growth while at the same time it helps the sum of things. At length, though at first slowly and partially, we learn to make the conscious sacrifice; even, in the end, we take joy to give ourselves and what we envisage as belonging to us in a spirit of love and devotion to That which appears for the moment other than ourselves and is certainly other than our limited personalities. The sacrifice and the divine return for our sacrifice then become a gladly accepted means towards our last perfection; for it is recognised now as the road to the fulfilment in us of the eternal purpose.

But, most often, the sacrifice is done unconsciously, egoistically and without knowledge or acceptance of the true meaning of the great world-rite. It is so that the vast majority of earth-creatures do it; and, when it is so done, the individual derives only a mechanical minimum of natural inevitable profit, achieves by it only a slow painful progress limited and tortured by the smallness and suffering of the ego. Only when the heart, the will and the mind of knowledge associate themselves with the law and gladly follow it, can there come the deep joy and the happy fruitfulness of divine sacrifice. The mind's knowledge of the law and the heart's gladness in it culminate in the perception that it is to our own Self and Spirit and the one Self and Spirit of all that we give. And this is true even when our self-offering is still to our fellow-creatures or to lesser Powers and Principles and not yet to the Supreme. "Not for the sake of the wife," says Yajnavalkya in the Upanishad, "but for the sake of the Self is the wife dear to us." This in the lower sense of the individual self is the hard fact behind the coloured and passionate professions of egoistic love; but in a higher sense it is the inner significance of that love too which is not egoistic but divine. All true love and all sacrifice are in their essence Nature's contradiction of the primary egoism and its separative error; it is her attempt to turn from a necessary first fragmentation towards a recovered oneness. All unity between creatures is in its essence a self-finding, a fusion with that from which we have separated, a discovery of one's self in others.

But it is only a divine love and unity that can possess in the light what the human forms of these things seek for in the darkness. For the true unity is not merely an association and agglomeration like that of physical cells joined by a life of common interests; it is not even an emotional understanding, sympathy, solidarity or close drawing together. Only then are we really unified with those separated from us by the divisions of Nature, when we annul the division and find ourselves in that which seemed to us not ourselves. Association is a vital and physical unity; its sacrifice is that of mutual aid and concessions. Nearness, sympathy, solidarity create a mental, moral and emotional unity; theirs is a sacrifice of mutual support and mutual gratifications. But the true unity is spiritual; its sacrifice is a mutual self-giving, an interfusion of our inner substance. The law of sacrifice travels in Nature towards its culmination in this complete and unreserved self-giving; it awakens the consciousness of one common self in the giver and the object of the sacrifice. This culmination of sacrifice is the height even of human love and devotion when it tries to become divine; for there too the highest peak of love points into a heaven of complete mutual self-giving, its summit is the rapturous fusing of two souls into one.

This profounder idea of the world-wide law is at the heart of the teaching about works given in the Gita; a spiritual union with the Highest by sacrifice, an unreserved self-giving to the Eternal is the core of its doctrine. The vulgar conception of sacrifice is an act of painful self-immolation, austere self-mortification, difficult self-effacement; this kind of sacrifice may go even as far as self-mutilation and self-torture. These things may be temporarily necessary in man's hard endeavour to exceed his natural self; if the egoism in his nature is violent and obstinate, it has to be met sometimes by an answering strong internal repression and counterbalancing violence. But the Gita discourages any excess of violence done to oneself; for the self within is really the Godhead evolving, it is Krishna, it is the Divine; it has not to be troubled and tortured as the Titans of the world trouble and torture it, but to be increased, fostered, cherished, luminously opened to a divine light and strength and joy and wideness. It is not one's self, but the band of the spirit's inner enemies that we have to discourage, expel, slay upon the altar of the growth of the spirit; these can be ruthlessly excised, whose names are desire, wrath, inequality, greed, attachment to outward pleasures and pains, the cohort of usurping demons that are the cause of the soul's errors and sufferings. These should be regarded not as part of oneself but as intruders and perverters of our self's real and diviner nature; these have to be sacrificed in the harsher sense of the word, whatever pain in going they may throw by reflection on the consciousness of the seeker.

But the true essence of sacrifice is not self-immolation, it is self-giving; its object not self-effacement, but self-fulfilment; its method not self-mortification, but a greater life, not self-mutilation, but a transformation of our natural human parts into divine members, not self-torture, but a passage from a lesser satisfaction to a greater Ananda. There is only one thing painful in the beginning to a raw or turbid part of the surface nature; it is the indispensable discipline demanded, the denial necessary for the merging of the incomplete ego. But for that there can be a speedy and enormous compensation in the discovery of a real greater or ultimate completeness in others, in all things, in the cosmic oneness, in the freedom of the transcendent Self and Spirit, in the rapture of the touch of the Divine. Our sacrifice is not a giving without any return or any fruitful acceptance from the other side; it is an interchange between the embodied soul and conscious Nature in us and the eternal Spirit. For even though no return is demanded, yet there is the knowledge deep within us that a marvellous return is inevitable. The soul knows that it does not give itself to God in vain; claiming nothing, it yet receives the infinite riches of the divine Power and Presence.

Last, there is to be considered the recipient of the sacrifice and the manner of the sacrifice. The sacrifice may be offered to others or it may be offered to divine Powers; it may be offered to the cosmic All or it may be offered to the transcendent Supreme. The worship given may take any shape from the dedication of a leaf or flower, a cup of water, a handful of rice, a loaf of bread, to consecration of all that we possess and the submission of all that we are. Whoever the recipient, whatever the gift, it is the Supreme, the Eternal in things, who receives and accepts it, even if it be rejected or ignored by the immediate recipient. For the Supreme who transcends the universe, is yet here too, however veiled, in us and in the world and in its happenings; he is there as the omniscient Witness and Receiver of all our works and their secret Master. All our actions, all our efforts, even our sins and stumblings and sufferings and struggles are obscurely or consciously, known to us and seen or else unknown and in a disguise, governed in their last result by the One. All is turned towards him in his numberless forms and offered through them to the single Omnipresence. In whatever form and with whatever spirit we approach him, in that form and with that spirit he receives the sacrifice.

And the fruit also of the sacrifice of works varies according to the work, according to the intention in the work and according to the spirit that is behind the intention. But all other sacrifices are partial, egoistic, mixed, temporal, incomplete, — even those offered to the highest Powers and Principles keep this character: the result too is partial, limited, temporal, mixed in its reactions, effective only for a minor or intermediate purpose. The one entirely acceptable sacrifice is a last and highest and uttermost self-giving, — it is that surrender made face to face, with devotion and knowledge, freely and without any reserve to One who is at once our immanent Self, the environing constituent All, the Supreme Reality beyond this or any manifestation and, secretly, all these together, concealed everywhere, the immanent Transcendence. For to the soul that wholly gives itself to him, God also gives himself altogether. Only the one who offers his whole nature, finds the Self. Only the one who can give everything, enjoys the Divine All everywhere. Only a supreme self-abandonment attains to the Supreme. Only the sublimation by sacrifice of all that we are, can enable us to embody the Highest and live here in the immanent consciousness of the transcendent Spirit.

*
* *

This, in short, is the demand made on us, that we should turn our whole life into a conscious sacrifice. Every moment and every movement of our being is to be resolved into a continuous and a devoted self-giving to the Eternal. All our actions, not less the smallest and most ordinary and trifling than the greatest and most uncommon and noble, must be performed as consecrated acts. Our individualised nature must live in the single consciousness of an inner and outer movement dedicated to Something that is beyond us and greater than our ego. No matter what the gift or to whom it is presented by us, there must be a consciousness in the act that we are presenting it to the one divine Being in all beings. Our commonest or most grossly material actions must assume this sublimated character; when we eat, we should be conscious that we are giving our food to that Presence in us; it must be a sacred offering in a temple and the sense of a mere physical need or self-gratification must pass away from us. In any great labour, in any high discipline, in any difficult or noble enterprise, whether undertaken for ourselves, for others or for the race, it will no longer be possible to stop short at the idea of the race, of ourselves or of others. The thing we are doing must be consciously offered as a sacrifice of works, not to these, but either through them or directly to the One Godhead; the Divine Inhabitant who was hidden by these figures must be no longer hidden but ever present to our soul, our mind, our sense. The workings and results of our acts must be put in the hands of that One in the feeling that that Presence is the Infinite and Most High by whom alone our labour and our aspiration are possible. For in his being all takes place; for him all labour and aspiration are taken from us by Nature and offered on his altar. Even in those things in which Nature is herself very plainly the worker and we only the witnesses of her working and its containers and supporters, there should be the same constant memory and insistent consciousness of a work and of its divine Master. Our very inspiration and respiration, our very heart-beats can and must be made conscious in us as the living rhythm of the universal sacrifice.

It is clear that a conception of this kind and its effective practice must carry in them three results that are of a central importance for our spiritual ideal. It is evident, to begin with, that, even if such a discipline is begun without devotion, it leads straight and inevitably towards the highest devotion possible; for it must deepen naturally into the completest adoration imaginable, the most profound God-love. There is bound up with it a growing sense of the Divine in all things, a deepening communion with the Divine in all our thought, will and action and at every moment of our lives, a more and more moved consecration to the Divine of the totality of our being. Now these implications of the Yoga of works are also of the very essence of an integral and absolute Bhakti. The seeker who puts them into living practice makes in himself continually a constant, active and effective representation of the very spirit of self-devotion, and it is inevitable that out of it there should emerge the most engrossing worship of the Highest to whom is given this service. An absorbing love for the Divine Presence to whom he feels an always more intimate closeness, grows upon the consecrated worker. And with it is born or in it is contained a universal love too for all these beings, living forms and creatures that are habitations of the Divine — not the brief restless grasping emotions of division, but the settled selfless love that is the deeper vibration of oneness. In all the seeker begins to meet the one Object of his adoration and service. The way of works turns by this road of sacrifice to meet the path of Devotion; it can be itself a devotion as complete, as absorbing, as integral as any the desire of the heart can ask for or the passion of the mind can imagine.

Next, the practice of this Yoga demands a constant inward remembrance of the one central liberating knowledge, and a constant active externalising of it in works comes in too to intensify the remembrance. In all is the one Self, the one Divine is all; all are in the Divine, all are the Divine and there is nothing else in the universe, — this thought or this faith is the whole background until it becomes the whole substance of the consciousness of the worker. A memory, a self-dynamising meditation of this kind, must and does in its end turn into a profound and uninterrupted vision and a vivid and all-embracing consciousness of that which we so powerfully remember or on which we so constantly meditate. For it compels a constant reference at each moment to the Origin of all being and will and action and there is at once an embracing and exceeding of all particular forms and appearances in That which is their cause and upholder. This way cannot go to its end without a seeing vivid and vital, as concrete in its way as physical sight, of the works of the universal Spirit everywhere. On its summits it rises into a constant living and thinking and willing and acting in the presence of the Supramental, the Transcendent. Whatever we see and hear, whatever we touch and sense, all of which we are conscious, has to be known and felt by us as That which we worship and serve; all has to be turned into an image of the Divinity, perceived as a dwelling-place of his Godhead, enveloped with the eternal Omnipresence. In its close, if not long before it, this way of works turns by communion with the Divine Presence, Will and Force into a way of Knowledge more complete and integral than any the mere creature intelligence can construct or the search of the intellect can discover.

Lastly, the practice of this Yoga of sacrifice compels us to renounce all the inner supports of egoism, casting them out of our mind and will and actions, and to eliminate its seed, its presence, its influence out of our nature. All must be done for the Divine; all must be directed towards the Divine. Nothing must be attempted for ourselves as a separate existence; nothing done for others, whether neighbours, friends, family, country or mankind or other creatures merely because they are connected with our personal life and thought and sentiment or because the ego takes a preferential interest in their welfare. In this way of doing and seeing all works and all life become only a daily dynamic worship and service of the Divine in the unbounded temple of his own vast cosmic existence. Life becomes more and more the sacrifice of the eternal in the individual constantly self-offered to the eternal Transcendence. It is offered in the wide sacrificial ground of the field of the eternal cosmic Spirit; and the Force too that offers it is the eternal Force, the omnipresent

Mother. Therefore is this way a way of union and communion by acts and by the spirit and knowledge in the act as complete and integral as any our Godward will can hope for or our soul's strength execute.

It has all the power of a way of works integral and absolute, but because of its law of sacrifice and self-giving to the Divine Self and Master, it is accompanied on its one side by the whole power of the path of Love and on the other by the whole power of the path of Knowledge. At its end all these three divine Powers work together, fused, united, completed, perfected by each other.

*
* *

The Divine, the Eternal is the Lord of our sacrifice of works and union with him in all our being and consciousness and in its expressive instruments is the one object of the sacrifice; the steps of the sacrifice of works must therefore be measured, first, by the growth in our nature of something that brings us nearer to divine Nature, but secondly also by an experience of the Divine, his presence, his manifestation to us, an increasing closeness and union with that Presence. But the Divine is in his essence infinite and his manifestation too is multitudinously infinite. If that is so, it is not likely that our true integral perfection in being and in nature can come by one kind of realisation alone; it must combine many different strands of divine experience. It cannot be reached by the exclusive pursuit of a single line of identity till that is raised to its absolute; it must harmonise many aspects of the Infinite. An integral consciousness with a multiform dynamic experience is essential for the complete transformation of our nature.

There is one fundamental perception indispensable towards any integral knowledge or many-sided experience of this Infinite. It is to realise the Divine in its essential self and truth unaltered by forms and phenomena. Otherwise we are likely to remain caught in the net of appearances or wander confusedly in a chaotic multitude of cosmic or particular aspects, and if we avoid this confusion, it will be at the price of getting chained to some mental formula or shut up in a limited personal experience. The one secure and all-reconciling truth which is the very foundation of the universe is this that life is the manifestation of an uncreated Self and Spirit, and the key to life's hidden secret is the true relation of this Spirit with its own created existences. There is behind all this life the look of an eternal Being upon its multitudinous becomings; there is around and everywhere in it the envelopment and penetration of a manifestation in time by an unmanifested timeless Eternal. But this knowledge is valueless for Yoga if it is only an intellectual and metaphysical notion void of life and barren of consequence; a mental realisation alone cannot be sufficient for the seeker. For what Yoga searches after is not truth of thought alone or truth of mind alone, but the dynamic truth of a living and revealing spiritual experience. There must awake in us a constant indwelling and enveloping nearness, a vivid perception, a close feeling and communion, a concrete sense and contact of a true and infinite Presence always and everywhere. That Presence must remain with us as the living, pervading Reality in which we and all things exist and move and act, and we must feel it always and everywhere, concrete, visible, inhabiting all things; it must be patent to us as their true Self, tangible as their imperishable Essence, met by us closely as their inmost Spirit. To see, to feel, to sense, to contact in every way and not merely to conceive this Self and Spirit here in all existences and to feel with the same vividness all existences in this Self and Spirit, is the fundamental experience which must englobe all other knowledge.

This infinite and eternal Self of things is an omnipresent Reality, one existence everywhere; it is a single unifying presence and not different in different creatures; it can be met, seen or felt in its completeness in each soul or each form in the universe. For its infinity is spiritual and essential and not merely a boundlessness in Space or an endlessness in Time; the Infinite can be felt in an infinitesimal atom or in a second of time as convincingly as in the stretch of the aeons or the stupendous enormity of the intersolar spaces. The knowledge or experience of it can begin anywhere and express itself through anything; for the Divine is in all, and all is the Divine.

This fundamental experience will yet begin differently for different natures and take long to develop all the Truth that it conceals in its thousand aspects. I see perhaps or feel in myself or as myself first the eternal Presence and afterwards only can extend the vision or sense of this greater self of mine to all creatures. I then see the world in me or as one with me. I perceive the universe as a scene in my being, the play of its processes as a movement of forms and souls and forces in my cosmic spirit; I meet myself and none else everywhere. Not, be it well noted, with the error of the Asura, the Titan, who lives in his own inordinately magnified shadow, mistakes ego for the self and spirit and tries to impose his fragmentary personality as the one dominant existence upon all his surroundings. For, having the knowledge, I have already seized this reality that my true self is the non-ego, so always my greater Self is felt by me either as an impersonal vastness or an essential Person containing yet beyond all personalities or as both these together; but in any case, whether Impersonal or illimitable Personal or both together, it is an ego-exceeding Infinite. If I have sought it out and found it first in the form of it I call myself rather than in others, it is only because there it is easiest for me, owing to the subjectivity of my consciousness, to find it, to know it at once and to realise it. But if the narrow instrumental ego does not begin to merge in this Self as soon as it is seen, if the smaller external mind-constructed I refuses to disappear into that greater permanent uncreated spiritual I, then my realisation is either not genuine or radically imperfect. There is somewhere in me an egoistic obstacle; some part of my nature has opposed a self-regarding and self-preserving denial to the all-swallowing truth of the Spirit.

On the other hand — and to some this is an easier way — I may see the Divinity first in the world outside me, not in myself but in others. I meet it there from the beginning as an indwelling and all-containing Infinite that is not bound up with all these forms, creatures and forces which it bears on its surface. Or else I see and feel it as a pure solitary Self and Spirit which contains all these powers and existences, and I lose my sense of ego in the silent Omnipresence around me. Afterwards it is this that begins to pervade and possess my instrumental being and out of it seem to proceed all my impulsions to action, all my light of thought and speech, all the formations of my consciousness and all its relations and impacts with other soul-forms of this one world-wide Existence. I am already no longer this little personal self, but That with something of itself put forward which sustains a selected form of its workings in the universe.

There is another basic realisation, the most extreme of all, that yet comes sometimes as the first decisive opening or an early turn of the Yoga. It is the awakening to an ineffable high transcendent Unknowable above myself and above this world in which I seem to move, a timeless and spaceless condition or entity which is at once, in some way compelling and convincing to an essential consciousness in me, the one thing that is to it overwhelmingly real. This experience is usually accompanied by an equally compelling sense either of the dreamlike or shadowy illusoriness of all things here or else of their temporary, derivative and only half-real character. For a time at least all around me may seem to be a moving of cinematographic shadow forms or surface figures and my own action may appear as a fluid formulation from some Source ungrasped as yet and perhaps unseizable above or outside me. To remain in this consciousness, to carry out this initiation or follow out this first suggestion of the character of things would be to proceed towards the goal of dissolution of self and world in the Unknowable, — Moksha, Nirvana. But this is not the only line of issue; it is possible, on the contrary, for me to wait till through the silence of this timeless unfilled liberation I begin to enter into relations with that yet ungrasped Source of myself and my actions; then the void begins to fill, there emerges out of it or there rushes into it all the manifold Truth of the Divine, all the aspects and man-ifestations and many levels of a dynamic Infinite. At first this experience imposes on the mind and then on all our being an absolute, a fathomless, almost an abysmal peace and silence. Overpowered and subjugated, stilled, liberated from itself, the mind accepts the Silence itself as the Supreme. But afterwards the seeker discovers that all is there for him contained or new-made in that silence or through it descends upon him from a greater concealed transcendent Existence. For this Transcendent, this Absolute is not a mere peace of signless emptiness; it has its own infinite contents and riches of which ours are debased and diminished values. If there were not that Source of all things, there could be no universe; all powers, all works and activities would be an illusion, all creation and manifestation would be impossible.

These are the three fundamental realisations, so fundamental that to the Yogin of the way of Knowledge they seem ultimate, sufficient in themselves, destined to overtop and replace all others. And yet for the integral seeker, whether accorded to him at an early stage suddenly and easily by a miraculous grace or achieved with difficulty after a long progress and endeavour, they are neither the sole truth nor the full and only clues to the integral truth of the Eternal, but rather the unfilled beginning, the vast foundation of a greater divine Knowledge. Other realisations there are that are imperatively needed and must be explored to the full limit of their possibilities; and if some of them appear to a first sight to cover only Divine Aspects that are instrumental to the activity of existence but not inherent in its essence, yet, when followed to their end through that activity to its everlasting Source, it is found that they lead to a disclosure of the Divine without which our knowledge of the Truth behind things would be left bare and incomplete. These seeming Instrumentals are the key to a secret without which the Fundamentals themselves would not unveil all their mystery. All the revelatory aspects of the Divine must be caught in the wide net of the integral Yoga.

*
* *

If a departure from the world and its activities, a supreme release and quietude were the sole aim of the seeker, the three great fundamental realisations would be sufficient for the fulfilment of his spiritual life: concentrated in them alone he could suffer all other divine or mundane knowledge to fall away from him and himself unencumbered, depart into the eternal Silence. But he has to take account of the world and its activities, learn what divine truth there may be behind them and reconcile that apparent opposition between the Divine Truth and the manifest creation which is the starting-point of most spiritual experience. Here, on each line of approach that he can take, he is confronted with a constant Duality, a separation between two terms of existence that seem to be opposites and their opposition to be the very root of the riddle of the universe. Later, he may and does discover that these are the two poles of One Being, connected by two simultaneous currents of energy negative and positive in relation to each other, their interaction the very condition for the manifestation of what is within the Being, their reunion the appointed means for the reconciliation of life's discords and for the discovery of the integral truth of which he is the seeker.

For on one side he is aware of this Self everywhere, this everlasting Spirit-Substance — Brahman, the Eternal — the same self-existence here in time behind each appearance he sees or senses and timeless beyond the universe. He has this strong overpowering experience of a Self that is neither our limited ego nor our mind, life or body, world-wide but not outwardly phenomenal, yet to some spirit-sense in him more concrete than any form or phenomenon, universal yet not dependent for its being on anything in the universe or on the whole totality of the universe; if all this were to disappear, its extinction would make no difference to this Eternal of his constant intimate experience. He is sure of an inexpressible Self-Existence which is the essence of himself and all things; he is intimately aware of an essential Consciousness of which thinking mind and life-sense and body-sense are only partial and diminished figures, a Consciousness with an illimitable Force in it of which all energies are the out-come, but which is yet not explained or accounted for by the sum or power or nature of all these energies together; he feels, he lives in an inalienable self-existent Bliss which is not this lesser

transient joy or happiness or pleasure. A changeless imperishable
infinity, a timeless eternity, a self-awareness which is not this
receptive and reactive or tentacular mental consciousness, but
is behind and above it and present too below it, even in what
we call Inconscience, a oneness in which there is no possibility
of any other existence, are the fourfold character of this settled
experience. Yet this eternal Self-Existence is seen by him also
as a conscious Time-Spirit bearing the stream of happenings, a
self-extended spiritual Space containing all things and beings,
a Spirit-Substance which is the very form and material of all
that seems non-spiritual, temporary and finite. For all that is
transitory, temporal, spatial, bounded, is yet felt by him to be in
its substance and energy and power no other than the One, the
Eternal, the Infinite.

And yet there is not only in him or before him this eternal
self-aware Existence, this spiritual Consciousness, this infinity of
self-illumined Force, this timeless and endless Beatitude. There is
too, constant also to his experience, this universe in measurable
Space and Time, some kind perhaps of boundless finite, and in it
all is transient, limited, fragmentary, plural, ignorant, exposed to
disharmony and suffering, seeking vaguely for some unrealised
yet inherent harmony of oneness, unconscious or half-conscious
or, even when most conscious, still tied to the original Ignorance
and Inconscience. He is not always in a trance of peace or bliss
and, even if he were, it would be no solution, for he knows
that this would still be going on outside him and yet within
some larger self of him as if for ever. At times these two states
of his spirit seem to exist for him alternately according to his
state of consciousness; at others they are there as two parts of
his being, disparate and to be reconciled, two halves, an upper
and a lower or an inner and an outer half of his existence.
He finds soon that this separation in his consciousness has an
immense liberative power; for by it he is no longer bound to
the Ignorance, the Inconscience; it no longer appears to him the
very nature of himself and things but an illusion which can be
overcome or at least a temporary wrong self-experience, Maya.
It is tempting to regard it as only a contradiction of the Divine,

an incomprehensible mystery-play, masque or travesty of the Infinite — and so it irresistibly seems to his experience at times, on one side the luminous verity of Brahman, on the other a dark illusion of Maya. But something in him will not allow him to cut existence thus permanently in two and, looking more closely, he discovers that in this half-light or darkness too is the Eternal — it is the Brahman who is here with this face of Maya.

This is the beginning of a growing spiritual experience which reveals to him more and more that what seemed to him dark incomprehensible Maya was all the time no other than the Consciousness-Puissance of the Eternal, timeless and illimitable beyond the universe, but spread out here under a mask of bright and dark opposites for the miracle of the slow manifestation of the Divine in Mind and Life and Matter. All the Timeless presses towards the play in Time; all in Time turns upon and around the timeless Spirit. If the separate experience was liberative, this unitive experience is dynamic and effective. For he now not only feels himself to be in his soul-substance part of the Eternal, in his essential self and spirit entirely one with the Eternal, but in his active nature an instrumentation of its omniscient and omnipotent Consciousness-Puissance. However bounded and relative its present play in him, he can open to a greater and greater consciousness and power of it and to that expansion there seems to be no assignable limit. A level spiritual and supramental of that Consciousness-Puissance seems even to reveal itself above him and lean to enter into contact, where there are not these trammels and limits, and its powers too are pressing upon the play in Time with the promise of a greater descent and a less disguised or no longer disguised manifestation of the Eternal. The once conflicting but now biune duality of Brahman-Maya stands revealed to him as the first great dynamic aspect of the Self of all selves, the Master of existence, the Lord of the world-sacrifice and of his sacrifice.

On another line of approach another Duality presents itself to the experience of the seeker. On one side he becomes aware of a witness recipient observing experiencing Consciousness which does not appear to act but for which all these activities inside and outside us seem to be undertaken and continue. On the other side he is aware at the same time of an executive Force or an energy of Process which is seen to constitute, drive and guide all conceivable activities and to create a myriad forms visible to us and invisible and use them as stable supports for its incessant flux of action and creation. Entering exclusively into the witness consciousness he becomes silent, untouched, immobile; he sees that he has till now passively reflected and appropriated to himself the movements of Nature and it is by this reflection that they acquired from the witness soul within him what seemed a spiritual value and significance. But now he has withdrawn that ascription or mirroring identification; he is conscious only of his silent self and aloof from all that is in motion around it; all activities are outside him and at once they cease to be intimately real; they appear now mechanical, detachable, endable. Entering exclusively into the kinetic move-ment, he has an opposite self-awareness; he seems to his own perception a mass of activities, a formation and result of forces; if there is an active consciousness, even some kind of kinetic being in the midst of it all, yet there is no longer a free soul in it anywhere. These two different and opposite states of being alternate in him or else stand simultaneously over against each other; one silent in the inner being observes but is unmoved and does not participate; the other active in some outer or surface self pursues its habitual movements. He has entered into an intense separative perception of the great duality, Soul-Nature, Purusha-Prakriti.

But as the consciousness deepens, he becomes aware that this is only a first frontal appearance. For he finds that it is by the silent support, permission or sanction of this witness soul in him that this executive nature can work intimately or persistently upon his being; if the soul withdraws its sanction, the movements of Nature in their action upon and within him become a wholly mechanical repetition, vehement at first as if seeking still to enforce their hold, but afterwards less and less dynamic and real. More actively using this power of sanction or refusal, he perceives that he can, slowly and uncertainly at first, more decisively afterwards, change the movements of Nature. Eventually in this witness soul or behind it is revealed to him the presence of a Knower and master Will in Nature, and all her activities more and more appear as an expression of what is known and either actively willed or passively permitted by this Lord of her existence. Prakriti herself now seems to be mechanical only in the carefully regulated appearance of her workings, but in fact a conscious Force with a soul within her, a self-aware significance in her turns, a revelation of a secret Will and Knowledge in her steps and figures. This Duality, in aspect separate, is inseparable. Wherever there is Prakriti, there is Purusha; wherever there is Purusha, there is Prakriti. Even in his inactivity he holds in himself all her force and energies ready for projection; even in the drive of her action she carries with her all his observing and mandatory consciousness as the whole support and sense of her creative purpose. Once more the seeker discovers in his experience the two poles of existence of One Being and the two lines or currents of their energy negative and positive in relation to each other which effect by their simultaneity the manifestation of all that is within it. Here too he finds that the separative aspect is liberative; for it releases him from the bondage of identification with the inadequate workings of Nature in the Ignorance. The unitive aspect is dynamic and effective; for it enables him to arrive at mastery and perfection; while rejecting what is less divine or seemingly undivine in her, he can rebuild her forms and movements in himself according to a nobler pattern and the law and rhythm of a greater existence. At a certain spiritual and supramental level the Duality becomes still more perfectly Two-in-one, the Master Soul with the Conscious Force within it, and its potentiality disowns all barriers and breaks through every limit. Thus this once separate, now biune Duality of Purusha-Prakriti is revealed to him in all its truth as the second great instrumental and effective aspect of the Soul of all souls, the Master of existence, the Lord of the Sacrifice.

On yet another line of approach the seeker meets another corresponding but in aspect distinct Duality in which the biune character is more immediately apparent, — the dynamic Duality of Ishwara-Shakti. On one side he is aware of an infinite and self-existent Godhead in being who contains all things in an ineffable potentiality of existence, a Self of all selves, a Soul of all souls, a spiritual Substance of all substances, an impersonal inexpressible Existence, but at the same time an illimitable Person who is here self-represented in numberless personality, a Master of Knowledge, a Master of Forces, a Lord of love and bliss and beauty, a single Origin of the worlds, a self-manifester and self-creator, a Cosmic Spirit, a universal Mind, a universal Life, the conscious and living Reality supporting the appearance which we sense as unconscious inanimate Matter. On the other side he becomes aware of the same Godhead in effectuating consciousness and power put forth as a self-aware Force that contains and carries all within her and is charged to manifest it in universal Time and Space. It is evident to him that here there is one supreme and infinite Being represented to us in two different sides of itself, obverse and reverse in relation to each other. All is either prepared or pre-existent in the Godhead in Being and issues from it and is upheld by its Will and Presence; all is brought out, carried in movement by the Godhead in power; all becomes and acts and develops by her and in her its individual or its cosmic purpose. It is again a Duality necessary for the manifestation, creating and enabling that double current of energy which seems always necessary for the world-workings, two poles of the same Being, but here closer to each other and always very evidently carrying each the powers of the other in its essence and its dynamic nature. At the same time by the fact that the two great elements of the divine Mystery, the Personal and the Impersonal, are here fused together, the seeker of the integral Truth feels in the duality of Ishwara-Shakti his closeness to a more intimate and ultimate secret of the divine Transcendence and the Manifestation than that offered to him by any other experience.

For the Ishwari Shakti, divine Conscious-Force and World-Mother, becomes a mediatrix between the eternal One and the manifested Many. On one side, by the play of the energies which she brings from the One, she manifests the multiple Divine in the

universe, involving and evolving its endless appearances out of
her revealing substance; on the other by the reascending current
of the same energies she leads back all towards That from which
they have issued so that the soul in its evolutionary manifestation
may more and more return towards the Divinity there or here put
on its divine character. There is not in her, although she devises
a cosmic mechanism, the character of an inconscient mechanical
Executrix which we find in the first physiognomy of Prakriti, the
Nature-Force; neither is there that sense of an Unreality, creatrix
of illusions or semi-illusions, which is attached to our first view
of Maya. It is at once clear to the experiencing soul that here is a
conscious Power of one substance and nature with the Supreme
from whom she came. If she seems to have plunged us into the
Ignorance and Inconscience in pursuance of a plan we cannot yet
interpret, if her forces present themselves as all these ambiguous
forces of the universe, yet it becomes visible before long that she
is working for the development of the Divine Consciousness in us
and that she stands above drawing us to her own higher entity,
revealing to us more and more the very essence of the Divine
Knowledge, Will and Ananda. Even in the movements of the
Ignorance the soul of the seeker becomes aware of her conscious
guidance supporting his steps and leading them slowly or swiftly,
straight or by many detours out of the darkness into the light
of a greater consciousness, out of mortality into immortality,
out of evil and suffering towards a highest good and felicity of
which as yet his human mind can form only a faint image. Thus
her power is at once liberative and dynamic, creative, effective,
— creative not only of things as they are, but of things that are
to be; for, eliminating the twisted and tangled movements of
his lower consciousness made of the stuff of the Ignorance, it
rebuilds and new-makes his soul and nature into the substance
and forces of a higher divine Nature.

In this Duality too there is possible a separative experience.
At one pole of it the seeker may be conscious only of the Master
of Existence putting forth on him His energies of knowledge,
power and bliss to liberate and divinise; the Shakti may appear
to him only an impersonal Force expressive of these things or

an attribute of the Ishwara. At the other pole he may encounter the World-Mother, creatrix of the universe, putting forth the Gods and the worlds and all things and existences out of her spirit-substance. Or even if he sees both aspects, it may be with an unequal separating vision, subordinating one to the other, regarding the Shakti only as a means for approaching the Ishwara. There results a one-sided tendency or a lack of balance, a power of effectuation not perfectly supported or a light of revelation not perfectly dynamic. It is when a complete union of the two sides of the Duality is effected and rules his consciousness that he begins to open to a fuller power that will draw him altogether out of the confused clash of Ideas and Forces here into a higher Truth and enable the descent of that Truth to illumine and deliver and act sovereignly upon this world of Ignorance. He has begun to lay his hand on the integral secret which in its fullness can be grasped only when he overpasses the double term that reigns here of Knowledge inextricably intertwined with an original Ignorance and crosses the border where spiritual mind disappears into supramental Gnosis. It is through this third and most dynamic dual aspect of the One that the seeker begins with the most integral completeness to enter into the deepest secret of the being of the Lord of the Sacrifice.

For it is behind the mystery of the presence of personality in an apparently impersonal universe — as in that of consciousness manifesting out of the Inconscient, life out of the inanimate, soul out of brute Matter — that is hidden the solution of the riddle of existence. Here again is another dynamic Duality more pervading than appears at first view and deeply necessary to the play of the slowly self-revealing Power. It is possible for the seeker in his spiritual experience, standing at one pole of the Duality, to follow Mind in seeing a fundamental Impersonality everywhere. The evolving soul in the material world begins from a vast impersonal Inconscience in which our inner sight yet perceives the presence of a veiled infinite Spirit; it proceeds with the emergence of a precarious consciousness and personality that even at their fullest have the look of an episode, but an episode that repeats itself in a constant series; it arises through experience of life out of mind into an infinite, impersonal and absolute Superconscience in which personality, mind-consciousness, life-consciousness seem all to disappear by a liberating annihilation, Nirvana. At a lower pitch he still experiences this fundamental impersonality as an immense liberating force everywhere. It releases his knowledge from the narrowness of personal mind, his will from the clutch of personal desire, his heart from the bondage of petty mutable emotions, his life from its petty personal groove, his soul from ego, and it allows them to embrace calm, equality, wideness, universality, infinity. A Yoga of works would seem to require Personality as its mainstay, almost its source, but here too the impersonal is found to be the most direct liberating force; it is through a wide egoless impersonality that one can become a free worker and a divine creator. It is not surprising that the overwhelming power of this experience from the impersonal pole of the Duality should have moved the sages to declare this to be the one way and an impersonal Superconscience to be the sole truth of the Eternal.

But still to the seeker standing at the opposite pole of the Duality another line of experience appears which justifies an intuition deeply-seated behind the heart and in our very life-force, that personality, like consciousness, life, soul, is not a brief-lived stranger in an impersonal Eternity, but contains the very meaning of existence. This fine flower of the cosmic Energy carries in it a forecast of the aim and a hint of the very motive of the universal labour. As an occult vision opens in him, he becomes aware of worlds behind in which consciousness and personality hold an enormous place and assume a premier value; even here in the material world to this occult vision the inconscience of Matter fills with a secret pervading consciousness, its inanimation harbours a vibrant life, its mechanism is the device of an indwelling Intelligence, God and soul are everywhere. Above all stands an infinite conscious Being who is variously self-expressed in all these worlds; impersonality is only a first means of that expression. It is a field of principles and forces, an equal basis of manifestation; but these forces express themselves through beings, have conscious spirits at their head and are the emanation of a One Conscious Being who is their source. A multiple innumerable personality expressing that One is the very sense and central aim of the manifestation and if now personality seems to be narrow, fragmentary, restrictive, it is only because it has not opened to its source or flowered into its own divine truth and fullness packing itself with the universal and the infinite. Thus the world-creation is no more an illusion, a fortuitous mechanism, a play that need not have happened, a flux without consequence; it is an intimate dynamism of the conscious and living Eternal.

This extreme opposition of view from the two poles of one Existence creates no fundamental difficulty for the seeker of the integral Yoga; for his whole experience has shown him the necessity of these double terms and their currents of Energy, negative and positive in relation to each other, for the manifestation of what is within the one Existence. For himself Personality and Impersonality have been the two wings of his spiritual ascension and he has the prevision that he will reach a height where their helpful interaction will pass into a fusion of their powers and disclose the integral Reality and release into action the original force of the Divine. Not only in the fundamental Aspects but in all the working of his sadhana he has felt their double truth and mutually complementary working. An impersonal Presence has dominated from above or penetrated and occupied his nature; a Light descending has suffused his mind, life-power, the very cells of his body, illumined them with knowledge, revealed him to himself down to his most disguised and unsuspected movements, exposing, purifying, destroying or brilliantly changing all that belonged to the Ignorance. A Force has poured into him in currents or like a sea, worked in his being and all its members, dissolved, new-made, reshaped, transfigured everywhere. A Bliss has invaded him and shown that it can make suffering and sorrow impossible and turn pain itself into divine pleasure. A Love without limits has joined him to all creatures or revealed to him a world of inseparable intimacy and unspeakable sweetness and beauty and begun to impose its law of perfection and its ecstasy even amidst the disharmony of terrestrial life. A spiritual

Truth and Right have convicted the good and evil of this world of imperfection or of falsehood and unveiled a supreme good and its clue of subtle harmony and its sublimation of action and feeling and knowledge. But behind all these and in them he has felt a Divinity who is all these things, a Bringer of Light, a Guide and All-Knower, a Master of Force, a Giver of Bliss, Friend, Helper, Father, Mother, Playmate in the world-game, an absolute Master of his being, his soul's Beloved and Lover. All relations known to human personality are there in the soul's contact with the Divine; but they rise towards superhuman levels and compel him towards a divine nature.

It is an integral knowledge that is being sought, an integral force, a total amplitude of union with the All and Infinite behind existence. For the seeker of the integral Yoga no single experience, no one Divine Aspect, — however overwhelming to the human mind, sufficient for its capacity, easily accepted as the sole or the ultimate reality, — can figure as the exclusive truth of the Eternal. For him the experience of the Divine Oneness carried to its extreme is more deeply embraced and amply fathomed by following out to the full the experience of the Divine Multiplicity. All that is true behind polytheism as well as behind monotheism falls within the scope of his seeking; but he passes beyond their superficial sense to human mind to grasp their mystic truth in the Divine. He sees what is aimed at by the jarring sects and philosophies and accepts each facet of the Reality in its own place, but rejects their narrownesses and errors and proceeds farther till he discovers the One Truth that binds them together. The reproach of anthropomorphism and anthropolatry cannot deter him, — for he sees them to be prejudices of the ignorant and arrogant reasoning intelligence, the abstracting mind turning on itself in its own cramped circle. If human relations as practised now by man are full of smallness and perversity and ignorance, yet are they disfigured shadows of something in the Divine and by turning them to the Divine he finds that of which they are a shadow and brings it down for manifestation in life. It is through the human exceeding itself and opening itself to a supreme plenitude that the Divine must manifest itself here, since that comes inevitably in the course and process of the spiritual evolution, and therefore he will not despise or blind himself to the Godhead because it is lodged in a human body, *mānuṣīm tanum āśritam*. Beyond the limited human conception of God, he will pass to the one divine Eternal, but also he will meet him in the faces of the Gods, his cosmic personalities supporting the World-Play, detect him behind the mask of the Vibhutis, embodied World-Forces or human Leaders, reverence and obey him in the Guru, worship him in the Avatar. This will be to him his exceeding good fortune if he can meet one who has realised or is becoming That which he seeks for and can by opening to it in this vessel of its manifestation himself realise it. For that is the most palpable sign of the growing fulfilment, the promise of the great mystery of the progressive Descent into Matter which is the secret sense of the material creation and the justification of terrestrial existence.

Thus reveals himself to the seeker in the progress of the sacrifice the Lord of the sacrifice. At any point this revelation can begin; in any aspect the Master of the Work can take up the work in him and more and more press upon him and it for the unfolding of his presence. In time all the Aspects disclose themselves, separate, combine, fuse, are unified together. At the end there shines through it all the supreme integral Reality, unknowable to Mind which is part of the Ignorance, but knowable because self-aware in the light of a spiritual consciousness and a supramental knowledge.

*
* *

This revelation of a highest Truth or a highest Being, Consciousness, Power, Bliss and Love, impersonal and personal at once and so taking up both sides of our own being, — since in us also is the ambiguous meeting of a Person and a mass of impersonal principles and forces, — is at once the first aim and the condition of the ultimate achievement of the sacrifice. The achievement itself takes the shape of a union of our own existence with That which is thus made manifest to our vision and experience, and the union has a threefold character. There is a union in spiritual essence, by identity; there is a union by the indwelling of our soul in this highest Being and Consciousness; there is a dynamic union of likeness or oneness of nature between That and our instrumental being here. The first is the liberation from the Ignorance and identification with the Real and Eternal, *mokṣa*, *sāyujya*, which is the characteristic aim of the Yoga of Knowledge. The second, the dwelling of the soul with or in the Divine, *sāmīpya*, *sālokya*, is the intense hope of all Yoga of love and beatitude. The third, identity in nature, likeness to the Divine, to be perfect as That is perfect, is the high intention of all Yoga of power and perfection or of divine works and service. The combined completeness of the three together, founded here on a multiple Unity of the self-manifesting Divine, is the complete result of the integral Yoga, the goal of its triple Path and the fruit of its triple sacrifice.

A union by identity may be ours, a liberation and change of our substance of being into that supreme Spirit-substance, of our consciousness into that divine Consciousness, of our soul-state into that ecstasy of spiritual beatitude or that calm eternal bliss of existence. A luminous indwelling in the Divine can be attained by us secure against any fall or exile into this lower consciousness of the darkness and the Ignorance, the soul ranging freely and firmly in its own natural world of light and joy and freedom and oneness. And since this is not merely to be attained in some other existence beyond but pursued and discovered here also, it can only be by a descent, by a bringing down of the Divine Truth, by the establishment here of the soul's native world of light, joy, freedom, oneness. A union of our instrumental being no less than of our soul and spirit must change our imperfect nature into the very likeness and image of Divine Nature; it must put off the blind, marred, mutilated, discordant movements of the Ignorance and put on the inherence of that light, peace, bliss, harmony, universality, mastery, purity, perfection; it must convert itself into a receptacle of divine knowledge, an instrument of divine Will-Power and Force of Being, a channel of divine Love, Joy and Beauty. This is the transformation to be effected, an integral transformation of all that we now are or seem to be, by the joining — Yoga — of the finite being in Time with the Eternal and Infinite.

All this difficult result can become possible only if there is an immense conversion, a total reversal of our consciousness, a supernormal entire transfiguration of the nature. There must be an ascension of the whole being, an ascension of spirit chained here and trammelled by its instruments and its environment to sheer Spirit free above, an ascension of soul towards some blissful Super-soul, an ascension of mind towards some luminous Supermind, an ascension of life towards some vast Super-life, an ascension of our very physicality to join its origin in some pure and plastic spirit-substance. And this cannot be a single swift upsoaring but, like the ascent of the sacrifice described in the Veda, a climbing from peak to peak in which from each summit one looks up to the much more that has still to be done. At the same time there must be a descent too to affirm below what we have gained above: on each height we conquer we have to turn to bring down its power and its illumination into the lower mortal movement; the discovery of the Light for ever radiant on high must correspond with the release of the same Light secret below in every part down to the deepest caves of subconscient Nature. And this pilgrimage of ascension and this descent for the labour of transformation must be inevitably a battle, a long war with ourselves and with opposing forces around us which, while it lasts, may well seem interminable. For all our old obscure and ignorant nature will contend repeatedly and obstinately with the transforming Influence, supported in its lagging unwillingness or its stark resistance by most of the established forces of environing universal Nature; the powers and principalities and the ruling beings of the Ignorance will not easily give up their empire.

At first there may have to be a prolonged, often tedious and painful period of preparation and purification of all our being till it is ready and fit for an opening to a greater Truth and Light or to the Divine Influence and Presence. Even when centrally fitted, prepared, open already, it will still be long before all our movements of mind, life and body, all the multiple and conflicting members and elements of our personality consent or, consenting, are able to bear the difficult and exacting process of the transformation. And hardest of all, even if all in us is willing, is the struggle we shall have to carry through against the universal forces attached to the present unstable creation when we seek to make the final supramental conversion and reversal of consciousness by which the Divine Truth must be established in us in its plenitude and not merely what they would more readily permit, an illumined Ignorance.

It is for this that a surrender and submission to That which is beyond us enabling the full and free working of its Power is indispensable. As that self-giving progresses, the work of the sacrifice becomes easier and more powerful and the prevention of the opposing Forces loses much of its strength, impulsion and substance. Two inner changes help most to convert what now seems difficult or impracticable into a thing possible and even sure. There takes place a coming to the front of some secret inmost soul within which was veiled by the restless activity of the mind, by the turbulence of our vital impulses and by the obscurity of the physical consciousness, the three powers which in their confused combination we now call our self. There will come about as a result a less impeded growth of a Divine Presence at the centre with its liberating Light and effective Force and an irradiation of it into all the conscious and subconscious ranges of our nature. These are the two signs, one marking our completed conversion and consecration to the great Quest, the other the final acceptance by the Divine of our sacrifice.

Chapter V

The Ascent of the Sacrifice – 1

The Works of Knowledge — The Psychic Being

THIS THEN is in its foundations the integral knowledge of the Supreme and Infinite to whom we offer our sacrifice, and this the nature of the sacrifice itself in its triple character, — a sacrifice of works, a sacrifice of love and adoration, a sacrifice of knowledge. For even when we speak of the sacrifice of works by itself, we do not mean the offering only of our outward acts, but of all that is active and dynamic in us; our internal movements no less than our external doings are to be consecrated on the one altar. The inner heart of all work that is made into a sacrifice is a labour of self-discipline and self-perfection by which we can hope to become conscious and luminous with a Light from above poured into all our movements of mind, heart, will, sense, life and body. An increasing light of divine consciousness will make us close in soul and one by identity in our inmost being and spiritual substance with the Master of the world-sacrifice, — the supreme object of existence proposed by the ancient Vedanta; but also it will tend to make us one in our becoming by resemblance to the Divine in our nature, the mystic sense of the symbol of sacrifice in the sealed speech of the seers of the Veda.

But if this is to be the character of the rapid evolution from a mental to a spiritual being contemplated by the integral Yoga, a question arises full of many perplexities but of great dynamic importance. How are we to deal with life and works as they now are, with the activities proper to our still unchanged human nature? An ascension towards a greater consciousness, an occupation of our mind, life and body by its powers has been accepted as the outstanding object of the Yoga: but still life here, not some other-life elsewhere, is proposed as the immediate field of the action of the Spirit, — a transformation, not an annihilation of our instrumental being and nature. What then becomes of the present activities of our being, activities of the mind turned towards knowledge and the expression of knowledge, activities of our emotional and sensational parts, activities of outward conduct, creation, production, the will turned towards mastery over men, things, life, the world, the forces of Nature? Are they to be abandoned and to be replaced by some other way of living in which a spiritualised consciousness can find its true expression and figure? Are they to be maintained as they are in their outward appearance, but transformed by an inner spirit in the act or enlarged in scope and liberated into new forms by a reversal of consciousness such as was seen on earth when man took up the vital activities of the animal to mentalise and extend and transfigure them by the infusion of reason, thinking will, refined emotion, an organised intelligence? Or is there to be an abandonment in part, a preservation only of such of them as can bear a spiritual change and, for the rest, the creation of a new life expressive, in its form no less than in its inspiration and motive-force, of the unity, wideness, peace, joy and harmony of the liberated spirit? It is this problem most of all that has exercised the minds of those who have tried to trace the paths that lead from the human to the Divine in the long journey of the Yoga.

Every kind of solution has been offered from the entire abandonment of works and life, so far as that is physically possible, to the acceptance of life as it is but with a new spirit animating and uplifting its movements, in appearance the same as they were but changed in the spirit behind them and therefore in their inner significance. The extreme solution insisted on by the world-shunning ascetic or the inward-turned ecstatical and self-oblivious mystic is evidently foreign to the purpose of an integral Yoga, — for if we are to realise the Divine in the world, it cannot be done by leaving aside the world-action and action itself altogether. At a less high pitch it was laid down by the religious mind in ancient times that one should keep only such actions as are in their nature part of the seeking, service or cult of the Divine and such others as are attached to these or, in addition, those that are indispensable to the ordinary setting of life but done in a religious spirit and according to the injunctions of traditional religion and Scripture. But this is too formalist a rule for the fulfilment of the free spirit in works, and it is besides professedly no more than a provisional solution for tiding over the transition from life in the world to a life in the Beyond which still remains the sole ultimate purpose. An integral Yoga must lean rather to the catholic injunction of the Gita that even the liberated soul, living in the Truth, should still do all the works of life so that the plan of the universal evolution under a secret divine leading may not languish or suffer. But if all works are to be done with the same forms and on the same lines as they are now done in the Ignorance, our gain is only inward and our life is in danger of becoming the dubious and ambiguous formula of an inner Light doing the works of an outer Twilight, the perfect Spirit expressing itself in a mould of imperfection foreign to its own divine nature. If no better can be done for a time, — and during a long period of transition something like this does inevitably happen, — then so it must remain till things are ready and the spirit within is powerful enough to impose its own forms on the life of the body and the world outside; but this can be accepted only as a transitional stage and not as our soul's ideal or the ultimate goal of the passage.

For the same reason the ethical solution is insufficient; for an ethical rule merely puts a bit in the mouth of the wild horses of Nature and exercises over them a difficult and partial control, but it has no power to transform Nature so that she may move in a secure freedom fulfilling the intuitions that proceed from a divine self-knowledge. At best its method is to lay down limits, to coerce the devil, to put the wall of a relative and very doubtful safety around us. This or some similar device of self-protection may be necessary for a time whether in ordinary life or in Yoga; but in Yoga it can only be the mark of a transition. A fundamental transformation and a pure wideness of spiritual life are the aim before us and, if we are to reach it, we must find a deeper solution, a surer supra-ethical dynamic principle. To be spiritual within, ethical in the outside life, this is the ordinary religious solution, but it is a compromise; the spiritualisation of both the inward being and the outward life and not a compromise between life and the spirit is the goal of which we are the seekers. Nor can the human confusion of values which obliterates the distinction between spiritual and moral and even claims that the moral is the only true spiritual element in our nature be of any use to us; for ethics is a mental control, and the limited erring mind is not and cannot be the free and ever-luminous spirit. It is equally impossible to accept the gospel that makes life the one aim, takes its elements fundamentally as they are and only calls in a half-spiritual or pseudo-spiritual light to flush and embellish it. Inadequate too is the very frequent attempt at a misalliance between the vital and the spiritual, a mystic experience within with an aestheticised intellectual and sensuous Paganism or ex-alted hedonism outside leaning upon it and satisfying itself in the glow of a spiritual sanction; for this too is a precarious and never successful compromise and it is as far from the divine Truth and its integrality as the puritanic opposite. These are all stumbling solutions of the fallible human mind groping for a transaction between the high spiritual summits and the lower pitch of the ordinary mind-motives and life-motives. Whatever partial truth may be hidden behind them, that truth can only be accepted when it has been raised to the spiritual level, tested in the supreme Truth-consciousness and extricated from the soil and error of the Ignorance.

In sum, it may be safely affirmed that no solution offered can be anything but provisional until a supramental Truth-consciousness is reached by which the appearances of things are put in their place and their essence revealed and that in them which derives straight from the spiritual essence. In the meanwhile our only safety is to find a guiding law of spiritual experience — or else to liberate a light within that can lead us on the way until that greater direct Truth-consciousness is reached above us or born within us. For all else in us that is only out-ward, all that is not a spiritual sense or seeing, the constructions, representations or conclusions of the intellect, the suggestions or instigations of the life-force, the positive necessities of physical things are sometimes half-lights, sometimes false lights that can at best only serve for a while or serve a little and for the rest either detain or confuse us. The guiding law of spiritual experience can only come by an opening of human consciousness to the Divine Consciousness; there must be the power to receive in us the working and command and dynamic presence of the Divine Shakti and surrender ourselves to her control; it is that surrender and that control which bring the guidance. But the surrender is not sure, there is no absolute certitude of the guidance so long as we are besieged by mind formations and life impulses and instigations of ego which may easily betray us into the hands of a false experience. This danger can only be countered by the opening of a now nine-tenths concealed inmost soul or psychic being that is already there but not commonly active within us. That is the inner light we must liberate; for the light of this inmost soul is our one sure illumination so long as we walk still amidst the siege of the Ignorance and the Truth-consciousness has not taken up the entire control of our Godward endeavour. The working of the Divine Force in us under the conditions of the transition and the light of the psychic being turning us always towards a conscious and seeing obedience to that higher impulsion and away from the demands and instigations of the Forces of the Ignorance, these between them create an ever progressive inner law of our action which continues till the spiritual and supramental can be established in our nature. In the transition there may well be a period in which we take up all life and action and offer them to the Divine for purification, change and deliverance of the truth within them, another period in which we draw back and build a spiritual wall around us admitting through its gates only such activities as consent to undergo the law of the spiritual transformation, a third in which a free and all-embracing action, but with new forms fit for the utter truth of the Spirit, can again be made possible. These things, however, will be decided by no mental rule but in the light of the soul within us and by the ordaining force and progressive guidance of the Divine Power that secretly or overtly first impels, then begins clearly to control and order and finally takes up the whole burden of the Yoga.

In accordance with the triple character of the sacrifice we may divide works too into a triple order, the works of Knowledge, the works of Love, the works of the Will-in-Life, and see how this more plastic spiritual rule applies to each province and effects the transition from the lower to the higher nature.

*
* *

It is natural from the point of view of the Yoga to divide into two categories the activities of the human mind in its pursuit of knowledge. There is the supreme supra-intellectual knowledge which concentrates itself on the discovery of the One and Infinite in its transcendence or tries to penetrate by intuition, contemplation, direct inner contact into the ultimate truths behind the appearances of Nature; there is the lower science which diffuses itself in an outward knowledge of phenomena, the disguises of the One and Infinite as it appears to us in or through the more exterior forms of the world-manifestation around us. These two, an upper and a lower hemisphere, in the form of them constructed or conceived by men within the mind's ignorant limits, have even there separated themselves, as they developed, with some sharpness.... Philosophy, sometimes spiritual or at least intuitive, sometimes abstract and intellectual, sometimes intellectualising spiritual experience or supporting with a logical apparatus the discoveries of the spirit, has claimed always to take the fixation of ultimate Truth as its province. But even when it did not separate itself on rarefied metaphysical heights from the knowledge that belongs to the practical world and the pursuit of ephemeral objects, intellectual Philosophy by its habit of abstraction has seldom been a power for life. It has been sometimes powerful for high speculation, pursuing mental Truth for its own sake without any ulterior utility or object, sometimes for a subtle gymnastic of the mind in a mistily bright cloud-land of words and ideas, but it has walked or acrobatised far from the more tangible realities of existence. Ancient

Philosophy in Europe was more dynamic, but only for the few; in India in its more spiritualised forms, it strongly influenced but without transforming the life of the race.... Religion did not attempt, like Philosophy, to live alone on the heights; its aim was rather to take hold of man's parts of life even more than his parts of mind and draw them Godwards; it professed to build a bridge between spiritual Truth and the vital and material human existence; it strove to subordinate and reconcile the lower to the higher, make life serviceable to God, Earth obedient to Heaven. It has to be admitted that too often this necessary effort had the opposite result of making Heaven a sanction for Earth's desires; for, continually, the religious idea has been turned into an excuse for the worship and service of the human ego. Religion, leaving constantly its little shining core of spiritual experience, has lost itself in the obscure mass of its ever extending ambiguous compromises with life: in attempting to satisfy the thinking mind, it more often succeeded in oppressing or fettering it with a mass of theological dogmas; while seeking to net the human heart, it fell itself into pits of pietistic emotionalism and sensationalism; in the act of annexing the vital nature of man to dominate it, it grew itself vitiated and fell a prey to all the fanaticism, homicidal fury, savage or harsh turn for oppression, pullulating falsehood, obstinate attachment to ignorance to which that vital nature is prone; its desire to draw the physical in man towards God betrayed it into chaining itself to ecclesiastic mechanism, hollow ceremony and lifeless ritual. The corruption of the best produced the worst by that strange chemistry of the power of life which generates evil out of good even as it can also generate good out of evil. At the same time in a vain effort at self-defence against this downward gravitation, Religion was driven to cut existence into two by a division of knowledge, works, art, life itself into two opposite categories, the spiritual and the worldly, religious and mundane, sacred and profane; but this defensive distinction itself became conventional and artificial and aggravated rather than healed the disease.... On their side Science and Art and the knowledge of Life, although at first they served or lived in the shadow of Religion, ended by emancipating themselves, became estranged or hostile, or have even recoiled with indifference, contempt or scepticism from what seem to them the cold, barren and distant or unsubstantial and illusory heights of unreality to which metaphysical Philosophy and Religion aspire. For a time the divorce has been as complete as the one-sided intolerance of the human mind could make it and threatened even to end in a complete extinction of all attempt at a higher or a more spiritual knowledge. Yet even in the earthward life a higher knowledge is indeed the one thing that is throughout needful, and without it the lower sciences and pursuits, however fruitful, however rich, free, miraculous in the abundance of their results, become easily a sacrifice offered without due order and to false gods; corrupting, hardening in the end the heart of man, limiting his mind's horizons, they confine in a stony material imprisonment or lead to a final baffling incertitude and disillusionment. A sterile agnosticism awaits us above the brilliant phosphorescence of a half-knowledge that is still the Ignorance.

A Yoga turned towards an all-embracing realisation of the Supreme will not despise the works or even the dreams, if dreams they are, of the Cosmic Spirit or shrink from the splendid toil and many-sided victory which he has assigned to himself in the human creature. But its first condition for this liberality is that our works in the world too must be part of the sacrifice offered to the Highest and to none else, to the Divine Shakti and to no other Power, in the right spirit and with the right knowledge, by the free soul and not by the hypnotised bondslave of material Nature. If a division of works has to be made, it is between those that are nearest to the heart of the sacred flame and those that are least touched or illumined by it because they are more at a distance, or between the fuel that burns strongly and brightly and the logs that if too thickly heaped on the altar may impede the ardour of the fire by their rather damp, heavy and diffused abundance. But, otherwise, apart from this division, all activities of knowledge that seek after or express Truth are in themselves rightful materials for a complete offering; none ought necessarily to be excluded from the wide framework of the divine life. The mental and physical sciences which examine into the laws and forms and processes of things, those which concern the life of men and animals, the social, political, linguistic and historical and those which seek to know and control the labours and activities by which man subdues and utilises his world and environment, and the noble and beautiful Arts which are at once work and knowledge, — for every well-made and significant poem, picture, statue or building is an act of creative knowledge, a living discovery of the consciousness, a figure of Truth, a dynamic form of mental and vital self-expression or world-expression, — all that seeks, all that finds, all that voices or figures is a realisation of something of the play of the Infinite and to that extent can be made a means of God-realisation or of divine formation. But the Yogin has to see that it is no longer done as part of an ignorant mental life; it can be accepted by him only if by the feeling, the remembrance, the dedication within it, it is turned into a movement of the spiritual consciousness and becomes a part of its vast grasp of comprehensive illuminating knowledge.

For all must be done as a sacrifice, all activities must have the One Divine for their object and the heart of their meaning. The Yogin's aim in the sciences that make for knowledge should be to discover and understand the workings of the Divine Consciousness-Puissance in man and creatures and things and forces, her creative significances, her execution of the mysteries, the symbols in which she arranges the manifestation. The Yogin's aim in the practical sciences, whether mental and physical or occult and psychic, should be to enter into the ways of the Divine and his processes, to know the materials and means for the work given to us so that we may use that knowledge for a conscious and faultless expression of the spirit's mastery, joy and self-fulfilment. The Yogin's aim in the Arts should not be a mere aesthetic, mental or vital gratification, but, seeing the Divine everywhere, worshipping it with a revelation of the meaning of its own works, to express that One Divine in ideal forms, the One Divine in principles and forces, the One Divine in gods and men and creatures and objects. The theory that sees an intimate connection between religious aspiration and the truest and greatest Art is in essence right; but we must substitute for the mixed and doubtful religious motive a spiritual aspiration, vision, interpreting experience. For the wider and more comprehensive the seeing, the more it contains in itself the sense of the hidden Divine in humanity and in all things and rises beyond a superficial religiosity into the spiritual life, the more luminous, flexible, deep and powerful will the Art be that springs from that high motive. The Yogin's distinction from other men is this that he lives in a higher and vaster spiritual consciousness; all his work of knowledge or creation must then spring from there: it must not be made in the mind, — for it is a greater truth and vision than mental man's that he has to express or rather that presses to express itself through him and mould his works, not for his personal satisfaction, but for a divine purpose.

At the same time the Yogin who knows the Supreme is not subject to any need or compulsion in these activities; for to him they are neither a duty nor a necessary occupation for the mind nor a high amusement, nor imposed even by the loftiest human purpose. He is not attached, bound and limited by any nor has he any personal motive of fame, greatness or personal satisfaction in these works; he can leave or pursue them as the Divine in him wills, but he need not otherwise abandon them in his pursuit of the higher integral knowledge. He will do these things just as the supreme Power acts and creates, for a certain spiritual joy in creation and expression or to help in the holding together and right ordering or leading of this world of God's workings. The Gita teaches that the man of knowledge shall by his way of life give to those who have not yet the spiritual consciousness, the love and habit of *all* works and not only of actions recognised as pious, religious or ascetic in their character; he should not draw men away from the world-action by his example. For the world must proceed in its great upward aspiring; men and nations must not be led to fall away from even an ignorant activity into a worse ignorance of inaction or to sink down into that miserable disintegration and tendency of dissolution which comes upon communities and peoples when there predominates the tamasic principle, the principle whether of obscure confusion and error or of weariness and inertia. "For I too," says the Lord in the Gita, "have no need to do works, since there is nothing I have not or must yet gain for myself; yet I do works in the world: for if I did not do works, all laws would fall into confusion, the worlds would sink towards chaos and I would be the destroyer of these peoples." The spiritual life does not need, for its purity, to destroy interest in all things except the Inexpressible or to cut at the roots of the Sciences, the Arts and Life. It may well be one of the effects of an integral spiritual knowledge and activity to lift them out of their limitations, substitute for our mind's ignorant, limited, tepid or trepidant pleasure in them a free, intense and uplifting urge of delight and supply a new source of creative spiritual power and illumination by which they can be carried more swiftly and profoundly towards their absolute light in knowledge and their yet undreamed possibilities and most dynamic energy of content and form and practice. The one thing needful must be pursued first and always; but all things else come with it as its outcome and have not so much to be added to us as recovered and reshaped in its self-light and as portions of its self-expressive force.

*
* *

This then is the true relation between divine and human knowledge; it is not a separation into disparate fields, sacred and profane, that is the heart of the difference, but the character of the consciousness behind the working. All is human knowledge that proceeds from the ordinary mental consciousness interested in the outside or upper layers of things, in process, in phenomena for their own sake or for the sake of some surface utility or mental or vital satisfaction of Desire or of the Intelligence. But the same activity of knowledge can become part of the Yoga if it proceeds from the spiritual or spiritualising consciousness which seeks and finds in all that it surveys or penetrates the presence of the timeless Eternal and the ways of manifestation of the Eternal in Time. It is evident that the need of a concentration indispensable for the transition out of the Ignorance may make it necessary for the seeker to gather together his energies and focus them only on that which will help the transition and to leave aside or subordinate for the time all that is not directly turned towards the one object. He may find that this or that pursuit of human knowledge with which he was accustomed to deal by the surface power of the mind still brings him by reason of this tendency or habit out of the depths to the surface or down from the heights which he has climbed or is nearing to lower levels. These activities then may have to be intermitted or put aside until, secure in a higher consciousness, he is able to turn its powers on all the mental fields; then, subjected to that light or taken up into it, they are turned, by the transformation of his consciousness, into a province of the spiritual and divine. All that cannot be so transformed or refuses to be part of a divine consciousness he will abandon without hesitation, but not from any preconceived prejudgment of its unfitness or its incapacity to be an element of the new inner life. There can be no fixed mental test or principle for these things; he will therefore follow no unalterable rule, but accept or repel an activity of the mind according to his feeling, insight or experience until the greater Power and Light are there to turn their unerring scrutiny on all that is below and choose or reject their material out of what the human evolution has prepared for the divine labour.

How precisely or by what stages this progression and change will take place must depend on the form, need and powers of the individual nature. In the spiritual domain the essence is always one, but there is yet an infinite variety and, at any rate in the integral Yoga, the rigidity of a strict and precise mental rule is seldom applicable; for, even when they walk in the same direction, no two natures proceed on exactly the same lines, in the same series of steps or with quite identical stages of their progress. It may yet be said that a logical succession of the states of progress would be very much in this order. First, there is a large turning in which all the natural mental activities proper to the individual nature are taken up or referred to a higher standpoint and dedicated by the soul in us, the psychic being, the priest of the sacrifice, to the divine service; next, there is an attempt at an ascent of the being and a bringing down of the Light and Power proper to some new height of consciousness gained by its upward effort into the whole action of the knowledge. Here there may be a strong concentration on the inward central change of the consciousness and an abandonment of a large part of the outward-going mental life or else its relegation to a small and subordinate place. At different stages it or parts of it may be taken up again from time to time to see how far the new inner psychic and spiritual consciousness can be brought into its movements; but that compulsion of the temperament or the nature which in human beings necessitates one kind of activity or another and makes it seem almost an indispensable portion of the existence, will diminish and eventually no attachment will be left, no lower compulsion or driving force felt anywhere. Only the Divine will matter, the Divine alone will be the one need of the whole being; if there is any compulsion to activity it will be not that of implanted desire or of force of Nature, but the luminous driving of some greater Consciousness-Force which is becoming more and more the sole motive power of the whole existence. On the other hand, it is possible at any period of the inner spiritual progress that one may experience an extension rather than a restriction of the activities; there may be an opening of new capacities of mental creation and new provinces of knowledge by the miraculous touch of the Yoga-Shakti. Aesthetic feeling, the power of artistic creation in one field or many fields together, talent or genius of literary expression, a faculty of metaphysical thinking, any power of eye or ear or hand or mind-power may awaken where none was apparent before. The Divine within may throw these latent riches out from the depths in which they were hidden or a Force from above may pour down its energies to equip the instrumental nature for the activity or the creation of which it is meant to be a channel or a builder. But, whatever may be the method or the course of development chosen by the hidden Master of the Yoga, the common culmination of this stage is the growing consciousness of him alone as the mover, decider, shaper of all the movements of the mind and all the activities of knowledge.

There are two signs of the transformation of the seeker's mind of knowledge and works of knowledge from the process of the Ignorance to the process of a liberated consciousness working partly, then wholly in the light of the Spirit. There is first a central change of the consciousness and a growing direct experience, vision, feeling of the Supreme and the cosmic existence, the Divine in itself and the Divine in all things; the mind will be taken up into a growing preoccupation with this first and foremost and will feel itself heightening, widening into a more and more illumined means of expression of the one fundamental knowledge. But also the central Consciousness in its turn will take up more and more the outer mental activities of knowledge and turn them into a parcel of itself or an annexed province; it will infuse into them its more authentic movement and make a more and more spiritualised and illumined mind its instrument in these surface fields, its new conquests, as well as in its own deeper spiritual empire. And this will be the second sign, the sign of a certain completion and perfection, that the Divine himself has become the Knower and all the inner movements, including the activities of what was once a purely human mental action, have become his field of knowledge. There will be less and less individual choice, opinion, preference, less and less of intellectualisation, mental weaving, cerebral galley-slave labour; a Light within will see all that has to be seen, know all that has to be known, develop, create, organise. It will be the Inner Knower who will do in the liberated and universalised mind of the individual the works of an all-comprehending knowledge.

These two changes are the signs of a first effectuation in which the activities of the mental nature are lifted up, spiritualised, widened, universalised, liberated, led to a consciousness of their true purpose as an instrumentation of the Divine creating and developing its manifestation in the temporal universe. But this cannot be the whole scope of the transformation; for it is not in these limits that the integral seeker can cease from his ascension or confine the widening of his nature. For, if it were so, knowledge would still remain a working of the mind, liberated, universalised, spiritualised, but still, as all mind must be, comparatively restricted, relative, imperfect in the very essence of its dynamism; it would reflect luminously great constructions of Truth, but not move in the domain where Truth is authentic, direct, sovereign and native. There is an ascension still to be made from this height, by which the spiritualised mind will exceed itself and transmute into a supramental power of knowledge. Already in the process of spiritualisation it will have begun to pass out of the brilliant poverty of the human intellect; it will mount successively into the pure broad reaches of a higher mind, and next into the gleaming belts of a still greater free Intelligence illumined with a Light from above. At this point it will begin to feel more freely, admit with a less mixed response the radiant beginnings of an Intuition, not illumined, but luminous in itself, true in itself, no longer entirely mental and therefore subjected to the abundant intrusion of error. Here too is not an end, for it must rise beyond into the very domain of that untruncated Intuition, the first direct light from the self-awareness of essential Being and, beyond it, attain that from which this light comes. For there is an Overmind behind Mind, a Power more original and dynamic which supports Mind, sees it as a diminished radiation from itself, uses it as a transmitting belt of passage downward or an instrument for the creations of the Ignorance. The last step of the ascension would be the surpassing of Overmind itself or its return into its own still greater origin, its conversion into the supramental light of the Divine Gnosis. For there in the supramental Light is the seat of a divine Truth-consciousness that has native in it, as no other consciousness below it can have, the power to organise the works of a Truth which is no longer tarnished by the shadow of the cosmic Inconscience and Ignorance. There to reach and thence to bring down a supramental dynamism that can transform the Ignorance is the distant but imperative supreme goal of the integral Yoga.

As the light of each of these higher powers is turned upon the human activities of knowledge, any distinction of sacred and profane, human and divine, begins more and more to fade until it is finally abolished as otiose; for whatever is touched and thoroughly penetrated by the Divine Gnosis is transfigured and becomes a movement of its own Light and Power, free from the turbidity and limitations of the lower intelligence. It is not a separation of some activities, but a transformation of them all by the change of the informing consciousness that is the way of liberation, an ascent of the sacrifice of knowledge to a greater and ever greater light and force. All the works of mind and intellect must be first heightened and widened, then illumined, lifted into the domain of a higher Intelligence, afterwards translated into workings of a greater non-mental Intuition, these again transformed into the dynamic outpourings of the Overmind radiance, and those transfigured into the full light and sovereignty of the supramental Gnosis. It is this that the evolution of consciousness in the world carries prefigured but latent in its seed and in the straining tense intention of its process; nor can that process, that evolution cease till it has evolved the instruments of a perfect in place of its now imperfect manifestation of the Spirit.

*
* *

If knowledge is the widest power of the consciousness and its function is to free and illumine, yet love is the deepest and most intense and its privilege is to be the key to the most profound and secret recesses of the Divine Mystery. Man, because he is a mental being, is prone to give the highest importance to the thinking mind and its reason and will and to its way of approach and effectuation of Truth and, even, he is inclined to hold that there is no other. The heart with its emotions and incalculable movements is to the eye of his intellect an obscure, uncertain and often a perilous and misleading power which needs to be kept in control by the reason and the mental will and intelligence. And yet there is in the heart or behind it a profounder mystic light which, if not what we call intuition, — for that, though not of the mind, yet descends through the mind, — has yet a direct touch upon Truth and is nearer to the Divine than the human intellect in its pride of knowledge. According to the ancient teaching the seat of the immanent Divine, the hidden Purusha, is in the mystic heart, — the secret heart-cave, *hṛdaye guhāyām,* as the Upanishads put it, — and, according to the experience of many Yogins, it is from its depths that there comes the voice or the breath of the inner oracle.

This ambiguity, these opposing appearances of depth and blindness are created by the double character of the human emotive being. For there is in front in man a heart of vital emotion similar to the animal's, if more variously developed; its emotions are governed by egoistic passion, blind instinctive affections and all the play of the life-impulses with their imperfections, perversions, often sordid degradations, — a heart besieged and given over to the lusts, desires, wraths, intense or fierce demands or little greeds and mean pettinesses of an obscure and fallen life-force and debased by its slavery to any and every impulse. This mixture of the emotive heart and the sensational hungering vital creates in man a false soul of desire; it is this that is the crude and dangerous element which the reason rightly distrusts and feels a need to control, even though the actual control or rather coercion it succeeds in establishing over our raw and insistent vital nature remains always very uncertain and deceptive. But the true soul of man is not there; it is in the true invisible heart hidden in some luminous cave of the nature: there under some infiltration of the divine Light is our soul, a silent inmost being of which few are even aware; for if all have a soul, few are conscious of their true soul or feel its direct impulse. There dwells the little spark of the Divine which supports the obscure mass of our nature and around it grows the psychic being, the formed soul or the real Man within us. It is as this psychic being in him grows and the movements of the heart reflect its divinations and impulsions that man becomes more and more aware of his soul, ceases to be a superior animal and, awakening to glimpses of the godhead within him, admits more and more its intimations of a deeper life and consciousness and an impulse towards things divine. It is one of the decisive moments of the integral Yoga when this psychic being, liberated, brought out from the veil to the front, can pour the full flood of its divinations, seeings and impulsions on the mind, life and body of man and begins to prepare the upbuilding of divinity in the earthly nature.

As in the works of knowledge, so in dealing with the workings of the heart, we are obliged to make a preliminary distinction between two categories of movements, those that are either moved by the true soul or aid towards its liberation and rule in the nature and those that are turned to the satisfaction of the unpurified vital nature. But the distinctions ordinarily laid down in this sense are of little use for the deeper spiritual purpose of Yoga. Thus a division can be made between religious emotions and mundane feelings and it can be laid down as a rule of spiritual life that the religious emotions alone should be cultivated and all worldly feelings and passions must be rejected and fall away from our existence. This in practice would mean the religious life of the saint or devotee, alone within with the Divine or linked only to others in a common God-love or at the most pouring out the fountains of a sacred, religious or pietistic love on the world outside. But religious emotion itself is too constantly invaded by the turmoil and obscurity of the vital movements and it is often either crude or narrow or fanatical or mixed with movements that are not signs of the spirit's perfection. It is evident besides that even at the best an intense figure of sainthood clamped in rigid hieratic lines is quite other than the wide ideal of an integral Yoga. A larger psychic and emotional relation with God and the world, more deep and plastic in its essence, more wide and embracing in its movements, more capable of taking up in its sweep the whole of life, is imperative.

A wider formula has been provided by the secular mind of man of which the basis is the ethical sense; for it distinguishes between the emotions sanctioned by the ethical sense and those that are egoistic and selfishly common and mundane. It is the works of altruism, philanthropy, compassion, benevolence, humanitarianism, service, labour for the well-being of man and all creatures that are to be our ideal; to shuffle off the coil of egoism and grow into a soul of self-abnegation that lives only or mainly for others or for humanity as a whole is the way of man's inner evolution according to this doctrine. Or if this is too secular and mental to satisfy the whole of our being, since there is a deeper religious and spiritual note there that is left out of account by the humanitarian formula, a religio-ethical foundation can be provided for it — and such was indeed its original basis. To the inner worship of the Divine or the Supreme by the devotion of the heart or to the pursuit of the Ineffable by the seeking of a highest knowledge can be added a worship through altruistic works or a preparation through acts of love, of benevolence, of service to mankind or to those around us. It is indeed by the religio-ethical sense that the law of universal goodwill or universal compassion or of love and service to the neighbour, the Vedantic, the Buddhistic, the Christian ideal, was created; only by a sort of secular refrigeration extinguishing the fervour of the religious element in it could the humanitarian ideal disengage itself and become the highest plane of a secular system of mental and moral ethics. For in the religious system this law of works is a means that ceases when its object is accomplished or a side issue; it is a part of the cult by which one adores and seeks the Divinity or it is a penultimate step of the excision of self in the passage to Nirvana. In the secular ideal it is promoted into an object in itself; it becomes a sign of the moral perfection of the human being, or else it is a condition for a happier state of man upon earth, a better society, a more united life of the race. But none of these things satisfy the demand of the soul that is placed before us by the integral Yoga.

Altruism, philanthropy, humanitarianism, service are flowers of the mental consciousness and are at best the mind's cold and pale imitation of the spiritual flame of universal Divine Love. Not truly liberative from ego-sense, they widen it at most and give it a higher and larger satisfaction; impotent in practice to change man's vital life and nature, they only modify and palliate its action and daub over its unchanged egoistic essence. Or if they are intensely followed with an entire sincerity of the will, it is by an exaggerated amplification of one side of our nature; in that exaggeration there can be no clue for the full and perfect divine evolution of the many sides of our individualised being towards the universal and transcendent Eternal. Nor can the religio-ethical ideal be a sufficient guide, — for this is a compromise or compact of mutual concessions for mutual support between a religious urge which seeks to get a closer hold on earth by taking into itself the higher turns of ordinary human nature and an ethical urge which hopes to elevate itself out of its own mental hardness and dryness by some touch of a religious fervour. In making this compact religion lowers itself to the mental level and inherits the inherent imperfections of mind and its inability to convert and transform life. The mind is the sphere of the dualities and, just as it is impossible for it to achieve any absolute Truth but only truths relative or mixed with error, so it is impossible for it to achieve any absolute good; for moral good exists as a counterpart and corrective to evil and has evil always for its shadow, complement, almost its reason for existence. But the spiritual consciousness belongs to a higher than the mental plane and there the dualities cease; for there falsehood confronted with the truth by which it profited through a usurping falsification of it and evil faced by the good of which it was a perversion or a lurid substitute, are obliged to perish for want of sustenance and to cease. The integral Yoga, refusing to rely upon the fragile stuff of mental and moral ideals, puts its whole emphasis in this field on three central dynamic processes, — the development of the true soul or psychic being to take the place of the false soul of desire, the sublimation of human into divine love, the elevation of consciousness from its mental to its spiritual and supramental plane by whose power alone both the soul and the life-force can be utterly delivered from the veils and prevarications of the Ignorance.

It is the very nature of the soul or the psychic being to turn towards the divine Truth as the sunflower to the sun; it accepts and clings to all that is divine or progressing towards divinity, and draws back from all that is a perversion or a denial of it, from all that is false and undivine. Yet the soul is at first but a spark and then a little flame of godhead burning in the midst of a great darkness; for the most part it is veiled in its inner sanctum and to reveal itself it has to call on the mind, the life-force and the physical consciousness and persuade them, as best they can, to express it; ordinarily, it succeeds at most in suffusing their outwardness with its inner light and modifying with its purifying fineness their dark obscurities or their coarser mixture. Even when there is a formed psychic being able to express itself with some directness in life, it is still in all but a few a smaller portion of the being — "no bigger in the mass of the body than the thumb of a man" was the image used by the ancient seers — and it is not always able to prevail against the obscurity or ignorant smallness of the physical consciousness, the mistaken surenesses of the mind or the arrogance and vehemence of the vital nature. This soul is obliged to accept the human mental, emotive, sensational life as it is, its relations, its activities, its cherished forms and figures; it has to labour to disengage and increase the divine element in all this relative truth mixed with a continual falsifying error, this love turned to the uses of the animal body or the satisfaction of the vital ego, this life of an average manhood shot with rare and pale glimpses of godhead and the darker luridities of the demon and the brute. Unerring in the essence of its will, it is obliged often under the pressure of its instruments to submit to mistakes of action, wrong placement of feeling, wrong choice of person, errors in the exact form of its will, in the circumstances of its expression of the infallible inner ideal. Yet is there a divination within it which makes it a surer guide than the reason or than even the highest desire, and through apparent errors and stumblings its voice can still lead better than the precise intellect and the considering mental judgment. This voice of the soul is not what we call conscience — for that is only a mental and often conventional erring substitute; it is a deeper and more seldom heard call; yet to follow it when heard is wisest: even, it is better to wander at the call of one's soul than to go apparently straight with the reason and the outward moral mentor. But it is only when the life turns towards the Divine that the soul can truly come forward and impose its power on the outer members; for, itself a spark of the Divine, to grow in flame towards the Divine is its true life and its very reason of existence.

At a certain stage in the Yoga when the mind is sufficiently quieted and no longer supports itself at every step on the sufficiency of its mental certitudes, when the vital has been steadied and subdued and is no longer constantly insistent on its own rash will, demand and desire, when the physical has been sufficiently altered not to bury altogether the inner flame under the mass of its outwardness, obscurity or inertia, an inmost being, long hidden within and felt only in its rare influences, is able to come forward and illumine the rest and take up the lead of the Sadhana. Its character is a one-pointed orientation towards the Divine or the Highest, one-pointed and yet plastic in action and movement; it does not create a rigidity of direction like the one-pointed intellect or a bigotry of the regnant idea or impulse like the one-pointed vital force; it is at every moment and with a supple sureness that it points the way to the Truth, automatically distinguishes the right step from the false, extricates the divine or Godward movement from the clinging mixture of the undivine. Its action is like a searchlight showing up all that has to be changed in the nature; it has in it a flame of will insistent on perfection, on an alchemic transmutation of all the inner and outer existence. It sees the divine essence everywhere but rejects the mere mask and the disguising figure. It insists on Truth, on will and strength and mastery, on Joy and Love and Beauty, but on a Truth of abiding Knowledge that surpasses the mere practical momentary truth of the Ignorance, on an inward joy and not on mere vital pleasure, — for it prefers rather a purifying suffering and sorrow to degrading satisfactions, — on love winged upward and not tied to the stake of egoistic craving or with its feet sunk in the mire, on beauty restored to its priesthood of interpretation of the Eternal, on strength and will and mastery as instruments not of the ego but of the Spirit. Its will is for the divinisation of life, the expression through it of a higher Truth, its dedication to the Divine and the Eternal.

But the most intimate character of the psychic is its pressure towards the Divine through a sacred love, joy and oneness. It is a divine Love that it seeks most, it is the love of the Divine that is its spur, its goal, its star of Truth shining over the luminous cave of the nascent or the still obscure cradle of the new-born godhead within us. In the first long stage of its growth and immature existence it has leaned on earthly love, affection,

tenderness, goodwill, compassion, benevolence, on all beauty
and gentleness and fineness and light and strength and courage,
on all that can help to refine and purify the grossness and com-
monness of human nature; but it knows how mixed are these
human movements at their best and at their worst how fallen
and stamped with the mark of ego and self-deceptive sentimental
falsehood and the lower self profiting by the imitation of a soul-
movement. At once, emerging, it is ready and eager to break
all the old ties and imperfect emotional activities and replace
them by a greater spiritual Truth of love and oneness. It may
still admit the human forms and movements, but on condition
that they are turned towards the One alone. It accepts only
the ties that are helpful, the heart's and mind's reverence for
the Guru, the union of the God-seekers, a spiritual compassion
for this ignorant human and animal world and its peoples, the
joy and happiness and satisfaction of beauty that comes from
the perception of the Divine everywhere. It plunges the nature
inward towards its meeting with the immanent Divine in the
heart's secret centre and, while that call is there, no reproach
of egoism, no mere outward summons of altruism or duty or
philanthropy or service will deceive or divert it from its sacred
longing and its obedience to the attraction of the Divinity within
it. It lifts the being towards a transcendent Ecstasy and is ready
to shed all the downward pull of the world from its wings in
its uprising to reach the One Highest; but it calls down also
this transcendent Love and Beatitude to deliver and transform
this world of hatred and strife and division and darkness and
jarring Ignorance. It opens to a universal Divine Love, a vast
compassion, an intense and immense will for the good of all,
for the embrace of the World-Mother enveloping or gathering
to her her children, the divine Passion that has plunged into
the night for the redemption of the world from the universal
Inconscience. It is not attracted or misled by mental imitations or
any vital misuse of these great deep-seated Truths of existence;
it exposes them with its detecting search-ray and calls down
the entire truth of divine Love to heal these malformations, to
deliver mental, vital, physical love from their insufficiencies or

their perversions and reveal to them their true abounding share of the intimacy and the oneness, the ascending ecstasy and the descending rapture.

All true Truth of love and of the works of love the psychic being accepts in their place: but its flame mounts always upward and it is eager to push the ascent from lesser to higher degrees of Truth, since it knows that only by the ascent to a highest Truth and the descent of that highest Truth can Love be delivered from the cross and placed upon the throne; for the cross is the sign of the Divine Descent barred and marred by the transversal line of a cosmic deformation which turns it into a stake of suffering and misfortune. Only by the ascent to the original Truth can the deformation be healed and all the works of love, as too all the works of knowledge and of life, be restored to a divine significance and become part of an integral spiritual existence.

Chapter VI

The Ascent of the Sacrifice – 2

The Works of Love — The Works of Life

IT IS therefore through the sacrifice of love, works and knowledge with the psychic being as the leader and priest of the sacrifice that life itself can be transformed into its own true spiritual figure. If the sacrifice of knowledge rightly done is easily the largest and purest offering we can bring to the Highest, the sacrifice of love is not less demanded of us for our spiritual perfection; it is even more intense and rich in its singleness and can be made not less vast and pure. This pure wideness is brought into the intensity of the sacrifice of love when into all our activities there is poured the spirit and power of a divine infinite joy and the whole atmosphere of our life is suffused with an engrossing adoration of the One who is the All and the Highest. For then does the sacrifice of love attain its utter perfection when, offered to the divine All, it becomes integral, catholic and boundless, and when, uplifted to the Supreme, it ceases to be the weak, superficial and transient movement men call love and becomes a pure and grand and deep uniting Ananda.

Although it is a divine love for the supreme and universal Divine that must be the rule of our spiritual existence, this does not exclude altogether all forms of individual love or the ties that draw soul to soul in manifested existence. A psychic change is demanded, a divestiture of the masks of the Ignorance, a purification of the egoistic mental, vital and physical movements that prolong the old inferior consciousness; each movement of love, spiritualised, must depend no longer on mental preference, vital passion or physical craving, but on the recognition of soul by soul, — love restored to its fundamental spiritual and psychic essence with the mind, the vital, the physical as manifesting instruments and elements of that greater oneness.

In this change the individual love also is converted by a natural heightening into a divine love for the Divine Inhabitant immanent in a mind and soul and body occupied by the One in all creatures.

All love, indeed, that is adoration has a spiritual force behind it, and even when it is offered ignorantly and to a limited object, something of that splendour appears through the poverty of the rite and the smallness of its issues. For love that is worship is at once an aspiration and a preparation: it can bring even within its small limits in the Ignorance a glimpse of a still more or less blind and partial but surprising realisation; for there are moments when it is not we but the One who loves and is loved in us, and even a human passion can be uplifted and glorified by a slight glimpse of this infinite Love and Lover. It is for this reason that the worship of the god, the worship of the idol, the human magnet or ideal are not to be despised; for these are steps through which the human race moves towards that blissful passion and ecstasy of the Infinite which, even in limiting it, they yet represent for our imperfect vision when we have still to use the inferior steps Nature has hewn for our feet and admit the stages of our progress. Certain idolatries are indispensable for the development of our emotional being, nor will the man who knows be hasty at any time to shatter the image unless he can replace it in the heart of the worshipper by the Reality it figures. Moreover, they have this power because there is always something in them that is greater than their forms and, even when we reach the supreme worship, that abides and becomes a prolongation of it or a part of its catholic wholeness. Our knowledge is still imperfect in us, love incomplete if even when we know That which surpasses all forms and manifestations, we cannot still accept the Divine in creature and object, in man, in the kind, in the animal, in the tree, in the flower, in the work of our hands, in the Nature-Force which is then no longer to us the blind action of a material machinery but a face and power of the universal Shakti: for in these things too is the presence of the Eternal.

An ultimate inexpressible adoration offered by us to the

Transcendent, to the Highest,[1] to the Ineffable, is yet no complete worship if it is not offered to him wherever he manifests or wherever even he hides his godhead — in man[2] and object and every creature. An Ignorance is there no doubt which imprisons the heart, distorts its feelings, obscures the significance of its offering; all partial worship, all religion which erects a mental or a physical idol is tempted to veil and protect the truth in it by a certain cloak of ignorance and easily loses the truth in its image. But the pride of exclusive knowledge is also a limitation and a barrier. For there is, concealed behind individual love, obscured by its ignorant human figure, a mystery which the mind cannot seize, the mystery of the body of the Divine, the secret of a mystic form of the Infinite which we can approach only through the ecstasy of the heart and the passion of the pure and sublimated sense, and its attraction which is the call of the divine Flute-player, the mastering compulsion of the All-Beautiful, can only be seized and seize us through an occult love and yearning which in the end makes one the Form and the Formless, and identifies Spirit and Matter. It is that which the spirit in Love is seeking here in the darkness of the Ignorance and it is that which it finds when individual human love is changed into the love of the Immanent Divine incarnate in the material universe.

As with individual, so with universal Love; all that widening of the self through sympathy, goodwill, universal benevolence and beneficence, love of mankind, love of creatures, the attraction of all the myriad forms and presences that surround us, by which mentally and emotionally man escapes from the first limits of his ego, has to be taken up into a unifying divine love for the universal Divine. Adoration fulfilled in love, love in Ananda, — the surpassing love, the self-wrapped ecstasy of transcendent delight in the Transcendent which awaits us at the end of the path of Devotion, — has for its wider result a universal love for all beings, the Ananda of all that is; we perceive behind every veil the Divine, spiritually embrace in all forms the All-Beautiful. A

---

[1] *param bhāvam.*   [2] *mānuṣīṁ tanum āśritam.*

universal delight in his endless manifestation flows through us, taking in its surge every form and movement, but not bound or stationary in any and always reaching out to a greater and more perfect expression. This universal love is liberative and dynamic for transformation; for the discord of forms and appearances ceases to affect the heart that has felt the one Truth behind them all and understood their perfect significance. The impartial equality of soul of the selfless worker and knower is transformed by the magic touch of divine Love into an all-embracing ecstasy and million-bodied beatitude. All things become bodies and all movements the playings of the divine Beloved in his infinite house of pleasure. Even pain is changed and in their reaction and even in their essence things painful alter; the forms of pain fall away, there are created in their place the forms of Ananda.

This is in its essence the nature of the change of consciousness which turns existence itself into a glorified field of a Divine Love and Ananda. In its essence it begins for the seeker when he passes from the ordinary to the spiritual level and looks with a new heart of luminous vision and feeling on the world and self and others. It reaches its height when the spiritual becomes also the supramental level and then also it is possible not only to feel it in essence but realise it dynamically as a Power for the transformation of the whole inner life and the whole outer existence.

*   *
*   *

It is not altogether difficult for the mind to envisage, even though it may be difficult for the human will with its many earth-ties to accept, this transformation of the spirit and nature of love from the character of a mixed and limited human emotion to a supreme and all-embracing divine passion. It is when we come to the works of love that a certain perplexity is likely to intervene. It is possible, as in a certain high exaggeration of the path of knowledge, to cut here also the knot of the problem, escape the difficulty of uniting the spirit of love with the crudities of the world-action by avoiding it; it is open to us, withdrawing from outward life and action altogether, to live alone with our adoration of the Divine in the heart's silence. It is possible too to admit only those acts that are either in themselves an expression of love for the Divine, prayer, praise, symbolic acts of worship or subordinate activities that may be attached to these things and partake of their spirit, and to leave aside all else; the soul turns away to satisfy its inner longing in the absorbed or the God-centred life of the saint and devotee. It is possible, again, to open the doors of life more largely and to spend one's love of the Divine in acts of service to those around us and to the race; one can do the works of philanthropy, benevolence and beneficence, charity and succour to man and beast and every creature, transfigure them by a kind of spiritual passion, at least bring into their merely ethical appearance the greater power of a spiritual motive. This is indeed the solution most commonly favoured by the religious mind of today and we see it confidently advanced on all sides as the proper field of action of the God-seeker or of the man whose life is founded on divine love and knowledge. But the integral Yoga pushed towards a complete union of the Divine with the earth-life cannot stop short in this narrow province or limit this union within the lesser dimensions of an ethical rule of philanthropy and beneficence. All action must be made in it part of the God-life, our acts of knowledge, our acts of power and production and creation, our acts of joy and beauty and the soul's pleasure, our acts of will and endeavour and struggle and not our acts only of love and beneficent service. Its way to do these things will be not outward and mental, but inward and spiritual, and to that end it will bring into all activities, whatever they are, the spirit of divine love, the spirit of adoration and worship, the spirit of happiness in the Divine and in the beauty of the Divine so as to make all life a sacrifice of the works of the soul's love to the Divine, its cult of the Master of its existence.

It is possible so to turn life into an act of adoration to the Supreme by the spirit in one's works; for, says the Gita, "He who gives to me with a heart of adoration a leaf, a flower, a fruit or a cup of water, I take and enjoy that offering of his devotion"; and it is not only any dedicated external gift that can be so offered with love and devotion, but all our thoughts, all our feelings and sensations, all our outward activities and their forms and objects can be such gifts to the Eternal. It is true that the special act or form of action has its importance, even a great importance, but it is the spirit in the act that is the essential factor; the spirit of which it is the symbol or materialised expression gives it its whole value and justifying significance. Or it may be said that a complete act of divine love and worship has in it three parts that are the expressions of a single whole, — a practical worship of the Divine in the act, a symbol of worship in the form of the act expressing some vision and seeking or some relation with the Divine, an inner adoration and longing for oneness or feeling of oneness in the heart and soul and spirit. It is so that life can be changed into worship, — by putting behind it the spirit of a transcendent and universal love, the seeking of oneness, the sense of oneness; by making each act a symbol, an expression of Godward emotion or a relation with the Divine; by turning all we do into an act of worship, an act of the soul's communion, the mind's understanding, the life's obedience, the heart's surrender.

In any cult the symbol, the significant rite or expressive figure is not only a moving and enriching aesthetic element, but a physical means by which the human being begins to make outwardly definite the emotion and aspiration of his heart, to confirm it and to dynamise it. For if without a spiritual aspiration worship is meaningless and vain, yet the aspiration also without the act and the form is a disembodied and, for life, an incompletely effective power. It is unhappily the fate of all forms in human life to become crystallised, purely formal and therefore effete, and although form and cult preserve always their power for the man who can still enter into their meaning, the majority come to use the ceremony as a mechanical rite and the symbol as a lifeless sign, and because that kills the soul of religion, cult and form have in the end to be changed or thrown aside altogether. There are those even to whom all cult and form are for this reason suspect and offensive; but few can dispense with the support of outward symbols and, even, a certain divine element in human nature demands them always for the completeness of its spiritual satisfaction. Always the symbol is legitimate in so far as it is true, sincere, beautiful and delightful, and even one may say that a spiritual consciousness without any aesthetic or emotional content is not entirely or at any rate not integrally spiritual. In the spiritual life the basis of the act is a spiritual consciousness perennial and renovating, moved to express itself always in new forms or able to renew the truth of a form always by the flow of the spirit, and to so express itself and make every action a living symbol of some truth of the soul is the very nature of its creative vision and impulse. It is so that the spiritual seeker must deal with life and transmute its form and glorify it in its essence.

A supreme divine Love is a creative Power and, even though it can exist in itself silent and unchangeable, yet rejoices in external form and expression and is not condemned to be a speechless and bodiless godhead. It has even been said that creation itself was an act of love or at least the building up of a field in which Divine Love could devise its symbols and fulfil itself in act of mutuality and self-giving, and, if not the initial nature of creation, this may well be its ultimate object and motive. It does not so appear now because, even if a Divine Love is there in the world upholding all this evolution of creatures, yet the stuff of life and its action is made up of an egoistic formation, a division, a struggle of life and consciousness to exist and survive in an apparently indifferent, inclement or even hostile world of inanimate and inconscient Matter. In the confusion and obscurity of this struggle all are thrown against each other with a will in each to assert its own existence first and foremost and only secondarily to assert itself in others and very partially for others; for even man's altruism remains essentially egoistic and must be so till the soul finds the secret of the divine Oneness. It is to discover that at its supreme source, to bring it from within and to radiate it out up to the extreme confines of life that is turned the effort of the Yoga. All action, all creation must be turned into a form, a symbol of the cult, the adoration, the sacrifice; it must carry something that makes it bear in it the stamp of a dedication, a reception and translation of the Divine Consciousness, a service of the Beloved, a self-giving, a surrender. This has to be done wherever possible in the outward body and form of the act; it must be done always in its inward emotion and an intensity that shows it to be an outflow from the soul towards the Eternal.

In itself the adoration in the act is a great and complete and powerful sacrifice that tends by its self-multiplication to reach the discovery of the One and make the radiation of the Divine possible. For devotion by its embodiment in acts not only makes its own way broad and full and dynamic, but brings at once into the harder way of works in the world the divinely passionate element of joy and love which is often absent in its beginning when it is only the austere spiritual Will that follows in a struggling uplifting tension the steep ascent, and the heart is still asleep or bound to silence. If the spirit of divine love can enter, the hardness of the way diminishes, the tension is lightened, there is a sweetness and joy even in the core of difficulty and struggle. The indispensable surrender of all our will and works and activities to the Supreme is indeed only perfect and perfectly effective when it is a surrender of love. All life turned into this cult, all actions done in the love of the Divine and in the love of the world and its creatures seen and felt as the Divine manifested in many disguises become by that very fact part of an integral Yoga.

It is the inner offering of the heart's adoration, the soul of it in the symbol, the spirit of it in the act, that is the very life of the sacrifice. If this offering is to be complete and universal, then a turning of all our emotions to the Divine is imperative. This is the intensest way of purification for the human heart, more powerful than any ethical or aesthetic catharsis could ever be by its half-power and superficial pressure. A psychic fire within must be lit into which all is thrown with the Divine Name upon it. In that fire all the emotions are compelled to cast off their grosser elements and those that are undivine perversions are burned away and the others discard their insufficiencies, till a spirit of largest love and a stainless divine delight arises out of the flame and smoke and frankincense. It is the divine love which so emerges that, extended in inward feeling to the Divine in man and all creatures in an active universal equality, will be more potent for the perfectibility of life and a more real instrument than the ineffective mental ideal of brotherhood can ever be. It is this poured out into acts that could alone create a harmony in the world and a true unity between all its creatures; all else strives in vain towards that end so long as Divine Love has not disclosed itself as the heart of the delivered manifestation in terrestrial Nature.

It is here that the emergence of the secret psychic being in us as the leader of the sacrifice is of the utmost importance; for this inmost being alone can bring with it the full power of the spirit in the act, the soul in the symbol. It alone can assure, even while the spiritual consciousness is incomplete, the perennial freshness and sincerity and beauty of the symbol and prevent it from becoming a dead form or a corrupted and corrupting magic; it alone can preserve for the act its power with its significance. All the other members of our being, mind, life-force, physical or body consciousness, are too much under the control of the Ignorance to be a sure instrumentation and much less can they be a guide or the source of an unerring impulse. Always the greater part of the motive and action of these powers clings to the old law, the deceiving tablets, the cherished inferior movements of Nature and they meet with reluctance, alarm or revolt or obstructing inertia the voices and the forces that call and impel us to exceed and transform ourselves into a greater being and a wider Nature. In their major part the response is either a resistance or a qualified or temporising acquiescence; for even if they follow the call, they yet tend — when not consciously, then by automatic habit — to bring into the spiritual action their own natural disabilities and errors. At every moment they are moved to take egoistic advantage of the psychic and spiritual influences and can be detected using the power, joy or light these bring into us for a lower life-motive. Afterwards too, even when the seeker has opened to the Divine Love transcendental, universal or immanent, yet if he tries to pour it into life, he meets the power of obscuration and perversion of these lower Nature-forces. Always they draw away towards pitfalls, pour into that higher intensity their diminishing elements, seek to capture the descending Power for themselves and their interests and degrade it into an aggrandised mental, vital or physical instrumentation for desire and ego. Instead of a Divine Love creator of a new heaven and a new earth of Truth and Light, they would hold it here prisoner as a tremendous sanction and glorifying force of sublimation to gild the mud of the old earth and colour with its rose and sapphire the old turbid unreal skies of sentimen-talising vital imagination and mental idealised chimera. If that falsification is permitted, the higher Light and Power and Bliss withdraw, there is a fall back to a lower status; or else the realisation remains tied to an insecure half-way and mixture or is covered and even submerged by an inferior exaltation that is not the true Ananda. It is for this reason that Divine Love which is at the heart of all creation and the most powerful of all redeeming and creative forces has yet been the least frontally present in earthly life, the least successfully redemptive, the least creative. Human nature has been unable to bear it in its purity for the very reason that it is the most powerful, pure, rare and intense of all the divine energies; what little could be seized has been corrupted at once into a vital pietistic ardour, a defenceless religious or ethical sentimentalism, a sensuous or even sensual erotic mysticism of the roseate coloured mind or passionately turbid life-impulse and with these simulations compensated its inability to house the Mystic Flame that could rebuild the world with its tongues of sacrifice. It is only the inmost psychic being unveiled and emerging in its full power that can lead the pilgrim sacrifice unscathed through these ambushes and pitfalls; at each moment it catches, exposes, repels the mind's and the life's false-hoods, seizes hold on the truth of the Divine Love and Ananda and separates it from the excitement of the mind's ardours and the blind enthusiasms of the misleading life-force. But all things that are true at their core in mind and life and the physical being it extricates and takes with it in the journey till they stand on the heights, new in spirit and sublime in figure.

And yet even the leading of the inmost psychic being is not found sufficient until it has succeeded in raising itself out of this mass of inferior Nature to the highest spiritual levels and the divine spark and flame descended here have rejoined themselves to their original fiery Ether. For there is there no longer a spiritual consciousness still imperfect and half lost to itself in the thick sheaths of human mind, life and body, but the full spiritual consciousness in its purity, freedom and intense wideness. There, as it is the eternal Knower that becomes the Knower in us and mover and user of all knowledge, so it is the eternal All-Blissful who is the Adored attracting to himself the eternal divine portion of his being and joy that has gone out into the play of the universe, the infinite Lover pouring himself out in the multiplicity of his own manifested selves in a happy Oneness. All Beauty in the world is there the beauty of the Beloved, and all forms of beauty have to stand under the light of that eternal Beauty and submit themselves to the sublimating and transfiguring power of the unveiled Divine Perfection. All Bliss and Joy are there of the All-Blissful, and all inferior forms of enjoyment, happiness or pleasure are subjected to the shock of the intensity of its floods or currents and either they are broken to pieces as inadequate things under its convicting stress or compelled to transmute themselves into the forms of the Divine Ananda. Thus for the individual consciousness a Force is manifested which can deal sovereignly in it with the diminutions and degradations of the values of the Ignorance. At last it begins to be possible to bring down into life the immense reality and intense concreteness of the love and joy that are of the Eternal. Or at any rate it will be possible for our spiritual consciousness to raise itself out of mind into the supramental Light and Force and Vastness; there in the light and potency of the supramental Gnosis are the splendour and joy of a power of divine self-expression and self-organisation which could rescue and re-create even the world of the Ignorance into a figure of the Truth of the Spirit.

There in the supramental Gnosis is the fulfilment, the culminating height, the all-embracing extent of the inner adoration, the profound and integral union, the flaming wings of Love upbearing the power and joy of a supreme Knowledge. For supramental Love brings an active ecstasy that surpasses the void passive peace and stillness which is the heaven of the liberated Mind and does not betray the deeper greater calm which is the beginning of the supramental silence. The unity of a love which is able to include in itself all differences without being diminished or abrogated by their present limitations and apparent dissonances is raised to its full potentiality on the supramental level. For there an intense oneness with all creatures founded on a profound oneness of the soul with the Divine can harmonise with a play of relations that only makes the oneness more perfect and absolute. The power of Love supramentalised can take hold of all living relations without hesitation or danger and turn them Godwards delivered from their crude, mixed and petty human settings and sublimated into the happy material of a divine life. For it is the very nature of the supramental experience that it can perpetuate the play of difference without forfeiting or in the least diminishing either the divine union or the infinite oneness. For a supramentalised consciousness it would be utterly possible to embrace all contacts with men and the world in a purified flame-force and with a transfigured significance, because the soul would then perceive always as the object of all emotion and all seeking for love or beauty the One Eternal and could spiritually use a wide and liberated life-urge to meet and join with that One Divine in all things and all creatures.

* * *

Into the third and last category of the works of sacrifice can be gathered all that is directly proper to the Yoga of works; for here is its direct field of effectuation and major province. It covers the entire range of life's more visible activities; under it fall the multiform energies of the Will-to-Life throwing itself outward to make the most of material existence. It is here that an ascetic or other-worldly spirituality feels an insurmountable denial of the Truth which it seeks after and is compelled to turn away from terrestrial existence, rejecting it as for ever the dark

playground of an incurable Ignorance. Yet it is precisely these
activities that are claimed for a spiritual conquest and divine
transformation by the integral Yoga. Abandoned altogether by
the more ascetic disciplines, accepted by others only as a field of
temporary ordeal or a momentary, superficial and ambiguous
play of the concealed spirit, this existence is fully embraced
and welcomed by the integral seeker as a field of fulfilment, a
field for divine works, a field of the total self-discovery of the
concealed and indwelling spirit. A discovery of the Divinity in
oneself is his first object, but a total discovery too of the Divinity
in the world behind the apparent denial offered by its scheme
and figures and, last, a total discovery of the dynamism of some
transcendent Eternal; for by its descent this world and self will
be empowered to break their disguising envelopes and become
divine in revealing form and manifesting process as they now
are secretly in their hidden essence.

This object of the integral Yoga must be accepted wholly
by those who follow it, but the acceptance must not be in ignorance of the immense stumbling-blocks that lie in the way of
the achievement; on the contrary we must be fully aware of the
compelling cause of the refusal of so many other disciplines to
regard even its possibility, much less its imperative character, as
the true meaning of terrestrial existence. For here in the works of
life in the earth-nature is the very heart of the difficulty that has
driven Philosophy to its heights of aloofness and turned away
even the eager eye of Religion from the malady of birth in a
mortal body to a distant Paradise or a silent peace of Nirvana.
A way of pure Knowledge is comparatively straightforward and
easy to the tread of the seeker in spite of our mental limitations
and the pitfalls of the Ignorance; a way of pure Love, although
it has its stumbling-blocks and its sufferings and trials, can in
comparison be as easy as the winging of a bird through the free
azure. For Knowledge and Love are pure in their essence and
become mixed and embarrassed, corrupted and degraded only
when they enter into the ambiguous movement of the life-forces
and are seized by them for the outward life's crude movements
and obstinately inferior motives. Alone of the three powers Life

or at least a certain predominant Will-in-Life has the appearance of something impure, accursed or fallen in its very essence. At its contact, wrapped in its dull sheaths or caught in its iridescent quagmires, the divinities themselves become common and muddy and hardly escape from being dragged downwards into its perversions and disastrously assimilated to the demon and the Asura. A principle of dark and dull inertia is at its base; all are tied down by the body and its needs and desires to a trivial mind, petty desires and emotions, an insignificant repetition of small worthless functionings, needs, cares, occupations, pains, pleasures that lead to nothing beyond themselves and bear the stamp of an ignorance that knows not its own why and whither. This physical mind of inertia believes in no divinity other than its own small earth-gods; it aspires perhaps to a greater comfort, order, pleasure, but asks for no uplifting and no spiritual deliverance. At the centre we meet a stronger Will of life with a greater gusto, but it is a blinded Daemon, a perverted spirit and exults in the very elements that make of life a striving turmoil and an unhappy imbroglio. It is a soul of human or Titanic desire clinging to the garish colour, disordered poetry, violent tragedy or stirring melodrama of this mixed flux of good and evil, joy and sorrow, light and darkness, heady rapture and bitter torture. It loves these things and would have more and more of them or, even when it suffers and cries out against them, can accept or joy in nothing else; it hates and revolts against higher things and in its fury would trample, tear or crucify any diviner Power that has the presumption to offer to make life pure, luminous and happy and snatch from its lips the fiery brew of that exciting mixture. Another Will-in-Life there is that is ready to follow the ameliorating ideal Mind and is allured by its offer to extract some harmony, beauty, light, nobler order out of life, but this is a smaller part of the vital nature and can be easily overpowered by its more violent or darker duller yoke-comrades; nor does it readily lend itself to a call higher than that of the Mind unless that call defeats itself, as Religion usually does, by lowering its demand to conditions more intelligible to our obscure vital nature. All these forces the spiritual seeker grows aware of in himself and finds all around him and has to struggle and combat incessantly to be rid of their grip and dislodge the long-entrenched mastery they have exercised over his own being as over the environing human existence. The difficulty is great; for their hold is so strong, so apparently invincible that it justifies the disdainful dictum which compares human nature to a dog's tail, — for, straighten it never so much by force of ethics, religion, reason or any other redemptive effort, it returns in the end always to the crooked curl of Nature. And so great is the vim, the clutch of that more agitated Life-Will, so immense the peril of its passions and errors, so subtly insistent or persistently invasive, so obstinate up to the very gates of Heaven the fury of its attack or the tedious obstruction of its obstacles that even the saint and the Yogin cannot be sure of their liberated purity or their trained self-mastery against its intrigue or its violence. All labour to straighten out this native crookedness strikes the struggling will as a futility; a flight, a withdrawal to happy Heaven or peaceful dissolution easily finds credit as the only wisdom and to find a way not to be born again gets established as the only remedy for the dull bondage or the poor shoddy delirium or the blinded and precarious happiness and achievement of earthly existence.

A remedy yet there should be and is, a way of redress and a chance of transformation for this troubled vital nature; but for that the cause of deviation must be found and remedied at the heart of Life itself and in its very principle, since Life too is a power of the Divine and not a creation of some malignant Chance or dark Titanic impulse, however obscure or perverted may be its actual appearance. In Life itself there is the seed of its own salvation, it is from the Life-Energy that we must get our leverage; for though there is a saving light in Knowledge, a redeeming and transforming force in Love, these cannot be effective here unless they secure the consent of Life and can use the instrumentation of some delivered energy at its centre for a sublimation of the erring human into a divine Life-Force. It is not possible to cut the difficulty by a splitting up of the works of sacrifice; we cannot escape it by deciding that we shall do only the works of Love and Knowledge and leave aside the works of will and power, possession and acquisition, production and fruitful expense of capacity, battle and victory and mastery, striking away from us the larger part of life because it seems to be made of the very stuff of desire and ego and therefore doomed to be a field of disharmony and mere conflict and disorder. For the division cannot really be made; or, if attempted, it must fail in its essential purpose, since it would isolate us from the total energies of the World-Power and sterilise an important part of integral Nature, just the one force in it that is a necessary instrument in any world-creative purpose. The Life-Force is an indispensable intermediary, the effectuating element in Nature here; mind needs its alliance if the works of mind are not to remain shining inner formations without a body; the spirit needs it to give an outer force and form to its manifested possibilities and arrive at a complete self-expression incarnated in Matter. If Life refuses the aid of its intermediary energy to the spirit's other workings or is itself refused, they are likely to be reduced for all the effect they can have here to a static seclusion or a golden impotence; or if anything is done, it will be a partial irradiation of our action more subjective than objective, modifying existence perhaps, but without force to change it. Yet if Life brings its forces to the spirit but unregenerate, a worse result may follow since it is likely to reduce the spiritual action of Love or Knowledge to diminished and corrupted motions or make them accomplices of its own inferior or perverse workings. Life is indispensable to the completeness of the creative spiritual realisation, but life released, transformed, uplifted, not the ordinary mentalised human-animal life, nor the demoniac or Titanic, nor even the divine and the undivine mixed together. Whatever may be done by other world-shunning or heaven-seeking disciplines, this is the difficult but unavoidable task of the integral Yoga; it cannot afford to leave unsolved the problem of the outward works of Life, it must find in them their native Divinity and ally it firmly and for ever to the divinities of Love and Knowledge.

It is no solution either to postpone dealing with the works of Life till Love and Knowledge have been evolved to a point

at which they can sovereignly and with safety lay hold on the
Life-Force to regenerate it; for we have seen that they have to
rise to immense heights before they can be secure from the vital
perversion which hampers or hamstrings their power to deliver.
If once our consciousness could reach the heights of a supramental Nature, then indeed these disabilities would disappear.
But here there is the dilemma that it is impossible to reach the
supramental heights with the burden of an unregenerated Life-
Force on our shoulders and equally impossible to regenerate
radically the Will-in-Life without bringing down the infallible
light and unconquerable power that belong to the spiritual and
supramental levels. The Supramental Consciousness is not only
a Knowledge, a Bliss, an intimate Love and Oneness, it is also
a Will, a principle of Power and Force, and it cannot descend
till the element of Will, of Power, of Force in this manifested
Nature is sufficiently developed and sublimated to receive and
bear it. But Will, Power, Force are the native substance of the
Life-Energy, and herein lies the justification for the refusal of Life
to acknowledge the supremacy of Knowledge and Love alone,
— for its push towards the satisfaction of something far more
unreflecting, headstrong and dangerous that can yet venture too
in its own bold and ardent way towards the Divine and Absolute. Love and Wisdom are not the only aspects of the Divine,
there is also its aspect of Power. As the mind gropes for Knowledge, as the heart feels out for Love, so the life-force, however
fumblingly or trepidantly, stumbles in search of Power and the
control given by Power. It is a mistake of the ethical or religious
mind to condemn Power as in itself a thing not to be accepted
or sought after because naturally corrupting and evil; in spite
of its apparent justification by a majority of instances, this is at
its core a blind and irrational prejudice. However corrupted and
misused, as Love and Knowledge too are corrupted and misused,
Power is divine and put here for a divine use. Shakti, Will, Power
is the driver of the worlds and, whether it be Knowledge-Force
or Love-Force or Life-Force or Action-Force or Body-Force, is
always spiritual in its origin and divine in its native character.
It is the use of it made in the Ignorance by brute, man or Titan

that has to be cast aside and replaced by its greater natural —
even if to us supernormal — action led by the Light of an inner
consciousness which is in tune with the Infinite and the Eternal.
The integral Yoga cannot reject the works of Life and be satisfied
with an inward experience only; it has to go inward in order to
change the outward, making the Life-Force a part and a working
of a Yoga-Energy which is in touch with the Divine and divine
in its guidance.

All the difficulty in dealing spiritually with the works of Life
arises because the Will-in-Life for its purposes in the Ignorance
has created a false soul of desire and substituted it for that spark
of the Divine which is the true psyche. All or most of the works
of life are at present or seem to be actuated and vitiated by this
soul of desire; even those that are ethical or religious, even those
that wear the guise of altruism, philanthropy, self-sacrifice, self-
denial, are shot through and through with the threads of its
making. This soul of desire is a separative soul of ego and all its
instincts are for a separative self-affirmation; it pushes always,
openly or under more or less shining masks, for its own growth,
for possession, for enjoyment, for conquest and empire. If the
curse of disquiet and disharmony and perversion is to be lifted
from Life, the true soul, the psychic being, must be given its
leading place and there must be a dissolution of the false soul
of desire and ego. But this does not mean that life itself must
be coerced and denied its native line of fulfilment; for behind
this outer life soul of desire there is in us an inner and true
vital being which has not to be dissolved but brought out into
prominence and released to its true working as a power of the
Divine Nature. The prominence of this true vital being under
the lead of the true inmost soul within us is the condition for the
divine fulfilment of the objects of the Life-Force. Those objects
will even remain the same in essence, but transformed in their
inner motive and outer character. The Divine Life-Power too will
be a will for growth, a force of self-affirmation, but affirmation
of the Divine within us, not of the little temporary personality on
the surface, — growth into the true divine Individual, the central
being, the secret imperishable Person who can emerge only by

the subordination and disappearance of the ego. This is life's true object: growth, but a growth of the spirit in Nature, affirming and developing itself in mind, life and body; possession, but a possession by the Divine of the Divine in all things, and not of things for their own sake by the desire of the ego; enjoyment, but an enjoyment of the divine Ananda in the universe; battle and conquest and empire in the shape of a victorious conflict with the Powers of Darkness, an entire spiritual self-rule and mastery over inward and outward Nature, a conquest by Knowledge, Love and Divine Will over the domains of the Ignorance.

These are the conditions and these must be the aims of the divine effectuation of the works of Life and their progressive transformation which is the third element of the triple sacrifice. It is not a rationalisation but a supramentalisation, not a moralising but a spiritualising of life that is the object of the Yoga. It is not a handling of externals or superficial psychological motives that is its main purpose, but a refounding of life and its action on their hidden divine element; for only such a refounding of life can bring about its direct government by the secret Divine Power above us and its transfiguration into a manifest expression of the Divinity, not as now a disguise and a disfiguring mask of the eternal Actor. It is a spiritual essential change of consciousness, not the surface manipulation which is the method of Mind and Reason, that can alone make Life other than it now is and rescue it out of its present distressed and ambiguous figure.

*
* *

It is then by a transformation of life in its very principle, not by an external manipulation of its phenomena, that the integral Yoga proposes to change it from a troubled and ignorant into a luminous and harmonious movement of Nature. There are three conditions which are indispensable for the achievement of this central inner revolution and new formation; none of them is altogether sufficient in itself, but by their united threefold power the uplifting can be done, the conversion made and completely made. For, first, life as it is is a movement of desire and it has built in us as its centre a desire-soul which refers to itself all the motions of life and puts in them its own troubled hue and pain of an ignorant, half-lit, baffled endeavour: for a divine living, desire must be abolished and replaced by a purer and firmer motive-power, the tormented soul of desire dissolved and in its stead there must emerge the calm, strength, happiness of a true vital being now concealed within us. Next, life as it is is driven or led partly by the impulse of the life-force, partly by a mind which is mostly a servant and abettor of the ignorant life-impulse, but in part also its uneasy and not too luminous or competent guide and mentor; for a divine life the mind and the life-impulse must cease to be anything but instruments and the inmost psychic being must take their place as the leader on the path and the indicator of a divine guidance. Last, life as it is is turned towards the satisfaction of the separative ego; ego must disappear and be replaced by the true spiritual person, the central being, and life itself must be turned towards the fulfilment of the Divine in terrestrial existence; it must feel a Divine Force awaking within it and become an obedient instrumentation of its purpose.

There is nothing that is not ancient and familiar in the first of these three transforming inner movements; for it has always been one of the principal objects of spiritual discipline. It has been best formulated in the already expressed doctrine of the Gita by which a complete renouncement of desire for the fruits as the motive of action, a complete annulment of desire itself, the complete achievement of a perfect equality are put forward as the normal status of a spiritual being. A perfect spiritual equality is the one true and infallible sign of the cessation of desire, — to be equal-souled to all things, unmoved by joy and sorrow, the pleasant and the unpleasant, success or failure, to look with an equal eye on high and low, friend and enemy, the virtuous and the sinner, to see in all beings the manifold manifestation of the One and in all things the multitudinous play or the slow masked evolution of the embodied Spirit. It is not a mental quiet, aloofness, indifference, not an inert vital quiescence, not a passivity of the physical consciousness consenting to no movement or to any movement that is the condition aimed at, though these things are sometimes mistaken for this spiritual condition, but a wide comprehensive unmoved universality such as that of the Witness Spirit behind Nature. For all here seems to be a mobile half-ordered half-confused organisation of forces, but behind them one can feel a supporting peace, silence, wideness, not inert but calm, not impotent but potentially omnipotent with a concentrated, stable, immobile energy in it capable of bearing all the motions of the universe. This Presence behind is equal-souled to all things: the energy it holds in it can be unloosed for any action, but no action will be chosen by any desire in the Witness Spirit; a Truth acts which is beyond and greater than the action itself or its apparent forms and impulses, beyond and greater than mind or life-force or body, although it may take for the immediate purpose a mental, a vital or a physical appearance. It is when there is this death of desire and this calm equal wideness in the consciousness everywhere, that the true vital being within us comes out from the veil and reveals its own calm, intense and potent presence. For such is the true nature of the vital being, *prāṇamaya puruṣa*; it is a projection of the Divine Purusha into life, — tranquil, strong, luminous, many-energied, obedient to the Divine Will, egoless, yet or rather therefore capable of all action, achievement, highest or largest enterprise. The true Life-Force too reveals itself as no longer this troubled harassed divided striving surface energy, but a great and radiant Divine Power, full of peace and strength and bliss, a wide-wayed Angel of Life with its wings of Might enfolding the universe.

And yet this transformation into a large strength and equality is insufficient; for if it opens to us the instrumentation of a Divine Life, it does not provide its government and initiative. It is here that the presence of the released psychic being intervenes; it does not give the supreme government and direction, — for that is not its function, — but it supplies during the transition from ignorance to a divine Knowledge a progressive guidance for the inner and outer life and action; it indicates at each moment the method, the way, the steps that will lead to that fulfilled spiritual condition in which a supreme dynamic initiative will be always there directing the activities of a divinised Life-Force.

The light it sheds illuminates the other parts of the nature which,
for want of any better guidance than their own confused and
groping powers, have been wandering in the rounds of the Ignorance; it gives to mind the intrinsic feeling of the thoughts
and perceptions, to life the infallible sense of the movements
that are misled or misleading and those that are well-inspired;
something like a quiet oracle from within discloses the causes of
our stumblings, warns in time against their repetition, extracts
from experience and intuition the law, not rigid but plastic,
of a just direction for our acts, a right stepping, an accurate
impulse. A will is created that becomes more in consonance
with evolving Truth rather than with the circling and dilatory
mazes of a seeking Error. A determined orientation towards the
greater Light to be, a soul-instinct, a psychic tact and insight
into the true substance, motion and intention of things, coming
always nearer and nearer to a spiritual vision, to a knowledge by
inner contact, inner sight and even identity, begin to replace the
superficial keenness of mental judgment and the eager graspings
of the life-force. The works of Life right themselves, escape from
confusion, substitute for the artificial or legal order imposed by
the intellect and for the arbitrary rule of desire the guidance
of the soul's inner insight, enter into the profound paths of the
Spirit. Above all, the psychic being imposes on life the law of
the sacrifice of all its works as an offering to the Divine and
the Eternal. Life becomes a call to that which is beyond Life; its
every smallest act enlarges with the sense of the Infinite.

   As an inner equality increases and with it the sense of the
true vital being waiting for the greater direction it has to serve,
as the psychic call too increases in all the members of our nature, That to which the call is addressed begins to reveal itself,
descends to take possession of the life and its energies and fills
them with the height, intimacy, vastness of its presence and its
purpose. In many, if not most, it manifests something of itself
even before the equality and the open psychic urge or guidance
are there. A call of the veiled psychic element oppressed by the
mass of the outer ignorance and crying for deliverance, a stress
of eager meditation and seeking for knowledge, a longing of the

heart, a passionate will ignorant yet but sincere may break the lid that shuts off that Higher from this Lower Nature and open the floodgates. A little of the Divine Person may reveal itself or some Light, Power, Bliss, Love out of the Infinite. This may be a momentary revelation, a flash or a brief-lived gleam that soon withdraws and waits for the preparation of the nature; but also it may repeat itself, grow, endure. A long and large and comprehensive working will then have begun, sometimes luminous or intense, sometimes slow and obscure. A Divine Power comes in front at times and leads and compels or instructs and enlightens; at others it withdraws into the background and seems to leave the being to its own resources. All that is ignorant, obscure, perverted or simply imperfect and inferior in the being is raised up, perhaps brought to its acme, dealt with, corrected, exhausted, shown its own disastrous results, compelled to call for its own cessation or transformation or expelled as worthless or incorrigible from the nature. This cannot be a smooth and even process; alternations there are of day and night, illumination and darkness, calm and construction or battle and upheaval, the presence of the growing Divine Consciousness and its absence, heights of hope and abysses of despair, the clasp of the Beloved and the anguish of its absence, the overwhelming invasion, the compelling deceit, the fierce opposition, the disabling mockery of hostile Powers or the help and comfort and communion of the Gods and the Divine Messengers. A great and long revolution and churning of the ocean of Life with strong emergences of its nectar and its poison is enforced till all is ready and the increasing Descent finds a being, a nature prepared and conditioned for its complete rule and its all-encompassing presence. But if the equality and the psychic light and will are already there, then this process, though it cannot be dispensed with, can still be much lightened and facilitated: it will be rid of its worst dangers; an inner calm, happiness, confidence will support the steps through all the difficulties and trials of the transformation and the growing Force profiting by the full assent of the nature will rapidly diminish and eliminate the power of the opposing forces. A sure guidance and protection will be present throughout, sometimes standing in front, sometimes working behind the veil, and the power of the end will be already there even in the beginning and in the long middle stages of the great endeavour. For at all times the seeker will be aware of the Divine Guide and Protector or the working of the supreme Mother-Force; he will know that all is done for the best, the progress assured, the victory inevitable. In either case the process is the same and unavoidable, a taking up of the whole nature, of the whole life, of the internal and of the external, to reveal and handle and transform its forces and their movements under the pressure of a diviner Life from above, until all here has been possessed by greater spiritual powers and made an instrumentation of a spiritual action and a divine purpose.

In this process and at an early stage of it it becomes evident that what we know of ourselves, our present conscious existence, is only a representative formation, a superficial activity, a changing external result of a vast mass of concealed existence. Our visible life and the actions of that life are no more than a series of significant expressions, but that which it tries to express is not on the surface; our existence is something much larger than this apparent frontal being which we suppose ourselves to be and which we offer to the world around us. This frontal and external being is a confused amalgam of mind-formations, life-movements, physical functionings of which even an exhaustive analysis into its component parts and machinery fails to reveal the whole secret. It is only when we go behind, below, above into the hidden stretches of our being that we can know it; the most thorough and acute surface scrutiny and manipulation cannot give us the true understanding or the completely effective control of our life, its purposes, its activities; that inability indeed is the cause of the failure of reason, morality and every other surface action to control and deliver and perfect the life of the human race. For below even our most obscure physical consciousness is a subconscious being in which as in a covering and supporting soil are all manner of hidden seeds that sprout up, unaccountably to us, on our surface and into which we are constantly throwing fresh seeds that prolong our past and will influence our future, — a subconscious being, obscure, small in its motions, capriciously

and almost fantastically subrational, but of an immense potency
for the earth-life. Again behind our mind, our life, our conscious
physical there is a larger subliminal consciousness, — there are
inner mental, inner vital, inner more subtle physical reaches
supported by an inmost psychic existence which is the animating
soul of all the rest; and in these hidden reaches too lie a mass
of numerous pre-existent personalities which supply the material, the motive-forces, the impulsions of our developing surface
existence. For in each one of us here there may be one central
person, but also a multitude of subordinate personalities created
by the past history of its manifestation or by expressions of it on
these inner planes which support its present play in this external
material cosmos. And while on our surface we are cut off from
all around us except through an exterior mind and sense contact
which delivers but little of us to our world or of our world to
us, in these inner reaches the barrier between us and the rest
of existence is thin and easily broken; there we can feel at once
— not merely infer from their results, but feel directly — the
action of the secret world-forces, mind-forces, life-forces, subtle
physical forces that constitute universal and individual existence;
we shall even be able, if we will but train ourselves to it, to lay
our hands on these world-forces that throw themselves on us or
surround us and more and more to control or at least strongly
modify their action on us and others, their formations, their very
movements. Yet again, above our human mind are still greater
reaches superconscient to it and from there secretly descend
influences, powers, touches which are the original determinants
of things here and, if they were called down in their fullness,
could altogether alter the whole make and economy of life in the
material universe. It is all this latent experience and knowledge
that the Divine Force working upon us by our opening to it in
the integral Yoga, progressively reveals to us, uses and works out
the consequences as means and steps towards a transformation
of our whole being and nature. Our life is thenceforth no longer
a little rolling wave on the surface, but interpenetrant if not
coincident with the cosmic life. Our spirit, our self rises not
only into an inner identity with some wide cosmic Self but into

some contact with that which is beyond, though aware of and dominant over the action of the universe.

It is thus by an integralisation of our divided being that the Divine Shakti in the Yoga will proceed to its object; for liberation, perfection, mastery are dependent on this integralisation, since the little wave on the surface cannot control its own movement, much less have any true control over the vast life around it. The Shakti, the power of the Infinite and the Eternal descends within us, works, breaks up our present psychological formations, shatters every wall, widens, liberates, presents us with always newer and greater powers of vision, ideation, perception and newer and greater life-motives, enlarges and new-models increasingly the soul and its instruments, confronts us with every imperfection in order to convict and destroy it, opens to a greater perfection, does in a brief period the work of many lives or ages so that new births and new vistas open constantly within us. Expansive in her action, she frees the consciousness from confinement in the body; it can go out in trance or sleep or even waking and enter into worlds or other regions of this world and act there or carry back its experience. It spreads out, feeling the body only as a small part of itself, and begins to contain what before contained it; it achieves the cosmic consciousness and extends itself to be commensurate with the universe. It begins to know inwardly and directly and not merely by external observation and contact the forces at play in the world, feels their movement, distinguishes their functioning and can operate immediately upon them as the scientist operates upon physical forces, accept their action and results in our mind, life, body or reject them or modify, change, reshape, create immense new powers and movements in place of the old small functionings of the nature. We begin to perceive the working of the forces of universal Mind and to know how our thoughts are created by that working, separate from within the truth and falsehood of our perceptions, enlarge their field, extend and illumine their significance, become master of our own minds and active to shape the movements of Mind in the world around us. We begin to perceive the flow and surge of the universal life-forces, detect the origin and law of our feelings, emotions, sensations, passions, are free to accept, reject, new-create, open to wider, rise to higher planes of Life-Power. We begin to perceive too the key to the enigma of Matter, follow the interplay of Mind and Life and Consciousness upon it, discover more and more its instrumental and resultant function and detect ultimately the last secret of Matter as a form not merely of Energy but of involved and arrested or unstably fixed and restricted consciousness and begin to see too the possibility of its liberation and plasticity of response to higher Powers, its possibilities for the conscious and no longer the more than half-inconscient incarnation and self-expression of the Spirit. All this and more becomes more and more possible as the working of the Divine Shakti increases in us and, against much resistance or labour to respond of our obscure consciousness, through much struggle and movement of progress and regression and renewed progress necessitated by the work of intensive transformation of a half-inconscient into a conscious substance, moves to a greater purity, truth, height, range. All depends on the psychic awakening in us, the completeness of our response to her and our growing surrender.

But all this can only constitute a greater inner life with a greater possibility of the outer action and is a transitional achievement; the full transformation can come only by the ascent of the sacrifice to its farthest heights and its action upon life with the power and light and beatitude of the divine supramental Gnosis. For then alone all the forces that are divided and express themselves imperfectly in life and its works are raised to their original unity, harmony, single truth, authentic absoluteness and entire significance. There Knowledge and Will are one, Love and Force a single movement; the opposites that afflict us here are resolved into their reconciled unity: good develops its absolute and evil divesting itself of its error returns to the good that was behind it; sin and virtue vanish in a divine purity and an infallible truth-movement; the dubious evanescence of pleasure disappears in a Bliss that is the play of an eternal and happy spiritual certitude, and pain in perishing discovers the touch of an Ananda which was betrayed by some dark perversion and incapacity of the will of the Inconscient to receive it. These things, to the Mind an imagination or a mystery, become evident and capable of experience as the consciousness rises out of limited embodied Matter-mind to the freedom and fullness of the higher and higher ranges of the super-intelligence; but they can become entirely true and normal only when the supramental becomes the law of the nature.

It is therefore on the accomplishment of this ascent and on the possibility of a full dynamism from these highest levels descending into earth-consciousness that is dependent the justification of Life, its salvation, its transformation into a Divine Life in a transfigured terrestrial Nature.

*
* *

The nature of the integral Yoga so conceived, so conditioned, progressing by these spiritual means, turning upon this integral transformation of the nature, determines of itself its answer to the question of the ordinary activities of life and their place in the Yoga.

There is not and cannot be here any ascetic or contemplative or mystic abandonment of works and life altogether, any gospel of an absorbed meditation and inactivity, any cutting away or condemnation of the Life-Force and its activities, any rejection of the manifestation in the earth-nature. It may be necessary for the seeker at any period to withdraw into himself, to remain plunged in his inner being, to shut out from him the noise and turmoil of the life of the Ignorance until a certain inner change has been accomplished or something achieved without which a further effective action on life has become difficult or impossible. But this can only be a period or an episode, a temporary necessity or a preparatory spiritual manoeuvre; it cannot be the rule of his Yoga or its principle.

A splitting up of the activities of human existence on a religious or an ethical basis or both together, a restriction to the works of worship only or to the works of philanthropy and beneficence only would be contrary to the spirit of the integral

Yoga. Any merely mental rule or merely mental acceptance or repudiation is alien to the purpose and method of its discipline. All must be taken to a spiritual height and placed upon a spiritual basis; the presence of an inner spiritual change and an outer transformation must be enforced upon the whole of life and not merely on a part of life; all must be accepted that is helpful towards this change or admits it, all must be rejected that is incapable or inapt or refuses to submit itself to the transforming movement. There must be no attachment to any form of things or of life, any object, any activity; all must be renounced if need be, all must be admitted that the Divine chooses as its material for the divine life. But what accepts or rejects must be neither mind nor open or camouflaged vital will of desire nor ethical sense, but the insistence of the psychic being, the command of the Divine Guide of the Yoga, the vision of the higher Self or Spirit, the illumined guidance of the Master. The way of the spirit is not a mental way; a mental rule or mental consciousness cannot be its determinant or its leader.

Equally, a combination or a compromise between two orders of consciousness, the spiritual and the mental or the spiritual and the vital or a mere sublimation from within of Life outwardly unchanged cannot be the law or the aim of the Yoga. All life must be taken up but all life must be transformed; all must become a part, a form, an adequate expression of a spiritual being in the supramental nature. This is the height and crowning movement of a spiritual evolution in the material world, and as the change from the vital animal to mental man made life another thing altogether in basic consciousness, scope, significance, so this change from the materialised mental being to the spiritual and supramental being using but not dominated by matter must take up life and make it another thing altogether than the flawed, imperfect limited human, quite other in its basic consciousness, scope, significance. All forms of life activity that cannot bear the change must disappear, all that can bear it will survive and enter into the kingdom of the spirit. A divine Force is at work and will choose at each moment what has to be done or has not to be done, what has to be momentarily or permanently taken up, momentarily or permanently abandoned. For provided we do not substitute for that our desire or our ego, and to that end the soul must be always awake, always on guard, alive to the divine guidance, resistant to the undivine misleading from within or without us, that Force is sufficient and alone competent and she will lead us to the fulfilment along ways and by means too large, too inward, too complex for the mind to follow, much less to dictate. It is an arduous and difficult and dangerous way, but there is none other.

Two rules alone there are that will diminish the difficulty and obviate the danger. One must reject all that comes from the ego, from vital desire, from the mere mind and its presumptuous reasoning incompetence, all that ministers to these agents of the Ignorance. One must learn to hear and follow the voice of the inmost soul, the direction of the Guru, the command of the Master, the working of the Divine Mother. Whoever clings to the desires and weaknesses of the flesh, the cravings and passions of the vital in its turbulent ignorance, the dictates of his personal mind unsilenced and unillumined by a greater knowledge, cannot find the true inner law and is heaping obstacles in the way of the divine fulfilment. Whoever is able to detect and renounce those obscuring agencies and to discern and follow the true Guide within and without will discover the spiritual law and reach the goal of the Yoga.

A radical and total change of consciousness is not only the whole meaning but, in an increasing force and by progressive stages, the whole method of the integral Yoga.

Chapter VII
Standards of Conduct and Spiritual Freedom

THE KNOWLEDGE on which the doer of works in Yoga has to found all his action and development has for the keystone of its structure a more and more concrete perception of unity, the living sense of an all-pervading oneness; he moves in the increasing consciousness of all existence as an indivisible whole: all work too is part of this divine indivisible whole. His personal action and its results can no longer be or seem a separate movement mainly or entirely determined by the egoistic "free" will of an individual, himself separate in the mass. Our works are part of an indivisible cosmic action; they are put or, more accurately, put themselves into their place in the whole out of which they arise and their outcome is determined by forces that overpass us. That world action in its vast totality and in every petty detail is the indivisible movement of the One who manifests himself progressively in the cosmos. Man too becomes progressively conscious of the truth of himself and the truth of things in proportion as he awakens to this One within him and outside him and to the occult, miraculous and significant process of its forces in the motion of Nature. This action, this movement, is not confined even in ourselves and those around us to the little fragmentary portion of the cosmic activities of which we in our superficial consciousness are aware; it is supported by an immense underlying environing existence subliminal to our minds or subconscious, and it is attracted by an immense transcending existence which is superconscious to our nature. Our action arises, as we ourselves have emerged, out of a universality of which we are not aware; we give it a shape by our personal temperament, personal mind and will of thought or force of impulse or desire; but the true truth of things, the true law of action exceeds these personal and human formations. Every standpoint, every man-made rule of action which ignores the indivisible totality of the cosmic movement, whatever its utility in external practice, is to the eye of spiritual Truth an imperfect view and a law of the Ignorance.

Even when we have arrived at some glimpse of this idea or succeeded in fixing it in our consciousness as a knowledge of the mind and a consequent attitude of the soul, it is difficult for us in our outward parts and active nature to square accounts between this universal standpoint and the claims of our personal opinion, our personal will, our personal emotion and desire. We are forced still to go on dealing with this indivisible movement as if it were a mass of impersonal material out of which we, the ego, the person, have to carve something according to our own will and mental fantasy by a personal struggle and effort. This is man's normal attitude towards his environment, actually false because our ego and its will are creations and puppets of the cosmic forces and it is only when we withdraw from ego into the consciousness of the divine Knowledge-Will of the Eternal who acts in them that we can be by a sort of deputation from above their master. And yet is this personal position the right attitude for man so long as he cherishes his individuality and has not yet fully developed it; for without this view-point and motive-force he cannot grow in his ego, cannot sufficiently develop and differentiate himself out of the subconscious or half-conscious universal mass-existence.

But the hold of this ego-consciousness upon our whole habit of existence is difficult to shake off when we have no longer need of the separative, the individualistic and aggressive stage of development, when we would proceed forward from this necessity of littleness in the child-soul to unity and universality, to the cosmic consciousness and beyond, to our transcendent spirit-stature. It is indispensable to recognise clearly, not only in our mode of thought but in our way of feeling, sensing, doing, that this movement, this universal action is not a helpless impersonal wave of being which lends itself to the will of any ego according to that ego's strength and insistence. It is the movement of a cosmic Being who is the Knower of his field, the steps of a Divinity who is the Master of his own progressive force of action. As the movement is one and indivisible, so he who is present in the movement is one, sole and indivisible. Not only all result is determined by him, but all initiation, action and process are dependent on the motion of his cosmic force and only belong secondarily and in their form to the creature.

But what then must be the spiritual position of the personal worker? What is his true relation in dynamic Nature to this one cosmic Being and this one total movement? He is a centre only — a centre of differentiation of the one personal consciousness, a centre of determination of the one total movement; his personality reflects in a wave of persistent individuality the one universal Person, the Transcendent, the Eternal. In the Ignorance it is always a broken and distorted reflection because the crest of the wave which is our conscious waking self throws back only an imperfect and falsified similitude of the divine Spirit. All our opinions, standards, formations, principles are only attempts to represent in this broken, reflecting and distorting mirror something of the universal and progressive total action and its many-sided movement towards some ultimate self-revelation of the Divine. Our mind represents it as best it can with a narrow approximation that becomes less and less inadequate in proportion as its thought grows in wideness and light and power; but it is always an approximation and not even a true partial figure. The Divine Will acts through the aeons to reveal progressively not only in the unity of the cosmos, not only in the collectivity of living and thinking creatures, but in the soul of each individual something of its divine Mystery and the hidden truth of the Infinite. Therefore there is in the cosmos, in the collectivity, in the individual, a rooted instinct or belief in its own perfectibility, a constant drive towards an ever increasing and more adequate and more harmonious self-development nearer to the secret truth of things. This effort is represented to the constructing mind of man by standards of knowledge, feeling, character, aesthesis and action, — rules, ideals, norms and laws that he essays to turn into universal dharmas.

* * *

If we are to be free in the spirit, if we are to be subject only to the supreme Truth, we must discard the idea that our mental or moral laws are binding on the Infinite or that there can be anything sacrosanct, absolute or eternal even in the highest of our existing standards of conduct. To form higher and higher temporary standards as long as they are needed is to serve the Divine in his world march; to erect rigidly an absolute standard is to attempt the erection of a barrier against the eternal waters in their onflow. Once the nature-bound soul realises this truth, it is delivered from the duality of good and evil. For good is all that helps the individual and the world towards their divine fullness, and evil is all that retards or breaks up that increasing perfection. But since the perfection is progressive, evolutive in Time, good and evil are also shifting quantities and change from time to time their meaning and value. This thing which is evil now and in its present shape must be abandoned was once helpful and necessary to the general and individual progress. That other thing which we now regard as evil may well become in another form and arrangement an element in some future perfection. And on the spiritual level we transcend even this distinction; for we discover the purpose and divine utility of all these things that we call good and evil. Then have we to reject the falsehood in them and all that is distorted, ignorant and obscure in that which is called good no less than in that which is called evil. For we have then to accept only the true and the divine, but to make no other distinction in the eternal processes.

To those who can act only on a rigid standard, to those who can feel only the human and not the divine values, this truth may seem to be a dangerous concession which is likely to destroy the very foundation of morality, confuse all conduct and establish only chaos. Certainly, if the choice must be between an eternal and unchanging ethics and no ethics at all, it would have that result for man in his ignorance. But even on the human level, if we have light enough and flexibility enough to recognise that a standard of conduct may be temporary and yet necessary for its time and to observe it faithfully until it can be replaced by a better, then we suffer no such loss, but lose only the fanaticism of an imperfect and intolerant virtue. In its place we gain openness and a power of continual moral progression, charity, the capacity to enter into an understanding sympathy with all this world of struggling and stumbling creatures and by that charity a better right and a greater strength to help it upon its way. In the end where the human closes and the divine commences, where the mental disappears into the supramental consciousness and the finite precipitates itself into the infinite, all evil disappears into a transcendent divine Good which becomes universal on every plane of consciousness that it touches.

This, then, stands fixed for us that all standards by which we may seek to govern our conduct are only our temporary, imperfect and evolutive attempts to represent to ourselves our stumbling mental progress in the universal self-realisation towards which Nature moves. But the divine manifestation cannot be bound by our little rules and fragile sanctities; for the consciousness behind it is too vast for these things. Once we have grasped this fact, disconcerting enough to the absolutism of our reason, we shall better be able to put in their right place in regard to each other the successive standards that govern the different stages in the growth of the individual and the collective march of mankind. At the most general of them we may cast a passing glance. For we have to see how they stand in relation to that other standardless spiritual and supramental mode of working for which Yoga seeks and to which it moves by the surrender of the individual to the divine Will and, more effectively, through his ascent by this surrender to the greater consciousness in which a certain identity with the dynamic Eternal becomes possible.

*
* *

There are four main standards of human conduct that make an ascending scale. The first is personal need, preference and desire;

the second is the law and good of the collectivity; the third is an ideal ethic; the last is the highest divine law of the nature.

Man starts on the long career of his evolution with only the first two of these four to enlighten and lead him; for they constitute the law of his animal and vital existence and it is as the vital and physical animal man that he begins his progress. The true business of man upon earth is to express in the type of humanity a growing image of the Divine; whether knowingly or unknowingly, it is to this end that Nature is working in him under the thick veil of her inner and outer processes. But the material or animal man is ignorant of the inner aim of life; he knows only its needs and its desires and he has necessarily no other guide to what is required of him than his own perception of need and his own stirrings and pointings of desire. To satisfy his physical and vital demands and necessities before all things else and, in the next rank, whatever emotional or mental cravings or imaginations or dynamic notions rise in him must be the first natural rule of his conduct. The sole balancing or overpowering law that can modify or contradict this pressing natural claim is the demand put on him by the ideas, needs and desires of his family, community or tribe, the herd, the pack of which he is a member.

If man could live to himself, — and this he could only do if the development of the individual were the sole object of the Divine in the world, — this second law would not at all need to come into operation. But all existence proceeds by the mutual action and reaction of the whole and the parts, the need for each other of the constituents and the thing constituted, the interdependence of the group and the individuals of the group. In the language of Indian philosophy the Divine manifests himself always in the double form of the separative and the collective being, *vyaṣṭi, samaṣṭi.* Man, pressing after the growth of his separate individuality and its fullness and freedom, is unable to satisfy even his own personal needs and desires except in conjunction with other men; he is a whole in himself and yet incomplete without others. This obligation englobes his personal law of conduct in a group-law which arises from the formation of a lasting group-entity with a collective mind and life of its own to which his own embodied mind and life are subordinated as a transitory unit. And yet is there something in him immortal and free, not bound to this group-body which outlasts his own embodied existence but cannot outlast or claim to chain by its law his eternal spirit.

In itself this seemingly larger and overriding law is no more than an extension of the vital and animal principle that governs the individual elementary man; it is the law of the pack or herd. The individual identifies partially his life with the life of a certain number of other individuals with whom he is associated by birth, choice or circumstance. And since the existence of the group is necessary for his own existence and satisfaction, in time, if not from the first, its preservation, the fulfilment of its needs and the satisfaction of its collective notions, desires, habits of living, without which it would not hold together, must come to take a primary place. The satisfaction of personal idea and feeling, need and desire, propensity and habit has to be constantly subordinated, by the necessity of the situation and not from any moral or altruistic motive, to the satisfaction of the ideas and feelings, needs and desires, propensities and habits, not of this or that other individual or number of individuals, but of the society as a whole. This social need is the obscure matrix of morality and of man's ethical impulse.

It is not actually known that in any primitive times man lived to himself or with only his mate as do some of the animals. All record of him shows him to us as a social animal, not an isolated body and spirit. The law of the pack has always overridden his individual law of self-development; he seems always to have been born, to have lived, to have been formed as a unit in a mass. But logically and naturally from the psychological viewpoint the law of personal need and desire is primary, the social law comes in as a secondary and usurping power. Man has in him two distinct master impulses, the individualistic and the communal, a personal life and a social life, a personal motive of conduct and a social motive of conduct. The possibility of their opposition and the attempt to find their equation lie at the very roots of human civilisation and persist in other figures when he has passed beyond the vital animal into a highly individualised mental and spiritual progress.

The existence of a social law external to the individual is at different times a considerable advantage and a heavy disadvantage to the development of the divine in man. It is an advantage at first when man is crude and incapable of self-control and self-finding, because it erects a power other than that of his personal egoism through which that egoism may be induced or compelled to moderate its savage demands, to discipline its irrational and often violent movements and even to lose itself sometimes in a larger and less personal egoism. It is a disadvantage to the adult spirit ready to transcend the human formula because it is an external standard which seeks to impose itself on him from outside, and the condition of his perfection is that he shall grow from within and in an increasing freedom, not by the suppression but by the transcendence of his perfected individuality, not any longer by a law imposed on him that trains and disciplines his members but by the soul from within breaking through all previous forms to possess with its light and transmute his members.

*
* *

In the conflict of the claims of society with the claims of the individual two ideal and absolute solutions confront one another. There is the demand of the group that the individual should subordinate himself more or less completely or even lose his independent existence in the community, — the smaller must be immolated or self-offered to the larger unit. He must accept the need of the society as his own need, the desire of the society as his own desire; he must live not for himself but for the tribe, clan, commune or nation of which he is a member. The ideal and absolute solution from the individual's standpoint would be a society that existed not for itself, for its all-overriding collective purpose, but for the good of the individual and his fulfilment, for the greater and more perfect life of all its members. Representing as far as possible his best self and helping him to realise it, it would respect the freedom of each of its members and maintain itself not by law and force but by the free and spontaneous consent of its constituent persons. An ideal society of either kind does not exist anywhere and would be most difficult to create, more difficult still to keep in precarious existence so long as individual man clings to his egoism as the primary motive of existence. A general but not complete domination of the society over the individual is the easier way and it is the system that Nature from the first instinctively adopts and keeps in equilibrium by rigorous law, compelling custom and a careful indoctrination of the still subservient and ill-developed intelligence of the human creature.

In primitive societies the individual life is submitted to rigid and immobile communal custom and rule; this is the ancient and would-be eternal law of the human pack that tries always to masquerade as the everlasting decree of the Imperishable, *esa dharmaḥ sanātanaḥ*. And the ideal is not dead in the human mind; the most recent trend of human progress is to establish an enlarged and sumptuous edition of this ancient turn of collective living towards the enslavement of the human spirit. There is here a serious danger to the integral development of a greater truth upon earth and a greater life. For the desires and free seekings of the individual, however egoistic, however false or perverted they may be in their immediate form, contain in their obscure shell the seed of a development necessary to the whole; his searchings and stumblings have behind them a force that has to be kept and transmuted into the image of the divine ideal. That force needs to be enlightened and trained but must not be suppressed or harnessed exclusively to society's heavy cart-wheels. Individualism is as necessary to the final perfection as the power behind the group-spirit; the stifling of the individual may well be the stifling of the god in man. And in the present balance of humanity there is seldom any real danger of exaggerated individualism breaking up the social integer. There is continually a danger that the exaggerated pressure of the social mass by its heavy unenlightened mechanical weight may suppress or unduly discourage the free development of the individual spirit. For man in the individual can be more easily enlightened, conscious, open to clear influences; man in the mass is still obscure, half-conscious, ruled by universal forces that escape its mastery and its knowledge.

Against this danger of suppression and immobilisation Nature in the individual reacts. It may react by an isolated resistance ranging from the instinctive and brutal revolt of the criminal to the complete negation of the solitary and ascetic. It may react by the assertion of an individualistic trend in the social idea, may impose it on the mass consciousness and establish a compromise between the individual and the social demand. But a compromise is not a solution; it only salves over the difficulty and in the end increases the complexity of the problem and multiplies its issues. A new principle has to be called in other and higher than the two conflicting instincts and powerful at once to override and to reconcile them. Above the natural individual law which sets up as our one standard of conduct the satisfaction of our individual needs, preferences and desires and the natural communal law which sets up as a superior standard the satisfaction of the needs, preferences and desires of the community as a whole, there had to arise the notion of an ideal moral law which is not the satisfaction of need and desire, but controls and even coerces or annuls them in the interests of an ideal order that is not animal, not vital and physical, but mental, a creation of the mind's seeking for light and knowledge and right rule and right movement and true order. The moment this notion becomes powerful in man, he begins to escape from the engrossing vital and material into the mental life; he climbs from the first to the second degree of the threefold ascent of Nature. His needs and desires themselves are touched with a more elevated light of purpose and the mental need, the aesthetic, intellectual and emotional desire begin to predominate over the demand of the physical and vital nature.

* *

The natural law of conduct proceeds from a conflict to an equilibrium of forces, impulsions and desires; the higher ethical law proceeds by the development of the mental and moral nature towards a fixed internal standard or else a self-formed ideal of absolute qualities, — justice, righteousness, love, right reason, right power, beauty, light. It is therefore essentially an individual standard; it is not a creation of the mass mind. The thinker is the individual; it is he who calls out and throws into forms that which would otherwise remain subconscious in the amorphous human whole. The moral striver is also the individual; self-discipline, not under the yoke of an outer law, but in obedience to an internal light, is essentially an individual effort. But by positing his personal standard as the translation of an absolute moral ideal the thinker imposes it, not on himself alone, but on all the individuals whom his thought can reach and penetrate. And as the mass of individuals come more and more to accept it in idea if only in an imperfect practice or no practice, society also is compelled to obey the new orientation. It absorbs the ideative influence and tries, not with any striking success, to mould its institutions into new forms touched by these higher ideals. But always its instinct is to translate them into binding law, into pattern forms, into mechanic custom, into an external social compulsion upon its living units.

For, long after the individual has become partially free, a moral organism capable of conscious growth, aware of an inward life, eager for spiritual progress, society continues to be external in its methods, a material and economic organism, mechanical, more intent upon status and self-preservation than on growth and self-perfection. The greatest present triumph of the thinking and progressive individual over the instinctive and static society has been the power he has acquired by his thought-will to compel it to think also, to open itself to the idea of social justice and righteousness, communal sympathy and mutual compassion, to feel after the rule of reason rather than blind custom as the test of its institutions and to look on the mental and moral assent of its individuals as at least one essential element in the validity of its laws. Ideally at least, to consider light rather than force as its sanction, moral development and not vengeance or restraint as the object even of its penal action, is becoming just possible to the communal mind. The greatest future triumph of the thinker will come when he can persuade the individual integer and the collective whole to rest their life-relation and its union and stability upon a free and harmonious consent and self-adaptation, and shape and govern the external by the internal truth rather than to constrain the inner spirit by the tyranny of the external form and structure.

But even this success that he has gained is rather a thing in potentiality than in actual accomplishment. There is always a disharmony and a discord between the moral law in the individual and the law of his needs and desires, between the moral law proposed to society and the physical and vital needs, desires, customs, prejudices, interests and passions of the caste, the clan, the religious community, the society, the nation. The moralist erects in vain his absolute ethical standard and calls upon all to be faithful to it without regard to consequences. To him the needs and desires of the individual are invalid if they are in conflict with the moral law, and the social law has no claims upon him if it is opposed to his sense of right and denied by his conscience. This is his absolute solution for the individual that he shall cherish no desires and claims that are not consistent with love, truth and justice. He demands from the community or nation that it shall hold all things cheap, even its safety and its most pressing interests, in comparison with truth, justice, humanity and the highest good of the peoples.

No individual rises to these heights except in intense moments, no society yet created satisfies this ideal. And in the present state of morality and of human development none perhaps can or ought to satisfy it. Nature will not allow it, Nature knows that it should not be. The first reason is that our moral ideals are themselves for the most part ill-evolved, ignorant and arbitrary, mental constructions rather than transcriptions of the eternal truths of the spirit. Authoritative and dogmatic, they assert certain absolute standards in theory, but in practice every existing system of ethics proves either in application unworkable or is in fact a constant coming short of the absolute standard to which the ideal pretends. If our ethical system is a compromise or a makeshift, it gives at once a principle of justification to the further sterilising compromises which society and the individual hasten to make with it. And if it insists on absolute love, justice, right with an uncompromising insistence, it soars above the head of human possibility and is professed with lip homage but ignored in practice. Even it is found that it ignores other elements in humanity which equally insist on survival but refuse to come within the moral formula. For just as the individual law of desire contains within it invaluable elements of the infinite whole which have to be protected against the tyranny of the absorbing social idea, the innate impulses too both of individual and of collective man contain in them invaluable elements which escape the limits of any ethical formula yet discovered and are yet necessary to the fullness and harmony of an eventual divine perfection.

Moreover, absolute love, absolute justice, absolute right reason in their present application by a bewildered and imperfect humanity come easily to be conflicting principles. Justice often demands what love abhors. Right reason dispassionately considering the facts of nature and human relations in search of a satisfying norm or rule is unable to admit without modification either any reign of absolute justice or any reign of absolute love. And in fact man's absolute justice easily turns out to be in practice a sovereign injustice; for his mind, one-sided and rigid in its constructions, puts forward a one-sided partial and rigorous scheme or figure and claims for it totality and absoluteness and an application that ignores the subtler truth of things and the plasticity of life. All our standards turned into action either waver on a flux of compromises or err by this partiality and unelastic structure. Humanity sways from one orientation to another; the race moves upon a zigzag path led by conflicting claims and, on the whole, works out instinctively what Nature intends, but with much waste and suffering, rather than either what it desires or what it holds to be right or what the highest light from above demands from the embodied spirit.

*
* *

The fact is that when we have reached the cult of absolute ethical qualities and erected the categorical imperative of an ideal
law, we have not come to the end of our search or touched
the truth that delivers. There is, no doubt, something here that
helps us to rise beyond limitation by the physical and vital man
in us, an insistence that overpasses the individual and collective
needs and desires of a humanity still bound to the living mud
of Matter in which it took its roots, an aspiration that helps to
develop the mental and moral being in us: this new sublimating
element has been therefore an acquisition of great importance;
its workings have marked a considerable step forward in the
difficult evolution of terrestrial Nature. And behind the inadequacy of these ethical conceptions something too is concealed
that does attach to a supreme Truth; there is here the glimmer
of a light and power that are part of a yet unreached divine
Nature. But the mental idea of these things is not that light and
the moral formulation of them is not that power. These are only
representative constructions of the mind that cannot embody
the divine spirit which they vainly endeavour to imprison in
their categorical formulas. Beyond the mental and moral being
in us is a greater divine being that is spiritual and supramental;
for it is only through a large spiritual plane where the mind's
formulas dissolve in a white flame of direct inner experience
that we can reach beyond mind and pass from its constructions
to the vastness and freedom of the supramental realities. There
alone can we touch the harmony of the divine powers that are
poorly mispresented to our mind or framed into a false figure
by the conflicting or wavering elements of the moral law. There
alone the unification of the transformed vital and physical and
the illumined mental man becomes possible in that supramental
Spirit which is at once the secret source and goal of our mind
and life and body. There alone is there any possibility of an
absolute justice, love and right — far other than that which we
imagine — at one with each other in the light of a supreme divine
knowledge. There alone can there be a reconciliation of the
conflict between our members.

   In other words there is, above society's external law and

man's moral law and beyond them, though feebly and ignorantly aimed at by something within them, a larger truth of a vast unbound consciousness, a law divine towards which both these blind and gross formulations are progressive faltering steps that try to escape from the natural law of the animal to a more exalted light or universal rule. That divine standard, since the godhead in us is our spirit moving towards its own concealed perfection, must be a supreme spiritual law and truth of our nature. Again, as we are embodied beings in the world with a common existence and nature and yet individual souls capable of direct touch with the Transcendent, this supreme truth of ourselves must have a double character. It must be a law and truth that discovers the perfect movement, harmony, rhythm of a great spiritualised collective life and determines perfectly our relations with each being and all beings in Nature's varied oneness. It must be at the same time a law and truth that discovers to us at each moment the rhythm and exact steps of the direct expression of the Divine in the soul, mind, life, body of the individual creature.[1] And we find in experience that this supreme light and force of action in its highest expression is at once an imperative law and an absolute freedom. It is an imperative law because it governs by immutable Truth our every inner and outer movement. And yet at each moment and in each movement the absolute freedom of the Supreme handles the perfect plasticity of our conscious and liberated nature.

The ethical idealist tries to discover this supreme law in his own moral data, in the inferior powers and factors that belong to the mental and ethical formula. And to sustain and organise them he selects a fundamental principle of conduct essentially unsound and constructed by the intellect — utility, hedonism, reason, intuitive conscience or any other generalised standard. All such efforts are foredoomed to failure. Our inner nature is the progressive expression of the eternal Spirit and too complex a power to be tied down by a single dominant mental or

---

[1] Therefore the Gita defines "dharma", an expression which means more than either religion or morality, as action controlled by our essential manner of self-being.

moral principle. Only the supramental consciousness can reveal to its differing and conflicting forces their spiritual truth and harmonise their divergences.

The later religions endeavour to fix the type of a supreme truth of conduct, erect a system and declare God's law through the mouth of Avatar or prophet. These systems, more powerful and dynamic than the dry ethical idea, are yet for the most part no more than idealistic glorifications of the moral principle sanctified by religious emotion and the label of a superhuman origin. Some, like the extreme Christian ethic, are rejected by Nature because they insist unworkably on an impracticable absolute rule. Others prove in the end to be evolutionary compromises and become obsolete in the march of Time. The true divine law, unlike these mental counterfeits, cannot be a system of rigid ethical determinations that press into their cast-iron moulds all our life-movements. The Law divine is truth of life and truth of the spirit and must take up with a free living plasticity and inspire with the direct touch of its eternal light each step of our action and all the complexity of our life issues. It must act not as a rule and formula but as an enveloping and penetrating conscious presence that determines all our thoughts, activities, feelings, impulsions of will by its infallible power and knowledge.

The older religions erected their rule of the wise, their dicta of Manu or Confucius, a complex Shastra in which they attempted to combine the social rule and moral law with the declaration of certain eternal principles of our highest nature in some kind of uniting amalgam. All three were treated on the same ground as equally the expression of everlasting verities, *sanātana dharma*. But two of these elements are evolutionary and valid for a time, mental constructions, human readings of the will of the Eternal; the third, attached and subdued to certain social and moral formulas, had to share the fortunes of its forms. Either the Shastra grows obsolete and has to be progressively changed or finally cast away or else it stands as a rigid barrier to the self-development of the individual and the race. The Shastra erects a collective and external standard; it ignores the inner nature of the individual, the indeterminable elements of a secret spiritual force within him. But the nature of the individual will not be ignored; its demand is inexorable. The unrestrained indulgence of his outer impulses leads to anarchy and dissolution, but the suppression and coercion of his soul's freedom by a fixed and mechanical rule spells stagnation or an inner death. Not this coercion or determination from outside, but the free discovery of his highest spirit and the truth of an eternal movement is the supreme thing that he has to discover.

The higher ethical law is discovered by the individual in his mind and will and psychic sense and then extended to the race. The supreme law also must be discovered by the individual in his spirit. Then only, through a spiritual influence and not by the mental idea, can it be extended to others. A moral law can be imposed as a rule or an ideal on numbers of men who have not attained that level of consciousness or that fineness of mind and will and psychic sense in which it can become a reality to them and a living force. As an ideal it can be revered without any need of practice. As a rule it can be observed in its outsides even if the inner sense is missed altogether. The supramental and spiritual life cannot be mechanised in this way, it cannot be turned into a mental ideal or an external rule. It has its own great lines, but these must be made real, must be the workings of an active Power felt in the individual's consciousness and the transcriptions of an eternal Truth powerful to transform mind, life and body. And because it is thus real, effective, imperative, the generalisation of the supramental consciousness and the spiritual life is the sole force that can lead to individual and collective perfection in earth's highest creatures. Only by our coming into constant touch with the divine Consciousness and its absolute Truth can some form of the conscious Divine, the dynamic Absolute, take up our earth-existence and transform its strife, stumbling, sufferings and falsities into an image of the supreme Light, Power and Ananda.

The culmination of the soul's constant touch with the Supreme is that self-giving which we call surrender to the divine Will and immergence of the separated ego in the One who is all. A vast universality of soul and an intense unity with all is the base and fixed condition of the supramental consciousness and spiritual life. In that universality and unity alone can we find the supreme law of the divine manifestation in the life of the embodied spirit; in that alone can we discover the supreme motion and right play of our individual nature. In that alone can all these lower discords resolve themselves into a victorious harmony of the true relations between manifested beings who are portions of the one Godhead and children of one universal Mother.

*
* *

All conduct and action are part of the movement of a Power, a Force infinite and divine in its origin and secret sense and will even though the forms of it we see seem inconscient or ignorant, material, vital, mental, finite, which is working to bring out progressively something of the Divine and Infinite in the obscurity of the individual and collective nature. This power is leading towards the Light, but still through the Ignorance. It leads man first through his needs and desires; it guides him next through enlarged needs and desires modified and enlightened by a mental and moral ideal. It is preparing to lead him to a spiritual realisation that overrides these things and yet fulfils and reconciles them in all that is divinely true in their spirit and purpose. It transforms the needs and desires into a divine Will and Ananda. It transforms the mental and moral aspiration into the powers of Truth and Perfection that are beyond them. It substitutes for the divided straining of the individual nature, for the passion and strife of the separate ego, the calm, profound, harmonious and happy law of the universalised person within us, the central being, the spirit that is a portion of the supreme Spirit. This true Person in us, because it is universal, does not seek its separate gratification but only asks in its outward expression in Nature its growth to its real stature, the expression of its inner divine self, that transcendent spiritual power and presence within it which is one with all and in sympathy with each thing and creature and with all the collective personalities and powers of the divine

existence, and yet it transcends them and is not bound by the
egoism of any creature or collectivity or limited by the ignorant
controls of their lower nature. This is the high realisation in front
of all our seeking and striving, and it gives the sure promise of
a perfect reconciliation and transmutation of all the elements
of our nature. A pure, total and flawless action is possible only
when that is effected and we have reached the height of this
secret Godhead within us.

The perfect supramental action will not follow any single
principle or limited rule. It is not likely to satisfy the standard
either of the individual egoist or of any organised group-mind.
It will conform to the demand neither of the positive practical
man of the world nor of the formal moralist nor of the pa-
triot nor of the sentimental philanthropist nor of the idealising
philosopher. It will proceed by a spontaneous outflowing from
the summits in the totality of an illumined and uplifted being,
will and knowledge and not by the selected, calculated and stan-
dardised action which is all that the intellectual reason or ethical
will can achieve. Its sole aim will be the expression of the divine
in us and the keeping together of the world and its progress
towards the Manifestation that is to be. This even will not be
so much an aim and purpose as a spontaneous law of the being
and an intuitive determination of the action by the Light of the
divine Truth and its automatic influence. It will proceed like the
action of Nature from a total will and knowledge behind her,
but a will and knowledge enlightened in a conscious supreme
Nature and no longer obscure in this ignorant Prakriti. It will
be an action not bound by the dualities but full and large in
the spirit's impartial joy of existence. The happy and inspired
movement of a divine Power and Wisdom guiding and impelling
us will replace the perplexities and stumblings of the suffering
and ignorant ego.

If by some miracle of divine intervention all mankind at
once could be raised to this level, we should have something on
earth like the Golden Age of the traditions, Satya Yuga, the Age
of Truth or true existence. For the sign of the Satya Yuga is that
the Law is spontaneous and conscious in each creature and does

its own works in a perfect harmony and freedom. Unity and universality, not separative division, would be the foundation of the consciousness of the race; love would be absolute; equality would be consistent with hierarchy and perfect in difference; absolute justice would be secured by the spontaneous action of the being in harmony with the truth of things and the truth of himself and others and therefore sure of true and right result; right reason, no longer mental but supramental, would be satisfied not by the observation of artificial standards but by the free automatic perception of right relations and their inevitable execution in the act. The quarrel between the individual and society or disastrous struggle between one community and another could not exist: the cosmic consciousness imbedded in embodied beings would assure a harmonious diversity in oneness.

In the actual state of humanity, it is the individual who must climb to this height as a pioneer and precursor. His isolation will necessarily give a determination and a form to his outward activities that must be quite other than those of a consciously divine collective action. The inner state, the root of his acts, will be the same; but the acts themselves may well be very different from what they would be on an earth liberated from ignorance. Nevertheless his consciousness and the divine mechanism of his conduct, if such a word can be used of so free a thing, would be such as has been described, free from that subjection to vital impurity and desire and wrong impulse which we call sin, unbound by that rule of prescribed moral formulas which we call virtue, spontaneously sure and pure and perfect in a greater consciousness than the mind's, governed in all its steps by the light and truth of the Spirit. But if a collectivity or group could be formed of those who had reached the supramental perfection, there indeed some divine creation could take shape; a new earth could descend that would be a new heaven, a world of supramental light could be created here amidst the receding darkness of this terrestrial ignorance.

Chapter VIII

The Supreme Will

IN THE light of this progressive manifestation of the Spirit, first apparently bound in the Ignorance, then free in the power and wisdom of the Infinite, we can better understand the great and crowning injunction of the Gita to the Karma-yogin, "Abandoning all dharmas, all principles and laws and rules of conduct, take refuge in me alone." All standards and rules are temporary constructions founded upon the needs of the ego in its transition from Matter to Spirit. These makeshifts have a relative imperativeness so long as we rest satisfied in the stages of transition, content with the physical and vital life, attached to the mental movement, or even fixed in the ranges of the mental plane that are touched by the spiritual lustres. But beyond is the unwalled wideness of a supramental infinite consciousness and there all temporary structures cease. It is not possible to enter utterly into the spiritual truth of the Eternal and Infinite if we have not the faith and courage to trust ourselves into the hands of the Lord of all things and the Friend of all creatures and leave utterly behind us our mental limits and measures. At one moment we must plunge without hesitation, reserve, fear or scruple into the ocean of the free, the infinite, the Absolute. After the Law, Liberty; after the personal, after the general, after the universal standards there is something greater, the impersonal plasticity, the divine freedom, the transcendent force and the supernal impulse. After the strait path of the ascent the wide plateaus on the summit.

There are three stages of the ascent, — at the bottom the bodily life enslaved to the pressure of necessity and desire, in the middle the mental, higher emotional and psychic rule that feels after greater interests, aspirations, experiences, at the summits first a deeper psychic and spiritual state and then a supramental eternal consciousness in which all our aspirations and seekings discover their own intimate significance. In the bodily life first desire and need and then the practical good of the individual and the society are the governing consideration, the dominant force. In the mental life ideas and ideals rule, ideas that are half-lights wearing the garb of Truth, ideals formed by the mind as a result of a growing but still imperfect intuition and experience. Whenever the mental life prevails and the bodily diminishes its brute insistence, man the mental being feels pushed by the urge of mental Nature to mould in the sense of the idea or the ideal the life of the individual, and in the end even the vaguer more complex life of the society is forced to undergo this subtle process. In the spiritual life, or when a higher power than Mind has manifested and taken possession of the nature, these limited motive-forces recede, dwindle, tend to disappear. The spiritual or supramental Self, the Divine Being, the supreme and immanent Reality, must be alone the Lord within us and shape freely our final development according to the highest, widest, most integral expression possible of the law of our nature. In the end that nature acts in the perfect Truth and its spontaneous freedom; for it obeys only the luminous power of the Eternal. The individual has nothing further to gain, no desire to fulfil; he has become a portion of the impersonality or the universal personality of the Eternal. No other object than the manifestation and play of the Divine Spirit in life and the maintenance and conduct of the world in its march towards the divine goal can move him to action. Mental ideas, opinions, constructions are his no more; for his mind has fallen into silence, it is only a channel for the Light and Truth of the divine knowledge. Ideals are too narrow for the vastness of his spirit; it is the ocean of the Infinite that flows through him and moves him for ever.

*
* *

Whoever sincerely enters the path of works, must leave behind him the stage in which need and desire are the first law of our acts. For whatever desires still trouble his being, he must, if he accepts the high aim of Yoga, put them away from him into the hands of the Lord within us. The supreme Power will deal with them for the good of the sadhaka and for the good of all. In effect, we find that once this surrender is done, — always provided the rejection is sincere, — egoistic indulgence of desire may for some time recur under the continued impulse of past nature but only in order to exhaust its acquired momentum and to teach the embodied being in his most unteachable part, his nervous, vital, emotional nature, by the reactions of desire, by its grief and unrest bitterly contrasted with calm periods of the higher peace or marvellous movements of divine Ananda, that egoistic desire is not a law for the soul that seeks liberation or aspires to its own original god-nature. Afterwards the element of desire in those impulsions will be thrown away or persistently eliminated by a constant denying and transforming pressure. Only the pure force of action in them (*pravṛtti*) justified by an equal delight in all work and result that is inspired or imposed from above will be preserved in the happy harmony of a final perfection. To act, to enjoy is the normal law and right of the nervous being; but to choose by personal desire its action and enjoyment is only its ignorant will, not its right. Alone the supreme and universal Will must choose; action must change into a dynamic movement of that Will; enjoyment must be replaced by the play of a pure spiritual Ananda. All personal will is either a temporary delegation from on high or a usurpation by the ignorant Asura.

The social law, that second term of our progress, is a means to which the ego is subjected in order that it may learn discipline by subordination to a wider collective ego. This law may be quite empty of any moral content and may express only the needs or the practical good of the society as each society conceives it. Or it may express those needs and that good, but modified and coloured and supplemented by a higher moral or ideal law. It is binding on the developing but not yet perfectly developed individual in the shape of social duty, family obligation, communal or national demand, so long as it is not in conflict with his growing sense of the higher Right. But the sadhaka of the Karmayoga will abandon this also to the Lord of works. After he has made this surrender, his social impulses and judgments will, like his desires, only be used for their exhaustion or, it may be, so far as they are still necessary for a time to enable him to identify his lower mental nature with mankind in general or with any grouping of mankind in its works and hopes and aspirations. But after that brief time is over, they will be withdrawn and a divine government will alone abide. He will be identified with the Divine and with others only through the divine consciousness and not through the mental nature.

For, even after he is free, the sadhaka will be in the world and to be in the world is to remain in works. But to remain in works without desire is to act for the good of the world in general or for the kind or the race or for some new creation to be evolved on the earth or some work imposed by the Divine Will within him. And this must be done either in the framework provided by the environment or the grouping in which he is born or placed or else in one which is chosen or created for him by a divine direction. Therefore in our perfection there must be nothing left in the mental being which conflicts with or prevents our sympathy and free self-identification with the kind, the group or whatever collective expression of the Divine he is meant to lead, help or serve. But in the end it must become a free self-identification through identity with the Divine and not a mental bond or moral tie of union or a vital association dominated by any kind of personal, social, national, communal or credal egoism. If any social law is obeyed, it will not be from physical necessity or from the sense of personal or general interest or for expediency or because of the pressure of the environment or from any sense of duty, but solely for the sake of the Lord of works and because it is felt or known to be the Divine Will that the social law or rule or relation as it stands can still be kept as a figure of the inner life and the minds of men must not be disturbed by its infringement. If, on the other hand, the social law, rule or relation is disregarded, that too will not be for the indulgence of desire, personal will or personal opinion, but because a greater rule is felt that expresses the law of the Spirit or because it is known that there must be in the march of the divine All-Will a movement towards the changing, exceeding or abolition of existing laws and forms for the sake of a freer larger life necessary to the world's progress.

There is still left the moral law or the ideal and these, even to many who think themselves free, appear for ever sacred and intangible. But the sadhaka, his gaze turned always to the heights, will abandon them to Him whom all ideals seek imperfectly and fragmentarily to express; all moral qualities are only a poor and rigid travesty of his spontaneous and illimitable perfection. The bondage to sin and evil passes away with the passing of nervous desire; for it belongs to the quality of vital passion, impulsion or drive of propensity in us (*rajoguṇa*) and is extinguished with the transformation of that mode of Nature. But neither must the aspirant remain subject to the gilded or golden chain of a conventional or a habitual or a mentally ordered or even a high or clear sattwic virtue. That will be replaced by something profounder and more essential than the minor inadequate thing that men call virtue. The original sense of the word was manhood and this is a much larger and deeper thing than the moral mind and its structures. The culmination of Karmayoga is a yet higher and deeper state that may perhaps be called "soulhood", — for the soul is greater than the man; a free soulhood spontaneously welling out in works of a supreme Truth and Love will replace human virtue. But this supreme Truth cannot be forced to inhabit the petty edifices of the practical reason or even confined in the more dignified constructions of the larger ideative reason that imposes its representations as if they were pure truth on the limited human intelligence. This supreme Love will not necessarily be consistent, much less will it be synonymous, with the partial and feeble, ignorant and emotion-ridden movements of human attraction, sympathy and pity. The petty law cannot bind the vaster movement; the mind's partial attainment cannot dictate its terms to the soul's supreme fulfilment.

At first, the higher Love and Truth will fulfil its movement in the sadhaka according to the essential law or way of his own nature. For that is the special aspect of the divine Nature, the particular power of the supreme Shakti, out of which his soul has emerged into the Play, not limited indeed by the forms of this law or way, for the soul is infinite. But still its stuff of nature bears that stamp, evolves fluently along those lines or turns around the spiral curves of that dominating influence. He will manifest the divine Truth-movement according to the temperament of the sage or the lion-like fighter or the lover and enjoyer or the worker and servant or in any combination of essential attributes (gunas) that may constitute the form given to his being by its own inner urge. It is this self-nature playing freely in his acts which men will see in him and not a conduct cut, chalked out, artificially regulated, by any lesser rule or by any law from outside.

But there is a yet higher attainment, there is an infinity (*ānantya*) in which even this last limitation is exceeded, because the nature is utterly fulfilled and its boundaries vanish. There the soul lives without any boundaries; for it uses all forms and moulds according to the divine Will in it, but it is not restrained, it is not tied down, it is not imprisoned in any power or form that it uses. This is the summit of the path of works and this the utter liberty of the soul in its actions. In reality, it has there no actions; for all its activities are a rhythm of the Supreme and sovereignly proceed from That alone like a spontaneous music out of the Infinite.

*
* *

The total surrender, then, of all our actions to a supreme and universal Will, an unconditioned and standardless surrender of all works to the government of something eternal within us which will replace the ordinary working of the ego-nature, is the way and end of Karmayoga. But what is this divine supreme Will and how can it be recognised by our deluded instruments and our blind prisoned intelligence?

Ordinarily, we conceive of ourselves as a separate "I" in the universe that governs a separate body and mental and moral nature, chooses in full liberty its own self-determined actions and is independent and therefore sole master of its works and responsible. It is not easy for the ordinary mind, the mind that has not thought nor looked deeply into its own constitution and constituents, it is difficult even for minds that have thought but have no spiritual vision and experience, to imagine how there can be anything else in us truer, deeper and more powerful than this apparent "I" and its empire. But the very first step towards self-knowledge as towards the true knowledge of phenomena is to get behind the apparent truth of things and find the real but masked, essential and dynamic truth which their appearances cover.

This ego or "I" is not a lasting truth, much less our essential part; it is only a formation of Nature, a mental form of thought-centralisation in the perceiving and discriminating mind, a vital form of the centralisation of feeling and sensation in our parts of life, a form of physical conscious reception centralising substance and function of substance in our bodies. All that we internally are is not ego, but consciousness, soul or spirit. All that we externally and superficially are and do is not ego but Nature. An executive cosmic force shapes us and dictates through our temperament and environment and mentality so shaped, through our individualised formulation of the cosmic energies, our actions and their results. Truly, we do not think, will or act but thought occurs in us, will occurs in us, impulse and act occur in us; our ego-sense gathers around itself, refers to itself all this flow of natural activities. It is cosmic Force, it is Nature that forms the thought, imposes the will, imparts the impulse. Our body, mind and ego are a wave of that sea of force in action and do not govern it, but by it are governed and directed. The sadhaka in his progress towards truth and self-knowledge must come to a point where the soul opens its eyes of vision and recognises this truth of ego and this truth of works. He gives up the idea of a mental, vital, physical "I" that acts or governs action; he recognises that Prakriti, Force of cosmic nature following her fixed modes, is the one and only worker in him and in all things and creatures.

But what has fixed the modes of Nature? Or who has originated and governs the movements of Force? There is a Consciousness — or a Conscient — behind that is the lord, witness, knower, enjoyer, upholder and source of sanction for her works;

this consciousness is Soul or Purusha. Prakriti shapes the action in us; Purusha in her or behind her witnesses, assents, bears and upholds it. Prakriti forms the thought in our minds; Purusha in her or behind her knows the thought and the truth in it. Prakriti determines the result of the action; Purusha in her or behind her enjoys or suffers the consequence. Prakriti forms mind and body, labours over them, develops them; Purusha upholds the formation and evolution and sanctions each step of her works. Prakriti applies the Will-force which works in things and men; Purusha sets that Will-force to work by his vision of that which should be done. This Purusha is not the surface ego, but a silent Self, a source of Power, an originator and receiver of Knowledge behind the ego. Our mental "I" is only a false reflection of this Self, this Power, this Knowledge. This Purusha or supporting Consciousness is therefore the cause, recipient and support of all Nature's works, but he is not himself the doer. Prakriti, Nature-Force, in front and Shakti, Conscious-Force, Soul-Force behind her, — for these two are the inner and outer faces of the universal Mother, — account for all that is done in the universe. The universal Mother, Prakriti-Shakti, is the one and only worker.

Purusha-Prakriti, Consciousness-Force, Soul supporting Nature, — for the two even in their separation are one and inseparable, — are at once a universal and a transcendent Power. But there is something in the individual too which is not the mental ego, something that is one in essence with this greater reality: it is a pure reflection or portion of the one Purusha; it is the Soul Person or the embodied being, the individual self, Jivatman; it is the Self that seems to limit its power and knowledge so as to support an individual play of transcendent and universal Nature. In deepest reality the infinitely One is also infinitely multiple; we are not only a reflection or portion of That but we are That; our spiritual individuality — unlike our ego — does not preclude our universality and transcendence. But at present the soul or self in us intent on individualisation in Nature allows itself to be confused with the idea of the ego; it has to get rid of this ignorance, it has to know itself as a reflection or portion or being of the supreme and universal Self and solely a centre of its consciousness in the world-action. But this Jiva Purusha too is not the doer of works any more than the ego or the supporting consciousness of the Witness and Knower. Again and always it is the transcendent and universal Shakti who is the sole doer. But behind her is the one Supreme who manifests through her as the dual power, Purusha-Prakriti, Ishwara-Shakti.[1] The Supreme becomes dynamic as the Shakti and is by her the sole originator and Master of works in the universe.

* * *

If this is the truth of works, the first thing the sadhaka has to do is to recoil from the egoistic forms of activity and get rid of the sense of an "I" that acts. He has to see and feel that everything happens in him by the plastic conscious or subconscious or sometimes superconscious automatism of his mental and bodily instruments moved by the forces of spiritual, mental, vital and physical Nature. There is a personality on his surface that chooses and wills, submits and struggles, tries to make good in Nature or prevail over Nature, but this personality is itself a construction of Nature and so dominated, driven, determined by her that it cannot be free. It is a formation or expression of the Self in her, — it is a self of Nature rather than a self of Self, his natural and processive, not his spiritual and permanent being, a temporary constructed personality, not the

---

[1] Ishwara-Shakti is not quite the same as Purusha-Prakriti; for Purusha and Prakriti are separate powers, but Ishwara and Shakti contain each other. Ishwara is Purusha who contains Prakriti and rules by the power of the Shakti within him. Shakti is Prakriti ensouled by Purusha and acts by the will of the Ishwara which is her own will and whose presence in her movement she carries always with her. The Purusha-Prakriti realisation is of the first utility to the seeker on the Way of Works; for it is the separation of the conscient being and the Energy and the subjection of the being to the mechanism of the Energy that are the efficient cause of our ignorance and imperfection; by this realisation the being can liberate himself from the mechanical action of the nature and become free and arrive at a first spiritual control over the nature. Ishwara-Shakti stands behind the relation of Purusha-Prakriti and its ignorant action and turns it to an evolutionary purpose. The Ishwara-Shakti realisation can bring participation in a higher dynamism and a divine working and a total unity and harmony of the being in a spiritual nature.

true immortal Person. It is that Person that he must become. He must succeed in being inwardly quiescent, detach himself as the observer from the outer active personality and learn the play of the cosmic forces in him by standing back from all blinding absorption in its turns and movements. Thus calm, detached, a student of himself and a witness of his nature, he realises that he is the individual soul who observes the works of Nature, accepts tranquilly her results and sanctions or withholds his sanction from the impulse to her acts. At present this soul or Purusha is little more than an acquiescent spectator, influencing perhaps the action and development of the being by the pressure of its veiled consciousness, but for the most part delegating its powers or a fragment of them to the outer personality, — in fact to Nature, for this outer self is not lord but subject to her, *aniśa*; but, once unveiled, it can make its sanction or refusal effective, become the master of the action, dictate sovereignly a change of Nature. Even if for a long time, as the result of fixed association and past storage of energy, the habitual movement takes place independent of the Purusha's assent and even if the sanctioned movement is persistently refused by Nature for want of past habit, still he will discover that in the end his assent or refusal prevails, — slowly with much resistance or quickly with a rapid accommodation of her means and tendencies she modifies herself and her workings in the direction indicated by his inner sight or volition. Thus he learns in place of mental control or egoistic will an inner spiritual control which makes him master of the Nature-forces that work in him and not their unconscious instrument or mechanic slave. Above and around him is the Shakti, the universal Mother and from her he can get all his inmost soul needs and wills if only he has a true knowledge of her ways and a true surrender to the divine Will in her. Finally, he becomes aware of that highest dynamic Self within him and within Nature which is the source of all his seeing and knowing, the source of the sanction, the source of the acceptance, the source of the rejection. This is the Lord, the Supreme, the One-in-all, Ishwara-Shakti, of whom his soul is a portion, a being of that Being and a power of that Power. The rest of our progress depends on our knowledge of the ways in which the Lord of works manifests his Will in the world and in us and executes them through the transcendent and universal Shakti.

The Lord sees in his omniscience the thing that has to be done. This seeing is his Will, it is a form of creative Power, and that which he sees the all-conscious Mother, one with him, takes into her dynamic self and embodies, and executive Nature-Force carries it out as the mechanism of their omnipotent omniscience. But this vision of what is to be and therefore of what is to be done arises out of the very being, pours directly out of the consciousness and delight of existence of the Lord, spontaneously, like light from the Sun. It is not our mortal attempt to see, our difficult arrival at truth of action and motive or just demand of Nature. When the individual soul is entirely at one in its being and knowledge with the Lord and directly in touch with the original Shakti, the transcendent Mother, the supreme Will can then arise in us too in the high divine manner as a thing that must be and is achieved by the spontaneous action of Nature. There is then no desire, no responsibility, no reaction; all takes place in the peace, calm, light, power of the supporting and enveloping and inhabiting Divine.

But even before that highest approach to identity is achieved, something of the supreme Will can manifest in us as an imperative impulsion, a God-driven action; we then act by a spontaneous self-determining Force but a fuller knowledge of meaning and aim arises only afterwards. Or the impulse to action may come as an inspiration or intuition, but rather in the heart and body than in the mind; here an effective sight enters in but the complete and exact knowledge is still deferred and comes, if at all, later. But the divine Will may descend too as a luminous single command or a total perception or a continuous current of perception of what is to be done into the will or into the thought or as a direction from above spontaneously fulfilled by the lower members. When the Yoga is imperfect, only some actions can be done in this way, or else a general action may so proceed but only during periods of exaltation and illumination. When the

Yoga is perfect, all action becomes of this character. We may indeed distinguish three stages of a growing progress by which, first, the personal will is occasionally or frequently enlightened or moved by a supreme Will or conscious Force beyond it, then constantly replaced and, last, identified and merged in that divine Power-action. The first is the stage when we are still governed by the intellect, heart and senses; these have to seek or wait for the divine inspiration and guidance and do not always find or receive it. The second is the stage when human intelligence is more and more replaced by a high illumined or intuitive spiritualised mind, the external human heart by the inner psychic heart, the senses by a purified and selfless vital force. The third is the stage when we rise even above spiritualised mind to the supramental levels.

In all three stages the fundamental character of the liberated action is the same, a spontaneous working of Prakriti no longer through or for the ego but at the will and for the enjoyment of the supreme Purusha. At a higher level this becomes the Truth of the absolute and universal Supreme expressed through the individual soul and worked out consciously through the nature, — no longer through a half-perception and a diminished or distorted effectuation by the stumbling, ignorant and all-deforming energy of lower nature in us but by the all-wise transcendent and universal Mother.

The Lord has veiled himself and his absolute wisdom and eternal consciousness in ignorant Nature-Force and suffers her to drive the individual being, with its complicity, as the ego; this lower action of Nature continues to prevail, often even in spite of man's half-lit imperfect efforts at a nobler motive and a purer self-knowledge. Our human effort at perfection fails, or progresses very incompletely, owing to the force of Nature's past actions in us, her past formations, her long-rooted associations; it turns towards a true and high-climbing success only when a greater Knowledge and Power than our own breaks through the lid of our ignorance and guides or takes up our personal will. For our human will is a misled and wandering ray that has parted from the supreme Puissance. The period of slow emergence out of this lower working into a higher light and purer force is the valley of the shadow of death for the striver after perfection; it is a dreadful passage full of trials, sufferings, sorrows, obscurations, stumblings, errors, pitfalls. To abridge and alleviate this ordeal or to penetrate it with the divine delight faith is necessary, an increasing surrender of the mind to the knowledge that imposes itself from within and, above all, a true aspiration and a right and unfaltering and sincere practice. "Practise unfalteringly," says the Gita, "with a heart free from despondency," the Yoga; for even though in the earlier stage of the path we drink deep of the bitter poison of internal discord and suffering, the last taste of this cup is the sweetness of the nectar of immortality and the honey-wine of an eternal Ananda.

Chapter IX

Equality and the Annihilation of Ego

AN ENTIRE self-consecration, a complete equality, an unsparing effacement of the ego, a transforming deliverance of the nature from its ignorant modes of action are the steps by which the surrender of all the being and nature to the Divine Will can be prepared and achieved, — a self-giving true, total and without reserve. The first necessity is an entire spirit of self-consecration in our works; it must become first the constant will, then the ingrained need in all the being, finally its automatic but living and conscious habit, the self-existent turn to do all action as a sacrifice to the Supreme and to the veiled Power present in us and in all beings and in all the workings of the universe. Life is the altar of this sacrifice, works are our offering; a transcendent and universal Power and Presence as yet rather felt or glimpsed than known or seen by us is the Deity to whom they are offered. This sacrifice, this self-consecration has two sides to it; there is the work itself and there is the spirit in which it is done, the spirit of worship to the Master of Works in all that we see, think and experience.

The work itself is at first determined by the best light we can command in our ignorance. It is that which we conceive as the thing that should be done. And whether it be shaped by our sense of duty, by our feeling for our fellow-creatures, by our idea of what is for the good of others or the good of the world or by the direction of one whom we accept as a human Master, wiser than ourselves and for us the representative of that Lord of all works in whom we believe but whom we do not yet know, the principle is the same. The essential of the sacrifice of works must be there and the essential is the surrender of all desire for the fruit of our works, the renunciation of all attachment to the result for which yet we labour. For so long as we work with attachment to the result, the sacrifice is offered not to the Divine, but to our ego.

We may think otherwise, but we are deceiving ourselves; we are making our idea of the Divine, our sense of duty, our feeling for our fellow-creatures, our idea of what is good for the world or others, even our obedience to the Master a mask for our egoistic satisfactions and preferences and a specious shield against the demand made on us to root all desire out of our nature.

At this stage of the Yoga and even throughout the Yoga this form of desire, this figure of the ego is the enemy against whom we have to be always on our guard with an unsleeping vigilance. We need not be discouraged when we find him lurking within us and assuming all sorts of disguises, but we should be vigilant to detect him in all his masks and inexorable in expelling his influence. The illumining Word of this movement is the decisive line of the Gita, "To action thou hast a right but never under any circumstances to its fruit." The fruit belongs solely to the Lord of all works; our only business with it is to prepare success by a true and careful action and to offer it, if it comes, to the divine Master. Afterwards even as we have renounced attachment to the fruit, we must renounce attachment to the work also; at any moment we must be prepared to change one work, one course or one field of action for another or abandon all works if that is the clear command of the Master. Otherwise we do the act not for his sake but for our satisfaction and pleasure in the work, from the kinetic nature's need of action or for the fulfilment of our propensities; but these are all stations and refuges of the ego. However necessary for our ordinary motion of life, they have to be abandoned in the growth of the spiritual consciousness and replaced by divine counterparts: an Ananda, an impersonal and God-directed delight will cast out or supplant the unillumined vital satisfaction and pleasure, a joyful driving of the Divine Energy the kinetic need; the fulfilment of the propensities will no longer be an object or a necessity, there will be instead the fulfilment of the Divine Will through the natural dynamic truth in action of a free soul and a luminous nature. In the end, as the attachment to the fruit of the work and to the work itself has been excised from the heart, so also the last clinging attachment to the idea and sense of ourselves as the doer has to be relinquished; the Divine Shakti must be known and felt above and within us as the true and sole worker.

* *
*

The renunciation of attachment to the work and its fruit is the beginning of a wide movement towards an absolute equality in the mind and soul which must become all-enveloping if we are to be perfect in the spirit. For the worship of the Master of works demands a clear recognition and glad acknowledgment of him in ourselves, in all things and in all happenings. Equality is the sign of this adoration; it is the soul's ground on which true sacrifice and worship can be done. The Lord is there equally in all beings, we have to make no essential distinctions between ourselves and others, the wise and the ignorant, friend and enemy, man and animal, the saint and the sinner. We must hate none, despise none, be repelled by none; for in all we have to see the One disguised or manifested at his pleasure. He is a little revealed in one or more revealed in another or concealed and wholly distorted in others according to his will and his knowledge of what is best for that which he intends to become in form in them and to do in works in their nature. All is ourself, one self that has taken many shapes. Hatred and disliking and scorn and repulsion, clinging and attachment and preference are natural, necessary, inevitable at a certain stage: they attend upon or they help to make and maintain Nature's choice in us. But to the Karmayogin they are a survival, a stumbling-block, a process of the Ignorance and, as he progresses, they fall away from his nature. The child-soul needs them for its growth; but they drop from an adult in the divine culture. In the God-nature to which we have to rise there can be an adamantine, even a destructive severity but not hatred, a divine irony but not scorn, a calm, clear-seeing and forceful rejection but not repulsion and dislike. Even what we have to destroy, we must not abhor or fail to recognise as a disguised and temporary movement of the Eternal.

And since all things are the one Self in its manifestation, we shall have equality of soul towards the ugly and the beautiful, the maimed and the perfect, the noble and the vulgar, the pleasant and the unpleasant, the good and the evil. Here also there will be no hatred, scorn and repulsion, but instead the equal eye that sees all things in their real character and their appointed place. For we shall know that all things express or disguise, develop or distort, as best they can or with whatever defect they must, under the circumstances intended for them, in the way possible to the immediate status or function or evolution of their nature, some truth or fact, some energy or potential of the Divine necessary by its presence in the progressive manifestation both to the whole of the present sum of things and for the perfection of the ultimate result. That truth is what we must seek and discover behind the transitory expression; undeterred by appearances, by the deficiencies or the disfigurements of the expression, we can then worship the Divine for ever unsullied, pure, beautiful and perfect behind his masks. All indeed has to be changed, not ugliness accepted but divine beauty, not imperfection taken as our resting-place but perfection striven after, the supreme good made the universal aim and not evil. But what we do has to be done with a spiritual understanding and knowledge, and it is a divine good, beauty, perfection, pleasure that has to be followed after, not the human standards of these things. If we have not equality, it is a sign that we are still pursued by the Ignorance, we shall truly understand nothing and it is more than likely that we shall destroy the old imperfection only to create another: for we are substituting the appreciations of our human mind and desire-soul for the divine values.

Equality does not mean a fresh ignorance or blindness; it does not call for and need not initiate a greyness of vision and a blotting out of all hues. Difference is there, variation of expression is there and this variation we shall appreciate, — far more justly than we could when the eye was clouded by a partial and erring love and hate, admiration and scorn, sympathy and antipathy, attraction and repulsion. But behind the variation we shall always see the Complete and Immutable who dwells within it and we shall feel, know or at least, if it is hidden from us, trust in the wise purpose and divine necessity of the particular manifestation, whether it appear to our human standards harmonious and perfect or crude and unfinished or even false and evil.

And so too we shall have the same equality of mind and soul towards all happenings, painful or pleasurable, defeat and success, honour and disgrace, good repute and ill-repute, good fortune and evil fortune. For in all happenings we shall see the will of the Master of all works and results and a step in the evolving expression of the Divine. He manifests himself, to those who have the inner eye that sees, in forces and their play and results as well as in things and in creatures. All things move towards a divine event; each experience, suffering and want no less than joy and satisfaction, is a necessary link in the carrying out of a universal movement which it is our business to understand and second. To revolt, to condemn, to cry out is the impulse of our unchastened and ignorant instincts. Revolt like everything else has its uses in the play and is even necessary, helpful, decreed for the divine development in its own time and stage; but the movement of an ignorant rebellion belongs to the stage of the soul's childhood or to its raw adolescence. The ripened soul does not condemn but seeks to understand and master, does not cry out but accepts or toils to improve and perfect, does not revolt inwardly but labours to obey and fulfil and transfigure. Therefore we shall receive all things with an equal soul from the hands of the Master. Failure we shall admit as a passage as calmly as success until the hour of the divine victory arrives. Our souls and minds and bodies will remain unshaken by acutest sorrow and suffering and pain if in the divine dispensation they come to us, unoverpowered by intensest joy and pleasure. Thus supremely balanced we shall continue steadily on our way meeting all things with an equal calm until we are ready for a more exalted status and can enter into the supreme and universal Ananda.

*
* *

This equality cannot come except by a protracted ordeal and patient self-discipline; so long as desire is strong, equality cannot come at all except in periods of quiescence and the fatigue of desire, and it is then more likely to be an inert indifference or desire's recoil from itself than the true calm and the positive spiritual oneness. Moreover, this discipline or this growth into equality of spirit has its necessary epochs and stages. Ordinarily we have to begin with a period of endurance; for we must learn to confront, to suffer and to assimilate all contacts. Each fibre in us must be taught not to wince away from that which pains and repels and not to run eagerly towards that which pleases and attracts, but rather to accept, to face, to bear and to conquer. All touches we must be strong to bear, not only those that are proper and personal to us but those born of our sympathy or our conflict with the worlds around, above or below us and with their peoples. We shall endure tranquilly the action and impact on us of men and things and forces, the pressure of the Gods and the assaults of Titans; we shall face and engulf in the unstirred seas of our spirit all that can possibly come to us down the ways of the soul's infinite experience. This is the stoical period of the preparation of equality, its most elementary and yet its heroic age. But this steadfast endurance of the flesh and heart and mind must be reinforced by a sustained sense of spiritual submission to a divine Will: this living clay must yield not only with a stern or courageous acquiescence, but with knowledge or with resignation, even in suffering, to the touch of the divine Hand that is preparing its perfection. A sage, a devout or even a tender stoicism of the God-lover is possible, and these are better than the merely pagan self-reliant endurance which may lend itself to a too great hardening of the vessel of God: for this kind prepares the strength that is capable of wisdom and of love; its tranquillity is a deeply moved calm that passes easily into bliss. The gain of this period of resignation and endurance is the soul's strength equal to all shocks and contacts.

There is next a period of high-seated impartiality and indifference in which the soul becomes free from exultation and depression and escapes from the snare of the eagerness of joy as from the dark net of the pangs of grief and suffering. All things and persons and forces, all thoughts and feelings and sensations and actions, one's own no less than those of others, are regarded from above by a spirit that remains intact and immutable and is not disturbed by these things. This is the philosophic period of the preparation of equality, a wide and august movement. But indifference must not settle into an inert turning away from action and experience; it must not be an aversion born of weariness, disgust and distaste, a recoil of disappointed or satiated desire, the sullenness of a baffled and dissatisfied egoism forced back from its passionate aims. These recoils come inevitably in the unripe soul and may in some way help the progress by a discouragement of the eager desire-driven vital nature, but they are not the perfection towards which we labour. The indifference or the impartiality that we must seek after is a calm superiority of the high-seated soul above the contacts of things;[1] it regards and accepts or rejects them but is not moved in the rejection and is not subjected by the acceptance. It begins to feel itself near, kin to, one with a silent Self and Spirit self-existent and separate from the workings of Nature which it supports and makes possible, part of or merged in the motionless calm Reality that transcends the motion and action of the universe. The gain of this period of high transcendence is the soul's peace unrocked and unshaken by the pleasant ripplings or by the tempestuous waves and billows of the world's movement.

If we can pass through these two stages of the inner change without being arrested or fixed in either, we are admitted to a greater divine equality which is capable of a spiritual ardour and tranquil passion of delight, a rapturous, all-understanding and all-possessing equality of the perfected soul, an intense and even wideness and fullness of its being embracing all things. This is the supreme period and the passage to it is through the joy of a total self-giving to the Divine and to the universal Mother. For strength is then crowned by a happy mastery, peace deepens into bliss, the possession of the divine calm is uplifted

---

[1] *udāsīna.*

and made the ground for the possession of the divine movement.
But if this greater perfection is to arrive, the soul's impartial
high-seatedness looking down from above on the flux of forms
and personalities and movements and forces must be modified
and change into a new sense of strong and calm submission
and a powerful and intense surrender. This submission will be
no longer a resigned acquiescence but a glad acceptance: for
there will be no sense of suffering or of the bearing of a burden
or cross; love and delight and the joy of self-giving will be its
brilliant texture. And this surrender will be not only to a divine
Will which we perceive and accept and obey, but to a divine
Wisdom in the Will which we recognise and a divine Love in it
which we feel and rapturously suffer, the wisdom and love of a
supreme Spirit and Self of ourselves and all with which we can
achieve a happy and perfect unity. A lonely power, peace and
stillness is the last word of the philosophic equality of the sage;
but the soul in its integral experience liberates itself from this
self-created status and enters into the sea of a supreme and all-
embracing ecstasy of the beginningless and endless beatitude of
the Eternal. Then we are at last capable of receiving all contacts
with a blissful equality, because we feel in them the touch of
the imperishable Love and Delight, the happiness absolute that
hides ever in the heart of things. The gain of this culmination
in a universal and equal rapture is the soul's delight and the
opening gates of the Bliss that is infinite, the Joy that surpasses
all understanding.

*
* *

Before this labour for the annihilation of desire and the conquest
of the soul's equality can come to its absolute perfection and
fruition, that turn of the spiritual movement must have been
completed which leads to the abolition of the sense of ego. But
for the worker the renunciation of the egoism of action is the
most important element in this change. For even when by giving
up the fruits and the desire of the fruits to the Master of the
Sacrifice we have parted with the egoism of rajasic desire, we

may still have kept the egoism of the worker. Still we are subject to the sense that we are ourselves the doer of the act, ourselves its source and ourselves the giver of the sanction. It is still the "I" that chooses and determines, it is still the "I" that undertakes the responsibility and feels the demerit or the merit.

An entire removal of this separative ego-sense is an essential aim of our Yoga. If any ego is to remain in us for a while, it is only a form of it which knows itself to be a form and is ready to disappear as soon as a true centre of consciousness is manifested or built in us. That true centre is a luminous formulation of the one Consciousness and a pure channel and instrument of the one Existence. A support for the individual manifestation and action of the universal Force, it gradually reveals behind it the true Person in us, the central eternal being, an everlasting being of the Supreme, a power and portion of the transcendent Shakti.[2]

Here too, in this movement by which the soul divests itself gradually of the obscure robe of the ego, there is a progress by marked stages. For not only the fruit of works belongs to the Lord alone, but our works also must be his; he is the true lord of our actions no less than of our results. This we must not see with the thinking mind only, it must become entirely true to our entire consciousness and will. The sadhaka has not only to think and know but to see and feel concretely and intensely even in the moment of the working and in its initiation and whole process that his works are not his at all, but are coming through him from the Supreme Existence. He must be always aware of a Force, a Presence, a Will that acts through his individual nature. But there is in taking this turn the danger that he may confuse his own disguised or sublimated ego or an inferior power with the Lord and substitute its demands for the supreme dictates. He may fall into a common ambush of this lower nature and distort his supposed surrender to a higher Power into an excuse for a magnified and uncontrolled indulgence of his own self-will and even of his desires and passions. A great sincerity is asked for and has to be imposed not only on the conscious mind but

---

[2] *aṁśaḥ sanātanaḥ, parā prakṛtir jīvabhūtā.*

still more on the subliminal part of us which is full of hidden movements. For there is there, especially in our subliminal vital nature, an incorrigible charlatan and actor. The sadhaka must first have advanced far in the elimination of desire and in the firm equality of his soul towards all workings and all happenings before he can utterly lay down the burden of his works on the Divine. At every moment he must proceed with a vigilant eye upon the deceits of the ego and the ambushes of the misleading Powers of Darkness who ever represent themselves as the one Source of Light and Truth and take on them a simulacrum of divine forms in order to capture the soul of the seeker.

Immediately he must take the further step of relegating himself to the position of the Witness. Aloof from the Prakriti, impersonal and dispassionate, he must watch the executive Nature-Force at work within him and understand its action; he must learn by this separation to recognise the play of her universal forces, distinguish her interweaving of light and night, the divine and the undivine, and detect her formidable Powers and Beings that use the ignorant human creature. Nature works in us, says the Gita, through the triple quality of Prakriti, the quality of light and good, the quality of passion and desire and the quality of obscurity and inertia. The seeker must learn to distinguish, as an impartial and discerning witness of all that proceeds within this kingdom of his nature, the separate and the combined action of these qualities; he must pursue the workings of the cosmic forces in him through all the labyrinth of their subtle unseen processes and disguises and know every intricacy of the maze. As he proceeds in this knowledge, he will be able to become the giver of the sanction and no longer remain an ignorant tool of Nature. At first he must induce the Nature-Force in its action on his instruments to subdue the working of its two lower qualities and bring them into subjection to the quality of light and good and, afterwards, he must persuade that again to offer itself so that all three may be transformed by a higher Power into their divine equivalents, supreme repose and calm, divine illumination and bliss, the eternal divine dynamis, Tapas. The first part of this discipline and change can be firmly done in principle by the will of the mental being in us; but its full execution and the subsequent transformation can be done only when the deeper psychic soul increases its hold on the nature and replaces the mental being as its ruler. When this happens, he will be ready to make, not only with an aspiration and intention and an initial and progressive self-abandonment but with the most intense actuality of dynamic self-giving, the complete renunciation of his works to the Supreme Will. By degrees his mind of an imperfect human intelligence will be replaced by a spiritual and illumined mind and that can in the end enter into the supramental Truth-Light; he will then no longer act from his nature of the Ignorance with its three modes of confused and imperfect activity, but from a diviner nature of spiritual calm, light, power and bliss. He will act not from an amalgam of an ignorant mind and will with the drive of a still more ignorant heart of emotion and the desire of the life-being and the urge and instinct of the flesh, but first from a spiritualised self and nature and, last, from a supramental Truth-consciousness and its divine force of supernature.

Thus are made possible the final steps when the veil of Nature is withdrawn and the seeker is face to face with the Master of all existence and his activities are merged in the action of a supreme Energy which is pure, true, perfect and blissful for ever. Thus can he utterly renounce to the supramental Shakti his works as well as the fruits of his works and act only as the conscious instrument of the eternal Worker. No longer giving the sanction, he will rather receive in his instruments and follow in her hands a divine mandate. No longer doing works, he will accept their execution through him by her unsleeping Force. No longer willing the fulfilment of his own mental constructions and the satisfaction of his own emotional desires, he will obey and participate in an omnipotent Will that is also an omniscient Knowledge and a mysterious, magical and unfathomable Love and a vast bottomless sea of the eternal Bliss of Existence.

Chapter X
The Three Modes of Nature

TO TRANSCEND the natural action of the lower Prakriti is indispensable to the soul, if it is to be free in its self and free in its works. Harmonious subjection to this actual universal Nature, a condition of good and perfect work for the natural instruments, is not an ideal for the soul, which should rather be subject to God and his Shakti, but master of its own nature. As agent or as channel of the Supreme Will it must determine by its vision and sanction or refusal the use that shall be made of the storage of energy, the conditions of environment, the rhythm of combined movement which are provided by Prakriti for the labour of the natural instruments, mind, life and body. But this inferior Nature can only be mastered if she is surmounted and used from above. And this can only be done by a transcendence of her forces, qualities and modes of action; otherwise we are subject to her conditions and helplessly dominated by her, not free in the spirit.

The idea of the three essential modes of Nature is a creation of the ancient Indian thinkers and its truth is not at once obvious, because it was the result of long psychological experiment and profound internal experience. Therefore without a long inner experience, without intimate self-observation and intuitive perception of the Nature-forces it is difficult to grasp accurately or firmly utilise. Still certain broad indications may help the seeker on the Way of Works to understand, analyse and control by his assent or refusal the combinations of his own nature. These modes are termed in the Indian books qualities, *guṇas*, and are given the names *sattva, rajas, tamas*. Sattwa is the force of equilibrium and translates in quality as good and harmony and happiness and light; rajas is the force of kinesis and translates in quality as struggle and effort, passion and action; tamas is the force of inconscience and inertia and translates in quality as obscurity and incapacity and inaction. Ordinarily used for psychological self-analysis, these distinctions are valid also in physical Nature. Each thing and every existence in the lower Prakriti contains them and its process and dynamic form are the result of the interaction of these qualitative powers.

Every form of things, whether animate or inanimate, is a constantly maintained poise of natural forces in motion and is subject to an unending stream of helpful, disturbing or disintegrating contacts from other combinations of forces that surround it. Our own nature of mind, life and body is nothing else than such a formative combination and poise. In the reception of the environing contacts and the reaction to them the three modes determine the temper of the recipient and the character of the response. Inert and inapt, he may suffer them without any responsive reaction, any motion of self-defence or any capacity of assimilation and adjustment; this is the mode of tamas, the way of inertia. The stigmata of tamas are blindness and unconsciousness and incapacity and unintelligence, sloth and indolence and inactivity and mechanical routine and the mind's torpor and the life's sleep and the soul's slumber. Its effect, if uncorrected by other elements, can be nothing but disintegration of the form or the poise of the nature without any new creation or new equilibrium or force of kinetic progress. At the heart of this inert impotence is the principle of ignorance and an inability or slothful unwillingness to comprehend, seize and manage the stimulating or assailing contact, the suggestion of environing forces and their urge towards fresh experience.

On the other hand, the recipient of Nature's contacts, touched and stimulated, solicited or assailed by her forces, may react to the pressure or against it. She allows, encourages, impels him to strive, to resist, to attempt, to dominate or engross his environment, to assert his will, to fight and create and conquer. This is the mode of rajas, the way of passion and action and the thirst of desire. Struggle and change and new creation, victory and defeat and joy and suffering and hope and disappointment are its children and build the many-coloured house of life in which it takes its pleasure. But its knowledge is an imperfect or a false knowledge and brings with it ignorant effort, error, a constant misadjustment, pain of attachment, disappointed desire, grief of loss and failure. The gift of rajas is kinetic force, energy, activity, the power that creates and acts and can overcome; but it moves in the wrong lights or the half-lights of the Ignorance and it is perverted by the touch of the Asura, Rakshasa and Pishacha. The arrogant ignorance of the human mind and its self-satisfied perversions and presumptuous errors, the pride and vanity and ambition, the cruelty and tyranny and beast wrath and violence, the selfishness and baseness and hypocrisy and treachery and vile meanness, the lust and greed and rapacity, the jealousy, envy and bottomless ingratitude that disfigure the earth-nature are the natural children of this indispensable but strong and dangerous turn of Nature.

But the embodied being is not limited to these two modes of Prakriti; there is a better and more enlightened way in which he can deal with surrounding impacts and the stream of the world-forces. There is possible a reception and reaction with clear comprehension, poise and balance. This way of natural being has the power that, because it understands, sympathises; it fathoms and controls and develops Nature's urge and her ways: it has an intelligence that penetrates her processes and her significances and can assimilate and utilise; there is a lucid response that is not overpowered but adjusts, corrects, adapts, harmonises, elicits the best in all things. This is the mode of sattwa, the turn of Nature that is full of light and poise, directed to good, to knowledge, to delight and beauty, to happiness, right understanding, right equilibrium, right order: its temperament is the opulence of a bright clearness of knowledge and a lucent warmth of sympathy and closeness. A fineness and enlighten-ment, a governed energy, an accomplished harmony and poise of the whole being is the consummate achievement of the sattwic nature.

No existence is cast entirely in the single mould of any of these three modes of the cosmic Force; all three are present in everyone and everywhere. There is a constant combining and separation of their shifting relations and interpenetrating influences, often a conflict, a wrestling of forces, a struggle to dominate each other. All have in great or in small extent or degree, even if sometimes in a hardly appreciable minimum, their sattwic states and clear tracts or inchoate tendencies of light, clarity and happiness, fine adaptation and sympathy with the environment, intelligence, poise, right mind, right will and feeling, right impulse, virtue, order. All have their rajasic moods and impulses and turbid parts of desire and passion and struggle, perversion and falsehood and error, unbalanced joy and sorrow, aggressive push to work and eager creation and strong or bold or fiery or fierce reactions to the pressure of the environment and to life's assaults and offers. All have their tamasic states and constant obscure parts, their moments or points of unconsciousness, their long habit or their temporary velleities of weak resignation or dull acceptance, their constitutional feeblenesses or movements of fatigue, negligence and indolence and their lapses into ignorance and incapacity, depression and fear and cowardly recoil or submission to the environment and to the pressure of men and events and forces. Each one of us is sattwic in some directions of his energy of Nature or in some parts of his mind or character, in others rajasic, tamasic in others. According as one or other of the modes usually dominates his general temperament and type of mind and turn of action, it is said of him that he is the sattwic, the rajasic or the tamasic man; but few are always of one kind and none is entire in his kind. The wise are not always or wholly wise, the intelligent are intelligent only in patches; the saint suppresses in himself many unsaintly movements and the evil are not entirely evil: the dullest has his unexpressed or unused and undeveloped capacities, the most timorous his moments or his way of courage, the helpless and the weakling a latent part of strength in his nature. The dominant gunas are not the essential soul-type of the embodied being but only the index of the formation he has made for this life or during his present existence and at a given moment of his evolution in Time.

*
* *

When the sadhaka has once stood back from the action of Prakriti within him or upon him and, not interfering, not amending or inhibiting, not choosing or deciding, allowed its play and analysed and watched the process, he soon discovers that her modes are self-dependent and work as a machine once put in action works by its own structure and propelling forces. The force and the propulsion come from Prakriti and not from the creature. Then he realises how mistaken was his impression that his mind was the doer of his works; his mind was only a small part of him and a creation and engine of Nature. Nature was acting all the while in her own modes moving the three general qualities about as a girl might play with her puppets. His ego was all along a tool and plaything; his character and intelligence, his moral qualities and mental powers, his creations and works and exploits, his anger and forbearance, his cruelty and mercy, his love and his hatred, his sin and his virtue, his light and his darkness, his passion of joy and his anguish of sorrow were the play of Nature to which the soul, attracted, won and subjected, lent its passive concurrence. And yet the determinism of Nature or Force is not all; the soul has a word to say in the matter, — but the secret soul, the Purusha, not the mind or the ego, since these are not independent entities, they are parts of Nature. For the soul's sanction is needed for the play and by an inner silent will as the lord and giver of the sanction it can determine the principle of the play and intervene in its combinations, although the execution in thought and will and act and impulse must still be Nature's part and privilege. The Purusha can dictate a harmony for Nature to execute, not by interfering in her functions but by a conscious regard on her which she transmutes at once or after much difficulty into translating idea and dynamic impetus and significant figure.

An escape from the action of the two inferior gunas is very evidently indispensable if we are to transmute our present nature into a power and form of the divine consciousness and an instrument of its forces. Tamas obscures and prevents the light of the divine knowledge from penetrating into the dark and dull corners of our nature. Tamas incapacitates and takes away the power to respond to divine impulse and the energy to change and the will to progress and make ourselves plastic to a greater Shakti. Rajas perverts knowledge, makes our reason the accomplice of falsehood and the abettor of every wrong movement, disturbs and twists our life-force and its impulses, oversets the balance and health of the body. Rajas captures all high-born ideas and high-seated movements and turns them to a false and egoistic use; even divine Truth and divine influences, when they descend into the earthly plane, cannot escape this misuse and seizure. Tamas unenlightened and rajas unconverted, no divine change or divine life is possible.

An exclusive resort to sattwa would seem to be the way of escape: but there is this difficulty that no one of the qualities can prevail by itself against its two companions and rivals. If, envisaging the quality of desire and passion as the cause of disturbance, suffering, sin and sorrow, we strain and labour to quell and subdue it, rajas sinks but tamas rises. For, the principle of activity dulled, inertia takes its place. A quiet peace, happiness, knowledge, love, right sentiment can be founded by the principle of light, but, if rajas is absent or completely suppressed, the quiet in the soul tends to become a tranquillity of inaction, not the firm ground of a dynamic change. Ineffectively right-thinking, right-doing, good, mild and even, the nature may become in its dynamic parts sattwa-tamasic, neutral, pale-tinted, uncreative or emptied of power. Mental and moral obscurity may be absent, but so are the intense springs of action, and this is a hampering limitation and another kind of incompetence. For tamas is a double principle; it contradicts rajas by inertia, it contradicts sattwa by narrowness, obscurity and ignorance and, if either is depressed, it pours in to occupy its place.

If we call in rajas again to correct this error and bid it ally itself to sattwa and by their united agency endeavour to get rid of the dark principle, we find that we have elevated our action, but that there is again subjection to rajasic eagerness, passion, disappointment, suffering, anger. These movements may be more exalted in their scope and spirit and action than before, but they are not the peace, the freedom, the power, the self-mastery at which we long to arrive. Wherever desire and ego harbour, passion and disturbance harbour with them and share their life. And if we seek a compromise between the three modes, sattwa leading, the others subordinate, still we have only arrived at a more temperate action of the play of Nature. A new poise has been reached, but a spiritual freedom and mastery are not in sight or else are still only a far-off prospect.

A radically different movement has to draw us back from the gunas and lift us above them. The error that accepts the action of the modes of Nature must cease; for as long as it is accepted, the soul is involved in their operations and subjected to their law. Sattwa must be transcended as well as rajas and tamas; the golden chain must be broken no less than the leaden fetters and the bond-ornaments of a mixed alloy. The Gita prescribes to this end a new method of self-discipline. It is to stand back in oneself from the action of the modes and observe this unsteady flux as the Witness seated above the surge of the forces of Nature. He is one who watches but is impartial and indifferent, aloof from them on their own level and in his native posture high above them. As they rise and fall in their waves, the Witness looks, observes, but neither accepts nor for the moment interferes with their course. First there must be the freedom of the impersonal Witness; afterwards there can be the control of the Master, the Ishwara.

*
* *

The initial advantage of this process of detachment is that one begins to understand one's own nature and all Nature. The detached Witness is able to see entirely without the least blinding by egoism the play of her modes of the Ignorance and to pursue it into all its ramifications, coverings and subtleties — for it is full of camouflage and disguise and snare and treachery and ruse. Instructed by long experience, conscious of all act and condition as their interaction, made wise of their processes, he cannot any longer be overcome by their assaults, surprised in their nets or deceived by their disguises. At the same time he perceives the ego to be nothing better than a device and the sustaining knot of their interaction and, perceiving it, he is delivered from the illusion of the lower egoistic Nature. He escapes from the sattwic egoism of the altruist and the saint and the thinker; he shakes off from its control on his life-impulses the rajasic egoism of the self-seeker and ceases to be the laborious caterer of self-interest and the pampered prisoner or toiling galley-slave of passion and desire; he slays with the light of knowledge the tamasic egoism of the ignorant or passive being, dull, unintelligent, attached to the common round of human life. Thus convinced and conscious of the essential vice of the ego-sense in all our personal action, he seeks no longer to find a means of self-correction and self-liberation in the rajasic or sattwic ego but looks above, beyond the instruments and the working of Nature, to the Master of works alone and his supreme Shakti, the supreme Prakriti. There alone all the being is pure and free and the rule of a divine Truth possible.

In this progression the first step is a certain detached superiority to the three modes of Nature. The soul is inwardly separated and free from the lower Prakriti, not involved in its coils, indifferent and glad above it. Nature continues to act in the triple round of her ancient habits, — desire, grief and joy attack the heart, the instruments fall into inaction and obscurity and weariness, light and peace come back into the heart and mind and body; but the soul stands unchanged and untouched by these changes. Observing and unmoved by the grief and desire of the lower members, smiling at their joys and their strainings, regarding and unoverpowered by the failing and the darknesses of the thought and the wildness or the weaknesses of the heart and nerves, uncompelled and unattached to the mind's illuminations and its relief and sense of ease or of power in the return of light and gladness, it throws itself into none of these things, but waits unmoved for the intimations of a higher Will and the intuitions of a greater luminous knowledge. Thus doing always, it becomes eventually free even in its nature parts from the strife of the three modes and their insufficient values and imprisoning limits. For now this lower Prakriti feels progressively a compulsion from a higher Shakti. The old habits to which it clung receive no further sanction and begin steadily to lose their frequency and force of recurrence. At last it understands that it is called to a higher action and a better state and, however slowly, however reluctantly, with whatever initial or prolonged ill-will and stumbling ignorance, it submits, turns and prepares itself for the change.

The static freedom of the soul, no longer witness only and knower, is crowned by a dynamic transformation of the nature. The constant mixture, the uneven operation of the three modes acting upon each other in our three instruments ceases from its normal confused, troubled and improper action and movement. Another action becomes possible, commences, grows, culminates, a working more truly right, more luminous, natural and normal to the deepest divine interplay of Purusha and Prakriti although supernatural and supernormal to our present imperfect nature. The body conditioning the physical mind insists no longer on its tamasic inertia that repeats always the same ignorant movement: it becomes a passive field and instrument of a greater force and light, it responds to every demand of the spirit's force, holds and supports every variety and intensity of new divine experience. Our kinetic and dynamic vital parts, our nervous and emotional and sensational and volitional being, expand in power and admit a tireless action and a blissful enjoyment of experience, but learn at the same time to stand on a foundation of wide self-possessed and self-poised calm, sublime in force, divine in rest, neither exulting and excited nor tortured by sorrow and pain, neither harried by desire and importunate impulses nor dulled by incapacity and indolence. The intelligence, the thinking, understanding and reflective mind, renounces its sattwic limitations and opens to an essential light and peace. An infinite knowledge offers to us its splendid ranges, a knowledge not made up of mental constructions, not bound by opinion and idea or dependent on a stumbling uncertain logic and the petty support of the senses, but self-sure, authentic, all-penetrating, all-comprehending; a boundless bliss and peace, not dependent on deliverance from the hampered strenuousness of creative energy and dynamic action, not constituted by a few limited felicities but self-existent and all-including, pour into ever-enlarging fields and through ever-widening and always more numerous channels to possess the nature. A higher force, bliss and knowledge from a source beyond mind and life and body seize on them to remould in a diviner image.

Here the disharmonies of the triple mode of our inferior existence are overpassed and there begins a greater triple mode of a divine Nature. There is no obscurity of tamas or inertia. Tamas is replaced by a divine peace and tranquil eternal repose out of which is released from a supreme matrix of calm concentration the play of action and knowledge. There is no rajasic kinesis, no desire, no joyful and sorrowful striving of action, creation and possession, no fruitful chaos of troubled impulse. Rajas is replaced by a self-possessed power and illimitable act of force, that even in its most violent intensities does not shake the immovable poise of the soul or stain the vast and profound heavens and luminous abysses of its peace. There is no constructing light of mind casting about to seize and imprison the Truth, no insecure or inactive ease. Sattwa is replaced by an illumination and a spiritual bliss identical with the depth and infinite existence of the soul and instinct with a direct and authentic knowledge that springs straight from the veiled glories of the secret Omniscience.

This is the greater consciousness into which our inferior consciousness has to be transformed, this nature of the Ignorance with its unquiet unbalanced activity of the three modes changed into this greater luminous supernature. At first we become free from the three gunas, detached, untroubled, *nistraigunya*; but this is the recovery of the native state of the soul, the self, the spirit free and watching in its motionless calm the motion of Prakriti in her force of the Ignorance. If on this basis the nature, the motion of Prakriti, is also to become free, it must be by a quiescence of action in a luminous peace and silence in which all necessary movements are done without any conscious reaction or participation or initiation of action by the mind or by the life-being, without any ripple of thought or eddy of the vital parts: it must be done under the impulsion, by the initiation, by the working of an impersonal cosmic or a transcendent Force. A cosmic Mind, Life, Substance must act, or a pure transcendent Self-Power and Bliss other than our own personal being or its building of Nature. This is a state of freedom which can come in the Yoga of works through renunciation of ego and desire and personal initiation and the surrender of the being to the cosmic Self or to the universal Shakti; it can come in the Yoga of knowledge by the cessation of thought, the silence of the mind, the opening of the whole being to the cosmic Consciousness, to the cosmic Self, the cosmic Dynamis or to the supreme Reality; it can come in the Yoga of devotion by the surrender of the heart and the whole nature into the hands of the All-Blissful as the adored Master of our existence. But the culminating change intervenes by a more positive and dynamic transcendence: there is a transference or transmutation into a superior spiritual status, *triguṇātīta*, in which we participate in a greater spiritual dynamisation; for the three lower unequal modes pass into an equal triune mode of eternal calm, light and force, the repose, kinesis, illumination of the divine Nature.

This supreme harmony cannot come except by the cessation of egoistic will and choice and act and the quiescence of our limited intelligence. The individual ego must cease to strive, the mind fall silent, the desire-will learn not to initiate. Our personality must join its source and all thought and initiation come from above. The secret Master of our activities will be slowly unveiled to us and from the security of the supreme Will and Knowledge give the sanction to the Divine Shakti who will do all works in us with a purified and exalted nature for her instrument; the individual centre of personality will be only the upholder of her works here, their recipient and channel, the reflector of her power and luminous participator in her light, joy and force. Acting it will not act and no reaction of the lower Prakriti will touch it. The transcendence of the three modes of Nature is the first condition, their transformation the decisive step of this change by which the Way of Works climbs out of the pit of narrowness of our darkened human nature into the unwalled wideness of the Truth and Light above us.

Chapter XI

The Master of the Work

THE MASTER and Mover of our works is the One, the Universal and Supreme, the Eternal and Infinite. He is the transcendent unknown or unknowable Absolute, the unexpressed and unmanifested Ineffable above us; but he is also the Self of all beings, the Master of all worlds, transcending all worlds, the Light and the Guide, the All-Beautiful and All-Blissful, the Beloved and the Lover. He is the Cosmic Spirit and all-creating Energy around us; he is the Immanent within us. All that is is he, and he is the More than all that is, and we ourselves, though we know it not, are being of his being, force of his force, conscious with a consciousness derived from his; even our mortal existence is made out of his substance and there is an immortal within us that is a spark of the Light and Bliss that are for ever. No matter whether by knowledge, works, love or any other means, to become aware of this truth of our being, to realise it, to make it effective here or elsewhere is the object of all Yoga.

*
* *

But the passage is long and the labour arduous before we can look on him with eyes that see true, and still longer and more arduous must be our endeavour if we would rebuild ourselves in his true image. The Master of the work does not reveal himself at once to the seeker. Always it is his Power that acts behind the veil, but it is manifest only when we renounce the egoism of the worker, and its direct movement increases in proportion as that renunciation becomes more and more complete. Only when our surrender to his Divine Shakti is absolute, shall we have the right to live in his absolute presence. And only then can we see our work throw itself naturally, completely and simply into the mould of the Divine Will.

There must, therefore, be stages and gradations in our approach to this perfection, as there are in the progress towards all other perfection on any plane of Nature. The vision of the full glory may come to us before, suddenly or slowly, once or often, but until the foundation is complete, it is a summary and concentrated, not a durable and all-enveloping experience, not a lasting presence. The amplitudes, the infinite contents of the Divine Revelation come afterwards and unroll gradually their power and their significance. Or, even, the steady vision can be there on the summits of our nature, but the perfect response of the lower members comes only by degrees. In all Yoga the first requisites are faith and patience. The ardours of the heart and the violences of the eager will that seek to take the kingdom of heaven by storm can have miserable reactions if they disdain to support their vehemence on these humbler and quieter auxiliaries. And in the long and difficult integral Yoga there must be an integral faith and an unshakable patience.

It is difficult to acquire or to practise this faith and steadfastness on the rough and narrow path of Yoga because of the impatience of both heart and mind and the eager but soon faltering will of our rajasic nature. The vital nature of man hungers always for the fruit of its labour and, if the fruit appears to be denied or long delayed, he loses faith in the ideal and in the guidance. For his mind judges always by the appearance of things, since that is the first ingrained habit of the intellectual reason in which he so inordinately trusts. Nothing is easier for us than to accuse God in our hearts when we suffer long or stumble in the darkness or to abjure the ideal that we have set before us. For we say, "I have trusted to the Highest and I am betrayed into suffering and sin and error." Or else, "I have staked my whole life on an idea which the stern facts of experience contradict and discourage. It would have been better to be as other men are who accept their limitations and walk on the firm ground of normal experience." In such moments — and they are sometimes frequent and long — all the higher experience is forgotten and the heart concentrates itself in its own bitterness. It is in these dark passages that it is possible to fall for good or to turn back from the divine labour.

If one has walked long and steadily in the path, the faith of the heart will remain under the fiercest adverse pressure; even if it is concealed or apparently overborne, it will take the first opportunity to re-emerge. For something higher than either heart or intellect upholds it in spite of the worst stumblings and through the most prolonged failure. But even to the experienced sadhaka such falterings or overcloudings bring a retardation of his progress and they are exceedingly dangerous to the novice. It is therefore necessary from the beginning to understand and accept the arduous difficulty of the path and to feel the need of a faith which to the intellect may seem blind, but yet is wiser than our reasoning intelligence. For this faith is a support from above; it is the brilliant shadow thrown by a secret light that exceeds the intellect and its data; it is the heart of a hidden knowledge that is not at the mercy of immediate appearances. Our faith, persevering, will be justified in its works and will be lifted and transfigured at last into the self-revelation of a divine knowledge. Always we must adhere to the injunction of the Gita, "Yoga must be continually applied with a heart free from despondent sinking." Always we must repeat to the doubting intellect the promise of the Master, "I will surely deliver thee from all sin and evil; do not grieve." At the end, the flickerings of faith will cease; for we shall see his face and feel always the Divine Presence.

*
* *

The Master of our works respects our nature even when he is transforming it; he works always through the nature and not by any arbitrary caprice. This imperfect nature of ours contains the materials of our perfection, but inchoate, distorted, misplaced, thrown together in disorder or a poor imperfect order. All this material has to be patiently perfected, purified, reorganised, new-moulded and transformed, not hacked and hewn and slain or mutilated, not obliterated by simple coercion and denial. This world and we who live in it are his creation and manifestation, and he deals with it and us in a way our narrow and ignorant mind cannot understand unless it falls silent and opens to a divine knowledge. In our errors is the substance of a truth which labours to reveal its meaning to our groping intelligence. The human intellect cuts out the error and the truth with it and replaces it by another half-truth half-error; but the Divine Wisdom suffers our mistakes to continue until we are able to arrive at the truth hidden and protected under every false cover. Our sins are the misdirected steps of a seeking Power that aims, not at sin, but at perfection, at something that we might call a divine virtue. Often they are the veils of a quality that has to be transformed and delivered out of this ugly disguise: otherwise, in the perfect providence of things, they would not have been suffered to exist or to continue. The Master of our works is neither a blunderer nor an indifferent witness nor a dallier with the luxury of unneeded evils. He is wiser than our reason and wiser than our virtue.

Our nature is not only mistaken in will and ignorant in knowledge but weak in power; but the Divine Force is there and will lead us if we trust in it and it will use our deficiencies and our powers for the divine purpose. If we fail in our immediate aim, it is because he has intended the failure; often our failure or ill-result is the right road to a truer issue than an immediate and complete success would have put in our reach. If we suffer, it is because something in us has to be prepared for a rarer possibility of delight. If we stumble, it is to learn in the end the secret of a more perfect walking. Let us not be in too furious a haste to acquire even peace, purity and perfection. Peace must be ours, but not the peace of an empty or devastated nature or of slain or mutilated capacities incapable of unrest because we have made them incapable of intensity and fire and force. Purity must be our aim, but not the purity of a void or of a bleak and rigid coldness. Perfection is demanded of us, but not the perfection that can exist only by confining its scope within narrow limits or putting an arbitrary full stop to the ever self-extending scroll of the Infinite. Our object is to change into the divine nature, but the divine nature is not a mental or moral but a spiritual condition, difficult to achieve, difficult even to conceive by our intelligence. The Master of our work and our Yoga knows the thing to be done, and we must allow him to do it in us by his own means and in his own manner.

The movement of the Ignorance is egoistic at its core and nothing is more difficult for us than to get rid of egoism while yet we admit personality and adhere to action in the half-light and half-force of our unfinished nature. It is easier to starve the ego by renouncing the impulse to act or to kill it by cutting away from us all movement of personality. It is easier to exalt it into self-forgetfulness immersed in a trance of peace or an ecstasy of divine Love. But our more difficult problem is to liberate the true Person and attain to a divine manhood which shall be the pure vessel of a divine force and the perfect instrument of a divine action. Step after step has to be firmly taken; difficulty after difficulty has to be entirely experienced and entirely mastered. Only the Divine Wisdom and Power can do this for us and it will do all if we yield to it in an entire faith and follow and assent to its workings with a constant courage and patience.

The first step on this long path is to consecrate all our works as a sacrifice to the Divine in us and in the world; this is an attitude of the mind and heart, not too difficult to initiate, but very difficult to make absolutely sincere and all-pervasive. The second step is to renounce attachment to the fruit of our works; for the only true, inevitable and utterly desirable fruit of sacrifice — the one thing needful — is the Divine Presence and the Divine Consciousness and Power in us, and if that is gained, all else will be added. This is a transformation of the egoistic will in our vital being, our desire-soul and desire-nature, and it is far more difficult than the other. The third step is to get rid of the central egoism and even the ego-sense of the worker. That is the most difficult transformation of all and it cannot be perfectly done if the first two steps have not been taken; but these first steps too cannot be completed unless the third comes in to crown the movement and, by the extinction of egoism, eradicates the very origin of desire. Only when the small ego-sense is rooted out from the nature can the seeker know his true person that stands above as a portion and power of the Divine and renounce all motive-force other than the will of the Divine Shakti.

*
* *

There are gradations in this last integralising movement; for it cannot be done at once or without long approaches that bring it progressively nearer and make it at last possible. The first attitude to be taken is to cease to regard ourselves as the worker and firmly to realise that we are only one instrument of the cosmic Force. At first it is not the one Force but many cosmic forces that seem to move us; but these may be turned into feeders of the ego and this vision liberates the mind but not the rest of the nature. Even when we become aware of all as the working of one cosmic Force and of the Divine behind it, that too need not liberate. If the egoism of the worker disappears, the egoism of the instrument may replace it or else prolong it in a disguise. The life of the world has been full of instances of egoism of this kind and it can be more engrossing and enormous than any other; there is the same danger in Yoga. A man becomes a leader of men or eminent in a large or lesser circle and feels himself full of a power that he knows to be beyond his own ego-force; he may be aware of a Fate acting through him or a Will mysterious and unfathomable or a Light within of great brilliance. There are extraordinary results of his thoughts, his actions or his creative genius. He effects some tremendous destruction that clears the path for humanity or some great construction that becomes its momentary resting-place. He is a scourge or he is a bringer of light and healing, a creator of beauty or a messenger of knowledge. Or, if his work and its effects are on a lesser scale and have a limited field, still they are attended by the strong sense that he is an instrument and chosen for his mission or his labour. Men who have this destiny and these powers come easily to believe and declare themselves to be mere instruments in the hand of God or of Fate: but even in the declaration we can see that there can intrude or take refuge an intenser and more exaggerated egoism than ordinary men have the courage to assert or the strength to house within them. And often if men of this kind speak of God, it is to erect an image of him which is really nothing but a huge shadow of themselves or their own nature, a sustaining Deific Essence of their own type of will and thought and quality and force. This magnified image of their ego is the Master whom they serve. This happens only too often in Yoga to strong but crude vital natures or minds too easily exalted when they allow ambition, pride or the desire of greatness to enter into their spiritual seeking and vitiate its purity of motive; a magnified ego stands between them and their true being and grasps for its own personal purpose the strength from a greater unseen Power, divine or undivine, acting through them of which they become vaguely or intensely aware. An intellectual perception or vital sense of a Force greater than ours and of ourselves as moved by it is not sufficient to liberate from the ego.

This perception, this sense of a greater Power in us or above and moving us, is not a hallucination or a megalomania. Those who thus feel and see have a larger sight than ordinary men and have advanced a step beyond the limited physical intelligence, but theirs is not the plenary vision or the direct experience. For, because they are not clear in mind and aware in the soul, because their awakening is more in the vital parts than into the spiritual substance of Self, they cannot be the conscious instruments of the Divine or come face to face with the Master, but are used through their fallible and imperfect nature. The most they see of the Divinity is a Fate or a cosmic Force or else they give his name to a limited Godhead or, worse, to a Titanic or demoniac Power that veils him. Even certain religious founders have erected the image of the God of a sect or a national God or a Power of terror and punishment or a Numen of sattwic love and mercy and virtue and seem not to have seen the One and Eternal. The Divine accepts the image they make of him and does his work in them through that medium, but, since the one Force is felt and acts in their imperfect nature but more intensely than in others, the motive principle of egoism too can be more intense in them than in others. An exalted rajasic or sattwic ego still holds them and stands between them and the integral Truth. Even this is something, a beginning, although far from the true and perfect experience. A much worse thing may befall those who break something of the human bonds but have not purity and have not the knowledge, for they may become instruments, but not of the Divine; too often, using his name, they serve unconsciously his Masks and black Contraries, the Powers of Darkness.

Our nature must house the cosmic Force but not in its lower aspect or in its rajasic or sattwic movement; it must serve the universal Will, but in the light of a greater liberating knowledge. There must be no egoism of any kind in the attitude of the instrument, even when we are fully conscious of the greatness of the Force within us. Every man is knowingly or unknowingly the instrument of a universal Power and, apart from the inner Presence, there is no such essential difference between one action and another, one kind of instrumentation and another as would warrant the folly of an egoistic pride. The difference between knowledge and ignorance is a grace of the Spirit; the breath of divine Power blows where it lists and fills today one and tomorrow another with the word or the puissance. If the potter shapes one pot more perfectly than another, the merit lies not in the vessel but the maker. The attitude of our mind must not be "This is my strength" or "Behold God's power in me", but rather "A Divine Power works in this mind and body and it is the same that works in all men and in the animal, in the plant and in the metal, in conscious and living things and in things apparently inconscient and inanimate." This large view of the One working in all and of the whole world as the equal instrument of a divine action and gradual self-expression, if it becomes our entire experience, will help to eliminate all rajasic egoism out of us and even the sattwic ego-sense will begin to pass away from our nature.

The elimination of this form of ego leads straight towards the true instrumental action which is the essence of a perfect Karmayoga. For while we cherish the instrumental ego, we may pretend to ourselves that we are conscious instruments of the Divine, but in reality we are trying to make of the Divine Shakti an instrument of our own desires or our egoistic purpose. And even if the ego is subjected but not eliminated, we may indeed be engines of the Divine Work, but we shall be imperfect tools and deflect or impair the working by our mental errors, our vital distortions or the obstinate incapacities of our physical nature. If this ego disappears, then we can truly become, not only pure instruments consciously consenting to every turn of the divine Hand that moves us, but aware of our true nature, conscious portions of the one Eternal and Infinite put out in herself for her works by the supreme Shakti.

*
* *

There is another greater step to be taken after the surrender of our instrumental ego to the Divine Shakti. It is not enough to know her as the one Cosmic Force that moves us and all creatures on the planes of mind, life and matter; for this is the lower Nature and, although the Divine Knowledge, Light, Power are there concealed and at work in this Ignorance and can break partly its veil and manifest something of their true character or descend from above and uplift these inferior workings, yet, even if we realise the One in a spiritualised mind, a spiritualised life-movement, a spiritualised body-consciousness, an imperfection remains in the dynamic parts. There is a stumbling response to the Supreme Power, a veil over the face of the Divine, a constant mixture of the Ignorance. It is only when we open to the Divine Shakti in the truth of her Force which transcends this lower Prakriti that we can be perfect instruments of her power and knowledge.

Not only liberation but perfection must be the aim of the Karmayoga. The Divine works through our nature and according to our nature; if our nature is imperfect, the work also will be imperfect, mixed, inadequate. Even it may be marred by gross errors, falsehoods, moral weaknesses, diverting influences. The work of the Divine will be done in us even then, but according to our weakness, not according to the strength and purity of its source. If ours were not an integral Yoga, if we sought only the liberation of the self within us or the motionless existence of Purusha separated from Prakriti, this dynamic imperfection might not matter. Calm, untroubled, not depressed, not elated, refusing to accept the perfection or imperfection, fault or merit, sin or virtue as ours, perceiving that it is the modes of Nature working in the field of her modes that make this mixture, we could withdraw into the silence of the spirit and, pure, untouched, witness only the workings of Prakriti. But in an integral realisation this can only be a step on the way, not our last resting-place. For we aim at the divine realisation not only in the immobility of the Spirit, but also in the movement of Nature. And this cannot be altogether until we can feel the presence and power of the Divine in every step, motion, figure of our activities, in every turn of our will, in every thought, feeling and impulse. No doubt, we can feel that in essence even in the nature of the Ignorance, but it is the divine Power and Presence in a disguise, a diminution, an inferior figure. Ours is a greater demand, that our nature shall be a power of the Divine in the Truth of the Divine, in the Light, in the force of the eternal self-conscient Will, in the wideness of the sempiternal Knowledge.

After the removal of the veil of ego, the removal of the veil of Nature and her inferior modes that govern our mind, life and body. As soon as the limits of the ego begin to fade, we see how that veil is constituted and detect the action of cosmic Nature in us, and in or behind cosmic Nature we sense the presence of the cosmic Self and the dynamis of the world-pervading Ishwara. The Master of the instrument stands behind all this working, and even within the working there is his touch and the drive of a great guiding or disposing Influence. It is no longer ego or ego-force that we serve; we obey the World-Master and his evolutionary impulse. At each step we can say in the language of the Sanskrit verse, "Even as I am appointed by Thee seated in my heart, so, O Lord, I act." But still this action may be of two very different kinds, one only illumined, the other transformed and uplifted into a greater supernature. For we may keep on in the way of action upheld and followed by our nature when by her and her illusion of egoism we were "turned as if mounted on a machine," but now with a perfect understanding of the mechanism and its utilisation for his world purposes by the Master of works whom we feel behind it. This is indeed as far as even many great Yogis have reached on the levels of spiritualised mind; but it need not be so always, for there is a greater supramental possibility. It is possible to rise beyond spiritualised mind and to act spontaneously in the living presence of the original divine Truth-Force of the Supreme Mother. Our motion one with her motion and merged in it, our will one with her will, our energy absolved in her energy, we shall feel her working through us as the Divine manifest in a supreme Wisdom-Power, and we shall be aware of the transformed mind, life and body only as the channels of a supreme Light and Force beyond them, infallible in its steps because transcendent and total in its knowledge. Of this Light and Force we shall not only be the recipients, channels, instruments, but become a part of it in a supreme uplifted abiding experience.

Already, before we reach this last perfection, we can have the union with the Divine in works in its extreme wideness, if not yet on its most luminous heights; for we perceive no longer merely Nature or the modes of Nature, but become conscious, in our physical movements, in our nervous and vital reactions, in our mental workings, of a Force greater than body, mind and life which takes hold of our limited instruments and drives all their motion. There is no longer the sense of ourselves moving, thinking or feeling but of that moving, feeling and thinking in us. This force that we feel is the universal Force of the Divine, which, veiled or unveiled, acting directly or permitting the use of its powers by beings in the cosmos, is the one Energy that alone exists and alone makes universal or individual action possible. For this force is the Divine itself in the body of its power; all is that, power of act, power of thought and knowledge, power of mastery and enjoyment, power of love. Conscious always and in everything, in ourselves and in others, of the Master of Works possessing, inhabiting, enjoying through this Force that is himself, becoming through it all existences and all happenings, we shall have arrived at the divine union through works and achieved by that fulfilment in works all that others have gained through absolute devotion or through pure knowledge. But there is still another step that calls us, an ascent out of this cosmic identity into the identity of the Divine Transcendence.

The Master of our works and our being is not merely a Godhead here within us, nor is he merely a cosmic Spirit or some kind of universal Power. The world and the Divine are not one and the same thing, as a certain kind of pantheistic thinking would like to believe. The world is an emanation; it depends upon something that manifests in it but is not limited by it: the Divine is not here alone; there is a Beyond, an eternal Transcendence. The individual being also in its spiritual part is not a formation in the cosmic existence — our ego, our mind, our life, our body are that; but the immutable spirit, the imperishable soul in us has come out of the Transcendence.

*

* *

A Transcendent who is beyond all world and all Nature and yet possesses the world and its nature, who has descended with something of himself into it and is shaping it into that which as yet it is not, is the Source of our being, the Source of our works and their Master. But the seat of the Transcendent Consciousness is above in an absoluteness of divine Existence — and there too is the absolute Power, Truth, Bliss of the Eternal — of which our mentality can form no conception and of which even our greatest spiritual experience is only a diminished reflection in the spiritualised mind and heart, a faint shadow, a thin derivate. Yet proceeding from it there is a sort of golden corona of Light, Power, Bliss and Truth — a divine Truth-Consciousness as the ancient mystics called it, a Supermind, a Gnosis, with which this world of a lesser consciousness proceeding by Ignorance is in secret relation and which alone maintains it and prevents it from falling into a disintegrated chaos. The powers we are now satisfied to call gnosis, intuition or illumination are only fainter lights of which that is the full and flaming source, and between the highest human intelligence and it there lie many levels of ascending consciousness, highest mental or overmental, which we would have to conquer before we arrived there or could bring down its greatness and glory here. Yet, however difficult, that ascent, that victory is the destiny of the human spirit and that luminous descent or bringing down of the divine Truth is the inevitable term of the troubled evolution of the earth-nature; that intended consummation is its *raison d'être*, our culminating state and the explanation of our terrestrial existence. For though the transcendental Divine is already here as the Purushottama in the secret heart of our mystery, he is veiled by many coats and disguises of his magic world-wide Yoga-Maya; it is only by the ascent and victory of the Soul here in the body that the disguises can fall away and the dynamis of the supreme Truth replace this tangled weft of half-truth that becomes creative error, this emergent Knowledge that is converted by its plunge into the inconscience of Matter and its slow partial return towards itself into an effective Ignorance.

For here in the world, though the Gnosis is there secretly behind existence, what acts is not the Gnosis but a magic of Knowledge-Ignorance, an incalculable yet apparently mechanical Overmind Maya. The Divine appears to us here in one view as an equal, inactive and impersonal Witness Spirit, an immobile consenting Purusha not bound by quality or Space or Time, whose support or sanction is given impartially to the play of all action and energies which the transcendent Will has once permitted and authorised to fulfil themselves in the cosmos. This Witness Spirit, this immobile Self in things, seems to will nothing and determine nothing; yet we become aware that his very passivity, his silent presence compels all things to travel even in their ignorance towards a divine goal and attracts through division towards a yet unrealised oneness. Yet no supreme infallible Divine Will seems to be there, only a widely deployed Cosmic Energy or a mechanical executive Process, Prakriti. This is one side of the cosmic Self; the other presents itself as a universal Divine, one in being, multiple in personality and power, who conveys to us, when we enter into the consciousness of his universal forces, a sense of infinite quality and will and act and world-wide knowledge and a one yet innumerable delight; for through him we become one with all existences not only in their essence but in their play of action, see ourself in all and all in ourself, perceive all knowledge and thought and feeling as motions of the one Mind and Heart, all energy and action as kinetics of the one Will in power, all Matter and form as particles of the one Body, all personalities as projections of the one Person, all egos as deformations of the one and sole real "I" in existence. In him we no longer stand separate, but lose our active ego in the universal movement, even as by the Witness who is without qualities and for ever unattached and unentangled, we lose our static ego in the universal peace.

And yet there remains a contradiction between these two terms, the aloof divine Silence and the all-embracing divine Action, which we may heal in ourselves in a certain manner, in a certain high degree which seems to us complete, yet is not complete because it cannot altogether transform and conquer. A universal Peace, Light, Power, Bliss is ours, but its effective expression is not that of the Truth-Consciousness, the divine Gnosis, but still, though wonderfully freed, uplifted and illumined, supports only the present self-expression of the Cosmic Spirit and does not transform, as would a transcendental Descent, the ambiguous symbols and veiled mysteries of a world of Ignorance. Ourselves are free, but the earth-consciousness remains in bondage; only a further transcendental ascent and descent can entirely heal the contradiction and transform and deliver.

For there is yet a third intensely close and personal aspect of the Master of Works which is a key to his sublimest hidden mystery and ecstasy; for he detaches from the secret of the hidden Transcendence and the ambiguous display of the cosmic Movement an individual Power of the Divine that can mediate between the two and bridge our passage from the one to the other. In this aspect the transcendent and universal person of the Divine conforms itself to our individualised personality and accepts a personal relation with us, at once identified with us as our supreme Self and yet close and different as our Master, Friend, Lover, Teacher, our Father and our Mother, our Playmate in the great world-game who has disguised himself throughout as friend and enemy, helper and opponent and, in all relations and in all workings that affect us, has led our steps towards our perfection and our release. It is through this more personal manifestation that we are admitted to some possibility of the complete transcendental experience; for in him we meet the One not merely in a liberated calm and peace, not merely with a passive or active submission in our works or through the mystery of union with a universal Knowledge and Power filling and guiding us, but with an ecstasy of divine Love and divine Delight that shoots up beyond silent Witness and active World-Power to some positive divination of a greater beatific secret. For it is not so much knowledge leading to some ineffable Absolute, not so much works lifting us beyond world-process to the originating supreme Knower and Master, but rather this thing most intimate to us, yet at present most obscure, which keeps for us wrapped in its passionate veil the deep and rapturous secret of the transcendent Godhead and some absolute positiveness of its perfect Being, its all-concentrating Bliss, its mystic Ananda.

But the individual relation with the Divine does not always or from the beginning bring into force a widest enlargement or a highest self-exceeding. At first this Godhead close to our being or immanent within us can be felt fully only in the scope of our personal nature and experience, a Leader and Master, a Guide and Teacher, a Friend and Lover, or else a spirit, power or presence, constituting and uplifting our upward and enlarging movement by the force of his intimate reality inhabiting the heart or presiding over our nature from above even our highest intelligence. It is our personal evolution that is his preoccupation, a personal relation with him that is our joy and fulfilment, the building of our nature into his divine image that is our self-finding and perfection. The outside world seems to exist only as a field for this growth and a provider of materials or of helping and opposing forces for its successive stages. Our works done in that world are his works, but even when they serve some temporary universal end, their main purpose for us is to make outwardly dynamic or give inward power to our relations with this immanent Divine. Many seekers ask for no more or see the continuation and fulfilment of this spiritual flowering only in heavens beyond; the union is consummated and made perpetual in an eternal dwelling-place of his perfection, joy and beauty. But this is not enough for the integral seeker; however intense and beautiful, a personal isolated achievement cannot be his sole aim or his entire experience. A time must come when the personal opens out into the universal; our very individuality, spiritual, mental, vital, physical even, becomes universalised: it is seen as a power of his universal force and cosmic spirit, or else it contains the universe in that ineffable wideness which comes to the individual consciousness when it breaks its bonds and flows upward towards the Transcendent and on every side into the Infinite.

*
*   *

In a Yoga lived entirely on the spiritualised mental plane it is possible and even usual for these three fundamental aspects of the Divine — the Individual or Immanent, the Cosmic and the Transcendent — to stand out as separate realisations. Each by itself then appears sufficient to satisfy the yearning of the seeker. Alone with the personal Divine in the inner heart's illumined secret chamber, he can build his being into the Beloved's image and ascend out of fallen Nature to dwell with him in some heaven of the Spirit. Absolved in the cosmic wideness, released from ego, his personality reduced to a point of working of the universal Force, himself calm, liberated, deathless in universality, motionless in the Witness Self even while outspread without limit in unending Space and Time, he can enjoy in the world the freedom of the Timeless. One-pointed towards some ineffable Transcendence, casting away his personality, shedding from him the labour and trouble of the universal Dynamis, he can escape into an inexpressible Nirvana, annul all things in an intolerant exaltation of flight into the Incommunicable.

But none of these achievements is enough for one who seeks the wide completeness of an integral Yoga. An individual salvation is not enough for him; for he finds himself opening to a cosmic consciousness which far exceeds by its breadth and vastness the narrower intensity of a limited individual fulfilment, and its call is imperative; driven by that immense compulsion, he must break through all separative boundaries, spread himself in world-Nature, contain the universe. Above too, there is urgent upon him a dynamic realisation pressing from the Supreme upon this world of beings, and only some encompassing and exceeding of the cosmic consciousness can release into manifestation here that yet unlavished splendour. But the cosmic consciousness too is not sufficient; for it is not all the Divine Reality, not integral. There is a divine secret behind personality that he must discover; there, waiting in it to be delivered here into Time, stands the mystery of the embodiment of the Transcendence. In the cosmic consciousness there remains at the end a hiatus, an unequal equation of a highest Knowledge that can liberate but not effectuate with a Power seeming to use a limited Knowledge or masking itself with a surface Ignorance that can create but creates imperfection or a perfection transient, limited and in fetters. On one side there is a free undynamic Witness and on the other side a bound Executrix of action who has not been given all the means of action. The reconciliation of these companions and opposites seems to be reserved, postponed, held back in an Unmanifest still beyond us. But, again, a mere escape into some absolute Transcendence leaves personality unfulfilled and the universal action inconclusive and cannot satisfy the integral seeker. He feels that the Truth that is for ever is a Power that creates as well as a stable Existence; it is not a Power solely of illusory or ignorant manifestation. The eternal Truth can manifest its truths in Time; it can create in Knowledge and not only in Inconscience and Ignorance. A divine Descent no less than an ascent to the Divine is possible; there is a prospect of the bringing down of a future perfection and a present deliverance. As his knowledge widens, it becomes for him more and more evident that it was this for which the Master of Works cast down the soul within him here as a spark of his fire into the darkness, that it might grow there into a centre of the Light that is for ever.

The Transcendent, the Universal, the Individual are three

powers overarching, underlying and penetrating the whole manifestation; this is the first of the Trinities. In the unfolding of
consciousness also, these are the three fundamental terms and
none of them can be neglected if we would have the experience
of the whole Truth of existence. Out of the individual we wake
into a vaster freer cosmic consciousness; but out of the universal
too with its complex of forms and powers we must emerge by
a still greater self-exceeding into a consciousness without limits
that is founded on the Absolute. And yet in this ascension we do
not really abolish but take up and transfigure what we seem to
leave; for there is a height where the three live eternally in each
other, on that height they are blissfully joined in a nodus of their
harmonised oneness. But that summit is above the highest and
largest spiritualised mentality, even if some reflection of it can
be experienced there; mind, to attain to it, to live there, must
exceed itself and be transformed into a supramental gnostic light,
power and substance. In this lower diminished consciousness a
harmony can indeed be attempted, but it must always remain
imperfect; a coordination is possible, not a simultaneous fused
fulfilment. An ascent out of the mind is, for any greater realisation, imperative. Or else, there must be, with the ascent or
consequent to it, a dynamic descent of the self-existent Truth
that exists always uplifted in its own light above Mind, eternal,
prior to the manifestation of Life and Matter.

For Mind is Maya, *sat-asat*: there is a field of embrace of
the true and the false, the existent and the non-existent, and it
is in that ambiguous field that Mind seems to reign; but even
in its own reign it is in truth a diminished consciousness, it is
not part of the original and supremely originating power of the
Eternal. Even if Mind is able to reflect some image of essential
Truth in its substance, yet the dynamic force and action of Truth
appears in it always broken and divided. All Mind can do is to
piece together the fragments or deduce a unity; truth of Mind is
only a half-truth or a portion of a puzzle. Mental knowledge is
always relative, partial and inconclusive, and its outgoing action
and creation come out still more confused in its steps or precise
only in narrow limits and by imperfect piecings together. Even

in this diminished consciousness the Divine manifests as a Spirit in Mind, just as he moves as a Spirit in Life or dwells still more obscurely as a Spirit in Matter; but not here is his full dynamic revelation, not here the perfect identities of the Eternal. Only when we cross the border into a larger luminous consciousness and self-aware substance where divine Truth is a native and not a stranger, will there be revealed to us the Master of our existence in the imperishable integral truth of his being and his powers and his workings. Only there, too, will his works in us assume the flawless movement of his unfailing supramental purpose.

*
* *

But that is the end of a long and difficult journey, and the Master of works does not wait till then to meet the seeker on the path of Yoga and put his secret or half-shown Hand upon him and upon his life and actions. Already he was there in the world as the Originator and Receiver of works behind the dense veils of the Inconscient, disguised in force of Life, visible to the Mind through symbol godheads and figures. It may well be in these disguises that he first meets the soul destined to the way of the integral Yoga. Or even, wearing still vaguer masks, he may be conceived by us as an Ideal or mentalised as an abstract Power of Love, Good, Beauty or Knowledge; or, as we turn our feet towards the Way, he may come to us veiled as the call of Humanity or a Will in things that drives towards the deliverance of the world from the grasp of Darkness and Falsehood and Death and Suffering — the great quaternary of the Ignorance. Then, after we have entered the path, he envelops us with his wide and mighty liberating Impersonality or moves near to us with the face and form of a personal Godhead. In and around us we feel a Power that upholds and protects and cherishes; we hear a Voice that guides; a conscious Will greater than ourselves rules us; an imperative Force moves our thought and actions and our very body; an ever-widening Consciousness assimilates ours, a living Light of Knowledge lights all within, or a Beatitude invades us; a Mightiness presses from above, concrete, massive and overpowering, and penetrates and pours itself into the very stuff of our nature; a Peace sits there, a Light, a Bliss, a Strength, a Greatness. Or there are relations, personal, intimate as life itself, sweet as love, encompassing like the sky, deep like deep waters. A Friend walks at our side; a Lover is with us in our heart's secrecy; a Master of the Work and the Ordeal points our way; a Creator of things uses us as his instrument; we are in the arms of the eternal Mother. All these more seizable aspects in which the Ineffable meets us are truths and not mere helpful symbols or useful imaginations; but as we progress, their first imperfect formulations in our experience yield to a larger vision of the one Truth that is behind them. At each step their mere mental masks are shed and they acquire a larger, a profounder, a more intimate significance. At last on the supramental borders all these Godheads combine their forces and, without at all ceasing to be, coalesce together. On this path the Divine Aspects are not revealed in order to be cast away; they are not temporary spiritual conveniences or compromises with an illusory Consciousness or dream-figures mysteriously cast upon us by the incommunicable superconscience of the Absolute; on the contrary, their power increases and their absoluteness reveals itself as they draw near to the Truth from which they issue.

For that now superconscient Transcendence is a Power as well as an Existence. The supramental Transcendence is not a vacant Wonder, but an Inexpressible which contains for ever all essential things that have issued from it; it holds them there in their supreme everlasting reality and their own characteristic absolutes. The diminution, division, degradation that create here the sense of an unsatisfactory puzzle, a mystery of Maya, themselves diminish and fall from us in our ascension, and the Divine Powers assume their real forms and appear more and more as the terms of a Truth in process of realisation here. A soul of the Divine is here slowly awaking out of its involution and concealment in the material Inconscience. The Master of our works is not a Master of illusions, but a supreme Reality who is working out his self-expressive realities delivered slowly from the cocoons of the Ignorance in which for the purposes of an evolutionary manifestation they were allowed for a while to slumber. For the supramental Transcendence is not a thing absolutely apart and unconnected with our present existence. It is a greater Light out of which all this has come for the adventure of the Soul lapsing into the Inconscience and emerging out of it, and, while that adventure proceeds, it waits superconscient above our minds till it can become conscious in us. Hereafter it will unveil itself and by the unveiling reveal to us all the significance of our own being and our works; for it will disclose the Divine whose fuller manifestation in the world will release and accomplish that covert significance.

In that disclosure the Transcendent Divine will be more and more made known to us as the Supreme Existence and the Perfect Source of all that we are; but equally we shall see him as a Master of works and creation prepared to pour out more and more of himself into the field of his manifestation. The cosmic consciousness and its action will appear no longer as a huge regulated Chance, but as a field of the manifestation; there the Divine is seen as a presiding and pervading Cosmic Spirit who receives all out of the Transcendence and develops what descends into forms that are now an opaque disguise or a baffling half-disguise, but destined to be a transparent revelation. The individual consciousness will recover its true sense and action; for it is the form of a Soul sent out from the Supreme and, in spite of all appearances, a nucleus or nebula in which the Divine Mother-Force is at work for the victorious embodiment of the timeless and formless Divine in Time and Matter. This will reveal itself slowly to our vision and experience as the will of the Master of works and as their own ultimate significance, which alone gives to world-creation and to our own action in the world a light and a meaning. To recognise that and to strive towards its effectuation is the whole burden of the Way of Divine Works in the integral Yoga.

Chapter XII

The Divine Work

ONE QUESTION remains for the seeker upon the way of works, when his quest is or seems to have come to its natural end, — whether any work or what work is left for the soul after liberation and to what purpose? Equality has been seated in the nature or governs the whole nature; there has been achieved a radical deliverance from the ego-idea, from the pervading ego-sense, from all feelings and impulsions of the ego and its self-will and desires. The entire self-consecration has been made not only in thought and heart but in all the complexities of the being. A complete purity or transcendence of the three gunas has been harmoniously established. The soul has seen the Master of its works and lives in his presence or is consciously contained in his being or is unified with him or feels him in the heart or above and obeys his dictates. It has known its true being and cast away the veil of the Ignorance. What work then remains for the worker in man and with what motive, to what end, in what spirit will it be done?

*
* *

There is one answer with which we are very familiar in India; no work at all remains, for the rest is quiescence. When the soul can live in the eternal presence of the Supreme or when it is unified with the Absolute, the object of our existence in the world, if it can be said to have an object, at once ceases. Man, released from the curse of self-division and the curse of Ignorance, is released too from that other affliction, the curse of works. All action would then be a derogation from the supreme state and a return into the Ignorance. This attitude towards life is supported by an idea founded on the error of the vital nature to which action is dictated only by one or all of three inferior motives, necessity, restless instinct and impulse or desire. The instinct or impulse quiescent, desire extinguished, what place is there for works? Some mechanical necessity might remain but no other, and even that would cease for ever with the fall of the body. But after all, even so, while life remains, action is unavoidable. Mere thinking or, in the absence of thought, mere living is itself an act and a cause of many effects. All existence in the world is work, force, potency, and has a dynamic effect in the whole by its mere presence, even the inertia of the clod, even the silence of the immobile Buddha on the verge of Nirvana. There is the question only of the manner of the action, the instruments that are used or that act of themselves, and the spirit and knowledge of the worker. For in reality, no man works, but Nature works through him for the self-expression of a Power within that proceeds from the Infinite. To know that and live in the presence and in the being of the Master of Nature, free from desire and the illusion of personal impulsion, is the one thing needful. That and not the bodily cessation of action is the true release; for the bondage of works at once ceases. A man might sit still and motionless for ever and yet be as much bound to the Ignorance as the animal or the insect. But if he can make this greater consciousness dynamic within him, then all the work of all the worlds could pass through him and yet he would remain at rest, absolute in calm and peace, free from all bondage. Action in the world is given us first as a means for our self-development and self-fulfilment; but even if we reached a last possible divine self-completeness, it would still remain as a means for the fulfilment of the divine intention in the world and of the larger universal self of which each being is a portion — a portion that has come down with it from the Transcendence.

In a certain sense, when his Yoga has reached a certain culmination, works cease for a man; for he has no further personal necessity of works, no sense of works being done by him; but there is no need to flee from action or to take refuge in a blissful inertia. For now he acts as the Divine Existence acts without any binding necessity and without any compelling ignorance. Even in doing works *he* does not work at all; he undertakes no personal initiative. It is the Divine Shakti that works in him through his nature; his action develops through the spontaneity of a supreme Force by which his instruments are possessed, of which he is a part, with whose will his will is identical and his power is her power. The spirit within him contains, supports and watches this action; it presides over it in knowledge but is not glued or clamped to the work by attachment or need, is not bound by desire of its fruit, is not enslaved to any movement or impulse.

It is a common error to suppose that action is impossible or at least meaningless without desire. If desire ceases, we are told, action also must cease. But this, like other too simply comprehensive generalisations, is more attractive to the cutting and defining mind than true. The major part of the work done in the universe is accomplished without any interference of desire; it proceeds by the calm necessity and spontaneous law of Nature. Even man constantly does work of various kinds by a spontaneous impulse, intuition, instinct or acts in obedience to a natural necessity and law of forces without either mental planning or the urge of a conscious vital volition or emotional desire. Often enough his act is contrary to his intention or his desire; it proceeds out of him in subjection to a need or compulsion, in submission to an impulse, in obedience to a force in him that pushes for self-expression or in conscious pursuance of a higher principle. Desire is an additional lure to which Nature has given a great part in the life of animated beings in order to produce a certain kind of rajasic action necessary for her intermediate ends; but it is not her sole or even her chief engine. It has its great use while it endures: it helps us to rise out of inertia, it contradicts many tamasic forces which would otherwise inhibit action. But the seeker who has advanced far on the way of works has passed beyond this intermediate stage in which desire is a helpful engine. Its push is no longer indispensable for his action, but is rather a terrible hindrance and source of stumbling, inefficiency and failure. Others are obliged to obey a personal choice or motive, but he has to learn to act with an impersonal or a universal mind or as a part or an instrument of an infinite Person. A calm indifference, a joyful impartiality or a blissful response to a divine Force, whatever its dictate, is the condition of his doing any effective work or undertaking any worth-while action. Not desire, not attachment must drive him, but a Will that stirs in a divine peace, a Knowledge that moves from the transcendent Light, a glad Impulse that is a force from the supreme Ananda.

*
* *

In an advanced stage of the Yoga it is indifferent to the seeker, in the sense of any personal preference, what action he shall do or not do; even whether he shall act or not, is not decided by his personal choice or pleasure. Always he is moved to do whatever is in consonance with the Truth or whatever the Divine demands through his nature. A false conclusion is sometimes drawn from this that the spiritual man, accepting the position in which Fate or God or his past Karma has placed him, content to work in the field and cadre of the family, clan, caste, nation, occupation which are his by birth and circumstance, will not and even perhaps ought not to make any movement to exceed them or to pursue any great mundane end. Since he has really no work to do, since he has only to use works, no matter what works, as long as he is in the body in order to arrive at liberation or, having arrived, only to obey the supreme Will and do whatever it dictates, the actual field given him is sufficient for the purpose. Once free, he has only to continue working in the sphere assigned to him by Fate and circumstances till the great hour arrives when he can at last disappear into the Infinite. To insist on any particular end or to work for some great mundane object is to fall into the illusion of works; it is to entertain the error that terrestrial life has an intelligible intention and contains objects worthy of pursuit. The great theory of Illusion, which is a practical denial of the Divine in the world, even when in idea it acknowledges the Presence, is once more before us. But the Divine is here in the world, — not only in status but in dynamis, not only as a spiritual self and presence but as power, force, energy, — and therefore a divine work in the world is possible.

There is no narrow principle, no field of cabined action that can be imposed on the Karmayogin as his rule or his province. This much is true that every kind of works, whether small to man's imagination or great, petty in scope or wide, can be equally used in the progress towards liberation or for self-discipline. This much is also true that after liberation a man may dwell in any sphere of life and in any kind of action and fulfil there his existence in the Divine. According as he is moved by the Spirit, he may remain in the sphere assigned to him by birth and circumstances or break that framework and go forth to an untrammelled action which shall be the fitting body of his greatened consciousness and higher knowledge. To the outward eyes of men the inner liberation may make no apparent difference in his outward acts; or, on the contrary, the freedom and infinity within may translate itself into an outward dynamic working so large and new that all regards are drawn by this novel force. If such be the intention of the Supreme within him, the liberated soul may be content with a subtle and limited action within the old human surroundings which will in no way seek to change their outward appearance. But it may too be called to a work which will not only alter the forms and sphere of its own external life but, leaving nothing around it unchanged or unaffected, create a new world or a new order.

*
* *

A prevalent idea would persuade us that the sole aim of liberation is to secure for the individual soul freedom from physical rebirth in the unstable life of the universe. If this freedom is once assured, there is no further work for it in life here or elsewhere or only that which the continued existence of the body demands or the unfulfilled effects of past lives necessitate. This little, rapidly exhausted or consumed by the fire of Yoga, will cease with the departure of the released soul from the body. The aim of escape from rebirth, now long fixed in the Indian mentality as the highest object of the soul, has replaced the enjoyment of a heaven beyond fixed in the mentality of the devout by many religions as their divine lure. Indian religion also upheld that earlier and lower call when the gross external interpretation of the Vedic hymns was the dominant creed, and the dualists in later India also have kept that as part of their supreme spiritual motive. Undoubtedly a release from the limitations of the mind and body into an eternal peace, rest, silence of the Spirit, makes a higher appeal than the offer of a heaven of mental joys or eternised physical pleasures, but this too after all is a lure; its insistence on the mind's world-weariness, the life-being's shrinking from the adventure of birth, strikes a chord of weakness and cannot be the supreme motive. The desire of personal salvation, however high its form, is an outcome of ego; it rests on the idea of our own individuality and its desire for its personal good or welfare, its longing for a release from suffering or its cry for the extinction of the trouble of becoming and makes that the supreme aim of our existence. To rise beyond the desire of personal salvation is necessary for the complete rejection of this basis of ego. If we seek the Divine, it should be for the sake of the Divine and for nothing else, because that is the supreme call of our being, the deepest truth of the spirit. The pursuit of liberation, of the soul's freedom, of the realisation of our true and highest self, of union with the Divine, is justified only because it is the highest law of our nature, because it is the attraction of that which is lower in us to that which is highest, because it is the Divine Will in us. That is its sufficient justification and its one truest reason; all other motives are excrescences, minor or incidental truths or useful lures which the soul must abandon, the moment their utility has passed and the state of oneness with the Supreme and with all beings has become our normal consciousness and the bliss of that state our spiritual atmosphere.

Often, we see this desire of personal salvation overcome by another attraction which also belongs to the higher turn of our nature and which indicates the essential character of the action the liberated soul must pursue. It is that which is implied in the great legend of the Amitabha Buddha who turned away when his spirit was on the threshold of Nirvana and took the vow never to cross it while a single being remained in the sorrow and the Ignorance. It is that which underlies the sublime verse of the Bhagavata Purana, "I desire not the supreme state with all its eight siddhis nor the cessation of rebirth; may I assume the sorrow of all creatures who suffer and enter into them so that they may be made free from grief." It is that which inspires a remarkable passage in a letter of Swami Vivekananda. "I have lost all wish for my salvation," wrote the great Vedantin, "may I be born again and again and suffer thousands of miseries so that I may worship the only God that exists, the only God I believe in, the sum-total of all souls, — and above all, my God the wicked, my God the miserable, my God the poor of all races, of all species is the special object of my worship. He who is the high and low, the saint and the sinner, the god and the worm, Him worship, the visible, the knowable, the real, the omnipresent; break all other idols. In whom there is neither past life nor future birth, nor death nor going nor coming, in whom we always have been and always will be one, Him worship; break all other idols."

The last two sentences contain indeed the whole gist of the matter. The true salvation or the true freedom from the chain of rebirth is not the rejection of terrestrial life or the individual's escape by a spiritual self-annihilation, even as the true renunciation is not the mere physical abandonment of family and society; it is the inner identification with the Divine in whom there is no limitation of past life and future birth but instead the eternal existence of the unborn Soul. He who is free inwardly, even doing actions, does nothing at all, says the Gita; for it is Nature that works in him under the control of the Lord of Nature. Equally, even if he assumes a hundred times the body, he is free from any chain of birth or mechanical wheel of existence since he lives in the unborn and undying spirit and not in the life of the body. Therefore attachment to the escape from rebirth is one of the idols which, whoever keeps, the sadhaka of the integral Yoga must break and cast away from him. For his Yoga is not limited to the realisation of the Transcendent beyond all world by the individual soul; it embraces also the realisation of the Universal, "the sum-total of all souls", and cannot therefore be confined to the movement of a personal salvation and escape.

Even in his transcendence of cosmic limitations he is still one with all in God; a divine work remains for him in the universe.

*
* *

That work cannot be fixed by any mind-made rule or human standard; for his consciousness has moved away from human law and limits and passed into the divine liberty, away from government by the external and transient into the self-rule of the inner and eternal, away from the binding forms of the finite into the free self-determination of the Infinite. "Howsoever he lives and acts," says the Gita, "he lives and acts in Me." The rules which the intellect of men lays down cannot apply to the liberated soul, — by the external criteria and tests which their mental associations and prejudgments prescribe, such a one cannot be judged; he is outside the narrow jurisdiction of these fallible tribunals. It is immaterial whether he wears the garb of the ascetic or lives the full life of the householder; whether he spends his days in what men call holy works or in the many-sided activities of the world; whether he devotes himself to the direct leading of men to the Light like Buddha, Christ or Shankara or governs kingdoms like Janaka or stands before men like Sri Krishna as a politician or a leader of armies; what he eats or drinks; what are his habits or his pursuits; whether he fails or succeeds; whether his work be one of construction or of destruction; whether he supports or restores an old order or labours to replace it by a new; whether his associates are those whom men delight to honour or those whom their sense of superior righteousness outcastes and reprobates; whether his life and deeds are approved by his contemporaries or he is condemned as a misleader of men and a fomenter of religious, moral or social heresies. He is not governed by the judgments of men or the laws laid down by the ignorant; he obeys an inner voice and is moved by an unseen Power. His real life is within and this is its description that he lives, moves and acts in God, in the Divine, in the Infinite.

But if his action is governed by no external rule, one rule it will observe that is not external; it will be dictated by no personal desire or aim, but will be a part of a conscious and eventually a well-ordered because self-ordered divine working in the world. The Gita declares that the action of the liberated man must be directed not by desire, but towards the keeping together of the world, its government, guidance, impulsion, maintenance in the path appointed to it. This injunction has been interpreted in the sense that the world being an illusion in which most men must be kept, since they are unfit for liberation, he must so act outwardly as to cherish in them an attachment to their customary works laid down for them by the social law. If so, it would be a poor and petty rule and every noble heart would reject it to follow rather the divine vow of Amitabha Buddha, the sublime prayer of the Bhagavata, the passionate aspiration of Vivekananda. But if we accept rather the view that the world is a divinely guided movement of Nature emerging in man towards God and that this is the work in which the Lord of the Gita declares that he is ever occupied although he himself has nothing ungained that he has yet to win, then a deep and true sense will appear for this great injunction. To participate in that divine work, to live for God in the world will be the rule of the Karmayogin; to live for God in the world and therefore so to act that the Divine may more and more manifest himself and the world go forward by whatever way of its obscure pilgrimage and move nearer to the divine ideal.

How he shall do this, in what particular way, can be decided by no general rule. It must develop or define itself from within; the decision lies between God and our self, the Supreme Self and the individual self that is the instrument of the work; even before liberation, it is from the inner self, as soon as we become conscious of it, that there rises the sanction, the spiritually determined choice. It is altogether from within that must come the knowledge of the work that has to be done. There is no particular work, no law or form or outwardly fixed or invariable way of works which can be said to be that of the liberated being. The phrase used in the Gita to express this work that has to be done has indeed been interpreted in the sense that we must do our duty without regard to the fruit. But this is a conception born of European culture which is ethical rather than spiritual and external rather than inwardly profound in its concepts. No such general thing as duty exists; we have only duties, often in conflict with each other, and these are determined by our environment, our social relations, our external status in life. They are of great value in training the immature moral nature and setting up a standard which discourages the action of selfish desire. It has already been said that so long as the seeker has no inner light, he must govern himself by the best light he has, and duty, a principle, a cause are among the standards he may temporarily erect and observe. But for all that, duties are external things, not stuff of the soul and cannot be the ultimate standard of action in this path. It is the duty of the soldier to fight when called upon, even to fire upon his own kith and kin; but such a standard or any akin to it cannot be imposed on the liberated man. On the other hand, to love or have compassion, to obey the highest truth of our being, to follow the command of the Divine are not duties; these things are a law of the nature as it rises towards the Divine, an outflowing of action from a soul-state, a high reality of the spirit. The action of the liberated doer of works must be even such an outflowing from the soul; it must come to him or out of him as a natural result of his spiritual union with the Divine and not be formed by an edifying construction of the mental thought and will, the practical reason or the social sense. In the ordinary life a personal, social or traditional constructed rule, standard or ideal is the guide; once the spiritual journey has begun, this must be replaced by an inner and outer rule or way of living necessary for our self-discipline, liberation and perfection, a way of living proper to the path we follow or enjoined by the spiritual guide and master, the Guru, or else dictated by a Guide within us. But in the last state of the soul's infinity and freedom all outward standards are replaced or laid aside and there is left only a spontaneous and integral obedience to the Divine with whom we are in union and an action spontaneously fulfilling the integral spiritual truth of our being and nature.

*
*   *

It is this deeper sense in which we must accept the dictum of the Gita that action determined and governed by the nature must be our law of works. It is not, certainly, the superficial temperament or the character or habitual impulses that are meant, but in the literal sense of the Sanskrit word our "own being", our essential nature, the divine stuff of our souls. Whatever springs from this root or flows from these sources is profound, essential, right; the rest — opinions, impulses, habits, desires — may be merely surface formations or casual vagaries of the being or impositions from outside. They shift and change, but this remains constant. It is not the executive forms taken by Nature in us that are ourselves or the abidingly constant and expressive shape of ourselves; it is the spiritual being in us — and this includes the soul-becoming of it — that persists through time in the universe.

We cannot, however, easily distinguish this true inner law of our being; it is kept screened from us so long as the heart and intellect remain unpurified from egoism: till then we follow superficial and impermanent ideas, impulses, desires, suggestions and impositions of all kinds from our environment or work out formations of our temporary mental, vital, physical personality — that passing experimental and structural self which has been made for us by an interaction between our being and the pressure of a lower cosmic Nature. In proportion as we are purified, the true being within declares itself more clearly; our will is less entangled in suggestions from outside or shut up in our own superficial mental constructions. Egoism renounced, the nature purified, action will come from the soul's dictates, from the depths or the heights of the spirit, or it will be openly governed by the Lord who was all the time seated secretly within our hearts. The supreme and final word of the Gita for the Yogin is that he should leave all conventional formulas of belief and action, all fixed and external rules of conduct, all constructions of the outward or surface Nature, *dharmas*, and take refuge in the Divine alone. Free from desire and attachment, one with all beings, living in the infinite Truth and Purity and acting out of the profoundest deeps of his inner consciousness, governed by his immortal, divine and highest Self, all his works will be directed by the Power within through that essential spirit and nature in us which, knowing, warring, working, loving, serving, is always divine, towards the fulfilment of God in the world, an expression of the Eternal in Time.

A divine action arising spontaneously, freely, infallibly from the light and force of our spiritual self in union with the Divine is the last state of this integral Yoga of Works. The truest reason why we must seek liberation is not to be delivered, individually, from the sorrow of the world, though that deliverance too will be given to us, but that we may be one with the Divine, the Supreme, the Eternal. The truest reason why we must seek perfection, a supreme status, purity, knowledge, strength, love, capacity, is not that personally we may enjoy the divine Nature or be even as the gods, though that enjoyment too will be ours, but because this liberation and perfection are the divine Will in us, the highest truth of our self in Nature, the always intended goal of a progressive manifestation in the universe. The divine Nature, free and perfect and blissful, must be manifested in the individual in order that it may manifest in the world. Even in the Ignorance the individual lives really in the universal and for the universal Purpose, for in the very act of pursuing the purposes and desires of his ego, he is forced by Nature to contribute by his egoistic action to her work and purpose in the worlds; but it is without conscious intention, imperfectly done, and his contribution is to her half-evolved and half-conscient, her imperfect and crude movement. To escape from ego and be united with the Divine is at once the liberation and the consummation of his individuality; so liberated, purified, perfected, the individual — the divine soul — lives consciously and entirely, as was from the first intended, in and for the cosmic and transcendent Divine and for his Will in the universe.

In the Way of Knowledge we may arrive at a point where we can leap out of personality and universe, escape from all thought and will and works and all way of Nature and, absorbed and taken up into Eternity, plunge into the Transcendence; that, though not obligatory on the God-knower, may be the soul's decision, the turn pursued by the self within us. In the Way of

Devotion we may reach through an intensity of adoration and joy union with the supreme All-Beloved and remain eternally in the ecstasy of his presence, absorbed in him alone, intimately in one world of bliss with him; that then may be our being's impulsion, its spiritual choice. But in the Way of Works another prospect opens; for travelling on that path, we can enter into liberation and perfection by becoming of one law and power of nature with the Eternal; we are identified with him in our will and dynamic self as much as in our spiritual status; a divine way of works is the natural outcome of this union, a divine living in a spiritual freedom the body of its self-expression. In the Integral Yoga these three lines of approach give up their exclusions, meet and coalesce or spring out of each other; liberated from the mind's veil over the self, we live in the Transcendence, enter by the adoration of the heart into the oneness of a supreme love and bliss, and all our forces of being uplifted into the one Force, our will and works surrendered into the one Will and Power, assume the dynamic perfection of the divine Nature.

Appendix
to Part I

The following chapter was left unfinished. It was not included in the edition of *The Synthesis of Yoga*, Part I, that was published during Sri Aurobindo's lifetime.

Chapter XIII

The Supermind and the Yoga of Works

AN INTEGRAL Yoga includes as a vital and indispensable element in its total and ultimate aim the conversion of the whole being into a higher spiritual consciousness and a larger divine existence. Our parts of will and action, our parts of knowledge, our thinking being, our emotional being, our being of life, all our self and nature must seek the Divine, enter into the Infinite, unite with the Eternal. But man's present nature is limited, divided, unequal, — it is easiest for him to concentrate in the strongest part of his being and follow a definite line of progress proper to his nature: only rare individuals have the strength to take a large immediate plunge straight into the sea of the Divine Infinity. Some therefore must choose as a starting-point a concentration in thought or contemplation or the mind's one-pointedness to find the eternal reality of the Self in them; others can more easily withdraw into the heart to meet there the Divine, the Eternal: yet others are predominantly dynamic and active; for these it is best to centre themselves in the will and enlarge their being through works. United with the Self and source of all by their surrender of their will into its infinity, guided in their works by the secret Divinity within or surrendered to the Lord of the cosmic action as the master and mover of all their energies of thought, feeling, act, becoming by this enlargement of being selfless and universal, they can reach by works some first fullness of a spiritual status. But the path, whatever its point of starting, must debouch into a vaster dominion; it must proceed in the end through a totality of integrated knowledge, emotion, will of dynamic action, perfection of the being and the entire nature. In the supramental consciousness, on the level of the supramental existence this integration becomes consummate;

there knowledge, will, emotion, the perfection of the self and the dynamic nature rise each to its absolute of itself and all to their perfect harmony and fusion with each other, to a divine integrality, a divine perfection. For the supermind is a Truth-Consciousness in which the Divine Reality, fully manifested, no longer works with the instrumentation of the Ignorance; a truth of status of being which is absolute becomes dynamic in a truth of energy and activity of the being which is self-existent and perfect. Every movement there is a movement of the self-aware truth of Divine Being and every part is in entire harmony with the whole. Even the most limited and finite action is in the Truth-Consciousness a movement of the Eternal and Infinite and partakes of the inherent absoluteness and perfection of the Eternal and Infinite. An ascent into the supramental Truth not only raises our spiritual and essential consciousness to that height but brings about a descent of this Light and Truth into all our being and all our parts of nature. All then becomes part of the Divine Truth, an element and means of the supreme union and oneness; this ascent and descent must be therefore an ultimate aim of this Yoga.

A union with the Divine Reality of our being and all being is the one essential object of the Yoga. It is necessary to keep this in mind; we must remember that our Yoga is not undertaken for the sake of the acquisition of supermind itself but for the sake of the Divine; we seek the supermind not for its own joy and greatness but to make the union absolute and complete, to feel it, possess it, dynamise it in every possible way of our being, in its highest intensities and largest widenesses and in every range and turn and nook and recess of our nature. It is a mistake to think, as many are apt to think, that the object of a supramental Yoga is to arrive at a mighty magnificence of supermanhood, a divine power and greatness, the self-fulfilment of a magnified individual personality. This is a false and disastrous conception, — disastrous because it is likely to raise the pride, vanity and ambition of the rajasic vital mind in us and that, if not overpassed and overcome, must lead to spiritual downfall, false because it is an egoistic conception and the first condition of the supramental change is to get rid of ego. It is most dangerous for the active and dynamic nature of the man of will and works which can easily be led away by the pursuit of power. Power comes inevitably by the supramental change, it is a necessary condition for a perfect action: but it is the Divine Shakti that comes and takes up the nature and the life, the power of the One acting through the spiritual individual; it is not an aggrandisement of the personal force, not the last crowning fulfilment of the separative mental and vital ego. Self-fulfilment is a result of the Yoga, but its aim is not the greatness of the individual. The sole aim is a spiritual perfection, a finding of the true self and a union with the Divine by putting on the divine consciousness and nature.[1] All the rest is constituent detail and attendant circumstance. Ego-centric impulses, ambition, desire of power and greatness, motives of self-assertion are foreign to this greater consciousness and would be an insuperable bar against any possibility of even a distant approach towards the supramental change. One must lose one's little lower self to find the greater self. Union with the Divine must be the master motive; even the discovery of the truth of one's own being and of all being, life in that truth and its greater consciousness, perfection of the nature are only the natural results of that movement. Indispensable conditions of its entire consummation, they are part of the central aim only because they are a necessary development and a major consequence.

It must also be kept in mind that the supramental change is difficult, distant, an ultimate stage; it must be regarded as the end of a far-off vista; it cannot be and must not be turned into a first aim, a constantly envisaged goal or an immediate objective. For it can only come into the view of possibility after much arduous self-conquest and self-exceeding, at the end of many long and trying stages of a difficult self-evolution of the nature. One must first acquire an inner Yogic consciousness and replace by it our ordinary view of things, natural movements, motives of life; one must revolutionise the whole present build of our being. Next, we have to go still deeper, discover our veiled psychic entity and

---

[1] *sādharmya mukti.*

in its light and under its government psychicise our inner and
outer parts, turn mind-nature, life-nature, body-nature and all
our mental, vital, physical action and states and movements
into a conscious instrumentation of the soul. Afterwards or
concurrently we have to spiritualise the being in its entirety by
a descent of a divine Light, Force, Purity, Knowledge, freedom
and wideness. It is necessary to break down the limits of the personal mind, life and physicality, dissolve the ego, enter into the
cosmic consciousness, realise the self, acquire a spiritualised and
universalised mind and heart, life-force, physical consciousness.
Then only the passage into supramental consciousness begins to
become possible, and even then there is a difficult ascent to make
each stage of which is a separate arduous achievement. Yoga is
a rapid and concentrated conscious evolution of the being, but
however rapid, even though it may effect in a single life what in
an unassisted Nature might take centuries and millenniums or
many hundreds of lives, still all evolution must move by stages;
even the greatest rapidity and concentration of the movement
cannot swallow up all the stages or reverse natural process and
bring the end near to the beginning. A hasty and ignorant mind,
a too eager force easily forget this necessity; they rush forward
to make the supermind an immediate aim and expect to pull it
down with a pitchfork from its highest heights in the Infinite.
This is not only an absurd expectation but full of danger. For the
vital desire may very well bring in an action of dark or vehement
vital powers which hold out before it a promise of immediate
fulfilment of its impossible longing; the consequence is likely to
be a plunge into many kinds of self-deception, a yielding to the
falsehoods and temptations of the forces of darkness, a hunt
for supernormal powers, a turning away from the Divine to the
Asuric nature, a fatal self-inflation into an unnatural unhuman
and undivine bigness of magnified ego. If the being is small, the
nature weak and incapable, there is not this large-scale disaster;
but a loss of balance, a mental unhinging and fall into unreason or a vital unhinging and consequent moral aberration or a
deviation into some kind of morbid abnormality of the nature
may be the untoward consequence. This is not a Yoga in which

abnormality of any kind, even if it be an exalted abnormality, can be admitted as a way to self-fulfilment or spiritual realisation. Even when one enters into supernormal and suprarational experience, there should be no disturbance of the poise which must be kept firm from the summit of the consciousness to its base; the experiencing consciousness must preserve a calm balance, an unfailing clarity and order in its observation, a sort of sublimated commonsense, an unfailing power of self-criticism, right discrimination, coordination and firm vision of things; a sane grasp on facts and a high spiritualised positivism must always be there. It is not by becoming irrational or infrarational that one can go beyond ordinary nature into supernature; it should be done by passing through reason to a greater light of superreason. This superreason descends into reason and takes it up into higher levels even while breaking its limitations; reason is not lost but changes and becomes its own true unlimited self, a coordinating power of the supernature.

Another error that has to be guarded against is also one to which our mentality is easily prone; it is to take some higher intermediate consciousness or even any kind of supernormal consciousness for the supermind. To reach supermind it is not enough to go above the ordinary movements of the human mind; it is not enough to receive a greater light, a greater power, a greater joy or to develop capacities of knowledge, sight, effective will that surpass the normal range of the human being. All light is not the light of the spirit, still less is all light the light of the supermind; the mind, the vital, the physical itself have lights of their own, as yet hidden, which can be very inspiring, exalting, informative, powerfully executive. A breaking out into the cosmic consciousness may also bring in an immense enlargement of the consciousness and power. An opening into the inner mind, inner vital, inner physical, any range of the subliminal consciousness, can liberate an activity of abnormal or supernormal powers of knowledge, action or experience which the uninstructed mind can easily mistake for spiritual revelations, inspirations, intuitions. An opening upward into the greater ranges of the higher mental being can bring down much light and force creating an intense activity of the intuitivised mind and life-power or an ascent into these ranges can bring a true but still incomplete light easily exposed to mixture, a light which is spiritual in its source though it does not always remain spiritual in its active character when it comes down into the lower nature. But none of these things is the supramental light, the supramental power; that can only be seen and grasped when we have reached the summits of mental being, entered into overmind and stand on the borders of an upper, a greater hemisphere of spiritual existence. There the ignorance, the inconscience, the original blank Nescience slowly awaking towards a half-knowledge, which are the basis of material Nature and which surround, penetrate and powerfully limit all our powers of mind and life, cease altogether; for an unmixed and unmodified Truth-consciousness is there the substance of all the being, its pure spiritual texture. To imagine that we have reached such a condition when we are still moving in the dynamics of the Ignorance, though it may be an enlightened or illumined Ignorance, is to lay ourselves open either to a disastrous misleading or to an arrest of the evolution of the being. For if it is some inferior state that we thus mistake for the supermind, it lays us open to all the dangers we have seen to attend a presumptuous egoistic haste in our demand for achievement. If it is one of the higher states that we presume to be the highest, we may, though we achieve much, yet fall short of the greater, more perfect goal of our being; for we shall remain content with an approximation and the supreme transformation will escape us. Even the achievement of a complete inner liberation and a high spiritual consciousness is not that supreme transformation; for we may have that achievement, a status perfect in itself, in essence, and still our dynamic parts may in their instrumentation belong to an enlightened spiritualised mind and may be in consequence, like all mind, defective even in its greater power and knowledge, still subject to a partial or local obscuration or a limitation by the original circumscribing nescience.

*
*   *

Part II

The Yoga of Integral Knowledge

Chapter I

The Object of Knowledge

ALL SPIRITUAL seeking moves towards an object of Knowledge to which men ordinarily do not turn the eye of the mind, to someone or something Eternal, Infinite, Absolute that is not the temporal things or forces of which we are sensible, although he or it may be in them or behind them or their source or creator. It aims at a state of knowledge by which we can touch, enter or know by identity this Eternal, Infinite and Absolute, a consciousness other than our ordinary consciousness of ideas and forms and things, a Knowledge that is not what we call knowledge but something self-existent, everlasting, infinite. And although it may or even necessarily must, since man is a mental creature, start from our ordinary instruments of knowledge, yet it must as necessarily go beyond them and use supra-sensuous and supramental means and faculties, for it is in search of something that is itself supra-sensuous and supramental and beyond the grasp of the mind and senses, even if through mind and sense there can come a first glimpse of it or a reflected image.

The traditional systems, whatever their other differences, all proceed on the belief or the perception that the Eternal and Absolute can only be or at least can only inhabit a pure transcendent state of non-cosmic existence or else a non-existence. All cosmic existence or all that we call existence is a state of ignorance. Even the highest individual perfection, even the most blissful cosmic condition is no better than a supreme ignorance. All that is individual, all that is cosmic has to be austerely renounced by the seeker of the absolute Truth. The supreme quiescent Self or else the absolute Nihil is the sole Truth, the only object of spiritual knowledge. The state of knowledge, the consciousness other than this temporal that we must attain is Nirvana, an extinction of ego, a cessation of all mental, vital and physical activities, of all activities whatsoever, a supreme illumined quiescence, the pure bliss of an impersonal tranquillity self-absorbed and ineffable. The means are meditation, a concentration excluding all things else, a total loss of the mind in its object. Action is permissible only in the first stages of the search in order to purify the seeker and make him morally and temperamentally a fit vessel for the knowledge. Even this action must either be confined to the performance of the rites of worship and the prescribed duties of life rigorously ordained by the Hindu Shastra or, as in the Buddhistic discipline, must be guided along the eightfold path to the supreme practice of the works of compassion which lead towards the practical annihilation of self in the good of others. In the end, in any severe and pure Jnanayoga, all works must be abandoned for an entire quiescence. Action may prepare salvation; it cannot give it. Any continued adherence to action is incompatible with the highest progress and may be an insuperable obstacle to the attainment of the spiritual goal. The supreme state of quiescence is the very opposite of action and cannot be attained by those who persist in works. And even devotion, love, worship are disciplines for the unripe soul, are at best the best methods of the Ignorance. For they are offered to something other, higher and greater than ourselves; but in the supreme knowledge there can be no such thing, since there is either only one self or no self at all and therefore either no one to do the worship and offer the love and devotion or no one to receive it. Even thought-activity must disappear in the sole consciousness of identity or of nothingness and by its own quiescence bring about the quiescence of the whole nature. The absolute Identical alone must remain or else the eternal Nihil.

This pure Jnanayoga comes by the intellect, although it ends in the transcendence of the intellect and its workings. The thinker in us separates himself from all the rest of what we phenomenally are, rejects the heart, draws back from the life and the senses, separates from the body that he may arrive at his own exclusive fulfilment in that which is beyond even himself and his function. There is a truth that underlies, as there is an experience that seems to justify this attitude. There is an Essence that is in its nature a quiescence, a supreme of Silence in the Being that is beyond its own developments and mutations, immutable and therefore superior to all activities of which it is at most a Witness. And in the hierarchy of our psychological functions the Thought is in a way nearest to this Self, nearest at least to its aspect of the all-conscious knower who regards all activities but can stand back from them all. The heart, will and other powers in us are fundamentally active, turn naturally towards action, find through it their fulfilment, — although they also may automatically arrive at a certain quiescence by fullness of satisfaction in their activities or else by a reverse process of exhaustion through perpetual disappointment and dissatisfaction. The thought too is an active power, but is more capable of arriving at quiescence by its own conscious choice and will. The thought is more easily content with the illumined intellectual perception of this silent Witness Self that is higher than all our activities and, that immobile Spirit once seen, is ready, deeming its mission of truth-finding accomplished, to fall at rest and become itself immobile. For in its most characteristic movement it is itself apt to be a disinterested witness, judge, observer of things more than an eager participant and passionate labourer in the work and can arrive very readily at a spiritual or philosophic calm and detached aloofness. And since men are mental beings, thought, if not truly their best and highest, is at least their most constant, normal and effective means for enlightening their ignorance. Armed with its functions of gathering and reflection, meditation, fixed contemplation, the absorbed dwelling of the mind on its object, *śravaṇa, manana, nididhyāsana*, it stands at our tops as an indispensable aid to our realisation of that which we pursue, and it is not surprising that it should claim to be the leader of the journey and the only available guide or at least the direct and innermost door of the temple.

In reality, thought is only a scout and pioneer; it can guide but not command or effectuate. The leader of the journey, the captain of the march, the first and most ancient priest of our sacrifice is the Will. This Will is not the wish of the heart or the demand or preference of the mind to which we often give the name. It is that inmost, dominant and often veiled conscious force of our being and of all being, Tapas, Shakti, Sraddha, that sovereignly determines our orientation and of which the intellect and the heart are more or less blind and automatic servants and instruments. The Self that is quiescent, at rest, vacant of things and happenings is a support and background to existence, a silent channel or a hypostasis of something Supreme: it is not itself the one entirely real existence, not itself the Supreme. The Eternal, the Supreme is the Lord and the all-originating Spirit. Superior to all activities and not bound by any of them, it is the source, sanction, material, efficient power, master of all activities. All activities proceed from this supreme Self and are determined by it; all are its operations, processes of its own conscious force and not of something alien to Self, some power other than the Spirit. In these activities is expressed the conscious Will or Shakti of the Spirit moved to manifest its being in infinite ways, a Will or Power not ignorant but at one with its own self-knowledge and its knowledge of all that it is put out to express. And of this Power a secret spiritual will and soul-faith in us, the dominant hidden force of our nature, is the individual instrument, more nearly in communication with the Supreme, a surer guide and enlightener, could we once get at it and hold it, because profounder and more intimately near to the Identical and Absolute than the surface activities of our thought powers. To know that will in ourselves and in the universe and follow it to its divine finalities, whatever these may be, must surely be the highest way and truest culmination for knowledge as for works, for the seeker in life and for the seeker in Yoga.

The thought, since it is not the highest or strongest part of Nature, not even the sole or deepest index to Truth, ought not to follow its own exclusive satisfaction or take that for the sign of its attainment to the supreme Knowledge. It is here as the guide, up to a certain point, of the heart, the life and the other members, but it cannot be a substitute for them; it has to see not only what is its own ultimate satisfaction but whether there is not an ultimate satisfaction intended also for these other members. An exclusive path of abstract thought would be justified, only if the object of the Supreme Will in the universe has been nothing more than a descent into the activity of the ignorance operated by the mind as blinding instrument and jailor through false idea and sensation and an ascent into the quiescence of knowledge equally operated by the mind through correct thought as enlightening instrument and saviour. But the chances are that there is an aim in the world less absurd and aimless, an impulse towards the Absolute less dry and abstract, a truth of the world more large and complex, a more richly infinite height of the Infinite. Certainly, an abstract logic must always arrive, as the old systems arrived, at an infinite empty Negation or an infinite equally vacant Affirmation; for, abstract it moves towards an absolute abstraction and these are the only two abstractions that are absolutely absolute. But a concrete ever deepening wisdom waiting on more and more riches of infinite experience and not the confident abstract logic of the narrow and incompetent human mind is likely to be the key to a divine suprahuman knowledge. The heart, the will, the life and even the body, no less than the thought, are forms of a divine Conscious-Being and indices of great significance. These too have powers by which the soul can return to its complete self-awareness or means by which it can enjoy it. The object of the Supreme Will may well be a culmination in which the whole being is intended to receive its divine satisfaction, the heights enlightening the depths, the material Inconscient revealed to itself as the Divine by the touch of the supreme Superconscience.

The traditional Way of Knowledge proceeds by elimination and rejects successively the body, the life, the senses, the heart, the very thought in order to merge into the quiescent Self or supreme Nihil or indefinite Absolute. The way of integral knowledge supposes that we are intended to arrive at an integral self-fulfilment and the only thing that is to be eliminated is our own unconsciousness, the Ignorance and the results of the Ignorance. Eliminate the falsity of the being which figures as the ego; then our true being can manifest in us. Eliminate the falsity of the life which figures as mere vital craving and the mechanical round of our corporeal existence; our true life in the power of the Godhead and the joy of the Infinite will appear. Eliminate the falsity of the senses with their subjection to material shows and to dual sensations; there is a greater sense in us that can open through these to the Divine in things and divinely reply to it. Eliminate the falsity of the heart with its turbid passions and desires and its dual emotions; a deeper heart in us can open with its divine love for all creatures and its infinite passion and yearning for the responses of the Infinite. Eliminate the falsity of the thought with its imperfect mental constructions, its arrogant assertions and denials, its limited and exclusive concentrations; a greater faculty of knowledge is behind that can open to the true Truth of God and the soul and Nature and the universe. An integral self-fulfilment, — an absolute, a culmination for the experiences of the heart, for its instinct of love, joy, devotion and worship; an absolute, a culmination for the senses, for their pursuit of divine beauty and good and delight in the forms of things; an absolute, a culmination for the life, for its pursuit of works, of divine power, mastery and perfection; an absolute, a culmination beyond its own limits for the thought, for its hunger after truth and light and divine wisdom and knowledge. Not something quite other than themselves from which they are all cast away is the end of these things in our nature, but something supreme in which they at once transcend themselves and find their own absolutes and infinitudes, their harmonies beyond measure.

Behind the traditional way of Knowledge, justifying its thought-process of elimination and withdrawal, stands an overmastering spiritual experience. Deep, intense, convincing, common to all who have overstepped a certain limit of the active mind-belt into horizonless inner space, this is the great experience of liberation, the consciousness of something within us that is behind and outside of the universe and all its forms, interests, aims, events and happenings, calm, untouched, unconcerned, illimitable, immobile, free, the uplook to something above us indescribable and unseizable into which by abolition of our personality we can enter, the presence of an omnipresent eternal witness Purusha, the sense of an Infinity or a Timelessness that looks down on us from an august negation of all our existence and is alone the one thing Real. This experience is the highest sublimation of spiritualised mind looking resolutely beyond its own existence. No one who has not passed through this liberation can be entirely free from the mind and its meshes, but one is not compelled to linger in this experience for ever. Great as it is, it is only the Mind's overwhelming experience of what is beyond itself and all it can conceive. It is a supreme negative experience, but beyond it is all the tremendous light of an infinite Consciousness, an illimitable Knowledge, an affirmative absolute Presence.

The object of spiritual knowledge is the Supreme, the Divine, the Infinite and Absolute. This Supreme has its relations to our individual being and its relations to the universe and it transcends both the soul and the universe. Neither the universe nor the individual are what they seem to be, for the report of them which our mind and our senses give us is, so long as they are unenlightened by a faculty of higher supramental and suprasensuous knowledge, a false report, an imperfect construction, an attenuated and erroneous figure. And yet that which the universe and the individual seem to be is still a figure of what they really are, a figure that points beyond itself to the reality behind it. Truth proceeds by a correction of the values our mind and senses give us, and first by the action of a higher intelligence that enlightens and sets right as far as may be the conclusions of the ignorant sense-mind and limited physical intelligence; that is the method of all human knowledge and science. But beyond it there is a knowledge, a Truth-consciousness, that exceeds our intellect and brings us into the true light of which it is a refracted ray. There the abstract terms of the pure reason and the constructions of the mind disappear or are converted into concrete soul-vision and the tremendous actuality of spiritual experience. This knowledge can turn away to the absolute Eternal and lose vision of the soul and the universe; but it can too see this existence from that Eternal. When that is done, we find that the ignorance of the mind and the senses and all the apparent futilities of human life were not a useless excursion of the conscious being, an otiose blunder. Here they were planned as a rough ground for the self-expression of the Soul that comes from the Infinite, a material foundation for its self-unfolding and self-possessing in the terms of the universe. It is true that in themselves they and all that is here have no significance and to build separate significances for them is to live in an illusion, Maya; but they have a supreme significance in the Supreme, an absolute Power in the Absolute and it is that that assigns to them and refers to that Truth their present relative values. This is the all-uniting experience that is the foundation of the deepest integral and most intimate self-knowledge and world-knowledge.

In relation to the individual the Supreme is our own true and highest self, that which ultimately we are in our essence, that of which we are in our manifested nature. A spiritual knowledge, moved to arrive at the true Self in us, must reject, as the traditional way of knowledge rejects, all misleading appearances. It must discover that the body is not our self, our foundation of existence; it is a sensible form of the Infinite. The experience of Matter as the world's sole foundation and the physical brain and nerves and cells and molecules as the one truth of all things in us, the ponderous inadequate basis of materialism, is a delusion, a half-view taken for the whole, the dark bottom or shadow of things misconceived as the luminous substance, the effective figure of zero for the Integer. The materialist idea mistakes a creation for the creative Power, a means of expression for That which is expressed and expresses. Matter and our physical brain and nerves and body are the field and foundation for one action of a vital force that serves to connect the Self with the form of its works and maintains them by its direct dynamis. The material movements are an exterior notation by which the soul represents its perceptions of certain truths of the Infinite and makes them effective in the terms of Substance. These things are a language, a notation, a hieroglyphic, a system of symbols, not themselves the deepest truest sense of the things they intimate.

Neither is the Life ourself, the vitality, the energy which plays in the brain, nerves and body; it is a power and not the whole power of the Infinite. The experience of a life-force instrumentalising Matter as the foundation, source and true sum of all things, the vibrating unsteady basis of vitalism, is a delusion, a half-view taken for the whole, a tide on a near shore misconceived as all the ocean and its waters. The vitalist idea takes something powerful but outward for the essence. Life-force is the dynamisation of a consciousness which exceeds it. That consciousness is felt and acts but does not become valid to us in intelligence until we arrive at the higher term of Mind, our present summit. Mind is here apparently a creation of Life, but it is really the ulterior — not the ultimate — sense of Life itself and what is behind it and a more conscious formulation of its secret; Mind is an expression not of Life, but of that of which Life itself is a less luminous expression.

And yet Mind also, our mentality, our thinking, understanding part, is not our Self, is not That, not the end or the beginning; it is a half-light thrown from the Infinite. The experience of mind as the creator of forms and things and of these forms and things existing in the Mind only, the thin subtle basis of idealism, is also a delusion, a half-view taken for the whole, a pale refracted light idealised as the burning body of the Sun and its splendour. This idealist vision also does not arrive at the essence of being, does not even touch it but only an inferior mode of Nature. Mind is the dubious outer penumbra of a conscious existence which is not limited by mentality but exceeds it. The method of the traditional way of knowledge, eliminating all these things, arrives at the conception and realisation of a pure conscious existence, self-aware, self-blissful, unconditioned by mind and life and body and to its ultimate positive experience that is Atman, the Self, the original and essential nature of our existence. Here at last there is something centrally true, but in its haste to arrive at it this knowledge assumes that there is nothing between the thinking mind and the Highest, *buddheḥ paratas tu saḥ*, and, shutting its eyes in Samadhi, tries to rush through all that actually intervenes without even seeing these great and luminous kingdoms of the Spirit. Perhaps it arrives at its object, but only to fall asleep in the Infinite. Or, if it remains awake, it is in the highest experience of the Supreme into which the self-annulling Mind can enter, but not in the supreme of the Supreme, Paratpara. The Mind can only be aware of the Self in a mentalised spiritual thinness, only of the mind-reflected Sachchidananda. The highest truth, the integral self-knowledge is not to be gained by this self-blinded leap into the Absolute but by a patient transit beyond the mind into the Truth-consciousness where the Infinite can be known, felt, seen, experienced in all the fullness of its unending riches. And there we discover this Self that we are to be not only a static tenuous vacant Atman but a great dynamic Spirit individual, universal and transcendent. That Self and Spirit cannot be expressed by the mind's abstract generalisations; all the inspired descriptions of the seers and mystics cannot exhaust its contents and its splendours.

In relation to the universe the Supreme is Brahman, the one Reality which is not only the spiritual material and conscious substance of all the ideas and forces and forms of the universe, but their origin, support and possessor, the cosmic and supracosmic Spirit. All the last terms to which we can reduce the universe, Force and Matter, Name and Form, Purusha and Prakriti, are still not entirely that which the universe really is, either in itself or its nature. As all that we are is the play and form, the mental, psychic, vital and physical expression of a supreme Self unconditioned by mind and life and body, the universe too is the play and form and cosmic soul-expression and nature-expression of a supreme Existence which is unconditioned by force and matter, unconditioned by idea and name and form, unconditioned by the fundamental distinction of Purusha and Prakriti. Our supreme Self and the supreme Existence which has become the universe are one Spirit, one self and one existence. The individual is in nature one expression of the universal Being, in spirit an emanation of the Transcendence. For if he finds his self, he finds too that his own true self is not this natural personality, this created individuality, but is a universal being in its relations with others and with Nature and in its upward term a portion or the living front of a supreme transcendental Spirit.

This supreme Existence is not conditioned by the individual

or by the universe. A spiritual knowledge can therefore surpass or even eliminate these two powers of the Spirit and arrive at the conception of something utterly Transcendent, something that is unnameable and mentally unknowable, a sheer Absolute. The traditional way of knowledge eliminates individual and universe. The Absolute it seeks after is featureless, indefinable, relationless, not this, not that, *neti neti*. And yet we can say of it that it is One, that it is Infinite, that it is ineffable Bliss, Consciousness, Existence. Although unknowable to the mind, yet through our individual being and through the names and forms of the universe we can approach the realisation of the supreme Self that is Brahman, and by the realisation of the self we come to a certain realisation also of this utter Absolute of which our true self is the essential form in our consciousness (*svarūpa*). These are the devices the human mind is compelled to use if it is to form to itself any conception at all of a transcendent and unconditioned Absolute. The system of negation is indispensable to it in order to get rid of its own definitions and limited experience; it is obliged to escape through a vague Indefinite into the Infinite. For it lives in a closed prison of constructions and representations that are necessary for its action but are not the self-existent truth either of Matter or Life or Mind or Spirit. But if we can once cross beyond the Mind's frontier twilight into the vast plane of supramental Knowledge, these devices cease to be indispensable. Supermind has quite another, a positive and direct and living experience of the supreme Infinite. The Absolute is beyond personality and beyond impersonality, and yet it is both the Impersonal and the supreme Person and all persons. The Absolute is beyond the distinction of unity and multiplicity, and yet it is the One and the innumerable Many in all the universes. It is beyond all limitation by quality and yet it is not limited by a qualitiless void but is too all infinite qualities. It is the individual soul and all souls and none of them; it is the formless Brahman and the universe. It is the cosmic and the supracosmic Spirit, the supreme Lord, the supreme Self, the supreme Purusha and supreme Shakti, the Ever Unborn who is endlessly born, the Infinite who is innumerably finite, the multitudinous

One, the complex Simple, the many-sided Single, the Word of the Silence Ineffable, the impersonal omnipresent Person, the Mystery translucent in highest consciousness to its own spirit, but to a lesser consciousness veiled in its own exceeding light and impenetrable for ever. These things are to the dimensional mind irreconcilable opposites, but to the constant vision and experience of the supramental Truth-consciousness they are so simply and inevitably the intrinsic nature of each other that even to think of them as contraries is an unimaginable violence. The walls constructed by the measuring and separating Intellect have disappeared and the Truth in its simplicity and beauty appears and reduces all to terms of its harmony and unity and light. Dimensions and distinctions remain but as figures for use, not a separative prison for the self-forgetting Spirit.

The consciousness of the transcendent Absolute with its consequence in individual and universe is the last, the eternal knowledge. Our minds may deal with it on various lines, may build upon it conflicting philosophies, may limit, modify, over-stress, understress sides of the knowledge, deduce from it truth or error; but our intellectual variations and imperfect statements make no difference to the ultimate fact that if we push thought and experience to their end, this is the knowledge in which they terminate. The object of a Yoga of spiritual knowledge can be nothing else than this eternal Reality, this Self, this Brahman, this Transcendent that dwells over all and in all and is manifest yet concealed in the individual, manifest yet disguised in the universe.

The culmination of the path of knowledge need not necessarily entail extinction of our world-existence. For the Supreme to whom we assimilate ourselves, the Absolute and Transcendent into whom we enter has always the complete and ultimate consciousness for which we are seeking and yet he supports by it his play in the world. Neither are we compelled to believe that our world-existence ends because by attaining to knowledge its object or consummation is fulfilled and therefore there is nothing more for us here afterwards. For what we gain at first with its release and immeasurable silence and quietude is only the eternal self-realisation by the individual in the essence of his conscious being; there will still remain on that foundation, unannulled by the silence, one with the release and freedom, the infinitely proceeding self-fulfilment of Brahman, its dynamic divine manifestation in the individual and by his presence, example and action in others and in the universe at large, — the work which the Great Ones remain to do. Our dynamic self-fulfilment cannot be worked out so long as we remain in the egoistic consciousness, in the mind's candle-lit darkness, in the bondage. Our present limited consciousness can only be a field of preparation, it can consummate nothing; for all that it manifests is marred through and through by an ego-ridden ignorance and error. The true and divine self-fulfilment of Brahman in the manifestation is only possible on the foundation of the Brahman-consciousness and therefore through the acceptance of life by the liberated soul, the Jivanmukta.

This is the integral knowledge; for we know that everywhere and in all conditions all to the eye that sees is One, to a divine experience all is one block of the Divine. It is only the mind which for the temporary convenience of its own thought and aspiration seeks to cut an artificial line of rigid division, a fiction of perpetual incompatibility between one aspect and another of the eternal oneness. The liberated knower lives and acts in the world not less than the bound soul and ignorant mind but more, doing all actions, *sarvakṛt*, only with a true knowledge and a greater conscient power. And by so doing he does not forfeit the supreme unity nor fall from the supreme consciousness and the highest knowledge. For the Supreme, however hidden now to us, is here in the world no less than he could be in the most utter and ineffable self-extinction, the most intolerant Nirvana.

Chapter II

The Status of Knowledge

THE SELF, the Divine, the Supreme Reality, the All, the Transcendent, — the One in all these aspects is then the object of Yogic knowledge. Ordinary objects, the external appearances of life and matter, the psychology of our thoughts and actions, the perception of the forces of the apparent world can be part of this knowledge, but only in so far as it is part of the manifestation of the One. It becomes at once evident that the knowledge for which Yoga strives must be different from what men ordinarily understand by the word. For we mean ordinarily by knowledge an intellectual appreciation of the facts of life, mind and matter and the laws that govern them. This is a knowledge founded upon our sense-perception and upon reasoning from our sense-perceptions and it is undertaken partly for the pure satisfaction of the intellect, partly for practical efficiency and the added power which knowledge gives in managing our lives and the lives of others, in utilising for human ends the overt or secret forces of Nature and in helping or hurting, in saving and ennobling or in oppressing and destroying our fellow-men. Yoga, indeed, is commensurate with all life and can include all these subjects and objects. There is even a Yoga[1] which can be used for self-indulgence as well as for self-conquest, for hurting others as well as for their salvation. But "all life" includes not only, not even mainly life as humanity now leads it. It envisages rather and regards as its one true object a higher truly conscious existence which our half-conscious humanity does not yet possess and can only arrive at by a self-exceeding spiritual ascension. It is this greater consciousness and higher existence

---

[1] Yoga develops power, it develops it even when we do not desire or consciously aim at it; and power is always a double-edged weapon which can be used to hurt or destroy as well as to help and save. Be it also noted that all destruction is not evil.

which is the peculiar and appropriate object of Yogic discipline.

This greater consciousness, this higher existence are not an enlightened or illumined mentality supported by a greater dynamic energy or supporting a purer moral life and character. Their superiority to the ordinary human consciousness is not in degree but in kind and essence. There is a change not merely of the surface or instrumental manner of our being but of its very foundation and dynamic principle. Yogic knowledge seeks to enter into a secret consciousness beyond mind which is only occultly here, concealed at the basis of all existence. For it is that consciousness alone that truly knows and only by its possession can we possess God and rightly know the world and its real nature and secret forces. All this world visible or sensible to us and all too in it that is not visible is merely the phenomenal expression of something beyond the mind and the senses. The knowledge which the senses and intellectual reasoning from the data of the senses can bring us, is not true knowledge; it is a science of appearances. And even appearances cannot be properly known unless we know first the Reality of which they are images. This Reality is their self and there is one self of all; when that is seized, all other things can then be known in their truth and no longer as now only in their appearance.

It is evident that however much we may analyse the physical and sensible, we cannot by that means arrive at the knowledge of the Self or of ourselves or of that which we call God. The telescope, the microscope, the scalpel, the retort and alembic cannot go beyond the physical, although they may arrive at subtler and subtler truths about the physical. If then we confine ourselves to what the senses and their physical aids reveal to us and refuse from the beginning to admit any other reality or any other means of knowledge, we are obliged to conclude that nothing is real except the physical and that there is no Self in us or in the universe, no God within and without, no ourselves even except this aggregate of brain, nerves and body. But this we are only obliged to conclude because we have assumed it firmly from the beginning and therefore cannot but circle round to our original assumption.

If, then, there is a Self, a Reality not obvious to the senses, it must be by other means than those of physical Science that it is to be sought and known. The intellect is not that means. Undoubtedly there are a number of suprasensuous truths at which the intellect is able to arrive in its own manner and which it is able to perceive and state as intellectual conceptions. The very idea of Force for instance on which Science so much insists, is a conception, a truth at which the intellect alone can arrive by going beyond its data; for we do not sense this universal force but only its results, and the force itself we infer as a necessary cause of these results. So also the intellect by following a certain line of rigorous analysis can arrive at the intellectual conception and the intellectual conviction of the Self and this conviction can be very real, very luminous, very potent as the beginning of other and greater things. Still, in itself intellectual analysis can only lead to an arrangement of clear conceptions, perhaps to a right arrangement of true conceptions; but this is not the knowledge aimed at by Yoga. For it is not in itself an effective knowledge. A man may be perfect in it and yet be precisely what he was before except in the mere fact of the greater intellectual illumination. The change of our being at which Yoga aims, may not at all take place.

It is true that intellectual deliberation and right discrimination are an important part of the Yoga of knowledge; but their object is rather to remove a difficulty than to arrive at the final and positive result of this path. Our ordinary intellectual notions are a stumbling-block in the way of knowledge; for they are governed by the error of the senses and they found themselves on the notion that matter and body are the reality, that life and force are the reality, that passion and emotion, thought and sense are the reality; and with these things we identify ourselves, and because we identify ourselves with these things we cannot get back to the real self. Therefore, it is necessary for the seeker of knowledge to remove this stumbling-block and to get right notions about himself and the world; for how shall we pursue by knowledge the real self if we have no notion of what it is and are on the contrary burdened with ideas quite opposite to the truth?

Therefore right thought is a necessary preliminary, and once the habit of right thought is established, free from sense-error and desire and old association and intellectual prejudgment, the understanding becomes purified and offers no serious obstacle to the farther process of knowledge. Still, right thought only becomes effective when in the purified understanding it is followed by other operations, by vision, by experience, by realisation.

What are these operations? They are not mere psychological self-analysis and self-observation. Such analysis, such observation are, like the process of right thought, of immense value and practically indispensable. They may even, if rightly pursued, lead to a right thought of considerable power and effectivity. Like intellectual discrimination by the process of meditative thought they will have an effect of purification; they will lead to self-knowledge of a certain kind and to the setting right of the disorders of the soul and the heart and even of the disorders of the understanding. Self-knowledge of all kinds is on the straight path to the knowledge of the real Self. The Upanishad tells us that the Self-existent has so set the doors of the soul that they turn outwards and most men look outward into the appearances of things; only the rare soul that is ripe for a calm thought and steady wisdom turns its eye inward, sees the Self and attains to immortality. To this turning of the eye inward psychological self-observation and analysis is a great and effective introduction. We can look into the inward of ourselves more easily than we can look into the inward of things external to us because there, in things outside us, we are in the first place embarrassed by the form and secondly we have no natural previous experience of that in them which is other than their physical substance. A purified or tranquillised mind may reflect or a powerful concentration may discover God in the world, the Self in Nature even before it is realised in ourselves, but this is rare and difficult.[2] And it is only in ourselves that we can observe and know the

---

[2] In one respect, however, it is easier, because in external things we are not so much hampered by the sense of the limited ego as in ourselves; one obstacle to the realisation of God is therefore removed.

process of the Self in its becoming and follow the process by which it draws back into self-being. Therefore the ancient counsel, know thyself, will always stand as the first word that directs us towards *the* knowledge. Still, psychological self-knowledge is only the experience of the modes of the Self, it is not the realisation of the Self in its pure being.

The status of knowledge, then, which Yoga envisages is not merely an intellectual conception or clear discrimination of the truth, nor is it an enlightened psychological experience of the modes of our being. It is a "realisation", in the full sense of the word; it is the making real to ourselves and in ourselves of the Self, the transcendent and universal Divine, and it is the subsequent impossibility of viewing the modes of being except in the light of that Self and in their true aspect as its flux of becoming under the psychical and physical conditions of our world-existence. This realisation consists of three successive movements, internal vision, complete internal experience and identity.

This internal vision, *dṛṣṭi*, the power so highly valued by the ancient sages, the power which made a man a Rishi or Kavi and no longer a mere thinker, is a sort of light in the soul by which things unseen become as evident and real to it — to the soul and not merely to the intellect — as do things seen to the physical eye. In the physical world there are always two forms of knowledge, the direct and the indirect, *pratyakṣa*, of that which is present to the eyes, and *parokṣa*, of that which is remote from and beyond our vision. When the object is beyond our vision, we are necessarily obliged to arrive at an idea of it by inference, imagination, analogy, by hearing the descriptions of others who have seen it or by studying pictorial or other representations of it if these are available. By putting together all these aids we can indeed arrive at a more or less adequate idea or suggestive image of the object, but we do not realise the thing itself; it is not yet to us the grasped reality, but only our conceptual representation of a reality. But once we have seen it with the eyes, — for no other sense is adequate, — we possess, we realise; it is there secure in our satisfied being, part of ourselves in knowledge.

Precisely the same rule holds good of psychical things and of the Self. We may hear clear and luminous teachings about the Self from philosophers or teachers or from ancient writings; we may by thought, inference, imagination, analogy or by any other available means attempt to form a mental figure or conception of it; we may hold firmly that conception in our mind and fix it by an entire and exclusive concentration;[3] but we have not yet realised it, we have not seen God. It is only when after long and persistent concentration or by other means the veil of the mind is rent or swept aside, only when a flood of light breaks over the awakened mentality, *jyotirmaya brahman*, and conception gives place to a knowledge-vision in which the Self is as present, real, concrete as a physical object to the physical eye, that we possess in knowledge; for we have seen. After that revelation, whatever fadings of the light, whatever periods of darkness may afflict the soul, it can never irretrievably lose what it has once held. The experience is inevitably renewed and must become more frequent till it is constant; when and how soon depends on the devotion and persistence with which we insist on the path and besiege by our will or our love the hidden Deity.

This inner vision is one form of psychological experience; but the inner experience is not confined to that seeing; vision only opens, it does not embrace. Just as the eye, though it is alone adequate to bring the first sense of realisation, has to call in the aid of experience by the touch and other organs of sense before there is an embracing knowledge, so the vision of the self ought to be completed by an experience of it in all our members. Our whole being ought to demand God and not only our illumined eye of knowledge. For since each principle in us is only a manifestation of the Self, each can get back to its reality and have the experience of it. We can have a mental experience of the Self and seize as concrete realities all those apparently abstract things that to the mind constitute existence — consciousness, force, delight and their manifold forms and workings: thus the

---

[3] This is the idea of the triple operation of Jnanayoga, *śravaṇa, manana, nididhyāsana,* hearing, thinking or mentalising and fixing in concentration.

mind is satisfied of God. We can have an emotional experience of the Self through Love and through emotional delight, love and delight of the Self in us, of the Self in the universal and of the Self in all with whom we have relations: thus the heart is satisfied of God. We can have an aesthetic experience of the Self in beauty, a delight-perception and taste of the absolute reality all-beautiful in everything whether created by ourselves or Nature in its appeal to the aesthetic mind and the senses; thus the sense is satisfied of God. We can have even the vital, nervous experience and practically the physical sense of the Self in all life and formation and in all workings of powers, forces, energies that operate through us or others or in the world: thus the life and the body are satisfied of God.

All this knowledge and experience are primary means of arriving at and of possessing identity. It is our self that we see and experience and therefore vision and experience are incomplete unless they culminate in identity, unless we are able to live in all our being the supreme Vedantic knowledge, He am I. We must not only see God and embrace Him, but become that Reality. We must become one with the Self in its transcendence of all form and manifestation by the resolution, the sublimation, the escape from itself of ego and all its belongings into That from which they proceed, as well as become the Self in all its manifested existences and becomings, one with it in the infinite existence, consciousness, peace, delight by which it reveals itself in us and one with it in the action, formation, play of self-conception with which it garbs itself in the world.

It is difficult for the modern mind to understand how we can do more than conceive intellectually of the Self or of God; but it may borrow some shadow of this vision, experience and becoming from that inner awakening to Nature which a great English poet has made a reality to the European imagination. If we read the poems in which Wordsworth expressed his realisation of Nature, we may acquire some distant idea of what realisation is. For, first, we see that he had the vision of something in the world which is the very Self of all things that it contains, a conscious force and presence other than its forms, yet cause of its forms and manifested in them. We perceive that he had not only the vision of this and the joy and peace and universality which its presence brings, but the very sense of it, mental, aesthetic, vital, physical; not only this sense and vision of it in its own being but in the nearest flower and simplest man and the immobile rock; and, finally, that he even occasionally attained to that unity, that becoming the object of his meditation, one phase of which is powerfully and profoundly expressed in the poem "A slumber did my spirit seal," where he describes himself as become one in his being with earth, "rolled round in its diurnal course with rocks and stones and trees." Exalt this realisation to a profounder Self than physical Nature and we have the elements of the Yogic knowledge. But all this experience is only the vestibule to that suprasensuous, supramental realisation of the Transcendent who is beyond all His aspects, and the final summit of knowledge can only be attained by entering into the superconscient and there merging all other experience into a supernal unity with the Ineffable. That is the culmination of all divine knowing; that also is the source of all divine delight and divine living.

That status of knowledge is then the aim of this path and indeed of all paths when pursued to their end, to which intellectual discrimination and conception and all concentration and psychological self-knowledge and all seeking by the heart through love and by the senses through beauty and by the will through power and works and by the soul through peace and joy are only keys, avenues, first approaches and beginnings of the ascent which we have to use and to follow till the wide and infinite levels are attained and the divine doors swing open into the infinite Light.

Chapter III

The Purified Understanding

THE DESCRIPTION of the status of knowledge to which we aspire, determines the means of knowledge which we shall use. That status of knowledge may be summed up as a supramental realisation which is prepared by mental representations through various mental principles in us and once attained again reflects itself more perfectly in all the members of the being. It is a re-seeing and therefore a remoulding of our whole existence in the light of the Divine and One and Eternal free from subjection to the appearances of things and the externalities of our superficial being.

Such a passage from the human to the divine, from the divided and discordant to the One, from the phenomenon to the eternal Truth, such an entire rebirth or new birth of the soul must necessarily involve two stages, one of preparation in which the soul and its instruments must become fit and another of actual illumination and realisation in the prepared soul through its fit instruments. There is indeed no rigid line of demarcation in sequence of Time between these two stages; rather they are necessary to each other and continue simultaneously. For in proportion as the soul becomes fit it increases in illumination and rises to higher and higher, completer and completer realisations, and in proportion as these illuminations and these realisations increase, becomes fit and its instruments more adequate to their task: there are soul-seasons of unillumined preparation and soul-seasons of illumined growth and culminating soul-moments more or less prolonged of illumined possession, moments that are transient like the flash of the lightning, yet change the whole spiritual future, moments also that extend over many human hours, days, weeks in a constant light or blaze of the Sun of Truth. And through all these the soul once turned Godwards grows towards the permanence and perfection of its new birth and real existence.

The first necessity of preparation is the purifying of all the members of our being; especially, for the path of knowledge, the purification of the understanding, the key that shall open the door of Truth; and a purified understanding is hardly possible without the purification of the other members. An unpurified heart, an unpurified sense, an unpurified life confuse the understanding, disturb its data, distort its conclusions, darken its seeing, misapply its knowledge; an unpurified physical system clogs or chokes up its action. There must be an integral purity. Here also there is an interdependence; for the purification of each member of our being profits by the clarifying of every other, the progressive tranquillisation of the emotional heart helping for instance the purification of the understanding while equally a purified understanding imposes calm and light on the turbid and darkened workings of the yet impure emotions. It may even be said that while each member of our being has its own proper principles of purification, yet it is the purified understanding that in man is the most potent cleanser of his turbid and disordered being and most sovereignly imposes their right working on his other members. Knowledge, says the Gita, is the sovereign purity; light is the source of all clearness and harmony even as the darkness of ignorance is the cause of all our stumblings. Love, for example, is the purifier of the heart and by reducing all our emotions into terms of divine love the heart is perfected and fulfilled; yet love itself needs to be clarified by divine knowledge. The heart's love of God may be blind, narrow and ignorant and lead to fanaticism and obscurantism; it may, even when otherwise pure, limit our perfection by refusing to see Him except in a limited personality and by recoiling from the true and infinite vision. The heart's love of man may equally lead to distortions and exaggerations in feeling, action and knowledge which have to be corrected and prevented by the purification of the understanding.

We must, however, consider deeply and clearly what we mean by the understanding and by its purification. We use the word as the nearest equivalent we can get in the English tongue to the Sanskrit philosophical term *buddhi*; therefore we exclude from it the action of the sense mind which merely consists of the recording of perceptions of all kinds without distinction whether they be right or wrong, true or mere illusory phenomena, penetrating or superficial. We exclude that mass of confused conception which is merely a rendering of these perceptions and is equally void of the higher principle of judgment and discrimination. Nor can we include that constant leaping current of habitual thought which does duty for understanding in the mind of the average unthinking man, but is only a constant repetition of habitual associations, desires, prejudices, prejudgments, received or inherited preferences, even though it may constantly enrich itself by a fresh stock of concepts streaming in from the environment and admitted without the challenge of the sovereign discriminating reason. Undoubtedly this is a sort of understanding which has been very useful in the development of man from the animal; but it is only one remove above the animal mind; it is a half-animal reason subservient to habit, to desire and the senses and is of no avail in the search whether for scientific or philosophical or spiritual knowledge. We have to go beyond it; its purification can only be effected either by dismissing or silencing it altogether or by transmuting it into the true understanding.

By the understanding we mean that which at once perceives, judges and discriminates, the true reason of the human being not subservient to the senses, to desire or to the blind force of habit, but working in its own right for mastery, for knowledge. Certainly, the reason of man as he is at present does not even at its best act entirely in this free and sovereign fashion; but so far as it fails, it fails because it is still mixed with the lower half-animal action, because it is impure and constantly hampered and pulled down from its characteristic action. In its purity it should not be involved in these lower movements, but stand back from the object, and observe disinterestedly, put it in its right place in the whole by force of comparison, contrast, analogy, reason from its rightly observed data by deduction, induction, inference and holding all its gains in memory and supplementing them by a chastened and rightly-guided imagination view all in the light of a trained and disciplined judgment. Such is the pure intellectual understanding of which disinterested observation, judgment and reasoning are the law and characterising action.

But the term *buddhi* is also used in another and profounder sense. The intellectual understanding is only the lower *buddhi*; there is another and a higher *buddhi* which is not intelligence but vision, is not understanding but rather an over-standing[1] in knowledge, and does not seek knowledge and attain it in subjection to the data it observes but possesses already the truth and brings it out in the terms of a revelatory and intuitional thought. The nearest the human mind usually gets to this truth-conscious knowledge is that imperfect action of illumined finding which occurs when there is a great stress of thought and the intellect electrified by constant discharges from behind the veil and yielding to a higher enthusiasm admits a considerable instreaming from the intuitive and inspired faculty of knowledge. For there is an intuitive mind in man which serves as a recipient and channel for these instreamings from a supramental faculty. But the action of intuition and inspiration in us is imperfect in kind as well as intermittent in action; ordinarily, it comes in response to a claim from the labouring and struggling heart or intellect and, even before its givings enter the conscious mind, they are already affected by the thought or aspiration which went up to meet them, are no longer pure but altered to the needs of the heart or intellect; and after they enter the conscious mind, they are immediately seized upon by the intellectual understanding and dissipated or broken up so as to fit in with our imperfect intellectual knowledge, or by the heart and remoulded to suit our blind or half-blind emotional longings and preferences, or even by the lower cravings and distorted to the vehement uses of our hungers and passions.

If this higher *buddhi* could act pure of the interference of

---

[1] The Divine Being is described as the *adhyakṣa*, he who seated over all in the supreme ether over-sees things, views and controls them from above.

these lower members, it would give pure forms of the truth; observation would be dominated or replaced by a vision which could see without subservient dependence on the testimony of the sense-mind and senses; imagination would give place to the self-assured inspiration of the truth, reasoning to the spontaneous discernment of relations and conclusion from reasoning to an intuition containing in itself those relations and not building laboriously upon them, judgment to a thought-vision in whose light the truth would stand revealed without the mask which it now wears and which our intellectual judgment has to penetrate; while memory too would take upon itself that larger sense given to it in Greek thought and be no longer a paltry selection from the store gained by the individual in his present life, but rather the all-recording knowledge which secretly holds and constantly gives from itself everything that we now seem painfully to acquire but really in this sense remember, a knowledge which includes the future[2] no less than the past. Certainly, we are intended to grow in our receptivity to this higher faculty of truth-conscious knowledge, but its full and unveiled use is as yet the privilege of the gods and beyond our present human stature.

We see then what we mean precisely by the understanding and by that higher faculty which we may call for the sake of convenience the ideal faculty and which stands to the developed intellect much in the same relation as that intellect stands to the half-animal reason of the undeveloped man. It becomes evident also what is the nature of the purification which is necessary before the understanding can fulfil rightly its part in the attainment of right knowledge. All impurity is a confusion of working, a departure from the *dharma*, the just and inherently right action of things which in that right action are pure and helpful to our perfection and this departure is usually the result of an ignorant confusion[3] of dharmas in which the function lends itself to the demand of other tendencies than those which are properly its own.

---

[2] In this sense the power of prophecy has been aptly called a memory of the future.
[3] *saṅkara*.

The first cause of impurity in the understanding is the inter-miscence of desire in the thinking functions, and desire itself is an impurity of the Will involved in the vital and emotional parts of our being. When the vital and emotional desires interfere with the pure will-to-know, the thought-function becomes sub-servient to them, pursues ends other than those proper to itself and its perceptions are clogged and deranged. The understanding must lift itself beyond the siege of desire and emotion and, in order that it may have perfect immunity, it must get the vital parts and the emotions themselves purified. The will to enjoy is proper to the vital being but not the choice or the reaching after the enjoyment which must be determined and acquired by higher functions; therefore the vital being must be trained to accept whatever gain or enjoyment comes to it in the right functioning of the life in obedience to the working of the divine Will and to rid itself of craving and attachment. Similarly the heart must be freed from subjection to the cravings of the life-principle and the senses and thus rid itself of the false emotions of fear, wrath, hatred, lust, etc. which constitute the chief impurity of the heart. The will to love is proper to the heart, but here also the choice and reaching after love have to be foregone or tranquillised and the heart taught to love with depth and intensity indeed, but with a calm depth and a settled and equal, not a troubled and disordered intensity. The tranquillisation and mastery[4] of these members is a first condition for the immunity of the understanding from error, ignorance and perversion. This purification spells an entire equality of the nervous being and the heart; equality, therefore, even as it was the first word of the path of works, so also is the first word of the path of knowledge.

The second cause of impurity in the understanding is the illusion of the senses and the intermiscence of the sense-mind in the thinking functions. No knowledge can be true knowledge which subjects itself to the senses or uses them otherwise than as first indices whose data have constantly to be corrected and over-passed. The beginning of Science is the examination of the truths

---

[4] *śama* and *dama*.

of the world-force that underlie its apparent workings such as our senses represent them to be; the beginning of philosophy is the examination of the principles of things which the senses mistranslate to us; the beginning of spiritual knowledge is the refusal to accept the limitations of the sense-life or to take the visible and sensible as anything more than phenomenon of the Reality.

Equally must the sense-mind be stilled and taught to leave the function of thought to the mind that judges and understands. When the understanding in us stands back from the action of the sense-mind and repels its intermiscence, the latter detaches itself from the understanding and can be watched in its separate action. It then reveals itself as a constantly swirling and eddying undercurrent of habitual concepts, associations, perceptions, desires without any real sequence, order or principle of light. It is a constant repetition in a circle unintelligent and unfruitful. Ordinarily the human understanding accepts this undercurrent and tries to reduce it to a partial order and sequence; but by so doing it becomes itself subject to it and partakes of that disorder, restlessness, unintelligent subjection to habit and blind purposeless repetition which makes the ordinary human reason a misleading, limited and even frivolous and futile instrument. There is nothing to be done with this fickle, restless, violent and disturbing factor but to get rid of it whether by detaching it and then reducing it to stillness or by giving a concentration and singleness to the thought by which it will of itself reject this alien and confusing element.

A third cause of impurity has its source in the understanding itself and consists in an improper action of the will to know. That will is proper to the understanding, but here again choice and unequal reaching after knowledge clog and distort. They lead to a partiality and attachment which makes the intellect cling to certain ideas and opinions with a more or less obstinate will to ignore the truth in other ideas and opinions, cling to certain fragments of a truth and shy against the admission of other parts which are yet necessary to its fullness, cling to certain predilections of knowledge and repel all knowledge that does not agree with the personal temperament of thought which has been acquired by the past of the thinker. The remedy lies in a perfect equality of the mind, in the cultivation of an entire intellectual rectitude and in the perfection of mental disinterestedness. The purified understanding as it will not lend itself to any desire or craving, so will not lend itself either to any predilection or distaste for any particular idea or truth, and will refuse to be attached even to those ideas of which it is the most certain or to lay on them such an undue stress as is likely to disturb the balance of truth and depreciate the values of other elements of a complete and perfect knowledge.

An understanding thus purified would be a perfectly flexible, entire and faultless instrument of intellectual thought and being free from the inferior sources of obstruction and distortion would be capable of as true and complete a perception of the truths of the Self and the universe as the intellect can attain. But for real knowledge something more is necessary, since real knowledge is by our very definition of it supra-intellectual. In order that the understanding may not interfere with our attainment to real knowledge, we have to reach to that something more and cultivate a power exceedingly difficult for the active intellectual thinker and distasteful to his proclivities, the power of intellectual passivity. The object served is double and therefore two different kinds of passivity have to be acquired.

In the first place we have seen that intellectual thought is in itself inadequate and is not the highest thinking; the highest is that which comes through the intuitive mind and from the supramental faculty. So long as we are dominated by the intellectual habit and by the lower workings, the intuitive mind can only send its messages to us subconsciously and subject to a distortion more or less entire before it reaches the conscious mind; or if it works consciously, then only with an inadequate rarity and a great imperfection in its functioning. In order to strengthen the higher knowledge-faculty in us we have to effect the same separation between the intuitive and intellectual elements of our thought as we have already effected between the understanding and the sense-mind; and this is no easy task, for not only do our intuitions come to us incrusted in the intellectual action, but there are a great number of mental workings which masquerade and ape the appearances of the higher faculty. The remedy is to train first the intellect to recognise the true intuition, to distinguish it from the false and then to accustom it, when it arrives at an intellectual perception or conclusion, to attach no final value to it, but rather look upward, refer all to the divine principle and wait in as complete a silence as it can command for the light from above. In this way it is possible to transmute a great part of our intellectual thinking into the luminous truth-conscious vision, — the ideal would be a complete transition, — or at least to increase greatly the frequency, purity and conscious force of the ideal knowledge working behind the intellect. The latter must learn to be subject and passive to the ideal faculty.

But for the knowledge of the Self it is necessary to have the power of a complete intellectual passivity, the power of dismissing all thought, the power of the mind to think not at all which the Gita in one passage enjoins. This is a hard saying for the occidental mind to which thought is the highest thing and which will be apt to mistake the power of the mind not to think, its complete silence for the incapacity of thought. But this power of silence is a capacity and not an incapacity, a power and not a weakness. It is a profound and pregnant stillness. Only when the mind is thus entirely still, like clear, motionless and level water, in a perfect purity and peace of the whole being and the soul transcends thought, can the Self which exceeds and originates all activities and becomings, the Silence from which all words are born, the Absolute of which all relativities are partial reflections manifest itself in the pure essence of our being. In a complete silence only is the Silence heard; in a pure peace only is its Being revealed. Therefore to us the name of That is the Silence and the Peace.

Chapter IV

Concentration

ALONG with purity and as a help to bring it about, concentration. Purity and concentration are indeed two aspects, feminine and masculine, passive and active, of the same status of being; purity is the condition in which concentration becomes entire, rightly effective, omnipotent; by concentration purity does its works and without it would only lead to a state of peaceful quiescence and eternal repose. Their opposites are also closely connected; for we have seen that impurity is a confusion of dharmas, a lax, mixed and mutually entangled action of the different parts of the being; and this confusion proceeds from an absence of right concentration of its knowledge on its energies in the embodied Soul. The fault of our nature is first an inert subjection to the impacts of things[1] as they come in upon the mind pell-mell without order or control and then a haphazard imperfect concentration managed fitfully, irregularly with a more or less chance emphasis on this or on that object according as they happen to interest, not the higher soul or the judging and discerning intellect, but the restless, leaping, fickle, easily tired, easily distracted lower mind which is the chief enemy of our progress. In such a condition purity, the right working of the functions, the clear, unstained and luminous order of the being is an impossibility; the various workings, given over to the chances of the environment and external influences, must necessarily run into each other and clog, divert, distract, pervert. Equally, without purity the complete, equal, flexible concentration of the being in right thought, right will, right feeling or secure status of spiritual experience is not possible. Therefore the two must proceed together, each helping the victory of the other, until we arrive at that eternal calm from which may proceed some

---

[1] *bāhyasparśa.*

partial image in the human being of the eternal, omnipotent and omniscient activity.

But in the path of knowledge as it is practised in India concentration is used in a special and more limited sense. It means that removal of the thought from all distracting activities of the mind and that concentration of it on the idea of the One by which the soul rises out of the phenomenal into the one Reality. It is by the thought that we dissipate ourselves in the phenomenal; it is by the gathering back of the thought into itself that we must draw ourselves back into the real. Concentration has three powers by which this aim can be effected. By concentration on anything whatsoever we are able to know that thing, to make it deliver up its concealed secrets; we must use this power to know not things, but the one Thing-in-itself. By concentration again the whole will can be gathered up for the acquisition of that which is still ungrasped, still beyond us; this power, if it is sufficiently trained, sufficiently single-minded, sufficiently sincere, sure of itself, faithful to itself alone, absolute in faith, we can use for the acquisition of any object whatsoever; but we ought to use it not for the acquisition of the many objects which the world offers to us, but to grasp spiritually that one object worthy of pursuit which is also the one subject worthy of knowledge. By concentration of our whole being on one status of itself, we can become whatever we choose; we can become, for instance, even if we were before a mass of weaknesses and fears, a mass instead of strength and courage, or we can become all a great purity, holiness and peace or a single universal soul of Love; but we ought, it is said, to use this power to become not even these things, high as they may be in comparison with what we now are, but rather to become that which is above all things and free from all action and attributes, the pure and absolute Being. All else, all other concentration can only be valuable for preparation, for previous steps, for a gradual training of the dissolute and self-dissipating thought, will and being towards their grand and unique object.

This use of concentration implies like every other a previous purification; it implies also in the end a renunciation, a cessation and lastly an ascent into the absolute and transcendent state of Samadhi from which if it culminates, if it endures, there is, except perhaps for one soul out of many thousands, no return. For by that we go to the "supreme state of the Eternal whence souls revert not" into the cyclic action of Nature;[2] and it is into this Samadhi that the Yogin who aims at release from the world seeks to pass away at the time of leaving his body. We see this succession in the discipline of the Rajayoga. For first the Rajayogin must arrive at a certain moral and spiritual purity; he must get rid of the lower or downward activities of his mind, but afterwards he must stop all its activities and concentrate himself in the one idea that leads from activity to the quiescence of status. The Rajayogic concentration has several stages, that in which the object is seized, that in which it is held, that in which the mind is lost in the status which the object represents or to which the concentration leads, and only the last is termed Samadhi in the Rajayoga although the word is capable, as in the Gita, of a much wider sense. But in the Rajayogic Samadhi there are different grades of status, — that in which the mind, though lost to outward objects, still muses, thinks, perceives in the world of thought, that in which the mind is still capable of primary thought-formations and that in which, all out-darting of the mind even within itself having ceased, the soul rises beyond thought into the silence of the Incommunicable and Ineffable. In all Yoga there are indeed many preparatory objects of thought-concentration, forms, verbal formulas of thought, significant names, all of which are supports[3] to the mind in this movement, all of which have to be used and transcended; the highest support according to the Upanishads is the mystic syllable AUM, whose three letters represent the Brahman or Supreme Self in its three degrees of status, the Waking Soul, the Dream Soul and the Sleep Soul, and the whole potent sound rises towards that which is beyond status as beyond activity.[4]

---

[2] *yato naiva nivartante tad dhāma paramaṁ mama.*   [3] *avalambana.*
[4] Mandukya Upanishad.

For of all Yoga of knowledge the final goal is the Transcendent.

We have, however, conceived as the aim of an integral Yoga something more complex and less exclusive — less exclusively positive of the highest condition of the soul, less exclusively negative of its divine radiations. We must aim indeed at the Highest, the Source of all, the Transcendent but not to the exclusion of that which it transcends, rather as the source of an established experience and supreme state of the soul which shall transform all other states and remould our consciousness of the world into the form of its secret Truth. We do not seek to excise from our being all consciousness of the universe, but to realise God, Truth and Self in the universe as well as transcendent of it. We shall seek therefore not only the Ineffable, but also His manifestation as infinite being, consciousness and bliss embracing the universe and at play in it. For that triune infinity is His supreme manifestation and that we shall aspire to know, to share in and to become; and since we seek to realise this Trinity not only in itself but in its cosmic play, we shall aspire also to knowledge of and participation in the universal divine Truth, Knowledge, Will, Love which are His secondary manifestation, His divine becoming. With this too we shall aspire to identify ourselves, towards this too we shall strive to rise and, when the period of effort is passed, allow it by our renunciation of all egoism to draw us up into itself in our being and to descend into us and embrace us in all our becoming. This not only as a means of approach and passage to His supreme transcendence, but as the condition, even when we possess and are possessed by the Transcendent, of a divine life in the manifestation of the cosmos.

In order that we may do this, the terms concentration and Samadhi must assume for us a richer and profound meaning. All our concentration is merely an image of the divine Tapas by which the Self dwells gathered in itself, by which it manifests within itself, by which it maintains and possesses its manifestation, by which it draws back from all manifestation into its supreme oneness. Being dwelling in consciousness upon itself for bliss, this is the divine Tapas; and a Knowledge-Will dwelling in force of consciousness on itself and its manifestations is the essence of the divine concentration, the Yoga of the Lord of Yoga. Given the self-differentiation of the Divine in which we dwell, concentration is the means by which the individual soul identifies itself with and enters into any form, state or psychological self-manifestation (*bhāva*) of the Self. To use this means for unification with the Divine is the condition for the attainment of divine knowledge and the principle of all Yoga of knowledge.

This concentration proceeds by the Idea, using thought, form and name as keys which yield up to the concentrating mind the Truth that lies concealed behind all thought, form and name; for it is through the Idea that the mental being rises beyond all expression to that which is expressed, to that of which the Idea itself is only the instrument. By concentration upon the Idea the mental existence which at present we are breaks open the barrier of our mentality and arrives at the state of consciousness, the state of being, the state of power of conscious-being and bliss of conscious-being to which the Idea corresponds and of which it is the symbol, movement and rhythm. Concentration by the Idea is, then, only a means, a key to open to us the superconscient planes of our existence; a certain self-gathered state of our whole existence lifted into that superconscient truth, unity and infinity of self-aware, self-blissful existence is the aim and culmination; and that is the meaning we shall give to the term Samadhi. Not merely a state withdrawn from all consciousness of the outward, withdrawn even from all consciousness of the inward into that which exists beyond both whether as seed of both or transcendent even of their seed-state; but a settled existence in the One and Infinite, united and identified with it, and this status to remain whether we abide in the waking condition in which we are conscious of the forms of things or we withdraw into the inward activity which dwells in the play of the principles of things, the play of their names and typal forms or we soar to the condition of static inwardness where we arrive at the principles themselves and at the principle of all principles, the seed of name and form.[5]

---

[5] The Waking, Dream and Sleep states of the soul.

For the soul that has arrived at the essential Samadhi and is settled in it (*samādhistha*) in the sense the Gita attaches to the word,
has that which is fundamental to all experience and cannot fall
from it by any experience however distracting to one who has
not yet ascended the summit. It can embrace all in the scope of
its being without being bound by any or deluded or limited.

When we arrive at this state, all our being and consciousness
being concentrated, the necessity of concentration in the Idea
ceases. For there in that supramental state the whole position of
things is reversed. The mind is a thing that dwells in diffusion,
in succession; it can only concentrate on one thing at a time
and when not concentrated runs from one thing to another very
much at random. Therefore it has to concentrate on a single
idea, a single subject of meditation, a single object of contemplation, a single object of will in order to possess or master it,
and this it must do to at least the temporary exclusion of all
others. But that which is beyond the mind and into which we
seek to rise is superior to the running process of the thought,
superior to the division of ideas. The Divine is centred in itself
and when it throws out ideas and activities does not divide itself
or imprison itself in them, but holds them and their movement
in its infinity; undivided, its whole self is behind each Idea and
each movement and at the same time behind all of them together.
Held by it, each spontaneously works itself out, not through a
separate act of will, but by the general force of consciousness
behind it; if to us there seems to be a concentration of divine Will
and Knowledge in each, it is a multiple and equal and not an
exclusive concentration, and the reality of it is rather a free and
spontaneous working in a self-gathered unity and infinity. The
soul which has risen to the divine Samadhi participates in the
measure of its attainment in this reversed condition of things, —
the true condition, for that which is the reverse of our mentality
is the truth. It is for this reason that, as is said in the ancient
books, the man who has arrived at Self-possession attains spontaneously without the need of concentration in thought and
effort the knowledge or the result which the Idea or the Will in
him moves out to embrace.

To arrive then at this settled divine status must be the object of our concentration. The first step in concentration must be always to accustom the discursive mind to a settled unwavering pursuit of a single course of connected thought on a single subject and this it must do undistracted by all lures and alien calls on its attention. Such concentration is common enough in our ordinary life, but it becomes more difficult when we have to do it inwardly without any outward object or action on which to keep the mind; yet this inward concentration is what the seeker of knowledge must effect.[6] Nor must it be merely the consecutive thought of the intellectual thinker, whose only object is to conceive and intellectually link together his conceptions. It is not, except perhaps at first, a process of reasoning that is wanted so much as a dwelling so far as possible on the fruitful essence of the idea which by the insistence of the soul's will upon it must yield up all the facets of its truth. Thus if it be the divine Love that is the subject of concentration, it is on the essence of the idea of God as Love that the mind should concentrate in such a way that the various manifestation of the divine Love should arise luminously, not only to the thought, but in the heart and being and vision of the sadhaka. The thought may come first and the experience afterwards, but equally the experience may come first and the knowledge arise out of the experience. Afterwards the thing attained has to be dwelt on and more and more held till it becomes a constant experience and finally the dharma or law of the being.

This is the process of concentrated meditation; but a more strenuous method is the fixing of the whole mind in concentration on the essence of the idea only, so as to reach not the thought-knowledge or the psychological experience of the subject, but the very essence of the thing behind the idea. In this process thought ceases and passes into the absorbed or ecstatic contemplation of the object or by a merging into it in an inner Samadhi. If this be the process followed, then subsequently the

[6] In the elementary stages of internal debate and judgment, *vitarka* and *vicāra*, for the correction of false ideas and arrival at the intellectual truth.

state into which we rise must still be called down to take possession of the lower being, to shed its light, power and bliss on our ordinary consciousness. For otherwise we may possess it, as many do, in the elevated condition or in the inward Samadhi, but we shall lose our hold of it when we awake or descend into the contacts of the world; and this truncated possession is not the aim of an integral Yoga.

A third process is neither at first to concentrate in a strenuous meditation on the one subject nor in a strenuous contemplation of the one object of thought-vision, but first to still the mind altogether. This may be done by various ways; one is to stand back from the mental action altogether not participating in but simply watching it until, tired of its unsanctioned leaping and running, it falls into an increasing and finally an absolute quiet. Another is to reject the thought-suggestions, to cast them away from the mind whenever they come and firmly hold to the peace of the being which really and always exists behind the trouble and riot of the mind. When this secret peace is unveiled, a great calm settles on the being and there comes usually with it the perception and experience of the all-pervading silent Brahman, everything else at first seeming to be mere form and eidolon. On the basis of this calm everything else may be built up in the knowledge and experience no longer of the external phenomena of things but of the deeper truth of the divine manifestation.

Ordinarily, once this state is obtained, strenuous concentration will be found no longer necessary. A free concentration of will[7] using thought merely for suggestion and the giving of light to the lower members will take its place. This Will will then insist on the physical being, the vital existence, the heart and the mind remoulding themselves in the forms of the Divine which reveal themselves out of the silent Brahman. By swifter or slower degrees according to the previous preparation and purification of the members, they will be obliged with more or less struggle to obey the law of the will and its thought-suggestion, so that

---

[7] This subject will be dealt with more in detail when we come to the Yoga of self-perfection.

eventually the knowledge of the Divine takes possession of our consciousness on all its planes and the image of the Divine is formed in our human existence even as it was done by the old Vedic Sadhakas. For the integral Yoga this is the most direct and powerful discipline.

Chapter V

Renunciation

IF DISCIPLINE of all the members of our being by purification and concentration may be described as the right arm of the body of Yoga, renunciation is its left arm. By discipline or positive practice we confirm in ourselves the truth of things, truth of being, truth of knowledge, truth of love, truth of works and replace with these the falsehoods that have overgrown and perverted our nature; by renunciation we seize upon the falsehoods, pluck up their roots and cast them out of our way so that they shall no longer hamper by their persistence, their resistance or their recurrence the happy and harmonious growth of our divine living. Renunciation is an indispensable instrument of our perfection.

How far shall this renunciation go? what shall be its nature? and in what way shall it be applied? There is an established tradition long favoured by great religious teachings and by men of profound spiritual experience that renunciation must not only be complete as a discipline but definite and final as an end and that it shall fall nothing short of the renunciation of life itself and of our mundane existence. Many causes have contributed to the growth of this pure, lofty and august tradition. There is first the profounder cause of the radical opposition between the sullied and imperfect nature of life in the world as it now is in the present stage of our human evolution and the nature of spiritual living; and this opposition has led to the entire rejection of world-existence as a lie, an insanity of the soul, a troubled and unhappy dream or at best a flawed, specious and almost worthless good or to its characterisation as a kingdom of the world, the flesh and the devil, and therefore for the divinely led and divinely attracted soul only a place of ordeal and preparation or at best a play of the All-existence, a game of cross-purposes which He tires of and abandons. A second cause is the soul's hunger for personal salvation, for escape into some farther or farthest height of unalloyed bliss and peace untroubled by the labour and the struggle; or else it is its unwillingness to return from the ecstasy of the divine embrace into the lower field of work and service. But there are other slighter causes incidental to spiritual experience, — strong feeling and practical proof of the great difficulty, which we willingly exaggerate into an impossibility, of combining the life of works and action with spiritual peace and the life of realisation; or else the joy which the mind comes to take in the mere act and state of renunciation, — as it comes indeed to take joy in anything that it has attained or to which it has inured itself, — and the sense of peace and deliverance which is gained by indifference to the world and to the objects of man's desire. Lowest causes of all are the weakness that shrinks from the struggle, the disgust and disappointment of the soul baffled by the great cosmic labour, the selfishness that cares not what becomes of those left behind us so long as we personally can be free from the monstrous ever-circling wheel of death and rebirth, the indifference to the cry that rises up from a labouring humanity.

For the sadhaka of an integral Yoga none of these reasons are valid. With weakness and selfishness, however spiritual in their guise or trend, he can have no dealings; a divine strength and courage and a divine compassion and helpfulness are the very stuff of that which he would be, they are that very nature of the Divine which he would take upon himself as a robe of spiritual light and beauty. The revolvings of the great wheel bring to him no sense of terror or giddiness; he rises above it in his soul and knows from above their divine law and their divine purpose. The difficulty of harmonising the divine life with human living, of being in God and yet living in man is the very difficulty that he is set here to solve and not to shun. He has learned that the joy, the peace and the deliverance are an imperfect crown and no real possession if they do not form a state secure in itself, inalienable to the soul, not dependent on aloofness and inaction but firm in the storm and the race and the battle, unsullied whether by the joy of the world or by its suffering. The ecstasy of the divine embrace will not abandon him because he obeys the impulse of divine love for God in humanity; or if it seems to draw back from him for a while, he knows by experience that it is to try and test him still farther so that some imperfection in his own way of meeting it may fall away from him. Personal salvation he does not seek except as a necessity for the human fulfilment and because he who is himself in bonds cannot easily free others, — though to God nothing is impossible; for a heaven of personal joys he has no hankerings even as a hell of personal sufferings has for him no terrors. If there is an opposition between the spiritual life and that of the world, it is that gulf which he is here to bridge, that opposition which he is here to change into a harmony. If the world is ruled by the flesh and the devil, all the more reason that the children of Immortality should be here to conquer it for God and the Spirit. If life is an insanity, then there are so many million souls to whom there must be brought the light of divine reason; if a dream, yet is it real within itself to so many dreamers who must be brought either to dream nobler dreams or to awaken; or if a lie, then the truth has to be given to the deluded. Nor, if it be said that only by the luminous example of escape from the world can we help the world, shall we accept that dogma, since the contrary example of great Avataras is there to show that not only by rejecting the life of the world as it is can we help, but also and more by accepting and uplifting it. And if it is a play of the All-Existence, then we may well consent to play out our part in it with grace and courage, well take delight in the game along with our divine Playmate.

But, most of all, the view we have taken of the world forbids the renunciation of world-existence so long as we can be anything to God and man in their working-out of its purposes. We regard the world not as an invention of the devil or a self-delusion of the soul, but as a manifestation of the Divine, although as yet a partial because a progressive and evolutionary manifestation. Therefore for us renunciation of life cannot be the goal of life nor rejection of the world the object for which the world was created. We seek to realise our unity with God, but for us that realisation involves a complete and absolute recognition of our unity with man and we cannot cut the two asunder. To use Christian language, the Son of God is also the Son of Man and both elements are necessary to the complete Christhood; or to use an Indian form of thought, the divine Narayana of whom the universe is only one ray is revealed and fulfilled in man; the complete man is Nara-Narayana and in that completeness he symbolises the supreme mystery of existence.

Therefore renunciation must be for us merely an instrument and not an object; nor can it be the only or the chief instrument since our object is the fulfilment of the Divine in the human being, a positive aim which cannot be reached by negative means. The negative means can only be for the removal of that which stands in the way of the positive fulfilment. It must be a renunciation, a complete renunciation of all that is other than and opposed to the divine self-fulfilment and a progressive renunciation of all that is a lesser or only a partial achievement. We shall have no attachment to our life in the world; if that attachment exists, we must renounce it and renounce utterly; but neither shall we have any attachment to the escape from the world, to salvation, to the great self-annihilation; if that attachment exists, that also we must renounce and renounce it utterly.

Again our renunciation must obviously be an inward renunciation; especially and above all, a renunciation of attachment and the craving of desire in the senses and the heart, of self-will in the thought and action and of egoism in the centre of the consciousness. For these things are the three knots by which we are bound to our lower nature and if we can renounce these utterly, there is nothing else that can bind us. Therefore attachment and desire must be utterly cast out; there is nothing in the world to which we must be attached, not wealth nor poverty, nor joy nor suffering, nor life nor death, nor greatness nor littleness, nor vice nor virtue, nor friend, nor wife, nor children, nor country, nor our work and mission, nor heaven nor earth, nor all that is within them or beyond them. And this does not mean that there is nothing at all that we shall love, nothing in which we shall take delight; for attachment is egoism in love and not love itself, desire is limitation and insecurity in a hunger for pleasure and satisfaction and not the seeking after the divine delight in things. A universal love we must have, calm and yet eternally intense beyond the brief vehemence of the most violent passion; a delight in things rooted in a delight in God that does not adhere to their forms but to that which they conceal in themselves and that embraces the universe without being caught in its meshes.[1]

Self-will in thought and action has, we have already seen, to be quite renounced if we would be perfect in the way of divine works; it has equally to be renounced if we are to be perfect in divine knowledge. This self-will means an egoism in the mind which attaches itself to its preferences, its habits, its past or present formations of thought and view and will because it regards them as itself or its own, weaves around them the delicate threads of "I-ness" and "my-ness" and lives in them like a spider in its web. It hates to be disturbed, as a spider hates attack on its web, and feels foreign and unhappy if transplanted to fresh view-points and formations as a spider feels foreign in another web than its own. This attachment must be entirely excised from the mind. Not only must we give up the ordinary attitude to the world and life to which the unawakened mind clings as its natural element; but we must not remain bound in any mental construction of our own or in any intellectual thought-system or arrangement of religious dogmas or logical conclusions; we must not only cut asunder the snare of the mind and the senses, but flee also beyond the snare of the thinker, the snare of the theologian and the church-builder, the meshes of the Word and the bondage of the Idea. All these are within us waiting to wall in the spirit with forms; but we must always go beyond, always renounce the lesser for the greater, the finite for the Infinite; we must be prepared to proceed from illumination to illumination, from experience to experience, from soul-state to soul-state so as to reach the utmost transcendence of the Divine and its utmost universality. Nor must we attach ourselves even

---

[1] *Nirlipta.* The divine Ananda in things is *niṣkāma* and *nirlipta*, free from desire and therefore not attached.

to the truths we hold most securely, for they are but forms and expressions of the Ineffable who refuses to limit himself to any form or expression; always we must keep ourselves open to the higher Word from above that does not confine itself to its own sense and the light of the Thought that carries in it its own opposites.

But the centre of all resistance is egoism and this we must pursue into every covert and disguise and drag it out and slay it; for its disguises are endless and it will cling to every shred of possible self-concealment. Altruism and indifference are often its most effective disguises; so draped, it will riot boldly in the very face of the divine spies who are missioned to hunt it out. Here the formula of the supreme knowledge comes to our help; we have nothing to do in our essential standpoint with these distinctions, for there is no I nor thou, but only one divine Self equal in all embodiments, equal in the individual and the group, and to realise that, to express that, to serve that, to fulfil that is all that matters. Self-satisfaction and altruism, enjoyment and indifference are not the essential thing. If the realisation, fulfilment, service of the one Self demands from us an action that seems to others self-service or self-assertion in the egoistic sense or seems egoistic enjoyment and self-indulgence, that action we must do; we must be governed by the guide within rather than by the opinions of men. The influence of the environment works often with great subtlety; we prefer and put on almost unconsciously the garb which will look best in the eye that regards us from outside and we allow a veil to drop over the eye within; we are impelled to drape ourselves in the vow of poverty, or in the garb of service, or in outward proofs of indifference and renunciation and a spotless sainthood because that is what tradition and opinion demand of us and so we can make best an impression on our environment. But all this is vanity and delusion. We may be called upon to assume these things, for that may be the uniform of our service; but equally it may not. The eye of man outside matters nothing; the eye within is all.

We see in the teaching of the Gita how subtle a thing is the freedom from egoism which is demanded. Arjuna is driven to fight by the egoism of strength, the egoism of the Kshatriya; he is turned from the battle by the contrary egoism of weakness, the shrinking, the spirit of disgust, the false pity that overcomes the mind, the nervous being and the senses, — not that divine compassion which strengthens the arm and clarifies the knowledge. But this weakness comes garbed as renunciation, as virtue: "Better the life of the beggar than to taste these blood-stained enjoyments; I desire not the rule of all the earth, no, nor the kingdom of the gods." How foolish of the Teacher, we might say, not to confirm this mood, to lose this sublime chance of adding one more great soul to the army of Sannyasins, one more shining example before the world of a holy renunciation. But the Guide sees otherwise, the Guide who is not to be deceived by words; "This is weakness and delusion and egoism that speak in thee. Behold the Self, open thy eyes to the knowledge, purify thy soul of egoism." And afterwards? "Fight, conquer, enjoy a wealthy kingdom." Or to take another example from ancient Indian tradition. It was egoism, it would seem, that drove Rama, the Avatara, to raise an army and destroy a nation in order to recover his wife from the King of Lanka. But would it have been a lesser egoism to drape himself in indifference and misusing the formal terms of the knowledge to say, "I have no wife, no enemy, no desire; these are illusions of the senses; let me cultivate the Brahman-knowledge and let Ravana do what he will with the daughter of Janaka"?

The criterion is within, as the Gita insists. It is to have the soul free from craving and attachment, but free from the attachment to inaction as well as from the egoistic impulse to action, free from attachment to the forms of virtue as well as from the attraction to sin. It is to be rid of "I-ness" and "my-ness" so as to live in the one Self and act in the one Self; to reject the egoism of refusing to work through the individual centre of the universal Being as well as the egoism of serving the individual mind and life and body to the exclusion of others. To live in the Self is not to dwell for oneself alone in the Infinite immersed and oblivious of all things in that ocean of impersonal self-delight; but it is to live as the Self and in the Self equal in this embodiment and all embodiments and beyond all embodiments. This is the integral knowledge.

It will be seen that the scope we give to the idea of renunciation is different from the meaning currently attached to it. Currently its meaning is self-denial, inhibition of pleasure, rejection of the objects of pleasure. Self-denial is a necessary discipline for the soul of man, because his heart is ignorantly attached; inhibition of pleasure is necessary because his sense is caught and clogged in the mud-honey of sensuous satisfactions; rejection of the objects of pleasure is imposed because the mind fixes on the object and will not leave it to go beyond it and within itself. If the mind of man were not thus ignorant, attached, bound even in its restless inconstancy, deluded by the forms of things, renunciation would not have been needed; the soul could have travelled on the path of delight, from the lesser to the greater, from joy to diviner joy. At present that is not practicable. It must give up from within everything to which it is attached in order that it may gain that which they are in their reality. The external renunciation is not the essential, but even that is necessary for a time, indispensable in many things and sometimes useful in all; we may even say that a complete external renunciation is a stage through which the soul must pass at some period of its progress, — though always it should be without those self-willed violences and fierce self-torturings which are an offence to the Divine seated within us. But in the end this renunciation or self-denial is always an instrument and the period for its use passes. The rejection of the object ceases to be necessary when the object can no longer ensnare us because what the soul enjoys is no longer the object as an object but the Divine which it expresses; the inhibition of pleasure is no longer needed when the soul no longer seeks pleasure but possesses the delight of the Divine in all things equally without the need of a personal or physical possession of the thing itself; self-denial loses its field when the soul no longer claims anything, but obeys consciously the will of the one Self in all beings. It is then that we are freed from the Law and released into the liberty of the Spirit.

We must be prepared to leave behind on the path not only

that which we stigmatise as evil, but that which seems to us to be good, yet is not the one good. There are things which were beneficial, helpful, which seemed perhaps at one time the one thing desirable, and yet once their work is done, once they are attained, they become obstacles and even hostile forces when we are called to advance beyond them. There are desirable states of the soul which it is dangerous to rest in after they have been mastered, because then we do not march on to the wider kingdoms of God beyond. Even divine realisations must not be clung to, if they are not the divine realisation in its utter essentiality and completeness. We must rest at nothing less than the All, nothing short of the utter transcendence. And if we can thus be free in the spirit, we shall find out all the wonder of God's workings; we shall find that in inwardly renouncing everything we have lost nothing. "By all this abandoned thou shalt come to enjoy the All." For everything is kept for us and restored to us but with a wonderful change and transfiguration into the All-Good and the All-Beautiful, the All-Light and the All-Delight of Him who is for ever pure and infinite and the mystery and the miracle that ceases not through the ages.

Chapter VI

The Synthesis of the Disciplines of Knowledge

IN THE last chapter we have spoken of renunciation in its most general scope, even as we spoke of concentration in all its possibilities; what has been said, applies therefore equally to the path of Works and the path of Devotion as to the path of Knowledge; for on all three concentration and renunciation are needed, though the way and spirit in which they are applied may vary. But we must now turn more particularly to the actual steps of the Path of Knowledge on which the double force of concentration and renunciation must aid us to advance. Practically, this path is a reascent up the great ladder of being down which the soul has descended into the material existence.

The central aim of Knowledge is the recovery of the Self, of our true self-existence, and this aim presupposes the admission that our present mode of being is not our true self-existence. No doubt, we have rejected the trenchant solutions which cut the knot of the riddle of the universe; we recognise it neither as a fiction of material appearance created by Force, nor as an unreality set up by the Mind, nor as a bundle of sensations, ideas and results of idea and sensation with a great Void or a great blissful Zero behind it to strive towards as our true truth of eternal non-existence. We accept the Self as a reality and the universe as a reality of the Self, a reality of its consciousness and not of mere material force and formation, but none the less or rather all the more for that reason a reality. Still, though the universe is a fact and not a fiction, a fact of the divine and universal and not a fiction of the individual self, our state of existence here is a state of ignorance, not the true truth of our being. We conceive of ourselves falsely, we see ourselves as we are not; we live in a false relation with our environment, because we know neither the universe nor ourselves for what they really are but with an imperfect view founded on a temporary fiction which the Soul and Nature have established between themselves for the convenience of the evolving ego. And this falsity is the root of a general perversion, confusion and suffering which besiege at every step both our internal life and our relations with our environment. Our personal life and our communal life, our commerce with ourselves and our commerce with our fellows are founded on a falsity and are therefore false in their recognised principles and methods, although through all this error a growing truth continually seeks to express itself. Hence the supreme importance to man of Knowledge, not what is called the practical knowledge of life, but of the profoundest knowledge of the Self and Nature[1] on which alone a true practice of life can be founded.

The error proceeds from a false identification. Nature has created within her material unity separate-seeming bodies which the Soul manifested in material Nature enfolds, inhabits, possesses, uses; the Soul forgetting itself experiences only this single knot in Matter and says "I am this body." It thinks of itself as the body, suffers with the body, enjoys with the body, is born with the body, is dissolved with the body; or so at least it views its self-existence. Again, Nature has created within her unity of universal life separate-seeming currents of life which form themselves into a whorl of vitality around and in each body, and the Soul manifested in vital Nature seizes on and is seized by that current, is imprisoned momentarily in that little whirling vortex of life. The Soul, still forgetting itself, says "I am this life"; it thinks of itself as the life, craves with its cravings or desires, wallows in its pleasures, bleeds with its wounds, rushes or stumbles with its movements. If it is still mainly governed by the body-sense, it identifies its own existence with that of the whorl and thinks "When this whorl is dissipated by the dissolution of the body round which it has formed itself, then *I* shall be no more." If it has been able to sense the current of life which has formed the vortex, it thinks of itself as that

---

[1] *ātmajñāna* and *tattvajñāna*.

current and says "I am this stream of life; I have entered upon the possession of this body, I shall leave it and enter upon the possession of other bodies: I am an immortal life revolving in a cycle of constant rebirth."

But again Nature has created within her mental unity, formed in the universal Mind separate-seeming dynamos as it were of mentality, constant centres for the generation, distribution and reabsorption of mental force and mental activities, stations as it were in a system of mental telegraphy where messages are conceived, written, sent, received, deciphered, and these messages and these activities are of many kinds, sensational, emotional, perceptual, conceptual, intuitional, all of which the Soul manifested in mental Nature accepts, uses for its outlook on the world and seems to itself to project and to receive their shocks, to suffer or to master their consequences. Nature instals the base of these dynamos in the material bodies she has formed, makes these bodies the ground for her stations and connects the mental with the material by a nerve-system full of the movement of vital currents through which the mind becomes conscious of the material world and, so far as it chooses, of the vital world of Nature. Otherwise the mind would be conscious of the mental world first and chiefly and would only indirectly glimpse the material. As it is, its attention is fixed on the body and the material world in which it has been installed and it is aware of the rest of existence only dimly, indirectly or subconsciously in that vast remainder of itself with regard to which superficially it has become irresponsive and oblivious.

The Soul identifies itself with this mental dynamo or station and says "I am this mind." And since the mind is absorbed in the bodily life, it thinks "I am a mind in a living body" or, still more commonly, "I am a body which lives and thinks." It identifies itself with the thoughts, emotions, sensations of the embodied mind and imagines that because when the body is dissolved all this will dissolve, itself also will cease to exist. Or if it becomes conscious of the current of persistence of mental personality, it thinks of itself as a mental soul occupying the body whether once or repeatedly and returning from earthly living to mental worlds beyond; the persistence of this mental being mentally enjoying or suffering sometimes in the body, sometimes on the mental or vital plane of Nature it calls its immortal existence. Or else, because the mind is a principle of light and knowledge, however imperfect, and can have some notion of what is beyond it, it sees the possibility of a dissolution of the mental being into that which is beyond, some Void or some eternal Existence, and it says, "There I, the mental soul, cease to be." Such dissolution it dreads or desires, denies or affirms according to its measure of attachment to or repulsion from this present play of embodied mind and vitality.

Now, all this is a mixture of truth and falsehood. Mind, Life, Matter exist and mental, vital, physical individualisation exists as facts in Nature, but the identification of the soul with these things is a false identification. Mind, Life and Matter are ourselves only in this sense that they are principles of being which the true self has evolved by the meeting and interaction of Soul and Nature in order to express a form of its one existence as the Cosmos. Individual mind, life and body are a play of these principles which is set up in the commerce of Soul and Nature as a means for the expression of that multiplicity of itself of which the one Existence is eternally capable and which it holds eternally involved in its unity. Individual mind, life and body are forms of ourselves in so far as we are centres of the multiplicity of the One; universal Mind, Life and Body are also forms of our self, because we are that One in our being. But the self is more than universal or individual mind, life and body and when we limit ourselves by identification with these things, we found our knowledge on a falsehood, we falsify our determining view and our practical experience not only of our self-being but of our cosmic existence and of our individual activities.

The Self is an eternal utter Being and pure existence of which all these things are becomings. From this knowledge we have to proceed; this knowledge we have to realise and make it the foundation of the inner and the outer life of the individual. The Yoga of Knowledge, starting from this primary truth, has conceived a negative and positive method of discipline by which we shall get rid of these false identifications and recoil back from them into true self-knowledge. The negative method is to say always "I am not the body" so as to contradict and root out the false idea "I am the body", to concentrate on this knowledge and by renunciation of the attachment of the soul to the physical get rid of the body-sense. We say again "I am not the life" and by concentration on this knowledge and renunciation of attachment to the vital movements and desires, get rid of the life-sense. We say, finally, "I am not the mind, the motion, the sense, the thought" and by concentration on this knowledge and renunciation of the mental activities, get rid of the mind-sense. When we thus constantly create a gulf between ourselves and the things with which we identified ourselves, their veils progressively fall away from us and the Self begins to be visible to our experience. Of that then we say "I am That, the pure, the eternal, the self-blissful" and by concentrating our thought and being upon it we become That and are able finally to renounce the individual existence and the Cosmos. Another positive method belonging rather to the Rajayoga is to concentrate on the thought of the Brahman and shut out from us all other ideas, so that this dynamo of mind shall cease to work upon our external or varied internal existence; by mental cessation the vital and physical play also shall fall to rest in an eternal samadhi, some inexpressible deepest trance of the being in which we shall pass into the absolute Existence.

This discipline is evidently a self-centred and exclusive inner movement which gets rid of the world by denying it in thought and shutting the eyes of the soul to it in vision. But the universe is there as a truth in God even though the individual soul may have shut its eyes to it and the Self is there in the universe really and not falsely, supporting all that we have rejected, truly immanent in all things, really embracing the individual in the universal as well as embracing the universe in that which exceeds and transcends it. What shall we do with this eternal Self in this persistent universe which we see encompassing us every time we come out of the trance of inner meditation? The ascetic Path of Knowledge has its solution and its discipline for the soul that looks out on the universe. It is to regard the immanent and all-encompassing and all-constituting Self in the image of the ether in which all forms are, which is in all forms, of which all forms are made. In that ether cosmic Life and Mind move as the Breath of things, an atmospheric sea in the ethereal, and constitute from it all these forms; but what they constitute are merely name and form and not realities; the form of the pot we see is a form of earth only and goes back into the earth, earth a form resolvable into the cosmic Life, the cosmic Life a movement that falls to rest in that silent immutable Ether. Concentrating on this knowledge, rejecting all phenomenon and appearance, we come to see the whole as an illusion of name and form in the ether that is Brahman; it becomes unreal to us; and the universe becoming unreal the immanence becomes unreal and there is only the Self upon which our mind has falsely imposed the name and form of the universe. Thus are we justified in the withdrawal of the individual self into the Absolute.

Still, the Self goes on with its imperishable aspect of immanence, its immutable aspect of divine envelopment, its endless trick of becoming each thing and all things; our detection of the cheat and our withdrawal do not seem to affect one tittle either the Self or the universe. Must we not then know also what it is that thus persists superior to our acceptance and rejection and too great, too eternal to be affected by it? Here too there must be some invincible reality at work and the integrality of Knowledge demands that we shall see and realise it; otherwise it may prove that our own knowledge and not the Lord in the universe was the cheat and the illusion. Therefore we must concentrate again and see and realise also this which persists so sovereignly and must know the Self as no other than the Supreme Soul which is the Lord of Nature, the upholder of cosmic existence by whose sanction it proceeds, whose will compels its multitudinous actions and determines its perpetual cycles. And we must yet concentrate once again and see and realise and must know the Self as the one Existence who is both the Soul of all and the Nature of all, at once Purusha and Prakriti and so able both to express himself in all these forms of things and to be all these formations. Otherwise we have excluded what the Self does not exclude and made a wilful choice in our knowledge.

The old ascetic Path of Knowledge admitted the unity of things and the concentration on all these aspects of the one Existence, but it made a distinction and a hierarchy. The Self that becomes all these forms of things is the Virat or universal Soul; the Self that creates all these forms is Hiranyagarbha, the luminous or creatively perceptive Soul; the Self that contains all these things involved in it is Prajna, the conscious Cause or originally determining Soul; beyond all these is the Absolute who permits all this unreality, but has no dealings with it. Into That we must withdraw and have no farther dealings with the universe, since Knowledge means the final Knowledge, and therefore these lesser realisations must fall away from us or be lost in That. But evidently from our point of view these are practical distinctions made by the mind which have a value for certain purposes, but no ultimate value. Our view of the world insists on unity; the universal Self is not different from the perceptive and creative, nor the perceptive from the causal, nor the causal from the Absolute, but it is one "Self-being which has become all becomings", and which is not any other than the Lord who manifests Himself as all these individual existences nor the Lord any other than the sole-existing Brahman who verily is all this that we can see, sense, live or mentalise. That Self, Lord, Brahman we would know that we may realise our unity with it and with all that it manifests and in that unity we would live. For we demand of knowledge that it shall unite; the knowledge that divides must always be a partial knowing good for certain practical purposes; the knowledge that unites is *the* knowledge.

Therefore our integral Yoga will take up these various disciplines and concentrations, but harmonise and if possible fuse them by a synthesis which removes their mutual exclusions. Not realising the Lord and the All only to reject them for silent Self or unknowable Absolute as would an exclusively transcendental, nor living for the Lord alone or in the All alone as would an exclusively theistic or an exclusively pantheistic Yoga, the seeker of integral knowledge will limit himself neither in his thought nor in his practice nor in his realisation by any religious creed or philosophical dogma. He will seek the Truth of existence in its completeness. The ancient disciplines he will not reject, for they rest upon eternal truths, but he will give them an orientation in conformity with his aim.

We must recognise that our primary aim in knowledge must be to realise our own supreme Self more than that Self in others or as the Lord of Nature or as the All; for that is the pressing need of the individual, to arrive at the highest truth of his own being, to set right its disorders, confusions, false identifications, to arrive at its right concentration and purity and to know and mount to its source. But we do this not in order to disappear into its source, but so that our whole existence and all the members of this inner kingdom may find their right basis, may live in our highest self, live for our highest self only and obey no other law than that which proceeds from our highest self and is given to our purified being without any falsification in the transmitting mentality. And if we do this rightly we shall discover that in finding this supreme Self we have found the one Self in all, the one Lord of our nature and of all Nature, the All of ourselves who is the All of the universe. For this that we see in ourselves we must necessarily see everywhere, since that is the truth of His unity. By discovering and using rightly the Truth of our being the barrier between our individuality and the universe will necessarily be forced open and cast away and the Truth that we realise in our own being cannot fail to realise itself to us in the universality which will then be our self. Realising in ourselves the "I am He" of the Vedanta, we cannot but realise in looking upon all around us the identical knowledge on its other side, "Thou art That." We have only to see how practically the discipline must be conducted in order that we may arrive successfully at this great unification.

Chapter VII

The Release from Subjection
to the Body

OUR FIRST step in this path of knowledge, having once determined in our intellect that what seems is not the Truth, that the self is not the body or life or mind; since these are only its forms, must be to set right our mind in its practical relation with the life and the body so that it may arrive at its own right relation with the Self. This it is easiest to do by a device with which we are already familiar, since it played a great part in our view of the Yoga of Works; it is to create a separation between the Prakriti and the Purusha. The Purusha, the soul that knows and commands has got himself involved in the workings of his executive conscious force, so that he mistakes this physical working of it which we call the body for himself; he forgets his own nature as the soul that knows and commands; he believes his mind and soul to be subject to the law and working of the body; he forgets that he is so much else besides that is greater than the physical form; he forgets that the mind is really greater than Matter and ought not to submit to its obscurations, reactions, habit of inertia, habit of incapacity; he forgets that he is more even than the mind, a Power which can raise the mental being above itself; that he is the Master, the Transcendent and it is not fit the Master should be enslaved to his own workings, the Transcendent imprisoned in a form which exists only as a trifle in its own being. All this forgetfulness has to be cured by the Purusha remembering his own true nature and first by his remembering that the body is only a working and only one working of Prakriti.

We say then to the mind "This is a working of Prakriti, this is neither thyself nor myself; stand back from it." We shall find, if we try, that the mind has this power of detachment and can stand back from the body not only in idea, but in act and as it were physically or rather vitally. This detachment of the mind must be strengthened by a certain attitude of indifference to the things of the body; we must not care essentially about its sleep or its waking, its movement or its rest, its pain or its pleasure, its health or ill-health, its vigour or its fatigue, its comfort or its discomfort, or what it eats or drinks. This does not mean that we shall not keep the body in right order so far as we can; we have not to fall into violent asceticisms or a positive neglect of the physical frame. But we have not either to be affected in mind by hunger or thirst or discomfort or ill-health or attach the importance which the physical and vital man attaches to the things of the body, or indeed any but a quite subordinate and purely instrumental importance. Nor must this instrumental importance be allowed to assume the proportions of a necessity; we must not for instance imagine that the purity of the mind depends on the things we eat or drink, although during a certain stage restrictions in eating and drinking are useful to our inner progress; nor on the other hand must we continue to think that the dependence of the mind or even of the life on food and drink is anything more than a habit, a customary relation which Nature has set up between these principles. As a matter of fact the food we take can be reduced by contrary habit and new relation to a minimum without the mental or vital vigour being in any way reduced; even on the contrary with a judicious development they can be trained to a greater potentiality of vigour by learning to rely on the secret fountains of mental and vital energy with which they are connected more than upon the minor aid of physical aliments. This aspect of self-discipline is however more important in the Yoga of self-perfection than here; for our present purpose the important point is the renunciation by the mind of attachment to or dependence on the things of the body.

Thus disciplined the mind will gradually learn to take up towards the body the true attitude of the Purusha. First of all, it will know the mental Purusha as the upholder of the body and not in any way the body itself; for it is quite other than the physical existence which it upholds by the mind through the agency of the vital force. This will come to be so much the normal attitude of the whole being to the physical frame that the latter will feel to us as if something external and detachable like the dress we wear or an instrument we happen to be carrying in our hand. We may even come to feel that the body is in a certain sense non-existent except as a sort of partial expression of our vital force and of our mentality. These experiences are signs that the mind is coming to a right poise regarding the body, that it is exchanging the false view-point of the mentality obsessed and captured by physical sensation for the view-point of the true truth of things.

Secondly, with regard to the movements and experiences of the body the mind will come to know the Purusha seated within it as, first, the witness or observer of the movements and, secondly, the knower or perceiver of the experiences. It will cease to consider in thought or feel in sensation these movements and experiences as its own but rather consider and feel them as not its own, as operations of Nature governed by the qualities of Nature and their interaction upon each other. This detachment can be made so normal and carried so far that there will be a kind of division between the mind and the body and the former will observe and experience the hunger, thirst, pain, fatigue, depression, etc. of the physical being as if they were experiences of some other person with whom it has so close a *rapport* as to be aware of all that is going on within him. This division is a great means, a great step towards mastery; for the mind comes to observe these things first without being overpowered and finally without being at all affected by them, dispassionately, with clear understanding but with perfect detachment. This is the initial liberation of the mental being from servitude to the body; for by right knowledge put steadily into practice liberation comes inevitably.

Finally, the mind will come to know the Purusha in the mind as the master of Nature whose sanction is necessary to her movements. It will find that as the giver of the sanction he can withdraw the original fiat from the previous habits of

Nature and that eventually the habit will cease or change in the direction indicated by the will of the Purusha; not at once, for the old sanction persists as an obstinate consequence of the past Karma of Nature until that is exhausted, and a good deal also depends on the force of the habit and the idea of fundamental necessity which the mind had previously attached to it; but if it is not one of the fundamental habits Nature has established for the relation of the mind, life and body and if the old sanction is not renewed by the mind or the habit willingly indulged, then eventually the change will come. Even the habit of hunger and thirst can be minimised, inhibited, put away; the habit of disease can be similarly minimised and gradually eliminated and in the meantime the power of the mind to set right the disorders of the body whether by conscious manipulation of vital force or by simple mental fiat will immensely increase. By a similar process the habit by which the bodily nature associates certain forms and degrees of activity with strain, fatigue, incapacity can be rectified and the power, freedom, swiftness, effectiveness of the work whether physical or mental which can be done with this bodily instrument marvellously increased, doubled, tripled, decupled.

This side of the method belongs properly to the Yoga of self-perfection; but it is as well to speak briefly of these things here both because we thereby lay a basis for what we shall have to say of self-perfection, which is a part of the integral Yoga, and because we have to correct the false notions popularised by materialistic Science. According to this Science the normal mental and physical states and the relations between mind and body actually established by our past evolution are the right, natural and healthy conditions and anything other, anything opposite to them is either morbid and wrong or a hallucination, self-deception and insanity. Needless to say, this conservative principle is entirely ignored by Science itself when it so diligently and successfully improves on the normal operations of physical Nature for the greater mastery of Nature by man. Suffice it to say here once for all that a change of mental and physical state and of relations between the mind and body which increases the purity and freedom of the being, brings a clear joy and peace and multiplies the power of the mind over itself and over the physical functions, brings about in a word man's greater mastery of his own nature, is obviously not morbid and cannot be considered a hallucination or self-deception since its effects are patent and positive. In fact, it is simply a willed advance of Nature in her evolution of the individual, an evolution which she will carry out in any case but in which she chooses to utilise the human will as her chief agent, because her essential aim is to lead the Purusha to conscious mastery over herself.

This being said, we must add that in the movement of the path of knowledge perfection of the mind and body are no consideration at all or only secondary considerations. The one thing necessary is to rise out of Nature to the Self by either the most swift or the most thorough and effective method possible; and the method we are describing, though not the swiftest, is the most thorough-going in its effectivity. And here there arises the question of physical action or inaction. It is ordinarily considered that the Yogin should draw away from action as much as possible and especially that too much action is a hindrance because it draws off the energies outward. To a certain extent this is true; and we must note farther that when the mental Purusha takes up the attitude of mere witness and observer, a tendency to silence, solitude, physical calm and bodily inaction grows upon the being. So long as this is not associated with inertia, incapacity or unwillingness to act, in a word, with the growth of the tamasic quality, all this is to the good. The power to do nothing, which is quite different from indolence, incapacity or aversion to action and attachment to inaction, is a great power and a great mastery; the power to rest absolutely from action is as necessary for the Jnanayogin as the power to cease absolutely from thought, as the power to remain indefinitely in sheer solitude and silence and as the power of immovable calm. Whoever is not willing to embrace these states is not yet fit for the path that leads towards the highest knowledge; whoever is unable to draw towards them, is as yet unfit for its acquisition.

At the same time it must be added that the power is enough;

the abstention from all physical action is not indispensable, the aversion to action mental or corporeal is not desirable. The seeker of the integral state of knowledge must be free from attachment to action and equally free from attachment to inaction. Especially must any tendency to mere inertia of mind or vitality or body be surmounted, and if that habit is found growing on the nature, the will of the Purusha must be used to dismiss it. Eventually, a state arrives when the life and the body perform as mere instruments the will of the Purusha in the mind without any strain or attachment, without their putting themselves into the action with that inferior, eager and often feverish energy which is the nature of their ordinary working; they come to work as forces of Nature work without the fret and toil and reaction characteristic of life in the body when it is not yet master of the physical. When we attain to this perfection, then action and inaction become immaterial, since neither interferes with the freedom of the soul or draws it away from its urge towards the Self or its poise in the Self. But this state of perfection arrives later in the Yoga and till then the law of moderation laid down by the Gita is the best for us; too much mental or physical action then is not good since excess draws away too much energy and reacts unfavourably upon the spiritual condition; too little also is not good since defect leads to a habit of inaction and even to an incapacity which has afterwards to be surmounted with difficulty. Still, periods of absolute calm, solitude and cessation from works are highly desirable and should be secured as often as possible for that recession of the soul into itself which is indispensable to knowledge.

While dealing thus with the body we have necessarily to deal also with the Prana or life-energy. For practical purposes we have to make a distinction between the life-energy as it acts in the body, the physical Prana, and the life-energy as it acts in support of the mental activities, the psychical Prana. For we lead always a double life, mental and physical, and the same life-energy acts differently and assumes a different aspect according as it lends itself to one or the other. In the body it produces those reactions of hunger, thirst, fatigue, health, disease, physical vigour, etc. which are the vital experiences of the physical frame. For the gross body of man is not like the stone or the earth; it is a combination of two sheaths, the vital and the "food" sheath and its life is a constant interaction of these two. Still the life-energy and the physical frame are two different things and in the withdrawal of the mind from the absorbing sense of the body we become increasingly sensible of the Prana and its action in the corporeal instrument and can observe and more and more control its operations. Practically, in drawing back from the body we draw back from the physical life-energy also, even while we distinguish the two and feel the latter nearer to us than the mere physical instrument. The entire conquest of the body comes in fact by the conquest of the physical life-energy.

Along with the attachment to the body and its works the attachment to life in the body is overcome. For when we feel the physical being to be not ourselves, but only a dress or an instrument, the repulsion to the death of the body which is so strong and vehement an instinct of the vital man must necessarily weaken and can be thrown away. Thrown away it must be and entirely. The fear of death and the aversion to bodily cessation are the stigma left by his animal origin on the human being. That brand must be utterly effaced.

Chapter VIII

The Release from the Heart and the Mind

BUT THE ascending soul has to separate itself not only from the life in the body but from the action of the life-energy in the mind; it has to make the mind say as the representative of the Purusha "I am not the Life; the Life is not the self of the Purusha, it is only a working and only one working of Prakriti." The characteristics of Life are action and movement, a reaching out to absorb and assimilate what is external to the individual and a principle of satisfaction or dissatisfaction in what it seizes upon or what comes to it, which is associated with the all-pervading phenomenon of attraction and repulsion. These three things are everywhere in Nature because Life is everywhere in Nature. But in us mental beings they are all given a mental value according to the mind which perceives and accepts them. They take the form of action, of desire and of liking and disliking, pleasure and pain. The Prana is everywhere in us supporting not only the action of our body, but of our sense-mind, our emotional mind, our thought-mind; and bringing its own law or dharma into all these, it confuses, it limits, it throws into discord their right action and creates that impurity of misplacement and that tangled confusion which is the whole evil of our psychological existence. In that confusion one law seems to reign, the law of desire. As the universal Divine Being, all-embracing and all-possessing, acts, moves, enjoys purely for the satisfaction of divine Delight, so the individual life acts, moves, enjoys and suffers predominantly for the satisfaction of desire. Therefore the psychic life-energy presents itself to our experience as a sort of desire-mind, which we have to conquer if we mean to get back to our true self.

Desire is at once the motive of our actions, our lever of

accomplishment and the bane of our existence. If our sense-mind, emotional mind, thought-mind could act free from the intrusions and importations of the life-energy, if that energy could be made to obey their right action instead of imposing its own yoke on our existence, all human problems would move harmoniously to their right solution. The proper function of the life-energy is to do what it is bidden by the divine principle in us, to reach to and enjoy what is given to it by that indwelling Divine and not to desire at all. The proper function of the sense-mind is to lie open passively, luminously to the contacts of Life and transmit their sensations and the *rasa* or right taste and principle of delight in them to the higher function; but interfered with by the attractions and repulsions, the acceptances and refusals, the satisfactions and dissatisfactions, the capacities and incapacities of the life-energy in the body it is, to begin with, limited in its scope and, secondly, forced in these limits to associate itself with all these discords of the life in Matter. It becomes an instrument for pleasure and pain instead of for delight of existence.

Similarly the emotional mind compelled to take note of all these discords and subject itself to their emotional reactions becomes a hurtling field of joy and grief, love and hatred, wrath, fear, struggle, aspiration, disgust, likes, dislikes, indifferences, content, discontent, hopes, disappointments, gratitude, revenge and all the stupendous play of passion which is the drama of life in the world. This chaos we call our soul. But the real soul, the real psychic entity which for the most part we see little of and only a small minority in mankind has developed, is an instrument of pure love, joy and the luminous reaching out to fusion and unity with God and our fellow-creatures. This psychic entity is covered up by the play of the mentalised Prana or desire-mind which we mistake for the soul; the emotional mind is unable to mirror the real soul in us, the Divine in our hearts, and is obliged instead to mirror the desire-mind.

So too the proper function of the thought-mind is to observe, understand, judge with a dispassionate delight in knowledge and open itself to messages and illuminations playing upon all that it observes and upon all that is yet hidden from it but must progressively be revealed, messages and illuminations that secretly flash down to us from the divine Oracle concealed in light above our mentality whether they seem to descend through the intuitive mind or arise from the seeing heart. But this it cannot do rightly because it is pinned to the limitations of the life-energy in the senses, to the discords of sensation and emotion, and to its own limitations of intellectual preference, inertia, straining, self-will which are the form taken in it by the interference of this desire-mind, this psychic Prana. As is said in the Upanishads, our whole mind-consciousness is shot through with the threads and currents of this Prana, this Life-energy that strives and limits, grasps and misses, desires and suffers, and only by its purification can we know and possess our real and eternal self.

It is true that the root of all this evil is the ego-sense and that the seat of the conscious ego-sense is the mind itself; but in reality the conscious mind only reflects an ego already created in the subconscious mind in things, the dumb soul in the stone and the plant which is present in all body and life and only finally delivered into voicefulness and wakefulness but not originally created by the conscious mind. And in this upward procession it is the life-energy which has become the obstinate knot of the ego, it is the desire-mind which refuses to relax the knot even when the intellect and the heart have discovered the cause of their ills and would be glad enough to remove it; for the Prana in them is the Animal who revolts and who obscures and deceives their knowledge and coerces their will by his refusal.

Therefore the mental Purusha has to separate himself from association and self-identification with this desire-mind. He has to say "I am not this thing that struggles and suffers, grieves and rejoices, loves and hates, hopes and is baffled, is angry and afraid and cheerful and depressed, a thing of vital moods and emotional passions. All these are merely workings and habits of Prakriti in the sensational and emotional mind." The mind then draws back from its emotions and becomes with these, as with the bodily movements and experiences, the observer or witness. There is again an inner cleavage. There is this emotional mind in which these moods and passions continue to occur according to the habit of the modes of Nature and there is the observing mind which sees them, studies and understands but is detached from them. It observes them as if in a sort of action and play on a mental stage of personages other than itself, at first with interest and a habit of relapse into identification, then with entire calm and detachment, and, finally, attaining not only to calm but to the pure delight of its own silent existence, with a smile at their unreality as at the imaginary joys and sorrows of a child who is playing and loses himself in the play. Secondly, it becomes aware of itself as master of the sanction who by his withdrawal of sanction can make this play to cease. When the sanction is withdrawn, another significant phenomenon takes place; the emotional mind becomes normally calm and pure and free from these reactions, and even when they come, they no longer rise from within but seem to fall on it as impressions from outside to which its fibres are still able to respond; but this habit of response dies away and the emotional mind is in time entirely liberated from the passions which it has renounced. Hope and fear, joy and grief, liking and disliking, attraction and repulsion, content and discontent, gladness and depression, horror and wrath and fear and disgust and shame and the passions of love and hatred fall away from the liberated psychic being.

What takes their place? It may be, if we will, an entire calm, silence and indifference. But although this is a stage through which the soul has usually to pass, it is not the final aim we have placed before us. Therefore the Purusha becomes also the master who wills and whose will it is to replace wrong by right enjoyment of the psychic existence. What he wills, Nature executes. What was fabric-stuff of desire and passion, is turned into reality of pure, equal and calmly intense love and joy and oneness. The real soul emerges and takes the place left vacant by the desire-mind. The cleansed and emptied cup is filled with the wine of divine love and delight and no longer with the sweet and bitter poison of passion. The passions, even the passion for good, misrepresent the divine nature. The passion of pity with its impure elements of physical repulsion and emotional inability to bear the suffering of others has to be rejected and replaced by the higher divine compassion which sees, understands, accepts the burden of others and is strong to help and heal, not with self-will and revolt against the suffering in the world and with ignorant accusation of the law of things and their source, but with light and knowledge and as an instrument of the Divine in its emergence. So too the love that desires and grasps and is troubled with joy and shaken with grief must be rejected for the equal, all-embracing love that is free from these things and has no dependence upon circumstances and is not modified by response or absence of response. So we shall deal with all the movements of the soul; but of these things we shall speak farther when we consider the Yoga of self-perfection.

As with action and inaction, so it is with this dual possibility of indifference and calm on the one side and active joy and love on the other. Equality, not indifference is the basis. Equal endurance, impartial indifference, calm submission to the causes of joy and grief without any reaction of either grief or joy are the preparation and negative basis of equality; but equality is not fulfilled till it takes its positive form of love and delight. The sense-mind must find the equal *rasa* of the All-Beautiful, the heart the equal love and Ananda for all, the psychic Prana the enjoyment of this *rasa*, love and Ananda. This, however, is the positive perfection that comes by liberation; our first object on the path of knowledge is rather the liberation that comes by detachment from the desire-mind and by the renunciation of its passions.

The desire-mind must also be rejected from the instrument of thought and this is best done by the detachment of the Purusha from thought and opinion itself. Of this we have already had occasion to speak when we considered in what consists the integral purification of the being. For all this movement of knowledge which we are describing is a method of purification and liberation whereby entire and final self-knowledge becomes possible, a progressive self-knowledge being itself the instrument of the purification and liberation. The method with the thought-mind will be the same as with all the rest of the being. The Purusha, having used the thought-mind for release from identification with the life and body and with the mind of desire and sensations and emotions, will turn round upon the thought-mind itself and will say "This too I am not; I am not the thought or the thinker; all these ideas, opinions, speculations, strivings of the intellect, its predilections, preferences, dogmas, doubts, self-corrections are not myself; all this is only a working of Prakriti which takes place in the thought-mind." Thus a division is created between the mind that thinks and wills and the mind that observes and the Purusha becomes the witness only; he sees, he understands the process and laws of his thought, but detaches himself from it. Then as the master of the sanction he withdraws his past sanction from the tangle of the mental undercurrent and the reasoning intellect and causes both to cease from their importunities. He becomes liberated from subjection to the thinking mind and capable of the utter silence.

For perfection there is necessary also the resumption by the Purusha of his position as the lord of his Nature and the will to replace the mere mental undercurrent and intellect by the truth-conscious thought that lightens from above. But the silence is necessary; in the silence and not in the thought we shall find the Self, we shall become aware of it, not merely conceive it, and we shall withdraw out of the mental Purusha into that which is the source of the mind. But for this withdrawal a final liberation is needed, the release from the ego-sense in the mind.

Chapter IX

The Release from the Ego

THE FORMATION of a mental and vital ego tied to the body-sense was the first great labour of the cosmic Life in its progressive evolution; for this was the means it found for creating out of matter a conscious individual. The dissolution of this limiting ego is the one condition, the necessary means for this very same Life to arrive at its divine fruition: for only so can the conscious individual find either his transcendent self or his true Person. This double movement is usually represented as a fall and a redemption or a creation and a destruction, — the kindling of a light and its extinction or the formation first of a smaller temporary and unreal self and a release from it into our true self's eternal largeness. For human thought falls apart towards two opposite extremes: one, mundane and pragmatic, regards the fulfilment and satisfaction of the mental, vital and physical ego-sense individual or collective as the object of life and looks no farther, while the other, spiritual, philosophic or religious, regards the conquest of the ego in the interests of the soul, spirit or whatever be the ultimate entity, as the one thing supremely worth doing. Even in the camp of the ego there are two divergent attitudes which divide the mundane or materialist theory of the universe. One tendency of this thought regards the mental ego as a creation of our mentality which will be dissolved with the dissolution of mind by the death of the body; the one abiding truth is eternal Nature working in the race — this or another — and her purpose should be followed, not ours, — the fulfilment of the race, the collective ego, and not that of the individual should be the rule of life. Another trend of thought, more vitalistic in its tendencies, fixes on the conscious ego as the supreme achievement of Nature, no matter how transitory, ennobles it into a human representative of the Will-to-be and holds up its greatness and satisfaction as the highest aim of our existence. In the more numerous systems that take their stand on some kind of religious thought or spiritual discipline there is a corresponding divergence. The Buddhist denies the existence of a real self or ego, admits no universal or transcendent Being. The Adwaitin declares the apparently individual soul to be none other than the supreme Self and Brahman, its individuality an illusion; the putting off of individual existence is the only true release. Other systems assert, in flat contradiction of this view, the eternal persistence of the human soul; a basis of multiple consciousness in the One or else a dependent but still separate entity, it is constant, real, imperishable.

Amidst these various and conflicting opinions the seeker of the Truth has to decide for himself which shall be for him the Knowledge. But if our aim is a spiritual release or a spiritual fulfilment, then the exceeding of this little mould of ego is imperative. In human egoism and its satisfaction there can be no divine culmination and deliverance. A certain purification from egoism is the condition even of ethical progress and elevation, for social good and perfection; much more is it indispensable for inner peace, purity and joy. But a much more radical deliverance, not only from egoism but from ego-idea and ego-sense, is needed if our aim is to raise human into divine nature. Experience shows that, in proportion as we deliver ourselves from the limiting mental and vital ego, we command a wider life, a larger existence, a higher consciousness, a happier soul-state, even a greater knowledge, power and scope. Even the aim which the most mundane philosophy pursues, the fulfilment, perfection, satisfaction of the individual, is best assured not by satisfying the narrow ego but by finding freedom in a higher and larger self. There is no happiness in smallness of the being, says the Scripture, it is with the large being that happiness comes. The ego is by its nature a smallness of being; it brings contraction of the consciousness and with the contraction limitation of knowledge, disabling ignorance, — confinement and a diminution of power and by that diminution incapacity and weakness, — scission of oneness and by that scission disharmony and failure of sympathy and love and understanding, — inhibition or fragmentation of delight of being and by that fragmentation pain and sorrow. To recover what is lost we must break out of the walls of ego. The ego must either disappear in impersonality or fuse into a larger I: it must fuse into the wider cosmic "I" which comprehends all these smaller selves or the transcendent of which even the cosmic self is a diminished image.

But this cosmic self is spiritual in essence and in experience; it must not be confused with the collective existence, with any group soul or the life and body of a human society or even of all mankind. The subordination of the ego to the progress and happiness of the human race is now a governing idea in the world's thought and ethics; but this is a mental and moral and not a spiritual ideal. For that progress is a series of constant mental, vital and physical vicissitudes, it has no firm spiritual content, and offers no sure standing-ground to the soul of man. The consciousness of collective humanity is only a larger comprehensive edition or a sum of individual egos. Made of the same substance, in the same mould of nature, it has not in it any greater light, any more eternal sense of itself, any purer source of peace, joy and deliverance. It is rather even more tortured, troubled and obscured, certainly more vague, confused and unprogressive. The individual is in this respect greater than the mass and cannot be called on to subordinate his more luminous possibilities to this darker entity. If light, peace, deliverance, a better state of existence are to come, they must descend into the soul from something wider than the individual, but also from something higher than the collective ego. Altruism, philanthropy, the service of mankind are in themselves mental or moral ideals, not laws of the spiritual life. If into the spiritual aim there enters the impulse to deny the personal self or to serve humanity or the world at large, it comes not from the ego nor from the collective sense of the race, but from something more occult and profound transcendent of both these things; for it is founded on a sense of the Divine in all and it works not for the sake of the ego or the race but for the sake of the Divine and its purpose in the person or group or collective. It is this transcendent Source which we must seek and serve, this vaster being and consciousness to which the race and the individual are minor terms of its existence.

There is indeed a truth behind the pragmatic impulse which an exclusive one-sided spirituality is apt to ignore or deny or belittle. It is this that since the individual and the universal are terms of that higher and vaster Being, their fulfilment must have some real place in the supreme Existence. There must be behind them some high purpose in the supreme Wisdom and Knowledge, some eternal strain in the supreme Delight: they cannot have been, they were not created in vain. But the perfection and satisfaction of humanity like the perfection and satisfaction of the individual, can only be securely compassed and founded upon a more eternal yet unseized truth and right of things. Minor terms of some greater Existence, they can fulfil themselves only when that of which they are the terms is known and possessed. The greatest service to humanity, the surest foundation for its true progress, happiness and perfection is to prepare or find the way by which the individual and the collective man can transcend the ego and live in its true self, no longer bound to ignorance, incapacity, disharmony and sorrow. It is by the pursuit of the eternal and not by living bound in the slow collective evolution of Nature that we can best assure even that evolutionary, collective, altruistic aim our modern thought and idealism have set before us. But it is in itself a secondary aim; to find, know and possess the Divine existence, consciousness and nature and to live in it for the Divine is our true aim and the one perfection to which we must aspire.

It is then in the way of the spiritual philosophies and religions, not in that of any earth-bound materialistic doctrine, that the seeker of the highest knowledge has to walk, even if with enriched aims and a more comprehensive spiritual purpose. But how far has he to proceed in the elimination of the ego? In the ancient way of knowledge we arrive at the elimination of the ego-sense which attaches itself to the body, to the life, to the mind and says of all or any of them, "This is I". Not only do we, as in the way of works, get rid of the "I" of the worker and see the Lord alone as the true source of all works and sanction of works and His executive Nature-power or else His supreme Shakti as the sole agent and worker, — but we get rid also of the ego-sense which mistakes the instruments or the expressions of our being for our true self and spirit. But even if all this has been done, something remains still; there remains a substratum of all these, a general sense of the separate I. This substratum ego is something vague, indefinable, elusive; it does not or need not attach itself to anything in particular as the self; it does not identify itself with anything collective; it is a sort of fundamental form or power of the mind which compels the mental being to feel himself as a perhaps indefinable but still a limited being which is not mind, life or body, but under which their activities proceed in Nature. The others were a qualified ego-idea and ego-sense supporting themselves on the play of the Prakriti; but this is the pure fundamental ego-power supporting itself on the consciousness of the mental Purusha. And because it seems to be above or behind the play and not in it, because it does not say "I am the mind, life or body," but "I am a being on whom the action of mind, life and body depends," many think themselves released and mistake this elusive Ego for the One, the Divine, the true Purusha or at the very least for the true Person within them, — mistaking the indefinable for the Infinite. But so long as this fundamental ego-sense remains, there is no absolute release. The egoistic life, even if diminished in force and intensity, can still continue well enough with this support. If there is the error in identification, the ego life may under that pretext get rather an exaggerated intensity and force. Even if there is no such error, the ego life may be wider, purer, more flexible and release may be now much easier to attain and nearer to accomplishment, but still there is as yet no definitive release. It is imperative to go farther, to get rid of this indefinable but fundamental ego-sense also and get back to the Purusha on whom it is supporting itself, of whom it is a shadow; the shadow has to disappear and by its disappearance reveal the spirit's unclouded substance.

That substance is the self of the man called in European thought the Monad, in Indian philosophy, Jiva or Jivatman, the living entity, the self of the living creature. This Jiva is not the mental ego-sense constructed by the workings of Nature for her temporary purpose. It is not a thing bound, as the mental being, the vital, the physical are bound, by her habits, laws or processes. The Jiva is a spirit and self, superior to Nature. It is true that it consents to her acts, reflects her moods and upholds the triple medium of mind, life and body through which she casts them upon the soul's consciousness; but it is itself a living reflection or a soul-form or a self-creation of the Spirit universal and transcendent. The One Spirit who has mirrored some of His modes of being in the world and in the soul, is multiple in the Jiva. That Spirit is the very Self of our self, the One and the Highest, the Supreme we have to realise, the infinite existence into which we have to enter. And so far the teachers walk in company, all agreeing that this is the supreme object of knowledge, of works and of devotion, all agreeing that if it is to be attained, the Jiva must release himself from the ego-sense which belongs to the lower Nature or Maya. But here they part company and each goes his own way. The Monist fixes his feet on the path of an exclusive Knowledge and sets for us as sole ideal an entire return, loss, immersion or extinction of the Jiva in the Supreme. The Dualist or the partial Monist turns to the path of Devotion and directs us to shed indeed the lower ego and material life, but to see as the highest destiny of the spirit of man, not the self-annihilation of the Buddhist, not the self-immersion of the Adwaitin, not a swallowing up of the many by the One, but an eternal existence absorbed in the thought, love and enjoyment of the Supreme, the One, the All-Lover.

For the disciple of an integral Yoga there can be no hesitation; as a seeker of knowledge it is the integral knowledge and not anything either half-way and attractive or high-pinnacled and exclusive he must seek. He must soar to the utmost height, but also circle and spread to the most all-embracing wideness, not binding himself to any rigid structure of metaphysical thought, but free to admit and combine all the soul's highest and greatest and fullest and most numerous experiences. If the highest height of spiritual experience, the sheer summit of all realisation is the absolute union of the soul with the Transcendent

who exceeds the individual and the universe, the widest scope
of that union is the discovery of that very Transcendent as the
source, support, continent, informing and constituent spirit and
substance of both these manifesting powers of the divine Essence
and the divine Nature. Whatever the path, this must be for him
the goal. The Yoga of Action also is not fulfilled, is not absolute,
is not victoriously complete until the seeker has felt and lives
in his essential and integral oneness with the Supreme. One he
must be with the Divine both in his highest and inmost and
in his widest being and consciousness, in his work, his will,
his power of action, his mind, body, life. Otherwise he is only
released from the illusion of individual works, but not released
from the illusion of separate being and instrumentality. As the
servant and instrument of the Divine he works, but the crown
of his labour and its perfect base or motive is oneness with
that which he serves and fulfils. The Yoga of devotion too is
complete only when the lover and the Beloved are unified and
difference is abolished in the ecstasy of a divine oneness; and
yet in the mystery of this unification there is the sole existence
of the Beloved but no extinction or absorption of the lover. It
is the highest unity which is the express direction of the path of
knowledge, the call to absolute oneness is its impulse, the experience of it its magnet, but it is this very highest unity which takes
as its field of manifestation in him the largest possible cosmic
wideness. Obeying the necessity to withdraw successively from
the practical egoism of our triple nature and its fundamental
ego-sense, we come to the realisation of the spirit, the self, lord
of this individual human manifestation, but our knowledge is
not integral if we do not make this self in the individual one
with the cosmic spirit and find their greater reality above in
an inexpressible but not unknowable Transcendence. The Jiva,
possessed of himself, must give himself up into the being of the
Divine. The self of the man must be made one with the Self
of all; the self of the finite individual must pour itself into the
boundless finite and that cosmic spirit too must be exceeded in
the transcendent Infinite.

This cannot be done without an uncompromising abolition

of the ego-sense at its very basis and source. In the path of Knowledge one attempts this abolition, negatively by a denial of the reality of the ego, positively by a constant fixing of the thought upon the idea of the One and the Infinite in itself or the One and Infinite everywhere. This, if persistently done, changes in the end the mental outlook on oneself and the whole world and there is a kind of mental realisation; but afterwards by degrees or perhaps rapidly and imperatively and almost at the beginning the mental realisation deepens into spiritual experience — a realisation in the very substance of our being. More and more frequent conditions come of something indefinable and illimitable, a peace, a silence, a joy, a bliss beyond expression, a sense of absolute impersonal Power, a pure existence, a pure consciousness, an all-pervading Presence. The ego persists in itself or in its habitual movements, but the place of the one becomes more and more loosened, the others are broken, crushed, more and more rejected, becoming weak in their intensity, limp or mechanical in their action. In the end there is a constant giving up of the whole consciousness into the being of the Supreme. In the beginning when the restless confusion and obscuring impurity of our outward nature is active, when the mental, vital, physical ego-sense are still powerful, this new mental outlook, these experiences may be found difficult in the extreme: but once that triple egoism is discouraged or moribund and the instruments of the Spirit are set right and purified, in an entirely pure, silent, clarified, widened consciousness the purity, infinity, stillness of the One reflects itself like the sky in a limpid lake. A meeting or a taking in of the reflected Consciousness by that which reflects it becomes more and more pressing and possible; the bridging or abolition of the atmospheric gulf between that immutable ethereal impersonal vastness and this once mobile whirl or narrow stream of personal existence is no longer an arduous improbability and may be even a frequent experience, if not yet an entirely permanent state. For even before complete purification, if the strings of the egoistic heart and mind are already sufficiently frayed and loosened, the Jiva can by a sudden snapping of the main cords escape, ascending like a bird freed into the spaces or widening like a liberated flood into the One and Infinite. There is first a sudden sense of a cosmic consciousness, a casting of oneself into the universal; from that universality one can aspire more easily to the Transcendent. There is a pushing back and rending or a rushing down of the walls that imprisoned our conscious being; there is a loss of all sense of individuality and personality, of all placement in Space or Time or action and law of Nature; there is no longer an ego, a person definite and definable, but only consciousness, only existence, only peace or bliss; one becomes immortality, becomes eternity, becomes infinity. All that is left of the personal soul is a hymn of peace and freedom and bliss vibrating somewhere in the Eternal.

When there is an insufficient purity in the mental being, the release appears at first to be partial and temporary; the Jiva seems to descend again into the egoistic life and the higher consciousness to be withdrawn from him. In reality, what happens is that a cloud or veil intervenes between the lower nature and the higher consciousness and the Prakriti resumes for a time its old habit of working under the pressure but not always with a knowledge or present memory of that high experience. What works in it then is a ghost of the old ego supporting a mechanical repetition of the old habits upon the remnants of confusion and impurity still left in the system. The cloud intervenes and disappears, the rhythm of ascent and descent renews itself until the impurity has been worked out. This period of alternations may easily be long in the integral Yoga; for there an entire perfection of the system is required; it must be capable at all times and in all conditions and all circumstances, whether of action or inaction, of admitting and then living in the consciousness of the supreme Truth. Nor is it enough for the sadhaka to have the utter realisation only in the trance of Samadhi or in a motionless quietude, but he must in trance or in waking, in passive reflection or energy of action be able to remain in the constant Samadhi of the firmly founded Brahmic consciousness.[1] But if

---

[1] Gita.

or when our conscious being has become sufficiently pure and clear, then there is a firm station in the higher consciousness. The impersonalised Jiva, one with the universal or possessed by the Transcendent, lives high-seated above[2] and looks down undisturbed at whatever remnants of the old working of Nature may revisit the system. He cannot be moved by the workings of the three modes of Prakriti in his lower being, nor can he be shaken from his station by the attacks even of grief and suffering. And finally, there being no veil between, the higher peace overpowers the lower disturbance and mobility. There is a settled silence in which the soul can take sovereign possession of itself above and below and altogether.

Such possession is not indeed the aim of the traditional Yoga of knowledge whose object is rather to get away from the above and the below and the all into the indefinable Absolute. But whatever the aim, the path of knowledge must lead to one first result, an absolute quietude; for unless the old action of Nature in us be entirely quieted, it is difficult if not impossible to found either any true soul-status or any divine activity. Our nature acts on a basis of confusion and restless compulsion to action, the Divine acts freely out of a fathomless calm. Into that abyss of tranquillity we must plunge and become that, if we are to annul the hold of this lower nature upon the soul. Therefore the universalised Jiva first ascends into the Silence; it becomes vast, tranquil, actionless. What action takes place, whether of body and these organs or any working whatever, the Jiva sees but does not take part in, authorise or in any way associate itself with it. There is action, but no personal actor, no bondage, no responsibility. If personal action is needed, then the Jiva has to keep or recover what has been called the form of the ego, a sort of mental image of an "I" that is the knower, devotee, servant or instrument, but an image only and not a reality. If even that is not there, still action can continue by the mere continued force of Prakriti, without any personal actor, without indeed there

---

[2] *Udāsīna*, the word for the spiritual "indifference", that is to say the unattached freedom of the soul touched by the supreme knowledge.

being any sense of an actor at all; for the Self into which the Jiva
has cast its being is the actionless, the fathomlessly still. The
path of works leads to the realisation of the Lord, but here even
the Lord is not known; there is only the silent Self and Prakriti
doing her works, even, as it seems at first, not with truly living
entities but with names and forms existing in the Self but which
the Self does not admit as real. The soul may go even beyond
this realisation; it may either rise to the Brahman on the other
side of all idea of Self as a Void of everything that is here, a Void
of unnameable peace and extinction of all, even of the Sat, even
of that Existent which is the impersonal basis of individual or
universal personality; or else it may unite with it as an ineffable
"That" of which nothing can be said; for the universe and all
that is does not even exist in That, but appears to the mind
as a dream more unsubstantial than any dream ever seen or
imagined, so that even the word dream seems too positive a
thing to express its entire unreality. These experiences are the
foundation of that lofty Illusionism which takes such firm hold
of the human mind in its highest overleapings of itself.

These ideas of dream and illusion are simply results in our
still existent mentality of the new poise of the Jiva and its denial
of the claim made upon it by its old mental associations and
view of life and existence. In reality, the Prakriti does not act for
itself or by its own motion, but with the Self as lord; for out of
that Silence wells all this action, that apparent Void looses out
as if into movement all these infinite riches of experience. To this
realisation the sadhaka of the integral Yoga must arrive by the
process that we shall hereafter describe. What then, when he so
resumes his hold upon the universe and views no longer himself
in the world but the cosmos in himself, will be the position of
the Jiva or what will fill in his new consciousness the part of
the ego-sense? There will be no ego-sense even if there is a sort
of individualisation for the purposes of the play of universal
consciousness in an individual mind and frame; and for this
reason that all will be unforgettably the One and every Person
or Purusha will be to him the One in many forms or rather in
many aspects and poises, Brahman acting upon Brahman, one

Nara-Narayana[3] everywhere. In that larger play of the Divine the joy of the relations of divine love also is possible without the lapse into the ego-sense, — just as the supreme state of human love likewise is described as the unity of one soul in two bodies. The ego-sense is not indispensable to the world-play in which it is so active and so falsifies the truth of things; the truth is always the One at work on itself, at play with itself, infinite in unity, infinite in multiplicity. When the individualised consciousness rises to and lives in that truth of the cosmic play, then even in full action, even in possession of the lower being the Jiva remains still one with the Lord, and there is no bondage and no delusion. He is in possession of Self and released from the ego.

---

[3] The Divine, Narayana, making itself one with humanity even as the human, Nara becomes one with the Divine.

Chapter X

The Realisation of the Cosmic Self

OUR FIRST imperative aim when we draw back from mind, life, body and all else that is not our eternal being, is to get rid of the false idea of self by which we identify ourselves with the lower existence and can realise only our apparent being as perishable or mutable creatures in a perishable or ever mutable world. We have to know ourselves as the self, the spirit, the eternal; we have to exist consciously in our true being. Therefore this must be our primary, if not our first one and all-absorbing idea and effort in the path of knowledge. But when we have realised the eternal self that we are, when we have become that inalienably, we have still a secondary aim, to establish the true relation between this eternal self that we are and the mutable existence and mutable world which till now we had falsely taken for our real being and our sole possible status.

In order that there should be any real relation, it must be a relation between two realities. Formerly we had thought the eternal self to be a remote concept far from our mundane existence if not an illusion and an unreality, because in the nature of things we could not conceive of ourselves as anything except this mind, life, body, changing and moving in the succession of Time. When we have once got rid of our confinement to this lower status, we are apt to seize on the other side of the same erroneous relation between self and world; we tend to regard this eternity which we increasingly are or in which we live as the sole reality and begin to look down from it upon the world and man as a remote illusion and unreality, because that is a status quite opposite to our new foundation in which we no longer place our roots of consciousness, from which we have been lifted up and transfigured and with which we seem to have no longer any binding link. Especially is this likely to happen if we have made the finding of the eternal Self not only our primary, but our one and absorbing objective in the withdrawal from the lower triplicity; for then we are likely to shoot at once from pure mind to pure spirit without treading the stairs between this middle and that summit and we tend to fix on our consciousness the profound sense of a gulf which we cannot bridge and can no longer cross over again except by a painful fall.

But the self and the world are in an eternal close relation and there is a connection between them, not a gulf that has to be overleaped. Spirit and material existence are highest and lowest rung of an orderly and progressive series. Therefore between the two there must be a real relation and principle of connection by which the eternal Brahman is able to be at once pure Spirit and Self and yet hold in himself the universe of himself; and it must be possible for the soul that is one with or in union with the Eternal to adopt the same poise of divine relation in place of our present ignorant immersion in the world. This principle of connection is the eternal unity between the Self and all existences; of that eternal unity the liberated soul must be capable, just as the ever free and unbound Divine is capable of it, and that we should realise equally with the pure self-existence at which we have first to aim. For integral self-possession we must be one not only with the Self, with God, but with all existences. We must take back in the right relation and in the poise of an eternal Truth the world of our manifested existence peopled by our fellow-beings from which we had drawn back because we were bound to them in a wrong relation and in the poise of a falsehood created in Time by the principle of divided consciousness with all its oppositions, discords and dualities. We have to take back all things and beings into our new consciousness but as one with all, not divided from them by an egoistic individuality.

In other words, besides the consciousness of the transcendent Self pure, self-existent, timeless, spaceless we have to accept and become the cosmic consciousness, we have to identify our being with the Infinite who makes himself the base and continent of the worlds and dwells in all existences. This is the realisation which the ancient Vedantins spoke of as seeing all existences in the self and the self in all existences; and in addition they speak of the crowning realisation of the man in whom the original miracle of existence has been repeated, self-being has become all these existences that belong to the worlds of the becoming.[1] In these three terms is expressed, fundamentally, the whole of that real relation between the self and the world which we have to substitute for the false relation created by the limiting ego. This is the new vision and sense of infinite being which we have to acquire, this the foundation of that unity with all which we have to establish.

For our real self is not the individual mental being, that is only a figure, an appearance; our real self is cosmic, infinite, it is one with all existence and the inhabitant of all existences. The self behind our mind, life and body is the same as the self behind the mind, life and body of all our fellow-beings, and if we come to possess it, we shall naturally, when we turn to look out again upon them, tend to become one with them in the common basis of our consciousness. It is true that the mind opposes any such identification and if we allow it to persist in its old habits and activities, it will rather strive to bring again its veil of dissonances over our new realisation and possession of self than to shape and subject itself to this true and eternal vision of things. But in the first place, if we have proceeded rightly on the path of our Yoga, we shall have attained to Self through a purified mind and heart, and a purified mind is one that is necessarily passive and open to the knowledge. Secondly, even the mind in spite of its tendency to limit and divide can be taught to think in the rhythm of the unifying Truth instead of the broken terms of the limiting appearance. We must therefore accustom it by meditation and concentration to cease to think of things and beings as separately existent in themselves and rather to think always of the One everywhere and of all things as the One. Although we have spoken hitherto of the withdrawing motion of the Jiva as the first necessity of knowledge and as if it were to be pursued alone and by itself, yet in fact it is better for the sadhaka of the integral Yoga to unite the two movements. By

---

[1] Isha Upanishad.

one he will find the self within, by the other he will find that self in all that seems to us at present to be outside us. It is possible indeed to begin with the latter movement, to realise all things in this visible and sensible existence as God or Brahman or Virat Purusha and then to go beyond to all that is behind the Virat. But this has its inconveniences and it is better, if that be found possible, to combine the two movements.

This realisation of all things as God or Brahman has, as we have seen, three aspects of which we can conveniently make three successive stages of experience. First, there is the Self in whom all beings exist. The Spirit, the Divine has manifested itself as infinite self-extended being, self-existent, pure, not subject to Time and Space, but supporting Time and Space as figures of its consciousness. It is more than all things and contains them all within that self-extended being and consciousness, not bound by anything that it creates, holds or becomes, but free and infinite and all-blissful. It holds them, in the old image, as the infinite ether contains in itself all objects. This image of the ethereal (Akasha) Brahman may indeed be of great practical help to the sadhaka who finds a difficulty in meditating on what seems to him at first an abstract and unseizable idea. In the image of the ether, not physical but an encompassing ether of vast being, consciousness and bliss, he may seek to see with the mind and to feel in his mental being this supreme existence and to identify it in oneness with the self within him. By such meditation the mind may be brought to a favourable state of predisposition in which, by the rending or withdrawing of the veil, the supramental vision may flood the mentality and change entirely all our seeing. And upon that change of seeing, as it becomes more and more potent and insistent and occupies all our consciousness, there will supervene eventually a change of becoming so that what we see we become. We shall be in our self-consciousness not so much cosmic as ultra-cosmic, infinite. Mind and life and body will then be only movements in that infinity which we have become, and we shall see that what exists is not world at all but simply this infinity of spirit in which move the mighty cosmic harmonies of its own images of self-conscious becoming.

But what then of all these forms and existences that make up the harmony? Shall they be to us only images, empty name and form without any informing reality, poor worthless things in themselves and however grandiose, puissant or beautiful they once seemed to our mental vision, now to be rejected and held of no value? Not so; although that would be the first natural result of a very intense absorption in the infinity of the all-containing Self to the exclusion of the infinities that it contains. But these things are not empty, not mere unreal name and form imagined by a cosmic Mind; they are, as we have said, in their reality self-conscious becomings of the Self, that is to say, the Self dwells within all of them even as within us, conscious of them, governing their motion, blissful in his habitation as in his embrace of all that he becomes. As the ether both contains and is as it were contained in the jar, so this Self both contains and inhabits all existences, not in a physical but in a spiritual sense, and is their reality. This indwelling State of the Self we have to realise; we have to see and ourselves to become in our consciousness the Self in all existences. We have, putting aside all vain resistance of the intellect and the mental associations, to know that the Divine inhabits all these becomings and is their true Self and conscious Spirit, and not to know it only intellectually but to know by a self-experience that shall compel into its own diviner mould all the habits of the mental consciousness.

This Self that we are has finally to become to our self-consciousness entirely one with all existences in spite of its exceeding them. We have to see it not only as that which contains and inhabits all, but that which is all, not only as indwelling spirit, but also as the name and form, the movement and the master of the movement, the mind and life and body. It is by this final realisation that we shall resume entirely in the right poise and the vision of the Truth all that we drew back from in the first movement of recoil and withdrawal. The individual mind, life and body which we recoiled from as not our true being, we shall recover as a true becoming of the Self, but no longer in a purely individual narrowness. We shall take up the mind not as a separate mentality imprisoned in a petty motion, but as a large movement of the universal mind, the life not as an egoistic activity of vitality and sensation and desire, but as a free movement of the universal life, the body not as a physical prison of the soul but as a subordinate instrument and detachable robe, realising that also as a movement of universal Matter, a cell of the cosmic Body. We shall come to feel all the consciousness of the physical world as one with our physical consciousness, feel all the energies of the cosmic life around as our own energies, feel all the heart-beats of the great cosmic impulse and seeking in our heart-beats set to the rhythm of the divine Ananda, feel all the action of the universal mind flowing into our mentality and our thought-action flowing out upon it as a wave into that wide sea. This unity embracing all mind, life and matter in the light of a supramental Truth and the pulse of a spiritual Bliss will be to us our internal fulfilment of the Divine in a complete cosmic consciousness.

But since we must embrace all this in the double term of the Being and the Becoming, the knowledge that we shall possess must be complete and integral. It must not stop with the realisation of the pure Self and Spirit, but include also all those modes of the Spirit by which it supports, develops and throws itself out into its cosmic manifestation. Self-knowledge and world-knowledge must be made one in the all-ensphering knowledge of the Brahman.

Chapter XI

The Modes of the Self

SINCE the Self which we come to realise by the path of knowledge is not only the reality which lies behind and supports the states and movements of our psychological being, but also that transcendent and universal Existence which has manifested itself in all the movements of the universal, the knowledge of the Self includes also the knowledge of the principles of Being, its fundamental modes and its relations with the principles of the phenomenal universe. This was what was meant by the Upanishad when it spoke of the Brahman as that which being known all is known.[1] It has to be realised first as the pure principle of Existence, afterwards, says the Upanishad, its essential modes become clear to the soul which realises it. We may indeed, before realisation, try to analyse by the metaphysical reason and even understand intellectually what Being is and what the world is, but such metaphysical understanding is not the Knowledge. Moreover, we may have the realisation in knowledge and vision, but this is incomplete without realisation in the entire soul-experience and the unity of all our being with that which we realise.[2] It is the science of Yoga to know and the art of Yoga to be unified with the Highest so that we may live in the Self and act from that supreme poise, becoming one not only in the conscious essence but in the conscious law of our being with the transcendent Divine whom all things and creatures, whether ignorantly or with partial knowledge and experience, seek to express through the lower law of their members. To know the highest Truth and to be in harmony with it is the condition of right being, to express it in

---

[1] *yasmin vijñāte sarvaṁ vijñātam.*
[2] This is the distinction made in the Gita between Sankhya and Yoga; both are necessary to an integral knowledge.

all that we are, experience and do is the condition of right living.

But rightly to know and express the Highest is not easy for man the mental being because the highest Truth and therefore the highest modes of existence are supramental. They repose on the essential unity of what seem to the intellect and mind and are to our mental experience of the world opposite poles of existence and idea and therefore irreconcilable opposites and contradictions, but to the supramental experience are complementary aspects of the same Truth. We have seen this already in the necessity of realising the Self as at once one and many; for we have to realise each thing and being as That; we have to realise the unity of all as That, both in the unity of sum and in the oneness of essence; and we have to realise That as the Transcendent who is beyond all this unity and this multiplicity which we see everywhere as the two opposite, yet companion poles of all existence. For every individual being is the Self, the Divine in spite of the outward limitations of the mental and physical form through which it presents itself at the actual moment, in the actual field of space, in the actual succession of circumstances that make up the web of inner state and outward action and event through which we know the individual. So, equally, every collectivity small or great is each the Self, the Divine similarly expressing itself in the conditions of this manifestation. We cannot really know any individual or any collectivity if we know it only as it appears inwardly to itself or outwardly to us, but only if we know it as the Divine, the One, our own Self employing its various essential modes and its occasional circumstances of self-manifestation. Until we have transformed the habits of our mentality so that it shall live entirely in this knowledge reconciling all differences in the One, we do not live in the real Truth, because we do not live in the real Unity. The accomplished sense of Unity is not that in which all are regarded as parts of one whole, waves of one sea, but that in which each as well as the All is regarded wholly as the Divine, wholly as our Self in a supreme identity.

And yet, so complex is the Maya of the Infinite, there is a sense in which the view of all as parts of the whole, waves of the sea or even as in a sense separate entities becomes a necessary part of the integral Truth and the integral Knowledge. For if the Self is always one in all, yet we see that for the purposes at least of the cyclic manifestation it expresses itself in perpetual soul-forms which preside over the movements of our personality through the worlds and the aeons. This persistent soul-existence is the real Individuality which stands behind the constant mutations of the thing we call our personality. It is not a limited ego but a thing in itself infinite; it is in truth the Infinite itself consenting from one plane of its being to reflect itself in a perpetual soul-experience. This is the truth which underlies the Sankhya theory of many Purushas, many essential, infinite, free and impersonal souls reflecting the movements of a single cosmic energy. It stands also, in a different way, behind the very different philosophy of qualified Monism which arose as a protest against the metaphysical excesses of Buddhistic Nihilism and illusionist Adwaita. The old semi-Buddhistic, semi-Sankhya theory which saw only the Quiescent and nothing else in the world except a constant combination of the five elements and the three modes of inconscient Energy lighting up their false activity by the consciousness of the Quiescent in which it is reflected, is not the whole truth of the Brahman. We are not a mere mass of changing mind-stuff, life-stuff, body-stuff taking different forms of mind and life and body from birth to birth, so that at no time is there any real self or conscious reason of existence behind all the flux or none except that Quiescent who cares for none of these things. There is a real and stable power of our being behind the constant mutation of our mental, vital and physical personality, and this we have to know and preserve in order that the Infinite may manifest Himself through it according to His will in whatever range and for whatever purpose of His eternal cosmic activity.

And if we regard existence from the standpoint of the possible eternal and infinite relations of this One from whom all things proceed, these Many of whom the One is the essence and the origin and this Energy, Power, or Nature through which the relations of the One and the Many are maintained, we shall see a certain justification even for the dualist philosophies and religions which seem to deny most energetically the unity of beings and to make an unbridgeable differentiation between the Lord and His creatures. If in their grosser forms these religions aim only at the ignorant joys of the lower heavens, yet there is a far higher and profounder sense in which we may appreciate the cry of the devotee poet when in a homely and vigorous metaphor he claimed the right of the soul to enjoy for ever the ecstasy of its embrace of the Supreme. "I do not want to become sugar," he wrote, "I want to eat sugar." However strongly we may found ourselves on the essential identity of the one Self in all, we need not regard that cry as the mere aspiration of a certain kind of spiritual sensuousness or the rejection by an attached and ignorant soul of the pure and high austerity of the supreme Truth. On the contrary, it aims in its positive part at a deep and mysterious truth of Being which no human language can utter, of which human reason can give no adequate account, to which the heart has the key and which no pride of the soul of knowledge insisting on its own pure austerity can abolish. But that belongs properly to the summit of the path of Devotion and there we shall have again to return to it.

The sadhaka of an integral Yoga will take an integral view of his goal and seek its integral realisation. The Divine has many essential modes of His eternal self-manifestation, possesses and finds Himself on many planes and through many poles of His being; to each mode its purpose, to each plane or pole its fulfilment both in the apex and the supreme scope of the eternal Unity. It is necessarily through the individual Self that we must arrive at the One, for that is the basis of all our experience. By Knowledge we arrive at identity with the One; for there is, in spite of the Dualist, an essential identity by which we can plunge into our Source and free ourselves from all bondage to individuality and even from all bondage to universality. Nor is the experience of that identity a gain for knowledge only or for the pure state of abstract being. The height of all our action also, we have seen, is the immersion of ourselves in the Lord through unity with the divine Will or Conscious-Power by the way of works; the height of love is the rapturous immersion of ourselves in unity of ecstatic delight with the object of our love and adoration. But again for divine works in the world the individual Self converts itself into a centre of consciousness through which the divine Will, one with the divine Love and Light, pours itself out in the multiplicity of the universe. We arrive in the same way at our unity with all our fellow-beings through the identity of this self with the Supreme and with the self in all others. At the same time in the action of Nature we preserve by it as soul-form of the One a differentiation which enables us to preserve relations of difference in Oneness with other beings and with the Supreme Himself. The relations will necessarily be very different in essence and spirit from those which we had when we lived entirely in the Ignorance and Oneness was a mere name or a struggling aspiration of imperfect love, sympathy or yearning. Unity will be the law, difference will be simply for the various enjoyment of that unity. Neither descending again into that plane of division which clings to the separation of the ego-sense nor attached to an exclusive seeking for pure identity which cannot have to do with any play of difference, we shall embrace and reconcile the two poles of being where they meet in the infinity of the Highest.

The Self, even the individual self, is different from our personality as it is different from our mental ego-sense. Our personality is never the same; it is a constant mutation and various combination. It is not a basic consciousness, but a development of forms of consciousness, — not a power of being, but a various play of partial powers of being, — not the enjoyer of the self-delight of our existence, but a seeking after various notes and tones of experience which shall more or less render that delight in the mutability of relations. This also is Purusha and Brahman, but it is the mutable Purusha, the phenomenon of the Eternal, not its stable reality. The Gita makes a distinction between three Purushas who constitute the whole state and action of the divine Being, the Mutable, the Immutable and the Highest which is beyond and embraces the other two. That Highest is the Lord in whom we have to live, the supreme Self in us and in all. The Immutable is the silent, actionless, equal, unchanging self which we reach when we draw back from activity to passivity, from the play of consciousness and force and the seeking of delight to the pure and constant basis of consciousness and force and delight through which the Highest, free, secure and unattached, possesses and enjoys the play. The Mutable is the substance and immediate motive of that changing flux of personality through which the relations of our cosmic life are made possible. The mental being fixed in the Mutable moves in its flux and has not possession of an eternal peace and power and self-delight; the soul fixed in the Immutable holds all these in itself but cannot act in the world; but the soul that can live in the Highest enjoys the eternal peace and power and delight and wideness of being, is not bound in its self-knowledge and self-power by character and personality or by forms of its force and habits of its consciousness and yet uses them all with a large freedom and power for the self-expression of the Divine in the world. Here again the change is not any alteration of the essential modes of the Self, but consists in our emergence into the freedom of the Highest and the right use of the divine law of our being.

Connected with this triple mode of the Self is that distinction which Indian philosophy has drawn between the Qualitied and the Qualitiless Brahman and European thought has made between the Personal and the Impersonal God. The Upanishad indicates clearly enough the relative nature of this opposition, when it speaks of the Supreme as the "Qualitied who is without qualities".[3] We have again two essential modes, two fundamental aspects, two poles of eternal being, both of them exceeded in the transcendent divine Reality. They correspond practically to the Silent and the Active Brahman. For the whole action of the universe may be regarded from a certain point of view as the expression and shaping out in various ways of the numberless and infinite qualities of the Brahman. His being assumes by conscious Will all kinds of properties, shapings of the stuff of conscious being, habits as it were of cosmic character and power of dynamic self-consciousness, *gunas*, into which all the

---

[3] *nirguṇo guṇī.*

cosmic action can be resolved. But by none of these nor by all of them nor by their utmost infinite potentiality is He bound; He is above all His qualities and on a certain plane of being rests free from them. The Nirguna or Unqualitied is not incapable of qualities, rather it is this very Nirguna or No-Quality who manifests Himself as Saguna, as Ananta-guna, infinite quality, since He contains all in His absolute capacity of boundlessly varied self-revelation. He is free from them in the sense of exceeding them; and indeed if He were not free from them they could not be infinite; God would be subject to His qualities, bound by His nature, Prakriti would be supreme and Purusha its creation and plaything. The Eternal is bound neither by quality nor absence of quality, neither by Personality nor by Impersonality; He is Himself, beyond all our positive and all our negative definitions.

But if we cannot define the Eternal, we can unify ourselves with it. It has been said that we can become the Impersonal, but not the personal God, but this is only true in the sense that no one can become individually the Lord of all the universes; we *can* free ourselves into the existence of the active Brahman as well as that of the Silence; we can live in both, go back to our being in both, but each in its proper way, by becoming one with the Nirguna in our essence and one with the Saguna in the liberty of our active being, in our nature.[4] The Supreme pours Himself out of an eternal peace, poise and silence into an eternal activity, free and infinite, freely fixing for itself its self-determinations, using infinite quality to shape out of it varied combination of quality. We have to go back to that peace, poise and silence and act out of it with the divine freedom from the bondage of qualities but still using qualities even the most opposite largely and flexibly for the divine work in the world. Only, while the Lord acts out of the centre of all things, we have to act by transmission of His will and power and self-knowledge through the individual centre, the soul-form of Him which we are. The Lord is subject to nothing; the individual soul-form is subject to its own highest

---

[4] *sādharmya-mukti.*

Self and the greater and more absolute is that subjection, the greater becomes its sense of absolute force and freedom.

The distinction between the Personal and the Impersonal is substantially the same as the Indian distinction, but the associations of the English words carry within them a certain limitation which is foreign to Indian thought. The personal God of the European religions is a Person in the human sense of the word, limited by His qualities though otherwise possessed of omnipotence and omniscience; it answers to the Indian special conceptions of Shiva or Vishnu or Brahma or of the Divine Mother of all, Durga or Kali. Each religion really erects a different personal Deity according to its own heart and thought to adore and serve. The fierce and inexorable God of Calvin is a different being from the sweet and loving God of St. Francis, as the gracious Vishnu is different from the terrible though always loving and beneficent Kali who has pity even in her slaying and saves by her destructions. Shiva, the God of ascetic renunciation who destroys all things seems to be a different being from Vishnu and Brahma, who act by grace, love, preservation of the creature or for life and creation. It is obvious that such conceptions can be only in a very partial and relative sense true descriptions of the infinite and omnipresent Creator and Ruler of the universe. Nor does Indian religious thought affirm them as adequate descriptions. The Personal God is not limited by His qualities, He is Ananta-guna, capable of infinite qualities and beyond them and lord of them to use them as He will, and He manifests Himself in various names and forms of His infinite godhead to satisfy the desire and need of the individual soul according to its own nature and personality. It is for this reason that the normal European mind finds it so difficult to understand Indian religion as distinct from Vedantic or Sankhya philosophy, because it cannot easily conceive of a personal God with infinite qualities, a personal God who is not a Person, but the sole real Person and the source of all personality. Yet that is the only valid and complete truth of the divine Personality.

The place of the divine Personality in our synthesis will best be considered when we come to speak of the Yoga of devotion;

it is enough here to indicate that it has its place and keeps it in the integral Yoga even when liberation has been attained. There are practically three grades of the approach to the personal Deity; the first in which He is conceived with a particular form or particular qualities as the name and form of the Godhead which our nature and personality prefers;[5] a second in which He is the one real Person, the All-Personality, the Ananta-guna; a third in which we get back to the ultimate source of all idea and fact of personality in that which the Upanishad indicates by the single word *He* without fixing any attributes. It is there that our realisations of the personal and the impersonal Divine meet and become one in the utter Godhead. For the impersonal Divine is not ultimately an abstraction or a mere principle or a mere state or power and degree of being any more than we ourselves are really such abstractions. The intellect first approaches it through such conceptions, but realisation ends by exceeding them. Through the realisation of higher and higher principles of being and states of conscious existence we arrive not at the annullation of all in a sort of positive zero or even an inexpressible state of existence, but at the transcendent Existence itself which is also the Existent who transcends all definition by personality and yet is always that which is the essence of personality.

When in That we live and have our being, we can possess it in both its modes, the Impersonal in a supreme state of being and consciousness, in an infinite impersonality of self-possessing power and bliss, the Personal by the divine nature acting through the individual soul-form and by the relation between that and its transcendent and universal Self. We may keep even our relation with the personal Deity in His forms and names; if, for instance, our work is predominantly a work of Love it is as the Lord of Love that we can seek to serve and express Him, but we shall have at the same time an integral realisation of Him in all His names and forms and qualities and not mistake the front of Him which is prominent in our attitude to the world for all the infinite Godhead.

[5] *iṣṭa-devatā.*

Chapter XII

The Realisation of Sachchidananda

THE MODES of the Self which we have dealt with in our last Chapter may seem at first to be of a highly metaphysical character, to be intellectual conceptions more fit for philosophical analysis than for practical realisation. But this is a false distinction made by the division of our faculties. It is at least a fundamental principle of the ancient wisdom, the wisdom of the East on which we are founding ourselves, that philosophy ought not to be merely a lofty intellectual pastime or a play of dialectical subtlety or even a pursuit of metaphysical truth for its own sake, but a discovery by all right means of the basic truths of all-existence which ought then to become the guiding principles of our own existence. Sankhya, the abstract and analytical realisation of truth, is one side of Knowledge. Yoga, the concrete and synthetic realisation of it in our experience, inner state, outer life is the other. Both are means by which man can escape out of falsehood and ignorance and live in and by the truth. And since it is always the highest he can know or be capable of that must be the aim of the thinking man, it is the highest truth which the soul must seek out by thought and by life accomplish.

Here lies the whole importance of the part of the Yoga of Knowledge which we are now considering, the knowledge[1] of those essential principles of Being, those essential modes of self-existence on which the absolute Divine has based its self-manifestation. If the truth of our being is an infinite unity in which alone there is perfect wideness, light, knowledge, power, bliss, and if all our subjection to darkness, ignorance, weakness, sorrow, limitation comes of our viewing existence as a clash of infinitely multiple separate existences, then obviously it is the

---

[1] *tattvajñāna.*

most practical and concrete and utilitarian as well as the most lofty and philosophical wisdom to find a means by which we can get away from the error and learn to live in the truth. So also, if that One is in its nature a freedom from bondage to this play of qualities which constitute our psychology and if from subjection to that play are born the struggle and discord in which we live, floundering eternally between the two poles of good and evil, virtue and sin, satisfaction and failure, joy and grief, pleasure and pain, then to get beyond the qualities and take our foundation in the settled peace of that which is always beyond them is the only practical wisdom. If attachment to mutable personality is the cause of our self-ignorance, of our discord and quarrel with ourself and with life and with others, and if there is an impersonal One in which no such discord and ignorance and vain and noisy effort exist because it is in eternal identity and harmony with itself, then to arrive in our souls at that impersonality and untroubled oneness of being is the one line and object of human effort to which our reason can consent to give the name of practicality.

There is such a unity, impersonality, freedom from the play of qualities which lifts us above the strife and surge of Nature in her eternal seeking through mind and body for the true key and secret of all her relations. And it is the ancient highest experience of mankind that only by arriving there, only by making oneself impersonal, one, still, self-gathered, superior to the mental and vital existence in that which is eternally superior to it, can a settled, because self-existent peace and internal freedom be acquired. Therefore this is the first, in a sense the characteristic and essential object of the Yoga of Knowledge. But, as we have insisted, this, if first, is not all; if the essential, it is not the complete object. Knowledge is not complete if it merely shows us how to get away from relations to that which is beyond relations, from personality to impersonality, from multiplicity to featureless unity. It must give us also that key, that secret of the whole play of relations, the whole variation of multiplicity, the whole clash and interaction of personalities for which cosmic existence is seeking. And knowledge is still incomplete if it gives us only an idea and cannot verify it in experience; we seek the key, the secret in order that we may govern the phenomenon by the reality it represents, heal its discords by the hidden principle of concord and unification behind them and arrive from the converging and diverging effort of the world to the harmony of its fulfilment. Not merely peace, but fulfilment is what the heart of the world is seeking and what a perfect and effective self-knowledge must give to it; peace can only be the eternal support, the infinite condition, the natural atmosphere of self-fulfilment.

Moreover, the knowledge that finds the true secret of multi-plicity, personality, quality, play of relations, must show us some real oneness in essence of being and intimate unity in power of being between the impersonal and the source of personality, the qualitiless and that which expresses itself in qualities, the unity of existence and its many-featured multiplicity. The knowledge that leaves a yawning gulf between the two, can be no ulti-mate knowledge, however logical it may seem to the analytical intellect or however satisfactory to a self-dividing experience. True knowledge must arrive at a oneness which embraces even though it exceeds the totality of things, not at a oneness which is incapable of it and rejects it. For there can be no such original unbridgeable chasm of duality either in the All-existence itself or between any transcendent Oneness and the All-existent. And as in knowledge, so in experience and self-fulfilment. The ex-perience which finds at the summit of things such an original unbridgeable chasm between two contrary principles and can at most succeed in overleaping it so that it has to live in one or the other, but cannot embrace and unify, is not the ultimate experience. Whether we seek to know by thought or by the vision of knowledge which surpasses thought or by that perfect self-experience in our own being which is the crown and fulfilment of realisation by knowledge, we must be able to think out, see, experience and live the all-satisfying unity. This is what we find in the conception, vision and experience of the One whose oneness does not cease or disappear from view by self-expression in the Many, who is free from bondage to qualities but is yet infinite quality, who contains and combines all relations, yet is ever absolute, who is no one person and yet all persons because He is all being and the one conscious Being. For the individual centre we call ourselves, to enter by its consciousness into this Divine and reproduce its nature in itself is the high and marvellous, yet perfectly rational and most supremely pragmatic and utilitarian goal before us. It is the fulfilment of our self-existence and at the same time the fulfilment of our cosmic existence, of the individual in himself and of the individual in his relation to the cosmic Many. Between these two terms there is no irreconcilable opposition: rather, our own self and the self of the cosmos having been discovered to be one, there must be between them an intimate unity.

In fact all these opposite terms are merely general conditions for the manifestation of conscious being in that Transcendent who is always one not only behind, but within all conditions however apparently opposite. And the original unifying spirit-stuff of them all and the one substantial mode of them all is that which has been described for the convenience of our thought as the trinity of Sachchidananda. Existence, Consciousness, Bliss, these are everywhere the three inseparable divine terms. None of them is really separate, though our mind and our mental experience can make not only the distinction, but the separation. Mind can say and think "I was, but unconscious" — for no being can say "I am, but unconscious" — and it can think and feel "I am, but miserable and without any pleasure in existence." In reality this is impossible. The existence we really are, the eternal "I am", of which it can never be true to say "It was", is nowhere and at no time unconscious. What we call unconsciousness is simply other-consciousness; it is the going in of this surface wave of our mental awareness of outer objects into our subliminal self-awareness and into our awareness too of other planes of existence. We are really no more unconscious when we are asleep or stunned or drugged or "dead" or in any other state, than when we are plunged in inner thought oblivious of our physical selves and our surroundings. For anyone who has advanced even a little way in Yoga, this is a most elementary proposition and one which offers no difficulty whatever to the thought because it is proved at every point by experience. It is more difficult to realise that existence and undelight of existence cannot go together. What we call misery, grief, pain, absence of delight is again merely a surface wave of the delight of existence which takes on to our mental experience these apparently opposite tints because of a certain trick of false reception in our divided being — which is not our existence at all but only a fragmentary formulation or discoloured spray of conscious-force tossed up by the infinite sea of our self-existence. In order to realise this we have to get away from our absorption in these surface habits, these petty tricks of our mental being, — and when we do get behind and away from them it is surprising how superficial they are, what ridiculously weak and little-penetrating pin-pricks they prove to be, — and we have to realise true existence, and true consciousness, and true experience of existence and consciousness, Sat, Chit and Ananda.

Chit, the divine Consciousness, is not our mental self-awareness; that we shall find to be only a form, a lower and limited mode or movement. As we progress and awaken to the soul in us and things, we shall realise that there is a consciousness also in the plant, in the metal, in the atom, in electricity, in everything that belongs to physical nature; we shall find even that it is not really in all respects a lower or more limited mode than the mental, on the contrary it is in many "inanimate" forms more intense, rapid, poignant, though less evolved towards the surface. But this also, this consciousness of vital and physical Nature is, compared with Chit, a lower and therefore a limited form, mode and movement. These lower modes of consciousness are the conscious-stuff of inferior planes in one indivisible existence. In ourselves also there is in our subconscious being an action which is precisely that of the "inanimate" physical Nature whence has been constituted the basis of our physical being, another which is that of plant-life, and another which is that of the lower animal creation around us. All these are so much dominated and conditioned by the thinking and reasoning conscious-being in us that we have no real awareness of these lower planes; we are unable to perceive in their own terms what these parts of us are doing, and receive it very imperfectly in the terms and values of the thinking and reasoning mind. Still we know well enough that there is an animal in us as well as that which is characteristically human, — something which is a creature of conscious instinct and impulse, not reflective or rational, as well as that which turns back in thought and will on its experience, meets it from above with the light and force of a higher plane and to some degree controls, uses and modifies it. But the animal in man is only the head of our subhuman being; below it there is much that is also sub-animal and merely vital, much that acts by an instinct and impulse of which the constituting consciousness is withdrawn behind the surface. Below this sub-animal being, there is at a further depth the subvital. When we advance in that ultra-normal self-knowledge and experience which Yoga brings with it, we become aware that the body too has a consciousness of its own; it has habits, impulses, instincts, an inert yet effective will which differs from that of the rest of our being and can resist it and condition its effectiveness. Much of the struggle in our being is due to this composite existence and the interaction of these varied and heterogeneous planes on each other. For man here is the result of an evolution and contains in himself the whole of that evolution up from the merely physical and subvital conscious being to the mental creature which at the top he is.

But this evolution is really a manifestation and just as we have in us these subnormal selves and subhuman planes, so are there in us above our mental being supernormal and superhuman planes. There Chit as the universal conscious-stuff of existence takes other poises, moves out in other modes, on other principles and by other faculties of action. There is above the mind, as the old Vedic sages discovered, a Truth-plane, a plane of self-luminous, self-effective Idea, which can be turned in light and force upon our mind, reason, sentiments, impulses, sensations and use and control them in the sense of the real Truth of things just as we turn our mental reason and will upon our sense-experience and animal nature to use and control them in the sense of our rational and moral perceptions. There

there is no seeking, but rather natural possession; no conflict or separation between will and reason, instinct and impulse, desire and experience, idea and reality, but all are in harmony, concomitant, mutually effective, unified in their origin, in their development and in their effectuation. But beyond this plane and attainable through it are others in which the very Chit itself becomes revealed, Chit the elemental origin and primal completeness of all this varied consciousness which is here used for various formation and experience. There will and knowledge and sensation and all the rest of our faculties, powers, modes of experience are not merely harmonious, concomitant, unified, but are one being of consciousness and power of consciousness. It is this Chit which modifies itself so as to become on the Truth-plane the supermind, on the mental plane the mental reason, will, emotion, sensation, on the lower planes the vital or physical instincts, impulses, habits of an obscure force not in superficially conscious possession of itself. All is Chit because all is Sat; all is various movement of the original Consciousness because all is various movement of the original Being.

When we find, see or know Chit, we find also that its essence is Ananda or delight of self-existence. To possess self is to possess self-bliss; not to possess self is to be in more or less obscure search of the delight of existence. Chit eternally possesses its self-bliss; and since Chit is the universal conscious-stuff of being, conscious universal being is also in possession of conscious self-bliss, master of the universal delight of existence. The Divine whether it manifests itself in All-Quality or in No-Quality, in Personality or Impersonality, in the One absorbing the Many or in the One manifesting its essential multiplicity, is always in possession of self-bliss and all-bliss because it is always Sachchidananda. For us also to know and possess our true Self in the essential and the universal is to discover the essential and the universal delight of existence, self-bliss and all-bliss. For the universal is only the pouring out of the essential existence, consciousness and delight; and wherever and in whatever form that manifests as existence, there the essential consciousness must be and therefore there must be an essential delight.

The individual soul does not possess this true nature of itself or realise this true nature of its experience, because it separates itself both from the essential and the universal and identifies itself with the separate accidents, with the unessential form and mode and with the separate aspect and vehicle. Thus it takes its mind, body, life-stream for its essential self. It tries to assert these for their own sake against the universal, against that of which the universal is the manifestation. It is right in trying to assert and fulfil itself in the universal for the sake of something greater and beyond, but wrong in attempting to do so against the universal and in obedience to a fragmentary aspect of the universal. This fragmentary aspect or rather collection of fragmentary experiences it combines around an artificial centre of mental experience, the mental ego, and calls that itself and it serves this ego and lives for its sake instead of living for the sake of that something greater and beyond of which all aspects, even the widest and most general are partial manifestations. This is the living in the false and not the true self; this is living for the sake of and in obedience to the ego and not for the sake of and in obedience to the Divine. The question how this fall has come about and for what purpose it has been done, belongs to the domain of Sankhya rather than of Yoga. We have to seize on the practical fact that to such self-division is due the self-limitation by which we have become unable to possess the true nature of being and experience and are therefore in our mind, life and body subject to ignorance, incapacity and suffering. Non-possession of unity is the root cause; to recover unity is the sovereign means, unity with the universal and with that which the universal is here to express. We have to realise the true self of ourselves and of all; and to realise the true self is to realise Sachchidananda.

Chapter XIII

The Difficulties of the Mental Being

W E HAVE come to this stage in our development of the path of Knowledge that we began by affirming the realisation of our pure self, pure existence above the terms of mind, life and body, as the first object of this Yoga, but we now affirm that this is not sufficient and that we must also realise the Self or Brahman in its essential modes and primarily in its triune reality as Sachchidananda. Not only pure existence, but pure consciousness and pure bliss of its being and consciousness are the reality of the Self and the essence of Brahman.

Further, there are two kinds of realisation of Self or Sachchidananda. One is that of the silent passive quietistic, self-absorbed, self-sufficient existence, consciousness and delight, one, impersonal, without play of qualities, turned away from the infinite phenomenon of the universe or viewing it with indifference and without participation. The other is that of the same existence, consciousness, delight sovereign, free, lord of things, acting out of an inalienable calm, pouring itself out in infinite action and quality out of an eternal self-concentration, the one supreme Person holding in himself all this play of personality in a vast equal impersonality, possessing the infinite phenomenon of the universe without attachment but without any inseparable aloofness, with a divine mastery and an innumerable radiation of his eternal luminous self-delight — as a manifestation which he holds, but by which he is not held, which he governs freely and by which therefore he is not bound. This is not the personal God of the religious or the qualified Brahman of the philosophers, but that in which personal and impersonal, quality and non-quality are reconciled. It is the Transcendent possessing them both in His being and employing them both as modes for His manifestation. This then is the object of realisation for the sadhaka of the integral Yoga.

We see at once that from this point of view the realisation of the pure quiescent self which we gain by withdrawing from mind, life and body, is for us only the acquisition of the necessary basis for this greater realisation. Therefore that process is not sufficient for our Yoga; something else is needed more embracingly positive. As we drew back from all that constitutes our apparent self and the phenomenon of the universe in which it dwells to the self-existent, self-conscious Brahman, so we must now repossess our mind, life and body with the all-embracing self-existence, self-consciousness and self-delight of the Brahman. We must not only have the possession of a pure self-existence independent of the world-play, but possess all existence as our own; not only know ourselves as an infinite unegoistic consciousness beyond all change in Time and Space, but become one with all the outpouring of consciousness and its creative force in Time and Space; not only be capable of a fathomless peace and quiescence, but also of a free and an infinite delight in universal things. For that and not only pure calm is Sachchidananda, is the Brahman.

If it were easily possible to elevate ourselves to the supramental plane and, dwelling securely there, realise world and being, consciousness and action, outgoing and incoming of conscious experience by the power and in the manner of the divine supramental faculties, this realisation would offer no essential difficulties. But man is a mental and not yet a supramental being. It is by the mind therefore that he has to aim at knowledge and realise his being, with whatever help he can get from the supramental planes. This character of our actually realised being and therefore of our Yoga imposes on us certain limitations and primary difficulties which can only be overcome by divine help or an arduous practice, and in reality only by the combination of both these aids. These difficulties in the way of the integral knowledge, the integral realisation, the integral becoming we have to state succinctly before we can proceed farther.

Realised mental being and realised spiritual being are really two different planes in the arrangement of our existence, the one superior and divine, the other inferior and human. To the former belong infinite being, infinite consciousness and will, infinite bliss and the infinite comprehensive and self-effective knowledge of supermind, four divine principles; to the latter belong mental being, vital being, physical being, three human principles. In their apparent nature the two are opposed; each is the reverse of the other. The divine is infinite and immortal being; the human is life limited in time and scope and form, life that is death attempting to become life that is immortality. The divine is infinite consciousness transcending and embracing all that it manifests within it; the human is consciousness rescued from a sleep of inconscience, subjected to the means it uses, limited by body and ego and attempting to find its relation to other consciousnesses, bodies, egos positively by various means of uniting contact and sympathy, negatively by various means of hostile contact and antipathy. The divine is inalienable self-bliss and inviolable all-bliss; the human is sensation of mind and body seeking for delight, but finding only pleasure, indifference and pain. The divine is supramental knowledge comprehending all and supramental will effecting all; the human is ignorance reaching out to knowledge by the comprehension of things in parts and parcels which it has to join clumsily together, and it is incapacity attempting to acquire force and will through a gradual extension of power corresponding to its gradual extension of knowledge; and this extension it can only bring about by a partial and parcelled exercise of will corresponding to the partial and parcelled method of its knowledge. The divine founds itself upon unity and is master of the transcendences and totalities of things; the human founds itself on separated multiplicity and is the subject even when the master of their division and fragmentations and their difficult solderings and unifyings. Between the two there are for the human being a veil and a lid which prevent the human not only from attaining but even from knowing the divine.

When, therefore, the mental being seeks to know the divine, to realise it, to become it, it has first to lift this lid, to put by this veil. But when it succeeds in that difficult endeavour, it sees the divine as something superior to it, distant, high, conceptually, vitally, even physically above it, to which it looks up from its own humble station and to which it has, if at all that be possible, to rise, or if it be not possible, to call that down to itself, to be subject to it and to adore. It sees the divine as a superior plane of being, and then it regards it as a supreme state of existence, a heaven or a Sat or a Nirvana according to the nature of its own conception or realisation. Or it sees it as a supreme Being other than itself or at least other than its own present self, and then it calls it God under one name or another, and views it as personal or impersonal, qualitied or without qualities, silent and indifferent Power or active Lord and Helper, again according to its own conception or realisation, its vision or understanding of some side or some aspect of that Being. Or it sees it as a supreme Reality of which its own imperfect being is a reflection or from which it has become detached, and then it calls it Self or Brahman and qualifies it variously, always according to its own conception or realisation, — Existence, Non-Existence, Tao, Nihil, Force, Unknowable.

If then we seek mentally to realise Sachchidananda, there is likely to be this first difficulty that we shall see it as something above, beyond, around even in a sense, but with a gulf between that being and our being, an unbridged or even an unbridgeable chasm. There is this infinite existence; but it is quite other than the mental being who becomes aware of it, and we cannot either raise ourselves to it and become it or bring it down to ourselves so that our own experience of our being and world-being shall be that of its blissful infinity. There is this great, boundless, unconditioned consciousness and force; but our consciousness and force stands apart from it, even if within it, limited, petty, discouraged, disgusted with itself and the world, but unable to participate in that higher thing which it has seen. There is this immeasurable and unstained bliss; but our own being remains the sport of a lower Nature of pleasure and pain and dull neutral sensation incapable of its divine delight. There is this perfect Knowledge and Will; but our own remains always the mental deformed knowledge and limping will incapable of sharing in or even being in tune with that nature of Godhead. Or else so long as we live purely in an ecstatic contemplation of that vision, we are delivered from ourselves; but the moment we again turn our consciousness upon our own being, we fall away from it and it disappears or becomes remote and intangible. The Divinity leaves us; the Vision vanishes; we are back again in the pettiness of our mortal existence.

Somehow this chasm has to be bridged. And here there are two possibilities for the mental being. One possibility is for it to rise by a great, prolonged, concentrated, all-forgetting effort out of itself into the Supreme. But in this effort the mind has to leave its own consciousness, to disappear into another and temporarily or permanently lose itself, if not quite abolish. It has to go into the trance of Samadhi. For this reason the Raja and other systems of Yoga give a supreme importance to the state of Samadhi or Yogic trance in which the mind withdraws not only from its ordinary interests and preoccupations, but first from all consciousness of outward act and sense and being and then from all consciousness of inward mental activities. In this its inward-gathered state the mental being may have different kinds of realisation of the Supreme in itself or in various aspects or on various levels, but the ideal is to get rid of mind altogether and, going beyond mental realisation, to enter into the absolute trance in which all sign of mind or lower existence ceases. But this is a state of consciousness to which few can attain and from which not all can return.

It is obvious, since mind-consciousness is the sole waking state possessed by mental being, that it cannot ordinarily quite enter into another without leaving behind completely both all our waking existence and all our inward mind. This is the necessity of the Yogic trance. But one cannot continually remain in this trance; or, even if one could persist in it for an indefinitely long period, it is always likely to be broken in upon by any strong or persistent call on the bodily life. And when one returns to the mental consciousness, one is back again in the lower being. Therefore it has been said that complete liberation from the human birth, complete ascension from the life of the mental being is impossible until the body and the bodily life are finally cast off. The ideal upheld before the Yogin who follows this method is to renounce all desire and every least velleity of the human life, of the mental existence, to detach himself utterly from the world and, entering more and more frequently and more and more deeply into the most concentrated state of Samadhi, finally to leave the body while in that utter in-gathering of the being so that it may depart into the supreme Existence. It is also by reason of this apparent incompatibility of mind and Spirit that so many religions and systems are led to condemn the world and look forward only to a heaven beyond or else a void Nirvana or supreme featureless self-existence in the Supreme.

But what under these circumstances is the human mind which seeks the divine to do with its waking moments? For if these are subject to all the disabilities of mortal mentality, if they are open to the attacks of grief, fear, anger, passion, hunger, greed, desire, it is irrational to suppose that by the mere concentration of the mental being in the Yogic trance at the moment of putting off the body, the soul can pass away without return into the supreme existence. For the man's normal consciousness is still subject to what the Buddhists call the chain or the stream of Karma; it is still creating energies which must continue and have their effect in a continued life of the mental being which is creating them. Or, to take another point of view, consciousness being the determining fact and not the bodily existence which is only a result, the man still belongs normally to the status of human, or at least mental activity and this cannot be abrogated by the fact of passing out of the physical body; to get rid of mortal body is not to get rid of mortal mind. Nor is it sufficient to have a dominant disgust of the world or an anti-vital indifference or aversion to the material existence; for this too belongs to the lower mental status and activity. The highest teaching is that even the desire for liberation with all its mental concomitants must be surpassed before the soul can be entirely free. Therefore not only must the mind be able to rise in abnormal states out of itself into a higher consciousness, but its waking mentality also must be entirely spiritualised.

This brings into the field the second possibility open to the mental being; for if its first possibility is to rise out of itself into a divine supramental plane of being, the other is to call down the divine into itself so that its mentality shall be changed into an image of the divine, shall be divinised or spiritualised. This may be done and primarily must be done by the mind's power of reflecting that which it knows, relates to its own consciousness, contemplates. For the mind is really a reflector and a medium and none of its activities originate in themselves, none exist *per se*. Ordinarily, the mind reflects the status of mortal nature and the activities of the Force which works under the conditions of the material universe. But if it becomes clear, passive, pure by the renunciation of these activities and of the characteristic ideas and outlook of mental nature, then as in a clear mirror or like the sky in clear water which is without ripple and unruffled by winds, the divine is reflected. The mind still does not entirely possess the divine or become divine, but is possessed by it or by a luminous reflection of it so long as it remains in this pure passivity. If it becomes active, it falls back into the disturbance of the mortal nature and reflects that and no longer the divine. For this reason an absolute quietism and a cessation first of all outer action and then of all inner movement is the ideal ordinarily proposed; here too, for the follower of the path of knowledge, there must be a sort of waking Samadhi. Whatever action is unavoidable, must be a purely superficial working of the organs of perception and motor action in which the quiescent mind takes eventually no part and from which it seeks no result or profit.

But this is insufficient for the integral Yoga. There must be a positive transformation and not merely a negative quiescence of the waking mentality. The transformation is possible because, although the divine planes are above the mental consciousness and to enter actually into them we have ordinarily to lose the mental in Samadhi, yet there are in the mental being divine planes superior to our normal mentality which reproduce the conditions of the divine plane proper, although modified by the conditions, dominant here, of mentality. All that belongs to the experience of the divine plane can there be seized, but in the mental way and in a mental form. To these planes of divine mentality it is possible for the developed human being to arise in the waking state; or it is possible for him to derive from them a stream of influences and experiences which shall eventually open to them and transform into their nature his whole waking existence. These higher mental states are the immediate sources, the large actual instruments, the inner stations[1] of his perfection.

But in arriving to these planes or deriving from them the limitations of our mentality pursue us. In the first place the mind is an inveterate divider of the indivisible and its whole nature is to dwell on one thing at a time to the exclusion of others or to stress it to the subordination of others. Thus in approaching Sachchidananda it will dwell on its aspect of the pure existence, Sat, and consciousness and bliss are compelled then to lose themselves or remain quiescent in the experience of pure, infinite being which leads to the realisation of the quietistic Monist. Or it will dwell on the aspect of consciousness, Chit, and existence and bliss become then dependent on the experience of an infinite transcendent Power and Conscious-Force, which leads to the realisation of the Tantric worshipper of Energy. Or it will dwell on the aspect of delight, Ananda, and existence and consciousness then seem to disappear into a bliss without basis of self-possessing awareness or constituent being, which leads to the realisation of the Buddhistic seeker of Nirvana. Or it will dwell on some aspect of Sachchidananda which comes to the mind from the supramental Knowledge, Will or Love, and then the infinite impersonal aspect of Sachchidananda is almost or quite lost in the experience of the Deity which leads to the realisations of the various religions and to the possession of some supernal world or divine status of the human soul in relation to God. And for those whose object is to depart anywhither from cosmic existence, this is enough, since they are able by the mind's immergence into or seizure upon any one of these principles or aspects to effect through status in the divine planes of their

---

[1] Called in the Veda variously seats, houses, placings or statuses, footings, earths, dwelling-places, *sadas, gṛha* or *kṣaya, dhāma, padam, bhūmi, kṣiti.*

mentality or the possession by them of their waking state this desired transit.

But the sadhaka of the integral Yoga has to harmonise all so that they may become a plenary and equal unity of the full realisation of Sachchidananda. Here the last difficulty of mind meets him, its inability to hold at once the unity and the multiplicity. It is not altogether difficult to arrive at and dwell in a pure infinite or even, at the same time, a perfect global experience of the Existence which is Consciousness which is Delight. The mind may even extend its experience of this Unity to the multiplicity so as to perceive it immanent in the universe and in each object, force, movement in the universe or at the same time to be aware of this Existence-Consciousness-Bliss containing the universe and enveloping all its objects and originating all its movements. It is difficult indeed for it to unite and harmonise rightly all these experiences; but still it can possess Sachchidananda at once in himself and immanent in all and the continent of all. But with this to unite the final experience of all this as Sachchidananda and possess objects, movements, forces, forms as no other than He, is the great difficulty for mind. Separately any of these things may be done; the mind may go from one to the other, rejecting one as it arrives at another and calling this the lower or that the higher existence. But to unify without losing, to integralise without rejecting is its supreme difficulty.

Chapter XIV

The Passive and the Active Brahman

THE DIFFICULTY which the mental being experiences in arriving at an integral realisation of true being and world-being may be met by following one or other of two different lines of his self-development. He may evolve himself from plane to plane of his own being and embrace on each successively his oneness with the world and with Sachchidananda realised as the Purusha and Prakriti, Conscious-Soul and Nature-Soul of that plane, taking into himself the action of the lower grades of being as he ascends. He may, that is to say, work out by a sort of inclusive process of self-enlargement and transformation the evolution of the material into the divine or spiritual man. This seems to have been the method of the most ancient sages of which we get some glimpse in the Rig Veda and some of the Upanishads.[1] He may, on the other hand, aim straight at the realisation of pure self-existence on the highest plane of mental being and from that secure basis realise spiritually under the conditions of his mentality the process by which the self-existent becomes all existences, but without that descent into the self-divided egoistic consciousness which is a circumstance of evolution in the Ignorance. Thus identified with Sachchidananda in the universal self-existence as the spiritualised mental being, he may then ascend beyond to the supramental plane of the pure spiritual existence. It is the latter method the stages of which we may now attempt to trace for the seeker by the path of knowledge.

When the sadhaka has followed the discipline of withdrawal from the various identifications of the self with the ego, the mind, the life, the body, he has arrived at realisation by knowledge of a pure, still, self-aware existence, one, undivided, peaceful,

---

[1] Notably, the Taittiriya Upanishad.

inactive, undisturbed by the action of the world. The only relation that this Self seems to have with the world is that of a disinterested Witness not at all involved in or affected or even touched by any of its activities. If this state of consciousness is pushed farther one becomes aware of a self even more remote from world-existence; all that is in the world is in a sense in that Self and yet at the same time extraneous to its consciousness, non-existent in its existence, existing only in a sort of unreal mind, — a dream therefore, an illusion. This aloof and transcendent Real Existence may be realised as an utter Self of one's own being; or the very idea of a self and of one's own being may be swallowed up in it, so that it is only for the mind an unknowable That, unknowable to the mental consciousness and without any possible kind of actual connection or commerce with world-existence. It can even be realised by the mental being as a Nihil, Non-Existence or Void, but a Void of all that is in the world, a Non-existence of all that is in the world and yet the only Reality. To proceed farther towards that Transcendence by concentration of one's own being upon it is to lose mental existence and world-existence altogether and cast oneself into the Unknowable.

The integral Yoga of knowledge demands instead a divine return upon world-existence and its first step must be to realise the Self as the All, *sarvam brahma*. First, concentrating on the Self-existent, we have to realise all of which the mind and senses are aware as a figure of things existing in this pure Self that we now are to our own consciousness. This vision of the pure self translates itself to the mind-sense and the mind-perception as an infinite Reality in which all exists merely as name and form, not precisely unreal, not a hallucination or a dream, but still only a creation of the consciousness, perceptual and subtly sensible rather than substantial. In this poise of the consciousness all seems to be, if not a dream, yet very much like a representation or puppet-show taking place in the calm, motionless, peaceful, indifferent Self. Our own phenomenal existence is part of this conceptual movement, a mechanical form of mind and body among other forms, ourselves a name of being among other names, automatically mobile in this Self with its all-encompassing, still self-awareness. The active consciousness of the world is not present in this state to our realisation, because thought has been stilled in us and therefore our own consciousness is perfectly still and inactive, — whatever we do, seems to be purely mechanical, not attended with any conscious origination by our active will and knowledge. Or if thought occurs, that also happens mechanically like the rest, like the movement of our body, moved by the unseen springs of Nature as in the plant and element and not by any active will of our self-existence. For this Self is the immobile and does not originate or take part in the action which it allows. This Self is the All in the sense only of being the infinite One who is immutably and contains all names and forms.

The basis of this status of consciousness is the mind's exclusive realisation of pure self-existence in which consciousness is at rest, inactive, widely concentrated in pure self-awareness of being, not active and originative of any kind of becoming. Its aspect of knowledge is at rest in the awareness of undifferentiated identity; its aspect of force and will is at rest in the awareness of unmodifiable immutability. And yet it is aware of names and forms, it is aware of movement; but this movement does not seem to proceed from the Self, but to go on by some inherent power of its own and only to be reflected in the Self. In other words, the mental being has put away from himself by exclusive concentration the dynamic aspect of consciousness, has taken refuge in the static and built a wall of non-communication between the two; between the passive and the active Brahman a gulf has been created and they stand on either side of it, the one visible to the other but with no contact, no touch of sympathy, no sense of unity between them. Therefore to the passive Self all conscious being seems to be passive in its nature, all activity seems to be non-conscious in itself and mechanical (*jaḍa*) in its movement. The realisation of this status is the basis of the ancient Sankhya philosophy which taught that the Purusha or Conscious-Soul is a passive, inactive, immutable entity, Prakriti or the Nature-Soul including even the mind and the understanding active, mutable, mechanical, but reflected in the Purusha which identifies itself with what is reflected in it and lends to it its own light of consciousness. When the Purusha learns not to identify himself, then Prakriti begins to fall away from its impulse of movement and returns towards equilibrium and rest. The Vedantic view of the same status led to the philosophy of the inactive Self or Brahman as the one reality and of all the rest as name and form imposed on it by a false activity of mental illusion which has to be removed by right knowledge of the immutable Self and refusal of the imposition.[2] The two views really differ only in their language and their viewpoint; substantially, they are the same intellectual generalisation from the same spiritual experience.

If we rest here, there are only two possible attitudes towards the world. Either we must remain as mere inactive witnesses of the world-play or act in it mechanically without any participation of the conscious self and by mere play of the organs of sense and motor-action.[3] In the former choice what we do is to approach as completely as possible to the inactivity of the passive and silent Brahman. We have stilled our mind and silenced the activity of the thought and the disturbances of the heart, we have arrived at an entire inner peace and indifference; we attempt now to still the mechanical action of the life and body, to reduce it to the most meagre minimum possible so that it may eventually cease entirely and for ever. This, the final aim of the ascetic Yoga which refuses life, is evidently not our aim. By the alternative choice we can have an activity perfect enough in outward appearance along with an entire inner passivity, peace, mental silence, indifference and cessation of the emotions, absence of choice in the will.

To the ordinary mind this does not seem possible. As, emotionally, it cannot conceive of activity without desire and emotional preference, so intellectually it cannot conceive of activity without thought-conception, conscious motive and energising of the will. But, as a matter of fact, we see that a large part of our

---

[2] *adhyāropa.*   [3] *kevalair indriyair.* Gita.

own action as well as the whole activity of inanimate and merely animate life is done by a mechanical impulse and movement in which these elements are not, openly at least, at work. It may be said that this is only possible of the purely physical and vital activity and not of those movements which ordinarily depend upon the functioning of the conceptual and volitional mind, such as speech, writing and all the intelligent action of human life. But this again is not true, as we find when we are able to go behind the habitual and normal process of our mental nature. It has been found by recent psychological experiment that all these operations can be effected without any conscious origination in the thought and will of the apparent actor; his organs of sense and action, including the speech, become passive instruments for a thought and will other than his.

Certainly, behind all intelligent action there must be an intelligent will, but it need not be the intelligence or the will of the conscious mind in the actor. In the psychological phenomena of which I have spoken, it is obviously in some of them the will and intelligence of other human beings that uses the organs, in others it is doubtful whether it is an influence or actuation by other beings or the emergence of a subconscious, subliminal mind or a mixed combination of both these agencies. But in this Yogic status of action by the mere organs, *kevalair indriyair*, it is the universal intelligence and will of Nature itself working from centres superconscious and subconscious as it acts in the mechanically purposeful energies of plant-life or of the inanimate material form, but here with a living instrument who is the conscious witness of the action and instrumentation. It is a remarkable fact that the speech, writing and intelligent actions of such a state may convey a perfect force of thought, luminous, faultless, logical, inspired, perfectly adapting means to ends, far beyond what the man himself could have done in his old normal poise of mind and will and capacity, yet all the time he himself perceives but does not conceive the thought that comes to him, observes in its works but does not appropriate or use the will that acts through him, witnesses but does not claim as his own the powers which play upon the world through him as through a passive channel. But this phenomenon is not really abnormal or contrary to the general law of things. For do we not see a perfect working of the secret universal Will and Intelligence in the apparently brute (*jaḍa*) action of material Nature? And it is precisely this universal Will and Intelligence which thus acts through the calm, indifferent and inwardly silent Yogin who offers no obstacle of limited and ignorant personal will and intelligence to its operations. He dwells in the silent Self; he allows the active Brahman to work through his natural instruments, accepting impartially, without participation, the formations of its universal force and knowledge.

This status of an inner passivity and an outer action independent of each other is a state of entire spiritual freedom. The Yogin, as the Gita says, even in acting does no actions, for it is not he, but universal Nature directed by the Lord of Nature which is at work. He is not bound by his works, nor do they leave any after effects or consequences in his mind, nor cling to or leave any mark on his soul;[4] they vanish and are dissolved[5] by their very execution and leave the immutable self unaffected and the soul unmodified. Therefore this would seem to be the poise the uplifted soul ought to take, if it has still to preserve any relations with human action in the world-existence, an unalterable silence, tranquillity, passivity within, an action without regulated by the universal Will and Wisdom which works, as the Gita says, without being involved in, bound by or ignorantly attached to its works. And certainly this poise of a perfect activity founded upon a perfect inner passivity is that which the Yogin has to possess, as we have seen in the Yoga of Works. But here in this status of self-knowledge at which we have arrived, there is an evident absence of integrality; for there is still a gulf, an unrealised unity or a cleft of consciousness between the passive and the active Brahman. We have still to possess consciously the active Brahman without losing the possession of the silent Self. We have to preserve the inner silence, tranquillity,

---

[4] *na karma lipyate nare*. Isha Upanishad.   [5] *pravilīyante karmāṇi*. Gita.

passivity as a foundation; but in place of an aloof indifference to the works of the active Brahman we have to arrive at an equal and impartial delight in them; in place of a refusal to participate lest our freedom and peace be lost we have to arrive at a conscious possession of the active Brahman whose joy of existence does not abrogate His peace, nor His lordship of all workings impair His calm freedom in the midst of His works.

The difficulty is created by the exclusive concentration of the mental being on its plane of pure existence in which consciousness is at rest in passivity and delight of existence at rest in peace of existence. It has to embrace also its plane of conscious force of existence in which consciousness is active as power and will and delight is active as joy of existence. Here the difficulty is that mind is likely to precipitate itself into the consciousness of Force instead of possessing it. The extreme mental state of precipitation into Nature is that of the ordinary man who takes his bodily and vital activity and the mind-movements dependent on them for his whole real existence and regards all passivity of the soul as a departure from existence and an approach towards nullity. He lives in the superficies of the active Brahman and while to the silent soul exclusively concentrated in the passive self all activities are mere name and form, to him they are the only reality and it is the Self that is merely a name. In one the passive Brahman stands aloof from the active and does not share in its consciousness; in the other the active Brahman stands aloof from the passive and does not share in its consciousness nor wholly possess its own. Each is to the other in these exclusivenesses an inertia of status or an inertia of mechanically active non-possession of self if not altogether an unreality. But the sadhaka who has once seen firmly the essence of things and tasted thoroughly the peace of the silent Self, is not likely to be content with any state which involves loss of self-knowledge or a sacrifice of the peace of the soul. He will not precipitate himself back into the mere individual movement of mind and life and body with all its ignorance and straining and disturbance. Whatever new status he may acquire, will only satisfy him if it is founded upon and includes that which he has already found to be indispensable to real self-knowledge, self-delight and self-possession.

Still there is the likelihood of a partial, superficial and temporary relapse into the old mental movement when he attempts again to ally himself to the activity of the world. To prevent this relapse or to cure it when it arrives, he has to hold fast to the truth of Sachchidananda and extend his realisation of the infinite One into the movement of the infinite multiplicity. He has to concentrate on and realise the one Brahman in all things as conscious force of being as well as pure awareness of conscious being. The Self as the All, not only in the unique essence of things, but in the manifold form of things, not only as containing all in a transcendent consciousness, but as becoming all by a constituting consciousness, this is the next step towards his true possession of existence. In proportion as this realisation is accomplished, the status of consciousness as well as the mental view proper to it will change. Instead of an immutable Self containing name and form, containing without sharing in them the mutations of Nature, there will be the consciousness of the Self immutable in essence, unalterable in its fundamental poise but constituting and becoming in its experience all these existences which the mind distinguishes as name and form. All formations of mind and body will be not merely figures reflected in the Purusha, but real forms of which Brahman, Self, conscious Being is the substance and, as it were, the material of their formation. The name attaching to the form will be not a mere conception of the mind answering to no real existence bearing the name, but there will be behind it a true power of conscious being, a true self-experience of the Brahman answering to something that it contained potential but unmanifest in its silence. And yet in all its mutations it will be realised as one, free and above them. The realisation of a sole Reality suffering the imposition of names and forms will give place to that of eternal Being throwing itself out into infinite becoming. All existences will be to the consciousness of the Yogin soul-forms and not merely idea-forms of the Self, of himself, one with him, contained in his universal existence. All the soul-life, mental, vital, bodily existence of all that exists will be to him one indivisible movement and activity of the Being who is the same forever. The Self will be realised as the all in its double aspect of immutable status and mutable activity and it is this that will be seen as the comprehensive truth of our existence.

Chapter XV

The Cosmic Consciousness

TO REALISE and unite oneself with the active Brahman is to exchange, perfectly or imperfectly according as the union is partial or complete, the individual for the cosmic consciousness. The ordinary existence of man is not only an individual but an egoistic consciousness; it is, that is to say, the individual soul or Jivatman identifying himself with the nodus of his mental, vital, physical experiences in the movement of universal Nature, that is to say, with his mind-created ego, and, less intimately, with the mind, life, body which receive the experiences. Less intimately, because of these he can say "my mind, life, body," he can regard them as himself, yet partly as not himself and something rather which he possesses and uses, but of the ego he says, "It is I." By detaching himself from all identification with mind, life and body, he can get back from his ego to the consciousness of the true Individual, the Jivatman, who is the real possessor of mind, life and body. Looking back from this Individual to that of which it is the representative and conscious figure, he can get back to the transcendent consciousness of pure Self, absolute Existence or absolute Non-being, three poises of the same eternal Reality. But between the movement of universal Nature and this transcendent Existence, possessor of the one and cosmic self of the other, is the cosmic consciousness, the universal Purusha of whom all Nature is the Prakriti or active conscious Force. We can arrive at that, become that whether by breaking the walls of the ego laterally, as it were, and identifying oneself with all existences in the One, or else from above by realising the pure Self or absolute Existence in its outgoing, immanent, all-embracing, all-constituting self-knowledge and self-creative power.

The immanent, silent Self in all is the foundation of this cosmic consciousness for the experience of the mental being. It is the Witness pure and omnipresent who as the silent Conscious Soul of the cosmos regards all the activity of the universe; it is Sachchidananda for whose delight universal Nature displays the eternal procession of her works. We are aware of an un-wounded Delight, a pure and perfect Presence, an infinite and self-contained Power present in ourselves and all things, not divided by their divisions, not affected by the stress and struggle of the cosmic manifestation; it is within it all, but it is superior to it all. Because of that all this exists, but that does not exist because of all this; it is too great to be limited by the movement in Time and Space which it inhabits and supports. This foundation enables us to possess in the security of the divine existence the whole universe within our own being. We are no longer limited and shut in by what we inhabit, but like the Divine contain in ourselves all that for the purpose of the movement of Nature we consent to inhabit. We are not mind or life or body, but the informing and sustaining Soul, silent, peaceful, eternal, which possesses them; and since we find this Soul everywhere sustaining and informing and possessing all lives and minds and bodies, we cease to regard it as a separate and individual being in our own. In it all this moves and acts; within all this it is stable and immutable. Having this, we possess our eternal self-existence at rest in its eternal consciousness and bliss.

Next we have to realise this silent Self as the Lord of all the action of universal Nature; we have to see that it is this same Self-existent who is displayed in the creative force of His eternal consciousness. All this action is only His power and knowledge and self-delight going abroad in His infinite being to do the works of His eternal wisdom and will. We shall realise the Divine, the eternal Self of all, first, as the source of all action and inaction, of all knowledge and ignorance, of all delight and suffering, of all good and evil, perfection and imperfection, of all force and form, of all the outgoing of Nature from the eternal divine Principle and of all the return of Nature towards the Divine. We shall realise it next as itself going abroad in its Power and Knowledge, — for the Power and Knowledge are itself, — not only the source of their works, but the creator and doer of their works, one in all existences; for the many souls of the universal manifestation are only faces of the one Divine, the many minds, lives, bodies are only His masks and disguises. We perceive each being to be the universal Narayana presenting to us many faces; we lose ourselves in that universality and perceive our own mind, life and body as only one presentation of the Self, while all whom we formerly conceived of as others, are now to our consciousness our self in other minds, lives and bodies. All force and idea and event and figure of things in the universe are only manifest degrees of this Self, values of the Divine in His eternal self-figuration. Thus viewing things and beings we may see them first as if they were parts and parcels of His divided being;[1] but the realisation and the knowledge are not complete unless we go beyond this idea of quality and space and division by which there comes the experience of less and more, large and small, part and whole, and see the whole Infinite everywhere; we must see the universe and each thing in the universe as in its existence and secret consciousness and power and delight the indivisible Divine in its entirety, however much the figure it makes to our minds may appear only as a partial manifestation. When we possess thus the Divine as at once the silent and sur-passing Witness and the active Lord and all-constituting Being without making any division between these aspects, we possess the whole cosmic Divine, embrace all of the universal Self and Reality, are awake to the cosmic consciousness.

What will be the relation of our individual existence to this cosmic consciousness to which we have attained? For since we have still a mind and body and human life, our individual exis-tence persists even though our separate individual consciousness has been transcended. It is quite possible to realise the cosmic consciousness without becoming that; we can see it, that is to say, with the soul, feel it and dwell in it; we can even be united with it without becoming wholly one with it; in a word, we may preserve the individual consciousness of the Jivatman within the cosmic consciousness of the universal Self. We may preserve a

---

[1] The Gita speaks of the Jiva as a portion of the Lord.

yet greater distinctness between the two and enjoy the relations
between them; we may remain, in a way, entirely the individual
self while participating in the bliss and infinity of the universal
Self. Or we may possess them both as a greater and lesser self,
one we feel pouring itself out in the universal play of the divine
consciousness and force, the other in the action of the same
universal Being through our individual soul-centre or soul-form
for the purposes of an individual play of mind, life and body. But
the summit of this cosmic realisation by knowledge is always the
power to dissolve the personality in universal being, to merge
the individual in the cosmic consciousness, to liberate even the
soul-form into the unity and universality of the Spirit. This is
the *laya*, dissolution, or *mokṣa*, liberation, at which the Yoga
of Knowledge aims. This may extend itself, as in the traditional
Yoga, to the dissolution of mind, life and body itself into the
silent Self or absolute Existence; but the essence of the liberation
is the merging of the individual in the Infinite. When the Yogin
no longer feels himself to be a consciousness situated in the body
or limited by the mind, but has lost the sense of division in the
boundlessness of an infinite consciousness, that which he set out
to do is accomplished. Afterwards the retaining or non-retaining
of the human life is a circumstance of no essential importance,
for it is always the formless One who acts through its many
forms of the mind and life and body and each soul is only one
of the stations from which it chooses to watch and receive and
actuate its own play.

That into which we merge ourselves in the cosmic consciousness is Sachchidananda. It is one eternal Existence that we
then are, one eternal Consciousness which sees its own works in
us and others, one eternal Will or Force of that Consciousness
which displays itself in infinite workings, one eternal Delight
which has the joy of itself and all its workings. It is itself stable,
immutable, timeless, spaceless, supreme and it is still itself in the
infinity of its workings, not changed by their variations, not broken up by their multiplicity, not increased or diminished by their
ebbings and flowings in the seas of Time and Space, not confused
by their apparent contrarieties or limited by their divinely-willed

limitations. Sachchidananda is the unity of the many-sidedness of manifested things, Sachchidananda is the eternal harmony of all their variations and oppositions, Sachchidananda is the infinite perfection which justifies their limitations and is the goal of their imperfections.

So much for the essential relation; but we have to see also the practical results of this internal transformation. It is evident that by dwelling in this cosmic consciousness our whole experience and valuation of everything in the universe will be radically changed. As individual egos we dwell in the Ignorance and judge everything by a broken, partial and personal standard of knowledge; we experience everything according to the capacity of a limited consciousness and force and are therefore unable to give a divine response or set the true value upon any part of cosmic experience. We experience limitation, weakness, incapacity, grief, pain, struggle and its contradictory emotions and we accept these things and their opposites as opposites in an eternal duality and cannot reconcile them in the eternity of an absolute good and happiness. We live by fragments of experience and judge by our fragmentary values each thing and the whole. When we try to arrive at absolute values we only promote some partial view of things to do duty for a totality in the divine workings; we then make believe that our fractions are integers and try to thrust our one-sided view-points into the catholicity of the all-vision of the Divine.

But by entering into the cosmic consciousness we begin to participate in that all-vision and see everything in the values of the Infinite and the One. Limitation itself, ignorance itself change their meaning for us. Ignorance changes into a particularising action of divine knowledge; strength and weakness and incapacity change into a free putting forth and holding back various measures of divine Force; joy and grief, pleasure and pain change into a mastering and a suffering of divine delight; struggle, losing its discords, becomes a balancing of forces and values in the divine harmony. We do not then suffer by the limitations of our mind, life and body; for we no longer live in these, even when we record and accept them, but in the infinity of the Spirit, and these we view in their right value and place and purpose in the manifestation, as degrees of the supreme being, conscious-force and delight of Sachchidananda veiling and manifesting Himself in the cosmos. We cease also to judge other men and things by their outward appearances and are delivered from hostile and contradictory ideas and emotions; for it is the soul that we see, the Divine that we seek and find in every thing and creature, and the rest has only a secondary value to us in a scheme of relations which exist now for us only as self-expressions of the Divine and not as having any absolute value in themselves. So too no event can disturb us, since the distinction of happy and unhappy, beneficent and maleficent happenings loses its force, and all is seen in its divine value and its divine purpose. Thus we arrive at a perfect liberation and an infinite equality. It is this consummation of which the Upanishad speaks when it says "He in whom the self has become all existences, how shall he have delusion, whence shall he have grief who knows entirely[2] and sees in all things oneness."

But this can be only when there is perfection in the cosmic consciousness, and that is difficult for the mental being. The mentality when it arrives at the idea or the realisation of the Spirit, the Divine, tends to break existence into two opposite halves, the lower and the higher existence. It sees on one side the Infinite, the Formless, the One, the Peace and Bliss, the Calm and Silence, the Absolute, the Vast and Pure; on the other it sees the finite, the world of forms, the jarring multiplicity, the strife and suffering and imperfect, unreal good, the tormented activity and futile success, the relative, the limited and vain and vile. To those who make this division and this opposition, complete liberation is only attainable in the peace of the One, in the featurelessness of the Infinite, in the non-becoming of the Absolute which is to them the only real being; to be free all values must be destroyed, all limitations not only transcended but abolished.

---

[2] *Vijānataḥ*. Vijnana is the knowledge of the One and the Many, by which the Many are seen in the terms of the One, in the infinite unifying Truth, Right, Vast of the divine existence.

They have the liberation of the divine rest, but not the liberty of the divine action; they enjoy the peace of the Transcendent, but not the cosmic bliss of the Transcendent. Their liberty depends upon abstention from the cosmic movement, it cannot dominate and possess cosmic existence itself. But it is also possible for them to realise and participate in the immanent as well as the transcendent peace. Still the division is not cured. The liberty they enjoy is that of the silent unacting Witness, not the liberty of the divine Master-consciousness which possesses all things, delights in all, casts itself into all forms of existence without fear of fall or loss or bondage or stain. All the rights of the Spirit are not yet possessed; there is still a denial, a limitation, a holding back from the entire oneness of all existence. The workings of Mind, Life, Body are viewed from the calm and peace of the spiritual planes of the mental being and are filled with that calm and peace; they are not possessed by and subjected to the law of the all-mastering Spirit.

All this is when the mental being takes its station in its own spiritual planes, in the mental planes of Sat, Chit, Ananda, and casts down their light and delight upon the lower existence. But there is possible the attempt at a kind of cosmic consciousness by dwelling on the lower planes themselves after breaking their limitations laterally, as we have said, and then calling down into them the light and largeness of the higher existence. Not only Spirit is one, but Mind, Life, Matter are one. There is one cosmic Mind, one cosmic Life, one cosmic Body. All the attempt of man to arrive at universal sympathy, universal love and the under-standing and knowledge of the inner soul of other existences is an attempt to beat thin, breach and eventually break down by the power of the enlarging mind and heart the walls of the ego and arrive nearer to a cosmic oneness. And if we can by the mind and heart get at the touch of the Spirit, receive the powerful inrush of the Divine into this lower humanity and change our nature into a reflection of the divine nature by love, by universal joy, by oneness of mind with all Nature and all beings, we can break down the walls. Even our bodies are not really separate entities and therefore our very physical consciousness is capable of oneness with the physical consciousness of others and of the cosmos. The Yogin is able to feel his body one with all bodies, to be aware of and even to participate in their affections; he can feel constantly the unity of all Matter and be aware of his physical being as only a movement in its movement.[3] Still more is it possible for him to feel constantly and normally the whole sea of the infinite life as his true vital existence and his own life as only a wave of that boundless surge. And more easily yet is it possible for him to unite himself in mind and heart with all existences, be aware of their desires, struggles, joys, sorrows, thoughts, impulses, in a sense as if they were his own, at least as occurring in his larger self hardly less intimately or quite as intimately as the movements of his own heart and mind. This too is a realisation of cosmic consciousness.

It may even seem as if it were the greatest oneness, since it accepts all that we can be sensible of in the mind-created world as our own. Sometimes one sees it spoken of as the highest achievement. Certainly, it is a great realisation and the path to a greater. It is that which the Gita speaks of as the accepting of all existences as if oneself whether in grief or in joy; it is the way of sympathetic oneness and infinite compassion which helps the Buddhist to arrive at his Nirvana. Still there are gradations and degrees. In the first stage the soul is still subject to the reactions of the duality, still subject therefore to the lower Prakriti; it is depressed or hurt by the cosmic suffering, elated by the cosmic joy. We suffer the joys of others, suffer their griefs; and this oneness can be carried even into the body, as in the story of the Indian saint who, seeing a bullock tortured in the field by its cruel owner, cried out with the creature's pain and the weal of the lash was found reproduced on his own flesh. But there must be a oneness with Sachchidananda in his freedom as well as with the subjection of the lower being to the reactions of Prakriti. This is achieved when the soul is free and superior to the cosmic reactions which are then felt only in the life, mind and body and as an inferior movement; the soul understands, accepts the

[3] *jagatyāṁ jagat.* Isha Upanishad.

experience, sympathises, but is not overpowered or affected, so that at last even the mind and body learn also to accept without being overpowered or even affected except on their surface. And the consummation of this movement is when the two spheres of existence are no longer divided and the mind, life and body obeying utterly the higher law grow into the spirit's freedom; free from the lower or ignorant response to the cosmic touches, their struggle and their subjection to the duality ceases. This does not mean insensibility to the subjection and struggles and sufferings of others, but it does mean a spiritual supremacy and freedom which enables one to understand perfectly, put the right values on things and heal from above instead of struggling from below. It does not inhibit the divine compassion and helpfulness, but it does inhibit the human and animal sorrow and suffering.

The link between the spiritual and the lower planes of the being is that which is called in the old Vedantic phraseology the *vijñāna* and which we may describe in our modern turn of language as the Truth-plane or the ideal mind or supermind. There the One and the Many meet and our being is freely open to the revealing light of the divine Truth and the inspiration of the divine Will and Knowledge. If we can break down the veil of the intellectual, emotional, sensational mind which our ordinary existence has built between us and the Divine, we can then take up through the Truth-mind all our mental, vital and physical experience and offer it up to the spiritual — this was the secret or mystic sense of the old Vedic "sacrifice" — to be converted into the terms of the infinite truth of Sachchidananda, and we can receive the powers and illuminations of the infinite Existence in forms of a divine knowledge, will and delight to be imposed on our mentality, vitality, physical existence till the lower members are transformed into the perfect vessel of the higher nature. This was the double Vedic movement of the descent and birth of the gods in the human creature and the ascent of the human powers that struggle towards the divine knowledge, power and delight and climb into the godheads, the result of which was the possession of the One, the infinite, the beatific existence, the union with God, the Immortality. By possession of this ideal plane we break down entirely the opposition of the lower and the higher existence, the false gulf created by the Ignorance between the finite and the Infinite, God and Nature, the One and the Many, open the gates of the Divine, fulfil the individual in the complete harmony of the cosmic consciousness and realise in the cosmic being the epiphany of the transcendent Sachchidananda. And these results, which obtained on the supramental plane itself or beyond, would be the highest perfection of the human being, we can attain to partially, in a very modified way, in a sort of mental figure by awakening into activity on the corresponding plane of the mental nature. We can get a luminous shadow of that perfect harmony and light. But this belongs to another part of our subject; it is the knowledge on which we must found our Yoga of self-perfection.

Chapter XVI

Oneness

WHEN, then, by the withdrawal of the centre of consciousness from identification with the mind, life and body, one has discovered one's true self, discovered the oneness of that self with the pure, silent, immutable Brahman, discovered in the immutable, in the Akshara Brahman, that by which the individual being escapes from his own personality into the impersonal, the first movement of the Path of Knowledge has been completed. It is the sole that is absolutely necessary for the traditional aim of the Yoga of Knowledge, for immergence, for escape from cosmic existence, for release into the absolute and ineffable Parabrahman who is beyond all cosmic being. The seeker of this ultimate release may take other realisations on his way, may realise the Lord of the universe, the Purusha who manifests Himself in all creatures, may arrive at the cosmic consciousness, may know and feel his unity with all beings; but these are only stages or circumstances of his journey, results of the unfolding of his soul as it approaches nearer the ineffable goal. To pass beyond them all is his supreme object. When on the other hand, having attained to the freedom and the silence and the peace, we resume possession by the cosmic consciousness of the active as well as the silent Brahman and can securely live in the divine freedom as well as rest in it, we have completed the second movement of the Path by which the integrality of self-knowledge becomes the station of the liberated soul.

The soul thus possesses itself in the unity of Sachchidananda upon all the manifest planes of its own being. This is the characteristic of the integral knowledge that it unifies all in Sachchidananda because not only is Being one in itself, but it is one everywhere, in all its poises and in every aspect, in its utmost appearance of multiplicity as in its utmost appearance of oneness. The traditional knowledge while it admits this truth in theory, yet reasons practically as if the oneness were not equal everywhere or could not be equally realised in all. It finds it in the unmanifest Absolute, but not so much in the manifestation, finds it purer in the Impersonal than in the Personal, complete in the Nirguna, not so complete in the Saguna, satisfyingly present in the silent and inactive Brahman, not so satisfyingly present in the active. Therefore it places all these other terms of the Absolute below their opposites in the scale of ascent and urges their final rejection as if it were indispensable to the utter realisation. The integral knowledge makes no such division; it arrives at a different kind of absoluteness in its vision of the unity. It finds the same oneness in the Unmanifest and the Manifest, in the Impersonal and the Personal, in Nirguna and Saguna, in the infinite depths of the universal silence and the infinite largeness of the universal action. It finds the same absolute oneness in the Purusha and the Prakriti; in the divine Presence and the works of the divine Power and Knowledge; in the eternal manifestness of the one Purusha and the constant manifestation of the many Purushas; in the inalienable unity of Sachchidananda keeping constantly real to itself its own manifold oneness and in the apparent divisions of mind, life and body in which oneness is constantly, if secretly real and constantly seeks to be realised. All unity is to it an intense, pure and infinite realisation, all difference an abundant, rich and boundless realisation of the same divine and eternal Being.

The complete realisation of unity is therefore the essence of the integral knowledge and of the integral Yoga. To know Sachchidananda one in Himself and one in all His manifestation is the basis of knowledge; to make that vision of oneness real to the consciousness in its status and in its action and to become that by merging the sense of separate individuality in the sense of unity with the Being and with all beings is its effectuation in Yoga of knowledge; to live, think, feel, will and act in that sense of unity is its effectuation in the individual being and the individual life. This realisation of oneness and this practice of oneness in difference is the whole of the Yoga.

Sachchidananda is one in Himself in whatever status or

whatever plane of existence. We have therefore to make that the basis of all effectuation whether of consciousness or force or being, whether of knowledge or will or delight. We have, as we have seen, to live in the consciousness of the Absolute transcendent and of the Absolute manifested in all relations, impersonal and manifest as all personalities, beyond all qualities and rich in infinite quality, a silence out of which the eternal Word creates, a divine calm and peace possessing itself in infinite joy and activity. We have to find Him knowing all, sanctioning all, governing all, containing, upholding and informing all as the Purusha and at the same time executing all knowledge, will and formation as Prakriti. We have to see Him as one Existence, Being gathered in itself and Being displayed in all existences; as one Consciousness concentrated in the unity of its existence, extended in universal nature and many-centred in innumerable beings; one Force static in its repose of self-gathered consciousness and dynamic in its activity of extended consciousness; one Delight blissfully aware of its featureless infinity and blissfully aware of all feature and force and forms as itself; one creative knowledge and governing Will, supramental, originative and determinative of all minds, lives and bodies; one Mind containing all mental beings and constituting all their mental activities; one Life active in all living beings and generative of their vital activities; one substance constituting all forms and objects as the visible and sensible mould in which mind and life manifest and act just as one pure existence is that ether in which all Conscious-Force and Delight exist unified and find themselves variously. For these are the seven principles of the manifest being of Sachchidananda.

The integral Yoga of knowledge has to recognise the double nature of this manifestation, — for there is the higher nature of Sachchidananda in which He is found and the lower nature of mind, life and body in which He is veiled, — and to reconcile and unite the two in the oneness of the illumined realisation. We have not to leave them separate so that we live a sort of double life, spiritual within or above, mental and material in our active and earthly living; we have to re-view and remould the lower living in the light, force and joy of the higher reality. We have to realise Matter as a sense-created mould of Spirit, a vehicle for all manifestation of the light, force and joy of Sachchidananda in the highest conditions of terrestrial being and activity. We have to see Life as a channel for the infinite Force divine and break the barrier of a sense-created and mind-created farness and division from it so that that divine Power may take possession of and direct and change all our life-activities until our vitality transfigured ceases in the end to be the limited life-force which now supports mind and body and becomes a figure of the all-blissful conscious-force of Sachchidananda. We have similarly to change our sensational and emotional mentality into a play of the divine Love and universal Delight; and we have to surcharge the intellect which seeks to know and will in us with the light of the divine Knowledge-Will until it is transformed into a figure of that higher and sublime activity.

This transformation cannot be complete or really executed without the awakening of the truth-mind which corresponds in the mental being to the Supermind and is capable of receiving mentally its illuminations. By the opposition of Spirit and Mind without the free opening of this intermediate power the two natures, higher and lower, stand divided, and though there may be communication and influence or the catching up of the lower into the higher in a sort of luminous or ecstatic trance, there cannot be a full and perfect transfiguration of the lower nature. We may feel imperfectly by the emotional mind, we may have a sense by the sense-mind or a conception and perception by the intelligent mind of the Spirit present in Matter and all its forms, the divine Delight present in all emotion and sensation, the divine Force behind all life-activities; but the lower will still keep its own nature and limit and divide in its action and modify in its character the influence from above. Even when that influence assumes its highest, widest, intensest power, it will be irregular and disorderly in activity and perfectly realised only in calm and stillness; we shall be subject to reactions and periods of obscuration when it is withdrawn from us; we shall be apt to forget it in the stress of ordinary life and its outward touches and the siege of its dualities and to be fully possessed of it only when alone with ourselves and God or else only in moments or periods of a heightened exaltation and ecstasy. For our mentality, a restricted instrument moving in a limited field and seizing things by fragments and parcels, is necessarily shifting, restless and mutable; it can find steadiness only by limiting its field of action and fixity only by cessation and repose.

Our direct truth-perceptions on the other hand come from that Supermind, — a Will that knows and a Knowledge that effects, — which creates universal order out of infinity. Its awakening into action brings down, says the Veda, the unrestricted downpour of the rain of heaven, — the full flowing of the seven rivers from a superior sea of light and power and joy. It reveals Sachchidananda. It reveals the Truth behind the scattered and ill-combined suggestions of our mentality and makes each to fall into its place in the unity of the Truth behind; thus it can transform the half-light of our minds into a certain totality of light. It reveals the Will behind all the devious and imperfectly regulated strivings of our mental will and emotional wishes and vital effort and makes each to fall into its place in the unity of the luminous Will behind; thus it can transform the half-obscure struggle of our life and mind into a certain totality of ordered force. It reveals the delight for which each of our sensations and emotions is groping and from which they fall back in movements of partially grasped satisfaction or of dissatisfaction, pain, grief or indifference, and makes each take its place in the unity of the universal delight behind; thus it can transform the conflict of our dualised emotions and sensations into a certain totality of serene, yet profound and powerful love and delight. Moreover, revealing the universal action, it shows the truth of being out of which each of its movements arises and to which each progresses, the force of effectuation which each carries with it and the delight of being for which and from which each is born, and it relates all to the universal being, consciousness, force and delight of Sachchidananda. Thus it harmonises for us all the oppositions, divisions, contrarieties of existence and shows us in them the One and the Infinite. Uplifted into this supramental light, pain and pleasure and indifference begin to be converted into joy of the one self-existent Delight; strength and weakness, success and failure turn into powers of the one self-effective Force and Will; truth and error, knowledge and ignorance change into light of the one infinite self-awareness and universal knowledge; increase of being and diminution of being, limitation and the overcoming of limitation are transfigured into waves of the one self-realising conscious existence. All our life as well as all our essential being is transformed into the possession of Sachchidananda.

By way of this integral knowledge we arrive at the unity of the aims set before themselves by the three paths of knowledge, works and devotion. Knowledge aims at the realisation of true self-existence; works are directed to the realisation of the divine Conscious-Will which secretly governs all works; devotion yearns for the realisation of the Bliss which enjoys as the Lover all beings and all existences, — Sat, Chit-Tapas and Ananda. Each therefore aims at possessing Sachchidananda through one or other aspect of his triune divine nature. By Knowledge we arrive always at our true, eternal, immutable being, the self-existent which every "I" in the universe obscurely represents, and we abrogate difference in the great realisation, So Aham, I am He, while we arrive also at our identity with all other beings.

But at the same time the integral knowledge gives us the awareness of that infinite existence as the conscious-force which creates and governs the worlds and manifests itself in their works; it reveals the Self-existent in his universal conscious-will as the Lord, the Ishwara. It enables us to unite our will with His, to realise His will in the energies of all existences and to perceive the fulfilment of these energies of others as part of our own universal self-fulfilment. Thus it removes the reality of strife and division and opposition and leaves only their appearances. By that knowledge therefore we arrive at the possibility of a divine action, a working which is personal to our nature, but impersonal to our being, since it proceeds from That which is beyond our ego and acts only by its universal sanction. We proceed in our works with equality, without bondage to works and their results, in unison with the Highest, in unison with the universal, free from separate responsibility for our acts and therefore unaffected by their reactions. This which we have seen to be the fulfilment of the path of Works becomes thus an annexe and result of the path of Knowledge.

The integral knowledge again reveals to us the Self-existent as the All-blissful who, as Sachchidananda manifesting the world, manifesting all beings, accepts their adoration, even as He accepts their works of aspiration and their seekings of knowledge, leans down to them and drawing them to Himself takes all into the joy of His divine being. Knowing Him as our divine Self, we become one with Him, as the lover and beloved become one, in the ecstasy of that embrace. Knowing Him too in all beings, perceiving the glory and beauty and joy of the Beloved everywhere, we transform our souls into a passion of universal delight and a wideness and joy of universal love. All this which, as we shall find, is the summit of the path of Devotion, becomes also an annexe and result of the path of Knowledge.

Thus by the integral knowledge we unify all things in the One. We take up all the chords of the universal music, strains sweet or discordant, luminous in their suggestion or obscure, powerful or faint, heard or suppressed, and find them all changed and reconciled in the indivisible harmony of Sachchidananda. The Knowledge brings also the Power and the Joy. "How shall he be deluded, whence shall he have sorrow who sees everywhere the Oneness?"

Chapter XVII

The Soul and Nature

THIS IS the result of the integral knowledge taken in its mass; its work is to gather up the different strands of our being into the universal oneness. If we are to possess perfectly the world in our new divinised consciousness as the Divine himself possesses it, we have to know also each thing in its absoluteness, first by itself, secondly in its union with all that completes it; for so has the Divine imaged out and seen its being in the world. To see things as parts, as incomplete elements is a lower analytic knowledge. The Absolute is everywhere; it has to be seen and found everywhere. Every finite is an infinite and has to be known and sensed in its intrinsic infiniteness as well as in its surface finite appearance. But so to know the world, so to perceive and experience it, it is not enough to have an intellectual idea or imagination that so it is; a certain divine vision, divine sense, divine ecstasy is needed, an experience of union of ourselves with the objects of our consciousness. In that experience not only the Beyond but all here, not only the totality, the All in its mass, but each thing in the All becomes to us our self, God, the Absolute and Infinite, Sachchidananda. This is the secret of complete delight in God's world, complete satisfaction of the mind and heart and will, complete liberation of the consciousness. It is the supreme experience at which art and poetry and all the various efforts of subjective and objective knowledge and all desire and effort to possess and enjoy objects are trying more or less obscurely to arrive; their attempt to seize the forms and properties and qualities of things is only a first movement which cannot give the deepest satisfaction unless by seizing them perfectly and absolutely they get the sense of the infinite reality of which these are the outer symbols. To the rational mind and the ordinary sense-experience this may well seem only a poetic fancy or a mystic hallucination; but the absolute satisfaction and sense of illumination which it gives and alone can give is really a proof of its greater validity; we get by that a ray from the higher consciousness and the diviner sense into which our subjective being is intended eventually, if we will only allow it, to be transfigured.

We have seen that this applies to the highest principles of the Divine Being. Ordinarily, the discriminating mind tells us that only what is beyond all manifestation is absolute, only the formless Spirit is infinite, only the timeless, spaceless, immutable, immobile Self in its repose is absolutely real; and if we follow and are governed in our endeavour by this conception, that is the subjective experience at which we shall arrive, all else seeming to us false or only relatively true. But if we start from the larger conception, a completer truth and a wider experience open to us. We perceive that the immutability of the timeless, spaceless existence is an absolute and an infinite, but that also the conscious-force and the active delight of the divine Being in its all-blissful possession of the outpouring of its powers, qualities, self-creations is an absolute and an infinite, — and indeed the same absolute and infinite, so much the same that we can enjoy simultaneously, equally the divine timeless calm and peace and the divine time-possessing joy of activity, freely, infinitely, without bondage or the lapse into unrest and suffering. So too we can have the same experience of all the principles of this activity which in the Immutable are self-contained and in a sense drawn in and concealed, in the cosmic are expressed and realise their infinite quality and capacity.

The first of these principles in importance is the duality — which resolves itself into a unity — of Purusha and Prakriti of which we have had occasion to speak in the Yoga of Works, but which is of equal importance for the Yoga of Knowledge. This division was made most clearly by the old Indian philosophies; but it bases itself upon the eternal fact of practical duality in unity upon which the world-manifestation is founded. It is given different names according to our view of the universe. The Vedantins spoke of the Self and Maya, meaning according to their predilections by the Self the Immutable and by Maya the power the Self has of imposing on itself the cosmic illusion, or by the Self the Divine Being and by Maya the nature of conscious-being and the conscious-force by which the Divine embodies himself in soul-forms and forms of things. Others spoke of Ishwara and Shakti, the Lord and His force, His cosmic power. The analytic philosophy of the Sankhyas affirmed their eternal duality without any possibility of oneness, accepting only relations of union and separation by which the cosmic action of Prakriti begins, proceeds or ceases for the Purusha; for the Purusha is an inactive conscious existence, — it is the Soul the same in itself and immutable forever, — Prakriti the active force of Nature which by its motion creates and maintains and by its sinking into rest dissolves the phenomenon of the cosmos. Leaving aside these philosophical distinctions, we come to the original psychological experience from which all really take their start, that there are two elements in the existence of living beings, of human beings at least if not of all cosmos, — a dual being, Nature and the soul.

This duality is self-evident. Without any philosophy at all, by the mere force of experience it is what we can all perceive, although we may not take the trouble to define. Even the most thoroughgoing materialism which denies the soul or resolves it into a more or less illusory result of natural phenomena acting upon some ill-explained phenomenon of the physical brain which we call consciousness or the mind, but which is really no more than a sort of complexity of nervous spasms, cannot get rid of the practical fact of this duality. It does not matter at all how it came about; the fact is not only there, it determines our whole existence, it is the one fact which is really important to us as human beings with a will and an intelligence and a subjective existence which makes all our happiness and our suffering. The whole problem of life resolves itself into this one question, — "What are we to do with this soul and nature set face to face with each other, — we who have as one side of our existence this Nature, this personal and cosmic activity, which tries to impress itself upon the soul, to possess, control, determine it, and as the other side this soul which feels that in some mysterious way it has a freedom, a control over itself, a responsibility for what it is and does, and tries therefore to turn upon Nature, its own and the world's, and to control, possess, enjoy, or even, it may be, reject and escape from her?" In order to answer that question we have to know, — to know what the soul can do, to know what it can do with itself, to know too what it can do with Nature and the world. The whole of human philosophy, religion, science is really nothing but an attempt to get at the right data upon which it will be possible to answer the question and solve, as satisfactorily as our knowledge will allow, the problem of our existence.

The hope of a complete escape from our present strife with and subjection to our lower and troubled nature and existence arises when we perceive what religion and philosophy affirm, but modern thought has tried to deny, that there are two poises of our soul-existence, a lower, troubled and subjected, a higher, supreme, untroubled and sovereign, one vibrant in Mind, the other tranquil in Spirit. The hope not only of an escape, but of a completely satisfying and victorious solution comes when we perceive what some religions and philosophies affirm, but others seem to deny, that there is also in the dual unity of soul and nature a lower, an ordinary human status and a higher, a divine; for it is in the divine alone that the conditions of the duality stand reversed; there the soul becomes that which now it only struggles and aspires to be, master of its nature, free and by union with the Divine possessor also of the world-nature. According to our idea of these possibilities will be the solution we shall attempt to realise.

Involved in mind, possessed by the ordinary phenomenon of mental thought, sensation, emotion, reception of the vital and physical impacts of the world and mechanical reaction to them, the soul is subject to Nature. Even its will and intelligence are determined by its mental nature, determined even more largely by the mental nature of its environment which acts upon, subtly as well as overtly, and overcomes the individual mentality. Thus its attempt to regulate, to control, to determine its own experience and action is pursued by an element of illusion, since when it thinks it is acting, it is really Nature that is acting and determining all it thinks, wills and does. If there were not this constant knowledge in it that it is, that it exists in itself, is not the body or life but something other which at least receives and accepts the cosmic experience if it does not determine it, it would be compelled in the end to suppose that Nature is all and the soul an illusion. This is the conclusion modern Materialism affirms and to that nihilistic Buddhism arrived; the Sankhyas, perceiving the dilemma, solved it by saying that the soul in fact only mirrors Nature's determinations and itself determines nothing, is not the lord, but can by refusing to mirror them fall back into eternal immobility and peace. There are too the other solutions which arrive at the same practical conclusion, but from the other end, the spiritual; for they affirm either that Nature is an illusion or that both the soul and Nature are impermanent and they point us to a state beyond in which their duality has no existence; either they cease by the extinction of both in something permanent and ineffable or their discordances end by the exclusion of the active principle altogether. Though they do not satisfy humanity's larger hope and deep-seated impulse and aspiration, these are valid solutions so far as they go; for they arrive at an Absolute in itself or at the separate absolute of the soul, even if they reject the many rapturous infinities of the Absolute which the true possession of Nature by the soul in its divine existence offers to the eternal seeker in man.

Uplifted into the Spirit the soul is no longer subject to Nature; it is above this mental activity. It may be above it in detachment and aloofness, *udāsīna*, seated above and indifferent, or attracted by and lost in the absorbing peace or bliss of its undifferentiated, its concentrated spiritual experience of itself; we must then transcend by a complete renunciation of Nature and cosmic existence, not conquer by a divine and sovereign possession. But the Spirit, the Divine is not only above Nature; it is master of Nature and cosmos; the soul rising into its spiritual poise must at least be capable of the same mastery by its unity with the Divine. It must be capable of controlling its own nature not only in calm or by forcing it to repose, but with a sovereign control of its play and activity.

To arrive by an intense spirituality at the absolute of the soul is our possibility on one side of our dual existence; to enjoy the absolute of Nature and of everything in Nature is our possibility on the other side of this eternal duality. To unify these highest aspirations in a divine possession of God and ourselves and the world, should be our happy completeness. In the lower poise this is not possible because the soul acts through the mind and the mind can only act individually and fragmentarily in a contented obedience or a struggling subjection to that universal Nature through which the divine knowledge and the divine Will are worked out in the cosmos. But the Spirit is in possession of knowledge and will, of which it is the source and cause and not a subject; therefore in proportion as the soul assumes its divine or spiritual being, it assumes also control of the movements of its nature. It becomes, in the ancient language, Swarat, free and a self-ruler over the kingdom of its own life and being. But also it increases in control over its environment, its world.

This it can only do entirely by universalising itself; for it is the divine and universal will that it must express in its action upon the world. It must first extend its consciousness and see the universe in itself instead of being like the mind limited by the physical, vital, sensational, emotional, intellectual outlook of the little divided personality. It must accept the world-truths, the world-energies, the world-tendencies, the world-purposes as its own instead of clinging to its own intellectual ideas, desires and endeavours, preferences, objects, intentions, impulses; these, so far as they remain, must be harmonised with the universal. It must then submit its knowledge and will at their very source to the divine Knowledge and the divine Will and so arrive through submission at immergence, losing its personal light in the divine Light and its personal initiative in the divine initiative. To be first in tune with the Infinite, in harmony with the Divine, and then to be unified with the Infinite, taken into the Divine is its condition of perfect strength and mastery, and this is precisely the very nature of the spiritual life and the spiritual existence.

The distinction made in the Gita between the Purusha and the Prakriti gives us the clue to the various attitudes which the soul can adopt towards Nature in its movement towards perfect freedom and rule. The Purusha is, says the Gita, witness, upholder, source of the sanction, knower, lord, enjoyer; Prakriti executes, it is the active principle and must have an operation corresponding to the attitude of the Purusha. The soul may assume, if it wishes, the poise of the pure witness, *sākṣī*; it may look on at the action of Nature as a thing from which it stands apart; it watches, but does not itself participate. We have seen the importance of this quietistic capacity; it is the basis of the movement of withdrawal by which we can say of everything, — body, life, mental action, thought, sensation, emotion, — "This is Prakriti working in the life, mind and body, it is not myself, it is not even mine," and thus come to the soul's separation from these things and to their quiescence. This may, therefore, be an attitude of renunciation or at least of non-participation, tamasic, with a resigned and inert endurance of the natural action so long as it lasts, rajasic, with a disgust, aversion and recoil from it, sattwic, with a luminous intelligence of the soul's separateness and the peace and joy of aloofness and repose; but also it may be attended by an equal and impersonal delight as of a spectator at a show, joyous but unattached and ready to rise up at any moment and as joyfully depart. The attitude of the Witness at its highest is the absolute of unattachment and freedom from affection by the phenomena of the cosmic existence.

As the pure Witness, the soul refuses the function of upholder or sustainer of Nature. The upholder, *bhartā*, is another, God or Force or Maya, but not the soul, which only admits the reflection of the natural action upon its watching consciousness, but not any responsibility for maintaining or continuing it. It does not say "All this is in me and maintained by me, an activity of my being," but at the most "This is imposed on me, but really external to myself." Unless there is a clear and real duality in existence, this cannot be the whole truth of the matter; the soul is the upholder also, it supports in its being the energy which unrolls the spectacle of the cosmos and which conducts its energies. When the Purusha accepts this upholding, it may do it still passively and without attachment, feeling that it contributes the energy, but not that it controls and determines it. The control is another, God or Force or the very nature of Maya; the soul only upholds indifferently so long as it must, so long perhaps as the force of its past sanction and interest in the energy continues and refuses to be exhausted. But if the attitude of the upholder is fully accepted, an important step forward has been taken towards identification with the active Brahman and his joy of cosmic being. For the Purusha has become the active giver of the sanction.

In the attitude of the Witness there is also a kind of sanction, but it is passive, inert and has no kind of absoluteness about it; but if he consents entirely to uphold, the sanction has become active, even though the soul may do no more than consent to reflect, support and thereby maintain in action all the energies of Prakriti. It may refuse to determine, to select, believing that it is God or Force itself or some Knowledge-Will that selects and determines, and the soul only a witness and upholder and thereby giver of the sanction, *anumantā*, but not the possessor and the director of the knowledge and the will, *jñātā īśvaraḥ*. Then there is a general sanction in the form of an active upholding of whatever is determined by God or universal Will, but there is not an active determination. But if the soul habitually selects and rejects in what is offered to it, it determines; the relatively passive has become an entirely active sanction and is on the way to be an active control.

This it becomes when the soul accepts its complete function as the knower, lord and enjoyer of Nature. As the knower the soul possesses the knowledge of the force that acts and determines, it sees the values of being which are realising themselves in cosmos, it is in the secret of Fate. For the force that acts is itself determined by the knowledge which is its origin and the source and standardiser of its valuations and effectuations of values. Therefore in proportion as the soul becomes again the knower, it gets the capacity of becoming also the controller of the action whether by spiritual force alone or by that force figuring itself in mental and physical activities. There may be in our soul life a perfect spiritual knowledge and understanding not only of all our internal activities but of all the unrolling of things, events, human, animal, natural activities around us, the world-vision of the Rishi. This may not be attended by an active putting forth of power upon the world, though that is seldom entirely absent; for the Rishi is not uninterested in the world or in his fellow-creatures, but one with them by sympathy or by accepting all creatures as his own self in many minds and bodies. The old forest-dwelling anchorites even are described continually as busily engaged in doing good to all creatures. This can only be done in the spiritual realisation, not by an effort, for effort is a diminution of freedom, but by a spiritual influence or by a spiritual mastery over the minds of men and the workings of Nature, which reflects the divine effective immanence and the divine effective mastery.

Nor can it do this without becoming the active enjoyer, *bhoktā*. In the lower being the enjoyment is of a twofold kind, positive and negative, which in the electricity of sensation translates itself into joy and suffering; but in the higher it is an actively equal enjoyment of the divine delight in self-manifestation. That enjoyment again may be limited to a silent spiritual delight or an integral divine joy possessing all things around us and all activities of all parts of our being.

There is no loss of freedom, no descent into an ignorant attachment. The man free in his soul is aware that the Divine is the lord of the action of Nature, that Maya is His Knowledge-Will determining and effecting all, that Force is the Will side of this double divine Power in which knowledge is always present and effectual. He is aware of himself also, even individually, as a centre of the divine existence, — a portion of the Lord, the Gita expresses it, — controlling so far the action of Nature which he views, upholds, sanctions, enjoys, knows and by the determinative power of knowledge controls. And when he universalises himself, his knowledge still reflects only the divine knowledge, his will effectuates only the divine will, he enjoys only the divine delight and not an ignorant personal satisfaction. Thus the Purusha preserves its freedom in its possession, renunciation of limited personality even in its representative enjoyment and delight of cosmic being. It has taken up fully in the higher poise the true relations of the soul and Nature.

Purusha and Prakriti in their union and duality arise from the being of Sachchidananda. Self-conscious existence is the essential nature of the Being; that is Sat or Purusha. The Power of self-aware existence, whether drawn into itself or acting in the works of its consciousness and force, its knowledge and its will, Chit and Tapas, Chit and its Shakti, — that is Prakriti. Delight of being, Ananda, is the eternal truth of the union of this conscious being and its conscious force whether absorbed in itself or else deployed in the inseparable duality of its two aspects. It unrolls the worlds as Prakriti and views them as Purusha; acts in them and upholds the action; executes works and gives the sanction without which the force of Nature cannot act; executes and controls the knowledge and the will and knows and controls the determinations of the knowledge-force and will-force; ministers to the enjoyment and enjoys; — all is the Soul possessor, observer, knower, lord of Nature and Nature expressing the being, executing the will, satisfying the self-knowledge, ministering to the delight of being of the soul. There we have, founded on the very nature of being, the supreme and the universal relation of Prakriti with Purusha. The relation in its imperfect, perverted or reverse terms is the world as we see it; but the perfect relation brings the absolute joy of the soul in itself and, based upon that, the absolute joy of the soul in Nature which is the divine fulfilment of world-existence.

Chapter XVIII

The Soul and Its Liberation

WE HAVE now to pause and consider to what this acceptance of the relations of Purusha and Prakriti commits us; for it means that the Yoga which we are pursuing has for end none of the ordinary aims of humanity. It neither accepts our earthly existence as it is, nor can be satisfied with some kind of moral perfection or religious ecstasy, with a heaven beyond or with some dissolution of our being by which we get satisfactorily done with the trouble of existence. Our aim becomes quite other; it is to live in the Divine, the Infinite, in God and not in any mere egoism and temporality, but at the same time not apart from Nature, from our fellow-beings, from earth and the mundane existence, any more than the Divine lives aloof from us and the world. He exists also in relation to the world and Nature and all these beings, but with an absolute and inalienable power, freedom and self-knowledge. Our liberation and perfection is to transcend ignorance, bondage and weakness and live in Him in relation to the world and Nature with the divine power, freedom and self-knowledge. For the highest relation of the Soul to existence is the Purusha's possession of Prakriti, when he is no longer ignorant and subject to his nature, but knows, transcends, enjoys and controls his manifested being and determines largely and freely what shall be his self-expression.

A oneness finding itself out in the variations of its own duality is the whole play of the soul with Nature in its cosmic birth and becoming. One Sachchidananda everywhere, self-existent, illimitable, a unity indestructible by the utmost infinity of its own variations, is the original truth of being for which our knowledge seeks and to that our subjective existence eventually arrives. From that all other truths arise, upon that they are based, by that they are at every moment made possible and in that they in the end can know themselves and each other, are reconciled, harmonised and justified. All relations in the world, even to its greatest and most shocking apparent discords, are relations of something eternal to itself in its own universal existence; they are not anywhere or at any time collisions of disconnected beings who meet fortuitously or by some mechanical necessity of cosmic existence. Therefore to get back to this eternal fact of oneness is our essential act of self-knowledge; to live in it must be the effective principle of our inner possession of our being and of our right and ideal relations with the world. That is why we have had to insist first and foremost on oneness as the aim and in a way the whole aim of our Yoga of knowledge.

But this unity works itself out everywhere and on every plane by an executive or practical truth of duality. The Eternal is the one infinite conscious Existence, Purusha, and not something inconscient and mechanical; it exists eternally in its delight of the force of its own conscious being founded in an equilibrium of unity; but it exists also in the no less eternal delight of its force of conscious being at play with various creative self-experience in the universe. Just as we ourselves are or can become aware of being always something timeless, nameless, perpetual which we call our self and which constitutes the unity of all that we are, and yet simultaneously we have the various experience of what we do, think, will, create, become, such too is the self-awareness of this Purusha in the world. Only we, being at present limited and ego-bound mental individuals, have usually this experience in the ignorance and do not live in the self, but only look back at it or draw back to it from time to time, while the Eternal has it in His infinite self-knowledge, is eternally this self and looks from the fullness of self-being at all this self-experience. He does not like us, bound prisoners of the mind, conceive of His being as either a sort of indefinite result and sum or else a high contradiction of self-experience. The old philosophical quarrel between Being and Becoming is not possible to the eternal self-knowledge.

An active force of conscious-being which realises itself in its powers of self-experience, its powers of knowledge, will, self-delight, self-formulation with all their marvellous variations, inversions, conservations and conversions of energy, even perversions, is what we call Prakriti or Nature, in ourselves as in the cosmos. But behind this force of variation is the eternal equilibrium of the same force in an equal unity which supports impartially, governs even as it has originated the variations and directs them to whatever aim of its self-delight the Being, the Purusha, has conceived in its consciousness and determined by its will or power of consciousness. That is the divine Nature into unity with which we have to get back by our Yoga of self-knowledge. We have to become the Purusha, Sachchidananda, delighting in a divine individual possession of its Prakriti and no longer mental beings subject to our egoistic nature. For that is the real man, the supreme and integral self of the individual, and the ego is only a lower and partial manifestation of ourselves through which a certain limited and preparatory experience becomes possible and is for a time indulged. But this indulgence of the lower being is not our whole possibility; it is not the sole or crowning experience for which we exist as human beings even in this material world.

This individual being of ours is that by which ignorance is possible to self-conscious mind, but it is also that by which liberation into the spiritual being is possible and the enjoyment of divine immortality. It is not the Eternal in His transcendence or in His cosmic being who arrives at this immortality; it is the individual who rises into self-knowledge, in him it is possessed and by him it is made effective. All life, spiritual, mental or material, is the play of the soul with the possibilities of its nature; for without this play there can be no self-expression and no relative self-experience. Even, then, in our realisation of all as our larger self and in our oneness with God and other beings, this play can and must persist, unless we desire to cease from all self-expression and all but a tranced and absorbed self-experience. But then it is in the individual being that this trance or this liberated play is realised; the trance is this mental being's immersion in the sole experience of unity, the liberated play is the taking up of his mind into the spiritual being for the free realisation and delight of oneness. For the nature of the divine existence is to possess always its unity, but to possess it also in an infinite experience, from many standpoints, on many planes, through many conscious powers or selves of itself, individualities — in our limited intellectual language — of the one conscious being. Each one of us is one of these individualities. To stand away from God in limited ego, limited mind is to stand away from ourselves, to be unpossessed of our true individuality, to be the apparent and not the real individual; it is our power of ignorance. To be taken up into the divine Being and be aware of our spiritual, infinite and universal consciousness as that in which we now live, is to possess our supreme and integral self, our true individuality; it is our power of self-knowledge.

By knowing the eternal unity of these three powers of the eternal manifestation, God, Nature and the individual self, and their intimate necessity to each other, we come to understand existence itself and all that in the appearances of the world now puzzles our ignorance. Our self-knowledge abolishes none of these things, it abolishes only our ignorance and those circumstances proper to the ignorance which made us bound and subject to the egoistic determinations of our nature. When we get back to our true being, the ego falls away from us; its place is taken by our supreme and integral self, the true individuality. As this supreme self it makes itself one with all beings and sees all world and Nature in its own infinity. What we mean by this is simply that our sense of separate existence disappears into a consciousness of illimitable, undivided, infinite being in which we no longer feel bound to the name and form and the particular mental and physical determinations of our present birth and becoming and are no longer separate from anything or anyone in the universe. This was what the ancient thinkers called the Non-birth or the destruction of birth or Nirvana. At the same time we continue to live and act through our individual birth and becoming, but with a different knowledge and quite another kind of experience; the world also continues, but we see it in our own being and not as something external to it and other than ourselves. To be able to live permanently in this new consciousness of our real, our integral being is to attain liberation and enjoy immortality.

Here there comes in the complication of the idea that immortality is only possible after death in other worlds, upon higher planes of existence or that liberation must destroy all possibility of mental or bodily living and annihilate the individual existence for ever in an impersonal infinity. These ideas derive their strength from a certain justification in experience and a sort of necessity or upward attraction felt by the soul when it shakes off the compelling ties of mind and matter. It is felt that these ties are inseparable from all earthly living or from all mental existence. Death is the king of the material world, for life seems to exist here only by submission to death, by a constant dying; immortality has to be conquered here with difficulty and seems to be in its nature a rejection of all death and therefore of all birth into the material world. The field of immortality must be in some immaterial plane, in some heavens where either the body does not exist or else is different and only a form of the soul or a secondary circumstance. On the other hand, it is felt by those who would go beyond immortality even, that all planes and heavens are circumstances of the finite existence and the infinite self is void of all these things. They are dominated by a necessity to disappear into the impersonal and infinite and an inability to equate in any way the bliss of impersonal being with the soul's delight in its becoming. Philosophies have been invented which justify to the intellect this need of immersion and disappearance; but what is really important and decisive is the call of the Beyond, the need of the soul, its delight — in this case — in a sort of impersonal existence or non-existence. For what decides is the determining delight of the Purusha, the relation which it wills to establish with its Prakriti, the experience at which it arrives as the result of the line it has followed in the development of its individual self-experience among all the various possibilities of its nature. Our intellectual justifications are only the account of that experience which we give to the reason and the devices by which we help the mind to assent to the direction in which the soul is moving.

The cause of our world-existence is not, as our present experience induces us to believe, the ego; for the ego is only a result and a circumstance of our mode of world-existence. It is a relation which the many-souled Purusha has set up between individualised minds and bodies, a relation of self-defence and mutual exclusion and aggression in order to have among all the dependences of things in the world upon each other a possibility of independent mental and physical experience. But there can be no absolute independence upon these planes; impersonality which rejects all mental and physical becoming is therefore the only possible culmination of this exclusive movement: so only can an absolutely independent self-experience be achieved. The soul then seems to exist absolutely, independently in itself; it is free in the sense of the Indian word, *svādhīna*, dependent only on itself, not dependent upon God and other beings. Therefore in this experience God, personal self and other beings are all denied, cast away as distinctions of the ignorance. It is the ego recognising its own insufficiency and abolishing both itself and its contraries that its own essential instinct of independent self-experience may be accomplished; for it finds that its effort to achieve it by relations with God and others is afflicted throughout with a sentence of illusion, vanity and nullity. It ceases to admit them because by admitting them it becomes dependent on them; it ceases to admit its own persistence, because the persistence of ego means the admission of that which it tries to exclude as not-self, of the cosmos and other beings. The self-annihilation of the Buddhist is in its nature absolute exclusion of all that the mental being perceives; the self-immersion of the Adwaitin in his absolute being is the self-same aim differently conceived: both are a supreme self-assertion of the soul of its exclusive independence of Prakriti.

The experience which we first arrive at by the sort of short-cut to liberation which we have described as the movement of withdrawal, assists this tendency. For it is a breaking of the ego and a rejection of the habits of the mentality we now possess; for that is subject to matter and the physical senses and conceives of things only as forms, objects, external phenomena and as names which we attach to those forms. We are not aware directly of the subjective life of other beings except by analogy from our own and by inference or derivative perception based upon their external signs of speech, action, etc., which our minds translate into the terms of our own subjectivity. When we break out from ego and physical mind into the infinity of the spirit, we still see the world and others as the mind has accustomed us to see them, as names and forms; only in our new experience of the direct and superior reality of spirit, they lose that direct objective reality and that indirect subjective reality of their own which they had to the mind. They seem to be quite the opposite of the truer reality we now experience; our mentality, stilled and indifferent, no longer strives to know and make real to itself those intermediate terms which exist in them as in us and the knowledge of which has for its utility to bridge over the gulf between the spiritual self and the objective phenomena of the world. We are satisfied with the blissful infinite impersonality of a pure spiritual existence; nothing else and nobody else any longer matters to us. What the physical senses show to us and what the mind perceives and conceives about them and so imperfectly and transiently delights in, seems now unreal and worthless; we are not and do not care to be in possession of the intermediate truths of being through which these things are enjoyed by the One and possess for Him that value of His being and delight which makes, as we might say, cosmic existence a thing beautiful to Him and worth manifesting. We can no longer share in God's delight in the world; on the contrary it looks to us as if the Eternal had degraded itself by admitting into the purity of its being the gross nature of Matter or had falsified the truth of its being by imagining vain names and unreal forms. Or else if we perceive at all that delight, it is with a far-off detachment which prevents us from participating in it with any sense of intimate possession, or it is with an attraction to the superior delight of an absorbed and exclusive self-experience which does not allow us to stay any longer in these lower terms than we are compelled to stay by the continuance of our physical life and body.

But if either in the course of our Yoga or as the result of a free return of our realised Self upon the world and a free repossession of its Prakriti by the Purusha in us, we become conscious not only of the bodies and outward self-expression of others, but intimately of their inner being, their minds, their souls and that in them of which their own surface minds are not aware, then we see the real Being in them also and we see them as selves of our Self and not as mere names and forms. They become to us realities of the Eternal. Our minds are no longer subject to the delusion of trivial unworthiness or the illusion of unreality. The material life loses indeed for us its old absorbing value, but finds the greater value which it has for the divine Purusha; regarded no longer as the sole term of our becoming, but as merely having a subordinate value in relation to the higher terms of mind and spirit, it increases by that diminution instead of losing in value. We see that our material being, life, nature are only one poise of the Purusha in relation to its Prakriti and that their true purpose and importance can only be appreciated when they are seen not as a thing in itself, but as dependent on higher poises by which they are supported; from those superior relations they derive their meaning and, therefore, by conscious union with them they can fulfil all their valid tendencies and aims. Life then becomes justified to us and no longer stultified by the possession of liberated self-knowledge.

This larger integral knowledge and freedom liberates in the end and fulfils our whole existence. When we possess it, we see why our existence moves between these three terms of God, ourselves and the world; we no longer see them or any of them in opposition to each other, inconsistent, incompatible, nor do we on the other hand regard them as terms of our ignorance which all disappear at last into a pure impersonal unity. We perceive their necessity as terms rather of our self-fulfilment which preserve their value after liberation or rather find then only their real value. We have no longer the experience of our existence as exclusive of the other existences which make up by our relations with them our experience of the world; in this new consciousness they are all contained in ourselves and we in them. They and we are no longer so many mutually exclusive egos each seeking its own independent fulfilment or self-transcendence and ultimately aiming at nothing else; they are all the Eternal and the self in each secretly embraces all in itself and seeks in various ways to make that higher truth of its unity apparent and effective in its terrestrial being. Not mutual exclusiveness, but mutual inclusiveness is the divine truth of our individuality, love the higher law and not an independent self-fulfilment.

The Purusha who is our real being is always independent and master of Prakriti and at this independence we are rightly seeking to arrive; that is the utility of the egoistic movement and its self-transcendence, but its right fulfilment is not in making absolute the ego's principle of independent existence, but in arriving at this other highest poise of the Purusha with regard to its Prakriti. There there is transcendence of Nature, but also possession of Nature, perfect fulfilment of our individuality, but also perfect fulfilment of our relations with the world and with others. Therefore an individual salvation in heavens beyond careless of the earth is not our highest objective; the liberation and self-fulfilment of others is as much our own concern, — we might almost say, our divine self-interest, — as our own liberation. Otherwise our unity with others would have no effective meaning. To conquer the lures of egoistic existence in this world is our first victory over ourselves; to conquer the lure of individual happiness in heavens beyond is our second victory; to conquer the highest lure of escape from life and a self-absorbed bliss in the impersonal infinity is the last and greatest victory. Then are we rid of all individual exclusiveness and possessed of our entire spiritual freedom.

The state of the liberated soul is that of the Purusha who is for ever free. Its consciousness is a transcendence and an all-comprehending unity. Its self-knowledge does not get rid of all the terms of self-knowledge, but unifies and harmonises all things in God and in the divine nature. The intense religious ecstasy which knows only God and ourselves and shuts out all else, is only to it an intimate experience which prepares it for sharing in the embrace of the divine Love and Delight around all creatures. A heavenly bliss which unites God and ourselves and the blest, but enables us to look with a remote indifference on the unblest and their sufferings is not possible to the perfect soul; for these also are its selves; free individually from suffering and ignorance, it must naturally turn to draw them also towards its freedom. On the other hand any absorption in the relations between self and others and the world to the exclusion of God and the Beyond is still more impossible, and therefore it cannot be limited by the earth or even by the highest and most altruistic relations of man with man. Its activity or its culmination is not to efface and utterly deny itself for the sake of others, but to fulfil itself in God-possession, freedom and divine bliss that in and by its fulfilment others too may be fulfilled. For it is in God alone, by the possession of the Divine only that all the discords of life can be resolved, and therefore the raising of men towards the Divine is in the end the one effective way of helping mankind. All the other activities and realisations of our self-experience have their use and power, but in the end these crowded side-tracks or these lonely paths must circle round to converge into the wideness of the integral way by which the liberated soul transcends all, embraces all and becomes the promise and the power of the fulfilment of all in their manifested being of the Divine.

Chapter XIX

The Planes of Our Existence

IF THE Purusha in us has thus to become by union with its highest self, the Divine Purusha, the knower, lord, free enjoyer of its Prakriti, it cannot be done, evidently, by dwelling on the present plane of our being; for that is the material plane in which the reign of Prakriti is complete; there the divine Purusha is entirely hidden in the blinding surge of her activities, in the gross pomp of her workings, and the individual soul emerging from her involution of spirit in matter, subject in all its activities to its entangling in the material and vital instruments is unable to experience the divine freedom. What it calls its freedom and mastery, is only the subtle subjection of mind to Prakriti which is lighter indeed, nearer to the possibility of liberty and rule than the gross subjection of vital and material things like the animal, plant and metal, but is still not real freedom and mastery. Therefore we have had to speak of different planes of our consciousness and of the spiritual planes of the mental being; for if these did not exist, the liberation of the embodied being would have been impossible here on earth. He would have had to wait and at most to prepare himself for seeking it in other worlds and in a different kind of physical or spiritual embodiment less obstinately sealed in its shell of material experience.

In the ordinary Yoga of knowledge it is only necessary to recognise two planes of our consciousness, the spiritual and the materialised mental; the pure reason standing between these two views them both, cuts through the illusions of the phenomenal world, exceeds the materialised mental plane, sees the reality of the spiritual; and then the will of the individual Purusha unifying itself with this poise of knowledge rejects the lower and draws back to the supreme plane, dwells there, loses mind and body, sheds life from it and merges itself in the supreme Purusha, is delivered from individual existence. It knows that this is not the whole truth of our existence, which is much more complex; it knows there are many planes, but it disregards them or pays little attention to them because they are not essential to this liberation. They indeed rather hamper it, because to live on them brings new attractive psychical experiences, psychical enjoyments, psychical powers, a new world of phenomenal knowledge the pursuit of which creates stumbling-blocks in the way of its one object, immergence in Brahman, and brings a succession of innumerable way-side snares on the road which leads to God. But since we accept world-existence, and for us all world-existence is Brahman and full of the presence of God, these things can have no terrors for us; whatever dangers of distraction there may be, we have to face and overcome them. If the world and our own existence are so complex, we must know and embrace their complexities in order that our self-knowledge and our knowledge of the dealings of Purusha with its Prakriti may be complete. If there are many planes, we have to possess them all for the Divine, even as we seek to possess spiritually and transform our ordinary poise of mind, life and body.

The ancient knowledge in all countries was full of the search after the hidden truths of our being and it created that large field of practice and inquiry which goes in Europe by the name of occultism, — we do not use any corresponding word in the East, because these things do not seem to us so remote, mysterious and abnormal as to the occidental mentality; they are nearer to us and the veil between our normal material life and this larger life is much thinner. In India,[1] Egypt, Chaldea, China, Greece, the Celtic countries they have formed part of various Yogic systems and disciplines which had once a great hold everywhere, but to the modern mind have seemed mere superstition and mysticism, although the facts and experiences on which they are founded are quite as real in their own field and as much governed by intelligible laws of their own as the facts and experiences of the material world. It is not our intention here to plunge into this

---

[1] For example, the Tantric in India.

vast and difficult field of psychical knowledge.[2] But it becomes necessary now to deal with certain broad facts and principles which form its framework, for without them our Yoga of knowledge cannot be complete. We find that in the various systems the facts dealt with are always the same, but there are considerable differences of theoretic and practical arrangement, as is natural and inevitable in dealing with a subject so large and difficult. Certain things are here omitted, there made all-important, here understressed, there over-emphasised; certain fields of experience which are in one system held to be merely subordinate provinces, are in others treated as separate kingdoms. But I shall follow here consistently the Vedic and Vedantic arrangement of which we find the great lines in the Upanishads, first because it seems to me at once the simplest and most philosophical and more especially because it was from the beginning envisaged from the point of view of the utility of these various planes to the supreme object of our liberation. It takes as its basis the three principles of our ordinary being, mind, life and matter, the triune spiritual principle of Sachchidananda and the link principle of *vijñāna*, supermind, the free or spiritual intelligence, and thus arranges all the large possible poises of our being in a tier of seven planes, — sometimes regarded as five only, because, only the lower five are wholly accessible to us, — through which the developing being can rise to its perfection.

But first we must understand what we mean by planes of consciousness, planes of existence. We mean a general settled poise or world of relations between Purusha and Prakriti, between the Soul and Nature. For anything that we can call world is and can be nothing else than the working out of a general relation which a universal existence has created or established between itself, or let us say its eternal fact or potentiality and the powers of its becoming. That existence in its relations with and its experience of the becoming is what we call soul or Purusha,

---

[2] We hope to deal with it hereafter; but our first concern in the *Arya* must be with spiritual and philosophical truths; it is only when these have been grasped that the approach to the psychical becomes safe and clear.

individual soul in the individual, universal soul in the cosmos; the principle and the powers of the becoming are what we call Nature or Prakriti. But since Being, conscious force and delight of being are always the three constituent terms of existence, the nature of a world is really determined by the way in which Prakriti is set to deal with these three primary things and the forms which it is allowed to give to them. For existence itself is and must always be the stuff of its own becoming; it must be shaped into the substance with which Force has to deal. Force again must be the power which works out that substance and works with it to whatever ends; Force is that which we ordinarily call Nature. Again the end, the object with which the worlds are created must be worked out by the consciousness inherent in all existence and all force and all their workings, and the object must be the possession of itself and of its delight of existence in the world. To that all the circumstances and aims of any world-existence must reduce themselves; it is existence developing its terms of being, its power of being, its conscious delight of being; if these are involved, their evolution; if they are veiled, their self-revelation.

Here the soul lives in a material universe; of that alone it is immediately conscious; the realisation of its potentialities in that is the problem with which it is concerned. But matter means the involution of the conscious delight of existence in self-oblivious force and in a self-dividing, infinitesimally disaggregated form of substance. Therefore the whole principle and effort of a material world must be the evolution of what is involved and the development of what is undeveloped. Here everything is shut up from the first in the violently working inconscient sleep of material force; therefore the whole aim of any material becoming must be the waking of consciousness out of the inconscient; the whole consummation of a material becoming must be the removal of the veil of matter and the luminous revelation of the entirely self-conscious Being to its own imprisoned soul in the becoming. Since Man is such an imprisoned soul, this luminous liberation and coming to self-knowledge must be his highest object and the condition of his perfection.

But the limitations of a material universe seem to be hostile to the proper accomplishment of this object which is yet so inevitably the highest aim of a mental being born into a physical body. First existence has formed itself here, fundamentally, as Matter; it has been objectivised, made sensible and concrete to its own self-experiencing conscious-force in the form of self-dividing material substance, and by the aggregation of this matter there has been built up for man a physical body separate, divided from others and subject to the fixed habits of process or, as we call them, the laws of inconscient material Nature. His force of being too is nature or Force working in matter, which has waked slowly out of inconscience to life and is always limited by form, always dependent on the body, always separated by it from the rest of Life and from other living beings, always hampered in its development, persistence, self-perfectioning by the laws of the Inconscience and the limitations of bodily living. Equally, his consciousness is a mentality emerging in a body and in a sharply individualised life; it is therefore limited in its workings and capacities and dependent on bodily organs of no great competence and on a very restricted vital force; it is separated from the rest of cosmic mind and shut out from the thoughts of other mental beings whose inner workings are a sealed book to man's physical mind except in so far as he can read them by the analogy of his own mentality and by their insufficient bodily signs and self-expressions. His consciousness is always falling back towards the inconscience in which a large part of it is always involved, his life towards death, his physical being towards disaggregation. His delight of being depends on the relations of this imperfect consciousness with its environment based upon physical sensations and the sense-mind, in other words on a limited mind trying to lay hold on a world external and foreign to it by means of a limited body, limited vital force, limited organs. Therefore its power for possession is limited, its force for delight is limited, and every touch of the world which exceeds its force, which that force cannot bear, cannot seize on, cannot assimilate and possess must turn to something else than delight, to pain, discomfort or grief. Or else it must be met by non-reception, insensibility, or, if received, put away by indifference. Moreover such delight of being as it possesses, is not possessed naturally and eternally like the self-delight of Sachchidananda, but by experience and acquisition in Time, and can therefore only be maintained and prolonged by repetition of experience and is in its nature precarious and transient.

All this means that the natural relations of Purusha to Prakriti in the material universe are the complete absorption of conscious being in the force of its workings, therefore the complete self-oblivion and self-ignorance of the Purusha, the complete domination of Prakriti and subjection of the soul to Nature. The soul does not know itself, it only knows, if anything, the workings of Prakriti. The emergence of the individual self-conscious soul in Man does not of itself abrogate these primary relations of ignorance and subjection. For this soul is living on a material plane of existence, a poise of Prakriti in which matter is still the chief determinant of its relations to Nature, and its consciousness being limited by Matter cannot be an entirely self-possessing consciousness. Even the universal soul, if limited by the material formula, could not be in entire possession of itself; much less can the individual soul to which the rest of existence becomes by bodily, vital and mental limitation and separation something external to it on which it is yet dependent for its life and its delight and its knowledge. These limitations of his power, knowledge, life, delight of existence are the whole cause of man's dissatisfaction with himself and the universe. And if the material universe were all and the material plane the only plane of his being, then man the individual Purusha could never arrive at perfection and self-fulfilment or indeed to any other life than that of the animals. There must be either worlds in which he is liberated from these incomplete and unsatisfactory relations of Purusha with Prakriti, or planes of his own being by ascending to which he can transcend them, or at the very least planes, worlds and higher beings from which he can receive or be helped to knowledge, powers, joys, a growth of his being otherwise impossible. All these things, the ancient knowledge asserts, exist, — other worlds, higher planes, the possibility of communication, of ascension, of growth by contact with and influence from that which is above him in the present scale of his realised being.

As there is a poise of the relations of Purusha with Prakriti in which Matter is the first determinant, a world of material existence, so there is another just above it in which Matter is not supreme, but rather Life-force takes its place as the first determinant. In this world forms do not determine the conditions of the life, but it is life which determines the form, and therefore forms are there much more free, fluid, largely and to our conceptions strangely variable than in the material world. This life-force is not inconscient material force, not even, except in its lowest movements, an elemental subconscient energy, but a conscious force of being which makes for formation, but much more essentially for enjoyment, possession, satisfaction of its own dynamic impulse. Desire and the satisfaction of impulse are therefore the first law of this world of sheer vital existence, this poise of relations between the soul and its nature in which the life-power plays with so much greater a freedom and capacity than in our physical living; it may be called the desire-world, for that is its principal characteristic. Moreover, it is not fixed in one hardly variable formula as physical life seems to be, but is capable of many variations of its poise, admits many sub-planes ranging from those which touch material existence and, as it were, melt into that, to those which touch at the height of the life-power the planes of pure mental and psychic existence and melt into them. For in Nature in the infinite scale of being there are no wide gulfs, no abrupt chasms to be overleaped, but a melting of one thing into another, a subtle continuity; out of that her power of distinctive experience creates the orderings, the definite ranges, the distinct gradations by which the soul variously knows and possesses its possibilities of world-existence. Again, enjoyment of one kind or another being the whole object of desire, that must be the trend of the desire-world; but since wherever the soul is not free, — and it cannot be free when subject to desire, — there must be the negative as well as the positive of all its experience, this world contains not only the possibility of large or intense or continuous enjoyments almost inconceivable to the limited physical mind, but also the possibility of equally enormous sufferings. It is here therefore that there are situated the lowest heavens and all the hells with the tradition and imagination of which the human mind has lured and terrified itself since the earliest ages. All human imaginations indeed correspond to some reality or real possibility, though they may in themselves be a quite inaccurate representation or couched in too physical images and therefore inapt to express the truth of supraphysical realities.

Nature being a complex unity and not a collection of unrelated phenomena, there can be no unbridgeable gulf between the material existence and this vital or desire world. On the contrary, they may be said in a sense to exist in each other and are at least interdependent to a certain extent. In fact, the material world is really a sort of projection from the vital, a thing which it has thrown out and separated from itself in order to embody and fulfil some of its desires under conditions other than its own, which are yet the logical result of its own most material longings. Life on earth may be said to be the result of the pressure of this life-world on the material, inconscient existence of the physical universe. Our own manifest vital being is also only a surface result of a larger and profounder vital being which has its proper seat on the life-plane and through which we are connected with the life-world. Moreover, the life-world is constantly acting upon us and behind everything in material existence there stand appropriate powers of the life-world; even the most crude and elemental have behind them elemental life-powers, elemental beings by which or by whom they are supported. The influences of the life-world are always pouring out on the material existence and producing there their powers and results which return again upon the life-world to modify it. From that the life-part of us, the desire-part is being always touched and influenced; there too are beneficent and malefic powers of good desire and evil desire which concern themselves with us even when we are ignorant of and unconcerned with them. Nor are these powers merely tendencies, inconscient forces, nor, except on the verges of Matter, subconscient, but conscious powers, beings, living influences. As we awaken to the higher planes of our existence, we become aware of them as friends or enemies, powers which seek to possess or which we can master, overcome, pass beyond and leave behind. It is this possible relation of the human being with the powers of the life-world which occupied to so large an extent European occultism, especially in the Middle Ages, as well as certain forms of Eastern magic and spiritualism. The "superstitions" of the past — much superstition there was, that is to say, much ignorant and distorted belief, false explanations and obscure and clumsy dealing with the laws of the beyond, — had yet behind them truths which a future Science, delivered from its sole preoccupation with the material world, may rediscover. For the supra-material is as much a reality as the existence of mental beings in the material universe.

But why then are we not normally aware of so much that is behind us and always pressing upon us? For the same reason that we are not aware of the inner life of our neighbour, although it exists as much as our own and is constantly exercising an occult influence upon us, — for a great part of our thoughts and feelings come into us from outside, from our fellow-men, both from individuals and from the collective mind of humanity; and for the same reason that we are not aware of the greater part of our own being which is subconscient or subliminal to our waking mind and is always influencing and in an occult manner determining our surface existence. It is because we use, normally, only our corporeal senses and live almost wholly in the body and the physical vitality and the physical mind, and it is not directly through these that the life-world enters into relations with us. That is done through other sheaths of our being, — so they are termed in the Upanishads, — other bodies, as they are called in a later terminology, the mental sheath or subtle body in which our true mental being lives and the life sheath or vital body which is more closely connected with the physical or food-sheath and forms with it the gross body of our complex existence. These possess powers, senses, capacities which are always secretly acting in us, are connected with and impinge upon our physical organs and the plexuses of our physical life and mentality. By self-development we can become aware of them, possess our life in them, get through them into conscious relation with the life-world and other worlds and use them also for a more subtle experience and more intimate knowledge of the truths, facts and happenings of even the material world itself. We can by this self-development live more or less fully on planes of our existence other than the material which is now all in all to us.

What has been said of the life-world applies with the necessary differences to still higher planes of the cosmic existence. For beyond that is a mental plane, a world of mental existence in which neither life, nor matter, but mind is the first determinant. Mind there is not determined by material conditions or by the life-force, but itself determines and uses them for its own satisfaction. There mind, that is to say, the psychical and the intellectual being, is free in a certain sense, free at least to satisfy and fulfil itself in a way hardly conceivable to our body-bound and life-bound mentality; for the Purusha there is the pure mental being and his relations with Prakriti are determined by that purer mentality, Nature there is mental rather than vital and physical. Both the life-world and indirectly the material are a projection from that, the result of certain tendencies of the mental Being which have sought a field, conditions, an arrangement of harmonies proper to themselves; and the phenomena of mind in this world may be said to be a result of the pressure of that plane first on the life-world and then on life in the material existence. By its modification in the life-world it creates in us the desire-mind; in its own right it awakes in us the purer powers of our psychical and intellectual existence. But our surface mentality is only a secondary result of a larger subliminal mentality whose proper seat is the mental plane. This world of mental existence also is constantly acting upon us and our world, has its powers and its beings, is related to us through our mental body. There we find the psychical and mental heavens to which the Purusha can ascend when it drops this physical body and can there sojourn till the impulse to terrestrial existence again draws it downward. Here too are many planes, the lowest converging upon and melting into the worlds below, the highest at the heights of the mind-power into the worlds of a more spiritual existence.

These highest worlds are therefore supramental; they belong to the principle of supermind, the free, spiritual or divine intelligence[3] or gnosis and to the triple spiritual principle of Sachchidananda. From them the lower worlds derive by a sort of fall of the Purusha into certain specific or narrow conditions of the play of the soul with its nature. But these also are divided from us by no unbridgeable gulf; they affect us through what are called the knowledge-sheath and the bliss-sheath, through the causal or spiritual body, and less directly through the mental body, nor are their secret powers absent from the workings of the vital and material existence. Our conscious spiritual being and our intuitive mind awaken in us as a result of the pressure of these highest worlds on the mental being in life and body. But this causal body is, as we may say, little developed in the majority of men and to live in it or to ascend to the supramental planes, as distinguished from corresponding sub-planes in the mental being, or still more to dwell consciously upon them is the most difficult thing of all for the human being. It can be done in the trance of Samadhi, but otherwise only by a new evolution of the capacities of the individual Purusha of which few are even willing to conceive. Yet is that the condition of the perfect self-consciousness by which alone the Purusha can possess the full conscious control of Prakriti; for there not even the mind determines, but the Spirit freely uses the lower differentiating principles as minor terms of its existence governed by the higher and reaching by them their own perfect capacity. That alone would be the perfect evolution of the involved and development of the undeveloped for which the Purusha has sought in the material universe, as if in a wager with itself, the conditions of the greatest difficulty.

---

[3] Called the *vijñāna* or *buddhi*, a word which may lead to some misunderstanding as it is also applied to the mental intelligence which is only a lower derivation from the divine gnosis.

Chapter XX

The Lower Triple Purusha

SUCH is the constituent principle of the various worlds of cosmic existence and the various planes of our being; they are as if a ladder plunging down into Matter and perhaps below it, rising up into the heights of the Spirit, even perhaps to the point at which existence escapes out of cosmic being into ranges of a supra-cosmic Absolute, — so at least it is averred in the world-system of the Buddhists. But to our ordinary materialised consciousness all this does not exist because it is hidden from us by our preoccupation with our existence in a little corner of the material universe and with the petty experiences of the little hour of time which is represented by our life in a single body upon this earth. To that consciousness the world is a mass of material things and forces thrown into some kind of shape and harmonised into a system of regulated movements by a number of fixed self-existent laws which we have to obey, by which we are governed and circumscribed and of which we have to get the best knowledge we can so as to make the most of this one brief existence which begins with birth, ends with death and has no second recurrence. Our own being is a sort of accident or at least a very small and minor circumstance in the universal life of Matter or the eternal continuity of the workings of material Force. Somehow or other a soul or mind has come to exist in a body and it stumbles about among things and forces which it does not very well understand, at first preoccupied with the difficulty of managing to live in a dangerous and largely hostile world and then with the effort to understand its laws and use them so as to make life as tolerable or as happy as possible so long as it lasts. If we were really nothing more than such a minor movement of individualised mind in Matter, existence would have nothing more to offer us; its best part would be at most this struggle of an ephemeral intellect and will with eternal

Matter and with the difficulties of Life supplemented and eased by a play of imagination and by the consoling fictions presented to us by religion and art and all the wonders dreamed of by the brooding mind and restless fancy of man.

But because he is a soul and not merely a living body, man can never for long remain satisfied that this first view of his existence, the sole view justified by the external and objective facts of life, is the real truth or the whole knowledge: his subjective being is full of hints and inklings of realities beyond, it is open to the sense of infinity and immortality, it is easily convinced of other worlds, higher possibilities of being, larger fields of experience for the soul. Science gives us the objective truth of existence and the superficial knowledge of our physical and vital being; but we feel that there are truths beyond which possibly through the cultivation of our subjective being and the enlargement of its powers may come to lie more and more open to us. When the knowledge of this world is ours, we are irresistibly impelled to seek for the knowledge of other states of existence beyond, and that is the reason why an age of strong materialism and scepticism is always followed by an age of occultism, of mystical creeds, of new religions and profounder seekings after the Infinite and the Divine. The knowledge of our superficial mentality and the laws of our bodily life is not enough; it brings us always to all that mysterious and hidden depth of subjective existence below and behind of which our surface consciousness is only a fringe or an outer court. We come to see that what is present to our physical senses is only the material shell of cosmic existence and what is obvious in our superficial mentality is only the margin of immense continents which lie behind unexplored. To explore them must be the work of another knowledge than that of physical science or of a superficial psychology.

Religion is the first attempt of man to get beyond himself and beyond the obvious and material facts of his existence. Its first essential work is to confirm and make real to him his subjective sense of an Infinite on which his material and mental being depends and the aspiration of his soul to come into its presence and live in contact with it. Its function is to assure him too of that possibility of which he has always dreamed, but of which his ordinary life gives him no assurance, the possibility of transcending himself and growing out of bodily life and mortality into the joy of immortal life and spiritual existence. It also confirms in him the sense that there are worlds or planes of existence other than that in which his lot is now cast, worlds in which this mortality and this subjection to evil and suffering are not the natural state, but rather bliss of immortality is the eternal condition. Incidentally, it gives him a rule of mortal life by which he shall prepare himself for immortality. He is a soul and not a body and his earthly life is a means by which he determines the future conditions of his spiritual being. So much is common to all religions; beyond this we get from them no assured certainty. Their voices vary; some tell us that one life on earth is all we have in which to determine our future existence, deny the past immortality of the soul and assert only its future immortality, threaten it even with the incredible dogma of a future of eternal suffering for those who miss the right path, while others more large and rational affirm successive existences by which the soul grows into the knowledge of the Infinite with a complete assurance for all of ultimate arrival and perfection. Some present the Infinite to us as a Being other than ourselves with whom we can have personal relations, others as an impersonal existence into which our separate being has to merge; some therefore give us as our goal worlds beyond in which we dwell in the presence of the Divine, others a cessation of world-existence by immergence in the Infinite. Most invite us to bear or to abandon earthly life as a trial or a temporary affliction or a vanity and fix our hopes beyond; in some we find a vague hint of a future triumph of the Spirit, the Divine in the body, upon this earth, in the collective life of man, and so justify not only the separate hope and aspiration of the individual but the united and sympathetic hope and aspiration of the race. Religion in fact is not knowledge, but a faith and aspiration; it is justified indeed both by an imprecise intuitive knowledge of large spiritual truths and by the subjective experience of souls that have risen beyond the ordinary life, but in itself it only gives us the hope and faith by which we may be induced to aspire to the intimate possession of the hidden tracts and larger realities of the Spirit. That we turn always the few distinct truths and the symbols or the particular discipline of a religion into hard and fast dogmas, is a sign that as yet we are only infants in the spiritual knowledge and are yet far from the science of the Infinite.

Yet behind every great religion, behind, that is to say, its exoteric side of faith, hope, symbols, scattered truths and limiting dogmas, there is an esoteric side of inner spiritual training and illumination by which the hidden truths may be known, worked out, possessed. Behind every exoteric religion there is an esoteric Yoga, an intuitive knowledge to which its faith is the first step, inexpressible realities of which its symbols are the figured expression, a deeper sense for its scattered truths, mysteries of the higher planes of existence of which even its dogmas and superstitions are crude hints and indications. What Science does for our knowledge of the material world, replacing first appearances and uses by the hidden truths and as yet occult powers of its great natural forces and in our own minds beliefs and opinions by verified experience and a profounder understanding, Yoga does for the higher planes and worlds and possibilities of our being which are aimed at by the religions. Therefore all this mass of graded experience existing behind closed doors to which the consciousness of man may find, if it wills, the key, falls within the province of a comprehensive Yoga of knowledge, which need not be confined to the seeking after the Absolute alone or the knowledge of the Divine in itself or of the Divine only in its isolated relations with the individual human soul. It is true that the consciousness of the Absolute is the highest reach of the Yoga of knowledge and that the possession of the Divine is its first, greatest and most ardent object and that to neglect it for an inferior knowledge is to afflict our Yoga with inferiority or even frivolity and to miss or fall away from its characteristic object; but, the Divine in itself being known, the Yoga of knowledge may well embrace also the knowledge of the Divine in its relations with ourselves and the world on the different planes of our existence. To rise to the pure Self being steadfastly held to as the summit of our subjective self-uplifting, we may from that height possess our lower selves even to the physical and the workings of Nature which belong to them.

We may seek this knowledge on two sides separately, the side of Purusha, the side of Prakriti; and we may combine the two for the perfect possession of the various relations of Purusha and Prakriti in the light of the Divine. There is, says the Upanishad, a fivefold soul in man and the world, the microcosm and the macrocosm. The physical soul, self or being, — Purusha, Atman, — is that of which we are all at first conscious, a self which seems to have hardly any existence apart from the body and no action vital or even mental independent of it. This physical soul is present everywhere in material Nature; it pervades the body, actuates obscurely its movements and is the whole basis of its experiences; it informs all things even that are not mentally conscious. But in man this physical being has become vitalised and mentalised; it has received something of the law and capacities of the vital and mental being and nature. But its possession of them is derivative, superimposed, as it were, on its original nature and exercised under subjection to the law and action of the physical existence and its instruments. It is this dominance of our mental and vital parts by the body and the physical nature which seems at first sight to justify the theory of the materialists that mind and life are only circumstances and results of physical force and all their operations explicable by the activities of that force in the animal body. In fact entire subjection of the mind and the life to the body is the characteristic of an undeveloped humanity, as it is in an even greater degree of the infra-human animal. According to the theory of reincarnation those who do not get beyond this stage in the earthly life, cannot rise after death to the mental or higher vital worlds, but have to return from the confines of a series of physical planes to increase their development in the next earthly existence. For the undeveloped physical soul is entirely dominated by material nature and its impressions and has to work them out to a better advantage before it can rise in the scale of being.

A more developed humanity allows us to make a better and

freer use of all the capacities and experiences that we derive from the vital and mental planes of being, to lean more for support upon these hidden planes, be less absorbed by the physical and to govern and modify the original nature of the physical being by greater vital forces and powers from the desire-world and greater and subtler mental forces and powers from the psychical and intellectual planes. By this development we are able to rise to higher altitudes of the intermediary existence between death and rebirth and to make a better and more rapid use of rebirth itself for a yet higher mental and spiritual development. But even so, in the physical being which still determines the greater part of our waking self, we act without definite consciousness of the worlds or planes which are the sources of our action. We are aware indeed of the life-plane and mind-plane of the physical being, but not of the life-plane and mind-plane proper or of the superior and larger vital and mental being which we are behind the veil of our ordinary consciousness. It is only at a high stage of development that we become aware of them and even then, ordinarily, only at the back of the action of our mentalised physical nature; we do not actually live on those planes, for if we did we could very soon arrive at the conscious control of the body by the life-power and of both by the sovereign mind; we should then be able to determine our physical and mental life to a very large extent by our will and knowledge as masters of our being and with a direct action of the mind on the life and body. By Yoga this power of transcending the physical self and taking possession of the higher selves may to a greater or less degree be acquired through a heightened and widened self-consciousness and self-mastery.

This may be done, on the side of Purusha, by drawing back from the physical self and its preoccupation with physical nature and through concentration of thought and will raising oneself into the vital and then into the mental self. By doing so we can become the vital being and draw up the physical self into that new consciousness so that we are only aware of the body, its nature and its actions as secondary circumstances of the Life-soul which we now are, used by it for its relations with the material world. A certain remoteness from physical being and then a superiority to it; a vivid sense of the body being a mere instrument or shell and easily detachable; an extraordinary effectivity of our desires on our physical being and life-environment; a great sense of power and ease in manipulating and directing the vital energy of which we now become vividly conscious, for its action is felt by us concretely, subtly physical in relation to the body, sensible in a sort of subtle density as an energy used by the mind; an awareness of the life-plane in us above the physical and knowledge and contact with the beings of the desire-world; a coming into action of new powers, — what are usually called occult powers or siddhis; a close sense of and sympathy with the Life-soul in the world and a knowledge or sensation of the emotions, desires, vital impulses of others; these are some of the signs of this new consciousness gained by Yoga.

But all this belongs to the inferior grades of spiritual experience and indeed is hardly more spiritual than the physical existence. We have in the same way to go yet higher and raise ourselves into the mental self. By doing so we can become the mental self and draw up the physical and vital being into it, so that life and body and their operations become to us minor circumstances of our being used by the Mind-soul which we now are for the execution of its lower purposes that belong to the material existence. Here too we acquire at first a certain remoteness from the life and the body and our real life seems to be on quite another plane than material man's, in contact with a subtler existence, a greater light of knowledge than the terrestrial, a far rarer and yet more sovereign energy; we are in touch in fact with the mental plane, aware of the mental worlds, can be in communication with its beings and powers. From that plane we behold the desire-world and the material existence as if below us, things that we can cast away from us if we will and in fact easily reject when we relinquish the body, so as to dwell in the mental or psychical heavens. But we can also, instead of being thus remote and detached, become rather superior to the life and body and the vital and material planes and act upon them with mastery from our new height of being. Another sort of dynamis than physical or vital energy, something that we may call pure mind-power and soul-force, which the developed human being uses indeed but derivatively and imperfectly, but which we can now use freely and with knowledge, becomes the ordinary process of our action, while desire-force and physical action fall into a secondary place and are only used with this new energy behind them and as its occasional channels. We are in touch and sympathy also with the Mind in cosmos, conscious of it, aware of the intentions, directions, thought-forces, struggle of subtle powers behind all happenings, which the ordinary man is ignorant of or can only obscurely infer from the physical happening, but which we can now see and feel directly before there is any physical sign or even vital intimation of their working. We acquire too the knowledge and sense of the mind-action of other beings whether on the physical plane or on those above it; and the higher capacities of the mental being, — occult powers or siddhis, but of a much rarer or subtler kind than those proper to the vital plane, — naturally awake in our consciousness.

All these however are circumstances of the lower triple world of our being, the *trailokya* of the ancient sages. Living on these we are, whatever the enlargement of our powers and our consciousness, still living within the limits of the cosmic gods and subject, though with a much subtler, easier and modified subjection, to the reign of Prakriti over Purusha. To achieve real freedom and mastery we have to ascend to a yet higher level of the many-plateaued mountain of our being.

Chapter XXI

The Ladder of Self-Transcendence

THE TRANSCENDENCE of this lower triple being and this lower triple world, to which ordinarily our consciousness and its powers and results are limited, — a transcendence described by the Vedic seers as an exceeding or breaking beyond the two firmaments of heaven and earth, — opens out a hierarchy of infinitudes to which the normal existence of man even in its highest and widest flights is still a stranger. Into that altitude, even to the lowest step of its hierarchy, it is difficult for him to rise. A separation, acute in practice though unreal in essence, divides the total being of man, the microcosm, as it divides also the world-being, the macrocosm. Both have a higher and a lower hemisphere, the *parārdha* and *aparārdha* of the ancient wisdom. The higher hemisphere is the perfect and eternal reign of the Spirit; for there it manifests without cessation or diminution its infinities, deploys the unconcealed glories of its illimitable existence, its illimitable consciousness and knowledge, its illimitable force and power, its illimitable beatitude. The lower hemisphere belongs equally to the Spirit; but here it is veiled, closely, thickly, by its inferior self-expression of limiting mind, confined life and dividing body. The Self in the lower hemisphere is shrouded in name and form; its consciousness is broken up by the division between the internal and external, the individual and universal; its vision and sense are turned outward; its force, limited by division of its consciousness, works in fetters; its knowledge, will, power, delight, divided by this division, limited by this limitation, are open to the experience of their contrary or perverse forms, to ignorance, weakness and suffering. We can indeed become aware of the true Self or Spirit in ourselves by turning our sense and vision inward; we can discover too the same Self or Spirit in the external world and its phenomena by plunging them there also inward through the veil of names and forms to that which dwells in these or else stands behind them. Our normal consciousness through this inward look may become by reflection aware of the infinite being, consciousness and delight of the Self and share in its passive or static infinity of these things. But we can only to a very limited extent share in its active or dynamic manifestation of knowledge, power and joy. Even this static identity by reflection cannot, ordinarily, be effected without a long and difficult effort and as the result of many lives of progressive self-development; for very firmly is our normal consciousness bound to the law of its lower hemisphere of being. To understand the possibility of transcending it at all, we must restate in a practical formula the relations of the worlds which constitute the two hemispheres.

All is determined by the Spirit, for all from subtlest existence to grossest matter is manifestation of the Spirit. But the Spirit, Self or Being determines the world it lives in and the experiences of its consciousness, force and delight in that world by some poise — among many possible — of the relations of Purusha and Prakriti, Soul and Nature, — some basic poise in one or other of its own cosmic principles. Poised in the principle of Matter, it becomes the physical self of a physical universe in the reign of a physical Nature. Spirit is then absorbed in its experience of Matter; it is dominated by the ignorance and inertia of the tamasic Power proper to physical existence. In the individual it becomes a materialised soul, *annamaya puruṣa*, whose life and mind have developed out of the ignorance and inertia of the material principle and are subject to their fundamental limitations. For life in Matter works in dependence on the body; mind in Matter works in dependence on the body and on the vital or nervous being; spirit itself in Matter is limited and divided in its self-relation and its powers by the limitations and divisions of this matter-governed and life-driven mind. This materialised soul lives bound to the physical body and its narrow superficial external consciousness, and it takes normally the experiences of its physical organs, its senses, its matter-bound life and mind, with at most some limited spiritual glimpses, as the whole truth of existence.

Man is a spirit, but a spirit that lives as a mental being in physical Nature; he is to his own self-consciousness a mind in a physical body. But at first he is this mental being materialised and he takes the materialised soul, *annamaya puruṣa*, for his real self. He is obliged to accept, as the Upanishad expresses it, Matter for the Brahman because his vision here sees Matter as that from which all is born, by which all lives and to which all return in their passing. His natural highest concept of Spirit is an Infinite, preferably an inconscient Infinite, inhabiting or pervading the material universe (which alone it really knows), and manifesting by the power of its presence all these forms around him. His natural highest conception of himself is a vaguely conceived soul or spirit, a soul manifested only by the physical life's experiences, bound up with physical phenomena and forced on its dissolution to return by an automatic necessity to the vast indeterminateness of the Infinite. But because he has the power of self-development, he can rise beyond these natural conceptions of the materialised soul; he can supplement them with a certain derivative experience drawn from supraphysical planes and worlds. He can concentrate in mind and develop the mental part of his being, usually at the expense of the fullness of his vital and physical life and in the end the mind predominates and can open to the Beyond. He can concentrate this self-liberating mind on the Spirit. Here too usually in the process he turns away more and more from his full mental and physical life; he limits or discourages their possibilities as much as his material foundation in nature will allow him. In the end his spiritual life predominates, destroys his earthward tendency and breaks its ties and limitations. Spiritualised, he places his real existence beyond in other worlds, in the heavens of the vital or mental plane; he begins to regard life on earth as a painful or troublesome incident or passage in which he can never arrive at any full enjoyment of his inner ideal self, his spiritual essence. Moreover, his highest conception of the Self or Spirit is apt to be more or less quietistic; for, as we have seen, it is its static infinity alone that he can entirely experience, the still freedom of Purusha unlimited by Prakriti, the Soul standing back from Nature. There may come indeed some divine dynamic manifestation in him, but it cannot rise entirely above the heavy limitations of physical Nature. The peace of the silent and passive Self is more easily attainable and he can more easily and fully hold it; too difficult for him is the bliss of an infinite activity, the dynamis of an immeasurable Power.

But the Spirit can be poised in the principle of Life, not in Matter. The Spirit so founded becomes the vital self of a vital world, the Life-soul of a Life-energy in the reign of a consciously dynamic Nature. Absorbed in the experiences of the power and play of a conscious Life, it is dominated by the desire, activity and passion of the rajasic principle proper to vital existence. In the individual this spirit becomes a vital soul, *prāṇamaya puruṣa*, in whose nature the life-energies tyrannise over the mental and physical principles. The physical element in a vital world readily shapes its activities and formations in response to desire and its imaginations, it serves and obeys the passion and power of life and their formations and does not thwart or limit them as it does here on earth where life is a precarious incident in inanimate Matter. The mental element too is moulded and limited by the life-power, obeys it and helps only to enrich and fulfil the urge of its desires and the energy of its impulses. This vital soul lives in a vital body composed of a substance much subtler than physical matter; it is a substance surcharged with conscious energy, capable of much more powerful perceptions, capacities, sense-activities than any that the gross atomic elements of earth-matter can offer. Man too has in himself behind his physical being, subliminal to it, unseen and unknown, but very close to it and forming with it the most naturally active part of his existence, this vital soul, this vital nature and this vital body; a whole vital plane connected with the life-world or desire-world is hidden in us, a secret consciousness in which life and desire find their untrammelled play and their easy self-expression and from there throw their influences and formations on our outer life.

In proportion as the power of this vital plane manifests itself in man and takes hold of his physical being, this son of earth becomes a vehicle of the life energy, forceful in his desires, vehement in his passions and emotions, intensely dynamic in his action, more and more the rajasic man. It is possible now for him to awaken in his consciousness to the vital plane and to become the vital soul, *prāṇamaya puruṣa*, put on the vital nature and live in the secret vital as well as the visible physical body. If he achieves this change with some fullness or one-pointedness — usually it is under great and salutary limitations or attended by saving complexities — and without rising beyond these things, without climbing to a supra-vital height from which they can be used, purified, uplifted, he becomes the lower type of Asura or Titan, a Rakshasa in nature, a soul of sheer power and life-energy, magnified or racked by a force of unlimited desire and passion, hunted and driven by an active capacity and colossal rajasic ego, but in possession of far greater and more various powers than those of the physical man in the ordinary more inert earth-nature. Even if he develops mind greatly on the vital plane and uses its dynamic energy for self-control as well as for self-satisfaction, it will still be with an Asuric energism (*tapasyā*) although of a higher type and directed to a more governed satisfaction of the rajasic ego.

But for the vital plane also it is possible, even as on the physical, to rise to a certain spiritual greatness in its own kind. It is open to the vital man to lift himself beyond the conceptions and energies natural to the desire-soul and the desire-plane. He can develop a higher mentality and, within the conditions of the vital being, concentrate upon some realisation of the Spirit or Self behind or beyond its forms and powers. In this spiritual realisation there would be a less strong necessity of quietism; for there would be a greater possibility of an active effectuation of the bliss and power of the Eternal, mightier and more self-satisfied powers, a richer flowering of the dynamic Infinite. Nevertheless that effectuality could never come anywhere near to a true and integral perfection; for the conditions of the desire-world are like those of the physical improper to the development of the complete spiritual life. The vital being too must develop spirit to the detriment of his fullness, activity and force of life in the lower hemisphere of our existence and turn in the end away from the vital formula, away from life either to the Silence or to an ineffable Power beyond him. If he does not withdraw from life, he must remain enchained by life, limited in his self-fulfilment by the downward pull of the desire-world and its dominant rajasic principle. On the vital plane also, in its own right alone, a perfect perfection is impossible; the soul that attains only so far would have to return to the physical life for a greater experience, a higher self-development, a more direct ascent to the Spirit.

Above matter and life stands the principle of mind, nearer to the secret Origin of things. The Spirit poised in mind becomes the mental self of a mental world and dwells there in the reign of its own pure and luminous mental Nature. There it acts in the intrinsic freedom of the cosmic Intelligence supported by the combined workings of a psycho-mental and a higher emotional mind-force, subtilised and enlightened by the clarity and happiness of the sattwic principle proper to the mental existence. In the individual the spirit so poised becomes a mental soul, *manomaya puruṣa*, in whose nature the clarity and luminous power of the mind acts in its own right independent of any limitation or oppression by the vital or corporeal instruments; it rather rules and determines entirely the forms of its body and the powers of its life. For mind in its own plane is not limited by life and obstructed by matter as it is here in the earth-process. This mental soul lives in a mental or subtle body which enjoys capacities of knowledge, perception, sympathy and interpenetration with other beings hardly imaginable by us and a free, delicate and extensive mentalised sense-faculty not limited by the grosser conditions of the life nature or the physical nature.

Man too has in himself, subliminal, unknown and unseen, concealed behind his waking consciousness and visible organism this mental soul, mental nature, mental body and a mental plane, not materialised, in which the principle of Mind is at home and not as here at strife with a world which is alien to it, obstructive to its freedom and corruptive of its purity and clearness. All the higher faculties of man, his intellectual and psycho-mental being and powers, his higher emotional life awaken and increase in proportion as this mental plane in him presses upon him. For the more it manifests, the more it influences the physical parts, the more it enriches and elevates the corresponding mental plane of the embodied nature. At a certain pitch of its increasing sovereignty it can make man truly man and not merely a reasoning animal; for it gives then its characteristic force to that mental being within us which our humanity is in the inwardly governing but still too hampered essence of its psychological structure.

It is possible for man to awaken to this higher mental consciousness, to become this mental being,[1] put on this mental nature and live not only in the vital and physical sheaths, but in this mental body. If there were a sufficient completeness in this transformation he would become capable of a life and a being at least half divine. For he would enjoy powers and a vision and perceptions beyond the scope of this ordinary life and body; he would govern all by the clarities of pure knowledge; he would be united to other beings by a sympathy of love and happiness; his emotions would be lifted to the perfection of the psycho-mental plane, his sensations rescued from grossness, his intellect subtle, pure and flexible, delivered from the deviations of the impure pranic energy and the obstructions of matter. And he would develop too the reflection of a wisdom and bliss higher than any mental joy and knowledge; for he could receive more fully and without our incompetent mind's deforming and falsifying mixture the inspirations and intuitions that are the arrows of the supramental Light and form his perfected mental existence in the mould and power of that vaster splendour. He could then realise too the self or Spirit in a much larger and more luminous and

---

[1] I include here in mind, not only the highest range of mind ordinarily known to man, but yet higher ranges to which he has either no current faculty of admission or else only a partial and mixed reception of some faint portion of their powers, — the illumined mind, the intuition and finally the creative Overmind or Maya which stands far above and is the source of our present existence. If mind is to be understood only as Reason or human intelligence, then the free mental being and its state would be something much more limited and very inferior to the description given here.

more intimate intensity than is now possible and with a greater play of its active power and bliss in the satisfied harmony of his existence.

And to our ordinary notions this may well seem to be a consummate perfection, something to which man might aspire in his highest flights of idealism. No doubt, it would be a sufficient perfection for the pure mental being in its own character; but it would still fall far below the greater possibilities of the spiritual nature. For here too our spiritual realisation would be subject to the limitations of the mind which is in the nature of a reflected, diluted and diffused or a narrowly intensive light, not the vast and comprehensive self-existent luminosity and joy of the Spirit. That vaster light, that profounder bliss are beyond the mental reaches. Mind indeed can never be a perfect instrument of the Spirit; a supreme self-expression is not possible in its movements because to separate, divide, limit is its very character. Even if mind could be free from all positive falsehood and error, even if it could be all intuitive and infallibly intuitive, it could still present and organise only half-truths or separate truths and these too not in their own body but in luminous representative figures put together to make an accumulated total or a massed structure. Therefore the self-perfecting mental being here must either depart into pure spirit by the shedding of its lower existence or return upon the physical life to develop in it a capacity not yet found in our mental and psychic nature. This is what the Upanishad expresses when it says that the heavens attained by the mind Purusha are those to which man is lifted by the rays of the sun, the diffused, separated, though intense beams of the supramental truth-consciousness, and from these it has to return to the earthly existence. But the illuminates who renouncing earth-life go beyond through the gateways of the sun, do not return hither. The mental being exceeding his sphere does not return because by that transition he enters a high range of existence peculiar to the superior hemisphere. He cannot bring down its greater spiritual nature into this lower triplicity; for here the mental being is the highest expression of the Self. Here the triple mental, vital and physical body provides almost the whole range of our capacity and cannot suffice for that greater consciousness; the vessel has not been built to contain a greater godhead or to house the splendours of this supramental force and knowledge.

This limitation is true only so long as man remains closed within the boundaries of the mental Maya. If he rises into the knowledge-self beyond the highest mental stature, if he becomes the knowledge-soul, the Spirit poised in gnosis, *vijñānamaya purusa*, and puts on the nature of its infinite truth and power, if he lives in the knowledge-sheath, the causal body as well as in these subtle mental, interlinking vital and grosser physical sheaths or bodies, then, but then only he will be able to draw down entirely into his terrestrial existence the fullness of the infinite spiritual consciousness; only then will he avail to raise his total being and even his whole manifested, embodied expressive nature into the spiritual kingdom. But this is difficult in the extreme; for the causal body opens itself readily to the consciousness and capacities of the spiritual planes and belongs in its nature to the higher hemisphere of existence, but it is either not developed at all in man or only as yet crudely developed and organised and veiled behind many intervening portals of the subliminal in us. It draws its stuff from the plane of the truth-knowledge and the plane of the infinite bliss and these pertain altogether to a still inaccessible higher hemisphere. Shedding upon this lower existence their truth and light and joy they are the source of all that we call spirituality and all that we call perfection. But this infiltration comes from behind thick coverings through which they arrive so tempered and weakened that they are entirely obscured in the materiality of our physical perceptions, grossly distorted and perverted in our vital impulses, perverted too though a little less grossly in our ideative seekings, minimised even in the comparative purity and intensity of the highest intuitive ranges of our mental nature. The supramental principle is secretly lodged in all existence. It is there even in the grossest materiality, it preserves and governs the lower worlds by its hidden power and law; but that power veils itself and that law works unseen through the shackled limitations and limping deformations of the lesser rule of our physical, vital, mental Nature. Yet its governing presence in the lowest forms assures us, because of the unity of all existence, that there is a possibility of their awakening, a possibility even of their perfect manifestation here in spite of every veil, in spite of all the mass of our apparent disabilities, in spite of the incapacity or unwillingness of our mind and life and body. And what is possible, must one day be, for that is the law of the omnipotent Spirit.

The character of these higher states of the soul and their greater worlds of spiritual Nature is necessarily difficult to seize. Even the Upanishads and the Veda only shadow them out by figures, hints and symbols. Yet it is necessary to attempt some account of their principles and practical effect so far as they can be grasped by the mind that stands on the border of the two hemispheres. The passage beyond that border would be the culmination, the completeness of the Yoga of self-transcendence by self-knowledge. The soul that aspires to perfection, draws back and upward, says the Upanishad, from the physical into the vital and from the vital into the mental Purusha, from the mental into the knowledge-soul and from that self of knowledge into the bliss Purusha. This self of bliss is the conscious foundation of perfect Sachchidananda and to pass into it completes the soul's ascension. The mind therefore must try to give to itself some account of this decisive transformation of the embodied consciousness, this radiant transfiguration and self-exceeding of our ever aspiring nature. The description mind can arrive at, can never be adequate to the thing itself, but it may point at least to some indicative shadow of it or perhaps some half-luminous image.

Chapter XXII

Vijnana or Gnosis

IN OUR perfect self-transcendence we pass out and up from the ignorance or half-enlightenment of our mental conscious-being into a greater wisdom-self and truth-power above it, there to dwell in the unwalled light of a divine knowledge. The mental man that we are is changed into the gnostic soul, the truth-conscious godhead, the *vijñānamaya* Purusha. Seated on that level of the hill of our ascension we are in a quite different plane from this material, this vital, this mental poise of the universal spirit, and with this change changes too all our view and experience of our soul-life and of the world around us. We are born into a new soul-status and put on a new nature; for according to the status of the soul is the status of the Prakriti. At each transition of the world-ascent, from matter to life, from life to mind, from mind bound to free intelligence, as the latent, half-manifested or already manifest soul rises to a higher and higher level of being, the nature also is elevated into a superior working, a wider consciousness, a vaster force and an intenser or larger range and joy of existence. But the transition from the mind-self to the knowledge-self is the great and the decisive transition in the Yoga. It is the shaking off of the last hold on us of the cosmic ignorance and our firm foundation in the Truth of things, in a consciousness infinite and eternal and inviolable by obscurity, falsehood, suffering or error.

This is the first summit which enters into the divine perfection, *sādharmya, sādṛśya*; for all the rest only look up to it or catch some rays of its significance. The highest heights of mind or of overmind come still within the belt of a mitigated ignorance; they can refract a divine Light but not pass it on in undiminished power to our lower members. For so long as we are within the triple stratum of mind, life and body, our active nature continues to work in the force of the ignorance even when the soul in Mind possesses something of the knowledge. And even if the soul were to reflect or to represent all the largeness of the knowledge in its mental consciousness, it would be unable to mobilise it rightly in force of action. The truth in its action might greatly increase, but it would still be pursued by a limitation, still condemned to a divisibility which would prevent it from working integrally in the power of the infinite. The power of a divinely illumined mind may be immense compared with ordinary powers, but it will still be subject to incapacity and there can be no perfect correspondence between the force of the effective will and the light of the idea which inspires it. The infinite Presence may be there in status, but the dynamis of the operations of nature still belongs to the lower Prakriti, must follow its triple modes of working and cannot give any adequate form to the greatness within it. This is the tragedy of ineffectivity, of the hiatus between ideal and effective will, of our constant incapacity to work out in living form and action the truth we feel in our inner consciousness that pursues all the aspiration of mind and life towards the divinity behind them. But the *vijñāna* or gnosis is not only truth but truth power, it is the very working of the infinite and divine nature; it is the divine knowledge one with the divine will in the force and delight of a spontaneous and luminous and inevitable self-fulfilment. By the gnosis, then, we change our human into a divine nature.

What then is this gnosis and how can we describe it? Two opposite errors have to be avoided, two misconceptions that disfigure opposite sides of the truth of gnosis. One error of intellect-bounded thinkers takes *vijñāna* as synonymous with the other Indian term *buddhi* and *buddhi* as synonymous with the reason, the discerning intellect, the logical intelligence. The systems that accept this significance, pass at once from a plane of pure intellect to a plane of pure spirit. No intermediate power is recognised, no diviner action of knowledge than the pure reason is admitted; the limited human means for fixing truth is taken for the highest possible dynamics of consciousness, its topmost force and original movement. An opposite error, a misconception of the mystics identifies *vijñāna* with the consciousness of the Infinite free from all ideation or else ideation packed into one essence of thought, lost to other dynamic action in the single and invariable idea of the One. This is the *caitanyaghana* of the Upanishad and is one movement or rather one thread of the many-aspected movement of the gnosis. The gnosis, the Vijnana, is not only this concentrated consciousness of the infinite Essence; it is also and at the same time an infinite knowledge of the myriad play of the Infinite. It contains all ideation (not mental but supramental), but it is not limited by ideation, for it far exceeds all ideative movement. Nor is the gnostic ideation in its character an intellectual thinking; it is not what we call the reason, not a concentrated intelligence. For the reason is mental in its methods, mental in its acquisitions, mental in its basis, but the ideative method of the gnosis is self-luminous, supramental, its yield of thought-light spontaneous, not proceeding by acquisition, its thought-basis a rendering of conscious identities, not a translation of the impressions born of indirect contacts. There is a relation and even a sort of broken identity between the two forms of thought; for one proceeds covertly from the other, mind is born from that which is beyond mind. But they act on different planes and reverse each other's process.

Even the purest reason, the most luminous rational intellectuality is not the gnosis. Reason or intellect is only the lower *buddhi*; it is dependent for its action on the percepts of the sense-mind and on the concepts of the mental intelligence. It is not like the gnosis, self-luminous, authentic, making the subject one with the object. There is, indeed, a higher form of the *buddhi* that can be called the intuitive mind or intuitive reason, and this by its intuitions, its inspirations, its swift revelatory vision, its luminous insight and discrimination can do the work of the reason with a higher power, a swifter action, a greater and spontaneous certitude. It acts in a self-light of the truth which does not depend upon the torch-flares of the sense-mind and its limited uncertain percepts; it proceeds not by intelligent but by visional concepts: it is a kind of truth-vision, truth-hearing, truth-memory, direct truth-discernment. This true and authentic intuition must be distinguished from a power of the ordinary mental reason which is too easily confused with it, the power of involved reasoning that reaches its conclusion by a bound and does not need the ordinary steps of the logical mind. The logical reason proceeds pace after pace and tries the sureness of each step like a man who is walking over unsafe ground and has to test by the hesitating touch of his foot each span of soil that he perceives with his eye. But this other supralogical process of the reason is a motion of rapid insight or swift discernment; it proceeds by a stride or leap, like a man who springs from one sure spot to another point of sure footing, — or at least held by him to be sure. He sees the space he covers in one compact and flashing view, but he does not distinguish or measure either by eye or touch its successions, features and circumstances. This movement has something of the sense of power of the intuition, something of its velocity, some appearance of its light and certainty, and we always are apt to take it for the intuition. But our assumption is an error and, if we trust to it, may lead us into grievous blunders.

It is even thought by the intellectualists that the intuition itself is nothing more than this rapid process in which the whole action of the logical mind is swiftly done or perhaps half-consciously or subconsciously done, not deliberately worked out in its reasoned method. In its nature, however, this proceeding is quite different from the intuition and it is not necessarily a truth-movement. The power of its leap may end in a stumble, its swiftness may betray, its certainty is too often a confident error. The validity of its conclusions must always depend on a subsequent verification or support from the evidence of the sense-perceptions or a rational linking of intelligent conceptions must intervene to explain to it its own certitudes. This lower light may indeed receive very readily a mixture of actual intuition into it and then a pseudo-intuitive or half-intuitive mind is created, very misleading by its frequent luminous successes palliating a whirl of intensely self-assured false certitudes. The true intuition on the contrary carries in itself its own guarantee of truth; it is sure and infallible within its limits. And so long as it is pure intuition and does not admit into itself any mixture of sense-error or intellectual ideation, it is never contradicted by experience: the intuition may be verified by the reason or the sense-perception afterwards, but its truth does not depend on that verification, it is assured by an automatic self-evidence. If the reason depending on its inferences contradicts the greater light, it will be found in the end on ampler knowledge that the intuitional conclusion was correct and that the more plausible rational and inferential conclusion was an error. For the true intuition proceeds from the self-existent truth of things and is secured by that self-existent truth and not by any indirect, derivatory or dependent method of arriving at knowledge.

But even the intuitive reason is not the gnosis; it is only an edge of light of the supermind finding its way by flashes of illumination into the mentality like lightnings in dim and cloudy places. Its inspirations, revelations, intuitions, self-luminous discernings are messages from a higher knowledge-plane that make their way opportunely into our lower level of consciousness. The very character of the intuitive mind sets a gulf of great difference between its action and the action of the self-contained gnosis. In the first place it acts by separate and limited illuminations and its truth is restricted to the often narrow reach or the one brief spot of knowledge lit up by that one lightning-flash with which its intervention begins and terminates. We see the action of the instinct in animals, — an automatic intuition in that vital or sense-mind which is the highest and surest instrument that the animal has to rely on, since it does not possess the human light of the reason, only a cruder and yet ill-formed intelligence. And we can observe at once that the marvellous truth of this instinct which seems so much surer than the reason, is limited in the bird, beast or insect to some particular and restricted utility it is admitted to serve. When the vital mind of the animal tries to act beyond that restricted limit, it blunders in a much blinder way than the reason of man and has to learn with difficulty by a succession of sense-experiences. The higher mental intuition of the human being is an inner visional, not a sense intuition; for it illumines the intelligence and not the sense-mind, it is self-conscious and luminous, not a half-subconscious blind light: it is freely self-acting, not mechanically automatic. But still, even when it is not marred by the imitative pseudo-intuition, it is restricted in man like the instinct in the animal, restricted to a particular purpose of will or knowledge as is the instinct to a particular life utility or Nature purpose. And when the intelligence, as is its almost invariable habit, tries to make use of it, to apply it, to add to it, it builds round the intuitive nucleus in its own characteristic fashion a mass of mixed truth and error. More often than not, by foisting an element of sense-error and conceptual error into the very substance of the intuition or by coating it up in mental additions and deviations, it not merely deflects but deforms its truth and converts it into a falsehood. At the best therefore the intuition gives us only a limited, though an intense light; at the worst, through our misuse of it or false imitations of it, it may lead us into perplexities and confusions which the less ambitious intellectual reason avoids by remaining satisfied with its own safe and plodding method, — safe for the inferior purposes of the reason, though never a satisfying guide to the inner truth of things.

It is possible to cultivate and extend the use of the intuitive mind in proportion as we rely less predominantly upon the reasoning intelligence. We may train our mentality not to seize, as it does now, upon every separate flash of intuitive illumination for its own inferior purposes, not to precipitate our thought at once into a crystallising intellectual action around it; we can train it to think in a stream of successive and connected intuitions, to pour light upon light in a brilliant and triumphant series. We shall succeed in this difficult change in proportion as we purify the interfering intelligence, — if we can reduce in it the element of material thought enslaved to the external appearances of things, the element of vital thought enslaved to the wishes, desires, impulses of the lower nature, the element of intellectual thought enslaved to our preferred, already settled or congenial ideas, conceptions, opinions, fixed operations of intelligence, if, having reduced to a minimum those elements, we can replace them by an intuitive vision and sense of things, an intuitive insight into appearances, an intuitive will, an intuitive ideation. This is hard enough for our consciousness naturally bound by the triple tie of mentality, vitality, corporeality to its own imperfection and ignorance, the upper, middle and lower cord in the Vedic parable of the soul's bondage, cords of the mixed truth and falsehood of appearances by which Shunahshepa was bound to the post of sacrifice.

But even if this difficult thing were perfectly accomplished, still the intuition would not be the gnosis; it would only be its thin prolongation into mind or its sharp edge of first entrance. The difference, not easy to define except by symbols, may be expressed if we take the Vedic image in which the Sun represents the gnosis and the sky, mid-air and earth the mentality, vitality, physicality of man and of the universe. Living on the earth, climbing into the mid-air or even winging in the sky, the mental being, the *manomaya* Purusha, would still live in the rays of the sun and not in its bodily light. And in those rays he would see things not as they are, but as reflected in his organ of vision, deformed by its faults or limited in their truth by its restrictions. But the *vijñānamaya* Purusha lives in the Sun itself, in the very body and blaze of the true light;[1] he knows this light to be his own self-luminous being and he sees besides all that dwells in the rays of the sun, sees the whole truth of the lower triplicity and each thing that is in it. He sees it not by reflection in a mental organ of vision, but with the Sun of gnosis itself as his eye, — for the Sun, says the Veda, is the eye of the gods. The mental being, even in the intuitive mind, can perceive the truth only by a brilliant reflection or limited communication and subject to the restrictions and the inferior capacity of the mental vision; but the supramental being sees it by the gnosis itself, from the very centre and outwelling fount of the truth, in its very form and by its own spontaneous and self-illumining process. For the Vijnana is a direct and divine as opposed to an indirect and human knowledge.

The nature of the gnosis can only be indicated to the intellect by contrasting it with the nature of the intellect, and even then

---

[1] So the Sun is called in the Veda, *ṛtaṁ jyotiḥ*.

the phrases we must use cannot illuminate unless aided by some amount of actual experience. For what language forged by the reason can express the suprarational? Fundamentally, this is the difference between these two powers that the mental reason proceeds with labour from ignorance to truth, but the gnosis has in itself the direct contact, the immediate vision, the easy and constant possession of the truth and has no need of seeking or any kind of procedure. The reason starts with appearances and labours, never or seldom losing at least a partial dependence on appearances, to arrive at the truth behind them; it shows the truth in the light of the appearances. The gnosis starts from the truth and shows the appearances in the light of the truth; it is itself the body of the truth and its spirit. The reason proceeds by inference, it concludes; but the gnosis proceeds by identity or vision, — it is, sees and knows. As directly as the physical vision sees and grasps the appearance of objects, so and far more directly the gnosis sees and grasps the truth of things. But where the physical sense gets into relation with objects by a veiled contact, the gnosis gets into identity with things by an unveiled oneness. Thus it is able to know all things as a man knows his own existence, simply, convincingly, directly. To the reason only what the senses give is direct knowledge, *pratyakṣa*, the rest of truth is arrived at indirectly; to the gnosis all its truth is direct knowledge, *pratyakṣa*. Therefore the truth gained by the intellect is an acquisition over which there hangs always a certain shadow of doubt, an incompleteness, a surrounding penumbra of night and ignorance or half-knowledge, a possibility of alteration or annullation by farther knowledge. The truth of the gnosis is free from doubt, self-evident, self-existent, irrefragable, absolute.

The reason has as its first instrument observation general, analytical and synthetic; it aids itself by comparison, contrast and analogy, — proceeds from experience to indirect knowledge by logical processes of deduction, induction, all kinds of inference, — rests upon memory, reaches out beyond itself by imagination, secures itself by judgment: all is a process of groping and seeking. The gnosis does not seek, it possesses. Or if it has to enlighten, it does not even then seek; it reveals, it illumines. In a consciousness transmuted from intelligence to gnosis, imagination would be replaced by truth-inspiration, mental judgment would give place to a self-luminous discerning. The slow and stumbling logical process from reasoning to conclusion would be pushed out by a swift intuitive proceeding; the conclusion or fact would be seen at once in its own right, by its own self-sufficient witness, and all the evidence by which we arrive at it would be seen too at once, along with it, in the same comprehensive figure, not as its evidence, but as its intimate conditions, connections and relations, its constituent parts or its wings of circumstance. Mental and sense observation would be changed into an inner vision using the instruments as channels, but not dependent on them as the mind in us is blind and deaf without the physical senses, and this vision would see not merely the thing, but all its truth, its forces, powers, the eternities within it. Our uncertain memory would fall away and there would come in its place a luminous possession of knowledge, the divine memory that is not a store of acquisition, but holds all things always contained in the consciousness, a memory at once of past, present and future.

For while the reason proceeds from moment to moment of time and loses and acquires and again loses and again acquires, the gnosis dominates time in a one view and perpetual power and links past, present and future in their indivisible connections, in a single continuous map of knowledge, side by side. The gnosis starts from the totality which it immediately possesses; it sees parts, groups and details only in relation to the totality and in one vision with it: the mental reason cannot really see the totality at all and does not know fully any whole except by starting from an analysis and synthesis of its parts, masses and details; otherwise its whole-view is always a vague apprehension or an imperfect comprehension or a confused summary of indistinct features. The reason deals with constituents and processes and properties; it tries in vain to form by them an idea of the thing in itself, its reality, its essence. But the gnosis sees the thing in itself first, penetrates to its original and eternal nature, adjoins its processes and properties only as a self-expression of its nature. The reason dwells in the diversity and is its prisoner: it deals with things separately and treats each as a separate existence, as it deals with sections of Time and divisions of Space; it sees unity only in a sum or by elimination of diversity or as a general conception and a vacant figure. But the gnosis dwells in the unity and knows by it all the nature of the diversities; it starts from the unity and sees diversities only of a unity, not diversities constituting the one, but a unity constituting its own multitudes. The gnostic knowledge, the gnostic sense does not recognise any real division; it does not treat things separately as if they were independent of their true and original oneness. The reason deals with the finite and is helpless before the infinite: it can conceive of it as an indefinite extension in which the finite acts, but the infinite in itself it can with difficulty conceive and cannot at all grasp or penetrate. But the gnosis is, sees and lives in the infinite; it starts always from the infinite and knows finite things only in their relation to the infinite and in the sense of the infinite.

If we would describe the gnosis as it is in its own awareness, not thus imperfectly as it is to us in contrast with our own reason and intelligence, it is hardly possible to speak of it except in figures and symbols. And first we must remember that the gnostic level, Mahat, Vijnana, is not the supreme plane of our consciousness, but a middle or link plane. Interposed between the triune glory of the utter Spirit, the infinite existence, consciousness and bliss of the Eternal and our lower triple being and nature, it is as if it stood there as the mediating, formulated, organising and creative wisdom, power and joy of the Eternal. In the gnosis Sachchidananda gathers up the light of his unseizable existence and pours it out on the soul in the shape and power of a divine knowledge, a divine will and a divine bliss of existence. It is as if infinite light were gathered up into the compact orb of the sun and lavished on all that depends upon the sun in radiances that continue for ever. But the gnosis is not only light, it is force; it is creative knowledge, it is the self-effective truth of the divine Idea. This idea is not creative imagination, not something that constructs in a void, but light and power of eternal substance, truth-light full of truth-force; and it brings out what is latent in being, it does not create a fiction that never was in being. The ideation of the gnosis is radiating light-stuff of the consciousness of the eternal Existence; each ray is a truth. The will in the gnosis is a conscious force of eternal knowledge; it throws the consciousness and substance of being into infallible forms of truth-power, forms that embody the idea and make it faultlessly effective, and it works out each truth-power and each truth-form spontaneously and rightly according to its nature. Because it carries this creative force of the divine Idea, the Sun, the lord and symbol of the gnosis, is described in the Veda as the Light which is the father of all things, Surya Savitri, the Wisdom-Luminous who is the bringer-out into manifest existence. This creation is inspired by the divine delight, the eternal Ananda; it is full of the joy of its own truth and power, it creates in bliss, creates out of bliss, creates that which is blissful. Therefore the world of the gnosis, the supramental world is the true and the happy creation, *ṛtam, bhadram,* since all in it shares in the perfect joy that made it. A divine radiance of undeviating knowledge, a divine power of unfaltering will and a divine ease of unstumbling bliss are the nature or Prakriti of the soul in supermind, in *vijñāna.*

The stuff of the gnostic or supramental plane is made of the perfect absolutes of all that is here imperfect and relative and its movement of the reconciled interlockings and happy fusions of all that here are opposites. For behind the appearance of these opposites are their truths and the truths of the Eternal are not in conflict with each other; our mind's and life's opposites transformed in the supermind into their own true spirit link together and are seen as tones and colourings of an eternal Reality and everlasting Ananda. Supermind or Gnosis is the supreme Truth, the supreme Thought, the supreme Word, the supreme Sight, the supreme Will-Idea; it is the inner and outer extension of the Infinite who is beyond Space, the unfettered Time of the Eternal who is timeless, the supernal harmony of all absolutes of the Absolute.

To the envisaging mind there are three powers of the Vijnana. Its supreme power knows and receives into it from above all the infinite existence, consciousness and bliss of the Ishwara;

it is in its highest height the absolute knowledge and force of eternal Sachchidananda. Its second power concentrates the Infinite into a dense luminous consciousness, *caitanyaghana* or *cidghana*, the seed-state of the divine consciousness in which are contained living and concrete all the immutable principles of the divine being and all the inviolable truths of the divine conscious-idea and nature. Its third power brings or looses out these things by the effective ideation, vision, authentic identities of the divine knowledge, movement of the divine will-force, vibration of the divine delight intensities into a universal harmony, an illimitable diversity, a manifold rhythm of their powers, forms and interplay of living consequences. The mental Purusha rising into the *vijñānamaya* must ascend into these three powers. It must turn by conversion of its movements into the movements of the gnosis its mental perception, ideation, will, pleasure into radiances of the divine knowledge, pulsations of the divine will-force, waves and floods of the divine delight-seas. It must convert its conscious stuff of mental nature into the *cidghana* or dense self-luminous consciousness. It must transform its conscious substance into a gnostic self or Truth-self of infinite Sachchidananda. These three movements are described in the Isha Upanishad, the first as *vyūha*, the marshalling of the rays of the Sun of gnosis in the order of the Truth-consciousness, the second as *samūha*, the gathering together of the rays into the body of the Sun of gnosis, the third as the vision of that Sun's fairest form of all in which the soul most intimately possesses its oneness with the infinite Purusha.[2] The Supreme above, in him, around, everywhere and the soul dwelling in the Supreme and one with it, — the infinite power and truth of the Divine concentrated in his own concentrated luminous soul nature, —

---

[2] *Sūrya raśmīn vyūha samūha tejo yat te kalyāṇatamaṁ rūpaṁ tat te paśyāmi yo 'sāv asau puruṣaḥ so 'ham asmi.* The Veda describes the *vijñāna* plane as *ṛtaṁ satyaṁ bṛhat*, the Right, Truth, Vast, the same triple idea differently expressed. *Ṛtam* is the action of the divine knowledge, will and joy in the lines of the truth, the play of the truth-consciousness. *Satyam* is the truth of being which so acts, the dynamic essence of the truth-consciousness. *Bṛhat* is the infinity of Sachchidananda out of which the other two proceed and in which they are founded.

a radiant activity of the divine knowledge, will and joy perfect in the natural action of the Prakriti, — this is the fundamental experience of the mental being transformed and fulfilled and sublimated in the perfection of the gnosis.

Chapter XXIII

The Conditions of Attainment to the Gnosis

KNOWLEDGE is the first principle of the Vijnana, but knowledge is not its only power. The Truth-consciousness, like every other plane, founds itself upon that particular principle which is naturally the key of all its motions; but it is not limited by it, it contains all the other powers of existence. Only the character and working of these other powers is modified and moulded into conformity with its own original and dominant law; intelligence, life, body, will, consciousness, bliss are all luminous, awake, instinct with divine knowledge. This is indeed the process of Purusha-Prakriti everywhere; it is the key-movement of all the hierarchy and graded harmonies of manifested existence.

In the mental being mind-sense or intelligence is the original and dominant principle. The mental being in the mind-world where he is native is in his central and determining nature intelligence; he is a centre of intelligence, a massed movement of intelligence, a receptive and radiating action of intelligence. He has the intelligent sense of his own existence, the intelligent sense of other existence than his own, the intelligent sense of his own nature and activities and the activities of others, the intelligent sense of the nature of things and persons and their relations with himself and each other. That makes up his experience of existence. He has no other knowledge of existence, no knowledge of life and matter except as they make themselves sensible to him and capable of being seized by his mental intelligence; what he does not sense and conceive, is to him practically non-existent, or at least alien to his world and his nature.

Man is in his principle a mental being, but not one living in a mind world, but in a dominantly physical existence; his is a mind cased in Matter and conditioned by Matter. Therefore he has to start with the action of the physical senses which are all channels of material contact; he does not start with the mind-sense. But even so he does not and cannot make free use of anything conveyed by these physical organs until and unless they are taken hold of by the mind-sense and turned into stuff and value of his intelligent being. What is in the lower subhuman submental world a pranic, a nervous, a dynamic action and reaction that proceeds very well without any need of translation into mind-terms or government by mind, has in him to be raised and offered to some kind of intelligence. In order to be characteristically human it has to become first a sense of force, sense of desire, sense of will, sense of intelligent will-action or mentally conscious sense of force-action. His lower delight of being translates itself into a sense of mental or mentalised vital or physical pleasure and its perversion pain, or into a mental or mentalised feeling-sensation of liking and disliking, or into an intelligence of delight and failure of delight, — all phenomena of the intelligent mind-sense. So too that which is above him and that which is around him and in which he lives, — God, the universal being, the cosmic Forces, — are non-existent and unreal to him until his mind awakes to them and gets, not yet their true truth, but some idea, observation, inference, imagination of things supersensuous, some mental sense of the Infinite, some intelligent interpreting consciousness of the forces of the superself above and around him.

All changes when we pass from mind to gnosis; for there a direct inherent knowledge is the central principle. The gnostic (*vijñānamaya*) being is in its character a truth-consciousness, a centre and circumference of the truth-vision of things, a massed movement or subtle body of gnosis. Its action is a self-fulfilling and radiating action of the truth-power of things according to the inner law of their deepest truest self and nature. This truth of things at which we must arrive before we can enter into the gnosis, — for in that all exists and from that all originates on the gnostic plane, — is, first of all, a truth of unity, of oneness, but of unity originating diversity, unity in multiplicity and still unity always, an indefeasible oneness. State of gnosis, the condition of *vijñānamaya* being, is impossible without an ample and close self-identification of ourselves with all existence and with all existences, a universal pervasiveness, a universal comprehension or containing, a certain all-in-allness. The gnostic Purusha has normally the consciousness of itself as infinite, normally too the consciousness of containing the world in itself and exceeding it; it is not like the divided mental being normally bound to a consciousness that feels itself contained in the world and a part of it. It follows that a deliverance from the limiting and imprisoning ego is the first elementary step towards the being of the gnosis; for so long as we live in the ego, it is idle to hope for this higher reality, this vast self-consciousness, this true self-knowledge. The least reversion to ego-thought, ego-action, ego-will brings back the consciousness tumbling out of such gnostic Truth as it has attained into the falsehoods of the divided mind-nature. A secure universality of being is the very basis of this luminous higher consciousness. Abandoning all rigid separateness (but getting instead a certain transcendent overlook or independence) we have to feel ourselves one with all things and beings, to identify ourselves with them, to become aware of them as ourselves, to feel their being as our own, to admit their consciousness as part of ours, to contact their energy as intimate to our energy, to learn how to be one self with all. That oneness is not indeed all that is needed, but it is a first condition and without it there is no gnosis.

This universality is impossible to achieve in its completeness so long as we continue to feel ourselves, as we now feel, a consciousness lodged in an individual mind, life and body. There has to be a certain elevation of the Purusha out of the physical and even out of the mental into the *vijñānamaya* body. No longer can the brain nor its corresponding mental "lotus" remain the centre of our thinking, no longer the heart nor its corresponding "lotus" the originating centre of our emotional and sensational being. The conscious centre of our being, our thought, our will and action, even the original force of our sensations and emotions rise out of the body and mind and take a free station above them. No longer have we the sensation of living in the body, but are above it as its lord, possessor or Ishwara and at the same time encompass it with a wider consciousness than that of the imprisoned physical sense. Now we come to realise with a very living force of reality, normal and continuous, what the sages meant when they spoke of the soul carrying the body or when they said that the soul is not in the body, but the body in the soul. It is from above the body and not from the brain that we shall ideate and will; the brain-action will become only a response and movement of the physical machinery to the shock of the thought-force and will-force from above. All will be originated from above; from above, all that corresponds in gnosis to our present mental activity takes place.[1]

But this centre and this action are free, not bound, not dependent on the physical machine, not clamped to a narrow ego-sense. It is not involved in body; it is not shut up in a separated individuality feeling out for clumsy contacts with the world outside or groping inward for its own deeper spirit. For in this great transformation we begin to have a consciousness not shut up in a generating box, but diffused freely and extending self-existently everywhere; there is or may be a centre, but it is a convenience for individual action, not rigid, not constitutive or separative. The very nature of our conscious activities is henceforth universal; one with those of the universal being, it proceeds from universality to a supple and variable individual-isation. It has become the awareness of an infinite being who acts always universally though with emphasis on an individual formation of its energies. But this emphasis is differential rather than separative, and this formation is no longer what we now understand by individuality; there is no longer a petty limited constructed person shut up in the formula of his own mecha-nism. This state of consciousness is so abnormal to our present mode of being that to the rational man who does not possess it it may seem impossible or even a state of alienation; but once

---

[1] Many, if not all, of these conditions of the gnostic change can and indeed have to be attained long before we reach the gnosis, — but imperfectly at first as if by a reflection, — in higher mind itself, and more completely in what we may call an overmind consciousness between mentality and gnosis.

possessed it vindicates itself even to the mental intelligence by its greater calm, freedom, light, power, effectivity of will, verifiable truth of ideation and feeling. For this condition begins already on the higher levels of liberated mind, and can therefore be partly sensed and understood by mind-intelligence, but it rises to perfect self-possession only when it leaves behind the mental levels, only in the supramental gnosis.

In this state of consciousness the infinite becomes to us the primal, the actual reality, the one thing immediately and sensibly true. It becomes impossible for us to think of or realise the finite apart from our fundamental sense of the infinite, in which alone the finite can live, can form itself, can have any reality or duration. So long as this finite mind and body are to our consciousness the first fact of our existence and the foundation of all our thinking, feeling and willing and so long as things finite are the normal reality from which we can rise occasionally, or even frequently, to an idea and sense of the infinite, we are still very far away from the gnosis. In the plane of the gnosis the infinite is at once our normal consciousness of being, its first fact, our sensible substance. It is very concretely to us there the foundation from which everything finite forms itself and its boundless incalculable forces are the origination of all our thought, will and delight. But this infinite is not only an infinite of pervasion or of extension in which everything forms and happens. Behind that immeasurable extension the gnostic consciousness is always aware of a spaceless inner infinite. It is through this double infinite that we shall arrive at the essential being of Sachchidananda, the highest self of our own being and the totality of our cosmic existence. There is opened to us an illimitable existence which we feel as if it were an infinity above us to which we attempt to rise and an infinity around us into which we strive to dissolve our separate existence. Afterwards we widen into it and rise into it; we break out of the ego into its largeness and are that for ever. If this liberation is achieved, its power can take, if so we will, increasing possession of our lower being also until even our lowest and perversest activities are refashioned into the truth of the Vijnana.

This is the basis, this sense of the infinite and possession by the infinite, and only when it is achieved, can we progress towards some normality of the supramental ideation, perception, sense, identity, awareness. For even this sense of the infinite is only a first foundation and much more has to be done before the consciousness can become dynamically gnostic. The supramental knowledge is the play of a supreme light; there are many other lights, other levels of knowledge higher than human mind which can open in us and receive or reflect something of that effulgence even before we rise into the gnosis. But to command or wholly possess it we must first enter into and become the being of the supreme light, our consciousness must be transformed into that consciousness, its principle and power of self-awareness and all-awareness by identity must be the very stuff of our existence. For our means and ways of knowledge and action must necessarily be according to the nature of our consciousness and it is the consciousness that must radically change if we are to command and not only be occasionally visited by that higher power of knowledge. But it is not confined to a higher thought or the action of a sort of divine reason. It takes up all our present means of knowledge immensely extended, active and effective where they are now debarred, blind, infructuous, and turns them into a high and intense perceptive activity of the Vijnana. Thus it takes up our sense action and illumines it even in its ordinary field so that we get a true sense of things. But also it enables the mind-sense to have a direct perception of the inner as well as the outer phenomenon, to feel and receive or perceive, for instance, the thoughts, feelings, sensations, the nervous reactions of the object on which it is turned.[2] It uses the subtle senses as well as the physical and saves them from their errors. It gives us the knowledge, the experience of planes of existence other than the material to which our ordinary mentality is ignorantly attached and it enlarges the world for us. It transforms similarly the

---

[2] This power, says Patanjali, comes by "*saṁyama*" on an object. That is for the mentality, in the gnosis there is no need of *saṁyama*. For this kind of perception is the natural action of the Vijnana.

sensations and gives them their full intensity as well as their full holding-power; for in our normal mentality the full intensity is impossible because the power to hold and sustain vibrations beyond a certain point is denied to it, mind and body would both break under the shock or the prolonged strain. It takes up too the element of knowledge in our feelings and emotions, — for our feelings too contain a power of knowledge and a power of effectuation which we do not recognise and do not properly develop, — and delivers them at the same time from their limitations and from their errors and perversions. For in all things the gnosis is the Truth, the Right, the highest Law, *devānām adabdhāni vratāni.*

Knowledge and Force or Will — for all conscious force is will — are the twin sides of the action of consciousness. In our mentality they are divided. The idea comes first, the will comes stumbling after it or rebels against it or is used as its imperfect tool with imperfect results; or else the will starts up first with a blind or half-seeing idea in it and works out something in confusion of which we get the right understanding afterwards. There is no oneness, no full understanding between these powers in us; or else there is no perfect correspondence of initiation with effectuation. Nor is the individual will in harmony with the universal; it tries to reach beyond it or falls short of it or deviates from and strives against it. It knows not the times and seasons of the Truth, nor its degrees and measures. The Vijnana takes up the will and puts it first into harmony and then into oneness with the truth of the supramental knowledge. In this knowledge the idea in the individual is one with the idea in the universal, because both are brought back to the truth of the supreme Knowledge and the transcendent Will. The gnosis takes up not only our intelligent will, but our wishes, desires, even what we call the lower desires, the instincts, the impulses, the reachings out of sense and sensation and it transforms them. They cease to be wishes and desires, because they cease first to be personal and then cease to be that struggling after the ungrasped which we mean by craving and desire. No longer blind or half-blind reachings out of the instinctive or intelligent mentality, they are transformed into a various action of the Truth-will; and that will acts with an inherent knowledge of the right measures of its decreed action and therefore with an effectivity unknown to our mental willing. Therefore too in the action of the *vijñānamaya* will there is no place for sin; for all sin is an error of the will, a desire and act of the Ignorance.

When desire ceases entirely, grief and all inner suffering also cease. The Vijnana takes up not only our parts of knowledge and will, but our parts of affection and delight and changes them into action of the divine Ananda. For if knowledge and force are the twin sides or powers of the action of consciousness, delight, Ananda — which is something higher than what we call pleasure — is the very stuff of consciousness and the natural result of the interaction of knowledge and will, force and self-awareness. Both pleasure and pain, both joy and grief are deformations caused by the disturbance of harmony between our consciousness and the force it applies, between our knowledge and will, a breaking up of their oneness by a descent to a lower plane in which they are limited, divided in themselves, restrained from their full and proper action, at odds with other-force, other-consciousness, other-knowledge, other-will. The Vijnana sets this to rights by the power of its truth and a wholesale restoration to oneness and harmony, to the Right and the highest Law. It takes up all our emotions and turns them into various forms of love and delight, even our hatreds, repulsions, causes of suffering. It finds out or reveals the meaning they missed and by missing it became the perversions they are; it restores our whole nature to the eternal Good. It deals similarly with our perceptions and sensations and reveals all the delight that they seek, but in its truth, not in any perversion and wrong seeking and wrong reception; it teaches even our lower impulses to lay hold on the Divine and Infinite in the appearances after which they run. All this is done not in the values of the lower being, but by a lifting up of the mental, vital, material into the inalienable purity, the natural intensity, the continual ecstasy, one yet manifold, of the divine Ananda.

Thus the being of Vijnana is in all its activities a play of perfected knowledge-power, will-power, delight-power, raised to a higher than the mental, vital and bodily level. All-pervasive, universalised, freed from egoistic personality and individuality, it is the play of a higher Self, a higher consciousness and therefore a higher force and higher delight of being. All that acts in the Vijnana in the purity, in the right, in the truth of the superior or divine Prakriti. Its powers may often seem to be what are called in ordinary Yogic parlance siddhis, by the Europeans occult powers, shunned and dreaded by devotees and by many Yogins as snares, stumbling-blocks, diversions from the true seeking after the Divine. But they have that character and are dangerous here because they are sought in the lower being, abnormally, by the ego for an egoistic satisfaction. In the Vijnana they are neither occult nor siddhis, but the open, unforced and normal play of its nature. The Vijnana is the Truth-power and Truth-action of the divine Being in its divine identities, and, when this acts through the individual lifted to the gnostic plane, it fulfils itself unperverted, without fault or egoistic reaction, without diversion from the possession of the Divine. There the individual is no longer the ego, but the free Jiva domiciled in the higher divine nature of which he is a portion, *parā prakṛtir jīvabhūtā*, the nature of the supreme and universal Self seen indeed in the play of multiple individuality but without the veil of ignorance, with self-knowledge, in its multiple oneness, in the truth of its divine Shakti.

In the Vijnana the right relation and action of Purusha and Prakriti are found, because there they become unified and the Divine is no longer veiled in Maya. All is his action. The Jiva no longer says "I think, I act, I desire, I feel"; he does not even say like the sadhaka striving after unity but before he has reached it, "As appointed by Thee seated in my heart, I act." For the heart, the centre of the mental consciousness is no longer the centre of origination but only a blissful channel. He is rather aware of the Divine seated above, lord of all, *adhiṣṭhita*, as well as acting within him. And seated himself in that higher being, *parārdhe, paramasyāṁ parāvati*, he can say truly and boldly, "God himself by his Prakriti knows, acts, loves, takes delight through my individuality and its figures and fulfils there in its higher and divine measures the multiple *līlā* which the Infinite for ever plays in the universality which is himself for ever."

Chapter XXIV

Gnosis and Ananda

THE ASCENT to the gnosis, the possession of something of the gnostic consciousness must elevate the soul of man and sublimate his life in the world into a glory of light and power and bliss and infinity that can seem in comparison with the lame action and limited realisations of our present mental and physical existence the very status and dynamis of a perfection final and absolute. And it is a true perfection, such as nothing before it has yet been in the ascension of the spirit. For even the highest spiritual realisation on the plane of mentality has in it something top-heavy, one-sided and exclusive; even the widest mental spirituality is not wide enough and it is marred too by its imperfect power of self-expression in life. And yet in comparison with what is beyond it, this too, this first gnostic splendour is only a bright passage to a more perfect perfection. It is the secure and shining step from which we can happily mount still upwards into the absolute infinities which are the origin and the goal of the incarnating spirit. In this farther ascension the gnosis does not disappear, but reaches rather its own supreme Light out of which it has descended to mediate between mind and the supreme Infinite.

The Upanishad tells us that after the knowledge-self above the mental is possessed and all the lower selves have been drawn up into it, there is another and last step of all still left to us — though one might ask, is it eternally the last or only the last practically conceivable or at all necessary for us now? — to take up our gnostic existence into the Bliss-Self and there complete the spiritual self-discovery of the divine Infinite. Ananda, a supreme Bliss eternal, far other and higher in its character than the highest human joy or pleasure, is the essential and original nature of the spirit. In Ananda our spirit will find its true self, in Ananda its essential consciousness, in Ananda the absolute power of its existence. The embodied soul's entry into this highest absolute, unlimited, unconditional bliss of the spirit is the infinite liberation and the infinite perfection. It is true that something of this bliss can be enjoyed by reflection, by a qualified descent even on the lower planes where the Purusha plays with his modified and qualified Nature. There can be the experience of a spiritual and boundless Ananda on the plane of matter, on the plane of life, on the plane of mind as well as on the gnostic truth-plane of knowledge and above it. And the Yogin who enters into these lesser realisations, may find them so complete and compelling that he will imagine there is nothing greater, nothing beyond it. For each of the divine principles contains in itself the whole potentiality of all the other six notes of our being; each plane of Nature can have its own perfection of these notes under its own conditions. But the integral perfection can come only by a mounting ascent of the lowest into the highest and an incessant descent of the highest into the lowest till all becomes one at once solid block and plastic sea-stuff of the Truth infinite and eternal.

The very physical consciousness in man, the *annamaya purusa*, can without this supreme ascent and integral descent yet reflect and enter into the self of Sachchidananda. It can do it either by a reflection of the Soul in physical Nature, its bliss, power and infinity secret but still present here, or by losing its separate sense of substance and existence in the Self within or without it. The result is a glorified sleep of the physical mind in which the physical being forgets itself in a kind of conscious Nirvana or else moves about like a thing inert in the hands of Nature, *jadavat*, like a leaf in the wind, or otherwise a state of pure happy and free irresponsibility of action, *balavat*, a divine childhood. But this comes without the higher glories of knowledge and delight which belong to the same status upon a more exalted level. It is an inert realisation of Sachchidananda in which there is neither any mastery of the Prakriti by the Purusha nor any sublimation of Nature into her own supreme power, the infinite glories of the Para Shakti. Yet these two, this mastery and this sublimation, are the two gates of perfection, the splendid doors into the supreme Eternal.

The life soul and life consciousness in man, *prāṇamaya purusa*, can in the same way directly reflect and enter into the self of Sachchidananda by a large and splendid and blissful reflection of the Soul in universal Life or by losing its separate sense of life and existence in the vast Self within or without it. The result is either a profound state of sheer self-oblivion or else an action driven irresponsibly by the life nature, an exalted enthusiasm of self-abandonment to the great world-energy in its vitalistic dance. The outer being lives in a God-possessed frenzy careless of itself and the world, *unmattavat*, or with an entire disregard whether of the conventions and proprieties of fitting human action or of the harmony and rhythms of a greater Truth. It acts as the unbound vital being, *piśācavat*, the divine maniac or else the divine demoniac. Here too there is no mastery or supreme sublimation of nature. There is only a joyful static possession by the Self within us and an unregulated dynamic possession by the physical and the vital Nature without us.

The mind soul and mind consciousness in man, *manomaya purusa*, can in the same direct way reflect and enter into Sachchidananda by a reflection of the Soul as it mirrors itself in the nature of pure universal mind luminous, unwalled, happy, plastic, illimitable, or by absorption in the vast free unconditioned uncentred Self within it and without it. The result is either the immobile cessation of all mind and action or a desire-free unbound action watched by the unparticipating inner Witness. The mental being becomes the eremite soul alone in the world and careless of all human ties or the saint soul that lives in a rapturous God-nearness or felicitous identity and in joyful relations of pure love and ecstasy towards all creatures. The mental being may even realise the Self in all three planes together. Then he is all these things alternately, successively or at once. Or he may transform the lower forms into manifestations of the higher state; he may draw upward the childlikeness or the inert irresponsibility of the free physical mind or the free vital mind's divine madness and carelessness of all rules, proprieties, harmonies and colour or disguise with them the ecstasy of the saint or the solitary liberty of the wandering eremite. Here again there is no mastery, no sublimation of the Nature by the soul in the world, but a double possession, by the freedom and delight of the mental-spiritual infinite within and without by the happy, natural and unregulated play of the mind-Nature. But since the mental being is capable of receiving the gnosis in a way in which the life soul and physical soul cannot receive it, since he can accept it with knowledge though only the limited knowledge of a mental response, he may to a certain extent govern by its light his outer action or, if not that, at least bathe and purify in it his will and his thinkings. But Mind can arrive only at a compromise between the infinite within and the finite nature without; it cannot pour the infinity of the inner being's knowledge and power and bliss with any sense of fullness into its external action which remains always inadequate. Still it is content and free because it is the Lord within who takes up the responsibility of the action adequate or inadequate, assumes its guidance and fixes its consequence.

But the gnostic soul, the *vijñānamaya puruṣa*, is the first to participate not only in the freedom, but in the power and sovereignty of the Eternal. For it receives the fullness, it has the sense of plenitude of the Godhead in its action; it shares the free, splendid and royal march of the Infinite, is a vessel of the original knowledge, the immaculate power, the inviolable bliss, transmutes all life into the eternal Light and the eternal Fire and the eternal Wine of the nectar. It possesses the infinite of the Self and it possesses the infinite of Nature. It does not so much lose as find its nature self in the self of the Infinite. On the other planes to which the mental being has easier access, man finds God in himself and himself in God; he becomes divine in essence rather than in person or nature. In the gnosis, even the mentalised gnosis, the Divine Eternal possesses, changes and stamps the human symbol, envelops and partly finds himself in the person and nature. The mental being at most receives or reflects that which is true, divine and eternal; the gnostic soul reaches a true identity, possesses the spirit and power of the truth-Nature. In the gnosis the dualism of Purusha and Prakriti, Soul and Nature, two separate powers complementary to each other, the great truth of the Sankhyas founded on the practical truth of our present natural existence, disappears in their biune entity, the dynamic mystery of the occult Supreme. The Truth-being is the Hara-Gauri[1] of the Indian iconological symbol; it is the double Power masculine-feminine born from and supported by the supreme Shakti of the Supreme.

Therefore the truth-soul does not arrive at self-oblivion in the Infinite; it comes to an eternal self-possession in the Infinite. Its action is not irregular; it is a perfect control in an infinite freedom. In the lower planes the soul is naturally subject to Nature and the regulating principle is found in the lower nature; all regulation there depends on the acceptance of a strict subjection to the law of the finite. If the soul on these planes withdraws from that law into the liberty of the infinite, it loses its natural centre and becomes centreless in a cosmic infinitude; it forfeits the living harmonic principle by which its external being was till then regulated and it finds no other. The personal nature or what is left of it merely continues mechanically for a while its past movements, or it dances in the gusts and falls of the universal energy that acts on the individual system rather than in that system, or it strays in the wild steps of an irresponsible ecstasy, or it remains inert and abandoned by the breath of the Spirit that was within it. If on the other hand the soul moves in its impulse of freedom towards the discovery of another and divine centre of control through which the Infinite can consciously govern its own action in the individual, it is moving towards the gnosis where that centre pre-exists, the centre of an eternal harmony and order. It is when he ascends above mind and life to the gnosis that the Purusha becomes the master of his own nature because subject only to supreme Nature. For there force or will is the exact counterpart, the perfect dynamis of the divine knowledge. And that knowledge is not merely the eye of the Witness, it is the immanent and compelling gaze of the Ishwara. Its luminous governing power, a power not to be hedged in or denied, imposes its self-expressive force on all the

---

[1] The biune body of the Lord and his Spouse, Ishwara and Shakti, the right half male, the left half female.

action and makes true and radiant and authentic and inevitable every movement and impulse.

The gnosis does not reject the realisations of the lower planes; for it is not an annihilation or extinction, not a Nirvana but a sublime fulfilment of our manifested Nature. It possesses the first realisations under its own conditions after it has transformed them and made them elements of a divine order. The gnostic soul is the child, but the king-child;[2] here is the royal and eternal childhood whose toys are the worlds and all universal Nature is the miraculous garden of the play that tires never. The gnosis takes up the condition of divine inertia; but this is no longer the inertia of the subject soul driven by Nature like a fallen leaf in the breath of the Lord. It is the happy passivity bearing an unimaginable intensity of action and Ananda of the Nature-Soul at once driven by the bliss of the mastering Purusha and aware of herself as the supreme Shakti above and around him and mastering and carrying him blissfully on her bosom for ever. This biune being of Purusha-Prakriti is as if a flaming Sun and body of divine Light self-carried in its orbit by its own inner consciousness and power at one with the universal, at one with a supreme Transcendence. Its madness is a wise madness of Ananda, the incalculable ecstasy of a supreme consciousness and power vibrating with an infinite sense of freedom and intensity in its divine life-movements. Its action is supra-rational and therefore to the rational mind which has not the key it seems a colossal madness. And yet this that seems madness is a wisdom in action that only baffles the mind by the liberty and richness of its contents and the infinite complexity in fundamental simplicity of its motions, it is the very method of the Lord of the worlds, a thing no intellectual interpretation can fathom, — a dance this also, a whirl of mighty energies, but the Master of the dance holds the hands of His energies and keeps them to the rhythmic order, the self-traced harmonic circles of his Rasa-lila. The gnostic soul is not bound any more than the divine demoniac by the petty conventions and proprieties of the

---

[2] So Heraclitus, "The kingdom is of the child."

normal human life or the narrow rules through which it makes some shift to accommodate itself with the perplexing dualities of the lower nature and tries to guide its steps among the seeming contradictions of the world, to avoid its numberless stumbling-blocks and to foot with gingerly care around its dangers and pitfalls. The gnostic supramental life is abnormal to us because it is free to all the hardihoods and audacious delights of a soul dealing fearlessly and even violently with Nature, but yet is it the very normality of the infinite and all governed by the law of the Truth in its exact unerring process. It obeys the law of a self-possessed Knowledge, Love, Delight in an innumerable Oneness. It seems abnormal only because its rhythm is not measurable by the faltering beats of the mind, but yet it steps in a wonderful and transcendent measure.

And what then is the necessity of a still higher step and what difference is there between the soul in gnosis and the soul in the Bliss? There is no essential difference, but yet a difference, because there is a transfer to another consciousness and a certain reversal in position, — for at each step of the ascent from Matter to the highest Existence there is a reversal of consciousness. The soul no longer looks up to something beyond it, but is in it and from it looks down on all that it was before. On all planes indeed the Ananda can be discovered, because everywhere it exists and is the same. Even there is a repetition of the Ananda plane in each lower world of consciousness. But in the lower planes not only is it reached by a sort of dissolution into it of the pure mind or the life-sense or the physical awareness, but it is, as it were, itself diluted by the dissolved form of mind, life or matter, held in the dilution and turned into a poor thinness wonderful to the lower consciousness but not comparable to its true intensities. The gnosis has on the contrary a dense light of essential consciousness[3] in which the intense fullness of the Ananda can be. And when the form of gnosis is dissolved into the Ananda, it is not annulled altogether, but undergoes a natural change by which the soul is carried up into its last and absolute

---

[3] *cidghana.*

freedom; for it casts itself into the absolute existence of the spirit and is enlarged into its own entirely self-existent bliss infinitudes. The gnosis has the infinite and absolute as the conscious source, accompaniment, condition, standard, field and atmosphere of all its activities, it possesses it as its base, fount, constituent material, indwelling and inspiring Presence; but in its action it seems to stand out from it as its operation, as the rhythmical working of its activities, as a divine Maya[4] or Wisdom-Formation of the Eternal. Gnosis is the divine Knowledge-Will of the divine Consciousness-Force; it is harmonic consciousness and action of Prakriti-Purusha full of the delight of the divine existence. In the Ananda the knowledge goes back from these willed harmonies into pure self-consciousness, the will dissolves into pure transcendent force and both are taken up into the pure delight of the Infinite. The basis of the gnostic existence is the self-stuff and self-form of the Ananda.

This in the ascension takes place because there is here completed the transition to the absolute unity of which the gnosis is the decisive step, but not the final resting-place. In the gnosis the soul is aware of its infinity and lives in it, yet it lives also in a working centre for the individual play of the Infinite. It realises its identity with all existences, but it keeps a distinction without difference by which it can have also the contact with them in a certain diverseness. This is that distinction for the joy of contact which in the mind becomes not only difference, but in its self-experience division from our other selves, in its spiritual being a sense of loss of self one with us in others and a reaching after the felicity it has forfeited, in life a compromise between egoistic self-absorption and a blind seeking out for the lost oneness. In its infinite consciousness, the gnostic soul creates a sort of voluntary limitation for its own wisdom-purposes; it has even its particular luminous aura of being in which it moves, although beyond that it enters into all things and identifies itself with all being and all existences. In the Ananda all is reversed,

---

[4] Not in the sense of illusion, but in the original Vedic significance of the word Maya. All in the gnostic existence is real, spiritually concrete, eternally verifiable.

the centre disappears. In the bliss nature there is no centre, nor any voluntary or imposed circumference, but all is, all are one equal being, one identical spirit. The bliss soul finds and feels itself everywhere; it has no mansion, is *aniketa*, or has the all for its mansion, or, if it likes, it has all things for its many mansions open to each other for ever. All other selves are entirely its own selves, in action as well as in essence. The joy of contact in diverse oneness becomes altogether the joy of absolute identity in innumerable oneness. Existence is no longer formulated in the terms of the Knowledge, because the known and knowledge and the knower are wholly one self here and, since all possesses all in an intimate identity beyond the closest closeness, there is no need of what we call knowledge. All the consciousness is of the bliss of the Infinite, all power is power of the bliss of the Infinite, all forms and activities are forms and activities of the bliss of the Infinite. In this absolute truth of its being the eternal soul of Ananda lives, here deformed by contrary phenomena, there brought back and transfigured into their reality.

The soul lives: it is not abolished, it is not lost in a featureless Indefinite. For on every plane of our existence the same principle holds; the soul may fall asleep in a trance of self-absorption, dwell in an ineffable intensity of God-possession, live in the highest glory of its own plane, — the Anandaloka, Brahmaloka, Vaikuntha, Goloka of various Indian systems, — even turn upon the lower worlds to fill them with its own light and power and beatitude. In the eternal worlds and more and more in all worlds above Mind these states exist in each other. For they are not separate; they are coexistent, even coincident powers of the consciousness of the Absolute. The Divine on the Ananda plane is not incapable of a world-play or self-debarred from any expression of its glories. On the contrary, as the Upanishad insists, the Ananda is the true creative principle. For all takes birth from this divine Bliss;[5] all is pre-existent in it as an absolute truth of existence which the Vijnana brings out and subjects to

---

[5] Therefore the world of the Ananda is called the Janaloka, in the double sense of birth and delight.

voluntary limitation by the Idea and the law of the Idea. In the Ananda all law ceases and there is an absolute freedom without binding term or limit. It is superior to all principles and in one and the same motion the enjoyer of all principles; it is free from all gunas and the enjoyer of its own infinite gunas; it is above all forms and the builder and enjoyer of all its self-forms and figures. This unimaginable completeness is what the spirit is, the spirit transcendent and universal, and to be one in bliss with the transcendent and universal spirit is for the soul too to be that and nothing less. Necessarily, since there is on this plane the absolute and the play of absolutes, it is ineffable by any of the conceptions of our mind or by signs of the phenomenal or ideal realities of which mind-conceptions are the figures in our intelligence. These realities are themselves indeed only relative symbols of those ineffable absolutes. The symbol, the expressive reality, may give an idea, a perception, sense, vision, contact even of the thing itself to us, but at last we get beyond it to the thing it symbolises, transcend idea, vision, contact, pierce through the ideal and pass to the real realities, the identical, the supreme, the timeless and eternal, the infinitely infinite.

Our first absorbing impulse when we become inwardly aware of something entirely beyond what we now are and know and are powerfully attracted to it, is to get away from the present actuality and dwell in that higher reality altogether. The extreme form of this attraction when we are drawn to the supreme Existence and the infinite Ananda is the condemnation of the lower and the finite as an illusion and an aspiration to Nirvana in the beyond, — the passion for dissolution, immersion, extinction in the Spirit. But the real dissolution, the true *nirvāṇa* is the release of all that is bindingly characteristic of the lower into the larger being of the Higher, the conscious possession of the living symbol by the living Real. We discover in the end that not only is that higher Reality the cause of all the rest, not only it embraces and exists in all the rest, but as more and more we possess it, all this rest is transformed in our soul-experience into a superior value and becomes the means of a richer expression of the Real, a more many-sided communion with the Infinite, a larger ascent to the Supreme. Finally, we get close to the absolute and its supreme values which are the absolutes of all things. We lose the passion for release, *mumukṣutva*, which till then actuated us, because we are now intimately near to that which is ever free, that which is neither attracted into attachment by what binds us now nor afraid of what to us seems to be bondage. It is only by the loss of the bound soul's exclusive passion for its freedom that there can come an absolute liberation of our nature. The Divine attracts the soul of man to him by various lures; all of them are born of its own relative and imperfect conceptions of bliss; all are its ways of seeking for the Ananda, but, if clung to till the end, miss the inexpressible truth of those surpassing felicities. First in order comes the lure of an earthly reward, a prize of material, intellectual, ethical or other joy in the terrestrial mind and body. A second remoter greater version of the same fruitful error is the hope of a heavenly bliss, far exceeding these earthly rewards; the conception of heaven rises in altitude and purity till it reaches the pure idea of the eternal presence of God or an unending union with the Eternal. And last we get the subtlest of all lures, an escape from these worldly or heavenly joys and from all pains and sorrows, effort and trouble and from all phenomenal things, a Nirvana, a self-dissolution in the Absolute, an Ananda of cessation and ineffable peace. In the end all these toys of the mind have to be transcended. The fear of birth and the desire of escape from birth must entirely fall away from us. For, to repeat the ancient language, the soul that has realised oneness has no sorrow or shrinking; the spirit that has entered into the bliss of the Spirit has nought to fear from anyone or anything whatsoever. Fear, desire and sorrow are diseases of the mind; born of its sense of division and limitation, they cease with the falsehood that begot them. The Ananda is free from these maladies; it is not the monopoly of the ascetic, it is not born from the disgust of existence.

The bliss soul is not bound to birth or to non-birth; it is not driven by desire of the Knowledge or harassed by fear of the Ignorance. The supreme bliss Soul has already the Knowledge and transcends all need of knowledge. Not limited in consciousness by the form and the act, it can play with the manifestation without being imbued with the Ignorance. Already it is taking its part above in the mystery of an eternal manifestation and here, when the time comes, it will descend into birth without being the slave of Ignorance chained to the revolutions of the wheel of Nature. For it knows that the purpose and law of the birth-series is for the soul in the body to rise from plane to plane and substitute always the rule of the higher for the rule of the lower play even down to the material field. The bliss-soul neither disdains to help that ascent from above nor fears to descend down the stairs of God into the material birth and there contribute the power of its own bliss nature to the upward pull of the divine forces. The time for that marvellous hour of the evolving Time-Spirit is not yet come. Man, generally, cannot yet ascend to the bliss nature; he has first to secure himself on the higher mental altitudes, to ascend from them to the gnosis. Still less can he bring down all the Bliss-Power into this terrestrial Nature; he must first cease to be mental man and become superhuman. All he can do now is to receive something of its power into his soul in greater or less degree, by a diminishing transmission through an inferior consciousness; but even that gives him the sense of an ecstasy and an unsurpassable beatitude.

And what will be the bliss nature when it manifests in a new supramental race? The fully evolved soul will be one with all beings in the status and dynamic effects of experience of a bliss-consciousness intense and illimitable. And since love is the effective power and soul-symbol of bliss-oneness he will approach and enter into this oneness by the gate of universal love, a sublimation of human love at first, a divine love afterwards, at its summits a thing of beauty, sweetness and splendour now to us inconceivable. He will be one in bliss-consciousness with all the world-play and its powers and happenings and there will be banished for ever the sorrow and fear, the hunger and pain of our poor and darkened mental and vital and physical existence. He will get that power of the bliss-freedom in which all the conflicting principles of our being shall be unified in their absolute values. All evil shall perforce change itself into good; the universal beauty of the All-beautiful will take possession of its fallen kingdoms; every darkness will be converted into a pregnant glory of light and the discords which the mind creates between Truth and Good and Beauty, Power and Love and Knowledge will disappear on the eternal summit, in the infinite extensions where they are always one.

The Purusha in mind, life and body is divided from Nature and in conflict with her. He labours to control and coerce what he can embody of her by his masculine force and is yet subject to her afflicting dualities and in fact her plaything from top to bottom, beginning to end. In the gnosis he is biune with her, finds as master of his own nature their reconciliation and harmony by their essential oneness even while he accepts an infinite blissful subjection, the condition of his mastery and his liberties, to the Supreme in his sovereign divine Nature. In the tops of the gnosis and in the Ananda he is one with the Prakriti and no longer solely biune with her. There is no longer the baffling play of Nature with the soul in the Ignorance; all is the conscious play of the soul with itself and all its selves and the Supreme and the divine Shakti in its own and the infinite bliss nature. This is the supreme mystery, the highest secret, simple to its own experience, however difficult and complex to our mental conceptions and the effort of our limited intelligence to understand what is beyond it. In the free infinity of the self-delight of Sachchidananda there is a play of the divine Child, a *rāsa līlā* of the infinite Lover and its mystic soul-symbols repeat themselves in characters of beauty and movements and harmonies of delight in a timeless forever.

Chapter XXV

The Higher and the Lower Knowledge

WE HAVE now completed our view of the path of Knowledge and seen to what it leads. First, the end of Yoga of Knowledge is God-possession, it is to possess God and be possessed by him through consciousness, through identification, through reflection of the divine Reality. But not merely in some abstraction away from our present existence, but here also; therefore to possess the Divine in himself, the Divine in the world, the Divine within, the Divine in all things and all beings. It is to possess oneness with God and through that to possess also oneness with the universal, with the cosmos and all existences; therefore to possess the infinite diversity also in the oneness, but on the basis of oneness and not on the basis of division. It is to possess God in his personality and his impersonality; in his purity free from qualities and in his infinite qualities; in time and beyond time; in his action and in his silence; in the finite and in the infinite. It is to possess him not only in pure self, but in all self; not only in self, but in Nature; not only in spirit, but in supermind, mind, life and body; to possess him with the spirit, with the mind, with the vital and the physical consciousness; and it is again for all these to be possessed by him, so that our whole being is one with him, full of him, governed and driven by him. It is, since God is oneness, for our physical consciousness to be one with the soul and the nature of the material universe; for our life, to be one with all life; for our mind, to be one with the universal mind; for our spirit, to be identified with the universal spirit. It is to merge in him in the absolute and find him in all relations.

Secondly, it is to put on the divine being and the divine nature. And since God is Sachchidananda, it is to raise our being into the divine being, our consciousness into the divine consciousness, our energy into the divine energy, our delight of existence into the divine delight of being. And it is not only to lift ourselves into this higher consciousness, but to widen into it in all our being, because it is to be found on all the planes of our existence and in all our members, so that our mental, vital, physical existence shall become full of the divine nature. Our intelligent mentality is to become a play of the divine knowledge-will, our mental soul-life a play of the divine love and delight, our vitality a play of the divine life, our physical being a mould of the divine substance. This God-action in us is to be realised by an opening of ourselves to the divine gnosis and divine Ananda and, in its fullness, by an ascent into and a permanent dwelling in the gnosis and the Ananda. For though we live physically on the material plane and in normal outward-going life the mind and soul are preoccupied with material existence, this externality of our being is not a binding limitation. We can raise our internal consciousness from plane to plane of the relations of Purusha with Prakriti, and even become, instead of the mental being dominated by the physical soul and nature, the gnostic being or the bliss-self and assume the gnostic or the bliss nature. And by this raising of the inner life we can transform our whole outward-going existence; instead of a life dominated by matter we shall then have a life dominated by spirit with all its circumstances moulded and determined by the purity of being, the consciousness infinite even in the finite, the divine energy, the divine joy and bliss of the spirit.

This is the goal; we have seen also what are the essentials of the method. But here we have first to consider briefly one side of the question of method which we have hitherto left untouched. In the system of an integral Yoga the principle must be that all life is a part of the Yoga; but the knowledge which we have been describing seems to be not the knowledge of what is ordinarily understood as life, but of something behind life. There are two kinds of knowledge, that which seeks to understand the apparent phenomenon of existence externally, by an approach from outside, through the intellect, — this is the lower knowledge, the knowledge of the apparent world; secondly, the knowledge which seeks to know the truth of existence from within, in its source and reality, by spiritual realisation. Ordinarily, a sharp distinction is drawn between the two, and it is supposed that when we get to the higher knowledge, the God-knowledge, then the rest, the world-knowledge, becomes of no concern to us: but in reality they are two sides of one seeking. All knowledge is ultimately the knowledge of God, through himself, through Nature, through her works. Mankind has first to seek this knowledge through the external life; for until its mentality is sufficiently developed, spiritual knowledge is not really possible, and in proportion as it is developed, the possibilities of spiritual knowledge become richer and fuller.

Science, art, philosophy, ethics, psychology, the knowledge of man and his past, action itself are means by which we arrive at the knowledge of the workings of God through Nature and through life. At first it is the workings of life and forms of Nature which occupy us, but as we go deeper and deeper and get a completer view and experience, each of these lines brings us face to face with God. Science at its limits, even physical Science, is compelled to perceive in the end the infinite, the universal, the spirit, the divine intelligence and will in the material universe. Still more easily must this be the end with the psychic sciences which deal with the operations of higher and subtler planes and powers of our being and come into contact with the beings and the phenomena of the worlds behind which are unseen, not sensible by our physical organs, but ascertainable by the subtle mind and senses. Art leads to the same end; the aesthetic human being intensely preoccupied with Nature through aesthetic emotion must in the end arrive at spiritual emotion and perceive not only the infinite life, but the infinite presence within her; preoccupied with beauty in the life of man he must in the end come to see the divine, the universal, the spiritual in humanity. Philosophy dealing with the principles of things must come to perceive the Principle of all these principles and investigate its nature, attributes and essential workings. So ethics must eventually perceive that the law of good which it seeks is the law of God and depends on the being and nature of the Master of the law. Psychology leads from the study of mind and the soul in living beings to the perception of the one soul and one mind in all things and beings. The history and study of man like the history and study of Nature lead towards the perception of the eternal and universal Power and Being whose thought and will work out through the cosmic and human evolution. Action itself forces us into contact with the divine Power which works through, uses, overrules our actions. The intellect begins to perceive and understand, the emotions to feel and desire and revere, the will to turn itself to the service of the Divine without whom Nature and man cannot exist or move and by conscious knowledge of whom alone we can arrive at our highest possibilities.

It is here that Yoga steps in. It begins by using knowledge, emotion and action for the possession of the Divine. For Yoga is the conscious and perfect seeking of union with the Divine towards which all the rest was an ignorant and imperfect moving and seeking. At first, then, Yoga separates itself from the action and method of the lower knowledge. For while this lower knowledge approaches God indirectly from outside and never enters his secret dwelling-place, Yoga calls us within and approaches him directly; while that seeks him through the intellect and becomes conscious of him from behind a veil, Yoga seeks him through realisation, lifts the veil and gets the full vision; where that only feels the presence and the influence, Yoga enters into the presence and fills itself with the influence; where that is only aware of the workings and through them gets some glimpse of the Reality, Yoga identifies our inner being with the Reality and sees from that the workings. Therefore the methods of Yoga are different from the methods of the lower knowledge.

The method of Yoga in knowledge must always be a turning of the eye inward and, so far as it looks upon outer things, a penetrating of the surface appearances to get at the one eternal reality within them. The lower knowledge is preoccupied with the appearances and workings; it is the first necessity of the higher to get away from them to the Reality of which they are the appearances and the Being and Power of conscious existence of which they are the workings. It does this by three movements each necessary to each other, by each of which the others become complete, — purification, concentration, identification. The object of purification is to make the whole mental being a clear mirror in which the divine reality can be reflected, a clear vessel and an unobstructing channel into which the divine presence and through which the divine influence can be poured, a subtilised stuff which the divine nature can take possession of, new-shape and use to divine issues. For the mental being at present reflects only the confusions created by the mental and physical view of the world, is a channel only for the disorders of the ignorant lower nature and full of obstructions and impurities which prevent the higher from acting; therefore the whole shape of our being is deformed and imperfect, indocile to the highest influences and turned in its action to ignorant and inferior utilities. It reflects even the world falsely; it is incapable of reflecting the Divine.

Concentration is necessary, first, to turn the whole will and mind from the discursive divagation natural to them, following a dispersed movement of the thoughts, running after many-branching desires, led away in the track of the senses and the outward mental response to phenomena: we have to fix the will and the thought on the eternal and real behind all, and this demands an immense effort, a one-pointed concentration. Secondly, it is necessary in order to break down the veil which is erected by our ordinary mentality between ourselves and the truth; for outer knowledge can be picked up by the way, by ordinary attention and reception, but the inner, hidden and higher truth can only be seized by an absolute concentration of the mind on its object, an absolute concentration of the will to attain it and, once attained, to hold it habitually and securely unite oneself with it. For identification is the condition of complete knowledge and possession; it is the intense result of a habitual purified reflecting of the reality and an entire concentration on it; and it is necessary in order to break down entirely that division and separation of ourselves from the divine being and the eternal reality which is the normal condition of our unregenerate ignorant mentality.

None of these things can be done by the methods of the lower knowledge. It is true that here also they have a preparing action, but up to a certain point and to a certain degree of intensity only, and it is where their action ceases that the action of Yoga takes up our growth into the Divine and finds the means to complete it. All pursuit of knowledge, if not vitiated by a too earthward tendency, tends to refine, to subtilise, to purify the being. In proportion as we become more mental, we attain to a subtler action of our whole nature which becomes more apt to reflect and receive higher thoughts, a purer will, a less physical truth, more inward influences. The power of ethical knowledge and the ethical habit of thought and will to purify is obvious. Philosophy not only purifies the reason and predisposes it to the contact of the universal and the infinite, but tends to stabilise the nature and create the tranquillity of the sage; and tranquillity is a sign of increasing self-mastery and purity. The preoccupation with universal beauty even in its aesthetic forms has an intense power for refining and subtilising the nature, and at its highest it is a great force for purification. Even the scientific habit of mind and the disinterested preoccupation with cosmic law and truth not only refine the reasoning and observing faculty, but have, when not counteracted by other tendencies, a steadying, elevating and purifying influence on the mind and moral nature which has not been sufficiently noticed.

The concentration of the mind and the training of the will towards the reception of the truth and living in the truth is also an evident result, a perpetual necessity of these pursuits; and at the end or in their highest intensities they may and do lead first to an intellectual, then to a reflective perception of the divine Reality which may culminate in a sort of preliminary identification with it. But all this cannot go beyond a certain point. The systematic purification of the whole being for an integral reflection and taking in of the divine reality can only be done by the special methods of Yoga. Its absolute concentration has to take the place of the dispersed concentrations of the lower knowledge; the vague and ineffective identification which is all the lower knowledge can bring, has to be replaced by the complete, intimate, imperative and living union which Yoga brings.

Nevertheless, Yoga does not either in its path or in its attainment exclude and throw away the forms of the lower knowledge, except when it takes the shape of an extreme asceticism or a mysticism altogether intolerant of this other divine mystery of the world-existence. It separates itself from them by the intensity, largeness and height of its objective and the specialisation of its methods to suit its aim; but it not only starts from them, but for a certain part of the way carries them with it and uses them as auxiliaries. Thus it is evident how largely ethical thought and practice, — not so much external as internal conduct, — enter into the preparatory method of Yoga, into its aim at purity. Again the whole method of Yoga is psychological; it might almost be termed the consummate practice of a perfect psychological knowledge. The data of philosophy are the supports from which it begins in the realisation of God through the principles of his being; only it carries the intelligent understanding which is all philosophy gives, into an intensity which carries it beyond thought into vision and beyond understanding into realisation and possession; what philosophy leaves abstract and remote, it brings into a living nearness and spiritual concreteness. The aesthetic and emotional mind and aesthetic forms are used by Yoga as a support for concentration even in the Yoga of knowledge and are, sublimated, the whole means of the Yoga of love and delight, as life and action, sublimated, are the whole means of the Yoga of works. Contemplation of God in Nature, contemplation and service of God in man and in the life of man and of the world in its past, present and future, are equally elements of which the Yoga of knowledge can make use to complete the realisation of God in all things. Only, all is directed to the one aim, directed towards God, filled with the idea of the divine, infinite, universal existence so that the outward-going, sensuous, pragmatical preoccupation of the lower knowledge with phenomena and forms is replaced by the one divine preoccupation. After attainment the same character remains. The Yogin continues to know and see God in the finite and be a channel of God-consciousness and God-action in the world; therefore the knowledge of the world and the enlarging and uplifting of all that appertains to life comes within his scope. Only, in all he sees God, sees the supreme reality, and his motive of work is to help mankind towards the knowledge of God and the possession of the supreme reality. He sees God through the data of science, God through the conclusions of philosophy, God through the forms of Beauty and the forms of Good, God in all the activities of life, God in the past of the world and its effects, in the present and its tendencies, in the future and its great progression. Into any or all of these he can bring his illumined vision and his liberated power of the spirit. The lower knowledge has been the step from which he has risen to the higher; the higher illumines for him the lower and makes it part of itself, even if only its lower fringe and most external radiation.

Chapter XXVI

Samadhi

INTIMATELY connected with the aim of the Yoga of Knowledge which must always be the growth, the ascent or the withdrawal into a higher or a divine consciousness not now normal to us, is the importance attached to the phenomenon of Yogic trance, to Samadhi. It is supposed that there are states of being which can only be gained in trance; that especially is to be desired in which all action of awareness is abolished and there is no consciousness at all except the pure supramental immersion in immobile, timeless and infinite being. By passing away in this trance the soul departs into the silence of the highest Nirvana without possibility of return into any illusory or inferior state of existence. Samadhi is not so all-important in the Yoga of devotion, but it still has its place there as the swoon of being into which the ecstasy of divine love casts the soul. To enter into it is the supreme step of the ladder of Yogic practice in Rajayoga and Hathayoga. What then is the nature of Samadhi or the utility of its trance in an integral Yoga? It is evident that where our objective includes the possession of the Divine in life, a state of cessation of life cannot be the last consummating step or the highest desirable condition: Yogic trance cannot be an aim, as in so many Yogic systems, but only a means, and a means not of escape from the waking existence, but to enlarge and raise the whole seeing, living and active consciousness.

The importance of Samadhi rests upon the truth which modern knowledge is rediscovering, but which has never been lost in Indian psychology, that only a small part whether of world-being or of our own being comes into our ken or into our action. The rest is hidden behind in subliminal reaches of being which descend into the profoundest depths of the subconscient and rise to highest peaks of superconscience, or which surround the little field of our waking self with a wide circumconscient existence of which our mind and sense catch only a few indications. The old Indian psychology expressed this fact by dividing consciousness into three provinces, waking state, dream-state, sleep-state, *jāgrat*, *svapna*, *suṣupti*; and it supposed in the human being a waking self, a dream-self, a sleep-self, with the supreme or absolute self of being, the fourth or Turiya, beyond, of which all these are derivations for the enjoyment of relative experience in the world.

If we examine the phraseology of the old books, we shall find that the waking state is the consciousness of the material universe which we normally possess in this embodied existence dominated by the physical mind. The dream-state is a consciousness corresponding to the subtler life-plane and mind-plane behind, which to us, even when we get intimations of them, have not the same concrete reality as the things of the physical existence. The sleep-state is a consciousness corresponding to the supramental plane proper to the gnosis, which is beyond our experience because our causal body or envelope of gnosis is not developed in us, its faculties not active, and therefore we are in relation to that plane in a condition of dreamless sleep. The Turiya beyond is the consciousness of our pure self-existence or our absolute being with which we have no direct relations at all, whatever mental reflections we may receive in our dream or our waking or even, irrecoverably, in our sleep consciousness. This fourfold scale corresponds to the degrees of the ladder of being by which we climb back towards the absolute Divine. Normally therefore we cannot get back from the physical mind to the higher planes or degrees of consciousness without receding from the waking state, without going in and away from it and losing touch with the material world. Hence to those who desire to have the experience of these higher degrees, trance becomes a desirable thing, a means of escape from the limitations of the physical mind and nature.

Samadhi or Yogic trance retires to increasing depths according as it draws farther and farther away from the normal or waking state and enters into degrees of consciousness less and less communicable to the waking mind, less and less ready to receive a summons from the waking world. Beyond a certain point the trance becomes complete and it is then almost or quite impossible to awaken or call back the soul that has receded into them; it can only come back by its own will or at most by a violent shock of physical appeal dangerous to the system owing to the abrupt upheaval of return. There are said to be supreme states of trance in which the soul persisting for too long a time cannot return; for it loses its hold on the cord which binds it to the consciousness of life, and the body is left, maintained indeed in its set position, not dead by dissolution, but incapable of recovering the ensouled life which had inhabited it. Finally, the Yogin acquires at a certain stage of development the power of abandoning his body definitively without the ordinary phenomena of death, by an act of will,[1] or by a process of withdrawing the pranic life-force through the gate of the upward life-current (*udāna*), opening for it a way through the mystic *brahmarandhra* in the head. By departure from life in the state of Samadhi he attains directly to that higher status of being to which he aspires.

In the dream-state itself there are an infinite series of depths; from the lighter recall is easy and the world of the physical senses is at the doors, though for the moment shut out; in the deeper it becomes remote and less able to break in upon the inner absorption, the mind has entered into secure depths of trance. There is a complete difference between Samadhi and normal sleep, between the dream-state of Yoga and the physical state of dream. The latter belongs to the physical mind; in the former the mind proper and subtle is at work liberated from the immixture of the physical mentality. The dreams of the physical mind are an incoherent jumble made up partly of responses to vague touches from the physical world round which the lower mind-faculties disconnected from the will and reason, the *buddhi*, weave a web of wandering phantasy, partly of disordered associations from the brain-memory, partly of reflections from the soul travelling on the mental plane, reflections which are, ordinarily, received

---

[1] *icchā-mṛtyu.*

without intelligence or coordination, wildly distorted in the reception and mixed up confusedly with the other dream elements, with brain-memories and fantastic responses to any sensory touch from the physical world. In the Yogic dream-state, on the other hand, the mind is in clear possession of itself, though not of the physical world, works coherently and is able to use either its ordinary will and intelligence with a concentrated power or else the higher will and intelligence of the more exalted planes of mind. It withdraws from experience of the outer world, it puts its seals upon the physical senses and their doors of communication with material things; but everything that is proper to itself, thought, reasoning, reflection, vision, it can continue to execute with an increased purity and power of sovereign concentration free from the distractions and unsteadiness of the waking mind. It can use too its will and produce upon itself or upon its environment mental, moral and even physical effects which may continue and have their after consequences on the waking state subsequent to the cessation of the trance.

To arrive at full possession of the powers of the dream-state, it is necessary first to exclude the attack of the sights, sounds etc. of the outer world upon the physical organs. It is quite possible indeed to be aware in the dream-trance of the outer physical world through the subtle senses which belong to the subtle body; one may be aware of them just so far as one chooses and on a much wider scale than in the waking condition: for the subtle senses have a far more powerful range than the gross physical organs, a range which may be made practically unlimited. But this awareness of the physical world through the subtle senses is something quite different from our normal awareness of it through the physical organs; the latter is incompatible with the settled state of trance, for the pressure of the physical senses breaks the Samadhi and calls back the mind to live in their normal field where alone they have power. But the subtle senses have power both upon their own planes and upon the physical world, though this is to them more remote than their own world of being. In Yoga various devices are used to seal up the doors of the physical sense, some of them physical devices; but the one all-sufficient means is a force of concentration by which the mind is drawn inward to depths where the call of physical things can no longer easily attain to it. A second necessity is to get rid of the intervention of physical sleep. The ordinary habit of the mind when it goes in away from contact with physical things is to fall into the torpor of sleep or its dreams, and therefore when called in for the purposes of Samadhi, it gives or tends to give, at the first chance, by sheer force of habit, not the response demanded, but its usual response of physical slumber. This habit of the mind has to be got rid of; the mind has to learn to be awake in the dream-state, in possession of itself, not with the outgoing, but with an ingathered wakefulness in which, though immersed in itself, it exercises all its powers.

The experiences of the dream-state are infinitely various. For not only has it sovereign possession of the usual mental powers, reasoning, discrimination, will, imagination, and can use them in whatever way, on whatever subject, for whatever purpose it pleases, but it is able to establish connection with all the worlds to which it has natural access or to which it chooses to acquire access, from the physical to the higher mental worlds. This it does by various means open to the subtlety, flexibility and comprehensive movement of this internalised mind liberated from the narrow limitations of the physical outward-going senses. It is able first to take cognizance of all things whether in the material world or upon other planes by aid of perceptible images, not only images of things visible, but of sounds, touch, smell, taste, movement, action, of all that makes itself sensible to the mind and its organs. For the mind in Samadhi has access to the inner space called sometimes the *cidākāśa*, to depths of more and more subtle ether which are heavily curtained from the physical sense by the grosser ether of the material universe, and all things sensible, whether in the material world or any other, create reconstituting vibrations, sensible echoes, reproductions, recurrent images of themselves which that subtler ether receives and retains.

It is this which explains many of the phenomena of clairvoyance, clairaudience, etc.; for these phenomena are only the exceptional admission of the waking mentality into a limited sensitiveness to what might be called the image memory of the subtle ether, by which not only the signs of all things past and present, but even those of things future can be seized; for things future are already accomplished to knowledge and vision on higher planes of mind and their images can be reflected upon mind in the present. But these things which are exceptional to the waking mentality, difficult and to be perceived only by the possession of a special power or else after assiduous training, are natural to the dream-state of trance consciousness in which the subliminal mind is free. And that mind can also take cognizance of things on various planes not only by these sensible images, but by a species of thought perception or of thought reception and impression analogous to that phenomenon of consciousness which in modern psychical science has been given the name of telepathy. But the powers of the dream-state do not end here. It can by a sort of projection of ourselves, in a subtle form of the mental body, actually enter into other planes and worlds or into distant places and scenes of this world, move among them with a sort of bodily presence and bring back the direct experience of their scenes and truths and occurrences. It may even project actually the mental or vital body for the same purpose and travel in it, leaving the physical body in a profoundest trance without sign of life until its return.

The greatest value of the dream-state of Samadhi lies, however, not in these more outward things, but in its power to open up easily higher ranges and powers of thought, emotion, will by which the soul grows in height, range and self-mastery. Especially, withdrawing from the distraction of sensible things, it can, in a perfect power of concentrated self-seclusion, prepare itself by a free reasoning, thought, discrimination, or more intimately, more finally, by an ever deeper vision and identification, for access to the Divine, the supreme Self, the transcendent Truth, both in its principles and powers and manifestations and in its highest original Being. Or it can by an absorbed inner joy and emotion, as in a sealed and secluded chamber of the soul, prepare itself for the delight of union with the divine Beloved, the Master of all bliss, rapture and Ananda.

For the integral Yoga this method of Samadhi may seem to have the disadvantage that when it ceases, the thread is broken and the soul returns into the distraction and imperfection of the outward life, with only such an elevating effect upon that outer life as the general memory of these deeper experiences may produce. But this gulf, this break is not inevitable. In the first place, it is only in the untrained psychic being that the experiences of the trance are a blank to the waking mind; as it becomes the master of its Samadhi, it is able to pass without any gulf of oblivion from the inner to the outer waking. Secondly, when this has been once done, what is attained in the inner state, becomes easier to acquire by the waking consciousness and to turn into the normal experience, powers, mental status of the waking life. The subtle mind which is normally eclipsed by the insistence of the physical being, becomes powerful even in the waking state, until even there the enlarging man is able to live in his several subtle bodies as well as in his physical body, to be aware of them and in them, to use their senses, faculties, powers, to dwell in possession of supraphysical truth, consciousness and experience.

The sleep-state ascends to a higher power of being, beyond thought into pure consciousness, beyond emotion into pure bliss, beyond will into pure mastery; it is the gate of union with the supreme state of Sachchidananda out of which all the activities of the world are born. But here we must take care to avoid the pitfalls of symbolic language. The use of the words dream and sleep for these higher states is nothing but an image drawn from the experience of the normal physical mind with regard to planes in which it is not at home. It is not the truth that the Self in the third status called perfect sleep, *suṣupti*, is in a state of slumber. The sleep self is on the contrary described as Prajna, the Master of Wisdom and Knowledge, Self of the Gnosis, and as Ishwara, the Lord of being. To the physical mind a sleep, it is to our wider and subtler consciousness a greater waking. To the normal mind all that exceeds its normal experience but still comes into its scope, seems a dream; but at the point where it borders on things quite beyond its scope, it can no longer see truth even as in a dream, but passes into the blank incomprehension and non-reception of slumber. This border-line varies with the power of the individual consciousness, with the degree and height of its enlightenment and awakening. The line may be pushed up higher and higher until it may pass even beyond the mind. Normally indeed the human mind cannot be awake, even with the inner waking of trance, on the supramental levels; but this disability can be overcome. Awake on these levels the soul becomes master of the ranges of gnostic thought, gnostic will, gnostic delight, and if it can do this in Samadhi, it may carry its memory of experience and its power of experience over into the waking state. Even on the yet higher level open to us, that of the Ananda, the awakened soul may become similarly possessed of the Bliss-Self both in its concentration and in its cosmic comprehension. But still there may be ranges above from which it can bring back no memory except that which says, "somehow, indescribably, I was in bliss," the bliss of an unconditioned existence beyond all potentiality of expression by thought or description by image or feature. Even the sense of being may disappear in an experience in which the word existence loses its sense and the Buddhistic symbol of Nirvana seems alone and sovereignly justified. However high the power of awakening goes, there seems to be a beyond in which the image of sleep, of *suṣupti*, will still find its application.

Such is the principle of the Yogic trance, Samadhi, — into its complex phenomena we need not now enter. It is sufficient to note its double utility in the integral Yoga. It is true that up to a point difficult to define or delimit almost all that Samadhi can give, can be acquired without recourse to Samadhi. But still there are certain heights of spiritual and psychic experience of which the direct as opposed to a reflecting experience can only be acquired deeply and in its fullness by means of the Yogic trance. And even for that which can be otherwise acquired, it offers a ready means, a facility which becomes more helpful, if not indispensable, the higher and more difficult of access become the planes on which the heightened spiritual experience is sought. Once attained there, it has to be brought as much as possible into the waking consciousness. For in a Yoga which embraces all life completely and without reserve, the full use of Samadhi comes only when its gains can be made the normal possession and experience for an integral waking of the embodied soul in the human being.

Chapter XXVII

Hathayoga

THERE are almost as many ways of arriving at Samadhi as there are different paths of Yoga. Indeed so great is the importance attached to it, not only as a supreme means of arriving at the highest consciousness, but as the very condition and status of that highest consciousness itself, in which alone it can be completely possessed and enjoyed while we are in the body, that certain disciplines of Yoga look as if they were only ways of arriving at Samadhi. All Yoga is in its nature an attempt and an arriving at unity with the Supreme, — unity with the being of the Supreme, unity with the consciousness of the Supreme, unity with the bliss of the Supreme, — or, if we repudiate the idea of absolute unity, at least at some kind of union, even if it be only for the soul to live in one status and periphery of being with the Divine, *sālokya*, or in a sort of indivisible proximity, *sāmīpya*. This can only be gained by rising to a higher level and intensity of consciousness than our ordinary mentality possesses. Samadhi, as we have seen, offers itself as the natural status of such a higher level and greater intensity. It assumes naturally a great importance in the Yoga of knowledge, because there it is the very principle of its method and its object to raise the mental consciousness into a clarity and concentrated power by which it can become entirely aware of, lost in, identified with true being. But there are two great disciplines in which it becomes of an even greater importance. To these two systems, to Rajayoga and Hathayoga, we may as well now turn; for in spite of the wide difference of their methods from that of the path of knowledge, they have this same principle as their final justification. At the same time, it will not be necessary for us to do more than regard the spirit of their gradations in passing; for in a synthetic and integral Yoga they take a secondary importance; their aims have indeed to be included, but their methods can either altogether be dispensed with or used only for a preliminary or else a casual assistance.

Hathayoga is a powerful, but difficult and onerous system whose whole principle of action is founded on an intimate connection between the body and the soul. The body is the key, the body the secret both of bondage and of release, of animal weakness and of divine power, of the obscuration of the mind and soul and of their illumination, of subjection to pain and limitation and of self-mastery, of death and of immortality. The body is not to the Hathayogin a mere mass of living matter, but a mystic bridge between the spiritual and the physical being; one has even seen an ingenious exegete of the Hathayogic discipline explain the Vedantic symbol OM as a figure of this mystic human body. Although, however, he speaks always of the physical body and makes that the basis of his practices, he does not view it with the eye of the anatomist or physiologist, but describes and explains it in language which always looks back to the subtle body behind the physical system. In fact the whole aim of the Hathayogin may be summarised from our point of view, though he would not himself put it in that language, as an attempt by fixed scientific processes to give to the soul in the physical body the power, the light, the purity, the freedom, the ascending scales of spiritual experience which would naturally be open to it, if it dwelt here in the subtle and the developed causal vehicle.

To speak of the processes of Hathayoga as scientific may seem strange to those who associate the idea of science only with the superficial phenomena of the physical universe apart from all that is behind them; but they are equally based on definite experience of laws and their workings and give, when rightly practised, their well-tested results. In fact, Hathayoga is, in its own way, a system of knowledge; but while the proper Yoga of knowledge is a philosophy of being put into spiritual practice, a psychological system, this is a science of being, a psycho-physical system. Both produce physical, psychic and spiritual results; but because they stand at different poles of the same truth, to one the psycho-physical results are of small importance, the pure psychic and spiritual alone matter, and even the pure psychic are only accessories of the spiritual which absorb all the attention; in the other the physical is of immense importance, the psychical a considerable fruit, the spiritual the highest and consummating result, but it seems for a long time a thing postponed and remote, so great and absorbing is the attention which the body demands. It must not be forgotten, however, that both do arrive at the same end. Hathayoga, also, is a path, though by a long, difficult and meticulous movement, *duhkham āptum*, to the Supreme.

All Yoga proceeds in its method by three principles of practice; first, purification, that is to say, the removal of all aberrations, disorders, obstructions brought about by the mixed and irregular action of the energy of being in our physical, moral and mental system; secondly, concentration, that is to say, the bringing to its full intensity and the mastered and self-directed employment of that energy of being in us for a definite end; thirdly, liberation, that is to say, the release of our being from the narrow and painful knots of the individualised energy in a false and limited play, which at present are the law of our nature. The enjoyment of our liberated being which brings us into unity or union with the Supreme, is the consummation; it is that for which Yoga is done. Three indispensable steps and the high, open and infinite levels to which they mount; and in all its practice Hathayoga keeps these in view.

The two main members of its physical discipline, to which the others are mere accessories, are *āsana*, the habituating of the body to certain attitudes of immobility, and *prāṇāyāma*, the regulated direction and arrestation by exercises of breathing of the vital currents of energy in the body. The physical being is the instrument; but the physical being is made up of two elements, the physical and the vital, the body which is the apparent instrument and the basis, and the life energy, *prāṇa*, which is the power and the real instrument. Both of these instruments are now our masters. We are subject to the body, we are subject to the life energy; it is only in a very limited degree that we can, though souls, though mental beings, at all pose as their masters. We are bound by a poor and limited physical nature, we are bound consequently by a poor and limited life-power which is all that the body can bear or to which it can give scope. Moreover, the action of each and both in us is subject not only to the narrowest limitations, but to a constant impurity, which renews itself every time it is rectified, and to all sorts of disorders, some of which are normal, a violent order, part of our ordinary physical life, others abnormal, its maladies and disturbances. With all this Hathayoga has to deal; all this it has to overcome; and it does it mainly by these two methods, complex and cumbrous in action, but simple in principle and effective.

The Hathayogic system of Asana has at its basis two profound ideas which bring with them many effective implications. The first is that of control by physical immobility, the second is that of power by immobility. The power of physical immobility is as important in Hathayoga as the power of mental immobility in the Yoga of knowledge, and for parallel reasons. To the mind unaccustomed to the deeper truths of our being and nature they would both seem to be a seeking after the listless passivity of inertia. The direct contrary is the truth; for Yogic passivity, whether of mind or body, is a condition of the greatest increase, possession and continence of energy. The normal activity of our minds is for the most part a disordered restlessness, full of waste and rapidly tentative expenditure of energy in which only a little is selected for the workings of the self-mastering will, — waste, be it understood, from this point of view, not that of universal Nature in which what is to us waste, serves the purposes of her economy. The activity of our bodies is a similar restlessness.

It is the sign of a constant inability of the body to hold even the limited life energy that enters into or is generated in it, and consequently of a general dissipation of this Pranic force with a quite subordinate element of ordered and well-economised activity. Moreover in the consequent interchange and balancing between the movement and interaction of the vital energies normally at work in the body and their interchange with those which act upon it from outside, whether the energies of others or of the general Pranic force variously active in the environment, there is a constant precarious balancing and adjustment which may at any moment go wrong. Every obstruction, every defect, every excess,.every lesion creates impurities and disorders. Nature manages it all well enough for her own purposes, when left to herself; but the moment the blundering mind and will of the human being interfere with her habits and her vital instincts and intuitions, especially when they create false or artificial habits, a still more precarious order and frequent derangement become the rule of the being. Yet this interference is inevitable, since man lives not for the purposes of the vital Nature in him alone, but for higher purposes which she had not contemplated in her first balance and to which she has with difficulty to adjust her operations. Therefore the first necessity of a greater status or action is to get rid of this disordered restlessness, to still the activity and to regulate it. The Hathayogin has to bring about an abnormal poise of status and action of the body and the life energy, abnormal not in the direction of greater disorder, but of superiority and self-mastery.

The first object of the immobility of the Asana is to get rid of the restlessness imposed on the body and to force it to hold the Pranic energy instead of dissipating and squandering it. The experience in the practice of Asana is not that of a cessation and diminution of energy by inertia, but of a great increase, inpouring, circulation of force. The body, accustomed to work off superfluous energy by movement, is at first ill able to bear this increase and this retained inner action and betrays it by violent tremblings; afterwards it habituates itself and, when the Asana is conquered, then it finds as much ease in the posture, however originally difficult or unusual to it, as in its easiest attitudes sedentary or recumbent. It becomes increasingly capable of holding whatever amount of increased vital energy is brought to bear upon it without needing to spill it out in movement, and this increase is so enormous as to seem illimitable, so that the body of the perfected Hathayogin is capable of feats of endurance, force, unfatigued expenditure of energy of which the normal physical powers of man at their highest would be incapable. For it is not only able to hold and retain this energy, but to bear its possession of the physical system and its more complete movement through it. The life energy, thus occupying and operating in a powerful, unified movement on the tranquil and passive body, freed from the restless balancing between the continent power and the contained, becomes a much greater and more effective force. In fact, it seems then rather to contain and possess and use the body than to be contained, possessed and used by it, — just as the restless active mind seems to seize on and use irregularly and imperfectly whatever spiritual force comes into it, but the tranquillised mind is held, possessed and used by the spiritual force.

The body, thus liberated from itself, purified from many of its disorders and irregularities, becomes, partly by Asana, completely by combined Asana and Pranayama, a perfected instrument. It is freed from its ready liability to fatigue; it acquires an immense power of health; its tendencies of decay, age and death are arrested. The Hathayogin even at an age advanced beyond the ordinary span maintains the unimpaired vigour, health and youth of the life in the body; even the appearance of physical youth is sustained for a longer time. He has a much greater power of longevity, and from his point of view, the body being the instrument, it is a matter of no small importance to preserve it long and to keep it for all that time free from impairing deficiencies. It is to be observed, also, that there are an enormous variety of Asanas in Hathayoga, running in their fullness beyond the number of eighty, some of them of the most complicated and difficult character. This variety serves partly to increase the results already noted, as well as to give a greater freedom and flexibility to the use of the body, but it serves also to alter the relation of the physical energy in the body to the earth energy with which it is related. The lightening of the heavy hold of the latter, of which the overcoming of fatigue is the first sign and the phenomenon of *utthāpana* or partial levitation the last, is one result. The gross body begins to acquire something of the nature of the subtle body and to possess something of its relations with the life-energy; that becomes a greater force more powerfully felt and yet capable of a lighter and freer and more resolvable physical action, powers which culminate in the Hathayogic *siddhis* or extraordinary powers of *garimā*, *mahimā*, *aṇimā* and *laghimā*.

Moreover, the life ceases to be entirely dependent on the action of the physical organs and functionings, such as the heart-beats and the breathing. These can in the end be suspended without cessation of or lesion to the life.

All this, however, the result in its perfection of Asana and Pranayama, is only a basic physical power and freedom. The higher use of Hathayoga depends more intimately on Pranayama. Asana deals more directly with the more material part of the physical totality, though here too it needs the aid of the other; Pranayama, starting from the physical immobility and self-holding which is secured by Asana, deals more directly with the subtler vital parts, the nervous system. This is done by various regulations of the breathing, starting from equality of respiration and inspiration and extending to the most diverse rhythmic regulations of both with an interval of inholding of the breath. In the end the keeping in of the breath, which has first to be done with some effort, and even its cessation become as easy and seem as natural as the constant taking in and throwing out which is its normal action. But the first objects of the Pranayama are to purify the nervous system, to circulate the life-energy through all the nerves without obstruction, disorder or irregularity, and to acquire a complete control of its functionings, so that the mind and will of the soul inhabiting the body may be no longer subject to the body or life or their combined limitations. The power of these exercises of breathing to bring about a purified and unobstructed state of the nervous system is a known and well-established fact of our physiology. It helps also to clear the physical system, but is not entirely effective at first on all its canals and openings; therefore the Hathayogin uses supplementary physical methods for clearing them out regularly of all their accumulations. The combination of these with Asana, — particular Asanas have even an effect in destroying particular diseases, — and with Pranayama maintains perfectly the health of the body. But the principal gain is that by this purification the vital energy can be directed anywhere, to any part of the body and in any way or with any rhythm of its movement.

The mere function of breathing into and out of the lungs is

only the most sensible, outward and seizable movement of the Prana, the Breath of Life in our physical system. The Prana has according to Yogic science a fivefold movement pervading all the nervous system and the whole material body and determining all its functionings. The Hathayogin seizes on the outward movement of respiration as a sort of key which opens to him the control of all these five powers of the Prana. He becomes sensibly aware of their inner operations, mentally conscious of his whole physical life and action. He is able to direct the Prana through all the *nāḍīs* or nerve-channels of his system. He becomes aware of its action in the six *cakras* or ganglionic centres of the nervous system, and is able to open it up in each beyond its present limited, habitual and mechanical workings. He gets, in short, a perfect control of the life in the body in its most subtle nervous as well as in its grossest physical aspects, even over that in it which is at present involuntary and out of the reach of our observing consciousness and will. Thus a complete mastery of the body and the life and a free and effective use of them established upon a purification of their workings is founded as a basis for the higher aims of Hathayoga.

All this, however, is still a mere basis, the outward and inward physical conditions of the two instruments used by Hathayoga. There still remains the more important matter of the psychical and spiritual effects to which they can be turned. This depends on the connection between the body and the mind and spirit and between the gross and the subtle body on which the system of Hathayoga takes its stand. Here it comes into line with Rajayoga, and a point is reached at which a transition from the one to the other can be made.

Chapter XXVIII

Rajayoga

A S THE body and the Prana are the key of all the closed doors of the Yoga for the Hathayogin, so is the mind the key in Rajayoga. But since in both the dependence of the mind on the body and the Prana is admitted, in the Hathayoga totally, in the established system of Rajayoga partially, therefore in both systems the practice of Asana and Pranayama is included; but in the one they occupy the whole field, in the other each is limited only to one simple process and in their unison they are intended to serve only a limited and intermediate office. We can easily see how largely man, even though in his being an embodied soul, is in his earthly nature the physical and vital being and how, at first sight at least, his mental activities seem to depend almost entirely on his body and his nervous system. Modern Science and psychology have even held, for a time, this dependence to be in fact an identity; they have tried to establish that there is no such separate entity as mind or soul and that all mental operations are in reality physical functionings. Even otherwise, apart from this untenable hypothesis, the dependence is so exaggerated that it has been supposed to be an altogether binding condition, and any such thing as the control of the vital and bodily functionings by the mind or its power to detach itself from them has long been treated as an error, a morbid state of the mind or a hallucination. Therefore the dependence has remained absolute, and Science neither finds nor seeks for the real key of the dependence and therefore can discover for us no secret of release and mastery.

The psycho-physical science of Yoga does not make this mistake. It seeks for the key, finds it and is able to effect the release; for it takes account of the psychical or mental body behind of which the physical is a sort of reproduction in gross form, and is able to discover thereby secrets of the physical body which do not appear to a purely physical enquiry. This mental or psychical body, which the soul keeps even after death, has also a subtle pranic force in it corresponding to its own subtle nature and substance, — for wherever there is life of any kind, there must be the pranic energy and a substance in which it can work, — and this force is directed through a system of numerous channels, called *nāḍī*, — the subtle nervous organisation of the psychic body, — which are gathered up into six (or really seven) centres called technically lotuses or circles, *cakra*, and which rise in an ascending scale to the summit where there is the thousand-petalled lotus from which all the mental and vital energy flows. Each of these lotuses is the centre and the storing-house of its own particular system of psychological powers, energies and operations, — each system corresponding to a plane of our psychological existence, — and these flow out and return in the stream of the pranic energies as they course through the *nāḍīs*.

This arrangement of the psychic body is reproduced in the physical with the spinal column as a rod and the ganglionic centres as the chakras which rise up from the bottom of the column, where the lowest is attached, to the brain and find their summit in the *brahmarandhra* at the top of the skull. These chakras or lotuses, however, are in physical man closed or only partly open, with the consequence that only such powers and only so much of them are active in him as are sufficient for his ordinary physical life, and so much mind and soul only is at play as will accord with its need. This is the real reason, looked at from the mechanical point of view, why the embodied soul seems so dependent on the bodily and nervous life, — though the dependence is neither so complete nor so real as it seems. The whole energy of the soul is not at play in the physical body and life, the secret powers of mind are not awake in it, the bodily and nervous energies predominate. But all the while the supreme energy is there, asleep; it is said to be coiled up and slumbering like a snake, — therefore it is called the *kuṇḍalinī śakti*, — in the lowest of the chakras, in the *mūlādhāra*. When by Pranayama the division between the upper and lower prana currents in the body is dissolved, this Kundalini is struck and awakened, it uncoils itself and begins to rise upward like a fiery serpent breaking open each lotus as it ascends until the Shakti meets the Purusha in the *brahmarandhra* in a deep samadhi of union.

Put less symbolically, in more philosophical though perhaps less profound language, this means that the real energy of our being is lying asleep and inconscient in the depths of our vital system, and is awakened by the practice of Pranayama. In its expansion it opens up all the centres of our psychological being in which reside the powers and the consciousness of what would now be called perhaps our subliminal self; therefore as each centre of power and consciousness is opened up, we get access to successive psychological planes and are able to put ourselves in communication with the worlds or cosmic states of being which correspond to them; all the psychic powers abnormal to physical man, but natural to the soul develop in us. Finally, at the summit of the ascension, this arising and expanding energy meets with the superconscient self which sits concealed behind and above our physical and mental existence; this meeting leads to a profound samadhi of union in which our waking consciousness loses itself in the superconscient. Thus by the thorough and unremitting practice of Pranayama the Hathayogin attains in his own way the psychic and spiritual results which are pursued through more directly psychical and spiritual methods in other Yogas. The one mental aid which he conjoins with it, is the use of the mantra, sacred syllable, name or mystic formula which is of so much importance in the Indian systems of Yoga and common to them all. This secret of the power of the mantra, the six chakras and the Kundalini Shakti is one of the central truths of all that complex psycho-physical science and practice of which the Tantric philosophy claims to give us a rationale and the most complete compendium of methods. All religions and disciplines in India which use largely the psycho-physical method, depend more or less upon it for their practices.

Rajayoga also uses the Pranayama and for the same principal psychic purposes as the Hathayoga, but being in its whole principle a psychical system, it employs it only as one stage in the series of its practices and to a very limited extent, for three or four large utilities. It does not start with Asana and Pranayama, but insists first on a moral purification of the mentality. This preliminary is of supreme importance; without it the course of the rest of the Rajayoga is likely to be troubled, marred and full of unexpected mental, moral and physical perils.[1] This moral purification is divided in the established system under two heads, five *yamas* and five *niyamas*. The first are rules of moral self-control in conduct such as truth-speaking, abstinence from injury or killing, from theft etc.; but in reality these must be regarded as merely certain main indications of the general need of moral self-control and purity. *Yama* is, more largely, any self-discipline by which the rajasic egoism and its passions and desires in the human being are conquered and quieted into perfect cessation. The object is to create a moral calm, a void of the passions, and so prepare for the death of egoism in the rajasic human being. The *niyamas* are equally a discipline of the mind by regular practices of which the highest is meditation on the divine Being, and their object is to create a sattwic calm, purity and preparation for concentration upon which the secure pursuance of the rest of the Yoga can be founded.

It is here, when this foundation has been secured, that the practice of Asana and Pranayama come in and can then bear their perfect fruits. By itself the control of the mind and moral being only puts our normal consciousness into the right preliminary condition; it cannot bring about that evolution or manifestation of the higher psychic being which is necessary for the greater aims of Yoga. In order to bring about this manifestation the present nodus of the vital and physical body with the mental being has to be loosened and the way made clear for the ascent through the greater psychic being to the union with the superconscient Purusha. This can be done by Pranayama.

---

[1] In modern India people attracted to Yoga, but picking up its processes from books or from persons only slightly acquainted with the matter, often plunge straight into Pranayama of Rajayoga, frequently with disastrous results. Only the very strong in spirit can afford to make mistakes in this path.

Asana is used by the Rajayoga only in its easiest and most natural position, that naturally taken by the body when seated and gathered together, but with the back and head strictly erect and in a straight line, so that there may be no deflection of the spinal cord. The object of the latter rule is obviously connected with the theory of the six chakras and the circulation of the vital energy between the *mūlādhāra* and the *brahmarandhra*. The Rajayogic Pranayama purifies and clears the nervous system; it enables us to circulate the vital energy equally through the body and direct it also where we will according to need, and thus maintain a perfect health and soundness of the body and the vital being; it gives us control of all the five habitual operations of the vital energy in the system and at the same time breaks down the habitual divisions by which only the ordinary mechanical processes of the vitality are possible to the normal life. It opens entirely the six centres of the psycho-physical system and brings into the waking consciousness the power of the awakened Shakti and the light of the unveiled Purusha on each of the ascending planes. Coupled with the use of the mantra it brings the divine energy into the body and prepares for and facilitates that concentration in Samadhi which is the crown of the Rajayogic method.

Rajayogic concentration is divided into four stages; it commences with the drawing both of the mind and senses from outward things, proceeds to the holding of the one object of concentration to the exclusion of all other ideas and mental activities, then to the prolonged absorption of the mind in this object, finally, to the complete ingoing of the consciousness by which it is lost to all outward mental activity in the oneness of Samadhi. The real object of this mental discipline is to draw away the mind from the outward and the mental world into union with the divine Being. Therefore in the first three stages use has to be made of some mental means or support by which the mind, accustomed to run about from object to object, shall fix on one alone, and that one must be something which represents the idea of the Divine. It is usually a name or a form or a mantra by which the thought can be fixed in the sole knowledge or adoration of the Lord. By this concentration on the idea the mind enters from the idea into its reality, into which it sinks silent, absorbed, unified. This is the traditional method. There are, however, others which are equally of a Rajayogic character, since they use the mental and psychical being as key. Some of them are directed rather to the quiescence of the mind than to its immediate absorption, as the discipline by which the mind is simply watched and allowed to exhaust its habit of vagrant thought in a purposeless running from which it feels all sanction, purpose and interest withdrawn, and that, more strenuous and rapidly effective, by which all outward-going thought is excluded and the mind forced to sink into itself where in its absolute quietude it can only reflect the pure Being or pass away into its superconscient existence. The method differs, the object and the result are the same.

Here, it might be supposed, the whole action and aim of Rajayoga must end. For its action is the stilling of the waves of consciousness, its manifold activities, *cittavṛtti*, first, through a habitual replacing of the turbid rajasic activities by the quiet and luminous sattwic, then, by the stilling of all activities; and its object is to enter into silent communion of soul and unity with the Divine. As a matter of fact we find that the system of Rajayoga includes other objects, — such as the practice and use of occult powers, — some of which seem to be unconnected with and even inconsistent with its main purpose. These powers or siddhis are indeed frequently condemned as dangers and distractions which draw away the Yogin from his sole legitimate aim of divine union. On the way, therefore, it would naturally seem as if they ought to be avoided; and once the goal is reached, it would seem that they are then frivolous and superfluous. But Rajayoga is a psychic science and it includes the attainment of all the higher states of consciousness and their powers by which the mental being rises towards the superconscient as well as its ultimate and supreme possibility of union with the Highest. Moreover, the Yogin, while in the body, is not always mentally inactive and sunk in Samadhi, and an account of the powers and states which are possible to him on the higher planes of his being is necessary to the completeness of the science.

These powers and experiences belong, first, to the vital and mental planes above this physical in which we live, and are natural to the soul in the subtle body; as the dependence on the physical body decreases, these abnormal activities become possible and even manifest themselves without being sought for. They can be acquired and fixed by processes which the science gives, and their use then becomes subject to the will; or they can be allowed to develop of themselves and used only when they come, or when the Divine within moves us to use them; or else, even though thus naturally developing and acting, they may be rejected in a single-minded devotion to the one supreme goal of the Yoga. Secondly, there are fuller, greater powers belonging to the supramental planes which are the very powers of the Divine in his spiritual and supramentally ideative being. These cannot be acquired at all securely or integrally by personal effort, but can only come from above, or else can become natural to the man if and when he ascends beyond mind and lives in the spiritual being, power, consciousness and ideation. They then become, not abnormal and laboriously acquired siddhis, but simply the very nature and method of his action, if he still continues to be active in the world-existence.

On the whole, for an integral Yoga the special methods of Rajayoga and Hathayoga may be useful at times in certain stages of the progress, but are not indispensable. It is true that their principal aims must be included in the integrality of the Yoga; but they can be brought about by other means. For the methods of the integral Yoga must be mainly spiritual, and dependence on physical methods or fixed psychic or psycho-physical processes on a large scale would be the substitution of a lower for a higher action. We shall have occasion to touch upon this question later when we come to the final principle of synthesis in method to which our examination of the different Yogas is intended to lead.

THE SYNTHESIS OF YOGA

PARTS III and IV

Part III

The Yoga of Divine Love

Chapter I

Love and the Triple Path

WILL, KNOWLEDGE and love are the three divine powers in human nature and the life of man, and they point to the three paths by which the human soul rises to the divine. The integrality of them, the union of man with God in all the three, must therefore, as we have seen, be the foundation of an integral Yoga.

Action is the first power of life. Nature begins with force and its works which, once conscious in man, become will and its achievements; therefore it is that by turning his action God-wards the life of man best and most surely begins to become divine. It is the door of first access, the starting-point of the initiation. When the will in him is made one with the divine will and the whole action of the being proceeds from the Divine and is directed towards the Divine, the union in works is perfectly accomplished. But works fulfil themselves in knowledge; all the totality of works, says the Gita, finds its rounded culmination in knowledge, *sarvaṁ karmākhilaṁ jñāne parisamāpyate*. By union in will and works we become one in the omnipresent conscious being from whom all our will and works have their rise and draw their power and in whom they fulfil the round of their energies. And the crown of this union is love; for love is the delight of conscious union with the Being in whom we live, act and move, by whom we exist, for whom alone we learn in the end to act and to be. That is the trinity of our powers, the union of all three in God to which we arrive when we start from works as our way of access and our line of contact.

Knowledge is the foundation of a constant living in the Divine. For consciousness is the foundation of all living and being, and knowledge is the action of the consciousness, the light by which it knows itself and its realities, the power by which, starting from action, we are able to hold the inner results of thought and act in a firm growth of our conscious being until it accomplishes itself, by union, in the infinity of the divine being. The Divine meets us in many aspects and to each of them knowledge is the key, so that by knowledge we enter into and possess the infinite and divine in every way of his being, *sarvabhāvena*,[1] and receive him into us and are possessed by him in every way of ours.

Without knowledge we live blindly in him with the blindness of the power of Nature intent on its works, but forgetful of its source and possessor, undivinely therefore, deprived of the real, the full delight of our being. By knowledge arriving at conscious oneness with that which we know, — for by identity alone can complete and real knowledge exist, — the division is healed and the cause of all our limitation and discord and weakness and discontent is abolished. But knowledge is not complete without works; for the Will in being also is God and not the being or its self-aware silent existence alone, and if works find their culmination in knowledge, knowledge also finds its fulfilment in works. And, here too, love is the crown of knowledge; for love is the delight of union, and unity must be conscious of joy of union to find all the riches of its own delight. Perfect knowledge indeed leads to perfect love, integral knowledge to a rounded and multitudinous richness of love. "He who knows me" says the Gita "as the supreme Purusha," — not only as the immutable oneness, but in the many-souled movement of the divine and as that, superior to both, in which both are divinely held, — "he, because he has the integral knowledge, seeks me by love in every way of his being." This is the trinity of our powers, the union of all three in God to which we arrive when we start from knowledge.

Love is the crown of all being and its way of fulfilment, that by which it rises to all intensity and all fullness and the ecstasy of utter self-finding. For if the Being is in its very nature conscious-ness and by consciousness we become one with it, therefore by perfect knowledge of it fulfilled in identity, yet is delight the

[1] Gita.

nature of consciousness and of the acme of delight love is the key and the secret. And if will is the power of conscious being by which it fulfils itself and by union in will we become one with the Being in its characteristic infinite power, yet all the works of that power start from delight, live in the delight, have delight for their aim and end; love of the Being in itself and in all of itself that its power of consciousness manifests, is the way to the perfect wideness of the Ananda. Love is the power and passion of the divine self-delight and without love we may get the rapt peace of its infinity, the absorbed silence of the Ananda, but not its absolute depth of richness and fullness. Love leads us from the suffering of division into the bliss of perfect union, but without losing that joy of the act of union which is the soul's greatest discovery and for which the life of the cosmos is a long preparation. Therefore to approach God by love is to prepare oneself for the greatest possible spiritual fulfilment.

Love fulfilled does not exclude knowledge, but itself brings knowledge; and the completer the knowledge, the richer the possibility of love. "By Bhakti" says the Lord in the Gita "shall a man know Me in all my extent and greatness and as I am in the principles of my being, and when he has known Me in the principles of my being, then he enters into Me." Love without knowledge is a passionate and intense, but blind, crude, often dangerous thing, a great power, but also a stumbling-block; love, limited in knowledge, condemns itself in its fervour and often by its very fervour to narrowness; but love leading to perfect knowledge brings the infinite and absolute union. Such love is not inconsistent with, but rather throws itself with joy into divine works; for it loves God and is one with him in all his being, and therefore in all beings, and to work for the world is then to feel and fulfil multitudinously one's love for God. This is the trinity of our powers, the union of all three in God to which we arrive when we start on our journey by the path of devotion with Love for the Angel of the Way to find in the ecstasy of the divine delight of the All-Lover's being the fulfilment of ours, its secure home and blissful abiding-place and the centre of its universal radiation.

Since then in the union of these three powers lies our base of perfection, the seeker of an integral self-fulfilment in the Divine must avoid or throw away, if he has them at all, the misunderstanding and mutual depreciation which we often find existent between the followers of the three paths. Those who have the cult of knowledge seem often, if not to despise, yet to look downward from their dizzy eminence on the path of the devotee as if it were a thing inferior, ignorant, good only for souls that are not yet ready for the heights of the Truth. It is true that devotion without knowledge is often a thing raw, crude, blind and dangerous, as the errors, crimes, follies of the religious have too often shown. But this is because devotion in them has not found its own path, its own real principle, has not therefore really entered on the path, but is fumbling and feeling after it, is on one of the bypaths that lead to it; and knowledge too at this stage is as imperfect as devotion, dogmatic, schismatic, intolerant, bound up in the narrowness of some single and exclusive principle, even that being usually very imperfectly seized. When the devotee has grasped the power that shall raise him, has really laid hold on love, that in the end purifies and enlarges him as effectively as knowledge can; they are equal powers, though their methods of arriving at the same goal are different. The pride of the philosopher looking down on the passion of the devotee arises, as does all pride, from a certain deficiency of his nature; for the intellect too exclusively developed misses what the heart has to offer. The intellect is not in every way superior to the heart; if it opens more readily doors at which the heart is apt to fumble in vain, it is, itself, apt to miss truths which to the heart are very near and easy to hold. And if when the way of thought deepens into spiritual experience, it arrives readily at the etherial heights, pinnacles, skiey widenesses, it cannot without the aid of the heart fathom the intense and rich abysses and oceanic depths of the divine being and the divine Ananda.

The way of Bhakti is supposed often to be necessarily inferior because it proceeds by worship which belongs to that stage of spiritual experience where there is a difference, an insufficient unity between the human soul and the Divine, because its very principle is love and love means always two, the lover and the beloved, a dualism therefore, while oneness is the highest spiritual experience, and because it seeks after the personal God while the Impersonal is the highest and the eternal truth, if not even the sole Reality. But worship is only the first step on the path of devotion. Where external worship changes into the inner adoration, real Bhakti begins; that deepens into the intensity of divine love; that love leads to the joy of closeness in our relations with the Divine; the joy of closeness passes into the bliss of union. Love too as well as knowledge brings us to a highest oneness and it gives to that oneness its greatest possible depth and intensity. It is true that love returns gladly upon a difference in oneness, by which the oneness itself becomes richer and sweeter. But here we may say that the heart is wiser than the thought, at least than that thought which fixes upon opposite ideas of the Divine and concentrates on one to the exclusion of the other which seems its contrary, but is really its complement and a means of its greatest fulfilment. This is the weakness of the mind that it limits itself by its thoughts, its positive and negative ideas, the aspects of the Divine Reality that it sees, and tends too much to pit one against the other.

Thought in the mind, *vicāra*, the philosophic trend by which mental knowledge approaches the Divine, is apt to lend a greater importance to the abstract over the concrete, to that which is high and remote over that which is intimate and near. It finds a greater truth in the delight of the One in itself, a lesser truth or even a falsehood in the delight of the One in the Many and of the Many in the One, a greater truth in the impersonal and the Nirguna, a lesser truth or a falsehood in the personal and the Saguna. But the Divine is beyond our oppositions of ideas, beyond the logical contradictions we make between his aspects. He is not, we have seen, bound and restricted by exclusive unity; his oneness realises itself in infinite variation and to the joy of that love has the completest key, without therefore missing the joy of the unity. The highest knowledge and highest spiritual experience by knowledge find his oneness as perfect in his various relations with the Many as in his self-absorbed delight. If to thought the Impersonal seems the wider and higher truth, the Personal a narrower experience, the spirit finds both of them to be aspects of a Reality which figures itself in both, and if there is a knowledge of that Reality to which thought arrives by insistence on the infinite Impersonality, there is also a knowledge of it to which love arrives by insistence on the infinite Personality. The spiritual experience of each leads, if followed to the end, to the same ultimate Truth. By Bhakti as by knowledge, as the Gita tells us, we arrive at unity with the Purushottama, the Supreme who contains in himself the impersonal and numberless personalities, the qualitiless and infinite qualities, pure being, consciousness and delight and the endless play of their relations.

The devotee on the other hand tends to look down on the sawdust dryness of mere knowledge. And it is true that philosophy by itself without the rapture of spiritual experience is something as dry as it is clear and cannot give all the satisfaction we seek, that its spiritual experience even, when it has not left its supports of thought and shot up beyond the mind, lives too much in an abstract delight and that what it reaches, is not indeed the void it seems to the passion of the heart, but still has the limitations of the peaks. On the other hand, love itself is not complete without knowledge. The Gita distinguishes between three initial kinds of Bhakti, that which seeks refuge in the Divine from the sorrows of the world, *ārta*, that which, desiring, approaches the Divine as the giver of its good, *arthārthī*, and that which attracted by what it already loves, but does not yet know, yearns to know this divine Unknown, *jijñāsu*; but it gives the palm to the Bhakti that knows. Evidently the intensity of passion which says, "I do not understand, I love," and, loving, cares not to understand, is not love's last self-expression, but its first, nor is it its highest intensity. Rather as knowledge of the Divine grows, delight in the Divine and love of it must increase. Nor can mere rapture be secure without the foundation of knowledge; to live in what we love, gives that security, and to live in it means to be one with it in consciousness, and oneness of consciousness is the perfect condition of knowledge. Knowledge of the Divine gives to love of the Divine its firmest security, opens to it its own widest joy of experience, raises it to its highest pinnacles of outlook.

If the mutual misunderstandings of these two powers are an ignorance, no less so is the tendency of both to look down on the way of works as inferior to their own loftier pitch of spiritual achievement. There is an intensity of love, as there is an intensity of knowledge, to which works seem something outward and distracting. But works are only thus outward and distracting when we have not found oneness of will and consciousness with the Supreme. When once that is found, works become the very power of knowledge and the very outpouring of love. If knowledge is the very state of oneness and love its bliss, divine works are the living power of its light and sweetness. There is a movement of love, as in the aspiration of human love, to separate the lover and the loved in the enjoyment of their exclusive oneness away from the world and from all others, shut up in the nuptial chambers of the heart. That is perhaps an inevitable movement of this path. But still the widest love fulfilled in knowledge sees the world not as something other and hostile to this joy, but as the being of the Beloved and all creatures as his being, and in that vision divine works find their joy and their justification.

This is the knowledge in which an integral Yoga must live. We have to start Godward from the powers of the mind, the intellect, the will, the heart, and in the mind all is limited. Limitations, exclusiveness there can hardly fail to be at the beginning and for a long time on the way. But an integral Yoga will wear these more loosely than more exclusive ways of seeking, and it will sooner emerge from the mental necessity. It may commence with the way of love, as with the way of knowledge or of works; but where they meet, is the beginning of its joy of fulfilment. Love it cannot miss, even if it does not start from it; for love is the crown of works and the flowering of knowledge.

Chapter II

The Motives of Devotion

ALL RELIGION begins with the conception of some
Power or existence greater and higher than our limited
and mortal selves, a thought and act of worship done to
that Power, and an obedience offered to its will, its laws or its
demands. But Religion, in its beginnings, sets an immeasurable
gulf between the Power thus conceived, worshipped and obeyed
and the worshipper. Yoga in its culmination abolishes the gulf;
for Yoga is union. We arrive at union with it through knowledge;
for as our first obscure conceptions of it clarify, enlarge, deepen,
we come to recognise it as our own highest self, the origin and
sustainer of our being and that towards which it tends. We arrive
at union with it through works; for from simply obeying we
come to identify our will with its Will, since only in proportion
as it is identified with this Power that is its source and ideal, can
our will become perfect and divine. We arrive at union with it
also by worship; for the thought and act of a distant worship
develops into the necessity of close adoration and this into the
intimacy of love, and the consummation of love is union with
the Beloved. It is from this development of worship that the
Yoga of devotion starts and it is by this union with the Beloved
that it finds its highest point and consummation.

All our instincts and the movements of our being begin by
supporting themselves on the ordinary motives of our lower
human nature, — mixed and egoistic motives at first, but afterwards they purify and elevate themselves, they become an intense
and special need of our higher nature quite apart from the results
our actions bring with them; finally they exalt themselves into
a sort of categorical imperative of our being, and it is through
our obedience to this that we arrive at that supreme something
self-existent in us which was all the time drawing us towards it,
first by the lures of our egoistic nature, then by something much

higher, larger, more universal, until we are able to feel its own direct attraction which is the strongest and most imperative of all. In the transformation of ordinary religious worship into the Yoga of pure Bhakti we see this development from the motived and interested worship of popular religion into a principle of motiveless and self-existent love. This last is in fact the touchstone of the real Bhakti and shows whether we are really in the central way or are only upon one of the bypaths leading to it. We have to throw away the props of our weakness, the motives of the ego, the lures of our lower nature before we can deserve the divine union.

Faced with the sense of a Power or perhaps a number of Powers greater and higher than himself by whom his life in Nature is overshadowed, influenced, governed, man naturally applies to it or to them the first primitive feelings of the natural being among the difficulties, desires and dangers of that life, — fear and interest. The enormous part played by these motives in the evolution of the religious instinct, is undeniable, and in fact, man being what he is, it could hardly have been less; and even when religion has advanced fairly far on its road, we see these motives still surviving, active, playing a sufficiently large part, justified and appealed to by Religion herself in support of her claims on man. The fear of God, it is said, — or, it may be added for the sake of historical truth, the fear of the Gods, — is the beginning of religion, a half-truth upon which scientific research, trying to trace the evolution of religion, ordinarily in a critical and often a hostile rather than in a sympathetic spirit, has laid undue emphasis. But not the fear of God only, for man does not act, even most primitively, from fear alone, but from twin motives, fear and desire, fear of things unpleasant and maleficent and desire of things pleasant and beneficent, — therefore from fear and interest. Life to him is primarily and engrossingly, — until he learns to live more in his soul and only secondarily in the action and reaction of outward things, — a series of actions and results, things to be desired, pursued and gained by action and things to be dreaded and shunned, yet which may come upon him as a result of action. And it is not only by his own action but by that also of others and of Nature around him that these things come to him. As soon, then, as he comes to sense a Power behind all this which can influence or determine action and result, he conceives of it as a dispenser of boons and sufferings, able and under certain conditions willing to help him or hurt, save and destroy.

In the most primitive parts of his being he conceives of it as a thing of natural egoistic impulses like himself, beneficent when pleased, maleficent when offended; worship is then a means of propitiation by gifts and a supplication by prayer. He gets God on his side by praying to him and flattering him. With a more advanced mentality, he conceives of the action of life as reposing on a certain principle of divine justice, which he reads always according to his own ideas and character, as a sort of enlarged copy of his human justice; he conceives the idea of moral good and evil and looks upon suffering and calamity and all things unpleasant as a punishment for his sins and upon happiness and good fortune and all things pleasant as a reward of his virtue. God appears to him as a king, judge, legislator, executor of justice. But still regarding him as a sort of magnified Man, he imagines that as his own justice can be deflected by prayers and propitiation, so the divine justice can also be deflected by the same means. Justice is to him reward and punishment, and the justice of punishment can be modified by mercy to the suppliant, while rewards can be supplemented by special favours and kindness such as Power when pleased can always bestow on its adherents and worshippers. Moreover God like ourselves is capable of wrath and revenge, and wrath and revenge can be turned by gifts and supplication and atonement; he is capable too of partiality, and his partiality can be attracted by gifts, by prayer and by praise. Therefore instead of relying solely on the observation of the moral law, worship as prayer and propitiation is still continued.

Along with these motives there arises another development of personal feeling, first of the awe which one naturally feels for something vast, powerful and incalculable beyond our nature by a certain inscrutability in the springs and extent of its action, and of the veneration and adoration which one feels for that which is higher in its nature or its perfection than ourselves. For, even while preserving largely the idea of a God endowed with the qualities of human nature, there still grows up along with it, mixed up with it or superadded, the conception of an omniscience, an omnipotence and a mysterious perfection quite other than our nature. A confused mixture of all these motives, variously developed, often modified, subtilised or glossed over, is what constitutes nine tenths of popular religion; the other tenth is a suffusion of the rest by the percolation into it of nobler, more beautiful and profounder ideas of the Divine which minds of a greater spirituality have been able to bring into the more primitive religious concepts of mankind. The result is usually crude enough and a ready target for the shafts of scepticism and unbelief, — powers of the human mind which have their utility even for faith and religion, since they compel a religion to purify gradually what is crude or false in its conceptions. But what we have to see is how far in purifying and elevating the religious instinct of worship any of these earlier motives need to survive and enter into the Yoga of devotion which itself starts from worship. That depends on how far they correspond to any truth of the divine Being and its relations with the human soul; for we seek by Bhakti union with the Divine and true relation with it, with its truth and not with any mirage of our lower nature and of its egoistic impulses and ignorant conceptions.

The ground on which sceptical unbelief assails Religion, namely, that there is in fact no conscient Power or Being in the universe greater and higher than ourselves or in any way influencing or controlling our existence, is one which Yoga cannot accept, as that would contradict all spiritual experience and make Yoga itself impossible. Yoga is not a matter of theory or dogma, like philosophy or popular religion, but a matter of experience. Its experience is that of a conscient universal and supracosmic Being with whom it brings us into union, and this conscious experience of union with the Invisible, always renewable and verifiable, is as valid as our conscious experience of a physical world and of visible bodies with whose invisible minds we daily communicate. Yoga proceeds by conscious union, the conscious being is its instrument, and a conscious union with the Inconscient cannot be. It is true that it goes beyond the human consciousness and in Samadhi becomes superconscient, but this is not an annullation of our conscious being, it is only its self-exceeding, the going beyond its present level and normal limits.

So far, then, all Yogic experience is agreed. But Religion and the Yoga of Bhakti go farther; they attribute to this Being a Personality and human relations with the human being. In both the human being approaches the Divine by means of his humanity, with human emotions, as he would approach a fellow-being, but with more intense and exalted feelings; and not only so, but the Divine also responds in a manner answering to these emotions. In that possibility of response lies the whole question; for if the Divine is impersonal, featureless and relationless, no such response is possible and all human approach to it becomes an absurdity; we must rather dehumanise, depersonalise, annul ourselves in so far as we are human beings or any kind of beings; on no other conditions and by no other means can we approach it. Love, fear, prayer, praise, worship of an Impersonality which has no relation with us or with anything in the universe and no feature that our minds can lay hold of, are obviously an irrational foolishness. On such terms religion and devotion become out of the question. The Adwaitin in order to find a religious basis for his bare and sterile philosophy, has to admit the practical existence of God and the gods and to delude his mind with the language of Maya. Buddhism only became a popular religion when Buddha had taken the place of the supreme Deity as an object of worship.

Even if the Supreme be capable of relations with us but only of impersonal relations, religion is robbed of its human vitality and the Path of Devotion ceases to be effective or even possible. We may indeed apply our human emotions to it, but in a vague and imprecise fashion, with no hope of a human response: the only way in which it can respond to us, is by stilling our emotions and throwing upon us its own impersonal calm and immutable equality; and this is what in fact happens when we approach the pure impersonality of the Godhead. We can obey it as a Law, lift our souls to it in aspiration towards its tranquil being, grow into it by shedding from us our emotional nature; the human being in us is not satisfied, but it is quieted, balanced, stilled. But the Yoga of devotion, agreeing in this with Religion, insists on a closer and warmer worship than this impersonal aspiration. It aims at a divine fulfilment of the humanity in us as well as of the impersonal part of our being; it aims at a divine satisfaction of the emotional being of man. It demands of the Supreme acceptance of our love and a response in kind; as we delight in Him and seek Him, so it believes that He too delights in us and seeks us. Nor can this demand be condemned as irrational, for if the supreme and universal Being did not take any delight in us, it is not easy to see how we could have come into being or could remain in being, and if He does not at all draw us towards him, — a divine seeking of us, — there would seem to be no reason in Nature why we should turn from the round of our normal existence to seek Him.

Therefore that there may be at all any possibility of a Yoga of devotion, we must assume first that the supreme Existence is not an abstraction or a state of existence, but a conscious Being; secondly, that he meets us in the universe and is in some way immanent in it as well as its source, — otherwise, we should have to go out of cosmic life to meet him; thirdly, that he is capable of personal relations with us and must therefore be not incapable of personality; finally, that when we approach him by our human emotions, we receive a response in kind. This does not mean that the nature of the Divine is precisely the same as our human nature though upon a larger scale, or that it is that nature pure of certain perversions and God a magnified or else an ideal Man. God is not and cannot be an ego limited by his qualities as we are in our normal consciousness. But on the other hand our human consciousness must certainly originate and have been derived from the Divine; though the forms which it takes in us may and must be other than the divine because we are limited by ego, not universal, not superior to our nature, not greater than our qualities and their workings, as he is, still our human emotions and impulses must have behind them a Truth in him of which they are the limited and very often, therefore, the perverse or even the degraded forms. By approaching him through our emotional being we approach that Truth, it comes down to us to meet our emotions and lift them towards it; through it our emotional being is united with him.

Secondly, this supreme Being is also the universal Being and our relations with the universe are all means by which we are prepared for entering into relation with him. All the emotions with which we confront the action of the universal existence upon us, are really directed towards him, in ignorance at first, but it is by directing them in growing knowledge towards him that we enter into more intimate relations with him, and all that is false and ignorant in them will fall away as we draw nearer towards unity. To all of them he answers, taking us in the stage of progress in which we are; for if we met no kind of response or help to our imperfect approach, the more perfect relations could never be established. Even as men approach him, so he accepts them and responds too by the divine Love to their bhakti, *tathaiva bhajate.* Whatever form of being, whatever qualities they lend to him, through that form and those qualities he helps them to develop, encourages or governs their advance and in their straight way or their crooked draws them towards him. What they see of him is a truth, but a truth represented to them in the terms of their own being and consciousness, partially, distortedly, not in the terms of its own higher reality, not in the aspect which it assumes when we become aware of the complete Divinity. This is the justification of the cruder and more primitive elements of religion and also their sentence of transience and passing. They are justified because there is a truth of the Divine behind them and only so could that truth of the Divine be approached in that stage of the developing human consciousness and be helped forward; they are condemned, because to persist always in these crude conceptions and relations with the Divine is to miss that closer union towards which these crude beginnings are the first steps, however faltering.

All life, we have said, is a Yoga of Nature; here in this material world life is her reaching out from her first inconscience towards a return to union with the conscient Divine from whom she proceeded. In religion the mind of man, her accomplished instrument, becomes aware of her goal in him, responds to her aspiration. Even popular religion is a sort of ignorant Yoga of devotion. But it does not become what we specifically call Yoga until the motive becomes in a certain degree clairvoyant, until it sees that union is its object and that love is the principle of union, and until therefore it tries to realise love and lose its separative character in love. When that has been accomplished, then the Yoga has taken its decisive step and is sure of its fruition. Thus the motives of devotion have first to direct themselves engrossingly and predominantly towards the Divine, then to transform themselves so that they are rid of their more earthy elements and finally to take their stand in pure and perfect love. All those that cannot coexist with the perfect union of love, must eventually fall away, while only those that can form themselves into expressions of divine love and into means of enjoying divine love, can remain. For love is the one emotion in us which can be entirely motiveless and self-existent; love need have no other motive than love. For all our emotions arise either from the seeking after delight and the possession of it, or from the baffling of the search, or from the failure of the delight we have possessed or had thought to grasp; but love is that by which we can enter directly into possession of the self-existent delight of the divine Being. Divine love is indeed itself that possession and, as it were, the body of the Ananda.

These are the truths which condition our approach to this Yoga and our journey on this path. There are subsidiary questions which arise and trouble the intellect of man, but, though we may have yet to deal with them they are not essential. Yoga of Bhakti is a matter of the heart and not of the intellect. For even for the knowledge which comes on this way, we set out from the heart and not from the intelligence. The truth of the motives of the heart's devotion and their final arrival and in some sort their disappearance into the supreme and unique self-existent motive of love, is therefore all that initially and essentially concerns us. Such difficult questions there are as whether the Divine has an original supraphysical form or power of form from which all forms proceed or is eternally formless; all we need at present say is that the Divine does at least accept the various forms which the devotee gives to him and through them meets him in love, while the mixing of our spirits with his spirit is essential to the fruition of Bhakti. So too, certain religions and religious philosophies seek to bind down devotion by a conception of an eternal difference between the human soul and the Divine, without which they say love and devotion cannot exist, while that philosophy which considers that One alone exists, consigns love and devotion to a movement in the ignorance, necessary perhaps or at the least useful as a preparatory movement while yet the ignorance lasts, but impossible when all difference is abolished and therefore to be transcended and discarded. We may hold, however, the truth of the one existence in this sense that all in Nature is the Divine even though God be more than all in Nature, and love becomes then a movement by which the Divine in Nature and man takes possession of and enjoys the delight of the universal and the supreme Divine. In any case, love has necessarily a twofold fulfilment by its very nature, that by which the lover and the beloved enjoy their union in difference and all too that enhances the joy of various union, and that by which they throw themselves into each other and become one Self. That truth is quite sufficient to start with, for it is the very nature of love, and since love is the essential motive of this Yoga, as is the whole nature of love, so will be too the crown and fulfilment of the movement of the Yoga.

Chapter III

The Godward Emotions

THE PRINCIPLE of Yoga is to turn Godward all or any of the powers of the human consciousness so that through that activity of the being there may be contact, relation, union. In the Yoga of Bhakti it is the emotional nature that is made the instrument. Its main principle is to adopt some human relation between man and the Divine Being by which through the ever intenser flowing of the heart's emotions towards him the human soul may at last be wedded to and grow one with him in a passion of divine Love. It is not ultimately the pure peace of oneness or the power and desireless will of oneness, but the ecstatic joy of union which the devotee seeks by his Yoga. Every feeling that can make the heart ready for this ecstasy the Yoga admits; everything that detracts from it must increasingly drop away as the strong union of love becomes closer and more perfect.

All the feelings with which religion approaches the worship, service and love of God, the Yoga admits, if not as its final accompaniments, yet as preparatory movements of the emotional nature. But there is one feeling with which the Yoga, at least as practised in India, has very little dealing. In certain religions, in most perhaps, the idea of the fear of God plays a very large part, sometimes the largest, and the Godfearing man is the typical worshipper of these religions. The sentiment of fear is indeed perfectly consistent with devotion of a certain kind and up to a certain point; at its highest it rises into a worship of the divine Power, the divine Justice, divine Law, divine Righteousness, and ethical obedience, an awed reverence for the almighty Creator and Judge. Its motive is therefore ethico-religious and it belongs not so strictly to the devotee, but to the man of works moved by a devotion to the divine ordainer and judge of his works. It regards God as the King and does not approach too near the glory of his throne unless justified by righteousness or led there by a mediator who will turn away the divine wrath for sin. Even when it draws nearest, it keeps an awed distance between itself and the high object of its worship. It cannot embrace the Divine with all the fearless confidence of the child in his mother or of the lover in his beloved or with that intimate sense of oneness which perfect love brings with it.

The origin of this divine fear was crude enough in some of the primitive popular religions. It was the perception of powers in the world greater than man, obscure in their nature and workings, which seemed always ready to strike him down in his prosperity and to smite him for any actions which displeased them. Fear of the gods arose from man's ignorance of God and his ignorance of the laws that govern the world. It attributed to the higher powers caprice and human passion; it made them in the image of the great ones of the earth, capable of whim, tyranny, personal enmity, jealous of any greatness in man which might raise him above the littleness of terrestrial nature and bring him too near to the divine nature. With such notions no real devotion could arise, except that doubtful kind which the weaker may feel for the stronger whose protection he can buy by worship and gifts and propitiation and obedience to such laws as he may have laid upon those beneath him and may enforce by rewards and punishments, or else the submissive and prostrate reverence and adoration which one may feel for a greatness, glory, wisdom, sovereign power which is above the world and is the source or at any rate the regulator of all its laws and happenings.

A nearer approach to the beginnings of the way of devotion becomes possible when this element of divine Power disengages itself from these crudities and fixes on the idea of a divine ruler, creator of the world and master of the Law who governs the earth and heavens and is the guide and helper and saviour of his creatures. This larger and higher idea of the divine Being long kept many elements and still keeps some elements of the old crudity. The Jews who brought it forward most prominently and from whom it overspread a great part of the world, could believe in a God of righteousness who was exclusive, arbitrary, wrathful, jealous, often cruel and even wantonly sanguinary. Even now it is possible for some to believe in a Creator who has made heaven and hell, an eternal hell, the two poles of his creation, and has even according to some religions predestined the souls he has created not only to sin and punishment, but to an eternal damnation. But even apart from these extravagances of a childish religious belief, the idea of the almighty Judge, Legislator, King, is a crude and imperfect idea of the Divine, when taken by itself, because it takes an inferior and an external truth for the main truth and it tends to prevent a higher approach to a more intimate reality. It exaggerates the importance of the sense of sin and thereby prolongs and increases the soul's fear and self-distrust and weakness. It attaches the pursuit of virtue and the shunning of sin to the idea of rewards and punishment, though given in an after life, and makes them dependent on the lower motives of fear and interest instead of the higher spirit which should govern the ethical being. It makes hell and heaven and not the Divine himself the object of the human soul in its religious living. These crudities have served their turn in the slow education of the human mind, but they are of no utility to the Yogin who knows that whatever truth they may represent belongs rather to the external relations of the developing human soul with the external law of the universe than any intimate truth of the inner relations of the human soul with the Divine; but it is these which are the proper field of Yoga.

Still out of this conception there arise certain developments which bring us nearer to the threshold of the Yoga of devotion. First, there can emerge the idea of the Divine as the source and law and aim of our ethical being and from this there can come the knowledge of him as the highest Self to which our active nature aspires, the Will to which we have to assimilate our will, the eternal Right and Purity and Truth and Wisdom into harmony with which our nature has to grow and towards whose being our being is attracted. By this way we arrive at the Yoga of works, and this Yoga has a place for personal devotion to the Divine, for the divine Will appears as the Master of our works to whose voice we must listen, whose divine impulsion we must obey and whose work it is the sole business of our active life and will to do. Secondly, there emerges the idea of the divine Spirit, the father of all who extends his wings of benignant protection and love over all his creatures, and from that grows between the soul and the Divine the relation of father and child, a relation of love, and as a result the relation of brotherhood with our fellow-beings. These relations of the Divine into the calm pure light of whose nature we have to grow and the Master whom we approach through works and service, the Father who responds to the love of the soul that approaches him as the child, are admitted elements of the Yoga of devotion.

The moment we come well into these developments and their deeper spiritual meaning, the motive of the fear of God becomes otiose, superfluous and even impossible. It is of importance chiefly in the ethical field when the soul has not yet grown sufficiently to follow good for its own sake and needs an authority above it whose wrath or whose stern passionless judgment it can fear and found upon that fear its fidelity to virtue. When we grow into spirituality, this motive can no longer remain except by the lingering on of some confusion in the mind, some persistence of the old mentality. Moreover, the ethical aim in Yoga is different from that of the external idea of virtue. Ordinarily, ethics is regarded as a sort of machinery of right action, the act is everything and how to do the right act is the whole question and the whole trouble. But to the Yogin action is chiefly important not for its own sake, but rather as a means for the growth of the soul Godward. Therefore what Indian spiritual writings lay stress upon is not so much the quality of the action to be done as the quality of the soul from which the action flows, upon its truth, fearlessness, purity, love, compassion, benevolence, absence of the will to hurt, and upon the actions as their outflowings. The old western idea that human nature is intrinsically bad and virtue is a thing to be followed out in despite of our fallen nature to which it is contrary, is foreign to the Indian mentality trained from ancient times in the ideas of the Yogins. Our nature contains, as well as its passionate rajasic and its downward-tending tamasic quality, a purer sattwic element and it is the encouragement of this, its highest part, which is the business of ethics. By it we increase the divine nature, *daivī prakṛti*, which is present in us and get rid of the Titanic and demoniac elements. Not therefore the Hebraic righteousness of the Godfearing man, but the purity, love, beneficence, truth, fearlessness, harmlessness of the saint and the God-lover are the goal of the ethical growth according to this notion. And, speaking more largely, to grow into the divine nature is the consummation of the ethical being. This can be done best by realising God as the higher Self, the guiding and uplifting Will or the Master whom we love and serve. Not fear of him, but love of him and aspiration to the freedom and eternal purity of his being must be the motive.

Certainly, fear enters into the relations of the master and the servant and even of the father and the child, but only when they are on the human level, when control and subjection and punishment figure predominantly in them and love is obliged to efface itself more or less behind the mask of authority. The Divine even as the Master does not punish anybody, does not threaten, does not force obedience. It is the human soul that has freely to come to the Divine and offer itself to his overpowering force that he may seize and uplift it towards his own divine levels, and give it that joy of mastery of the finite nature by the Infinite and of service to the Highest by which there comes freedom from the ego and the lower nature. Love is the key of this relation, and this service, *dāsyam*, is in Indian Yoga the happy service of the divine Friend or the passionate service to the divine Beloved. The Master of the worlds who in the Gita demands of his servant, the bhakta, to be nothing more in life than his instrument, makes this claim as the friend, the guide, the higher Self, and describes himself as the Lord of all the worlds who is the friend of all creatures, *sarvalokamaheśvaraṁ suhṛdaṁ sarvabhūtānām*; the two relations in fact must go together and neither can be perfect without the other. So too it is not the fatherhood of God as the Creator who demands obedience because he is the maker of our being, but the fatherhood of love which leads us towards the closer soul-union of Yoga. Love is the real key in both, and perfect love is inconsistent with the admission of the motive of fear. Closeness of the human soul to the Divine is the object, and fear sets always a barrier and a distance; even awe and reverence for the divine Power are a sign of distance and division and they disappear in the intimacy of the union of love. Moreover, fear belongs to the lower nature, to the lower self, and in approaching the higher Self must be put aside before we can enter into its presence.

This relation of the divine fatherhood and the closer relation with the Divine as the Mother-Soul of the universe have their springs in another early religious motive. One type of the Bhakta, says the Gita, is the devotee who comes to the Divine as the giver of his wants, the giver of his good, the satisfier of the needs of his inner and his outer being. "I bring to my bhakta" says the Lord "his getting and his having of good, *yogakṣemaṁ vahāmyaham.*" The life of man is a life of wants and needs and therefore of desires, not only in his physical and vital, but in his mental and spiritual being. When he becomes conscious of a greater Power governing the world, he approaches it through prayer for the fulfilment of his needs, for help in his rough journey, for protection and aid in his struggle. Whatever crudities there may be in the ordinary religious approach to God by prayer, and there are many, especially that attitude which imagines the Divine as if capable of being propitiated, bribed, flattered into acquiescence or indulgence by praise, entreaty and gifts and has often little regard to the spirit in which he is approached, still this way of turning to the Divine is an essential movement of our religious being and reposes on a universal truth.

The efficacy of prayer is often doubted and prayer itself supposed to be a thing irrational and necessarily superfluous and ineffective. It is true that the universal will executes always its aim and cannot be deflected by egoistic propitiation and entreaty, it is true of the Transcendent who expresses himself in the universal order that being omniscient his larger knowledge must foresee the thing to be done and it does not need direction or stimulation by human thought and that the individual's desires are not and cannot be in any world-order the true determining factor. But neither is that order or the execution of the universal will altogether effected by mechanical Law, but by powers and forces of which for human life at least human will, aspiration and faith are not among the least important. Prayer is only a particular form given to that will, aspiration and faith. Its forms are very often crude and not only childlike, which is in itself no defect, but childish; but still it has a real power and significance. Its power and sense is to put the will, aspiration and faith of man into touch with the divine Will as that of a conscious Being with whom we can enter into conscious and living relations. For our will and aspiration can act either by our own strength and endeavour, which can no doubt be made a thing great and effective whether for lower or higher purposes, — and there are plenty of disciplines which put it forward as the one force to be used, — or it can act in dependence upon and with subordination to the divine or the universal Will. And this latter way again may either look upon that Will as responsive indeed to our aspiration, but almost mechanically, by a sort of law of energy, or at any rate quite impersonally, or else it may look upon it as responding consciously to the divine aspiration and faith of the human soul and consciously bringing to it the help, the guidance, the protection and fruition demanded, *yogakṣemaṁ vahāmyaham.*

Prayer helps to prepare this relation for us at first on the lower plane even while it is there consistent with much that is mere egoism and self-delusion; but afterwards we can draw towards the spiritual truth which is behind it. It is not then the giving of the thing asked for that matters, but the relation itself, the contact of man's life with God, the conscious interchange. In spiritual matters and in the seeking of spiritual gains, this conscious relation is a great power; it is a much greater power than our own entirely self-reliant struggle and effort and it brings a fuller spiritual growth and experience. Necessarily in the end prayer either ceases in the greater thing for which it prepared us, — in fact the form we call prayer is not itself essential so long as the faith, the will, the aspiration are there, — or remains only for the joy of the relation. Also its objects, the *artha* or interest it seeks to realise, become higher and higher until we reach the highest motiveless devotion, which is that of divine love pure and simple without any other demand or longing.

The relations which arise out of this attitude towards the Divine, are that of the divine Father and the Mother with the child and that of the divine Friend. To the Divine as these things the human soul comes for help, for protection, for guidance, for fruition, — or if knowledge be the aim, to the Guide, Teacher, Giver of light, for the Divine is the Sun of knowledge, — or it comes in pain and suffering for relief and solace and deliverance, it may be deliverance either from the suffering itself or from the world-existence which is the habitat of the suffering or from all its inner and real causes.[1] In these things we find there is a certain gradation. For the relation of fatherhood is always less close, intense, passionate, intimate, and therefore it is less resorted to in the Yoga which seeks for the closest union. That of the divine Friend is a thing sweeter and more intimate, admits of an equality and intimacy even in inequality and the beginning of mutual self-giving; at its closest when all idea of other giving and taking disappears, when this relation becomes motiveless except for the one sole all-sufficing motive of love, it turns into the free and happy relation of the playmate in the Lila of existence. But closer and more intimate still is the relation of the Mother and the child, and that therefore plays a very large part wherever the religious impulse is most richly fervent and springs most warmly from the heart of man. The soul goes to the Mother-Soul in all its desires and troubles and the divine Mother wishes that it should be so, so that she may pour out her heart of love. It turns to her too because of the self-existent nature of this love and because that points us to the home towards which we turn from our wanderings in the world and to the bosom in which we find our rest.

---

[1] These are three of the four classes of devotee which are recognised by the Gita, *ārta, arthārthī, jijñāsu,* the distressed, the seeker of personal objects and the seeker of God-knowledge.

But the highest and the greatest relation is that which starts from none of the ordinary religious motives, but is rather of the very essence of Yoga, springs from the very nature of love itself; it is the passion of the Lover and the Beloved. Wherever there is the desire of the soul for its utter union with God, this form of the divine yearning makes its way even into religions which seem to do without it and give it no place in their ordinary system. Here the one thing asked for is love, the one thing feared is the loss of love, the one sorrow is the sorrow of separation of love; for all other things either do not exist for the lover or come in only as incidents or as results and not as objects or conditions of love. All love is indeed in its nature self-existent because it springs from a secret oneness in being and a sense of that oneness or desire of oneness in the heart between souls that are yet able to conceive of themselves as different from each other and divided. Therefore all these other relations too can arrive at their self-existent motiveless joy of being for the sake of love alone. But still they start from and to the end they to some extent find a satisfaction of their play in other motives. But here the beginning is love and the end is love and the whole aim is love. There is indeed the desire of possession, but even this is overcome in the fullness of the self-existent love and the final demand of the Bhakta is simply that his bhakti may never cease nor diminish. He does not ask for heaven or for liberation from birth or for any other object, but only that his love may be eternal and absolute.

Love is a passion and it seeks for two things, eternity and intensity, and in the relation of the Lover and Beloved the seeking for eternity and for intensity is instinctive and self-born. Love is a seeking for mutual possession, and it is here that the demand for mutual possession becomes absolute. Passing beyond desire of possession which means a difference, it is a seeking for oneness, and it is here that the idea of oneness, of two souls merging into each other and becoming one finds the acme of its longing and the utterness of its satisfaction. Love, too, is a yearning for beauty, and it is here that the yearning is eternally satisfied in the vision and the touch and the joy of the All-beautiful. Love is a child and a seeker of Delight, and it is here that it finds the highest possible ecstasy both of the heart-consciousness and of every fibre of the being. Moreover, this relation is that which as between human being and human being demands the most and, even while reaching the greatest intensities, is still the least satisfied, because only in the Divine can it find its real and its utter satisfaction. Therefore it is here most that the turning of human emotion Godwards finds its full meaning and discovers all the truth of which love is the human symbol, all its essential instincts divinised, raised, satisfied in the bliss from which our life was born and towards which by oneness it returns in the Ananda of the divine existence where love is absolute, eternal and unalloyed.

Chapter IV

The Way of Devotion

BHAKTI in itself is as wide as the heart-yearning of the soul for the Divine and as simple and straightforward as love and desire going straight towards their object. It cannot therefore be fixed down to any systematic method, cannot found itself on a psychological science like the Rajayoga, or a psycho-physical like the Hathayoga, or start from a definite intellectual process like the ordinary method of the Jnanayoga. It may employ various means or supports, and man, having in him a tendency towards order, process and system, may try to methodise his resort to these auxiliaries: but to give an account of their variations one would have to review almost all man's numberless religions upon their side of inner approach to the Deity. Really, however, the more intimate yoga of Bhakti resolves itself simply into these four movements, the desire of the Soul when it turns towards God and the straining of its emotion towards him, the pain of love and the divine return of love, the delight of love possessed and the play of that delight, and the eternal enjoyment of the divine Lover which is the heart of celestial bliss. These are things that are at once too simple and too profound for methodising or for analysis. One can at best only say, here are these four successive elements, steps, if we may so call them, of the siddhi, and here are, largely, some of the means which it uses, and here again are some of the aspects and experiences of the sadhana of devotion. We need only trace broadly the general line they follow before we turn to consider how the way of devotion enters into a synthetic and integral Yoga, what place it takes there and how its principle affects the other principles of divine living.

All Yoga is a turning of the human mind and the human soul, not yet divine in realisation, but feeling the divine impulse and attraction in it, towards that by which it finds its greater being. Emotionally, the first form which this turning takes must be that of adoration. In ordinary religion this adoration wears the form of external worship and that again develops a most external form of ceremonial worship. This element is ordinarily necessary because the mass of men live in their physical minds, cannot realise anything except by the force of a physical symbol and cannot feel that they are living anything except by the force of a physical action. We might apply here the Tantric gradation of *sādhana*, which makes the way of the *paśu*, the herd, the animal or physical being, the lowest stage of its discipline, and say that the purely or predominantly ceremonial adoration is the first step of this lowest part of the way. It is evident that even real religion, — and Yoga is something more than religion, — only begins when this quite outward worship corresponds to something really felt within the mind, some genuine submission, awe or spiritual aspiration, to which it becomes an aid, an outward expression and also a sort of periodical or constant reminder helping to draw back the mind to it from the preoccupations of ordinary life. But so long as it is only an idea of the Godhead to which one renders reverence or homage, we have not yet got to the beginning of Yoga. The aim of Yoga being union, its beginning must always be a seeking after the Divine, a longing after some kind of touch, closeness or possession. When this comes on us, the adoration becomes always primarily an inner worship; we begin to make ourselves a temple of the Divine, our thoughts and feelings a constant prayer of aspiration and seeking, our whole life an external service and worship. It is as this change, this new soul-tendency grows, that the religion of the devotee becomes a Yoga, a growing contact and union. It does not follow that the outward worship will necessarily be dispensed with, but it will increasingly become only a physical expression or outflowing of the inner devotion and adoration, the wave of the soul throwing itself out in speech and symbolic act.

Adoration, before it turns into an element of the deeper Yoga of devotion, a petal of the flower of love, its homage and self-uplifting to its sun, must bring with it, if it is profound, an increasing consecration of the being to the Divine who is adored.

And one element of this consecration must be a self-purifying so as to become fit for the divine contact, or for the entrance of the Divine into the temple of our inner being, or for his self-revelation in the shrine of the heart. This purifying may be ethical in its character, but it will not be merely the moralist's seeking for the right and blameless action or even, when once we reach the stage of Yoga, an obedience to the law of God as revealed in formal religion; but it will be a throwing away, *katharsis*, of all that conflicts whether with the idea of the Divine in himself or of the Divine in ourselves. In the former case it becomes in habit of feeling and outer act an imitation of the Divine, in the latter a growing into his likeness in our nature. What inner adoration is to ceremonial worship, this growing into the divine likeness is to the outward ethical life. It culminates in a sort of liberation by likeness to the Divine,[1] a liberation from our lower nature and a change into the divine nature.

Consecration becomes in its fullness a devoting of all our being to the Divine; therefore also of all our thoughts and our works. Here the Yoga takes into itself the essential elements of the Yoga of works and the Yoga of knowledge, but in its own manner and with its own peculiar spirit. It is a sacrifice of life and works to the Divine, but a sacrifice of love more than a tuning of the will to the divine Will. The bhakta offers up his life and all that he is and all that he has and all that he does to the Divine. This surrender may take the ascetic form, as when he leaves the ordinary life of men and devotes his days solely to prayer and praise and worship or to ecstatic meditation, gives up his personal possessions and becomes the monk or the mendicant whose one and only possession is the Divine, gives up all actions in life except those only which help or belong to the communion with the Divine and communion with other devotees, or at most keeps the doing from the secure fortress of the ascetic life of those services to men which seem peculiarly the outflowing of the divine nature of love, compassion and good. But there is the wider self-consecration, proper to any integral Yoga, which,

---

[1] *sādṛśya-mukti.*

accepting the fullness of life and the world in its entirety as the play of the Divine, offers up the whole being into his possession; it is a holding of all one is and has as belonging to him only and not to ourselves and a doing of all works as an offering to him. By this comes the complete active consecration of both the inner and the outer life, the unmutilated self-giving.

There is also the consecration of the thoughts to the Divine. In its inception this is the attempt to fix the mind on the object of adoration, — for naturally the restless human mind is occupied with other objects and, even when it is directed upwards, constantly drawn away by the world, — so that in the end it habitually thinks of him and all else is only secondary and thought of only in relation to him. This is done often with the aid of a physical image or, more intimately and characteristically, of a mantra or a divine name through which the divine being is realised. There are supposed by those who systematise to be three stages of the seeking through the devotion of the mind, first, the constant hearing of the divine name, qualities and all that has been attached to them, secondly, the constant thinking on them or on the divine being or personality, thirdly, the settling and fixing of the mind on the object; and by this comes the full realisation. And by these, too, there comes when the accompanying feeling or the concentration is very intense, the Samadhi, the ecstatic trance in which the consciousness passes away from outer objects. But all this is really incidental; the one thing essential is the intense devotion of the thought in the mind to the object of adoration. Although it seems akin to the contemplation of the way of knowledge, it differs from that in its spirit. It is in its real nature not a still, but an ecstatic contemplation; it seeks not to pass into the being of the Divine, but to bring the Divine into ourselves and to lose ourselves in the deep ecstasy of his presence or of his possession; and its bliss is not the peace of unity, but the ecstasy of union. Here, too, there may be the separative self-consecration which ends in the giving up of all other thought of life for the possession of this ecstasy, eternal afterwards in planes beyond, or the comprehensive consecration in which all the thoughts are full of the Divine and even in the occupations of life every thought remembers him. As in the other Yogas, so in this, one comes to see the Divine everywhere and in all and to pour out the realisation of the Divine in all one's inner activities and outward actions. But all is supported here by the primary force of the emotional union: for it is by love that the entire self-consecration and the entire possession is accomplished, and thought and action become shapes and figures of the divine love which possesses the spirit and its members.

This is the ordinary movement by which what may be at first a vague adoration of some idea of the Divine takes on the hue and character and then, once entered into the path of Yoga, the inner reality and intense experience of divine love. But there is the more intimate Yoga which from the first consists in this love and attains only by the intensity of its longing without other process or method. All the rest comes, but it comes out of this, as leaf and flower out of the seed; other things are not the means of developing and fulfilling love, but the radiations of love already growing in the soul. This is the way that the soul follows when, while occupied perhaps with the normal human life, it has heard the flute of the Godhead behind the near screen of secret woodlands and no longer possesses itself, can have no satisfaction or rest till it has pursued and seized and possessed the divine fluteplayer. This is in essence the power of love itself in the heart and soul turning from earthly objects to the spiritual source of all beauty and delight. There live in this seeking all the sentiment and passion, all the moods and experiences of love concentrated on a supreme object of desire and intensified a hundredfold beyond the highest acme of intensity possible to a human love. There is the disturbance of the whole life, the illumination by an unseized vision, the unsatisfied yearning for a single object of the heart's desire, the intense impatience of all that distracts from the one preoccupation, the intense pain of the obstacles that stand in the way of possession, the perfect vision of all beauty and delight in a single form. And there are all the many moods of love, the joy of musing and absorption, the delight of the meeting and fulfilment and embrace, the pain of separation, the wrath of love, the tears of longing, the increased delight of reunion. The heart is the scene of this supreme idyll of the inner consciousness, but a heart which undergoes increasingly an intense spiritual change and becomes the radiantly unfolding lotus of the spirit. And as the intensity of its seeking is beyond the highest power of the normal human emotions, so also the delight and the final ecstasy are beyond the reach of the imagination and beyond expression by speech. For this is the delight of the Godhead that passes human understanding.

Indian bhakti has given to this divine love powerful forms, poetic symbols which are not in reality so much symbols as intimate expressions of truth which can find no other expression. It uses human relations and sees a divine person, not as mere figures, but because there are divine relations of supreme Delight and Beauty with the human soul of which human relations are the imperfect but still the real type, and because that Delight and Beauty are not abstractions or qualities of a quite impalpable metaphysical entity, but the very body and form of the supreme Being. It is a living Soul to which the soul of the bhakta yearns; for the source of all life is not an idea or a conception or a state of existence, but a real Being. Therefore in the possession of the divine Beloved all the life of the soul is satisfied and all the relations by which it finds and in which it expresses itself, are wholly fulfilled; therefore, too, by any and all of them can the Beloved be sought, though those which admit the greatest intensity, are always those by which he can be most intensely pursued and possessed with the profoundest ecstasy. He is sought within in the heart and therefore apart from all by an inward-gathered concentration of the being in the soul itself; but he is also seen and loved everywhere where he manifests his being. All the beauty and joy of existence is seen as his joy and beauty; he is embraced by the spirit in all beings; the ecstasy of love enjoyed pours itself out in a universal love; all existence becomes a radiation of its delight and even in its very appearances is transformed into something other than its outward appearance. The world itself is experienced as a play of the divine Delight, a Lila, and that in which the world loses itself is the heaven of beatitude of the eternal union.

Chapter V

The Divine Personality

ONE QUESTION rises immediately in a synthetic Yoga which must not only comprise but unify knowledge and devotion, the difficult and troubling question of the divine Personality. All the trend of modern thought has been towards the belittling of personality; it has seen behind the complex facts of existence only a great impersonal force, an obscure becoming, and that too works itself out through impersonal forces and impersonal laws, while personality presents itself only as a subsequent, subordinate, partial, transient phenomenon upon the face of this impersonal movement. Granting even to this Force a consciousness, that seems to be impersonal, indeterminate, void in essence of all but abstract qualities or energies; for everything else is only a result, a minor phenomenon. Ancient Indian thought starting from quite the other end of the scale arrived on most of its lines at the same generalisation. It conceived of an impersonal existence as the original and eternal truth; personality is only an illusion or at best a phenomenon of the mind.

On the other hand, the way of devotion is impossible if the personality of the Divine cannot be taken as a reality, a real reality and not a hypostasis of the illusion. There can be no love without a lover and beloved. If our personality is an illusion and the Personality to whom our adoration rises only a primary aspect of the illusion, and if we believe that, then love and adoration must at once be killed, or can only survive in the illogical passion of the heart denying by its strong beats of life the clear and dry truths of the reason. To love and adore a shadow of our minds or a bright cosmic phenomenon which vanishes from the eye of Truth, may be possible, but the way of salvation cannot be built upon a foundation of wilful self-deception. The bhakta indeed does not allow these doubts of the intellect to come in his way; he has the divinations of his heart, and these are to him sufficient. But the sadhaka of the integral Yoga has to know the eternal and ultimate Truth and not to persist to the end in the delight of a Shadow. If the impersonal is the sole enduring truth, then a firm synthesis is impossible. He can at most take the divine personality as a symbol, a powerful and effective fiction, but he will have in the end to overpass it and to abandon devotion for the sole pursuit of the ultimate knowledge. He will have to empty being of all its symbols, values, contents in order to arrive at the featureless Reality.

We have said, however, that personality and impersonality, as our minds understand them, are only aspects of the Divine and both are contained in his being; they are one thing which we see from two opposite sides and into which we enter by two gates. We have to see this more clearly in order to rid ourselves of any doubts with which the intellect may seek to afflict us as we follow the impulse of devotion and the intuition of love or to pursue us into the joy of the divine union. They fall away indeed from that joy, but if we are too heavily weighted with the philosophical mind, they may follow us almost up to its threshold. It is well therefore to discharge ourselves of them as early as may be by perceiving the limits of the intellect, the rational philosophic mind, in its peculiar way of approaching the truth and the limits even of the spiritual experience which sets out from the approach through the intellect, to see that it need not be the whole integrality of the highest and widest spiritual experience. Spiritual intuition is always a more luminous guide than the discriminating reason, and spiritual intuition addresses itself to us not only through the reason, but through the rest of our being as well, through the heart and the life also. The integral knowledge will then be that which takes account of all and unifies their diverse truths. The intellect itself will be more deeply satisfied if it does not confine itself to its own data, but accepts truth of the heart and the life also and gives to them their absolute spiritual value.

The nature of the philosophical intellect is to move among ideas and to give them a sort of abstract reality of their own apart from all their concrete representations which affect our life and personal consciousness. Its bent is to reduce these representations to their barest and most general terms and to subtilise even these if possible into some final abstraction. The pure intellectual direction travels away from life. In judging things it tries to get back from their effects on our personality and to arrive at whatever general and impersonal truth may be behind them; it is inclined to treat that kind of truth as the only real truth of being or at least as the one superior and permanent power of reality. Therefore it is bound by its own nature to end in its extremes at an absolute impersonality and an absolute abstraction. This is where the ancient philosophies ended. They reduced everything to three abstractions, existence, consciousness and bliss of being, and they tended to get rid of the two of these three which seemed dependent on the first and most abstract, and to throw all back into a pure featureless existence from which everything else had been discharged, all representations, all values, except the one infinite and timeless fact of being. But the intellect had still one farther possible step to take and it took it in Buddhistic philosophy. It found that even this final fact of existence was only a representation; it abstracted that also and got to an infinite zero which might be either a void or an eternal inexpressible.

The heart and life, as we know, have an exactly opposite law. They cannot live with abstractions; they can find their satisfaction only in things that are concrete or can be made seizable; whether physically, mentally or spiritually, their object is not something which they seek to discriminate and arrive at by intellectual abstraction; a living becoming of it or a conscious possession and joy of their object is what they seek. Nor is it the satisfaction of an abstract mind or impersonal existence to which they respond, but the joy and the activity of a being, a conscious Person in us, whether finite or infinite, to whom the delights and powers of his existence are a reality. Therefore when the heart and life turn towards the Highest and the Infinite, they arrive not at an abstract existence or non-existence, a Sat or else a Nirvana, but at an existent, a Sat Purusha, not merely at a consciousness, but at a conscious Being, a Chaitanya Purusha, not merely at a purely impersonal delight of the Is, but at an infinite I Am of bliss, an Anandamaya Purusha; nor can they immerge and lose his consciousness and bliss in featureless existence, but must insist on all three in one, for delight of existence is their highest power and without consciousness delight cannot be possessed. That is the sense of the supreme figure of the intensest Indian religion of love, Sri Krishna, the All-blissful and All-beautiful.

The intelligence can also follow this trend, but it ceases then to be the pure intellect; it calls in its power of imagination to its aid, it becomes the image-maker, the creator of symbols and values, a spiritual artist and poet. Therefore the severest intellectual philosophy admits the Saguna, the divine Person, only as the supreme cosmic symbol; go beyond it to reality and you will arrive, it says, at last to the Nirguna, the pure Impersonal. The rival philosophy asserts the superiority of the Saguna; that which is impersonal is, it will perhaps say, only the material, the stuff of his spiritual nature out of which he manifests the powers of his being, consciousness and bliss, all that expresses him; the impersonal is the apparent negative out of which he looses the temporal variations of his eternal positive of personality. There are evidently here two instincts, or, if we hesitate to apply that word to the intellect, two innate powers of our being which are dealing each in its own manner with the same Reality.

Both the ideas of the intellect, its discriminations, and the aspirations of the heart and life, their approximations, have behind them realities at which they are the means of arriving. Both are justified by spiritual experience; both arrive at the divine absolute of that which they are seeking. But still each tends, if too exclusively indulged, to be hampered by the limitations of its innate quality and its characteristic means. We see that in our earthly living, where the heart and life followed exclusively failed to lead to any luminous issue, while an exclusive intellectuality becomes either remote, abstract and impotent or a sterile critic or dry mechanist. Their sufficient harmony and just reconciliation is one of the great problems of our psychology and our action.

The reconciling power lies beyond in the intuition. But there is an intuition which serves the intellect and an intuition which serves the heart and the life, and if we follow either of these exclusively, we shall not get much farther than before; we shall only make more intimately real to us, but still separately, the things at which the other and less seeing powers are aiming. But the fact that it can lend itself impartially to all parts of our being, — for even the body has its intuitions, — shows that the intuition is not exclusive, but an integral truth-finder. We have to question the intuition of our whole being, not only separately in each part of it, nor in a sum of their findings, but beyond all these lower instruments, beyond even their first spiritual correspondents, by rising into the native home of the intuition which is the native home of the infinite and illimitable Truth, *ṛtasya sve dame*, where all existence discovers its unity. That is what the ancient Veda meant when it cried, "There is a firm truth hidden by truth (the eternal truth concealed by this other of which we have here these lower intuitions); there the ten hundred rays of light stand together; that is One." *Ṛtena ṛtam apihitaṁ dhruvaṁ . . . daśa śatā saha tasthus, tad ekam.*

The spiritual intuition lays hold always upon the reality; it is the luminous harbinger of spiritual realisation or else its illuminative light; it sees that which the other powers of our being are labouring to explore; it gets at the firm truth of the abstract representations of the intellect and the phenomenal representations of the heart and life, a truth which is itself neither remotely abstract nor outwardly concrete, but something else for which these are only two sides of its psychological manifestation to us. What the intuition of our integral being perceives, when its members no longer dispute among themselves but are illumined from above, is that the whole of our being aims at the one reality. The impersonal is a truth, the personal too is a truth; they are the same truth seen from two sides of our psychological activity; neither by itself gives the total account of the Reality, and yet by either we can approach it.

Looked at from one side, it would seem as if an impersonal Thought were at work and created the fiction of the thinker for the convenience of its action, an impersonal Power at work creating the fiction of the doer, an impersonal existence in operation which uses the fiction of a personal being who has a conscious personality and a personal delight. Looked at from the other side, it is the thinker who expresses himself in thoughts which without him could not exist and our general notion of thought symbolises simply the power of the nature of the thinker; the Ishwara expresses himself by will and power and force; the Existent extends himself in all the forms integral and partial, direct, inverse and perverse of his existence, consciousness and bliss, and our abstract general notion of these things is only an intellectual representation of the triple power of his nature of being. All impersonality seems in its turn to become a fiction and existence in its every movement and its every particle nothing but the life, the consciousness, the power, the delight of the one and yet innumerable Personality, the infinite Godhead, the self-aware and self-unfolding Purusha. Both views are true, except that the idea of fiction, which is borrowed from our own intellectual processes, has to be exiled and each must be given its proper validity. The integral seeker has to see in this light that he can reach one and the same Reality on both lines, either successively or simultaneously, as if on two connected wheels travelling on parallel lines, but parallel lines which in defiance of intellectual logic but in obedience to their own inner truth of unity do meet in infinity.

We have to look at the divine Personality from this standpoint. When we speak of personality, we mean by it at first something limited, external and separative, and our idea of a personal God assumes the same imperfect character. Our personality is to us at first a separate creature, a limited mind, body, character which we conceive of as the person we are, a fixed quantity; for although in reality it is always changing, yet there is a sufficient element of stability to give a kind of practical justification to this notion of fixedness. We conceive of God as such a person, only without body, a separate person different from all others with a mind and character limited by certain qualities. At first in our primitive conceptions his deity is a thing of much inconstancy, freak and caprice, an enlarged edition of our human character; but afterwards we conceive of the divine nature of personality as a quite fixed quantity and we attribute to it those qualities alone which we regard as divine and ideal, while all the others are eliminated. This limitation compels us to account for all the rest by attributing them to a Devil, or by lending to man an original creative capacity for all that we consider evil, or else, when we perceive that this will not quite do, by erecting a power which we call Nature and attributing to that all the lower quality and mass of action for which we do not wish to make the Divine responsible. At a higher pitch the attribution of mind and character to God becomes less anthropomorphic and we regard him as an infinite Spirit, but still a separate person, a spirit with certain fixed divine qualities as his attributes. So are conceived the ideas of the divine Personality, the personal God which vary so much in various religions.

All this may seem at first sight to be an original anthropomorphism terminating in an intellectual notion of the Deity which is very much at variance with the actualities of the world as we see it. It is not surprising that the philosophical and sceptical mind should have found little difficulty in destroying it all intellectually, whether in the direction of the denial of a personal God and the assertion of an impersonal Force or Becoming or in that of an impersonal Being or an ineffable denial of existence with all the rest as only symbols of Maya or phenomenal truths of the Time-consciousness. But these are only the personifications of monotheism. Polytheistic religions, less exalted perhaps, but wider and more sensitive in their response to cosmic life, have felt that all in the cosmos has a divine origin; therefore they conceived of the existence of many divine personalities with a vague sense of an indefinable Divine behind, whose relations with the personal gods were not very clearly conceived. And in their more exoteric forms these gods were crudely anthropomorphic; but where the inner sense of spiritual things became clearer, the various godheads assumed the appearance of personalities of the one Divine, — that is the declared point of view of the ancient Veda. This Divine might be a supreme

Being who manifests himself in various divine personalities or an impersonal existence which meets the human mind in these forms; or both views might be held simultaneously without any intellectual attempt to reconcile them, since both were felt to be true to spiritual experience.

If we subject these notions of the divine Personality to the discrimination of the intellect, we shall be inclined to reduce them, according to our bent, to fictions of the imagination or to psychological symbols, in any case, the response of our sensitive personality to something which is not this at all, but is purely impersonal. We may say that That is in reality the very opposite of our humanity and our personality and therefore in order to enter into relations with it we are impelled to set up these human fictions and these personal symbols so as to make it nearer to us. But we have to judge by spiritual experience, and in a total spiritual experience we shall find that these things are not fictions and symbols, but truths of divine being in their essence, however imperfect may have been our representations of them. Even our first idea of our own personality is not an absolute error, but only an incomplete and superficial view beset by many mental errors. Greater self-knowledge shows us that we are not fundamentally the particular formulation of form, powers, properties, qualities with a conscious I identifying itself with them, which we at first appear to be. That is only a temporary fact, though still a fact, of our partial being on the surface of our active consciousness. We find within an infinite being with the potentiality of all qualities, of infinite quality, *ananta-guna*, which can be combined in any number of possible ways, and each combination is a revelation of our being. For all this personality is the self-manifestation of a Person, that is to say of a being who is conscious of his manifestation.

But we see too that this being does not seem to be composed even of infinite quality, but has a status of his complex reality in which he seems to stand back from it and to become an indefinable conscious existence, *anirdeśyam*. Even consciousness seems to be drawn back and leave merely a timeless pure existence. And again even this pure self of our being seems at a certain pitch to deny its own reality, or to be a projection from a self-less[1] baseless unknowable, which we may conceive of either as a nameless somewhat, or as a Nihil. It is when we would fix upon this exclusively and forget all that it has withdrawn into itself that we speak of pure impersonality or the void Nihil as the highest truth. But a more integral vision shows us that it is the Person and the personality and all that it had manifested which has thus cast itself upward into its own unexpressed absolute. And if we carry up our heart as well as our reasoning mind to the Highest, we shall find that we can reach it through the absolute Person as well as through an absolute impersonality. But all this self-knowledge is only the type within ourselves of the corresponding truth of the Divine in his universality. There too we meet him in various forms of divine personality; in formulations of quality which variously express him to us in his nature; in infinite quality, the Ananta-guna; in the divine Person who expresses himself through infinite quality; in absolute impersonality, an absolute existence or an absolute non-existence, which is yet all the time the unexpressed Absolute of this divine Person, this conscious Being who manifests himself through us and through the universe.

Even on the cosmic plane we are constantly approaching the Divine on either of these sides. We may think, feel and say that God is Truth, Justice, Righteousness, Power, Love, Delight, Beauty; we may see him as a universal force or as a universal consciousness. But this is only the abstract way of experience. As we ourselves are not merely a number of qualities or powers or a psychological quantity, but a being, a person who so expresses his nature, so is the Divine a Person, a conscious Being who thus expresses his nature to us. And we can adore him through different forms of this nature, a God of righteousness, a God of love and mercy, a God of peace and purity; but it is evident that there are other things in the divine nature which we have put outside the form of personality in which we are thus worshipping him. The courage of an unflinching spiritual vision and experience

---

[1] *anātmyam anilayanam.* Taittiriya Upanishad.

can meet him also in more severe or in terrible forms. None of these are all the Divinity; yet these forms of his personality are real truths of himself in which he meets us and seems to deal with us, as if the rest had been put away behind him. He is each separately and all altogether. He is Vishnu, Krishna, Kali; he reveals himself to us in humanity as the Christ personality or the Buddha personality. When we look beyond our first exclusively concentrated vision, we see behind Vishnu all the personality of Shiva and behind Shiva all the personality of Vishnu. He is the Ananta-guna, infinite quality and the infinite divine Personality which manifests itself through it. Again he seems to withdraw into a pure spiritual impersonality or beyond all idea even of impersonal Self and to justify a spiritualised atheism or agnosticism; he becomes to the mind of man an indefinable, *anirdeśyam*. But out of this unknowable the conscious Being, the divine Person, who has manifested himself here, still speaks, "This too is I; even here beyond the view of mind, I am He, the Purushottama."

For beyond the divisions and contradictions of the intellect there is another light and there the vision of a truth reveals itself which we may thus try to express to ourselves intellectually. There all is one truth of all these truths; for there each is present and justified in all the rest. In that light our spiritual experience becomes united and integralised; no least hair's breadth of real division is left, no shade of superiority and inferiority remains between the seeking of the Impersonal and the adoration of the divine Personality, between the way of knowledge and the way of devotion.

Chapter VI

The Delight of the Divine

THIS THEN is the way of devotion and this its justification to the highest and the widest, the most integral knowledge, and we can now perceive what form and place it will take in an integral Yoga. Yoga is in essence the union of the soul with the immortal being and consciousness and delight of the Divine, effected through the human nature with a result of development into the divine nature of being, whatever that may be, so far as we can conceive it in mind and realise it in spiritual activity. Whatever we see of this Divine and fix our concentrated effort upon it, that we can become or grow into some kind of unity with it or at the lowest into tune and harmony with it. The old Upanishad put it trenchantly in its highest terms, "Whoever envisages it as the Existence becomes that existence and whoever envisages it as the Non-existence, becomes that non-existence;" so too it is with all else that we see of the Divine, — that, we may say, is at once the essential and the pragmatic truth of the Godhead. It is something beyond us which is indeed already within us, but which we as yet are not or are only initially in our human existence; but whatever of it we see, we can create or reveal in our conscious nature and being and can grow into it, and so to create or reveal in ourselves individually the Godhead and grow into its universality and transcendence is our spiritual destiny. Or if this seem too high for the weakness of our nature, then at least to approach, reflect and be in secure communion with it is a near and possible consummation.

The aim of this synthetic or integral Yoga which we are considering, is union with the being, consciousness and delight of the Divine through every part of our human nature separately or simultaneously, but all in the long end harmonised and unified, so that the whole may be transformed into a divine nature of being. Nothing less than this can satisfy the integral seer, because what he sees must be that which he strives to possess spiritually and, so far as may be, become. Not with the knower in him alone, nor with the will alone, nor with the heart alone, but with all these equally and also with the whole mental and vital being in him he aspires to the Godhead and labours to convert their nature into its divine equivalents. And since God meets us in many ways of his being and in all tempts us to him even while he seems to elude us, — and to see divine possibility and overcome its play of obstacles constitutes the whole mystery and greatness of human existence, — therefore in each of these ways at its highest or in the union of all, if we can find the key of their oneness, we shall aspire to track out and find and possess him. Since he withdraws into impersonality, we follow after his impersonal being and delight, but since he meets us also in our personality and through personal relations of the Divine with the human, that too we shall not deny ourselves; we shall admit both the play of the love and the delight and its ineffable union.

By knowledge we seek unity with the Divine in his conscious being: by works we seek also unity with the Divine in his conscious being, not statically, but dynamically, through conscious union with the divine Will; but by love we seek unity with him in all the delight of his being. For that reason the way of love, however narrow it may seem in some of its first movements, is in the end more imperatively all-embracing than any other motive of Yoga. The way of knowledge tends easily towards the impersonal and the absolute, may very soon become exclusive. It is true that it need not do so; since the conscious being of the Divine is universal and individual as well as transcendent and absolute, here too there may be and should be a tendency to integral realisation of unity and we can arrive by it at a spiritual oneness with God in man and God in the universe not less complete than any transcendent union. But still this is not quite imperative. For we may plead that there is a higher and a lower knowledge, a higher self-awareness and a lower self-awareness, and that here the apex of knowledge is to be pursued to the exclusion of the mass of knowledge, the way of exclusion preferred to the integral way. Or we may discover a theory of illusion to justify our rejection of all connection with our fellow-men and with the cosmic action. The way of works leads us to the Transcendent whose power of being manifests itself as a will in the world one in us and all, by identity with which we come, owing to the conditions of that identity, into union with him as the one self in all and as the universal self and Lord in the cosmos. And this might seem to impose a certain comprehensiveness in our realisation of the unity. But still this too is not quite imperative. For this motive also may lean towards an entire impersonality and, even if it leads to a continued participation in the activities of the universal Godhead, may be entirely detached and passive in its principle. It is only when delight intervenes that the motive of integral union becomes quite imperative.

This delight which is so entirely imperative, is the delight in the Divine for his own sake and for nothing else, for no cause or gain whatever beyond itself. It does not seek God for anything that he can give us or for any particular quality in him, but simply and purely because he is our self and our whole being and our all. It embraces the delight of the transcendence, not for the sake of transcendence, but because he is the transcendent; the delight of the universal, not for the sake of universality, but because he is the universal; the delight of the individual not for the sake of individual satisfaction, but because he is the individual. It goes behind all distinctions and appearances and makes no calculations of more or less in his being, but embraces him wherever he is and therefore everywhere, embraces him utterly in the seeming less as in the seeming more, in the apparent limitation as in the revelation of the illimitable; it has the intuition and the experience of his oneness and completeness everywhere. To seek after him for the sake of his absolute being alone is really to drive at our own individual gain, the gain of absolute peace. To possess him absolutely indeed is necessarily the aim of this delight in his being, but this comes when we possess him utterly and are utterly possessed by him and need be limited to no particular status or condition. To seek after him in some heaven of bliss is to seek him not for himself, but for the bliss of heaven; when we have all the true delight of his being, then heaven is within ourselves, and wherever he is and we are, there we have the joy of his kingdom. So too to seek him only in ourselves and for ourselves, is to limit both ourselves and our joy in him. The integral delight embraces him not only within our own individual being, but equally in all men and in all beings. And because in him we are one with all, it seeks him not only for ourselves, but for all our fellows. A perfect and complete delight in the Divine, perfect because pure and self-existent, complete because all-embracing as well as all-absorbing, is the meaning of the way of Bhakti for the seeker of the integral Yoga.

Once it is active in us, all other ways of Yoga convert themselves, as it were, to its law and find by it their own richest significance. This integral devotion of our being to God does not turn away from knowledge; the bhakta of this path is the God-lover who is also the God-knower, because by knowledge of his being comes the whole delight of his being; but it is in delight that knowledge fulfils itself, the knowledge of the transcendent in the delight of the Transcendent, the knowledge of the universal in the delight of the universal Godhead, the knowledge of the individual manifestation in the delight of God in the individual, the knowledge of the impersonal in the pure delight of his impersonal being, the knowledge of the personal in the full delight of his personality, the knowledge of his qualities and their play in the delight of the manifestation, the knowledge of the quality-less in the delight of his colourless existence and non-manifestation.

So too this God-lover will be the divine worker, not for the sake of works or for a self-regarding pleasure in action, but because in this way God expends the power of his being and in his powers and their signs we find him, because the divine Will in works is the outflowing of the Godhead in the delight of its power, of divine Being in the delight of divine Force. He will feel perfect joy in the works and acts of the Beloved, because in them too he finds the Beloved; he will himself do all works because through those works too the Lord of his being expresses his divine joy in him: when he works, he feels that he is expressing in act and power his oneness with that which he loves and adores;

he feels the rapture of the will which he obeys and with which all the force of his being is blissfully identified. So too, again, this God-lover will seek after perfection, because perfection is the nature of the Divine and the more he grows into perfection, the more he feels the Beloved manifest in his natural being. Or he will simply grow in perfection like the blossoming of a flower because the Divine is in him and the joy of the Divine, and as that joy expands in him, soul and mind and life too expand naturally into their godhead. At the same time, because he feels the Divine in all, perfect within every limiting appearance, he will not have the sorrow of his imperfection.

Nor will the seeking of the Divine through life and the meeting of him in all the activities of his being and of the universal being be absent from the scope of his worship. All Nature and all life will be to him at once a revelation and a fine trysting-place. Intellectual and aesthetic and dynamic activities, science and philosophy and life, thought and art and action will assume for him a diviner sanction and a greater meaning. He will seek them because of his clear sight of the Divine through them and because of the delight of the Divine in them. He will not be indeed attached to their appearances, for attachment is an obstacle to the Ananda; but because he possesses that pure, powerful and perfect Ananda which obtains everything but is dependent on nothing, and because he finds in them the ways and acts and signs, the becomings and the symbols and images of the Beloved, he draws from them a rapture which the normal mind that pursues them for themselves cannot attain or even dream. All this and more becomes part of the integral way and its consummation.

The general power of Delight is love and the special mould which the joy of love takes is the vision of beauty. The God-lover is the universal lover and he embraces the All-blissful and All-beautiful. When universal love has seized on his heart, it is the decisive sign that the Divine has taken possession of him; and when he has the vision of the All-beautiful everywhere and can feel at all times the bliss of his embrace, that is the decisive sign that he has taken possession of the Divine. Union is the consummation of love, but it is this mutual possession that gives it at once the acme and the largest reach of its intensity. It is the foundation of oneness in ecstasy.

Chapter VII

The Ananda Brahman

THE WAY of devotion in the integral synthetic Yoga will take the form of a seeking after the Divine through love and delight and a seizing with joy on all the ways of his being. It will find its acme in a perfect union of love and a perfect enjoyment of all the ways of the soul's intimacy with God. It may start from knowledge or it may start from works, but it will then turn knowledge into a joy of luminous union with the being of the Beloved and turn works into a joy of the active union of our being with the will and the power of being of the Beloved. Or it may start directly from love and delight; it will then take both these other things into itself and will develop them as part of the complete joy of oneness.

The beginning of the heart's attraction to the Divine may be impersonal, the touch of an impersonal joy in something universal or transcendent that has revealed itself directly or indirectly to our emotional or our aesthetic being or to our capacity of spiritual felicity. That which we thus grow aware of is the Ananda Brahman, the bliss existence. There is an adoration of an impersonal Delight and Beauty, of a pure and an infinite perfection to which we can give no name or form, a moved attraction of the soul to some ideal and infinite Presence, Power, existence in the world or beyond it, which in some way becomes psychologically or spiritually sensible to us and then more and more intimate and real. That is the call, the touch of the bliss existence upon us. Then to have always the joy and nearness of its presence, to know what it is, so as to satisfy the intellect and the intuitional mind of its constant reality, to put our passive and, so far as we can manage it, our active, our inner immortal and even our outer mortal being into perfect harmony with it, grow into a necessity of our living. And to open ourselves to it is what we feel to be the one true happiness, to live into it the sole real perfection.

A transcendent Bliss, unimaginable and inexpressible by the mind and speech, is the nature of the Ineffable. That broods immanent and secret in the whole universe and in everything in the universe. Its presence is described as a secret ether of the bliss of being, of which the Scripture says that, if this were not, none could for a moment breathe or live. And this spiritual bliss is here also in our hearts. It is hidden in from the toil of the surface mind which catches only at weak and flawed translations of it into various mental, vital and physical forms of the joy of existence. But if the mind has once grown sufficiently subtle and pure in its receptions and not limited by the grosser nature of our outward responses to existence, we can take a reflection of it which will wear perhaps wholly or predominantly the hue of whatever is strongest in our nature. It may present itself first as a yearning for some universal Beauty which we feel in Nature and man and in all that is around us; or we may have the intuition of some transcendent Beauty of which all apparent beauty here is only a symbol. That is how it may come to those in whom the aesthetic being is developed and insistent and the instincts which, when they find form of expression, make the poet and artist, are predominant. Or it may be the sense of a divine spirit of love or else a helpful and compassionate infinite Presence in the universe or behind or beyond it which responds to us when we turn the need of our spirit towards it. So it may first show itself when the emotional being is intensely developed. It may come near to us in other ways, but always as a Power or Presence of delight, beauty, love or peace which touches the mind, but is beyond the forms these things take ordinarily in the mind.

For all joy, beauty, love, peace, delight are outflowings from the Ananda Brahman, — all delight of the spirit, the intellect, the imagination, aesthetic sense, ethical aspiration and satisfaction, action, life, the body. And through all ways of our being the Divine can touch us and make use of them to awaken and liberate the spirit. But to reach the Ananda Brahman in itself the mental reception of it must be subtilised, spiritualised, universalised, discharged of everything that is turbid and limiting. For when we draw quite near or enter into it, it is by an awakened spiritual sense of a transcendent and a universal Delight which exists within and yet behind and beyond the contradictions of the world and to which we can unite ourselves through a growing universal and spiritual or a transcendental ecstasy.

Ordinarily, the mind is satisfied with reflecting this Infinity we perceive or with feeling the sense of it within and without us, as an experience which, however frequent, yet remains exceptional. It seems in itself so satisfying and wonderful when it comes and our ordinary mind and the active life which we have to lead may seem to us so incompatible with it, that we may think it excessive to expect anything more. But the very spirit of Yoga is this, to make the exceptional normal, and to turn that which is above us and greater than our normal selves into our own constant consciousness. Therefore we should not hesitate to open ourselves more steadily to whatever experience of the Infinite we have, to purify and intensify it, to make it our object of constant thought and contemplation, till it becomes the originating power that acts in us, the Godhead we adore and embrace, our whole being is put into tune with it and it is made the very self of our being.

Our experience of it has to be purified of any mental alloy in it, otherwise it departs, we cannot hold it. And part of this purification is that it shall cease to be dependent on any cause or exciting condition of mind; it must become its own cause and self-existent, source of all other delight, which will exist only by it, and not attached to any cosmic or other image or symbol through which we first came into contact with it. Our experience of it has to be constantly intensified and made more concentrated; otherwise we shall only reflect it in the mirror of the imperfect mind and not reach that point of uplifting and transfiguration by which we are carried beyond the mind into the ineffable bliss. Object of our constant thought and contemplation, it will turn all that is into itself, reveal itself as the universal Ananda Brahman and make all existence its outpouring. If we wait upon it for the inspiration of all our inner and our outer acts, it will become the joy of the Divine pouring itself through us in light and love and power on life and all that lives. Sought by the adoration and love of the soul, it reveals itself as the Godhead, we see in it the face of God and know the bliss of our Lover. Tuning our whole being to it, we grow into a happy perfection of likeness to it, a human rendering of the divine nature. And when it becomes in every way the self of our self, we are fulfilled in being and we bear the plenitude.

Brahman always reveals himself to us in three ways, within ourselves, above our plane, around us in the universe. Within us, there are two centres of the Purusha, the inner Soul through which he touches us to our awakening; there is the Purusha in the lotus of the heart which opens upward all our powers and the Purusha in the thousand-petalled lotus whence descend through the thought and will, opening the third eye in us, the lightnings of vision and the fire of the divine energy. The bliss existence may come to us through either one of these centres. When the lotus of the heart breaks open, we feel a divine joy, love and peace expanding in us like a flower of light which irradiates the whole being. They can then unite themselves with their secret source, the Divine in our hearts, and adore him as in a temple; they can flow upwards to take possession of the thought and the will and break out upward towards the Transcendent; they stream out in thought and feeling and act towards all that is around us. But so long as our normal being offers any obstacle or is not wholly moulded into a response to this divine influence or an instrument of this divine possession, the experience will be intermittent and we may fall back constantly into our old mortal heart; but by repetition, *abhyāsa*, or by the force of our desire and adoration of the Divine, it will be progressively remoulded until this abnormal experience becomes our natural consciousness.

When the other upper lotus opens, the whole mind becomes full of a divine light, joy and power, behind which is the Divine, the Lord of our being on his throne with our soul beside him or drawn inward into his rays; all the thought and will become then a luminosity, power and ecstasy; in communication with the Transcendent, this can pour down towards our mortal members and flow by them outwards on the world. In this dawn too there are, as the Vedic mystics knew, our alternations of its day and night, our exiles from the light; but as we grow in the power to hold this new existence, we become able to look long on the sun from which this irradiation proceeds and in our inner being we can grow one body with it. Sometimes the rapidity of this change depends on the strength of our longing for the Divine thus revealed, and on the intensity of our force of seeking; but at others it proceeds rather by a passive surrender to the rhythms of his all-wise working which acts always by its own at first inscrutable method. But the latter becomes the foundation when our love and trust are complete and our whole being lies in the clasp of a Power that is perfect love and wisdom.

The Divine reveals himself in the world around us when we look upon that with a spiritual desire of delight that seeks him in all things. There is often a sudden opening by which the veil of forms is itself turned into a revelation. A universal spiritual Presence, a universal peace, a universal infinite Delight has manifested, immanent, embracing, all-penetrating. This Presence by our love of it, our delight in it, our constant thought of it returns and grows upon us; it becomes the thing that we see and all else is only its habitation, form and symbol. Even all that is most outward, the body, the form, the sound, whatever our senses seize, are seen as this Presence; they cease to be physical and are changed into a substance of spirit. This transformation means a transformation of our own inner consciousness; we are taken by the surrounding Presence into itself and we become part of it. Our own mind, life, body become to us only its habitation and temple, a form of its working and an instrument of its self-expression. All is only soul and body of this delight.

This is the Divine seen around us and on our own physical plane. But he may reveal himself above. We see or feel him as a high-uplifted Presence, a great infinite of Ananda above us, — or in it, our Father in heaven, — and do not feel or see him in ourselves or around us. So long as we keep this vision, the mortality in us is quelled by that Immortality; it feels the light, power and joy and responds to it according to its capacity; or it feels the descent of the spirit and it is then for a time transformed or else uplifted into some lustre of reflection of the light and power; it becomes a vessel of the Ananda. But at other times it lapses into the old mortality and exists or works dully or pettily in the ruck of its earthly habits. The complete redemption comes by the descent of the divine Power into the human mind and body and the remoulding of their inner life into the divine image, — what the Vedic seers called the birth of the Son by the sacrifice. It is in fact by a continual sacrifice or offering, a sacrifice of adoration and aspiration, of works, of thought and knowledge, of the mounting flame of the Godward will that we build ourselves into the being of this Infinite.

When we possess firmly this consciousness of the Ananda Brahman in all of these three manifestations, above, within, around, we have the full oneness of it and embrace all existences in its delight, peace, joy and love; then all the worlds become the body of this self. But we have not the richest knowledge of this Ananda if it is only an impersonal presence, largeness or immanence that we feel, if our adoration has not been intimate enough for this Being to reveal to us out of its wide-extended joy the face and body and make us feel the hands of the Friend and Lover. Its impersonality is the blissful greatness of the Brahman, but from that can look out upon us the sweetness and intimate control of the divine Personality. For Ananda is the presence of the Self and Master of our being and the stream of its outflowing can be the pure joy of his Lila.

Chapter VIII

The Mystery of Love

THE ADORATION of the impersonal Divine would not be strictly a Yoga of devotion according to the current interpretation; for in the current forms of Yoga it is supposed that the Impersonal can only be sought for a complete unity in which God and our own person disappear and there is none to adore or to be adored; only the delight of the experience of oneness and infinity remains. But in truth the miracles of spiritual consciousness are not to be subjected to so rigid a logic. When we first come to feel the presence of the infinite, as it is the finite personality in us which is touched by it, that may well answer to the touch and call with a sort of adoration. Secondly, we may regard the Infinite not so much as a spiritual status of oneness and bliss, or that only as its mould and medium of being, but rather as the presence of the ineffable Godhead to our consciousness, and then too love and adoration find their place. And even when our personality seems to disappear into unity with it, it may still be — and really is — the individual divine who is melting to the universal or the supreme by a union in which love and lover and loved are forgotten in a fusing experience of ecstasy, but are still there latent in the oneness and subconsciently persisting in it. All union of the self by love must necessarily be of this nature. We may even say, in a sense, that it is to have this joy of union as the ultimate crown of all the varied experiences of spiritual relation between the individual soul and God that the One became many in the universe.

Still, the more varied and most intimate experience of divine love cannot come by the pursuit of the impersonal Infinite alone; for that the Godhead we adore must become near and personal to us. It is possible for the Impersonal to reveal within itself all the riches of personality when we get into its heart, and one who sought only to enter into or to embrace the infinite Presence alone, may discover in it things he had not dreamed of; the being of the Divine has surprises for us which confound the ideas of the limiting intellect. But ordinarily the way of devotion begins from the other end; it starts from and it rises and widens to its issue by adoration of the divine Personality. The Divine is a Being and not an abstract existence or a status of pure timeless infinity; the original and universal existence is He, but that existence is inseparable from consciousness and bliss of being, and an existence conscious of its own being and its own bliss is what we may well call a divine infinite Person, — Purusha. Moreover all consciousness implies power, Shakti; where there is infinite consciousness of being, there is infinite power of being, and by that power all exists in the universe. All beings exist by this Being; all things are the faces of God; all thought and action and feeling and love proceed from him and return to him, all their results have him for source and support and secret goal. It is to this Godhead, this Being that the Bhakti of an integral Yoga will be poured out and uplifted. Transcendent, it will seek him in the ecstasy of an absolute union; universal, it will seek him in infinite quality and every aspect and in all beings with a universal delight and love; individual, it will enter into all human relations with him that love creates between person and person.

It may not be possible to seize from the beginning on all the complete integrality of that which the heart is seeking; in fact, it is only possible if the intelligence, the temperament, the emotional mind have already been developed into largeness and fineness by the trend of our previous living. That is what the experience of the normal life is meant to lead to by its widening culture of the intellect, the aesthetic and emotional mind and of our parts too of will and active experience. It widens and refines the normal being so that it may open easily to all the truth of That which was preparing it for the temple of its self-manifestation. Ordinarily, man is limited in all these parts of his being and he can grasp at first only so much of the divine truth as has some large correspondence to his own nature and its past development and associations. Therefore God meets us first in different limited affirmations of his divine qualities and nature; he presents himself to the seeker as an absolute of the things he can understand and to which his will and heart can respond; he discloses some name and aspect of his Godhead. This is what is called in Yoga the *iṣṭa-devatā*, the name and form elected by our nature for its worship. In order that the human being may embrace this Godhead with every part of himself, it is represented with a form that answers to its aspects and qualities and which becomes the living body of God to the adorer. These are those forms of Vishnu, Shiva, Krishna, Kali, Durga, Christ, Buddha, which the mind of man seizes on for adoration. Even the monotheist who worships a formless Godhead, yet gives to him some form of quality, some mental form or form of Nature by which he envisages and approaches him. But to be able to see a living form, a mental body, as it were, of the Divine gives to the approach a greater closeness and sweetness.

The way of the integral Yoga of bhakti will be to universalise this conception of the Deity, to personalise him intimately by a multiple and an all-embracing relation, to make him constantly present to all the being and to devote, give up, surrender the whole being to him, so that he shall dwell near to us and in us and we with him and in him. *Manana* and *darśana*, a constant thinking of him in all things and seeing of him always and everywhere is essential to this way of devotion. When we look on the things of physical Nature, in them we have to see the divine object of our love; when we look upon men and beings, we have to see him in them and in our relation with them to see that we are entering into relations with forms of him; when breaking beyond the limitation of the material world we know or have relations with the beings of other planes, still the same thought and vision has to be made real to our minds. The normal habit of our minds which are open only to the material and apparent form and the ordinary mutilated relation and ignore the secret Godhead within, has to yield by an unceasing habit of all-embracing love and delight to this deeper and ampler comprehension and this greater relation. In all godheads we have to see this one God whom we worship with our heart and all our being; they are forms of his divinity. So enlarging our spiritual embrace we reach a point at which all is he and the delight of this consciousness becomes to us our normal uninterrupted way of looking at the world. That brings us the outward or objective universality of our union with him.

Inwardly, the image of the Beloved has to become visible to the eye within, dwelling in us as in his mansion, informing our hearts with the sweetness of his presence, presiding over all our activities of mind and life as the friend, master and lover from the summit of our being, uniting us from above with himself in the universe. A constant inner communion is the joy to be made close and permanent and unfailing. This communion is not to be confined to an exceptional nearness and adoration when we retire quite into ourselves away from our normal preoccupations, nor is it to be sought by a putting away of our human activities. All our thoughts, impulses, feelings, actions have to be referred to him for his sanction or disallowance, or if we cannot yet reach this point, to be offered to him in our sacrifice of aspiration, so that he may more and more descend into us and be present in them all and pervade them with all his will and power, his light and knowledge, his love and delight. In the end all our thoughts, feelings, impulses, actions will begin to proceed from him and change into some divine seed and form of themselves; in our whole inner living we shall have grown conscious of ourselves as a part of his being till between the existence of the Divine whom we adore and our own lives there is no longer any division. So too in all happenings we have to come to see the dealings with us of the divine Lover and take such pleasure in them that even grief and suffering and physical pain become his gifts and turn to delight and disappear finally into delight, slain by the sense of the divine contact, because the touch of his hands is the alchemist of a miraculous transformation. Some reject life because it is tainted with grief and pain, but to the God-lover grief and pain become means of meeting with him, imprints of his pressure and finally cease as soon as our union with his nature becomes too complete for these masks of the universal delight at all to conceal it. They change into the Ananda.

All the relations by which this union comes about, become on this path intensely and blissfully personal. That which in the end contains, takes up or unifies them all, is the relation of lover and beloved, because that is the most intense and blissful of all and carries up all the rest into its heights and yet exceeds them. He is the teacher and guide and leads us to knowledge; at every step of the developing inner light and vision, we feel his touch like that of the artist moulding our clay of mind, his voice revealing the truth and its word, the thought he gives us to which we respond, the flashing of his spears of lightning which chase the darkness of our ignorance. Especially, in proportion as the partial lights of the mind become transformed into lights of gnosis, in whatever slighter or greater degree that may happen, we feel it as a transformation of our mentality into his and more and more he becomes the thinker and seer in us. We cease to think and see for ourselves, but think only what he wills to think for us and see only what he sees for us. And then the teacher is fulfilled in the lover; he lays hands on all our mental being to embrace and possess, to enjoy and use it.

He is the Master; but in this way of approach all distance and separation, all awe and fear and mere obedience disappear, because we become too close and united with him for these things to endure and it is the lover of our being who takes it up and occupies and uses and does with it whatever he wills. Obedience is the sign of the servant, but that is the lowest stage of this relation, *dāsya*. Afterwards we do not obey, but move to his will as the string replies to the finger of the musician. To be the instrument is this higher stage of self-surrender and submission. But this is the living and loving instrument and it ends in the whole nature of our being becoming the slave of God, rejoicing in his possession and its own blissful subjection to the divine grasp and mastery. With a passionate delight it does all he wills it to do without questioning and bears all he would have it bear, because what it bears is the burden of the beloved being.

He is the friend, the adviser, helper, saviour in trouble and distress, the defender from enemies, the hero who fights our battles for us or under whose shield we fight, the charioteer, the pilot of our ways. And here we come at once to a closer intimacy; he is the comrade and eternal companion, the playmate of the game of living. But still there is so far a certain division, however pleasant, and friendship is too much limited by the appearance of beneficence. The lover can wound, abandon, be wroth with us, seem to betray, yet our love endures and even grows by these oppositions; they increase the joy of reunion and the joy of possession; through them the lover remains the friend, and all that he does we find in the end has been done by the lover and helper of our being for our soul's perfection as well as for his joy in us. These contradictions lead to a greater intimacy. He is the father and mother too of our being, its source and protector and its indulgent cherisher and giver of our desires. He is the child born to our desire whom we cherish and rear. All these things the lover takes up; his love in its intimacy and oneness keeps in it the paternal and maternal care and lends itself to our demands upon it. All is unified in that deepest many-sided relation.

From the beginning even it is possible to have this closest relation of the lover and beloved, but it will not be as exclusive for the integral Yogin as for certain purely ecstatic ways of Bhakti. It will from the beginning take into itself something of the hues of the other relations, since he follows too knowledge and works and has need of the Divine as teacher, friend and master. The growing of the love of God must carry with it in him an expansion of the knowledge of God and of the action of the divine Will in his nature and living. The divine Lover reveals himself; he takes possession of the life. But still the essential relation will be that of love from which all things flow, love passionate, complete, seeking a hundred ways of fulfilment, every means of mutual possession, a million facets of the joy of union. All the distinctions of the mind, all its barriers and "cannot be"s, all the cold analyses of the reason are mocked at by this love or they are only used as the tests and fields and gates of union. Love comes to us in many ways; it may come as an awakening to the beauty of the Lover, by the sight of an ideal face and image of him, by his mysterious hints to us of himself behind the thousand faces of things in the world, by a slow or sudden need of the heart, by a vague thirst in the soul, by the sense of someone near us drawing us or pursuing us with love or of someone blissful and beautiful whom we must discover.

We may seek after him passionately and pursue the unseen beloved; but also the lover whom we think not of, may pursue us, may come upon us in the midst of the world and seize on us for his own whether at first we will or no. Even, he may come to us at first as an enemy, with the wrath of love, and our earliest relations with him may be those of battle and struggle. Where first there is love and attraction, the relations between the Divine and the soul may still for long be chequered with misunderstanding and offence, jealousy and wrath, strife and the quarrels of love, hope and despair and the pain of absence and separation. We throw up all the passions of the heart against him, till they are purified into a sole ecstasy of bliss and oneness. But that too is no monotony; it is not possible for the tongue of human speech to tell all the utter unity and all the eternal variety of the ananda of divine love. Our higher and our lower members are both flooded with it, the mind and life no less than the soul: even the physical body takes its share of the joy, feels the touch, is filled in all its limbs, veins, nerves with the flowing of the wine of the ecstasy, *amṛta*. Love and Ananda are the last word of being, the secret of secrets, the mystery of mysteries.

Thus universalised, personalised, raised to its intensities, made all-occupying, all-embracing, all-fulfilling, the way of love and delight gives the supreme liberation. Its highest crest is a supracosmic union. But for love complete union is *mukti*; liberation has to it no other sense; and it includes all kinds of *mukti* together, nor are they in the end, as some would have it, merely successive to each other and therefore mutually exclusive. We have the absolute union of the divine with the human spirit, *sāyujya*; in that reveals itself a content of all that depends here upon difference, — but there the difference is only a form of oneness, — ananda too of nearness and contact and mutual presence, *sāmīpya*, *sālokya*, ananda of mutual reflection, the thing that we call likeness, *sādṛśya*, and other wonderful things too for which language has as yet no name. There is nothing which is beyond the reach of the God-lover or denied to him; for he is the favourite of the divine Lover and the self of the Beloved.

Part IV

The Yoga of Self-Perfection

Chapter I

The Principle of the Integral Yoga

THE PRINCIPLE of Yoga is the turning of one or of all powers of our human existence into a means of reaching divine Being. In an ordinary Yoga one main power of being or one group of its powers is made the means, vehicle, path. In a synthetic Yoga all powers will be combined and included in the transmuting instrumentation.

In Hathayoga the instrument is the body and life. All the power of the body is stilled, collected, purified, heightened, concentrated to its utmost limits or beyond any limits by Asana and other physical processes; the power of the life too is similarly purified, heightened, concentrated by Asana and Pranayama. This concentration of powers is then directed towards that physical centre in which the divine consciousness sits concealed in the human body. The power of Life, Nature-power, coiled up with all its secret forces asleep in the lowest nervous plexus of the earth-being, — for only so much escapes into waking action in our normal operations as is sufficient for the limited uses of human life, — rises awakened through centre after centre and awakens, too, in its ascent and passage the forces of each successive nodus of our being, the nervous life, the heart of emotion and ordinary mentality, the speech, sight, will, the higher knowledge, till through and above the brain it meets with and it becomes one with the divine consciousness.

In Rajayoga the chosen instrument is the mind. Our ordinary mentality is first disciplined, purified and directed towards the divine Being, then by a summary process of Asana and Pranayama the physical force of our being is stilled and concentrated, the life-force released into a rhythmic movement capable of cessation and concentrated into a higher power of its upward action, the mind, supported and strengthened by this greater action and concentration of the body and life upon which it rests, is itself purified of all its unrest and emotion and its habitual thought-waves, liberated from distraction and dispersion, given its highest force of concentration, gathered up into a trance of absorption. Two objects, the one temporal, the other eternal, are gained by this discipline. Mind-power develops in another concentrated action abnormal capacities of knowledge, effective will, deep light of reception, powerful light of thought-radiation which are altogether beyond the narrow range of our normal mentality; it arrives at the Yogic or occult powers around which there has been woven so much quite dispensable and yet perhaps salutary mystery. But the one final end and the one all-important gain is that the mind, stilled and cast into a concentrated trance, can lose itself in the divine consciousness and the soul be made free to unite with the divine Being.

The triple way takes for its chosen instruments the three main powers of the mental soul-life of the human being. Knowledge selects the reason and the mental vision and it makes them by purification, concentration and a certain discipline of a God-directed seeking its means for the greatest knowledge and the greatest vision of all, God-knowledge and God-vision. Its aim is to see, know and be the Divine. Works, action selects for its instrument the will of the doer of works; it makes life an offering of sacrifice to the Godhead and by purification, concentration and a certain discipline of subjection to the divine Will a means for contact and increasing unity of the soul of man with the divine Master of the universe. Devotion selects the emotional and aesthetic powers of the soul and by turning them all Godward in a perfect purity, intensity, infinite passion of seeking makes them a means of God-possession in one or many relations of unity with the Divine Being. All aim in their own way at a union or unity of the human soul with the supreme Spirit.

Each Yoga in its process has the character of the instrument it uses; thus the Hathayogic process is psycho-physical, the Raja-yogic mental and psychic, the way of knowledge is spiritual and cognitive, the way of devotion spiritual, emotional and aesthetic, the way of works spiritual and dynamic by action. Each is guided in the ways of its own characteristic power. But all power is in the end one, all power is really soul-power. In the ordinary process of life, body and mind this truth is quite obscured by the dispersed, dividing and distributive action of Nature which is the normal condition of all our functionings, although even there it is in the end evident; for all material energy contains hidden the vital, mental, psychic, spiritual energy and in the end it must release these forms of the one Shakti, the vital energy conceals and liberates into action all the other forms, the mental supporting itself on the life and body and their powers and functionings contains undeveloped or only partially developed the psychic and the spiritual power of the being. But when by Yoga any of these powers is taken up from the dispersed and distributive action, raised to its highest degree, concentrated, it becomes manifest soul-power and reveals the essential unity. Therefore the Hathayogic process has too its pure psychic and spiritual result, the Rajayogic arrives by psychic means at a spiritual consummation. The triple way may appear to be altogether mental and spiritual in its way of seeking and its objectives, but it can be attended by results more characteristic of the other paths, which offer themselves in a spontaneous and involuntary flowering, and for the same reason, because soul-power is all-power and where it reaches its height in one direction its other possibilities also begin to show themselves in fact or in incipient potentiality. This unity at once suggests the possibility of a synthetic Yoga.

Tantric discipline is in its nature a synthesis. It has seized on the large universal truth that there are two poles of being whose essential unity is the secret of existence, Brahman and Shakti, Spirit and Nature, and that Nature is power of the spirit or rather is spirit as power. To raise nature in man into manifest power of spirit is its method and it is the whole nature that it gathers up for the spiritual conversion. It includes in its system of instrumentation the forceful Hathayogic process and especially the opening up of the nervous centres and the passage through them of the awakened Shakti on her way to her union with the Brahman, the subtler stress of the Rajayogic purification, meditation and concentration, the leverage of will-force, the motive power of devotion, the key of knowledge. But it does not stop short with an effective assembling of the different powers of these specific Yogas. In two directions it enlarges by its synthetic turn the province of the Yogic method. First, it lays its hand firmly on many of the main springs of human quality, desire, action and it subjects them to an intensive discipline with the soul's mastery of its motives as a first aim and their elevation to a diviner spiritual level as its final utility. Again, it includes in its objects of Yoga not only liberation,[1] which is the one all-mastering preoccupation of the specific systems, but a cosmic enjoyment[2] of the power of the Spirit, which the others may take incidentally on the way, in part, casually, but avoid making a motive or object. It is a bolder and larger system.

In the method of synthesis which we have been following, another clue of principle has been pursued which is derived from another view of the possibilities of Yoga. This starts from the method of Vedanta to arrive at the aim of the Tantra. In the Tantric method Shakti is all-important, becomes the key to the finding of spirit; in this synthesis spirit, soul is all-important, becomes the secret of the taking up of Shakti. The Tantric method starts from the bottom and grades the ladder of ascent upwards to the summit; therefore its initial stress is upon the action of the awakened Shakti in the nervous system of the body and its centres; the opening of the six lotuses is the opening up of the ranges of the power of Spirit. Our synthesis takes man as a spirit in mind much more than a spirit in body and assumes in him the capacity to begin on that level, to spiritualise his being by the power of the soul in mind opening itself directly to a higher spiritual force and being and to perfect by that higher force so possessed and brought into action the whole of his nature. For that reason our initial stress has fallen upon the utilisation of the powers of soul in mind and the turning of the triple key of knowledge, works and love in the locks of the spirit; the Hathayogic methods can be dispensed with, — though there is no objection to their partial use, — the Rajayogic will only enter

---

[1] Mukti.   [2] Bhukti.

in as an informal element. To arrive by the shortest way at the largest development of spiritual power and being and divinise by it a liberated nature in the whole range of human living is our inspiring motive.

The principle in view is a self-surrender, a giving up of the human being into the being, consciousness, power, delight of the Divine, a union or communion at all the points of meeting in the soul of man, the mental being, by which the Divine himself, directly and without veil master and possessor of the instrument, shall by the light of his presence and guidance perfect the human being in all the forces of the Nature for a divine living. Here we arrive at a farther enlargement of the objects of the Yoga. The common initial purpose of all Yoga is the liberation of the soul of man from its present natural ignorance and limitation, its release into spiritual being, its union with the highest self and Divinity. But ordinarily this is made not only the initial but the whole and final object: enjoyment of spiritual being there is, but either in a dissolution of the human and individual into the silence of self-being or on a higher plane in another existence. The Tantric system makes liberation the final, but not the only aim; it takes on its way a full perfection and enjoyment of the spiritual power, light and joy in the human existence, and even it has a glimpse of a supreme experience in which liberation and cosmic action and enjoyment are unified in a final overcoming of all oppositions and dissonances. It is this wider view of our spiritual potentialities from which we begin, but we add another stress which brings in a completer significance. We regard the spirit in man not as solely an individual being travelling to a transcendent unity with the Divine, but as a universal being capable of oneness with the Divine in all souls and all Nature and we give this extended view its entire practical consequence. The human soul's individual liberation and enjoyment of union with the Divine in spiritual being, consciousness and delight must always be the first object of the Yoga; its free enjoyment of the cosmic unity of the Divine becomes a second object; but out of that a third appears, the effectuation of the meaning of the divine unity with all beings by a sympathy and participation in the spiritual purpose of the Divine in humanity. The individual Yoga then turns from its separateness and becomes a part of the collective Yoga of the divine Nature in the human race. The liberated individual being, united with the Divine in self and spirit, becomes in his natural being a self-perfecting instrument for the perfect outflowering of the Divine in humanity.

This outflowering has its two terms; first, comes the growth out of the separative human ego into the unity of the spirit, then the possession of the divine nature in its proper and its higher forms and no longer in the inferior forms of the mental being which are a mutilated translation and not the authentic text of the original script of divine Nature in the cosmic individual. In other words, a perfection has to be aimed at which amounts to the elevation of the mental into the full spiritual and supramental nature. Therefore this integral Yoga of knowledge, love and works has to be extended into a Yoga of spiritual and gnostic self-perfection. As gnostic knowledge, will and ananda are a direct instrumentation of spirit and can only be won by growing into the spirit, into divine being, this growth has to be the first aim of our Yoga. The mental being has to enlarge itself into the oneness of the Divine before the Divine will perfect in the soul of the individual its gnostic outflowering. That is the reason why the triple way of knowledge, works and love becomes the key-note of the whole Yoga, for that is the direct means for the soul in mind to rise to its highest intensities where it passes upward into the divine oneness. That too is the reason why the Yoga must be integral. For if immergence in the Infinite or some close union with the Divine were all our aim, an integral Yoga would be superfluous, except for such greater satisfaction of the being of man as we may get by a self-lifting of the whole of it towards its Source. But it would not be needed for the essential aim, since by any single power of the soul-nature we can meet with the Divine; each at its height rises up into the infinite and absolute, each therefore offers a sufficient way of arrival, for all the hundred separate paths meet in the Eternal. But the gnostic being is a complete enjoyment and possession of the whole divine and spiritual nature; and it is a complete lifting of the whole nature of man into its power of a divine and spiritual existence. Integrality becomes then an essential condition of this Yoga.

At the same time we have seen that each of the three ways at its height, if it is pursued with a certain largeness, can take into itself the powers of the others and lead to their fulfilment. It is therefore sufficient to start by one of them and find the point at which it meets the other at first parallel lines of advance and melts into them by its own widenings. At the same time a more difficult, complex, wholly powerful process would be to start, as it were, on three lines together, on a triple wheel of soul-power. But the consideration of this possibility must be postponed till we have seen what are the conditions and means of the Yoga of self-perfection. For we shall see that this also need not be postponed entirely, but a certain preparation of it is part of and a certain initiation into it proceeds by the growth of the divine works, love and knowledge.

Chapter II

The Integral Perfection

A DIVINE perfection of the human being is our aim. We must know then first what are the essential elements that constitute man's total perfection; secondly, what we mean by a divine as distinguished from a human perfection of our being. That man as a being is capable of self-development and of some approach at least to an ideal standard of perfection which his mind is able to conceive, fix before it and pursue, is common ground to all thinking humanity, though it may be only the minority who concern themselves with this possibility as providing the one most important aim of life. But by some the ideal is conceived as a mundane change, by others as a religious conversion.

The mundane perfection is sometimes conceived of as something outward, social, a thing of action, a more rational dealing with our fellow-men and our environment, a better and more efficient citizenship and discharge of duties, a better, richer, kindlier and happier way of living, with a more just and more harmonious associated enjoyment of the opportunities of existence. By others again a more inner and subjective ideal is cherished, a clarifying and raising of the intelligence, will and reason, a heightening and ordering of power and capacity in the nature, a nobler ethical, a richer aesthetic, a finer emotional, a much healthier and better-governed vital and physical being. Sometimes one element is stressed, almost to the exclusion of the rest; sometimes, in wider and more well-balanced minds, the whole harmony is envisaged as a total perfection. A change of education and social institutions is the outward means adopted or an inner self-training and development is preferred as the true instrumentation. Or the two aims may be clearly united, the perfection of the inner individual, the perfection of the outer living.

But the mundane aim takes for its field the present life

and its opportunities; the religious aim on the contrary fixes before it the self-preparation for another existence after death, its commonest ideal is some kind of pure sainthood, its means a conversion of the imperfect or sinful human being by divine grace or through obedience to a law laid down by a scripture or else given by a religious founder. The aim of religion may include a social change, but it is then a change brought about by the acceptance of a common religious ideal and way of consecrated living, a brotherhood of the saints, a theocracy or kingdom of God reflecting on earth the kingdom of heaven.

The object of our synthetic Yoga must, in this respect too as in its other parts, be more integral and comprehensive, embrace all these elements or these tendencies of a larger impulse of self-perfection and harmonise them or rather unify, and in order to do that successfully it must seize on a truth which is wider than the ordinary religious and higher than the mundane principle. All life is a secret Yoga, an obscure growth of Nature towards the discovery and fulfilment of the divine principle hidden in her which becomes progressively less obscure, more self-conscient and luminous, more self-possessed in the human being by the opening of all his instruments of knowledge, will, action, life to the Spirit within him and in the world. Mind, life, body, all the forms of our nature are the means of this growth, but they find their last perfection only by opening out to something beyond them, first, because they are not the whole of what man is, secondly, because that other something which he is, is the key of his completeness and brings a light which discovers to him the whole high and large reality of his being.

Mind is fulfilled by a greater knowledge of which it is only a half-light, life discovers its meaning in a greater power and will of which it is the outward and as yet obscure functioning, body finds its last use as an instrument of a power of being of which it is a physical support and material starting-point. They have all themselves first to be developed and find out their ordinary possibilities; all our normal life is a trying of these possibilities and an opportunity for this preparatory and tentative self-training. But life cannot find its perfect self-fulfilment till it opens to that greater reality of being of which by this development of a richer power and a more sensitive use and capacity it becomes a well-prepared field of working.

Intellectual, volitional, ethical, emotional, aesthetic and physical training and improvement are all so much to the good, but they are only in the end a constant movement in a circle without any last delivering and illumining aim, unless they arrive at a point when they can open themselves to the power and presence of the Spirit and admit its direct workings. This direct working effects a conversion of the whole being which is the indispensable condition of our real perfection. To grow into the truth and power of the Spirit and by the direct action of that power to be made a fit channel of its self-expression, — a living of man in the Divine and a divine living of the Spirit in humanity, — will therefore be the principle and the whole object of an integral Yoga of self-perfection.

In the process of this change there must be by the very necessity of the effort two stages of its working. First, there will be the personal endeavour of the human being, as soon as he becomes aware by his soul, mind, heart of this divine possibility and turns towards it as the true object of life, to prepare himself for it and to get rid of all in him that belongs to a lower working, of all that stands in the way of his opening to the spiritual truth and its power, so as to possess by this liberation his spiritual being and turn all his natural movements into free means of its self-expression. It is by this turn that the self-conscious Yoga aware of its aim begins: there is a new awakening and an upward change of the life motive. So long as there is only an intellectual, ethical and other self-training for the now normal purposes of life which does not travel beyond the ordinary circle of working of mind, life and body, we are still only in the obscure and yet unillumined preparatory Yoga of Nature; we are still in pursuit of only an ordinary human perfection. A spiritual desire of the Divine and of the divine perfection, of a unity with him in all our being and a spiritual perfection in all our nature, is the effective sign of this change, the precursory power of a great integral conversion of our being and living.

By personal effort a precursory change, a preliminary conversion can be effected; it amounts to a greater or less spiritualising of our mental motives, our character and temperament, and a mastery, stilling or changed action of the vital and physical life. This converted subjectivity can be made the base of some communion or unity of the soul in mind with the Divine and some partial reflection of the divine nature in the mentality of the human being. That is as far as man can go by his unaided or indirectly aided effort, because that is an effort of mind and mind cannot climb beyond itself permanently: at most it arises to a spiritualised and idealised mentality. If it shoots up beyond that border, it loses hold of itself, loses hold of life, and arrives either at a trance of absorption or a passivity. A greater perfection can only be arrived at by a higher power entering in and taking up the whole action of the being. The second stage of this Yoga will therefore be a persistent giving up of all the action of the nature into the hands of this greater Power, a substitution of its influence, possession and working for the personal effort, until the Divine to whom we aspire becomes the direct master of the Yoga and effects the entire spiritual and ideal conversion of the being.

This double character of our Yoga raises it beyond the mundane ideal of perfection, while at the same time it goes too beyond the loftier, intenser, but much narrower religious formula. The mundane ideal regards man always as a mental, vital and physical being and it aims at a human perfection well within these limits, a perfection of mind, life and body, an expansion and refinement of the intellect and knowledge, of the will and power, of ethical character, aim and conduct, of aesthetic sensibility and creativeness, of emotional balanced poise and enjoyment, of vital and physical soundness, regulated action and just efficiency. It is a wide and full aim, but yet not sufficiently full and wide, because it ignores that other greater element of our being which the mind vaguely conceives as the spiritual element and leaves it either undeveloped or insufficiently satisfied as merely some high occasional or added derivatory experience, the result of the action of mind in its exceptional aspects or dependent upon mind for its presence and persistence. It can become a high aim when it seeks to develop the loftier and the larger reaches of our mentality, but yet not sufficiently high, because it does not aspire beyond mind to that of which our purest reason, our brightest mental intuition, our deepest mental sense and feeling, strongest mental will and power or ideal aim and purpose are only pale radiations. Its aim besides is limited to a terrestrial perfection of the normal human life.

A Yoga of integral perfection regards man as a divine spiritual being involved in mind, life and body; it aims therefore at a liberation and a perfection of his divine nature. It seeks to make an inner living in the perfectly developed spiritual being his constant intrinsic living and the spiritualised action of mind, life and body only its outward human expression. In order that this spiritual being may not be something vague and indefinable or else but imperfectly realised and dependent on the mental support and the mental limitations, it seeks to go beyond mind to the supramental knowledge, will, sense, feeling, intuition, dynamic initiation of vital and physical action, all that makes the native working of the spiritual being. It accepts human life, but takes account of the large supraterrestrial action behind the earthly material living, and it joins itself to the divine Being from whom the supreme origination of all these partial and lower states proceeds so that the whole of life may become aware of its divine source and feel in each action of knowledge, of will, of feeling, sense and body the divine originating impulse. It rejects nothing that is essential in the mundane aim, but enlarges it, finds and lives in its greater and its truer meaning now hidden from it, transfigures it from a limited, earthly and mortal thing to a figure of infinite, divine and immortal values.

The integral Yoga meets the religious ideal at several points, but goes beyond it in the sense of a greater wideness. The religious ideal looks, not only beyond this earth, but away from it to a heaven or even beyond all heavens to some kind of Nirvana. Its ideal of perfection is limited to whatever kind of inner or outer mutation will eventually serve the turning away of the soul from the human life to the beyond. Its ordinary idea of perfection is a religio-ethical change, a drastic purification of the active and the emotional being, often with an ascetic abrogation and rejection of the vital impulses as its completest reaching of excellence, and in any case a supraterrestrial motive and reward or result of a life of piety and right conduct. In so far as it admits a change of knowledge, will, aesthesis, it is in the sense of the turning of them to another object than the aims of human life and eventually brings a rejection of all earthly objects of aesthesis, will and knowledge. The method, whether it lays stress on personal effort or upon divine influence, on works and knowledge or upon grace, is not like the mundane a development, but rather a conversion; but in the end the aim is not a conversion of our mental and physical nature, but the putting on of a pure spiritual nature and being, and since that is not possible here on earth, it looks for its consummation by a transference to another world or a shuffling off of all cosmic existence.

But the integral Yoga founds itself on a conception of the spiritual being as an omnipresent existence, the fullness of which comes not essentially by a transference to other worlds or a cosmic self-extinction, but by a growth out of what we now are phenomenally into the consciousness of the omnipresent reality which we always are in the essence of our being. It substitutes for the form of religious piety its completer spiritual seeking of a divine union. It proceeds by a personal effort to a conversion through a divine influence and possession; but this divine grace, if we may so call it, is not simply a mysterious flow or touch coming from above, but the all-pervading act of a divine presence which we come to know within as the power of the highest Self and Master of our being entering into the soul and so possessing it that we not only feel it close to us and pressing upon our mortal nature, but live in its law, know that law, possess it as the whole power of our spiritualised nature. The conversion its action will effect is an integral conversion of our ethical being into the Truth and Right of the divine nature, of our intellectual into the illumination of divine knowledge, our emotional into the divine love and unity, our dynamic and volitional into a working of the divine power, our aesthetic into a plenary reception and a creative enjoyment of divine beauty, not excluding even in the end a divine conversion of the vital and physical being. It regards all the previous life as an involuntary and unconscious or half-conscious preparatory growing towards this change and Yoga as the voluntary and conscious effort and realisation of the change, by which all the aim of human existence in all its parts is fulfilled, even while it is transfigured. Admitting the supracosmic truth and life in worlds beyond, it admits too the terrestrial as a continued term of the one existence and a change of individual and communal life on earth as a strain of its divine meaning.

To open oneself to the supracosmic Divine is an essential condition of this integral perfection; to unite oneself with the universal Divine is another essential condition. Here the Yoga of self-perfection coincides with the Yogas of knowledge, works and devotion; for it is impossible to change the human nature into the divine or to make it an instrument of the divine knowledge, will and joy of existence, unless there is a union with the supreme Being, Consciousness and Bliss and a unity with its universal Self in all things and beings. A wholly separative possession of the divine nature by the human individual, as distinct from a self-withdrawn absorption in it, is not possible. But this unity will not be an inmost spiritual oneness qualified, so long as the human life lasts, by a separative existence in mind, life and body; the full perfection is a possession, through this spiritual unity, of unity too with the universal Mind, the universal Life, the universal Form which are the other constant terms of cosmic being. Moreover, since human life is still accepted as a self-expression of the realised Divine in man, there must be an action of the entire divine nature in our life; and this brings in the need of the supramental conversion which substitutes the native action of spiritual being for the imperfect action of the superficial nature and spiritualises and transfigures its mental, vital and physical parts by the spiritual ideality. These three elements, a union with the supreme Divine, unity with the universal Self, and a supramental life action from this transcendent origin and through this universality, but still with the individual as the soul-channel and natural instrument, constitute the essence of the integral divine perfection of the human being.

Chapter III

The Psychology of Self-Perfection

ESSENTIALLY, then, this divine self-perfection is a conversion of the human into a likeness of and a fundamental oneness with the divine nature, a rapid shaping of the image of God in man and filling in of its ideal outlines. It is what is ordinarily termed *sādṛśya-mukti*, a liberation into the divine resemblance out of the bondage of the human seeming, or, to use the expression of the Gita, *sādharmya-gati*, a coming to be one in law of being with the supreme, universal and indwelling Divine. To perceive and have a right view of our way to such a transformation we must form some sufficient working idea of the complex thing that this human nature at present is in the confused interminglings of its various principles, so that we may see the precise nature of the conversion each part of it must undergo and the most effective means for the conversion. How to disengage from this knot of thinking mortal matter the Immortal it contains, from this mentalised vital animal man the happy fullness of his submerged hints of Godhead, is the real problem of a human being and living. Life develops many first hints of the divinity without completely disengaging them; Yoga is the unravelling of the knot of Life's difficulty.

First of all we have to know the central secret of the psychological complexity which creates the problem and all its difficulties. But an ordinary psychology which only takes mind and its phenomena at their surface values, will be of no help to us; it will not give us the least guidance in this line of self-exploration and self-conversion. Still less can we find the clue in a scientific psychology with a materialistic basis which assumes that the body and the biological and physiological factors of our nature are not only the starting-point but the whole real foundation and regards human mind as only a subtle development from the life and the body. That may be the actual truth of the animal side of human nature and of the human mind in so far as it is limited and conditioned by the physical part of our being. But the whole difference between man and the animal is that the animal mind, as we know it, cannot get for one moment away from its origins, cannot break out from the covering, the close chrysalis which the bodily life has spun round the soul, and become something greater than its present self, a more free, magnificent and noble being; but in man mind reveals itself as a greater energy escaping from the restrictions of the vital and physical formula of being. But even this is not all that man is or can be: he has in him the power to evolve and release a still greater ideal energy which in its turn escapes out of the restrictions of the mental formula of his nature and discloses the supramental form, the ideal power of a spiritual being. In Yoga we have to travel beyond the physical nature and the superficial man and to discover the workings of the whole nature of the real man. In other words we must arrive at and use a psycho-physical knowledge with a spiritual foundation.

Man is in his real nature, — however obscure now this truth may be to our present understanding and self-consciousness, we must for the purposes of Yoga have faith in it, and we shall then find that our faith is justified by an increasing experience and a greater self-knowledge, — a spirit using the mind, life and body for an individual and a communal experience and self-manifestation in the universe. This spirit is an infinite existence limiting itself in apparent being for individual experience. It is an infinite consciousness which defines itself in finite forms of consciousness for joy of various knowledge and various power of being. It is an infinite delight of being expanding and contracting itself and its powers, concealing and discovering, formulating many terms of its joy of existence, even to an apparent obscuration and denial of its own nature. In itself it is eternal Sachchidananda, but this complexity, this knotting up and unravelling of the infinite in the finite is the aspect we see it assume in universal and in individual nature. To discover the eternal Sachchidananda, this essential self of our being within us, and live in it is the stable basis, to make its true nature evident and creative of a divine way of living in our instruments, supermind, mind, life and body, the active principle of a spiritual perfection.

Supermind, mind, life and body are the four instruments which the spirit uses for its manifestation in the workings of Nature. Supermind is spiritual consciousness acting as a self-luminous knowledge, will, sense, aesthesis, energy, self-creative and unveiling power of its own delight and being. Mind is the action of the same powers, but limited and only very indirectly and partially illumined. Supermind lives in unity though it plays with diversity; mind lives in a separative action of diversity, though it may open to unity. Mind is not only capable of ignorance, but, because it acts always partially and by limitation, it works characteristically as a power of ignorance: it may even and it does forget itself in a complete inconscience, or nescience, awaken from it to the ignorance of a partial knowledge and move from the ignorance towards a complete knowledge, — that is its natural action in the human being, — but it can never have by itself a complete knowledge. Supermind is incapable of real ignorance; even if it puts full knowledge behind it in the limitation of a particular working, yet all its working refers back to what it has put behind it and all is instinct with self-illumination; even if it involves itself in material nescience, it yet does there accurately the works of a perfect will and knowledge. Supermind lends itself to the action of the inferior instruments; it is always there indeed at the core as a secret support of their operations. In matter it is an automatic action and effectuation of the hidden idea in things; in life its most seizable form is instinct, an instinctive, subconscious or partly subconscious knowledge and operation; in mind it reveals itself as intuition, a swift, direct and self-effective illumination of intelligence, will, sense and aesthesis. But these are merely irradiations of the supermind which accommodate themselves to the limited functioning of the obscurer instruments: its own characteristic nature is a gnosis superconscient to mind, life and body. Supermind or gnosis is the characteristic, illumined, significant action of spirit in its own native reality.

Life is an energy of spirit subordinated to action of mind and body, which fulfils itself through mentality and physicality and acts as a link between them. It has its own characteristic operation but nowhere works independently of mind and body. All energy of the spirit in action works in the two terms of existence and consciousness, for the self-formation of existence and the play and self-realisation of consciousness, for the delight of existence and the delight of consciousness. In this inferior formulation of being in which we at present live, the spirit's energy of life works between the two terms of mind and matter, supporting and effecting the formulations of substance of matter and working as a material energy, supporting the formulations of consciousness of mind and the workings of mental energy, supporting the interaction of mind and body and working as a sensory and nervous energy. What we call vitality is for the purposes of our normal human existence power of conscious being emerging in matter, liberating from it and in it mind and the higher powers and supporting their limited action in the physical life, — just as what we call mentality is power of conscious being awaking in body to light of its own consciousness and to consciousness of all the rest of being immediately around it and working at first in the limited action set for it by life and body, but at certain points and at a certain height escaping from it to a partial action beyond this circle. But this is not the whole power whether of life or mentality; they have planes of conscious existence of their own kind, other than this material level, where they are freer in their characteristic action. Matter or body itself is a limiting form of substance of spirit in which life and mind and spirit are involved, self-hidden, self-forgetful by absorption in their own externalising action, but bound to emerge from it by a self-compelling evolution. But matter too is capable of refining to subtler forms of substance in which it becomes more apparently a formal density of life, of mind, of spirit. Man himself has, besides this gross material body, an encasing vital sheath, a mental body, a body of bliss and gnosis. But all matter, all body contains within it the secret powers of these higher principles; matter is a formation of life that has no real existence apart from the informing universal spirit which gives it its energy and substance.

This is the nature of spirit and its instruments. But to understand its operations and to get at a knowledge which will give to us a power of leverage in uplifting them out of the established groove in which our life goes spinning, we have to perceive that the Spirit has based all its workings upon two twin aspects of its being, Soul and Nature, Purusha and Prakriti. We have to treat them as different and diverse in power, — for in practice of consciousness this difference is valid, — although they are only two sides of the same reality, pole and pole of the one conscious being. Purusha or soul is spirit cognizant of the workings of its nature, supporting them by its being, enjoying or rejecting enjoyment of them in its delight of being. Nature is power of the spirit, and she is too working and process of its power formulating name and form of being, developing action of consciousness and knowledge, throwing itself up in will and impulsion, force and energy, fulfilling itself in enjoyment. Nature is Prakriti, Maya, Shakti. If we look at her on her most external side where she seems the opposite of Purusha, she is Prakriti, an inert and mechanical self-driven operation, inconscient or conscient only by the light of Purusha, elevated by various degrees, vital, mental, supramental, of his soul-illumination of her workings. If we look at her on her other internal side where she moves nearer to unity with Purusha, she is Maya, will of being and becoming or of cessation from being and becoming with all their results, apparent to the consciousness, of involution and evolution, existing and non-existing, self-concealment of spirit and self-discovery of spirit. Both are sides of one and the same thing, Shakti, power of being of the spirit which operates, whether superconsciously or consciously or subconsciously in a seeming inconscience, — in fact all these motions coexist at the same time and in the same soul, — as the spirit's power of knowledge, power of will, power of process and action, *jñāna-śakti, icchā-śakti, kriyā-śakti*. By this power the spirit creates all things in itself, hides and discovers all itself in the form and behind the veil of its manifestation.

Purusha is able by this power of its nature to take whatever poise it may will and to follow the law and form of being proper to any self-formulation. It is eternal soul and spirit in its own power of self-existence superior to and governing its manifestations; it is universal soul and spirit developed in power of becoming of its existence, infinite in the finite; it is individual soul and spirit absorbed in development of some particular course of its becoming, in appearance mutably finite in the infinite. All these things it can be at once, eternal spirit universalised in cosmos, individualised in its beings; it can too found the consciousness rejecting, governing or responding to the action of Nature in any one of them, put the others behind it or away from it, know itself as pure eternity, self-supporting universality or exclusive individuality. Whatever the formulation of its nature, soul can seem to become that and view itself as that only in the frontal active part of its consciousness; but it is never only what it seems to be; it is too the so much else that it can be; secretly, it is the all of itself that is yet hidden. It is not irrevocably limited by any particular self-formulation in Time, but can break through and beyond it, break it up or develop it, select, reject, new-create, reveal out of itself a greater self-formulation. What it believes itself to be by the whole active will of its consciousness in its instruments, that it is or tends to become, *yo yacchraddhaḥ sa eva saḥ*: what it believes it can be and has full faith in becoming, that it changes to in nature, evolves or discovers.

This power of the soul over its nature is of the utmost importance in the Yoga of self-perfection; if it did not exist, we could never get by conscious endeavour and aspiration out of the fixed groove of our present imperfect human being; if any greater perfection were intended, we should have to wait for Nature to effect it in her own slow or swift process of evolution. In the lower forms of being the soul accepts this complete subjection to Nature, but as it rises higher in the scale, it awakes to a sense of something in itself which can command Nature; but it is only when it arrives at self-knowledge that this free will and control becomes a complete reality. The change effects itself through process of nature, not therefore by any capricious magic, but an ordered development and intelligible process. When complete mastery is gained, then the process by its self-effective rapidity may seem a miracle to the intelligence, but it still proceeds by law of the truth of Spirit, — when the Divine within us by close union of our will and being with him takes up the Yoga and acts as the omnipotent master of the nature. For the Divine is our highest Self and the self of all Nature, the eternal and universal Purusha.

Purusha may establish himself in any plane of being, take any principle of being as the immediate head of his power and live in the working of its proper mode of conscious action. The soul may dwell in the principle of infinite unity of self-existence and be aware of all consciousness, energy, delight, knowledge, will, activity as conscious form of this essential truth, Sat or Satya. It may dwell in the principle of infinite conscious energy, Tapas, and be aware of it unrolling out of self-existence the works of knowledge, will and dynamic soul-action for the enjoyment of an infinite delight of the being. It may dwell in the principle of infinite self-existent delight and be aware of the divine Ananda creating out of its self-existence by its energy whatever harmony of being. In these three poises the consciousness of unity dominates; the soul lives in its awareness of eternity, universality, unity, and whatever diversity there is, is not separative, but only a multitudinous aspect of oneness. It may dwell too in the principle of supermind, in a luminous self-determining knowledge, will and action which develops some coordination of perfect delight of conscious being. In the higher gnosis unity is the basis, but it takes its joy in diversity; in lower fact of supermind diversity is the basis, but it refers back always to a conscious unity and it takes joy in unity. These ranges of consciousness are beyond our present level; they are superconscious to our normal mentality. That belongs to a lower hemisphere of being.

This lower being begins where a veil falls between soul and nature, between spirit in supermind and spirit in mind, life and body. Where this veil has not fallen, these instrumental powers are not what they are in us, but an enlightened part of the unified action of supermind and spirit. Mind gets to an independent idea of its own action when it forgets to refer back to the light from which it derives and becomes absorbed in the possibilities of its own separative process and enjoyment. The soul when it dwells in the principle of mind, not yet subject to but user of life and body, knows itself as a mental being working out its mental life and forces and images, bodies of the subtle mental substance, according to its individual knowledge, will and dynamis modified by its relation to other similar beings and powers in the universal mind. When it dwells in the principle of life, it knows itself as a being of the universal life working out action and consciousness by its desires under similar modifying conditions proper to a universal life-soul whose action is through many individual life-beings. When it dwells in the principle of matter, it knows itself as a consciousness of matter acting under a similar law of the energy of material being. In proportion as it leans towards the side of knowledge, it is aware of itself more or less clearly as a soul of mind, a soul of life, a soul of body viewing and acting in or acted upon by its nature; but where it leans towards the side of ignorance, it knows itself as an ego identified with nature of mind, of life or of body, a creation of Nature. But the native tendency of material being leads towards an absorption of the soul's energy in the act of formation and material movement and a consequent self-oblivion of the conscious being. The material universe begins from an apparent inconscience.

The universal Purusha dwells in all these planes in a certain simultaneity and builds upon each of these principles a world or series of worlds with its beings who live in the nature of that principle. Man, the microcosm, has all these planes in his own being, ranged from his subconscient to his superconscient existence. By a developing power of Yoga he can become aware of these concealed worlds hidden from his physical, materialised mind and senses which know only the material world, and then he becomes aware that his material existence is not a thing apart and self-existent, as the material universe in which he lives is also not a thing apart and self-existent, but is in constant relation to the higher planes and acted on by their powers and beings. He can open up and increase the action of these higher planes in himself and enjoy some sort of participation in the life of the other worlds, — which, for the rest, are or can be his dwelling-place, that is to say, the station of his awareness, *dhāma*, after death or between death and rebirth in a material body. But his most important capacity is that of developing the powers of the higher principles in himself, a greater power of life, a purer light of mind, the illumination of supermind, the infinite being, consciousness and delight of spirit. By an ascending movement he can develop his human imperfection towards that greater perfection.

But whatever his aim, however exalted his aspiration, he has to begin from the law of his present imperfection, to take full account of it and see how it can be converted to the law of a possible perfection. This present law of his being starts from the inconscience of the material universe, an involution of the soul in form and subjection to material nature; and, though in this matter life and mind have developed their own energies, yet they are limited and bound up in the action of the lower material, which is to the ignorance of his practical surface consciousness his original principle. Mind in him, though he is an embodied mental being, has to bear the control of the body and the physical life and can only by some more or less considerable effort of energy and concentration consciously control life and body. It is only by increasing that control that he can move towards perfection, — and it is only by developing soul-power that he can reach it. Nature-power in him has to become more and more completely a conscious act of soul, a conscious expression of all the will and knowledge of spirit. Prakriti has to reveal itself as shakti of the Purusha.

Chapter IV

The Perfection of the Mental Being

THE FUNDAMENTAL idea of a Yoga of self-perfection must be, under these conditions, a reversal of the present relations of the soul of man to his mental, vital and physical nature. Man is at present a partly self-conscious soul subject to and limited by mind, life and body, who has to become an entirely self-conscious soul master of his mind, life and body. Not limited by their claims and demands, a perfect self-conscious soul would be superior to and a free possessor of its instruments. This effort of man to be master of his own being has been the sense of a large part of his past spiritual, intellectual and moral strivings.

In order to be possessor of his being with any complete reality of freedom and mastery, man must find out his highest self, the real man or highest Purusha in him, which is free and master in its own inalienable power. He must cease to be the mental, vital, physical ego; for that is always the creation, instrument and subject of mental, vital, physical Nature. This ego is not his real self, but an instrumentation of Nature by which it has developed a sense of limited and separate individual being in mind, life and body. By this instrumentation he acts as if he were a separate existence in the material universe. Nature has evolved certain habitual limiting conditions under which that action takes place; self-identification of the soul with the ego is the means by which she induces the soul to consent to this action and accept these habitual limiting conditions. While the identification lasts, there is a self-imprisonment in this habitual round and narrow action, and, until it is transcended, there can be no free use by the soul of its individual living, much less a real self-exceeding. For this reason an essential movement of the Yoga is to draw back from the outward ego sense by which we are identified with the action of mind, life and body and live inwardly in the soul. The liberation from an externalised ego sense is the first step towards the soul's freedom and mastery.

When we thus draw back into the soul, we find ourselves to be not the mind, but a mental being who stands behind the action of the embodied mind, not a mental and vital personality, — personality is a composition of Nature, — but a mental Person, *manomaya puruṣa*. We become aware of a being within who takes his stand upon mind for self-knowledge and world-knowledge and thinks of himself as an individual for self-experience and world-experience, for an inward action and an outward-going action, but is yet different from mind, life and body. This sense of difference from the vital actions and the physical being is very marked; for although the Purusha feels his mind to be involved in life and body, yet he is aware that even if the physical life and body were to cease or be dissolved, he would still go on existing in his mental being. But the sense of difference from the mind is more difficult and less firmly distinct. But still it is there; it is characterised by any or all of three intuitions in which this mental Purusha lives and becomes by them aware of his own greater existence.

First, he has the intuition of himself as someone observing the action of the mind; it is something which is going on in him and yet before him as an object of his regarding knowledge. This self-awareness is the intuitive sense of the witness Purusha, *sākṣī*. Witness Purusha is a pure consciousness who watches Nature and sees it as an action reflected upon the consciousness and enlightened by that consciousness, but in itself other than it. To mental Purusha Nature is only an action, a complex action of discriminating and combining thought, of will, of sense, of emotion, of temperament and character, of ego feeling, which works upon a foundation of vital impulses, needs and cravings in the conditions imposed by the physical body. But it is not limited by them, since it can not only give them new directions and much variation, refining and extension, but is able to act in thought and imagination and a mental world of much more subtle and flexible creations. But also there is an intuition in the mental Purusha of something larger and greater than this present action in which he lives, a range of experience of which it is only a frontal scheme or a narrow superficial selection. By this intuition he stands upon the threshold of a subliminal self with a more extended possibility than this superficial mentality opens to his self-knowledge. A last and greatest intuition is an inner awareness of something which he more essentially is, something as high above mind as mind is above the physical life and body. This inner awareness is his intuition of his supramental and spiritual being.

The mental Purusha can at any time involve himself again in the superficial action from which he has drawn back, live for a while entirely identified with the mechanism of mind, life and body and absorbedly repeat its recurrent normal action. But once that separative movement has been made and lived in for some time, he can never be to himself quite what he was before. The involution in the outward action becomes now only a recurrent self-oblivion from which there is a tendency in him to draw back again to himself and to pure self-experience. It may be noted too that the Purusha by drawing back from the normal action of this outward consciousness which has created for him his present natural form of self-experience, is able to take two other poises. He can have an intuition of himself as a soul in body, which puts forth life as its activity and mind as the light of that activity. This soul in body is the physical conscious being, *annamaya puruṣa*, which uses life and mind characteristically for physical experience, — all else being regarded as a consequence of physical experience, — does not look beyond the life of the body and, so far as it feels anything beyond its physical individuality, is aware only of the physical universe and at most its oneness with the soul of physical Nature. But he can have too an intuition of himself as a soul of life, self-identified with a great movement of becoming in Time, which puts forth body as a form or basic sense-image and mind as a conscious activity of life-experience. This soul in life is the vital conscious being, *prāṇamaya puruṣa*, which is capable of looking beyond the duration and limits of the physical body, of feeling an eternity of life behind and in front, an identity with a universal Life-being, but does not look beyond a constant vital becoming in Time. These three Purushas are soul-forms of the Spirit by which it identifies its conscious existence with and founds its action upon any of these three planes or principles of its universal being.

But man is characteristically a mental being. Moreover, mentality is his highest present status in which he is nearest to his real self, most easily and largely aware of spirit. His way to perfection is not to involve himself in the outward or superficial existence, nor is it to place himself in the soul of life or the soul of body, but to insist on the three mental intuitions by which he can lift himself eventually above the physical, vital and mental levels. This insistence may take two quite different forms, each with its own object and way of proceeding. It is quite possible for him to accentuate it in a direction away from existence in Nature, a detachment, a withdrawal from mind, life and body. He may try to live more and more as the witness Purusha, regarding the action of Nature, without interest in it, without sanction to it, detached, rejecting the whole action, withdrawing into pure conscious existence. This is the Sankhya liberation. He may go inward into that larger existence of which he has the intuition and away from the superficial mentality into a dream-state or sleep-state which admits him into wider or higher ranges of consciousness. By passing away into these ranges he may put away from him the terrestrial being. There is even, it was supposed in ancient times, a transition to supramental worlds from which a return to earthly consciousness was either not possible or not obligatory. But the definite and sure finality of this kind of liberation depends on the elevation of the mental being into that spiritual self of which he becomes aware when he looks away and upward from all mentality. That is given as the key to entire cessation from terrestrial existence whether by immergence in pure being or a participation in supracosmic being.

But if our aim is to be not only free by self-detachment from Nature, but perfected in mastery, this type of insistence can no longer suffice. We have to regard our mental, vital and physical action of Nature, find out the knots of its bondage and the loosing-points of liberation, discover the keys of its imperfection and lay our finger on the key of perfection. When the regarding soul, the witness Purusha stands back from his action of nature and observes it, he sees that it proceeds of its own impulsion by the power of its mechanism, by force of continuity of movement, continuity of mentality, continuity of life impulse, continuity of an involuntary physical mechanism. At first the whole thing seems to be the recurrent action of an automatic machinery, although the sum of that action mounts constantly into a creation, development, evolution. He was as if seized in this wheel, attached to it by the ego sense, whirled round and onward in the circling of the machinery. A complete mechanical determinism or a stream of determinations of Nature to which he lent the light of his consciousness, is the natural aspect of his mental, vital and physical personality once it is regarded from this stable detached standpoint and no longer by a soul caught up in the movement and imagining itself to be a part of the action.

But on a farther view we find that this determinism is not so complete as it seemed; action of Nature continues and is what it is because of the sanction of the Purusha. The regarding Purusha sees that he supports and in some way fills and pervades the action with his conscious being. He discovers that without him it could not continue and that where he persistently withdraws this sanction, the habitual action becomes gradually enfeebled, flags and ceases. His whole active mentality can be thus brought to a complete stillness. There is yet a passive mentality which mechanically continues, but this too can be stilled by his withdrawal into himself out of the action. Even then the life action in its most mechanical parts continues; but that too can be stilled into cessation. It would appear then that he is not only the upholding (*bhartṛ*) Purusha, but in some way the master of his nature, Ishwara. It was the consciousness of this sanctioning control, this necessity of his consent, which made him in the ego-sense conceive of himself as a soul or mental being with a free will determining all his own becomings. Yet the free-will seems to be imperfect, almost illusory, since the actual will itself is a machinery of Nature and each separate willing determined by the stream of past action and the sum of conditions it created,

— although, because the result of the stream, the sum, is at each moment a new development, a new determination, it may seem to be a self-born willing, virginally creative at each moment. What he contributed all the while was a consent behind, a sanction to what Nature was doing. He does not seem able to rule her entirely, but only choose between certain well-defined possibilities: there is in her a power of resistance born of her past impetus and a still greater power of resistance born of the sum of fixed conditions she has created, which she presents to him as a set of permanent laws to be obeyed. He cannot radically alter her way of proceeding, cannot freely effect his will from within her present movement, nor, while standing in the mentality, get outside or above her in such a way as to exercise a really free control. There is a duality of dependence, her dependence on his consent, his dependence on her law and way and limits of action, determination denied by a sense of free-will, free-will nullified by the actuality of natural determination. He is sure that she is his power, but yet he seems to be subject to her. He is the sanctioning (*anumantṛ*) Purusha, but does not seem to be the absolute lord, Ishwara.

Nevertheless, there is somewhere an absolute control, a real Ishwara. He is aware of it and knows that if he can find it, he will enter into control, become not only the passive sanctioning witness and upholding soul of her will, but the free powerful user and determiner of her movements. But this control seems to belong to another poise than the mentality. Sometimes he finds himself using it, but as a channel or instrument; it comes to him from above. It is clear then that it is supramental, a power of the Spirit greater than mental being which he already knows himself to be at the summit and in the secret core of his conscious being. To enter into identity with that Spirit must then be his way to control and lordship. He can do it passively by a sort of reflection and receiving in his mental consciousness, but then he is only a mould, channel or instrument, not a possessor or participant in the power. He can arrive at identity by an absorption of his mentality in inner spiritual being, but then the conscious action ceases in a trance of identity. To be active master of the nature he must evidently rise to some higher supramental poise where there is possible not only a passive, but an active identity with the controlling spirit. To find the way of rising to this greater poise and be self-ruler, Swarat, is a condition of his perfection. The difficulty of the ascent is due to a natural ignorance. He is the Purusha, witness of mental and physical Nature, *sākṣī*, but not a complete knower of self and Nature, *jñātṛ*. Knowledge in the mentality is enlightened by his consciousness; he is the mental knower; but he finds that this is not a real knowledge, but only a partial seeking and partial finding, a derivative uncertain reflection and narrow utilisation for action from a greater light beyond which is the real knowledge. This light is the self-awareness and all-awareness of Spirit. The essential self-awareness he can arrive at even on the mental plane of being, by reflection in the soul of mind or by its absorption in spirit, as indeed it can be arrived at by another kind of reflection or absorption in soul of life and soul of body. But for participation in an effective all-awareness with this essential self-awareness as the soul of its action he must rise to supermind. To be lord of his being, he must be knower of self and Nature, *jñātā īśvaraḥ*. Partially this may be done on a higher level of mind where it responds directly to supermind, but really and completely this perfection belongs not to the mental being, but to the ideal or knowledge Soul, *vijñānamaya puruṣa*. To draw up the mental into the greater knowledge being and that into the Bliss-Self of the spirit, *ānandamaya puruṣa*, is the uttermost way of this perfection.

But no perfection, much less this perfection can be attained without a very radical dealing with the present nature and the abrogation of much that seems to be the fixed law of its complex nexus of mental, vital and physical being. The law of this nexus has been created for a definite and limited end, the temporary maintenance, preservation, possession, aggrandisement, enjoyment, experience, need, action of the mental ego in the living body. Other resultant uses are served, but this is the immediate and fundamentally determining object and utility. To arrive at a higher utility and freer instrumentation this nexus must be partly broken up, exceeded, transformed into a larger harmony of action. The Purusha sees that the law created is that of a partly stable, partly unstable selective determination of habitual, yet developing experiences out of a first confused consciousness of self and not-self, subjective being and external universe. This determination is managed by mind, life and body acting upon each other, in harmony and correspondence, but also in discord and divergence, mutual interference and limitation. There is a similar mixed harmony and discord between various activities of the mind in itself, as also between activities of the life in itself and of the physical being. The whole is a sort of disorderly order, an order evolved and contrived out of a constantly surrounding and invading confusion.

This is the first difficulty the Purusha has to deal with, a mixed and confused action of Nature, — an action without clear self-knowledge, distinct motive, firm instrumentation, only an attempt at these things and a general relative success of effec-tuality, — a surprising effect of adaptation in some directions, but also much distress of inadequacy. That mixed and confused action has to be mended; purification is an essential means towards self-perfection. All these impurities and inadequacies result in various kinds of limitation and bondage: but there are two or three primary knots of the bondage, — ego is the prin-cipal knot, — from which the others derive. These bonds must be got rid of; purification is not complete till it brings about liberation. Besides, after a certain purification and liberation has been effected, there is still the conversion of the purified instruments to the law of a higher object and utility, a large, real and perfect order of action. By the conversion man can arrive at a certain perfection of fullness of being, calm, power and knowledge, even a greater vital action and more perfect physical existence. One result of this perfection is a large and perfected delight of being, Ananda. Thus purification, liberation, perfection, delight of being are four constituent elements of the Yoga, — *śuddhi, mukti, siddhi, bhukti.*

But this perfection cannot be attained or cannot be secure

and entire in its largeness if the Purusha lays stress on individuality. To abandon identification with the physical, vital and mental ego, is not enough; he must arrive in soul also at a true, universalised, not separative individuality. In the lower nature man is an ego making a clean cut in conception between himself and all other existence; the ego is to him self, but all the rest not self, external to his being. His whole action starts from and is founded upon this self-conception and world-conception. But the conception is in fact an error. However sharply he individualises himself in mental idea and mental or other action, he is inseparable from the universal being, his body from universal force and matter, his life from the universal life, his mind from universal mind, his soul and spirit from universal soul and spirit. The universal acts on him, invades him, overcomes him, shapes itself in him at every moment; he in his reaction acts on the universal, invades, tries to impose himself on it, shape it, overcome its attack, rule and use its instrumentation.

This conflict is a rendering of the underlying unity, which assumes the aspect of struggle by a necessity of the original separation; the two pieces into which mind has cut the oneness, rush upon each other to restore the oneness and each tries to seize on and take into itself the separated portion. Universe seems to be always trying to swallow up man, the infinite to resume this finite which stands on its self-defence and even replies by aggression. But in real fact the universal being through this apparent struggle is working out its purpose in man, though the key and truth of the purpose and working is lost to his superficial conscious mind, only held obscurely in an underlying subconscient and only known luminously in an overruling superconscient unity. Man also is impelled towards unity by a constant impulse of extension of his ego, which identifies itself as best it can with other egos and with such portions of the universe as he can physically, vitally, mentally get into his use and possession. As man aims at knowledge and mastery of his own being, so also he aims at knowledge and mastery of the environmental world of nature, its objects, its instrumentation, its beings. First he tries to effect this aim by egoistic possession, but, as he develops, the element of sympathy born of the secret oneness grows in him and he arrives at the idea of a widening cooperation and oneness with other beings, a harmony with universal Nature and universal being.

The witness Purusha in the mind observes that the inadequacy of his effort, all the inadequacy in fact of man's life and nature arises from the separation and the consequent struggle, want of knowledge, want of harmony, want of oneness. It is essential for him to grow out of separative individuality, to universalise himself, to make himself one with the universe. This unification can be done only through the soul by making our soul of mind one with the universal Mind, our soul of life one with the universal Life-soul, our soul of body one with the universal soul of physical Nature. When this can be done, in proportion to the power, intensity, depth, completeness, permanence with which it can be done, great effects are produced upon the natural action. Especially there grows an immediate and profound sympathy and immixture of mind with mind, life with life, a lessening of the body's insistence on separateness, a power of direct mental and other intercommunication and effective mutual action which helps out now the inadequate indirect communication and action that was till now the greater part of the conscious means used by embodied mind. But still the Purusha sees that in mental, vital, physical nature, taken by itself, there is always a defect, inadequacy, confused action, due to the mechanically unequal interplay of the three modes or gunas of Nature. To transcend it he has in the universality too to rise to the supramental and spiritual, to be one with the supramental soul of cosmos, the universal spirit. He arrives at the larger light and order of a higher principle in himself and the universe which is the characteristic action of the divine Sachchidananda. Even, he is able to impose the influence of that light and order, not only on his own natural being, but, within the radius and to the extent of the Spirit's action in him, on the world he lives in, on that which is around him. He is *svarāṭ*, self-knower, self-ruler, but he begins to be also through this spiritual oneness and transcendence *samrāṭ*, a knower and master of his environing world of being.

In this self-development the soul finds that it has accomplished on this line the object of the whole integral Yoga, union with the Supreme in its self and in its universalised individuality. So long as he remains in the world-existence, this perfection must radiate out from him, — for that is the necessity of his oneness with the universe and its beings, — in an influence and action which help all around who are capable of it to rise to or advance towards the same perfection, and for the rest in an influence and action which help, as only the self-ruler and master man can help, in leading the human race forward spiritually towards this consummation and towards some image of a greater divine truth in their personal and communal existence. He becomes a light and power of the Truth to which he has climbed and a means for others' ascension.

Chapter V

The Instruments of the Spirit

IF THERE is to be an active perfection of our being, the first necessity is a purification of the working of the instruments which it now uses for a music of discords. The being itself, the spirit, the divine Reality in man stands in no need of purification; it is for ever pure, not affected by the faults of its instrumentation or the stumblings of mind and heart and body in their work, as the sun, says the Upanishad, is not touched or stained by the faults of the eye of vision. Mind, heart, the soul of vital desire, the life in the body are the seats of impurity; it is they that must be set right if the working of the spirit is to be a perfect working and not marked by its present greater or less concession to the devious pleasure of the lower nature. What is ordinarily called purity of the being, is either a negative whiteness, a freedom from sin gained by a constant inhibition of whatever action, feeling, idea or will we think to be wrong, or else, the highest negative or passive purity, the entire God-content, inaction, the complete stilling of the vibrant mind and the soul of desire, which in quietistic disciplines leads to a supreme peace; for then the spirit appears in all the eternal purity of its immaculate essence. That gained, there would be nothing farther to be enjoyed or done. But here we have the more difficult problem of a total, unabated, even an increased and more powerful action founded on perfect bliss of the being, the purity of the soul's instrumental as well as the spirit's essential nature. Mind, heart, life, body are to do the works of the Divine, all the works which they do now and yet more, but to do them divinely, as now they do not do them. This is the first appearance of the problem before him on which the seeker of perfection has to lay hold, that it is not a negative, prohibitory, passive or quietistic, but a positive, affirmative, active purity which is his object. A divine quietism discovers the immaculate eternity of the Spirit, a divine kinetism adds to it the right pure undeviating action of the soul, mind and body.

Moreover, it is a total purification of all the complex instrumentality in all the parts of each instrument that is demanded of us by the integral perfection. It is not, ultimately, the narrower moral purification of the ethical nature. Ethics deals only with the desire-soul and the active outward dynamical part of our being; its field is confined to character and action. It prohibits and inhibits certain actions, certain desires, impulses, propensities, — it inculcates certain qualities in the act, such as truthfulness, love, charity, compassion, chastity. When it has got this done and assured a base of virtue, the possession of a purified will and blameless habit of action, its work is finished. But the Siddha of the integral perfection has to dwell in a larger plane of the Spirit's eternal purity beyond good and evil. By this phrase it is not meant, as the rash hastily concluding intellect would be prone to imagine, that he will do good and evil indifferently and declare that to the spirit there is no difference between them, which would be in the plane of individual action an obvious untruth and might serve to cover a reckless self-indulgence of the imperfect human nature. Neither is it meant that since good and evil are in this world inextricably entangled together, like pain and pleasure, — a proposition which, however true at the moment and plausible as a generalisation, need not be true of the human being's greater spiritual evolution, — the liberated man will live in the spirit and stand back from the mechanical continued workings of a necessarily imperfect nature. This, however possible as a stage towards a final cessation of all activity, is evidently not a counsel of active perfection. But it is meant that the Siddha of the active integral perfection will live dynamically in the working of the transcendent power of the divine Spirit as a universal will through the supermind individualised in him for action. His works will therefore be the works of an eternal Knowledge, an eternal Truth, an eternal Might, an eternal Love, an eternal Ananda; but the truth, knowledge, force, love, delight will be the whole essential spirit of whatever work he will do and will not depend on its form; they will determine his action from the spirit within and the action will not determine the spirit or subject it to a fixed standard or rigid mould of working. He will have no dominant mere habit of character, but only a spiritual being and will with at the most a free and flexible temperamental mould for the action. His life will be a direct stream from the eternal fountains, not a form cut to some temporary human pattern. His perfection will not be a sattwic purity, but a thing uplifted beyond the gunas of Nature, a perfection of spiritual knowledge, spiritual power, spiritual delight, unity and harmony of unity; the outward perfection of his works will be freely shaped as the self-expression of this inner spiritual transcendence and universality. For this change he must make conscient in him that power of spirit and supermind which is now superconscient to our mentality. But that cannot work in him so long as his present mental, vital, physical being is not liberated from its actual inferior working. This purification is the first necessity.

In other words, purification must not be understood in any limited sense of a selection of certain outward kinetic movements, their regulation, the inhibition of other action or a liberation of certain forms of character or particular mental and moral capacities. These things are secondary signs of our derivative being, not essential powers and first forces. We have to take a wider psychological view of the primary forces of our nature. We have to distinguish the formed parts of our being, find out their basic defect of impurity or wrong action and correct that, sure that the rest will then come right naturally. We have not to doctor symptoms of impurity, or that only secondarily, as a minor help, — but to strike at its roots after a deeper diagnosis. We then find that there are two forms of impurity which are at the root of the whole confusion. One is a defect born of the nature of our past evolution, which has been a nature of separative ignorance; this defect is a radically wrong and ignorant form given to the proper action of each part of our instrumental being. The other impurity is born of the successive process of an evolution, where life emerges in and depends on body, mind emerges in and depends on life in the body, supermind emerges in and lends itself to instead of governing mind, soul itself is apparent only as a circumstance of the bodily life of the mental being and veils up the spirit in the lower imperfections. This second defect of our nature is caused by this dependence of the higher on the lower parts; it is an immixture of functions by which the impure working of the lower instrument gets into the characteristic action of the higher function and gives to it an added imperfection of embarrassment, wrong direction and confusion.

Thus the proper function of the life, the vital force, is enjoyment and possession, both of them perfectly legitimate, because the Spirit created the world for Ananda, enjoyment and possession of the many by the One, of the One by the many and of the many too by the many; but, — this is an instance of the first kind of defect, — the separative ignorance gives to it the wrong form of desire and craving which vitiates the whole enjoyment and possession and imposes on it its opposites, want and suffering. Again, because mind is entangled in life from which it evolves, this desire and craving get into the action of the mental will and knowledge; that makes the will a will of craving, a force of desire instead of a rational will and a discerning force of intelligent effectuation, and it distorts the judgment and reason so that we judge and reason according to our desires and prepossessions and not with the disinterested impartiality of a pure judgment and the rectitude of a reason which seeks only to distinguish truth and understand rightly the objects of its workings. That is an example of immixture. These two kinds of defect, wrong form of action and illegitimate mixture of action, are not limited to these signal instances, but belong to each instrument and to each combination of their functionings. They pervade the whole economy of our nature. They are fundamental defects of our lower instrumental nature, and if we can set them right, we shall get our instrumental being into a state of purity, enjoy the clarity of a pure will, a pure heart of emotion, a pure enjoyment of our vitality, a pure body. That will be a preliminary, a human perfection, but it can be made the basis and open out in its effort of self-attainment into the greater, the divine perfection.

Mind, life and body are the three powers of our lower

nature. But they cannot be taken quite separately because the life acts as a link and gives its character to body and to a great extent to our mentality. Our body is a living body; the life-force mingles in and determines all its functionings. Our mind too is largely a mind of life, a mind of physical sensation; only in its higher functions is it normally capable of something more than the workings of a physical mentality subjected to life. We may put it in this ascending order. We have first a body supported by the physical life-force, the physical prana which courses through the whole nervous system and gives its stamp to our corporeal action, so that all is of the character of the action of a living and not an inert mechanical body. Prana and physicality together make the gross body, *sthūla śarīra*. This is only the outer instrument, the nervous force of life acting in the form of body with its gross physical organs. Then there is the inner instrument, *antaḥkaraṇa*, the conscious mentality. This inner instrument is divided by the old system into four powers; *citta* or basic mental consciousness; *manas*, the sense mind; *buddhi*, the intelligence; *ahaṅkāra*, the ego-idea. The classification may serve as a starting-point, though for a greater practicality we have to make certain farther distinctions. This mentality is pervaded by the life-force, which becomes here an instrument for psychic consciousness of life and psychic action on life. Every fibre of the sense mind and basic consciousness is shot through with the action of this psychic prana, it is a nervous or vital and physical mentality. Even the buddhi and ego are overpowered by it, although they have the capacity of raising the mind beyond subjection to this vital, nervous and physical psychology. This combination creates in us the sensational desire-soul which is the chief obstacle to a higher human as well as to the still greater divine perfection. Finally, above our present conscious mentality is a secret supermind which is the proper means and native seat of that perfection.

Chitta, the basic consciousness, is largely subconscient; it has, open and hidden, two kinds of action, one passive or receptive, the other active or reactive and formative. As a passive power it receives all impacts, even those of which the mind is unaware or to which it is inattentive, and it stores them in an immense reserve of passive subconscient memory on which the mind as an active memory can draw. But ordinarily the mind draws only what it had observed and understood at the time, — more easily what it had observed well and understood carefully, less easily what it had observed carelessly or ill understood; at the same time there is a power in consciousness to send up to the active mind for use what that mind had not at all observed or attended to or even consciously experienced. This power only acts observably in abnormal conditions, when some part of the subconscious chitta comes as it were to the surface or when the subliminal being in us appears on the threshold and for a time plays some part in the outer chamber of mentality where the direct intercourse and commerce with the external world takes place and our inner dealings with ourselves develop on the surface. This action of memory is so fundamental to the entire mental action that it is sometimes said, memory is the man. Even in the submental action of the body and life, which is full of this subconscient chitta, though not under the control of the conscious mind, there is a vital and physical memory. The vital and physical habits are largely formed by this submental memory. For this reason they can be changed to an indefinite extent by a more powerful action of conscious mind and will, when that can be developed and can find means to communicate to the subconscient chitta the will of the spirit for a new law of vital and physical action. Even, the whole constitution of our life and body may be described as a bundle of habits formed by the past evolution in Nature and held together by the persistent memory of this secret consciousness. For chitta, the primary stuff of consciousness, is like prana and body universal in Nature, but is subconscient and mechanical in nature of Matter.

But in fact all action of the mind or inner instrument arises out of this chitta or basic consciousness, partly conscient, partly subconscient or subliminal to our active mentality. When it is struck by the world's impacts from outside or urged by the reflective powers of the subjective inner being, it throws up certain habitual activities, the mould of which has been determined by our evolution. One of these forms of activity is the emotional mind, — the heart, as we may call it for the sake of a convenient brevity. Our emotions are the waves of reaction and response which rise up from the basic consciousness, *citta-vṛtti*. Their action too is largely regulated by habit and an emotive memory. They are not imperative, not laws of Necessity; there is no really binding law of our emotional being to which we must submit without remedy; we are not obliged to give responses of grief to certain impacts upon the mind, responses of anger to others, to yet others responses of hatred or dislike, to others responses of liking or love. All these things are only habits of our affective mentality; they can be changed by the conscious will of the spirit; they can be inhibited; we may even rise entirely above all subjection to grief, anger, hatred, the duality of liking and disliking. We are subject to these things only so long as we persist in subjection to the mechanical action of the chitta in the emotive mentality, a thing difficult to get rid of because of the power of past habit and especially the importunate insistence of the vital part of mentality, the nervous life-mind or psychic prana. This nature of the emotive mind as a reaction of chitta with a certain close dependence upon the nervous life sensations and the responses of the psychic prana is so characteristic that in some languages it is called chitta and prana, the heart, the life soul; it is indeed the most directly agitating and powerfully insistent action of the desire-soul which the immixture of vital desire and responsive consciousness has created in us. And yet the true emotive soul, the real psyche in us, is not a desire-soul, but a soul of pure love and delight; but that, like the rest of our true being, can only emerge when the deformation created by the life of desire is removed from the surface and is no longer the characteristic action of our being. To get that done is a necessary part of our purification, liberation, perfection.

The nervous action of the psychic prana is most obvious in our purely sensational mentality. This nervous mentality pursues indeed all the action of the inner instrument and seems often to form the greater part of things other than sensation. The emotions are especially assailed and have the pranic stamp; fear is more even of a nervous sensation than an emotion, anger is largely or often a sensational response translated into terms of emotion. Other feelings are more of the heart, more inward, but they ally themselves to the nervous and physical longings or outward-going impulses of the psychic prana. Love is an emotion of the heart and may be a pure feeling, — all mentality, since we are embodied minds, must produce, even thought produces, some kind of life effect and some response in the stuff of body, but they need not for that reason be of a physical nature, — but the heart's love allies itself readily with a vital desire in the body. This physical element may be purified of that subjection to physical desire which is called lust, it may become love using the body for a physical as well as a mental and spiritual nearness; but love may, too, separate itself from all, even the most innocent physical element, or from all but a shadow of it, and be a pure movement to union of soul with soul, psyche with psyche. Still the proper action of the sensational mind is not emotion, but conscious nervous response and nervous feeling and affection, impulse of the use of physical sense and body for some action, conscious vital craving and desire. There is a side of receptive response, a side of dynamic reaction. These things get their proper normal use when the higher mind is not mechanically subject to them, but controls and regulates their action. But a still higher state is when they undergo a certain transformation by the conscious will of the spirit which gives its right and no longer its wrong or desire form of characteristic action to the psychic prana.

Manas, the sense mind, depends in our ordinary consciousness on the physical organs of receptive sense for knowledge and on the organs of the body for action directed towards the objects of sense. The superficial and outward action of the senses is physical and nervous in its character, and they may easily be thought to be merely results of nerve-action; they are sometimes called in the old books *prānas*, nervous or life activities. But still the essential thing in them is not the nervous excitation, but the consciousness, the action of the chitta, which makes use of the organ and of the nervous impact of which it is the channel. Manas, sense-mind, is the activity, emerging from the basic consciousness, which makes up the whole essentiality of what we call sense. Sight, hearing, taste, smell, touch are really properties of the mind, not of the body; but the physical mind which we ordinarily use, limits itself to a translation into sense of so much of the outer impacts as it receives through the nervous system and the physical organs. But the inner Manas has also a subtle sight, hearing, power of contact of its own which is not dependent on the physical organs. And it has, moreover, a power not only of direct communication of mind with object — leading even at a high pitch of action to a sense of the contents of an object within or beyond the physical range, — but direct communication also of mind with mind. Mind is able too to alter, modify, inhibit the incidence, values, intensities of sense impacts. These powers of the mind we do not ordinarily use or develop; they remain subliminal and emerge sometimes in an irregular and fitful action, more readily in some minds than in others, or come to the surface in abnormal states of the being. They are the basis of clairvoyance, clairaudience, transference of thought and impulse, telepathy, most of the more ordinary kinds of occult powers, — so called, though these are better described less mystically as powers of the now subliminal action of the Manas. The phenomena of hypnotism and many others depend upon the action of this subliminal sense-mind; not that it alone constitutes all the elements of the phenomena, but it is the first supporting means of intercourse, communication and response, though much of the actual operation belongs to an inner Buddhi. Mind physical, mind supraphysical, — we have and can use this double sense mentality.

Buddhi is a construction of conscious being which quite exceeds its beginnings in the basic chitta; it is the intelligence with its power of knowledge and will. Buddhi takes up and deals with all the rest of the action of the mind and life and body. It is in its nature thought-power and will-power of the Spirit turned into the lower form of a mental activity. We may distinguish three successive gradations of the action of this intelligence. There is first an inferior perceptive understanding which simply takes up, records, understands and responds to the communications of the sense-mind, memory, heart and sensational mentality. It creates by their means an elementary thinking mind which does not go beyond their data, but subjects itself to their mould and rings out their repetitions, runs round and round in the habitual circle of thought and will suggested by them or follows, with an obedient subservience of the reason to the suggestions of life, any fresh determinations which may be offered to its perception and conception. Beyond this elementary understanding, which we all use to an enormous extent, there is a power of arranging or selecting reason and will-force of the intelligence which has for its action and aim an attempt to arrive at a plausible, sufficient, settled ordering of knowledge and will for the use of an intellectual conception of life.

In spite of its more purely intellectual character this secondary or intermediate reason is really pragmatic in its intention. It creates a certain kind of intellectual structure, frame, rule into which it tries to cast the inner and outer life so as to use it with a certain mastery and government for the purposes of some kind of rational will. It is this reason which gives to our normal intellectual being our set aesthetic and ethical standards, our structures of opinion and our established norms of idea and purpose. It is highly developed and takes the primacy in all men of an at all developed understanding. But beyond it there is a reason, a highest action of the buddhi which concerns itself disinterestedly with a pursuit of pure truth and right knowledge; it seeks to discover the real Truth behind life and things and our apparent selves and to subject its will to the law of Truth. Few, if any of us, can use this highest reason with any purity, but the attempt to do it is the topmost capacity of the inner instrument, the *antaḥkaraṇa*.

Buddhi is really an intermediary between a much higher Truth-mind not now in our active possession, which is the direct instrument of Spirit, and the physical life of the human mind evolved in body. Its powers of intelligence and will are drawn from this greater direct Truth-mind or supermind. Buddhi centres its mental action round the ego-idea, the idea that I am this mind, life and body or am a mental being determined by their action. It serves this ego-idea whether limited by what we call egoism or extended by sympathy with the life around us. An ego-sense is created which reposes on the separate action of the body, of the individualised life, of the mind-responses, and the ego-idea in the buddhi centralises the whole action of this ego's thought, character, personality. The lower understanding and the intermediary reason are instruments of its desire of experience and self-enlargement. But when the highest reason and will develop, we can turn towards that which these outward things mean to the higher spiritual consciousness. The "I" can then be seen as a mental reflection of the Self, the Spirit, the Divine, the one existence transcendent, universal, individual in its multiplicity; the consciousness in which these things meet, become aspects of one being and assume their right relations, can then be unveiled out of all these physical and mental coverings. When the transition to supermind takes place, the powers of the Buddhi do not perish, but have all to be converted to their supramental values. But the consideration of the supermind and the conversion of the buddhi belongs to the question of the higher siddhi or divine perfection. At present we have to consider the purification of the normal being of man, preparatory to any such conversion, which leads to the liberation from the bonds of our lower nature.

Chapter VI

Purification — The Lower Mentality

WE HAVE to deal with the complex action of all these instruments and set about their purification. And the simplest way will be to fasten on the two kinds of radical defect in each, distinguish clearly in what they consist and set them right. But there is also the question where we are to begin. For the entanglement is great, the complete purification of one instrument depends on the complete purification too of all the others, and that is a great source of difficulty, disappointment and perplexity, — as when we think we have got the intelligence purified, only to find that it is still subject to attack and overclouding because the emotions of the heart and the will and sensational mind are still affected by the many impurities of the lower nature and they get back into the enlightened buddhi and prevent it from reflecting the pure truth for which we are seeking. But we have on the other hand this advantage that one important instrument sufficiently purified can be used as a means for the purification of the others, one step firmly taken makes easier all the others and gets rid of a host of difficulties. Which instrument then by its purification and perfection will bring about most easily and effectively or can aid with a most powerful rapidity the perfection of the rest?

Since we are the spirit enveloped in mind, a soul evolved here as a mental being in a living physical body, it must naturally be in the mind, the *antaḥkaraṇa*, that we must look for this desideratum. And in the mind it is evidently by the buddhi, the intelligence and the will of the intelligence that the human being is intended to do whatever work is not done for him by the physical or nervous nature as in the plant and the animal. Pending the evolution of any higher supramental power the intelligent will must be our main force for effectuation and to purify it becomes a very primary necessity. Once our intelligence and will are well purified of all that limits them and gives them a wrong action or wrong direction, they can easily be perfected, can be made to respond to the suggestions of Truth, understand themselves and the rest of the being, see clearly and with a fine and scrupulous accuracy what they are doing and follow out the right way to do it without any hesitating or eager error or stumbling deviation. Eventually their response can be opened up to the perfect discernings, intuitions, inspirations, revelations of the supermind and proceed by a more and more luminous and even infallible action. But this purification cannot be effected without a preliminary clearing of its natural obstacles in the other lower parts of the *antaḥkaraṇa*, and the chief natural obstacle running through the whole action of the *antaḥkaraṇa*, through the sense, the mental sensation, emotion, dynamic impulse, intelligence, will, is the intermiscence and the compelling claim of the psychic prana. This then must be dealt with, its dominating intermiscence ruled out, its claim denied, itself quieted and prepared for purification.

Each instrument has, it has been said, a proper and legitimate action and also a deformation or wrong principle of its proper action. The proper action of the psychic prana is pure possession and enjoyment, *bhoga*. To enjoy thought, will, action, dynamic impulse, result of action, emotion, sense, sensation, to enjoy too by their means objects, persons, life, the world, is the activity for which this prana gives us a psycho-physical basis. A really perfect enjoyment of existence can only come when what we enjoy is not the world in itself or for itself, but God in the world, when it is not things, but the Ananda of the spirit in things that forms the real, essential object of our enjoying and things only as form and symbol of the spirit, waves of the ocean of Ananda. But this Ananda can only come at all when we can get at and reflect in our members the hidden spiritual being, and its fullness can only be had when we climb to the supramental ranges. Meanwhile there is a just and permissible, a quite legitimate human enjoyment of these things, which is, to speak in the language of Indian psychology, predominantly sattwic in its nature. It is an enlightened enjoyment principally by the perceptive, aesthetic and emotive mind, secondarily only by the sensational, nervous and physical being, but all subject to the clear government of the buddhi, to a right reason, a right will, a right reception of the life impacts, a right order, a right feeling of the truth, law, ideal sense, beauty, use of things. The mind gets the pure taste of enjoyment of them, *rasa*, and rejects whatever is perturbed, troubled and perverse. Into this acceptance of the clear and limpid *rasa*, the psychic prana has to bring in the full sense of life and the occupying enjoyment by the whole being, *bhoga*, without which the acceptance and possession by the mind, *rasa-grahaṇa*, would not be concrete enough, would be too tenuous to satisfy altogether the embodied soul. This contribution is its proper function.

The deformation which enters in and prevents the purity, is a form of vital craving; the grand deformation which the psychic prana contributes to our being, is desire. The root of desire is the vital craving to seize upon that which we feel we have not, it is the limited life's instinct for possession and satisfaction. It creates the sense of want, — first the simpler vital craving of hunger, thirst, lust, then these psychical hungers, thirsts, lusts of the mind which are a much greater and more instant and pervading affliction of our being, the hunger which is infinite because it is the hunger of an infinite being, the thirst which is only temporarily lulled by satisfaction, but is in its nature insatiable. The psychic prana invades the sensational mind and brings into it the unquiet thirst of sensations, invades the dynamic mind with the lust of control, having, domination, success, fulfilment of every impulse, fills the emotional mind with the desire for the satisfaction of liking and disliking, for the wreaking of love and hate, brings the shrinkings and panics of fear and the strainings and disappointments of hope, imposes the tortures of grief and the brief fevers and excitements of joy, makes the intelligence and intelligent will the accomplices of all these things and turns them in their own kind into deformed and lame instruments, the will into a will of craving and the intelligence into a partial, a stumbling and an eager pursuer of limited, impatient, militant prejudgment and opinion. Desire is the root of all sorrow, disappointment, affliction, for though it has a feverish joy of pursuit and satisfaction, yet because it is always a straining of the being, it carries into its pursuit and its getting a labour, hunger, struggle, a rapid subjection to fatigue, a sense of limitation, dissatisfaction and early disappointment with all its gains, a ceaseless morbid stimulation, trouble, disquiet, *aśānti*. To get rid of desire is the one firm indispensable purification of the psychical prana, — for so we can replace the soul of desire with its pervading immiscence in all our instruments by a mental soul of calm delight and its clear and limpid possession of ourselves and world and Nature which is the crystal basis of the mental life and its perfection.

The psychical prana interferes in all the higher operations to deform them, but its defect is itself due to its being interfered with and deformed by the nature of the physical workings in the body which Life has evolved in its emergence from matter. It is that which has created the separation of the individual life in the body from the life of the universe and stamped on it the character of want, limitation, hunger, thirst, craving for what it has not, a long groping after enjoyment and a hampered and baffled need of possession. Easily regulated and limited in the purely physical order of things, it extends itself in the psychical prana immensely and becomes, as the mind grows, a thing with difficulty limited, insatiable, irregular, a busy creator of disorder and disease. Moreover, the psychical prana leans on the physical life, limits itself by the nervous force of the physical being, limits thereby the operations of the mind and becomes the link of its dependence on the body and its subjection to fatigue, incapacity, disease, disorder, insanity, the pettiness, the precariousness and even the possible dissolution of the workings of the physical mentality. Our mind instead of being a thing powerful in its own strength, a clear instrument of conscious spirit, free and able to control, use and perfect the life and body, appears in the result a mixed construction; it is a predominantly physical mentality limited by its physical organs and subject to the demands and to the obstructions of the life in the body. This can only be got rid of by a sort of practical, inward psychological operation of analysis by which we become aware of the mentality as a separate power, isolate it for a free working, distinguish too the psychical and the physical prana and make them no longer a link for dependence, but a transmitting channel for the Idea and Will in the buddhi, obedient to its suggestions and commands; the prana then becomes a passive means of effectuation for the mind's direct control of the physical life. This control, however abnormal to our habitual poise of action, is not only possible, — it appears to some extent in the phenomena of hypnosis, though these are unhealthily abnormal, because there it is a foreign will which suggests and commands, — but must become the normal action when the higher Self within takes up the direct command of the whole being. This control can be exercised perfectly, however, only from the supramental level, for it is there that the true effective Idea and Will reside and the mental thought-mind, even spiritualised, is only a limited, though it may be made a very powerful deputy.

Desire, it is thought, is the real motive power of human living and to cast it out would be to stop the springs of life; satisfaction of desire is man's only enjoyment and to eliminate it would be to extinguish the impulse of life by a quietistic asceticism. But the real motive power of the life of the soul is Will; desire is only a deformation of will in the dominant bodily life and physical mind. The essential turn of the soul to possession and enjoyment of the world consists in a will to delight, and the enjoyment of the satisfaction of craving is only a vital and physical degradation of the will to delight. It is essential that we should distinguish between pure will and desire, between the inner will to delight and the outer lust and craving of the mind and body. If we are unable to make this distinction practically in the experience of our being, we can only make a choice between a life-killing asceticism and the gross will to live or else try to effect an awkward, uncertain and precarious compromise between them. This is in fact what the mass of men do; a small minority trample down the life instinct and strain after an ascetic perfection; most obey the gross will to live with such modifications and restraints as society imposes or the normal social man has been trained to impose on his own mind and actions;

others set up a balance between ethical austerity and temperate indulgence of the desiring mental and vital self and see in this balance the golden mean of a sane mind and healthy human living. But none of these ways gives the perfection which we are seeking, the divine government of the will in life. To tread down altogether the prana, the vital being, is to kill the force of life by which the large action of the embodied soul in the human being must be supported; to indulge the gross will to live is to remain satisfied with imperfection; to compromise between them is to stop half way and possess neither earth nor heaven. But if we can get at the pure will undeformed by desire, — which we shall find to be a much more free, tranquil, steady and effective force than the leaping, smoke-stifled, soon fatigued and baffled flame of desire, — and at the calm inner will of delight not afflicted or limited by any trouble of craving, we can then transform the prana from a tyrant, enemy, assailant of the mind into an obedient instrument. We may call these greater things, too, by the name of desire, if we choose, but then we must suppose that there is a divine desire other than the vital craving, a God-desire of which this other and lower phenomenon is an obscure shadow and into which it has to be transfigured. It is better to keep distinct names for things which are entirely different in their character and inner action.

To rid the prana of desire and incidentally to reverse the ordinary poise of our nature and turn the vital being from a troublesomely dominant power into the obedient instrument of a free and unattached mind, is then the first step in purification. As this deformation of the psychical prana is corrected, the purification of the rest of the intermediary parts of the *antaḥkaraṇa* is facilitated, and when that correction is completed, their purification too can be easily made absolute. These intermediary parts are the emotional mind, the receptive sensational mind and the active sensational mind or mind of dynamic impulse. They all hang together in a strongly knotted interaction. The deformation of the emotional mind hinges upon the duality of liking and disliking, *rāga-dveṣa*, emotional attraction and repulsion. All the complexity of our emotions and their tyranny over the soul arise from the habitual responses of the soul of desire in the emotions and sensations to these attractions and repulsions. Love and hatred, hope and fear, grief and joy all have their founts in this one source. We like, love, welcome, hope for, joy in whatever our nature, the first habit of our being, or else a formed (often perverse) habit, the second nature of our being, presents to the mind as pleasant, *priyam*; we hate, dislike, fear, have repulsion from or grief of whatever it presents to us as unpleasant, *apriyam*. This habit of the emotional nature gets into the way of the intelligent will and makes it often a helpless slave of the emotional being or at least prevents it from exercising a free judgment and government of the nature. This deformation has to be corrected. By getting rid of desire in the psychic prana and its intermiscence in the emotional mind, we facilitate the correction. For then attachment which is the strong bond of the heart, falls away from the heart-strings; the involuntary habit of *rāga-dveṣa* remains, but, not being made obstinate by attachment, it can be dealt with more easily by the will and the intelligence. The restless heart can be conquered and get rid of the habit of attraction and repulsion.

But then if this is done, it may be thought, as with regard to desire, that this will be the death of the emotional being. It will certainly be so, if the deformation is eliminated but not replaced by the right action of the emotional mind; the mind will then pass into a neutral condition of blank indifference or into a luminous state of peaceful impartiality with no stir or wave of emotion. The former state is in no way desirable; the latter may be the perfection of a quietistic discipline, but in the integral perfection which does not reject love or shun various movement of delight, it can be no more than a stage which has to be overpassed, a preliminary passivity admitted as a first basis for a right activity. Attraction and repulsion, liking and disliking are a necessary mechanism for the normal man, they form a first principle of natural instinctive selection among the thousand flattering and formidable, helpful and dangerous impacts of the world around him. The buddhi starts with this material to work on and tries to correct the natural and instinctive by a wiser reasoned and willed selection; for obviously the pleasant is not always the right thing, the object to be preferred and selected, nor the unpleasant the wrong thing, the object to be shunned and rejected; the pleasant and the good, *preyas* and *śreyas*, have to be distinguished, and right reason has to choose and not the caprice of emotion. But this it can do much better when the emotional suggestion is withdrawn and the heart rests in a luminous passivity. Then too the right activity of the heart can be brought to the surface; for we find then that behind this emotion-ridden soul of desire there was waiting all the while a soul of love and lucid joy and delight, a pure psyche, which was clouded over by the deformations of anger, fear, hatred, repulsion and could not embrace the world with an impartial love and joy. But the purified heart is rid of anger, rid of fear, rid of hatred, rid of every shrinking and repulsion: it has a universal love, it can receive with an untroubled sweetness and clarity the various delight which God gives it in the world. But it is not the lax slave of love and delight; it does not desire, does not attempt to impose itself as the master of the actions. The selective process necessary to action is left principally to the buddhi and, when the buddhi has been overpassed, to the spirit in the supramental will, knowledge and Ananda.

The receptive sensational mind is the nervous mental basis of the affections; it receives mentally the impacts of things and gives to them the responses of mental pleasure and pain which are the starting-point of the duality of emotional liking and disliking. All the heart's emotions have a corresponding nervous-mental accompaniment, and we often find that when the heart is freed of any will to the dualities, there still survives a root of disturbance of nervous mind, or a memory in physical mind which falls more and more away to a quite physical character, the more it is repelled by the will in the buddhi. It becomes finally a mere suggestion from outside to which the nervous chords of the mind still occasionally respond until a complete purity liberates them into the same luminous universality of delight which the pure heart already possesses. The active dynamic mind of impulse is the lower organ or channel of responsive action; its deformation is a subjection to the suggestions of the impure emotional and sensational mentality and the desire of the prana, to impulses to action dictated by grief, fear, hatred, desire, lust, craving, and the rest of the unquiet brood. Its right form of action is a pure dynamic force of strength, courage, temperamental power, not acting for itself or in obedience to the lower members, but as an impartial channel for the dictates of the pure intelligence and will or the supramental Purusha. When we have got rid of these deformations and cleared the mentality for these truer forms of action, the lower mentality is purified and ready for perfection. But that perfection depends on the possession of a purified and enlightened buddhi; for the buddhi is the chief power in the mental being and the chief mental instrument of the Purusha.

Chapter VII

Purification — Intelligence and Will

TO PURIFY the buddhi we must first understand its rather complex composition. And first we have to make clear the distinction, ignored in ordinary speech, between the *manas*, mind, and *buddhi*, the discerning intelligence and the enlightened will. Manas is the sense mind. Man's initial mentality is not at all a thing of reason and will; it is an animal, physical or sense mentality which constitutes its whole experience from the impressions made on it by the external world and by its own embodied consciousness which responds to the outward stimulus of this kind of experience. The buddhi only comes in as a secondary power which has in the evolution taken the first place, but is still dependent on the inferior instrument it uses; it depends for its workings on the sense mind and does what it can on its own higher range by a difficult, elaborate and rather stumbling extension of knowledge and action from the physical or sense basis. A half-enlightened physical or sense mentality is the ordinary type of the mind of man.

In fact the manas is a development from the external chitta; it is a first organising of the crude stuff of the consciousness excited and aroused by external contacts, *bāhya-sparśa*. What we are physically is a soul asleep in matter which has evolved to the partial wakefulness of a living body pervaded by a crude stuff of external consciousness more or less alive and attentive to the outward impacts of the external world in which we are developing our conscious being. In the animal this stuff of externalised consciousness organises itself into a well-regulated mental sense or organ of perceiving and acting mind. Sense is in fact the mental contact of the embodied consciousness with its surroundings. This contact is always essentially a mental phenomenon; but in fact it depends chiefly upon the development of certain physical organs of contact with objects and with their properties to whose images it is able by habit to give their mental values. What we call the physical senses have a double element, the physical-nervous impression of the object and the mental-nervous value we give to it, and the two together make up our seeing, hearing, smell, taste, touch with all those varieties of sensation of which they, and the touch chiefly, are the starting-point or first transmitting agency. But the manas is able to receive sense impressions and draw results from them by a direct transmission not dependent on the physical organ. This is more distinct in the lower creation. Man, though he has really a greater capacity for this direct sense, the sixth sense in the mind, has let it fall into abeyance by an exclusive reliance on the physical senses supplemented by the activity of the buddhi.

The manas is therefore in the first place an organiser of sense experience; in addition it organises the natural reactions of the will in the embodied consciousness and uses the body as an instrument, uses, as it is ordinarily put, the organs of action. This natural action too has a double element, a physico-nervous impulse and behind it a mental-nervous power-value of instinctive will-impulse. That makes up the nexus of first perceptions and actions which is common to all developing animal life. But in addition there is in the manas or sense-mind a first resulting thought-element which accompanies the operations of animal life. Just as the living body has a certain pervading and possessing action of consciousness, *citta*, which forms into this sense-mind, so the sense-mind has in it a certain pervading and possessing power which mentally uses the sense data, turns them into perceptions and first ideas, associates experience with other experiences, and in some way or other thinks and feels and wills on the sense basis.

This sensational thought-mind which is based upon sense, memory, association, first ideas and resultant generalisations or secondary ideas, is common to all developed animal life and mentality. Man indeed has given it an immense development and range and complexity impossible to the animal, but still, if he stopped there, he would only be a more highly effective animal. He gets beyond the animal range and height because he has been able to disengage and separate to a greater or less extent his thought action from the sense mentality, to draw back from the latter and observe its data and to act on it from above by a separated and partially freed intelligence. The intelligence and will of the animal are involved in the sense-mind and therefore altogether governed by it and carried on its stream of sensations, sense-perceptions, impulses; it is instinctive. Man is able to use a reason and will, a self-observing, thinking and all-observing, an intelligently willing mind which is no longer involved in the sense-mind, but acts from above and behind it in its own right, with a certain separateness and freedom. He is reflective, has a certain relative freedom of intelligent will. He has liberated in himself and has formed into a separate power the buddhi.

But what is this buddhi? From the point of view of Yogic knowledge we may say that it is that instrument of the soul, of the inner conscious being in nature, of the Purusha, by which it comes into some kind of conscious and ordered possession both of itself and its surroundings. Behind all the action of the chitta and manas there is this soul, this Purusha; but in the lower forms of life it is mostly subconscient, asleep or half-awake, absorbed in the mechanical action of Nature; but it becomes more and more awake and comes more and more forward as it rises in the scale of life. By the activity of the buddhi it begins the process of an entire awakening. In the lower actions of the mind the soul suffers Nature rather than possesses her; for it is there entirely a slave to the mechanism which has brought it into conscious embodied experience. But in the buddhi we get to something, still a natural instrumentation, by which yet Nature seems to be helping and arming the Purusha to understand, possess and master her.

Neither understanding, possession nor mastery is complete, either because the buddhi in us is itself still incomplete, only yet half developed and half formed, or because it is in its nature only an intermediary instrument and before we can get complete knowledge and mastery, we must rise to something greater than the buddhi. Still it is a movement by which we come to the knowledge that there is a power within us greater than the animal life, a truth greater than the first truths or appearances perceived by the sense-mind, and can try to get at that truth and to labour towards a greater and more successful power of action and control, a more effective government both of our own nature and the nature of things around us, a higher knowledge, a higher power, a higher and larger enjoyment, a more exalted range of being. What then is the final object of this trend? Evidently, it must be for the Purusha to get to the highest and fullest truth of itself and of things, greatest truth of soul or self and greatest truth of Nature, and to an action and a status of being which shall be the result of or identical with that Truth, the power of this greatest knowledge and the enjoyment of that greatest being and consciousness to which it opens. This must be the final result of the evolution of the conscious being in Nature.

To arrive then at the whole truth of our self and Spirit and the knowledge, greatness, bliss of our free and complete being must be the object of the purification, liberation and perfection of the buddhi. But it is a common idea that this means not the full possession of Nature by the Purusha, but a rejection of Nature. We are to get at self by the removal of the action of Prakriti. As the buddhi, coming to the knowledge that the sense-mind only gives us appearances in which the soul is subject to Nature, discovers more real truths behind them, the soul must arrive at this knowledge that the buddhi too, when turned upon Nature, can give us only appearances and enlarge the subjection, and must discover behind them the pure truth of the Self. The Self is something quite other than Nature and the buddhi must purify itself of attachment to and preoccupation with natural things; so only can it discern and separate from them the pure Self and Spirit: the knowledge of the pure Self and Spirit is the only real knowledge, Ananda of the pure Self and Spirit is the only spiritual enjoyment, the consciousness and being of the pure Self and Spirit are the only real consciousness and being. Action and will must cease because all action is of the Nature; the will to be pure Self and Spirit means the cessation of all will to action.

But while the possession of the being, consciousness, delight, power of the Self is the condition of perfection, — for it is only by knowing and possessing and living in the truth of itself that the soul can become free and perfect, — we hold that Nature is an eternal action and manifestation of the Spirit; Nature is not a devil's trap, a set of misleading appearances created by desire, sense, life and mental will and intelligence, but these phenomena are hints and indications and behind all of them is a truth of Spirit which exceeds and uses them. We hold that there must be an inherent spiritual gnosis and will by which the secret Spirit in all knows its own truth, wills, manifests and governs its own being in Nature; to arrive at that, at communion with it or participation in it, must be part of our perfection. The object of the purification of the buddhi will then be to arrive at the possession of our own truth of self-being, but also at the possession of the highest truth of our being in Nature. For that purpose we must first purify the buddhi of all that makes it subject to the sense-mind and, that once done, purify it from its own limitations and convert its inferior mental intelligence and will into the greater action of a spiritual will and knowledge.

The movement of the buddhi to exceed the limits of the sense-mind is an effort already half accomplished in the human evolution; it is part of the common operation of Nature in man. The original action of the thought-mind, the intelligence and will in man, is a subject action. It accepts the evidence of the senses, the commands of the life-cravings, instincts, desires, emotions, the impulses of the dynamic sense-mind and only tries to give them a more orderly direction and effective success. But the man whose reason and will are led and dominated by the lower mind, is an inferior type of human nature, and the part of our conscious being which consents to this domination is the lowest part of our manhood. The higher action of the buddhi is to exceed and control the lower mind, not indeed to get rid of it, but to raise all the action of which it is the first suggestion into the nobler plane of will and intelligence. The impressions of the sense-mind are used by a thought which exceeds them and which arrives at truths they do not give, ideative truths of thought, truths of philosophy and science; a thinking, discovering, philo- sophic mind overcomes, rectifies and dominates the first mind of sense impressions. The impulsive reactive sensational mentality, the life-cravings and the mind of emotional desire are taken up by the intelligent will and are overcome, are rectified and dominated by a greater ethical mind which discovers and sets over them a law of right impulse, right desire, right emotion and right action. The receptive, crudely enjoying sensational mentality, the emotional mind and life mind are taken up by the intelligence and are overcome, rectified and dominated by a deeper, happier aesthetic mind which discovers and sets above them a law of true delight and beauty. All these new formations are used by a general Power of the intellectual, thinking and willing man in a soul of governing intellect, imagination, judgment, memory, volition, discerning reason and ideal feeling which uses them for knowledge, self-development, experience, discovery, creation, effectuation, aspires, strives, inwardly attains, endeavours to make a higher thing of the life of the soul in Nature. The primitive desire-soul no longer governs the being. It is still a desire-soul, but it is repressed and governed by a higher power, something which has manifested in itself the godheads of Truth, Will, Good, Beauty and tries to subject life to them. The crude desire-soul and mind is trying to convert itself into an ideal soul and mind, and the proportion in which some effect and harmony of this greater conscious being has been found and enthroned, is the measure of our increasing humanity.

But this is still a very incomplete movement. We find that it progresses towards a greater completeness in proportion as we arrive at two kinds of perfection; first, a greater and greater detachment from the control of the lower suggestions; secondly, an increasing discovery of a self-existent Being, Light, Power and Ananda which surpasses and transforms the normal humanity. The ethical mind becomes perfect in proportion as it detaches itself from desire, sense suggestion, impulse, customary dictated action and discovers a self of Right, Love, Strength and Purity in which it can live accomplished and make it the foundation of all its actions. The aesthetic mind is perfected in proportion as it detaches itself from all its cruder pleasures and from outward conventional canons of the aesthetic reason and discovers a self-existent self and spirit of pure and infinite Beauty and Delight which gives its own light and joy to the material of the aesthesis. The mind of knowledge is perfected when it gets away from impression and dogma and opinion and discovers a light of self-knowledge and intuition which illumines all the workings of the sense and reason, all self-experience and world-experience. The will is perfected when it gets away from and behind its impulses and its customary ruts of effectuation and discovers an inner power of the Spirit which is the source of an intuitive and luminous action and an original harmonious creation. The movement of perfection is away from all domination by the lower nature and towards a pure and powerful reflection of the being, power, knowledge and delight of the Spirit and Self in the buddhi.

The Yoga of self-perfection is to make this double movement as absolute as possible. All immiscence of desire in the buddhi is an impurity. The intelligence coloured by desire is an impure intelligence and it distorts Truth; the will coloured by desire is an impure will and it puts a stamp of distortion, pain and imperfection upon the soul's activity. All immiscence of the emotions of the soul of desire is an impurity and similarly distorts both the knowledge and the action. All subjection of the buddhi to the sensations and impulses is an impurity. The thought and will have to stand back detached from desire, troubling emotion, distracting or mastering impulse and to act in their own right until they can discover a greater guide, a Will, Tapas or divine Shakti which will take the place of desire and mental will and impulse, an Ananda or pure delight of the spirit and an illumined spiritual knowledge which will express themselves in the action of that Shakti. This complete detachment, impossible without an entire self-government, equality, calm, *śama*, *samatā*, *śānti*, is the surest step towards the purification of the buddhi. A calm, equal and detached mind can alone reflect the peace or base the action of the liberated spirit.

The buddhi itself is burdened with a mixed and impure action. When we reduce it to its own proper forms, we find that it has three stages or elevations of its functioning. First, its lowest basis is a habitual, customary action which is a link between the higher reason and the sense-mind, a kind of current understanding. This understanding is in itself dependent on the witness of the senses and the rule of action which the reason deduces from the sense-mind's perception of and attitude to life. It is not capable of itself forming pure thought and will, but it takes the workings of the higher reason and turns them into coin of opinion and customary standard of thought or canon of action. When we perform a sort of practical analysis of the thinking mind, cut away this element and hold back the higher reason free, observing and silent, we find that this current understanding begins to run about in a futile circle, repeating all its formed opinions and responses to the impressions of things, but incapable of any strong adaptation and initiation. As it feels more and more the refusal of sanction from the higher reason, it begins to fail, to lose confidence in itself and its forms and habits, to distrust the intellectual action and to fall into weakness and silence. The stilling of this current, running, circling, repeating thought-mind is the principal part of that silencing of the thought which is one of the most effective disciplines of Yoga.

But the higher reason itself has a first stage of dynamic, pragmatic intellectuality in which creation, action and will are the real motive and thought and knowledge are employed to form basic constructions and suggestions which are used principally for effectuation. To this pragmatic reason truth is only a formation of the intellect effective for the action of the inner and the outer life. When we cut it away from the still higher reason which seeks impersonally to reflect Truth rather than to create personally effective truth, we find then that this pragmatic reason can originate, progress, enlarge the experience by dynamic knowledge, but it has to depend on the current understanding as a pedestal and base and put its whole weight on life and becoming. It is in itself therefore a mind of the Will to life and action, much more a mind of Will than a mind of knowledge: it does not live in any assured and constant and eternal Truth, but in progressing and changing aspects of Truth which serve the shifting forms of our life and becoming or, at the highest, help life to grow and progress. By itself this pragmatic mind can give us no firm foundation and no fixed goal; it lives in the truth of the hour, not in any truth of eternity. But when purified of dependence on the customary understanding, it is a great creator and in association with the highest mental reason it becomes a strong channel and bold servant for the effectuation of Truth in life. The value of its work will depend on the value and the power of the highest truth-seeking reason. But by itself it is a sport of Time and a bondslave of Life. The seeker of the Silence has to cast it away from him; the seeker of the integral Divinity has to pass beyond it, to replace and transform this thinking mind intent on Life by a greater effectuating spiritual Will, the Truth-Will of the spirit.

The third and noblest stage of the intellectual will and reason is an intelligence which seeks for some universal reality or for a still higher self-existent Truth for its own sake and tries to live in that Truth. This is primarily a mind of knowledge and only secondarily a mind of Will. In its excess of tendency it often becomes incapable of Will except the one will to know; for action it is dependent on the aid of the pragmatic mind and therefore man tends in action to fall away from the purity of the Truth his highest knowledge holds into a mixed, inferior, inconstant and impure effectuation. The disparity, even when it is not an opposition, between knowledge and will is one of the principal defects of the human buddhi. But there are other inherent limitations of all human thinking. This highest Buddhi does not work in man in its own purity; it is assailed by the defects of the lower mentality, continually clouded by it, distorted, veiled, and prevented or lamed in its own proper action. Purified as much as may be from that habit of mental degradation, the human buddhi is still a power that searches for the Truth, but is never in full or direct possession of it; it can only reflect truth of the spirit and try to make it its own by giving it a limited mental value and a distinct mental body. Nor does it reflect integrally, but seizes either an uncertain totality or else a sum of limited particulars. First it seizes on this or that partial reflection and by subjection to the habit of customary mind turns it into a fixed imprisoning opinion; all new truth it judges from the standpoint it has thus formed and therefore puts on it the colour of a limiting prejudgment. Release it as much as possible from this habit of limiting opinion, still it is subject to another affliction, the demand of the pragmatic mind for immediate effectuation, which gives it no time to proceed to larger truth, but fixes it by the power of effective realisation in whatever it has already judged, known and lived. Freed from all these chains, the buddhi can become a pure and flexible reflector of Truth, adding light to light, proceeding from realisation to realisation. It is then limited only by its own inherent limitations.

These limitations are mainly of two kinds. First, its realisations are only mental realisations; to get to the Truth itself we have to go beyond the mental buddhi. Again, the nature of the mind prevents it from making an effective unification of the truths it seizes. It can only put them side by side and see oppositions or effect some kind of partial, executive and practical combination. But it finds finally that the aspects of the Truth are infinite and that none of its intellectual forms are quite valid, because the spirit is infinite and in the spirit all is true, but nothing in the mind can give the whole truth of the spirit. Either then the buddhi becomes a pure mirror of many reflections, reflecting all truth that falls on it, but ineffective and when turned to action either incapable of decision or chaotic, or it has to make a selection and act as if that partiality were the whole truth, though it knows otherwise. It acts in a helpless limitation of Ignorance, though it may hold a Truth far greater than its action. On the other hand, it may turn away from life and thought and seek to exceed itself and pass into the Truth beyond it. This it may do by seizing on some aspect, some principle, some symbol or suggestion of reality and pushing that to its absolute, all-absorbing, all-excluding term of realisation or by seizing on and realising some idea of indeterminate Being or Non-Being from which all thought and life fall away into cessation. The buddhi casts itself into a luminous sleep and the soul passes away into some ineffable height of spiritual being.

Therefore in dealing with the buddhi, we must either take

one of these choices or else try the rarer adventure of lifting the soul from the mental being into the spiritual gnosis to see what we can find in the very core of that supernal light and power. This gnosis contains the sun of the divine Knowledge-Will burning in the heavens of the supreme conscious Being, to which the mental intelligence and will are only a focus of diffused and deflected rays and reflections. That possesses the divine unity and yet or rather therefore can govern the multiplicity and diversity: whatever selection, self-limitation, combination it makes is not imposed on it by Ignorance, but is self-developed by a power of self-possessing divine Knowledge. When the gnosis is gained, it can then be turned on the whole nature to divinise the human being. It is impossible to rise into it at once; if that could be done, it would mean a sudden and violent overshooting, a breaking or slipping through the gates of the Sun, *sūryasya dvārā*, without near possibility of return. We have to form as a link or bridge an intuitive or illuminated mind, which is not the direct gnosis, but in which a first derivative body of the gnosis can form. This illumined mind will first be a mixed power which we shall have to purify of all its mental dependence and mental forms so as to convert all willing and thinking into thought-sight and truth-seeing will by an illumined discrimination, intuition, inspiration, revelation. That will be the final purification of the intelligence and the preparation for the siddhi of the gnosis.

Chapter VIII

The Liberation of the Spirit

THE PURIFICATION of the mental being and the psychic prana — we will leave aside for the time the question of the physical purification, that of the body and physical prana, though that too is necessary to an integral perfection, — prepares the ground for a spiritual liberation. *Śuddhi* is the condition for *mukti*. All purification is a release, a delivery; for it is a throwing away of limiting, binding, obscuring imperfections and confusions: purification from desire brings the freedom of the psychic prana, purification from wrong emotions and troubling reactions the freedom of the heart, purification from the obscuring limited thought of the sense mind the freedom of the intelligence, purification from mere intellectuality the freedom of the gnosis. But all this is an instrumental liberation. The freedom of the soul, *mukti*, is of a larger and more essential character; it is an opening out of mortal limitation into the illimitable immortality of the Spirit.

For certain ways of thinking liberation is a throwing off of all nature, a silent state of pure being, a nirvana or extinction, a dissolution of the natural existence into some indefinable Absolute, *mokṣa*. But an absorbed and immersed bliss, a wideness of actionless peace, a release of self-extinction or a self-drowning in the Absolute is not our aim. We shall give to the idea of liberation, *mukti*, only the connotation of that inner change which is common to all experience of this kind, essential to perfection and indispensable to spiritual freedom. We shall find that it then implies always two things, a rejection and an assumption, a negative and a positive side; the negative movement of freedom is a liberation from the principal bonds, the master-knots of the lower soul-nature, the positive side an opening or growth into the higher spiritual existence. But what are these master-knots — other and deeper twistings than the instrumental knots of the mind, heart, psychic life-force? We find them pointed out for us and insisted on with great force and a constant emphatic repetition in the Gita; they are four, desire, ego, the dualities and the three gunas of Nature; for to be desireless, ego-less, equal of mind and soul and spirit and *nistraigunya*, is in the idea of the Gita to be free, *mukta*. We may accept this description; for everything essential is covered by its amplitude. On the other hand, the positive sense of freedom is to be universal in soul, transcendently one in spirit with God, possessed of the highest divine nature, — as we may say, like to God, or one with him in the law of our being. This is the whole and full sense of liberation and this is the integral freedom of the spirit.

We have already had to speak of purification from the psychic desire of which the craving of the prana is the evolutionary or, as we may put it, the practical basis. But this is in the mental and psychic nature; spiritual desirelessness has a wider and more essential meaning: for desire has a double knot, a lower knot in the prana, which is a craving in the instruments, and a very subtle knot in the soul itself with the buddhi as its first support or *pratiṣṭhā*, which is the inmost origin of this mesh of our bondage. When we look from below, desire presents itself to us as a craving of the life force which subtilises in the emotions into a craving of the heart and is farther subtilised in the intelligence into a craving, preference, passion of the aesthetic, ethical, dynamic or rational turn of the buddhi. This desire is essential to the ordinary man; he cannot live or act as an individual without knotting up all his action into the service of some kind of lower or higher craving, preference or passion. But when we are able to look at desire from above, we see that what supports this instrumental desire is a will of the spirit. There is a will, *tapas*, *śakti*, by which the secret spirit imposes on its outer members all their action and draws from it an active delight of its being, an ananda, in which they very obscurely and imperfectly, if at all consciously, partake. This tapas is the will of the transcendent spirit who creates the universal movement, of the universal spirit who supports and informs it, of the free individual spirit who is the soul centre of its multiplicities. It is one will, free in all these at once, comprehensive, harmonious, unified; we find it, when we live and act in the spirit, to be an effortless and desireless, a spontaneous and illumined, a self-fulfilling and self-possessing, a satisfied and blissful will of the spiritual delight of being.

But the moment the individual soul leans away from the universal and transcendent truth of its being, leans towards ego, tries to make this will a thing of its own, a separate personal energy, that will changes its character: it becomes an effort, a straining, a heat of force which may have its fiery joys of effectuation and of possession, but has also its afflicting recoils and pain of labour. It is this that turns in each instrument into an intellectual, emotional, dynamic, sensational or vital will of desire, wish, craving. Even when the instruments *per se* are purified of their own apparent initiative and particular kind of desire, this imperfect tapas may still remain, and so long as it conceals the source or deforms the type of the inner action, the soul has not the bliss of liberty, or can only have it by refraining from all action; even, if allowed to persist, it will rekindle the pranic or other desires or at least throw a reminiscent shadow of them on the being. This spiritual seed or beginning of desire too must be expelled, renounced, cast away: the sadhaka must either choose an active peace and complete inner silence or lose individual initiation, *saṅkalpārambha*, in a unity with the universal will, the tapas of the divine Shakti. The passive way is to be inwardly immobile, without effort, wish, expectation or any turn to action, *niśceṣṭa, anīha, nirapekṣa, nivṛtta*; the active way is to be thus immobile and impersonal in the mind, but to allow the supreme Will in its spiritual purity to act through the purified instruments. Then, if the soul abides on the level of the spiritualised mentality, it becomes an instrument only, but is itself without initiative or action, *niṣkriya, sarvārambha-parityāgī*. But if it rises to the gnosis, it is at once an instrument and a participant in the bliss of the divine action and the bliss of the divine Ananda; it unifies in itself the *prakṛti* and the *puruṣa*.

The ego turn, the separative turn of the being, is the fulcrum of the whole embarrassed labour of the ignorance and the bondage. So long as one is not free from the ego sense, there can be no real freedom. The seat of the ego is said to be in the buddhi; it is an ignorance of the discriminating mind and reason which discriminate wrongly and take the individuation of mind, life and body for a truth of separative existence and are turned away from the greater reconciling truth of the oneness of all existence. At any rate in man it is the ego idea which chiefly supports the falsehood of a separative existence; to get rid of this idea, to dwell on the opposite idea of unity, of the one self, the one spirit, the one being of nature is therefore an effective remedy; but it is not by itself absolutely effective. For the ego, though it supports itself by this ego idea, *aham-buddhi*, finds its most powerful means for a certain obstinacy or passion of persistence in the normal action of the sense-mind, the prana and the body. To cast out of us the ego idea is not entirely possible or not entirely effective until these instruments have undergone purification; for, their action being persistently egoistic and separative, the buddhi is carried away by them, — as a boat by winds on the sea, says the Gita, — the knowledge in the intelligence is being constantly obscured or lost temporarily and has to be restored again, a very labour of Sisyphus. But if the lower instruments have been purified of egoistic desire, wish, will, egoistic passion, egoistic emotion and the buddhi itself of egoistic idea and preference, then the knowledge of the spiritual truth of oneness can find a firm foundation. Till then, the ego takes all sorts of subtle forms and we imagine ourselves to be free from it, when we are really acting as its instruments and all we have attained is a certain intellectual poise which is not the true spiritual liberation. Moreover, to throw away the active sense of ego is not enough; that may merely bring an inactive state of the mentality, a certain passive inert quietude of separate being may take the place of the kinetic egoism, which is also not the true liberation. The ego sense must be replaced by a oneness with the transcendental Divine and with universal being.

This necessity arises from the fact that the buddhi is only a *pratiṣṭhā* or chief support of the ego-sense in its manifold play, *ahaṅkāra*; but in its source it is a degradation or deformation of a truth of our spiritual being. The truth of being is that there is a transcendent existence, supreme self or spirit, a timeless soul of existence, an eternal, a Divine, or even we may speak of it in relation to current mental ideas of the Godhead as a supra-Divine, which is here immanent, all-embracing, all-initiating and all-governing, a great universal Spirit; and the individual is a conscious power of being of the Eternal, capable eternally of relations with him, but one with him too in the very core of reality of its own eternal existence. This is a truth which the intelligence can apprehend, can, when once purified, reflect, transmit, hold in a derivative fashion, but it can only be entirely realised, lived and made effective in the spirit. When we live in the spirit, then we not only know, but are this truth of our being. The individual then enjoys in the spirit, in the bliss of the spirit, his oneness with the universal existence, his oneness with the timeless Divine and his oneness with all other beings and that is the essential sense of a spiritual liberation from the ego. But the moment the soul leans towards the mental limitation, there is a certain sense of spiritual separativeness which has its joys, but may at any moment lapse into the entire ego-sense, ignorance, oblivion of oneness. To get rid of this separativeness an attempt is made to absorb oneself in the idea and realisation of the Divine, and this takes in certain forms of spiritual askesis the turn of a strain towards the abolition of all individual being and a casting away, in the trance of immersion, of all individual or universal relations with the Divine, in others it becomes an absorbed dwelling in him and not in this world or a continual absorbed or intent living in his presence, *sāyujya, sālokya, sāmīpya mukti*. The way proposed for the integral Yoga is a lifting up and surrender of the whole being to him, by which not only do we become one with him in our spiritual existence, but dwell too in him and he in us, so that the whole nature is full of his presence and changed into the divine nature; we become one spirit and consciousness and life and substance with the Divine and at the same time we live and move in and have a various joy of that oneness. This integral liberation from the ego into the divine spirit and nature can only be relatively complete on our present level, but it begins to become absolute as we open to and mount into the gnosis. This is the liberated perfection.

The liberation from ego, the liberation from desire together found the central spiritual freedom. The sense, the idea, the experience that I am a separately self-existent being in the universe, and the forming of consciousness and force of being into the mould of that experience are the root of all suffering, ignorance and evil. And it is so because that falsifies both in practice and in cognition the whole real truth of things; it limits the being, limits the consciousness, limits the power of our being, limits the bliss of being; this limitation again produces a wrong way of existence, wrong way of consciousness, wrong way of using the power of our being and consciousness, and wrong, perverse and contrary forms of the delight of existence. The soul limited in being and self-isolated in its environment feels itself no longer in unity and harmony with its Self, with God, with the universe, with all around it; but rather it finds itself at odds with the universe, in conflict and disaccord with other beings who are its other selves, but whom it treats as not-self; and so long as this disaccord and disagreement last, it cannot possess its world and it cannot enjoy the universal life, but is full of unease, fear, afflictions of all kinds, in a painful struggle to preserve and increase itself and possess its surroundings, — for to possess its world is the nature of infinite spirit and the necessary urge in all being. The satisfactions it gets from this labour and effort are of a stinted, perverse and unsatisfying kind: for the one real satisfaction it has is that of growth, of an increasing return towards itself, of some realisation of accord and harmony, of successful self-creation and self-realisation, but the little of these things that it can achieve on the basis of ego-consciousness is always limited, insecure, imperfect, transitory. It is at war too with its own self, — first because, since it is no longer in possession of the central harmonising truth of its own being, it cannot properly control its natural members or accord their tendencies, powers and demands; it has not the secret of harmony, because it has not the secret of its own unity and self-possession; and, secondly, not being in possession of its highest self, it has to struggle towards that, is not allowed to be at peace till it is in possession of its own true highest being. All this means that it is not at one with God; for to be at one with God is to be at one with oneself, at one with the universe and at one with all beings. This oneness is the secret of a right and a divine existence. But the ego cannot have it, because it is in its very nature separative and because even with regard to ourselves, to our own psychological existence it is a false centre of unity; for it tries to find the unity of our being in an identification with a shifting mental, vital, physical personality, not with the eternal self of our total existence. Only in the spiritual self can we possess the true unity; for there the individual enlarges to his own total being and finds himself one with universal existence and with the transcending Divinity.

All the trouble and suffering of the soul proceeds from this wrong egoistic and separative way of existence. The soul not in possession of its free self-existence, *anātmavān*, because it is limited in its consciousness, is limited in knowledge; and this limited knowledge takes the form of a falsifying knowledge. The struggle to return to a true knowing is imposed upon it, but the ego in the separative mind is satisfied with shows and fragments of knowledge which it pieces together into some false or some imperfect total or governing notion, and this knowledge fails it and has to be abandoned for a fresh pursuit of the one thing to be known. That one thing is the Divine, the Self, the Spirit in whom universal and individual being find at last their right foundation and their right harmonies. Again, because it is limited in force, the ego-prisoned soul is full of many incapacities; wrong knowledge is accompanied by wrong will, wrong tendencies and impulses of the being, and the acute sense of this wrongness is the root of the human consciousness of sin. This deficiency of its nature it tries to set right by standards of conduct which will help it to remove the egoistic consciousness and satisfactions of sin by the egoistic consciousness and self-satisfaction of virtue, the rajasic by the sattwic egoism. But the original sin has to be cured, the separation of its being and will from the divine Being and the divine Will; when it returns to unity with the divine Will and Being, it rises beyond sin and virtue to the infinite self-existent purity and the security of its own divine nature.

Its incapacities it tries to set right by organising its imperfect knowledge and disciplining its half-enlightened will and force and directing them by some systematic effort of the reason; but the result must always be a limited, uncertain, mutable and stumbling way and standard of capacity in action. Only when it returns again to the large unity of the free spirit, *bhūmā*, can the action of its nature move perfectly as the instrument of the infinite Spirit and in the steps of the Right and Truth and Power which belong to the free soul acting from the supreme centre of its existence. Again, because it is limited in the delight of being, it is unable to lay hold on the secure, self-existent perfect bliss of the spirit or the delight, the Ananda of the universe which keeps the world in motion, but is only able to move in a mixed and shifting succession of pleasures and pains, joys and sorrows, or must take refuge in some conscient inconscience or neutral indifference. The ego mind cannot do otherwise, and the soul which has externalised itself in ego, is subjected to this unsatisfactory, secondary, imperfect, often perverse, troubled or annulled enjoyment of existence; yet all the time the spiritual and universal Ananda is within, in the self, in the spirit, in its secret unity with God and existence. To cast away the chain of ego and go back to free self, immortal spiritual being is the soul's return to its own eternal divinity.

The will to the imperfect separative being, that wrong Tapas which makes the soul in Nature attempt to individualise itself, to individualise its being, consciousness, force of being, delight of existence in a separative sense, to have these things as its own, in its own right, and not in the right of God and of the universal oneness, is that which brings about this wrong turn and creates the ego. To turn from this original desire is therefore essential, to get back to the will without desire whose whole enjoyment of being and whole will in being is that of a free universal and unifying Ananda. These two things are one, liberation from the will that is of the nature of desire and liberation from the ego, and the oneness which is brought about by the happy loss of the will of desire and the ego, is the essence of Mukti.

Chapter IX

The Liberation of the Nature

THE TWO sides of our being, conscious experiencing soul and executive Nature continuously and variously offering to the soul her experiences, determine in their meeting all the affections of our inner status and its responses. Nature contributes the character of the happenings and the forms of the instruments of experience, the soul meets it by an assent to the natural determinations of the response to these happenings or by a will to other determination which it imposes upon the nature. The acceptance of the instrumental ego consciousness and the will to desire are the initial consent of the self to the lapse into the lower ranges of experience in which it forgets its divine nature of being; the rejection of these things, the return to free self and the will of the divine delight in being is the liberation of the spirit. But on the other side stand the contributions of Nature herself to the mixed tangle, which she imposes on the soul's experience of her doings and makings when once that first initial consent has been given and made the law of the whole outward transaction. Nature's essential contributions are two, the gunas and the dualities. This inferior action of Nature in which we live has certain essential qualitative modes which constitute the whole basis of its inferiority. The constant effect of these modes on the soul in its natural powers of mind, life and body is a discordant and divided experience, a strife of opposites, *dvandva*, a motion in all its experience and an oscillation between or a mixture of constant pairs of contraries, of combining positives and negatives, dualities. A complete liberation from the ego and the will of desire must bring with it a superiority to the qualitative modes of the inferior Nature, *traiguṇyātītya*, a release from this mixed and discordant experience, a cessation or solution of the dual action of Nature. But on this side too there are two kinds of freedom. A liberation from Nature in a quiescent bliss of the spirit is the first form of release. A farther liberation of the Nature into a divine quality and spiritual power of world-experience fills the supreme calm with the supreme kinetic bliss of knowledge, power, joy and mastery. A divine unity of supreme spirit and its supreme nature is the integral liberation.

Nature, because she is a power of spirit, is essentially qualitative in her action. One may almost say that Nature is only the power in being and the development in action of the infinite qualities of the spirit, *anantaguṇa*. All else belongs to her outward and more mechanical aspects; but this play of quality is the essential thing, of which the rest is the result and mechanical combination. Once we have set right the working of the essential power and quality, all the rest becomes subject to the control of the experiencing Purusha. But in the inferior nature of things the play of infinite quality is subject to a limited measure, a divided and conflicting working, a system of opposites and discords between which some practical mobile system of concords has to be found and to be kept in action; this play of concorded discords, conflicting qualities, disparate powers and ways of experience compelled to some just manageable, partial, mostly precarious agreement, an unstable mutable equilibrium, is managed by a fundamental working in three qualitative modes which conflict and combine together in all her creations. These three modes have been given in the Sankhya system, which is generally adopted for this purpose by all the schools of philosophic thought and of Yoga in India, the three names, *sattva*, *rajas* and *tamas*.[1] Tamas is the principle and power of inertia; rajas is the principle of kinesis, passion, endeavour, struggle, initiation (*ārambha*); sattwa the principle of assimilation, equilibrium and harmony. The metaphysical bearing of this classification does not concern us; but in its psychological and spiritual bearing it is of immense practical importance, because these three principles enter into all things, combine to give them their turn of active nature, result, effectuation, and their unequal working in the

---

[1] This subject has been treated in the Yoga of Works. It is restated here from the point of view of the general type of nature and the complete liberation of the being.

soul-experience is the constituent force of our active personality, our temperament, type of nature and cast of psychological response to experience. All character of action and experience in us is determined by the predominance and by the proportional interaction of these three qualities or modes of Nature. The soul in its personality is obliged, as it were, to run into their moulds; mostly, too, it is controlled by them rather than has any free control of them. The soul can only be free by rising above and rejecting the tormented strife of their unequal action and their insufficient concords and combinations and precarious harmonies, whether in the sense of a complete quiescence from the half-regulated chaos of their action or in the sense of a superiority to this lower turn of nature and a higher control or transformation of their working. There must be either an emptiness of the gunas or a superiority to the gunas.

The gunas affect every part of our natural being. They have indeed their strongest relative hold in the three different members of it, mind, life and body. Tamas, the principle of inertia, is strongest in material nature and in our physical being. The action of this principle is of two kinds, inertia of force and inertia of knowledge. Whatever is predominantly governed by Tamas, tends in its force to a sluggish inaction and immobility or else to a mechanical action which it does not possess, but is possessed by obscure forces which drive it in a mechanical round of energy; equally in its consciousness it turns to an inconscience or enveloped subconscience or to a reluctant, sluggish or in some way mechanical conscious action which does not possess the idea of its own energy, but is guided by an idea which seems external to it or at least concealed from its active awareness. Thus the principle of our body is in its nature inert, subconscient, incapable of anything but a mechanical and habitual self-guidance and action: though it has like everything else a principle of kinesis and a principle of equilibrium of its state and action, an inherent principle of response and a secret consciousness, the greatest portion of its rajasic motions are contributed by the life-power and all the overt consciousness by the mental being. The principle of rajas has its strongest hold on the vital nature. It is the Life within us that is the strongest kinetic motor power, but the life-power in earthly beings is possessed by the force of desire, therefore rajas turns always to action and desire; desire is the strongest human and animal initiator of most kinesis and action, predominant to such an extent that many consider it the father of all action and even the originator of our being. Moreover, rajas finding itself in a world of matter which starts from the principle of inconscience and a mechanical driven inertia, has to work against an immense contrary force; therefore its whole action takes on the nature of an effort, a struggle, a besieged and an impeded conflict for possession which is distressed in its every step by a limiting incapacity, disappointment and suffering: even its gains are precarious and limited and marred by the reaction of the effort and an aftertaste of insufficiency and transience. The principle of sattwa has its strongest hold in the mind; not so much in the lower parts of the mind which are dominated by the rajasic life-power, but mostly in the intelligence and the will of the reason. Intelligence, reason, rational will are moved by the nature of their predominant principle towards a constant effort of assimilation, assimilation by knowledge, assimilation by a power of understanding will, a constant effort towards equilibrium, some stability, rule, harmony of the conflicting elements of natural happening and experience. This satisfaction it gets in various ways and in various degrees of acquisition. The attainment of assimilation, equilibrium and harmony brings with it always a relative but more or less intense and satisfying sense of ease, happiness, mastery, security, which is other than the troubled and vehement pleasures insecurely bestowed by the satisfaction of rajasic desire and passion. Light and happiness are the characteristics of the sattwic guna. The whole nature of the embodied living mental being is determined by these three gunas.

But these are only predominant powers in each part of our complex system. The three qualities mingle, combine and strive in every fibre and in every member of our intricate psychology. The mental character is made by them, the character of our reason, the character of our will, the character of our moral, aesthetic, emotional, dynamic, sensational being. Tamas brings in all the ignorance, inertia, weakness, incapacity which afflicts our nature, a clouded reason, nescience, unintelligence, a clinging to habitual notions and mechanical ideas, the refusal to think and know, the small mind, the closed avenues, the trotting round of mental habit, the dark and the twilit places. Tamas brings in the impotent will, want of faith and self-confidence and initiative, the disinclination to act, the shrinking from endeavour and aspiration, the poor and little spirit, and in our moral and dynamic being the inertia, the cowardice, baseness, sloth, lax subjection to small and ignoble motives, the weak yielding to our lower nature. Tamas brings into our emotional nature insensibility, indifference, want of sympathy and openness, the shut soul, the callous heart, the soon spent affection and languor of the feelings, into our aesthetic and sensational nature the dull aesthesis, the limited range of response, the insensibility to beauty, all that makes in man the coarse, heavy and vulgar spirit. Rajas contributes our normal active nature with all its good and evil; when unchastened by a sufficient element of sattwa, it turns to egoism, self-will and violence, the perverse, obstinate or exaggerating action of the reason, prejudice, attachment to opinion, clinging to error, the subservience of the intelligence to our desires and preferences and not to the truth, the fanatic or the sectarian mind, self-will, pride, arrogance, selfishness, ambition, lust, greed, cruelty, hatred, jealousy, the egoisms of love, all the vices and passions, the exaggerations of the aesthesis, the morbidities and perversions of the sensational and vital being. Tamas in its own right produces the coarse, dull and ignorant type of human nature, rajas the vivid, restless, kinetic man, driven by the breath of action, passion and desire. Sattwa produces a higher type. The gifts of sattwa are the mind of reason and balance, clarity of the disinterested truth-seeking open intelligence, a will subordinated to the reason or guided by the ethical spirit, self-control, equality, calm, love, sympathy, refinement, measure, fineness of the aesthetic and emotional mind, in the sensational being delicacy, just acceptivity, moderation and poise, a vitality subdued and governed by the mastering intelligence. The accomplished types of the sattwic man are the philosopher, saint and sage, of the rajasic man the statesman, warrior, forceful man of action. But in all men there is in greater or less proportions a mingling of the gunas, a multiple personality and in most a good deal of shifting and alternation from the predominance of one to the prevalence of another guna; even in the governing form of their nature most human beings are of a mixed type. All the colour and variety of life is made of the intricate pattern of the weaving of the gunas.

But richness of life, even a sattwic harmony of mind and nature does not constitute spiritual perfection. There is a relative possible perfection, but it is a perfection of incompleteness, some partial height, force, beauty, some measure of nobility and greatness, some imposed and precariously sustained balance. There is a relative mastery, but it is a mastery of the body by life or of the life by mind, not a free possession of the instruments by the liberated and self-possessing spirit. The gunas have to be transcended if we would arrive at spiritual perfection. Tamas evidently has to be overcome, inertia and ignorance and incapacity cannot be elements of a true perfection; but it can only be overcome in Nature by the force of rajas aided by an increasing force of sattwa. Rajas has to be overcome, egoism, personal desire and self-seeking passion are not elements of the true perfection; but it can only be overcome by force of sattwa enlightening the being and force of tamas limiting the action. Sattwa itself does not give the highest or the integral perfection; sattwa is always a quality of the limited nature; sattwic knowledge is the light of a limited mentality; sattwic will is the government of a limited intelligent force. Moreover, sattwa cannot act by itself in Nature, but has to rely for all action on the aid of rajas, so that even sattwic action is always liable to the imperfections of rajas; egoism, perplexity, inconsistency, a one-sided turn, a limited and exaggerated will, exaggerating itself in the intensity of its limitations, pursue the mind and action even of the saint, philosopher and sage. There is a sattwic as well as a rajasic or tamasic egoism, at the highest an egoism of knowledge or virtue; but the mind's egoism of whatever type is incompatible with liberation. All the three gunas have to be transcended. Sattwa may bring us near to the Light, but its limited clarity falls away from us when we enter into the luminous body of the divine Nature.

This transcendence is usually sought by a withdrawal from the action of the lower nature. That withdrawal brings with it a stressing of the tendency to inaction. Sattwa when it wishes to intensify itself, seeks to get rid of rajas and calls in the aid of the tamasic principle of inaction; that is the reason why a certain type of highly sattwic men live intensely in the inward being, but hardly at all in the outward life of action, or else are there incompetent and ineffective. The seeker of liberation goes farther in this direction, strives by imposing an enlightened tamas on his natural being, a tamas which by this saving enlightenment is more of a quiescence than an incapacity, to give the sattwic guna freedom to lose itself in the light of the spirit. A quietude and stillness is imposed on the body, on the active life-soul of desire and ego, on the external mind, while the sattwic nature by stress of meditation, by an exclusive concentration of adoration, by a will turned inward to the Supreme, strives to merge itself in the spirit. But if this is sufficient for a quietistic release, it is not sufficient for the freedom of an integral perfection. This liberation depends upon inaction and is not entirely self-existent and absolute; the moment the soul turns to action, it finds that the activity of the nature is still the old imperfect motion. There is a liberation of the soul from the nature which is gained by inaction, but not a liberation of the soul in nature perfect and self-existent whether in action or in inaction. The question then arises whether such a liberation and perfection are possible and what may be the condition of this perfect freedom.

The ordinary idea is that it is not possible because all action is of the lower gunas, necessarily defective, *sadoṣam*, caused by the motion, inequality, want of balance, unstable strife of the gunas; but when these unequal gunas fall into perfect equilib-rium, all action of Nature ceases and the soul rests in its quietude. The divine Being, we may say, may either exist in his silence or act in Nature through her instrumentation, but in that case must put on the appearance of her strife and imperfection. That may be true of the ordinary deputed action of the Divine in the human spirit with its present relations of soul to nature in an embodied imperfect mental being, but it is not true of the divine nature of perfection. The strife of the gunas is only a representation in the imperfection of the lower nature; what the three gunas stand for are three essential powers of the Divine which are not merely existent in a perfect equilibrium of quietude, but unified in a perfect consensus of divine action. Tamas in the spiritual being becomes a divine calm, which is not an inertia and incapacity of action, but a perfect power, *śakti*, holding in itself all its capacity and capable of controlling and subjecting to the law of calm even the most stupendous and enormous activity: rajas becomes a self-effecting initiating sheer Will of the spirit, which is not desire, endeavour, striving passion, but the same perfect power of being, *śakti*, capable of an infinite, imperturbable and blissful action. Sattwa becomes not the modified mental light, *prakāśa*, but the self-existent light of the divine being, *jyotiḥ*, which is the soul of the perfect power of being and illumines in their unity the divine quietude and the divine will of action. The ordinary liberation gets the still divine light in the divine quietude, but the integral perfection will aim at this greater triune unity.

When this liberation of the nature comes, there is a liberation also of all the spiritual sense of the dualities of Nature. In the lower nature the dualities are the inevitable effect of the play of the gunas on the soul affected by the formations of the sattwic, rajasic and tamasic ego. The knot of this duality is an ignorance which is unable to seize on the spiritual truth of things and concentrates on the imperfect appearances, but meets them not with a mastery of their inner truth, but with a strife and a shifting balance of attraction and repulsion, capacity and incapacity, liking and disliking, pleasure and pain, joy and sorrow, acceptance and repugnance; all life is represented to us as a tangle of these things, of the pleasant and the unpleasant, the beautiful and the unbeautiful, truth and falsehood, fortune and misfortune, success and failure, good and evil, the inextricable double web of Nature. Attachment to its likings and repugnances keeps the soul bound in this web of good and evil, joys and sorrows. The seeker of liberation gets rid of attachment, throws away from his soul the dualities, but as the dualities appear to be the whole act, stuff and frame of life, this release would seem to be most easily compassed by a withdrawal from life, whether a physical withdrawal, so far as that is possible while in the body, or an inner retirement, a refusal of sanction, a liberating distaste, *vairāgya*, for the whole action of Nature. There is a separation of the soul from Nature. Then the soul watches seated above and unmoved, *udāsīna*, the strife of the gunas in the natural being and regards as an impassive witness the pleasure and pain of the mind and body. Or it is able to impose its indifference even on the outer mind and watches with the impartial calm or the impartial joy of the detached spectator the universal action in which it has no longer an active inner participation. The end of this movement is the rejection of birth and a departure into the silent self, *mokṣa*.

But this rejection is not the last possible word of liberation. The integral liberation comes when this passion for release, *mumukṣutva*, founded on distaste or *vairāgya*, is itself transcended; the soul is then liberated both from attachment to the lower action of nature and from all repugnance to the cosmic action of the Divine. This liberation gets its completeness when the spiritual gnosis can act with a supramental knowledge and reception of the action of Nature and a supramental luminous will in initiation. The gnosis discovers the spiritual sense in Nature, God in things, the soul of good in all things that have the contrary appearance; that soul is delivered in them and out of them, the perversions of the imperfect or contrary forms fall away or are transformed into their higher divine truth, — even as the gunas go back to their divine principles, — and the spirit lives in a universal, infinite and absolute Truth, Good, Beauty, Bliss which is the supramental or ideal divine Nature. The liberation of the Nature becomes one with the liberation of the spirit, and there is founded in the integral freedom the integral perfection.

Chapter X

The Elements of Perfection

WHEN the self is purified of the wrong and confused action of the instrumental Nature and liberated into its self-existent being, consciousness, power and bliss and the Nature itself liberated from the tangle of this lower action of the struggling gunas and the dualities into the high truth of the divine calm and the divine action, then spiritual perfection becomes possible. Purification and freedom are the indispensable antecedents of perfection. A spiritual self-perfection can only mean a growing into oneness with the nature of divine being, and therefore according to our conception of divine being will be the aim, effort and method of our seeking after this perfection. To the Mayavadin the highest or rather the only real truth of being is the impassive, impersonal, self-aware Absolute and therefore to grow into an impassive calm, impersonality and pure self-awareness of spirit is his idea of perfection and a rejection of cosmic and individual being and a settling into silent self-knowledge is his way. To the Buddhist for whom the highest truth is a negation of being, a recognition of the impermanence and sorrow of being and the disastrous nullity of desire and a dissolution of egoism, of the upholding associations of the Idea and the successions of Karma are the perfect way. Other ideas of the Highest are less negative; each according to its own idea leads towards some likeness to the Divine, *sādṛśya*, and each finds its own way, such as the love and worship of the Bhakta and the growing into the likeness of the Divine by love. But for the integral Yoga perfection will mean a divine spirit and a divine nature which will admit of a divine relation and action in the world; it will mean also in its entirety a divinising of the whole nature, a rejection of all its wrong knots of being and action, but no rejection of any part of our being or of any field of our action. The approach to perfection must be therefore a large and complex movement and its results and workings will have an infinite and varied scope. We must fix in order to find a clue and method on certain essential and fundamental elements and requisites of perfection, *siddhi*; for if these are secured, all the rest will be found to be only their natural development or particular working. We may cast these elements into six divisions, interdependent on each other to a great extent but still in a certain way naturally successive in their order of attainment. The movement will start from a basic equality of the soul and mount to an ideal action of the Divine through our perfected being in the largeness of the Brahmic unity.

The first necessity is some fundamental poise of the soul both in its essential and its natural being regarding and meeting the things, impacts and workings of Nature. This poise we shall arrive at by growing into a perfect equality, *samatā*. The self, spirit or Brahman is one in all and therefore one to all; it is, as is said in the Gita which has developed fully this idea of equality and indicated its experience on at least one side of equality, the equal Brahman, *samaṁ brahma*; the Gita even goes so far in one passage as to identify equality and yoga, *samatvaṁ yoga ucyate*. That is to say, equality is the sign of unity with the Brahman, of becoming Brahman, of growing into an undisturbed spiritual poise of being in the Infinite. Its importance can hardly be exaggerated; for it is the sign of our having passed beyond the egoistic determinations of our nature, of our having conquered our enslaved response to the dualities, of our having transcended the shifting turmoil of the gunas, of our having entered into the calm and peace of liberation. Equality is a term of consciousness which brings into the whole of our being and nature the eternal tranquillity of the Infinite. Moreover, it is the condition of a securely and perfectly divine action; the security and largeness of the cosmic action of the Infinite is based upon and never breaks down or forfeits its eternal tranquillity. That too must be the character of the perfect spiritual action; to be equal and one to all things in spirit, understanding, mind, heart and natural consciousness, — even in the most physical consciousness, — and to make all their workings, whatever their outward adaptation to the thing to be done, always and imminuably full of the divine equality and calm must be its inmost principle. That may be said to be the passive or basic, the fundamental and receptive side of equality, but there is also an active and possessive side, an equal bliss which can only come when the peace of equality is founded and which is the beatific flower of its fullness.

The next necessity of perfection is to raise all the active parts of the human nature to that highest condition and working pitch of their power and capacity, *śakti*, at which they become capable of being divinised into true instruments of the free, perfect, spiritual and divine action. For practical purposes we may take the understanding, the heart, the prana and the body as the four members of our nature which have thus to be prepared, and we have to find the constituent terms of their perfection. Also there is the dynamical force in us (*vīrya*) of the temperament, character and soul nature, *svabhāva*, which makes the power of our members effective in action and gives them their type and direction; this has to be freed from its limitations, enlarged, rounded so that the whole manhood in us may become the basis of a divine manhood, when the Purusha, the real Man in us, the divine Soul, shall act fully in this human instrument and shine fully through this human vessel. To divinise the perfected nature we have to call in the divine Power or Shakti to replace our limited human energy so that this may be shaped into the image of and filled with the force of a greater infinite energy, *daivī prakṛti, bhāgavatī śakti*. This perfection will grow in the measure in which we can surrender ourselves, first, to the guidance and then to the direct action of that Power and of the Master of our being and our works to whom it belongs, and for this purpose faith is the essential, faith is the great motor-power of our being in our aspirations to perfection, — here, a faith in God and the Shakti which shall begin in the heart and understanding, but shall take possession of all our nature, all its consciousness, all its dynamic motive-force. These four things are the essentials of this second element of perfection, the full powers of the members of the instrumental nature, the perfected dynamis of the soul nature, the assumption of them into the action of the divine

Power, and a perfect faith in all our members to call and support that assumption, *śakti, vīrya, daivī prakṛti, śraddhā.*

But so long as this development takes place only on the highest level of our normal nature, we may have a reflected and limited image of perfection translated into the lower terms of the soul in mind, life and body, but not the possession of the divine perfection in the highest terms possible to us of the divine Idea and its Power. That is to be found beyond these lower principles in the supramental gnosis; therefore the next step of perfection will be the evolution of the mental into the gnostic being. This evolution is effected by a breaking beyond the mental limitation, a stride upward into the next higher plane or region of our being hidden from us at present by the shining lid of the mental reflections and a conversion of all that we are into the terms of this greater consciousness. In the gnosis itself, *vijñāna,* there are several gradations which open at their highest into the full and infinite Ananda. The gnosis once effectively called into action will progressively take up all the terms of intelligence, will, sense-mind, heart, the vital and sensational being and translate them by a luminous and harmonising conversion into a unity of the truth, power and delight of a divine existence. It will lift into that light and force and convert into their own highest sense our whole intellectual, volitional, dynamic, ethical, aesthetic, sensational, vital and physical being. It has the power also of overcoming physical limitations and developing a more perfect and divinely instrumental body. Its light opens up the fields of the superconscient and darts its rays and pours its luminous flood into the subconscient and enlightens its obscure hints and withheld secrets. It admits us to a greater light of the Infinite than is reflected in the paler luminosity even of the highest mentality. While it perfects the individual soul and nature in the sense of a diviner existence and makes a full harmony of the diversities of our being, it founds all its action upon the Unity from which it proceeds and takes up everything into that Unity. Personality and impersonality, the two eternal aspects of existence, are made one by its action in the spiritual being and Nature body of the Purushottama.

The gnostic perfection, spiritual in its nature, is to be accomplished here in the body and takes life in the physical world as one of its fields, even though the gnosis opens to us possession of planes and worlds beyond the material universe. The physical body is therefore a basis of action, *pratiṣṭhā*, which cannot be despised, neglected or excluded from the spiritual evolution: a perfection of the body as the outer instrument of a complete divine living on earth will be necessarily a part of the gnostic conversion. The change will be effected by bringing in the law of the gnostic Purusha, *vijñānamaya puruṣa*, and of that into which it opens, the Anandamaya, into the physical consciousness and its members. Pushed to its highest conclusion this movement brings in a spiritualising and illumination of the whole physical consciousness and a divinising of the law of the body. For behind the gross physical sheath of this materially visible and sensible frame there is subliminally supporting it and discoverable by a finer subtle consciousness a subtle body of the mental being and a spiritual or causal body of the gnostic and bliss soul in which all the perfection of a spiritual embodiment is to be found, a yet unmanifested divine law of the body. Most of the physical siddhis acquired by certain Yogins are brought about by some opening up of the law of the subtle or a calling down of something of the law of the spiritual body. The ordinary method is the opening up of the *cakras* by the physical processes of Hathayoga (of which something is also included in the Rajayoga) or by the methods of the Tantric discipline. But while these may be optionally used at certain stages by the integral Yoga, they are not indispensable; for here the reliance is on the power of the higher being to change the lower existence, a working is chosen mainly from above downward and not the opposite way, and therefore the development of the superior power of the gnosis will be awaited as the instrumentative change in this part of the Yoga.

There will remain, because it will then only be entirely possible, the perfect action and enjoyment of being on the gnostic basis. The Purusha enters into cosmic manifestation for the variations of his infinite existence, for knowledge, action and enjoyment; the gnosis brings the fullness of spiritual knowledge and it will found on that the divine action and cast the enjoyment of world and being into the law of the truth, the freedom and the perfection of the spirit. But neither action nor enjoyment will be the lower action of the gunas and consequent egoistic enjoyment mostly of the satisfaction of rajasic desire which is our present way of living. Whatever desire will remain, if that name be given, will be the divine desire, the will to delight of the Purusha enjoying in his freedom and perfection the action of the perfected Prakriti and all her members. The Prakriti will take up the whole nature into the law of her higher divine truth and act in that law offering up the universal enjoyment of her action and being to the Anandamaya Ishwara, the Lord of existence and works and Spirit of bliss, who presides over and governs her workings. The individual soul will be the channel of this action and offering, and it will enjoy at once its oneness with the Ishwara and its oneness with the Prakriti and will enjoy all relations with Infinite and finite, with God and the universe and beings in the universe in the highest terms of the union of the universal Purusha and Prakriti.

All the gnostic evolution opens up into the divine principle of Ananda, which is the foundation of the fullness of spiritual being, consciousness and bliss of Sachchidananda or eternal Brahman. Possessed at first by reflection in the mental experience, it will be possessed afterwards with a greater fullness and directness in the massed and luminous consciousness, *cidghana*, which comes by the gnosis. The Siddha or perfected soul will live in union with the Purushottama in this Brahmic consciousness, he will be conscious in the Brahman that is the All, *sarvaṁ brahma*, in the Brahman infinite in being and infinite in quality, *anantaṁ brahma*, in Brahman as self-existent consciousness and universal knowledge, *jñānaṁ brahma*, in Brahman as the self-existent bliss and its universal delight of being, *ānandaṁ brahma*. He will experience all the universe as the manifestation of the One, all quality and action as the play of his universal and infinite energy, all knowledge and conscious experience as the outflowing of that consciousness, and all in the terms of that one Ananda. His physical being will be one with all material Nature, his vital being with the life of the universe, his mind with the cosmic mind, his spiritual knowledge and will with the divine knowledge and will both in itself and as it pours itself through these channels, his spirit with the one spirit in all beings. All the variety of cosmic existence will be changed to him in that unity and revealed in the secret of its spiritual significance. For in this spiritual bliss and being he will be one with That which is the origin and continent and inhabitant and spirit and constituting power of all existence. This will be the highest reach of self-perfection.

Chapter XI

The Perfection of Equality

THE VERY first necessity for spiritual perfection is a perfect equality. Perfection in the sense in which we use it in Yoga, means a growth out of a lower undivine into a higher divine nature. In terms of knowledge it is a putting on the being of the higher self and a casting away of the darker broken lower self or a transforming of our imperfect state into the rounded luminous fullness of our real and spiritual personality. In terms of devotion and adoration it is a growing into a likeness of the nature or the law of the being of the Divine, to be united with whom we aspire, — for if there is not this likeness, this oneness of the law of the being, unity between that transcending and universal and this individual spirit is not possible. The supreme divine nature is founded on equality. This affirmation is true of it whether we look on the Supreme Being as a pure silent Self and Spirit or as the divine Master of cosmic existence. The pure Self is equal, unmoved, the witness in an impartial peace of all the happenings and relations of cosmic existence. While it is not averse to them, — aversion is not equality, nor, if that were the attitude of the Self to cosmic existence, could the universe come at all into being or proceed upon its cycles, — a detachment, the calm of an equal regard, a superiority to the reactions which trouble and are the disabling weakness of the soul involved in outward nature, are the very substance of the silent Infinite's purity and the condition of its impartial assent and support to the many-sided movement of the universe. But in that power too of the Supreme which governs and develops these motions, the same equality is a basic condition.

The Master of things cannot be affected or troubled by the reactions of things; if he were, he would be subject to them, not master, not free to develop them according to his sovereign will and wisdom and according to the inner truth and necessity of what is behind their relations, but obliged rather to act according to the claim of temporary accident and phenomenon. The truth of all things is in the calm of their depths, not in the shifting inconstant wave form on the surface. The supreme conscious Being in his divine knowledge and will and love governs their evolution — to our ignorance so often a cruel confusion and distraction — from these depths and is not troubled by the clamour of the surface. The divine nature does not share in our gropings and our passions; when we speak of the divine wrath or favour or of God suffering in man, we are using a human language which mistranslates the inner significance of the movement we characterise. We see something of the real truth of them when we rise out of the phenomenal mind into the heights of the spiritual being. For then we perceive that whether in the silence of self or in its action in the cosmos, the Divine is always Sachchidananda, an infinite existence, an infinite consciousness and self-founded power of conscious being, an infinite bliss in all his existence. We ourselves begin to dwell in an equal light, strength, joy — the psychological rendering of the divine knowledge, will and delight in self and things which are the active universal outpourings from those infinite sources. In the strength of that light, power and joy a secret self and spirit within us accepts and transforms always into food of its perfect experience the dual letters of the mind's transcript of life, and if there were not the hidden greater existence even now within us, we could not bear the pressure of the universal force or subsist in this great and dangerous world. A perfect equality of our spirit and nature is a means by which we can move back from the troubled and ignorant outer consciousness into this inner kingdom of heaven and possess the spirit's eternal kingdoms, *rājyam samṛddham*, of greatness, joy and peace. That self-elevation to the divine nature is the complete fruit and the whole occasion of the discipline of equality demanded from us by the self-perfecting aim in Yoga.

A perfect equality and peace of the soul is indispensable to change the whole substance of our being into substance of the self out of its present stuff of troubled mentality. It is equally indispensable if we aspire to replace our present confused and ignorant action by the self-possessed and luminous works of a free spirit governing its nature and in tune with universal being. A divine action or even a perfect human action is impossible if we have not equality of spirit and an equality in the motive-forces of our nature. The Divine is equal to all, an impartial sustainer of his universe, who views all with equal eyes, assents to the law of developing being which he has brought out of the depths of his existence, tolerates what has to be tolerated, depresses what has to be depressed, raises what has to be raised, creates, sustains and destroys with a perfect and equal understanding of all causes and results and working out of the spiritual and pragmatic meaning of all phenomena. God does not create in obedience to any troubled passion of desire or maintain and preserve through an attachment of partial preference or destroy in a fury of wrath, disgust or aversion. The Divine deals with great and small, just and unjust, ignorant and wise as the Self of all who, deeply intimate and one with the being, leads all according to their nature and need with a perfect understanding, power and justness of proportion. But through it all he moves things according to his large aim in the cycles and draws the soul upward in the evolution through its apparent progress and retrogression towards the higher and ever higher development which is the sense of the cosmic urge. The self-perfecting individual who seeks to be one in will with the Divine and make his nature an instrument of the divine purpose, must enlarge himself out of the egoistic and partial views and motives of the human ignorance and mould himself into an image of this supreme equality.

This equal poise in action is especially necessary for the sadhaka of the integral Yoga. First, he must acquire that equal assent and understanding which will respond to the law of the divine action without trying to impose on it a partial will and the violent claim of a personal aspiration. A wise impersonality, a quiescent equality, a universality which sees all things as the manifestations of the Divine, the one Existence, is not angry, troubled, impatient with the way of things or on the other hand excited, over-eager and precipitate, but sees that the law must be obeyed and the pace of time respected, observes and understands with sympathy the actuality of things and beings, but looks also behind the present appearance to their inner significances and forward to the unrolling of their divine possibilities, is the first thing demanded of those who would do works as the perfect instruments of the Divine. But this impersonal acquiescence is only the basis. Man is the instrument of an evolution which wears at first the mask of a struggle, but grows more and more into its truer and deeper sense of a constant wise adjustment and must take on in a rising scale the deepest truth and significance — now only underlying the adjustment and struggle — of a universal harmony. The perfected human soul must always be an instrument for the hastening of the ways of this evolution. For that a divine power acting with the royalty of the divine will in it must be in whatever degree present in the nature. But to be accomplished and permanent, steadfast in action, truly divine, it has to proceed on the basis of a spiritual equality, a calm, impersonal and equal self-identification with all beings, an understanding of all energies. The Divine acts with a mighty power in the myriad workings of the universe, but with the supporting light and force of an imperturbable oneness, freedom and peace. That must be the type of the perfected soul's divine works. And equality is the condition of the being which makes possible this changed spirit in the action.

But even a human perfection cannot dispense with equality as one of its chief elements and even its essential atmosphere. The aim of a human perfection must include, if it is to deserve the name, two things, self-mastery and a mastery of the surroundings; it must seek for them in the greatest degree of these powers which is at all attainable by our human nature. Man's urge of self-perfection is to be, in the ancient language, *svarāṭ* and *samrāṭ*, self-ruler and king. But to be self-ruler is not possible for him if he is subject to the attack of the lower nature, to the turbulence of grief and joy, to the violent touches of pleasure and pain, to the tumult of his emotions and passions, to the bondage of his personal likings and dislikings, to the strong chains of desire and attachment, to the narrowness of a personal and emotionally preferential judgment and opinion, to all the hundred touches of his egoism and its pursuing stamp on his thought, feeling and action. All these things are the slavery to the lower self which the greater "I" in man must put under his feet if he is to be king of his own nature. To surmount them is the condition of self-rule; but of that surmounting again equality is the condition and the essence of the movement. To be quite free from all these things, — if possible, or at least to be master of and superior to them, — is equality. Farther, one who is not self-ruler, cannot be master of his surroundings. The knowledge, the will, the harmony which is necessary for this outward mastery, can come only as a crown of the inward conquest. It belongs to the self-possessing soul and mind which follows with a disinterested equality the Truth, the Right, the universal Largeness to which alone this mastery is possible, — following always the great ideal they present to our imperfection while it understands and makes a full allowance too for all that seems to conflict with them and stand in the way of their manifestation. This rule is true even on the levels of our actual human mentality, where we can only get a limited perfection. But the ideal of Yoga takes up this aim of Swarajya and Samrajya and puts it on the larger spiritual basis. There it gets its full power, opens to the diviner degrees of the spirit; for it is by oneness with the Infinite, by a spiritual power acting upon finite things, that some highest integral perfection of our being and nature finds its own native foundation.

A perfect equality not only of the self, but in the nature is a condition of the Yoga of self-perfection. The first obvious step to it will be the conquest of our emotional and vital being, for here are the sources of greatest trouble, the most rampant forces of inequality and subjection, the most insistent claim of our imperfection. The equality of these parts of our nature comes by purification and freedom. We might say that equality is the very sign of liberation. To be free from the domination of the urge of vital desire and the stormy mastery of the soul by the passions is to have a calm and equal heart and a life-principle governed by the large and even view of a universal spirit. Desire is the impurity of the Prana, the life-principle, and its chain of bondage. A free Prana means a content and satisfied life-soul which fronts the contact of outward things without desire and receives them with an equal response; delivered, uplifted above the servile duality of liking and disliking, indifferent to the urgings of pleasure and pain, not excited by the pleasant, not troubled and overpowered by the unpleasant, not clinging with attachment to the touches it prefers or violently repelling those for which it has an aversion, it will be opened to a greater system of values of experience. All that comes to it from the world with menace or with solicitation, it will refer to the higher principles, to a reason and heart in touch with or changed by the light and calm joy of the spirit. Thus quieted, mastered by the spirit and no longer trying to impose its own mastery on the deeper and finer soul in us, this life-soul will be itself spiritualised and work as a clear and noble instrument of the diviner dealings of the spirit with things. There is no question here of an ascetic killing of the life-impulse and its native utilities and functions; not its killing is demanded, but its transformation. The function of the Prana is enjoyment, but the real enjoyment of existence is an inward spiritual Ananda, not partial and troubled like that of our vital, emotional or mental pleasure, degraded as they are now by the predominance of the physical mind, but universal, profound, a massed concentration of spiritual bliss possessed in a calm ecstasy of self and all existence. Possession is its function, by possession comes the soul's enjoyment of things, but this is the real possession, a thing large and inward, not dependent on the outward seizing which makes us subject to what we seize. All outward possession and enjoyment will be only an occasion of a satisfied and equal play of the spiritual Ananda with the forms and phenomena of its own world-being. The egoistic possession, the making things our own in the sense of the ego's claim on God and beings and the world, *parigraha*, must be renounced in order that this greater thing, this large, universal and perfect life, may come. *Tyaktena bhuñjīthāḥ*, by renouncing the egoistic sense of desire and possession, the soul enjoys divinely its self and the universe.

A free heart is similarly a heart delivered from the gusts and storms of the affections and the passions; the assailing touch of grief, wrath, hatred, fear, inequality of love, trouble of joy, pain of sorrow fall away from the equal heart, and leave it a thing large, calm, equal, luminous, divine. These things are not incumbent on the essential nature of our being, but the creations of the present make of our outward active mental and vital nature and its transactions with its surroundings. The ego-sense which induces us to act as separate beings who make their isolated claim and experience the test of the values of the universe, is responsible for these aberrations. When we live in unity with the Divine in ourselves and the spirit of the universe, these imperfections fall away from us and disappear in the calm and equal strength and delight of the inner spiritual existence. Always that is within us and transforms the outward touches before they reach it by a passage through a subliminal psychic soul in us which is the hidden instrument of its delight of being. By equality of the heart we get away from the troubled desire-soul on the surface, open the gates of this profounder being, bring out its responses and impose their true divine values on all that solicits our emotional being. A free, happy, equal and all-embracing heart of spiritual feeling is the outcome of this perfection.

In this perfection too there is no question of a severe ascetic insensibility, an aloof spiritual indifference or a strained rugged austerity of self-suppression. This is not a killing of the emotional nature but a transformation. All that presents itself here in our outward nature in perverse or imperfect forms has a significance and utility which come out when we get back to the greater truth of divine being. Love will be not destroyed, but perfected, enlarged to its widest capacity, deepened to its spiritual rapture, the love of God, the love of man, the love of all things as ourselves and as beings and powers of the Divine; a large, universal love, not at all incapable of various relation, will replace the clamant, egoistic, self-regarding love of little joys and griefs and insistent demands afflicted with all the chequered pattern of angers and jealousies and satisfactions, rushings to unity and movements of fatigue, divorce and separation on which we now place so high a value. Grief will cease to exist, but a universal, an equal love and sympathy will take its place, not a suffering sympathy, but a power which, itself delivered, is strong to sustain, to help, to liberate. To the free spirit wrath and hatred are impossible, but not the strong Rudra energy of the Divine which can battle without hatred and destroy without wrath because all the time aware of the things it destroys as parts of itself, its own manifestations and unaltered therefore in its sympathy and understanding of those in whom are embodied these manifestations. All our emotional nature will undergo this high liberating transformation; but in order that it may do so, a perfect equality is the effective condition.

The same equality must be brought into the rest of our being. Our whole dynamic being is acting under the influence of unequal impulses, the manifestations of the lower ignorant nature. These urgings we obey or partially control or place on them the changing and modifying influence of our reason, our refining aesthetic sense and mind and regulating ethical notions. A tangled strain of right and wrong, of useful and harmful, harmonious or disordered activity is the mixed result of our endeavour, a shifting standard of human reason and unreason, virtue and vice, honour and dishonour, the noble and the ignoble, things approved and things disapproved of men, much trouble of self-approbation and disapprobation or of self-righteousness and disgust, remorse, shame and moral depression. These things are no doubt very necessary at present for our spiritual evolution. But the seeker of a greater perfection will draw back from all these dualities, regard them with an equal eye and arrive through equality at an impartial and universal action of the dynamic Tapas, spiritual force, in which his own force and will are turned into pure and just instruments of a greater calm secret of divine working. The ordinary mental standards will be exceeded on the basis of this dynamic equality. The eye of his will must look beyond to a purity of divine being, a motive of divine will-power guided by divine knowledge of which his perfected nature will be the engine, *yantra*. That must remain impossible in entirety as long as the dynamic ego with its subservience to the emotional and vital impulses and the preferences of the personal judgment interferes in his action. A perfect equality of the will is the power which dissolves these knots of the lower impulsion to works. This equality will not respond to the lower impulses, but watch for a greater seeing impulsion from the Light above the mind, and will not judge and govern with the intellectual judgment, but wait for enlightenment and direction from a superior plane of vision. As it mounts upward to the supramental being and widens inward to the spiritual largeness, the dynamic nature will be transformed, spiritualised like the emotional and pranic, and grow into a power of the divine nature. There will be plenty of stumblings and errors and imperfections of adjustment of the instruments to their new working, but the increasingly equal soul will not be troubled overmuch or grieve at these things, since, delivered to the guidance of the Light and Power within self and above mind, it will proceed on its way with a firm assurance and await with growing calm the vicissitudes and completion of the process of transformation. The promise of the Divine Being in the Gita will be the anchor of its resolution, "Abandon all dharmas and take refuge in Me alone; I will deliver thee from all sin and evil; do not grieve."

The equality of the thinking mind will be a part and a very important part of the perfection of the instruments in the nature. Our present attractive self-justifying attachment to our intellectual preferences, our judgments, opinions, imaginations, limiting associations of the memory which makes the basis of our mentality, to the current repetitions of our habitual mind, to the insistences of our pragmatic mind, to the limitations even of our intellectual truth-mind, must go the way of other attachments and yield to the impartiality of an equal vision. The equal thought-mind will look on knowledge and ignorance and on truth and error, those dualities created by our limited nature of consciousness and the partiality of our intellect and its little stock of reasonings and intuitions, accept them both without being bound to either twine of the skein and await a luminous transcendence. In ignorance it will see a knowledge which is imprisoned and seeks or waits for delivery, in error a truth at work which has lost itself or got thrown by the groping mind into misleading forms. On the other side it will not hold itself bound and limited by its knowledge or forbidden by it to proceed to fresh illumination, nor lay too fierce a grasp on truth, even when using it to the full, or tyrannously chain it to its present formulations. This perfect equality of the thinking mind is indispensable because the objective of this progress is the greater light which belongs to a higher plane of spiritual cognizance. This equality is the most delicate and difficult of all, the least practised by the human mind; its perfection is impossible so long as the supramental light does not fall fully on the upward looking mentality. But an increasing will to equality in the intelligence is needed, before that light can work freely upon the mental substance. This too is not an abnegation of the seekings and cosmic purposes of the intelligence, not an indifference or impartial scepticism, nor yet a stilling of all thought in the silence of the Ineffable. A stilling of the mental thought may be part of the discipline, when the object is to free the mind from its own partial workings, in order that it may become an equal channel of a higher light and knowledge; but there must also be a transformation of the mental substance; otherwise the higher light cannot assume full possession and a compelling shape for the ordered works of the divine consciousness in the human being. The silence of the Ineffable is a truth of divine being, but the Word which proceeds from that silence is also a truth, and it is this Word which has to be given a body in the conscious form of the nature.

But, finally, all this equalisation of the nature is a preparation for the highest spiritual equality to take possession of the whole being and make a pervading atmosphere in which the light, power and joy of the Divine can manifest itself in man amid an increasing fullness. That equality is the eternal equality of Sachchidananda. It is an equality of the infinite being which is self-existent, an equality of the eternal spirit, but it will mould into its own mould the mind, heart, will, life, physical being. It is an equality of the infinite spiritual consciousness which will contain and base the blissful flowing and satisfied waves of a divine knowledge. It is an equality of the divine Tapas which will initiate a luminous action of the divine will in all the nature. It is an equality of the divine Ananda which will found the play of a divine universal delight, universal love and an illimitable aesthesis of universal beauty. The ideal equal peace and calm of the Infinite will be the wide ether of our perfected being, but the ideal, equal and perfect action of the Infinite through the nature working on the relations of the universe will be the untroubled outpouring of its power in our being. This is the meaning of equality in the terms of the integral Yoga.

Chapter XII

The Way of Equality

IT WILL appear from the description of the complete and perfect equality that this equality has two sides. It must therefore be arrived at by two successive movements. One will liberate us from the action of the lower nature and admit us to the calm peace of the divine being; the other will liberate us into the full being and power of the higher nature and admit us to the equal poise and universality of a divine and infinite knowledge, will of action, Ananda. The first may be described as a passive or negative equality, an equality of reception which fronts impassively the impacts and phenomena of existence and negates the dualities of the appearances and reactions which they impose on us. The second is an active, a positive equality which accepts the phenomena of existence, but only as the manifestation of the one divine being and with an equal response to them which comes from the divine nature in us and transforms them into its hidden values. The first lives in the peace of the one Brahman and puts away from it the nature of the active Ignorance. The second lives in that peace, but also in the Ananda of the Divine and imposes on the life of the soul in nature the signs of the divine knowledge, power and bliss of being. It is this double orientation united by the common principle which will determine the movement of equality in the integral Yoga.

The effort towards a passive or purely receptive equality may start from three different principles or attitudes which all lead to the same result and ultimate consequence, — endurance, indifference and submission. The principle of endurance relies on the strength of the spirit within us to bear all the contacts, impacts, suggestions of this phenomenal Nature that besieges us on every side without being overborne by them and compelled to bear their emotional, sensational, dynamic, intellectual reactions. The outer mind in the lower nature has not this strength.

Its strength is that of a limited force of consciousness which has to do the best it can with all that comes in upon it or besieges it from the greater whirl of consciousness and energy which environs it on this plane of existence. That it can maintain itself at all and affirm its individual being in the universe, is due indeed to the strength of the spirit within it, but it cannot bring forward the whole of that strength or the infinity of that force to meet the attacks of life; if it could, it would be at once the equal and master of its world. In fact, it has to manage as it can. It meets certain impacts and is able to assimilate, equate or master them partially or completely, for a time or wholly, and then it has in that degree the emotional and sensational reactions of joy, pleasure, satisfaction, liking, love, etc., or the intellectual and mental reactions of acceptance, approval, understanding, knowledge, preference, and on these its will seizes with attraction, desire, the attempt to prolong, to repeat, to create, to possess, to make them the pleasurable habit of its life. Other impacts it meets, but finds them too strong for it or too dissimilar and discordant or too weak to give it satisfaction; these are things which it cannot bear or cannot equate with itself or cannot assimilate, and it is obliged to give to them reactions of grief, pain, discomfort, dissatisfaction, disliking, disapproval, rejection, inability to understand or know, refusal of admission. Against them it seeks to protect itself, to escape from them, to avoid or minimise their recurrence; it has with regard to them movements of fear, anger, shrinking, horror, aversion, disgust, shame, would gladly be delivered from them, but it cannot get away from them, for it is bound to and even invites their causes and therefore the results; for these impacts are part of life, tangled up with the things we desire, and the inability to deal with them is part of the imperfection of our nature. Other impacts again the normal mind succeeds in holding at bay or neutralising and to these it has a natural reaction of indifference, insensibility or tolerance which is neither positive acceptance and enjoyment nor rejection or suffering. To things, persons, happenings, ideas, workings, whatever presents itself to the mind, there are always these three kinds of reaction. At the same time, in spite of their generality, there is nothing absolute about them; they form a scheme for a habitual scale which is not precisely the same for all or even for the same mind at different times or in different conditions. The same impact may arouse in it at one time and another the pleasurable or positive, the adverse or negative or the indifferent or neutral reactions.

The soul which seeks mastery may begin by turning upon these reactions the encountering and opposing force of a strong and equal endurance. Instead of seeking to protect itself from or to shun and escape the unpleasant impacts it may confront them and teach itself to suffer and to bear them with perseverance, with fortitude, an increasing equanimity or an austere or calm acceptance. This attitude, this discipline brings out three results, three powers of the soul in relation to things. First, it is found that what was before unbearable, becomes easy to endure; the scale of the power that meets the impact rises in degree; it needs a greater and greater force of it or of its protracted incidence to cause trouble, pain, grief, aversion or any other of the notes in the gamut of the unpleasant reactions. Secondly, it is found that the conscious nature divides itself into two parts, one of the normal mental and emotional nature in which the customary reactions continue to take place, another of the higher will and reason which observes and is not troubled or affected by the passion of this lower nature, does not accept it as its own, does not approve, sanction or participate. Then the lower nature begins to lose the force and power of its reactions, to submit to the suggestions of calm and strength from the higher reason and will, and gradually that calm and strength take possession of the mental and emotional, even of the sensational, vital and physical being. This brings the third power and result, the power by this endurance and mastery, this separation and rejection of the lower nature, to get rid of the normal reactions and even, if we will, to remould all our modes of experience by the strength of the spirit. This method is applied not only to the unpleasant, but also to the pleasant reactions; the soul refuses to give itself up to or be carried away by them; it endures with calm the impacts which bring joy and pleasure; refuses to be excited by them and replaces the joy and eager seeking of the mind after pleasant things by the calm of the spirit. It can be applied too to the thought-mind in a calm reception of knowledge and of limitation of knowledge which refuses to be carried away by the fascination of this attractive or repelled by dislike for that unaccustomed or unpalatable thought-suggestion and waits on the Truth with a detached observation which allows it to grow on the strong, disinterested, mastering will and reason. Thus the soul becomes gradually equal to all things, master of itself, adequate to meet the world with a strong front in the mind and an undisturbed serenity of the spirit.

The second way is an attitude of impartial indifference. Its method is to reject at once the attraction or the repulsion of things, to cultivate for them a luminous impassivity, an inhibiting rejection, a habit of dissociation and desuetude. This attitude reposes less on the will, though will is always necessary, than on the knowledge. It is an attitude which regards these passions of the mind as things born of the illusion of the outward mentality or inferior movements unworthy of the calm truth of the single and equal spirit or a vital and emotional disturbance to be rejected by the tranquil observing will and dispassionate intelligence of the sage. It puts away desire from the mind, discards the ego which attributes these dual values to things, and replaces desire by an impartial and indifferent peace and ego by the pure self which is not troubled, excited or unhinged by the impacts of the world. And not only is the emotional mind quieted, but the intellectual being also rejects the thoughts of the ignorance and rises beyond the interests of an inferior knowledge to the one truth that is eternal and without change. This way too develops three results or powers by which it ascends to peace.

First, it is found that the mind is voluntarily bound by the petty joys and troubles of life and that in reality these can have no inner hold on it, if the soul simply chooses to cast off its habit of helpless determination by external and transient things. Secondly, it is found that here too a division can be made, a psychological partition between the lower or outward mind still subservient to the old habitual touches and the higher reason and will which stand back to live in the indifferent calm of the spirit. There grows on us, in other words, an inner separate calm which watches the commotion of the lower members without taking part in it or giving it any sanction. At first the higher reason and will may be often clouded, invaded, the mind carried away by the incitation of the lower members, but eventually this calm becomes inexpugnable, permanent, not to be shaken by the most violent touches, *na duḥkhena guruṇāpi vicālyate*. This inner soul of calm regards the trouble of the outer mind with a detached superiority or a passing uninvolved indulgence such as might be given to the trivial joys and griefs of a child, it does not regard them as its own or as reposing on any permanent reality. And, finally, the outer mind too accepts by degrees this calm and indifferent serenity; it ceases to be attracted by the things that attracted it or troubled by the griefs and pains to which it had the habit of attaching an unreal importance. Thus the third power comes, an all-pervading power of wide tranquillity and peace, a bliss of release from the siege of our imposed fantastic self-torturing nature, the deep undisturbed exceeding happiness of the touch of the eternal and infinite replacing by its permanence the strife and turmoil of impermanent things, *brahmasaṁsparśam atyantaṁ sukham aśnute*. The soul is fixed in the delight of the self, *ātmaratiḥ*, in the single and infinite Ananda of the spirit and hunts no more after outward touches and their griefs and pleasures. It observes the world only as the spectator of a play or action in which it is no longer compelled to participate.

The third way is that of submission, which may be the Christian resignation founded on submission to the will of God, or an unegoistic acceptance of things and happenings as a manifestation of the universal Will in time, or a complete surrender of the person to the Divine, to the supreme Purusha. As the first was a way of the will and the second a way of knowledge, of the understanding reason, so this is a way of the temperament and heart and very intimately connected with the principle of Bhakti. If it is pushed to the end, it arrives at the same result of a perfect equality. For the knot of the ego is loosened and the personal claim begins to disappear, we find that we are no longer bound to joy in things pleasant or sorrow over the unpleasant; we bear them without either eager acceptance or troubled rejection, refer them to the Master of our being, concern ourselves less and less with their personal result to us and hold only one thing of importance, to approach God, or to be in touch and tune with the universal and infinite Existence, or to be united with the Divine, his channel, instrument, servant, lover, rejoicing in him and in our relation with him and having no other object or cause of joy or sorrow. Here too there may be for some time a division between the lower mind of habitual emotions and the higher psychical mind of love and self-giving, but eventually the former yields, changes, transforms itself, is swallowed up in the love, joy, delight of the Divine and has no other interests or attractions. Then all within is the equal peace and bliss of that union, the one silent bliss that passes understanding, the peace that abides untouched by the solicitation of lower things in the depths of our spiritual existence.

These three ways coincide in spite of their separate starting-points, first, by their inhibition of the normal reactions of the mind to the touches of outward things, *bāhya-sparśān*, secondly, by their separation of the self or spirit from the outward action of Nature. But it is evident that our perfection will be greater and more embracingly complete, if we can have a more active equality which will enable us not only to draw back from or confront the world in a detached and separated calm, but to return upon it and possess it in the power of the calm and equal Spirit. This is possible because the world, Nature, action are not in fact a quite separate thing, but a manifestation of the Self, the All-Soul, the Divine. The reactions of the normal mind are a degradation of the divine values which would but for this degradation make this truth evident to us, — a falsification, an ignorance which alters their workings, an ignorance which starts from the involution of the Self in a blind material nescience. Once we return to the full consciousness of Self, of God, we can then put a true divine value on things and receive and act on them with the calm, joy, knowledge, seeing will of the Spirit. When we begin to do that, then the soul begins to have an equal joy in the universe, an equal will dealing with all energies, an equal knowledge which takes possession of the spiritual truth behind all the phenomena of this divine manifestation. It possesses the world as the Divine possesses it, in a fullness of the infinite light, power and Ananda.

All this existence can therefore be approached by a Yoga of positive and active in place of the negative and passive equality. This requires, first, a new knowledge which is the knowledge of unity, — to see all things as oneself and to see all things in God and God in all things. There is then a will of equal acceptance of all phenomena, all events, all happenings, all persons and forces as masks of the Self, movements of the one energy, results of the one power in action, ruled by the one divine wisdom; and on the foundation of this will of greater knowledge there grows a strength to meet everything with an untroubled soul and mind. There must be an identification of myself with the self of the universe, a vision and a feeling of oneness with all creatures, a perception of all forces and energies and results as the movement of this energy of my self and therefore intimately my own; not, obviously, of my ego-self which must be silenced, eliminated, cast away, — otherwise this perfection cannot come, — but of a greater impersonal or universal self with which I am now one. For my personality is now only one centre of action of that universal self, but a centre intimately in relation and unison with all other personalities and also with all those other things which are to us only impersonal objects and forces: but in fact they also are powers of the one impersonal Person (Purusha), God, Self and Spirit. My individuality is his and is no longer a thing incompatible with or separated from universal being; it is itself universalised, a knower of the universal Ananda and one with and a lover of all that it knows, acts on and enjoys. For to the equal knowledge of the universe and equal will of acceptance of the universe will be added an equal delight in all the cosmic manifestation of the Divine.

Here too we may describe three results or powers of the method. First, we develop this power of equal acceptance in the spirit and in the higher reason and will which respond to the spiritual knowledge. But also we find that though the nature can be induced to take this general attitude, there is yet a struggle between that higher reason and will and the lower mental being which clings to the old egoistic way of seeing the world and reacting to its impacts. Then we find that these two, though at first confused, mingled together, alternating, acting on each other, striving for possession, can be divided, the higher spiritual disengaged from the lower mental nature. But in this stage, while the mind is still subject to reactions of grief, trouble, an inferior joy and pleasure, there is an increased difficulty which does not act to the same extent in a more sharply individualised Yoga. For not only does the mind feel its own troubles and difficulties, but it shares in the joys and griefs of others, vibrates to them in a poignant sympathy, feels their impacts with a subtle sensitiveness, makes them its own; not only so, but the difficulties of others are added to our own and the forces which oppose the perfection act with a greater persistence, because they feel this movement to be an attack upon and an attempt to conquer their universal kingdom and not merely the escape of an isolated soul from their empire. But finally, we find too that there comes a power to surmount these difficulties; the higher reason and will impose themselves on the lower mind, which sensibly changes into the vast types of the spiritual nature; it takes even a delight in feeling, meeting and surmounting all troubles, obstacles and difficulties until they are eliminated by its own transformation. Then the whole being lives in a final power, the universal calm and joy, the seeing delight and will of the Spirit in itself and its manifestation.

To see how this positive method works, we may note very briefly its principle in the three great powers of knowledge, will and feeling. All emotion, feeling, sensation is a way of the soul meeting and putting effective values on the manifestations of the Self in nature. But what the self feels is a universal delight, Ananda. The soul in the lower mind on the contrary gives it, as we have seen, three varying values of pain, pleasure and neutral indifference, which tone by gradations of less and more into each other, and this gradation depends on the power of the individualised consciousness to meet, sense, assimilate, equate, master all that comes in on it from all of the greater self which it has by separative individualisation put outside of it and made as if notself to its experience. But all the time, because of the greater Self within us, there is a secret soul which takes delight in all these things and draws strength from and grows by all that touches it, profits as much by adverse as by favourable experience. This can make itself felt by the outer desire soul, and that in fact is why we have a delight in existing and can even take a certain kind of pleasure in struggle, suffering and the harsher colours of existence. But to get the universal Ananda all our instruments must learn to take not any partial or perverse, but the essential joy of all things. In all things there is a principle of Ananda, which the understanding can seize on and the aesthesis feel as the taste of delight in them, their *rasa*; but ordinarily they put upon them instead arbitrary, unequal and contrary values: they have to be led to perceive things in the light of the spirit and to transform these provisional values into the real, the equal and essential, the spiritual *rasa*. The life-principle is there to give this seizing of the principle of delight, *rasa-grahaṇa*, the form of a strong possessing enjoyment, *bhoga*, which makes the whole life-being vibrate with it and accept and rejoice in it; but ordinarily it is not, owing to desire, equal to its task, but turns it into the three lower forms, — pain and pleasure, *sukha-bhoga duḥkha-bhoga*, and that rejection of both which we call insensibility or indifference. The prana or vital being has to be liberated from desire and its inequalities and to accept and turn into pure enjoyment the *rasa* which the understanding and aesthesis perceive. Then there is no farther obstacle in the instruments to the third step by which all is changed into the full and pure ecstasy of the spiritual Ananda.

In the matter of knowledge, there are again three reactions of the mind to things, ignorance, error and true knowledge. The positive equality will accept all three of them to start with as movements of a self-manifestation which evolves out of ignorance through the partial or distorted knowledge which is the cause of error to true knowledge. It will deal with the ignorance of the mind, as what it is psychologically, a clouded, veiled or wrapped-up state of the substance of consciousness in which the knowledge of the all-knowing Self is hidden as if in a dark sheath; it will dwell on it by the mind and by the aid of related truths already known, by the intelligence or by an intuitive concentration deliver the knowledge out of the veil of the ignorance. It will not attach itself only to the known or try to force all into its little frame, but will dwell on the known and the unknown with an equal mind open to all possibility. So too it will deal with error; it will accept the tangled skein of truth and error, but attach itself to no opinion, rather seeking for the element of truth behind all opinions, the knowledge concealed within the error, — for all error is a disfiguration of some misunderstood fragments of truth and draws its vitality from that and not from its misapprehension; it will accept, but not limit itself even by ascertained truths, but will always be ready for new knowledge and seek for a more and more integral, a more and more extended, reconciling, unifying wisdom. This can only come in its fullness by rising to the ideal supermind, and therefore the equal seeker of truth will not be attached to the intellect and its workings or think that all ends there, but be prepared to rise beyond, accepting each stage of ascent and the contributions of each power of his being, but only to lift them into a higher truth. He must accept everything, but cling to nothing, be repelled by nothing however imperfect or however subversive of fixed notions, but also allow nothing to lay hold on him to the detriment of the free working of the Truth-Spirit. This equality of the intelligence is an essential condition for rising to the higher supramental and spiritual knowledge.

The will in us, because it is the most generally forceful power of our being, — there is a will of knowledge, a will of life, a will of emotion, a will acting in every part of our nature, — takes many forms and returns various reactions to things, such as incapacity, limitation of power, mastery, or right will, wrong or perverted will, neutral volition, — in the ethical mind virtue, sin and non-ethical volition, — and others of the kind.

These too the positive equality accepts as a tangle of provisional values from which it must start, but which it must transform into universal mastery, into the will of the Truth and universal Right, into the freedom of the divine Will in action. The equal will need not feel remorse, sorrow or discouragement over its stumblings; if these reactions occur in the habitual mentality, it will only see how far they indicate an imperfection and the thing to be corrected, — for they are not always just indicators, — and so get beyond them to a calm and equal guidance. It will see that these stumblings themselves are necessary to experience and in the end steps towards the goal. Behind and within all that occurs in ourselves and in the world, it will look for the divine meaning and the divine guidance; it will look beyond imposed limitations to the voluntary self-limitation of the universal Power by which it regulates its steps and gradations, — imposed on our ignorance, self-imposed in the divine knowledge, — and go beyond to unity with the illimitable power of the Divine. All energies and actions it will see as forces proceeding from the one Existence and their perversions as imperfections, inevitable in the developing movement, of powers that were needed for that movement; it will therefore have charity for all imperfections, even while pressing steadily towards a universal perfection. This equality will open the nature to the guidance of the divine and universal Will and make it ready for that supramental action in which the power of the soul in us is luminously full of and one with the power of the supreme Spirit.

The integral Yoga will make use of both the passive and the active methods according to the need of the nature and the guidance of the inner spirit, the Antaryamin. It will not limit itself by the passive way, for that would lead only to some individual quietistic salvation or negation of an active and universal spiritual being which would be inconsistent with the totality of its aim. It will use the method of endurance, but not stop short with a detached strength and serenity, but move rather to a positive strength and mastery, in which endurance will no longer be needed, since the self will then be in a calm and powerful spontaneous possession of the universal energy and capable of determining easily and happily all its reactions in the oneness and the Ananda. It will use the method of impartial indifference, but not end in an aloof indifference to all things, but rather move towards a high-seated impartial acceptance of life strong to transform all experience into the greater values of the equal spirit. It will use too temporarily resignation and submission, but by the full surrender of its personal being to the Divine it will attain to the all-possessing Ananda in which there is no need of resignation, to the perfect harmony with the universal which is not merely an acquiescence, but an embracing oneness, to the perfect instrumentality and subjection of the natural self to the Divine by which the Divine also is possessed by the individual spirit. It will use fully the positive method, but will go beyond any individual acceptance of things which would have the effect of turning existence into a field only of the perfected individual knowledge, power and Ananda. That it will have, but also it will have the oneness by which it can live in the existence of others for their sake and not only for its own and for their assistance and as one of their means, an associated and helping force in the movement towards the same perfection. It will live for the Divine, not shunning world-existence, not attached to the earth or the heavens, not attached either to a supracosmic liberation, but equally one with the Divine in all his planes and able to live in him equally in the Self and in the manifestation.

Chapter XIII

The Action of Equality

THE DISTINCTIONS that have already been made, will have shown in sufficiency what is meant by the status of equality. It is not mere quiescence and indifference, not a withdrawal from experience, but a superiority to the present reactions of the mind and life. It is the spiritual way of replying to life or rather of embracing it and compelling it to become a perfect form of action of the self and spirit. It is the first secret of the soul's mastery of existence. When we have it in perfection, we are admitted to the very ground of the divine spiritual nature. The mental being in the body tries to compel and conquer life, but is at every turn compelled by it, because it submits to the desire reactions of the vital self. To be equal, not to be overborne by any stress of desire, is the first condition of real mastery, self-empire is its basis. But a mere mental equality, however great it may be, is hampered by the tendency of quiescence. It has to preserve itself from desire by self-limitation in the will and action. It is only the spirit which is capable of sublime undisturbed rapidities of will as well as an illimitable patience, equally just in a slow and deliberate or a swift and violent, equally secure in a safely lined and limited or a vast and enormous action. It can accept the smallest work in the narrowest circle of cosmos, but it can work too upon the whirl of chaos with an understanding and creative force; and these things it can do because by its detached and yet intimate acceptance it carries into both an infinite calm, knowledge, will and power. It has that detachment because it is above all the happenings, forms, ideas and movements it embraces in its scope; and it has that intimate acceptance because it is yet one with all things. If we have not this free unity, *ekatvam anupaśyataḥ*, we have not the full equality of the spirit.

The first business of the sadhaka is to see whether he has

the perfect equality, how far he has gone in this direction or else where is the flaw, and to exercise steadily his will on his nature or invite the will of the Purusha to get rid of the defect and its causes. There are four things that he must have; first, equality in the most concrete practical sense of the word, *samatā*, freedom from mental, vital, physical preferences, an even acceptance of all God's workings within and around him; secondly, a firm peace and absence of all disturbance and trouble, *śānti*; thirdly, a positive inner spiritual happiness and spiritual ease of the natural being which nothing can lessen, *sukham*; fourthly, a clear joy and laughter of the soul embracing life and existence. To be equal is to be infinite and universal, not to limit oneself, not to bind oneself down to this or that form of the mind and life and its partial preferences and desires. But since man in his present normal nature lives by his mental and vital formations, not in the freedom of his spirit, attachment to them and the desires and preferences they involve is also his normal condition. To accept them is at first inevitable, to get beyond them exceedingly difficult and not, perhaps, altogether possible so long as we are compelled to use the mind as the chief instrument of our action. The first necessity therefore is to take at least the sting out of them, to deprive them, even when they persist, of their greater insistence, their present egoism, their more violent claim on our nature.

The test that we have done this is the presence of an undisturbed calm in the mind and spirit. The sadhaka must be on the watch as the witnessing and willing Purusha behind or, better, as soon as he can manage it, above the mind, and repel even the least indices or incidence of trouble, anxiety, grief, revolt, disturbance in his mind. If these things come, he must at once detect their source, the defect which they indicate, the fault of egoistic claim, vital desire, emotion or idea from which they start and this he must discourage by his will, his spiritualised intelligence, his soul unity with the Master of his being. On no account must he admit any excuse for them, however natural, righteous in seeming or plausible, or any inner or outer justification. If it is the prana which is troubled and clamorous, he must separate himself from the troubled prana, keep seated his higher nature in the buddhi and by the buddhi school and reject the claim of the desire-soul in him; and so too if it is the heart of emotion that makes the clamour and the disturbance. If on the other hand it is the will and intelligence itself that is at fault, then the trouble is more difficult to command, because then his chief aid and instrument becomes an accomplice of the revolt against the divine Will and the old sins of the lower members take advantage of this sanction to raise their diminished heads. Therefore there must be a constant insistence on one main idea, the self-surrender to the Master of our being, God within us and in the world, the supreme Self, the universal Spirit. The buddhi dwelling always in this master idea must discourage all its own lesser insistences and preferences and teach the whole being that the ego whether it puts forth its claim through the reason, the personal will, the heart or the desire-soul in the prana, has no just claim of any kind and all grief, revolt, impatience, trouble is a violence against the Master of the being.

This complete self-surrender must be the chief mainstay of the sadhaka because it is the only way, apart from complete quiescence and indifference to all action, — and that has to be avoided, — by which the absolute calm and peace can come. The persistence of trouble, *asānti*, the length of time taken for this purification and perfection, itself must not be allowed to become a reason for discouragement and impatience. It comes because there is still something in the nature which responds to it, and the recurrence of trouble serves to bring out the presence of the defect, put the sadhaka upon his guard and bring about a more enlightened and consistent action of the will to get rid of it. When the trouble is too strong to be kept out, it must be allowed to pass and its return discouraged by a greater vigilance and insistence of the spiritualised buddhi. Thus persisting, it will be found that these things lose their force more and more, become more and more external and brief in their recurrence, until finally calm becomes the law of the being. This rule persists so long as the mental buddhi is the chief instrument; but when the supramental light takes possession of mind and heart, then there can be no trouble, grief or disturbance; for that brings with it a spiritual nature of illumined strength in which these things can have no place. There the only vibrations and emotions are those which belong to the *ānandamaya* nature of divine unity.

The calm established in the whole being must remain the same whatever happens, in health and disease, in pleasure and in pain, even in the strongest physical pain, in good fortune and misfortune, our own or that of those we love, in success and failure, honour and insult, praise and blame, justice done to us or injustice, everything that ordinarily affects the mind. If we see unity everywhere, if we recognise that all comes by the divine will, see God in all, in our enemies or rather our opponents in the game of life as well as our friends, in the powers that oppose and resist us as well as the powers that favour and assist, in all energies and forces and happenings, and if besides we can feel that all is undivided from our self, all the world one with us within our universal being, then this attitude becomes much easier to the heart and mind. But even before we can attain or are firmly seated in that universal vision, we have by all the means in our power to insist on this receptive and active equality and calm. Even something of it, *alpam api asya dharmasya*, is a great step towards perfection; a first firmness in it is the beginning of liberated perfection; its completeness is the perfect assurance of a rapid progress in all the other members of perfection. For without it we can have no solid basis; and by the pronounced lack of it we shall be constantly falling back to the lower status of desire, ego, duality, ignorance.

This calm once attained, vital and mental preference has lost its disturbing force; it only remains as a formal habit of the mind. Vital acceptance or rejection, the greater readiness to welcome this rather than that happening, the mental acceptance or rejection, the preference of this more congenial to that other less congenial idea or truth, the dwelling upon the will to this rather than to that other result, become a formal mechanism still necessary as an index of the direction in which the Shakti is meant to turn or for the present is made to incline by the Master of our being. But it loses its disturbing aspect of strong egoistic will, intolerant desire, obstinate liking. These appearances may remain for a while in a diminished form, but as the calm of equality increases, deepens, becomes more essential and compact, *ghana*, they disappear, cease to colour the mental and vital substance or occur only as touches on the most external physical mind, are unable to penetrate within, and at last even that recurrence, that appearance at the outer gates of mind ceases. Then there can come the living reality of the perception that all in us is done and directed by the Master of our being, *yathā prayukto 'smi, tathā karomi*, which was before only a strong idea and faith with occasional and derivative glimpses of the divine action behind the becomings of our personal nature. Now every movement is seen to be the form given by the Shakti, the divine power in us, to the indications of the Purusha, still no doubt personalised, still belittled in the inferior mental form, but not primarily egoistic, an imperfect form, not a positive deformation. We have then to get beyond this stage even. For the perfect action and experience is not to be determined by any kind of mental or vital preference, but by the revealing and inspiring spiritual will which is the Shakti in her direct and real initiation. When I say that as I am appointed, I work, I still bring in a limiting personal element and mental reaction. But it is the Master who will do his own work through myself as his instrument, and there must be no mental or other preference in me to limit, to interfere, to be a source of imperfect working. The mind must become a silent luminous channel for the revelations of the supramental Truth and of the Will involved in its seeing. Then shall the action be the action of that highest Being and Truth and not a qualified translation or mistranslation in the mind. Whatever limitation, selection, relation is imposed, will be self-imposed by the Divine on himself in the individual at the moment for his own purpose, not binding, not final, not an ignorant determination of the mind. The thought and will become then an action from a luminous Infinite, a formulation not excluding other formulations, but rather putting them into their just place in relation to itself, englobing or transforming them even and proceeding to larger formations of the divine knowledge and action.

The first calm that comes is of the nature of peace, the absence of all unquiet, grief and disturbance. As the equality becomes more intense, it takes on a fuller substance of positive happiness and spiritual ease. This is the joy of the spirit in itself, dependent on nothing external for its absolute existence, *nirāśraya*, as the Gita describes it, *antaḥ-sukho antarārāmaḥ*, an exceeding inner happiness, *brahmasaṁsparśam atyantaṁ sukham aśnute*. Nothing can disturb it, and it extends itself to the soul's view of outward things, imposes on them too the law of this quiet spiritual joy. For the base of it is still calm, it is an even and tranquil neutral joy, *ahaituka*. And as the supramental light grows, a greater Ananda comes, the base of the abundant ecstasy of the spirit in all it is, becomes, sees, experiences and of the laughter of the Shakti doing luminously the work of the Divine and taking his Ananda in all the worlds.

The perfected action of equality transforms all the values of things on the basis of the divine *ānandamaya* power. The outward action may remain what it was or may change, that must be as the Spirit directs and according to the need of the work to be done for the world, — but the whole inner action is of another kind. The Shakti in its different powers of knowledge, action, enjoyment, creation, formulation, will direct itself to the different aims of existence, but in another spirit; they will be the aims, the fruits, the lines of working laid down by the Divine from his light above, not anything claimed by the ego for its own separate sake. The mind, the heart, the vital being, the body itself will be satisfied with whatever comes to them from the dispensation of the Master of the being and in that find a subtlest and yet fullest spiritualised satisfaction and delight; but the divine knowledge and will above will work forward towards its farther ends. Here both success and failure lose their present meanings. There can be no failure; for whatever happens is the intention of the Master of the worlds, not final, but a step on his way, and if it appears as an opposition, a defeat, a denial, even for the moment a total denial of the aim set before the instrumental being, it is so only in appearance and afterwards it will appear in its right place in the economy of his action, — a fuller supramental vision may even see at once or beforehand its necessity and its true relation to the eventual result to which it seems so contrary and even perhaps its definite prohibition. Or, if — while the light is deficient — there has been a misinterpretation whether with regard to the aim or the course of the action and the steps of the result, the failure comes as a rectification and is calmly accepted without bringing discouragement or a fluctuation of the will. In the end it is found that there is no such thing as failure and the soul takes an equal passive or active delight in all happenings as the steps and formulations of the divine Will. The same evolution takes place with regard to good fortune and ill fortune, the pleasant and the unpleasant in every form, *mangala amangala, priya apriya*.

And as with happenings, so with persons, equality brings an entire change of the view and the attitude. The first result of the equal mind and spirit is to bring about an increasing charity and inner toleration of all persons, ideas, views, actions, because it is seen that God is in all beings and each acts according to his nature, his *svabhāva*, and its present formulations. When there is the positive equal Ananda, this deepens to a sympathetic understanding and in the end an equal universal love. None of these things need prevent various relations or different formulations of the inner attitude according to the need of life as determined by the spiritual will, or firm furtherings of this idea, view, action against that other for the same need and purpose by the same determination, or a strong outward or inward resistance, opposition and action against the forces that are impelled to stand in the way of the decreed movement. And there may be even the rush of the Rudra energy forcefully working upon or shattering the human or other obstacle, because that is necessary both for him and for the world purpose. But the essence of the equal inmost attitude is not altered or diminished by these more superficial formulations. The spirit, the fundamental soul remain the same, even while the Shakti of knowledge, will, action, love does its work and assumes the various forms needed for its work. And in the end all becomes a form of a luminous spiritual unity with all persons, energies, things in the being of God and in the luminous, spiritual, one and universal force, in which one's own action becomes an inseparable part of the action of all, is not divided from it, but feels perfectly every relation as a relation with God in all in the complex terms of his universal oneness. That is a plenitude which can hardly be described in the language of the dividing mental reason for it uses all its oppositions, yet escapes from them, nor can it be put in the terms of our limited mental psychology. It belongs to another domain of consciousness, another plane of our being.

Chapter XIV

The Power of the Instruments

THE SECOND member of the Yoga of self-perfection is the heightened, enlarged and rectified power of the instruments of our normal Nature. The cultivation of this second perfection need not wait for the security of the equal mind and spirit, but it is only in that security that it can become complete and act in the safety of the divine leading. The object of this cultivation is to make the nature a fit instrument for divine works. All work is done by power, by Shakti, and since the integral Yoga does not contemplate abandonment of works, but rather a doing of all works from the divine consciousness and with the supreme guidance, the characteristic powers of the instruments, mind, life and body, must not only be purified of defects, but raised to a capacity for this greater action. In the end they must undergo a spiritual and supramental transfiguration.

There are four members of this second part of the sadhana or discipline of self-perfection and the first of them is right shakti, the right condition of the powers of the intelligence, heart, vital mind and body. It will only be possible at present to suggest a preliminary perfection of the last of these four, for the full siddhi will have to be dealt with after I have spoken of the supermind and its influence on the rest of the being. The body is not only the necessary outer instrument of the physical part of action, but for the purposes of this life a base or pedestal also for all inner action. All working of mind or spirit has its vibration in the physical consciousness, records itself there in a kind of subordinate corporeal notation and communicates itself to the material world partly at least through the physical machine. But the body of man has natural limitations in this capacity which it imposes on the play of the higher parts of his being. And, secondly, it has a subconscient consciousness of its own in which it keeps with an obstinate fidelity the past habits and past nature of the mental and vital being and which automatically opposes and obstructs any very great upward change or at least prevents it from becoming a radical transformation of the whole nature. It is evident that if we are to have a free divine or spiritual and supramental action conducted by the force and fulfilling the character of a diviner energy, some fairly complete transformation must be effected in this outward character of the bodily nature. The physical being of man has always been felt by the seekers of perfection to be a great impediment and it has been the habit to turn from it with contempt, denial or aversion and a desire to suppress altogether or as far as may be the body and the physical life. But this cannot be the right method for the integral Yoga. The body is given us as one instrument necessary to the totality of our works and it is to be used, not neglected, hurt, suppressed or abolished. If it is imperfect, recalcitrant, obstinate, so are also the other members, the vital being, heart and mind and reason. It has like them to be changed and perfected and to undergo a transformation. As we must get ourselves a new life, new heart, new mind, so we have in a certain sense to build for ourselves a new body.

The first thing the will has to do with the body is to impose on it progressively a new habit of all its being, consciousness, force and outward and inward action. It must be taught an entire passivity in the hands first of the higher instruments, but eventually in the hands of the spirit and its controlling and informing Shakti. It must be accustomed not to impose its own limits on the nobler members, but to shape its action and its response to their demands, to develop, one might say, a higher notation, a higher scale of responses. At present the notation of the body and the physical consciousness has a very large determining power on the music made by this human harp of God; the notes we get from the spirit, from the psychic soul, from the greater life behind our physical life cannot come in freely, cannot develop their high, powerful and proper strain. This condition must be reversed; the body and the physical consciousness must develop the habit of admitting and shaping themselves to these higher strains and not they, but the nobler parts of the nature must determine the music of our life and being.

The control of the body and life by the mind and its thought and will is the first step towards this change. All Yoga implies the carrying of that control to a very high pitch. But afterwards the mind must itself give place to the spirit, to the spiritual force, the supermind and the supramental force. And finally the body must develop a perfect power to hold whatever force is brought into it by the spirit and to contain its action without spilling and wasting it or itself getting cracked. It must be capable of being filled and powerfully used by whatever intensity of spiritual or higher mind or life force without any part of the mechanical instrument being agitated, upset, broken or damaged by the inrush or pressure, — as the brain, vital health or moral nature are often injured in those who unwisely attempt Yogic practice without preparation or by undue means or rashly invite a power they are intellectually, vitally, morally unfit to bear, — and, thus filled, it must have the capacity to work normally, automatically, rightly according to the will of that spiritual or other now un- usual agent without distorting, diminishing or mistranslating its intention and stress. This faculty of holding, *dhāraṇa-śakti*, in the physical consciousness, energy and machinery is the most important siddhi or perfection of the body.

The result of these changes will be to make the body a perfect instrument of the spirit. The spiritual force will be able to do what it wills and as it wills in and through the body. It will be able to conduct an unlimited action of the mind or at a higher stage of the supermind without the body betraying the action by fatigue, incapacity, inaptitude or falsification. It will be able too to pour a full tide of the life-force into the body and conduct a large action and joy of the perfected vital being without that quarrel and disparity which is the relation of the normal life- instincts and life-impulses to the insufficient physical instrument they are obliged to use. And it will also be able to conduct a full action of the spiritualised psychic being not falsified, degraded or in any way marred by the lower instincts of the body and to use physical action and expression as a free notation of the higher psychical life. And in the body itself there will be a presence of a greatness of sustaining force, an abounding strength, energy and puissance of outgoing and managing force, a lightness, swiftness and adaptability of the nervous and physical being, a holding and responsive power in the whole physical machine and its driving springs[1] of which it is now even at its strongest and best incapable.

This energy will not be in its essence an outward, physical or muscular strength, but will be of the nature, first, of an unbounded life-power or pranic force, secondly, sustaining and using this pranic energy, a superior or supreme will-power acting in the body. The play of the pranic shakti in the body or form is the condition of all action, even of the most apparently inanimate physical action. It is the universal Prana, as the ancients knew, which in various forms sustains or drives material energy in all physical things from the electron and atom and gas up through the metal, plant, animal, physical man. To get this pranic shakti to act more freely and forcibly in the body is knowingly or unknowingly the attempt of all who strive for a greater perfection of or in the body. The ordinary man tries to command it mechanically by physical exercises and other corporeal means, the Hathayogin more greatly and flexibly, but still mechanically by Asana and Pranayama; but for our purpose it can be commanded by more subtle, essential and pliable means; first, by a will in the mind widely opening itself to and potently calling in the universal pranic shakti on which we draw and fixing its stronger presence and more powerful working in the body; secondly, by the will in the mind opening itself rather to the spirit and its power and calling in a higher pranic energy from above, a supramental pranic force; thirdly, the last step, by the highest supramental will of the spirit entering and taking up directly the task of the perfection of the body. In fact, it is always really a will within which drives and makes effective the pranic instrument even when it uses what seem to be purely physical means; but at first it is dependent on the inferior action. When we go higher, the relation is gradually reversed; it is then able to act in its own power or handle the rest only as a subordinate instrumentation.

---

[1] *mahattva, bala, laghutā, dhāraṇa-sāmarthya.*

Most men are not conscious of this pranic force in the body or cannot distinguish it from the more physical form of energy which it informs and uses for its vehicle. But as the consciousness becomes more subtle by practice of Yoga, we can come to be aware of the sea of pranic shakti around us, feel it with the mental consciousness, concretely with a mental sense, see its courses and movements, and direct and act upon it immediately by the will. But until we thus become aware of it, we have to possess a working or at least an experimental faith in its presence and in the power of the will to develop a greater command and use of this prana force. There is necessary a faith, *śraddhā*, in the power of the mind to lay its will on the state and action of the body, such as those have who heal disease by faith, will or mental action; but we must seek this control not only for this or any other limited use, but generally as a legitimate power of the inner and greater over the outer and lesser instrument. This faith is combated by our past habits of mind, by our actual normal experience of its comparative helplessness in our present imperfect system and by an opposing belief in the body and physical consciousness. For they too have a limiting *śraddhā* of their own which opposes the idea in the mind when it seeks to impose on the system the law of a higher yet unattained perfection. But as we persist and find this power giving evidence of itself to our experience, the faith in the mind will be able to found itself more firmly and grow in vigour and the opposing faith in the body will change, admit what it first denied and not only accept in its habits the new yoke but itself call for this higher action. Finally we shall realise the truth that this being we are is or can become whatever it has the faith and will to be, — for faith is only a will aiming at greater truth, — and cease to set limits to our possibility or deny the potential omnipotence of the Self in us, the divine Power working through the human instrument. That however, at least as a practical force, comes in at a later stage of high perfection.

The Prana is not only a force for the action of physical and vital energy, but supports also the mental and spiritual action. Therefore the full and free working of the pranic shakti is required not only for the lower but still necessary use, but also for the free and full operation of mind and supermind and spirit in the instrumentality of our complex human nature. That is the main sense of the use of exercises of Pranayama for control of the vital force and its motions which is so important and indispensable a part of certain systems of Yoga. The same mastery must be got by the seeker of the integral Yoga; but he may arrive at it by other means and in any case he must not be dependent on any physical or breathing exercise for its possession and maintenance, for that will at once bring in a limitation and subjection to Prakriti. Her instrumentation has to be used flexibly by the Purusha, but not to be a fixed control on the Purusha. The necessity of the pranic force, however, remains and will be evident to our self-study and experience. It is in the Vedic image the steed and conveyance of the embodied mind and will, *vāhana*. If it is full of strength and swiftness and a plenitude of all its powers, then the mind can go on the courses of its action with a plenary and unhampered movement. But if it is lame or soon tired or sluggish or weak, then an incapacity is laid on the effectuation of the will and activity of the mind. The same rule holds good of the supermind when it first comes into action. There are indeed states and activities in which the mind takes up the pranic shakti into itself and this dependence is not felt at all; but even then the force is there, though involved in the pure mental energy. The supermind, when it gets into full strength, can do pretty well what it likes with the pranic shakti, and we find that in the end this life power is transformed into the type of a supramentalised prana which is simply one motor power of that greater consciousness. But this belongs to a later stage of the siddhi of the Yoga.

Then again there is the psychic prana, pranic mind or desire soul; this too calls for its own perfection. Here too the first necessity is a fullness of the vital capacity in the mind, its power to do its full work, to take possession of all the impulsions and energies given to our inner psychic life for fulfilment in this existence, to hold them and to be a means for carrying them out with strength, freedom, perfection. Many of the things we need for our perfection, courage, will-power effective in life, all the elements of what we now call force of character and force of personality, depend very largely for their completest strength and spring of energetic action on the fullness of the psychic prana. But along with this fullness there must be an established gladness, clearness and purity in the psychic life-being. This dynamis must not be a troubled, perfervid, stormy, fitfully or crudely passionate strength; energy there must be, rapture of its action it must have, but a clear and glad and pure energy, a seated and firmly supported pure rapture. And as a third condition of its perfection it must be poised in a complete equality. The desire-soul must get rid of the clamour, insistence or inequality of its desires in order that its desires may be satisfied with justice and balance and in the right way and eventually must rid them of the character of desire altogether and change them into impulsions of the divine Ananda. To that end it must make no demands nor seek to impose itself on heart, mind or spirit, but accept with a strong passive and active equality whatever impulsion and command come into it from the spirit through the channel of a still mind and a pure heart. And it must accept too whatever result of the impulse, whatever enjoyment more or less, full or nil, is given to it by the Master of our being. At the same time, possession and enjoyment are its law, function, use, swadharma. It is not intended to be a slain or mortified thing, dull in its receptive power, dreary, suppressed, maimed, inert or null. It must have a full power of possession, a glad power of enjoyment, an exultant power of pure and divine passion and rapture. The enjoyment it will have will be in the essence a spiritual bliss, but one which takes up into itself and transforms the mental, emotional, dynamic, vital and physical joy; it must have therefore an integral capacity for these things and must not by incapacity or fatigue or inability to bear great intensities fail the spirit, mind, heart, will and body. Fullness, clear purity and gladness, equality, capacity for possession and enjoyment are the fourfold perfection of the psychic prana.[2]

---

2 *pūrṇatā, prasannatā, samatā, bhoga-sāmarthya.*

The next instrument which needs perfection is the *citta*, and within the complete meaning of this expression we may include the emotional and the pure psychical being. This heart and psychic being of man shot through with the threads of the life instincts is a thing of mixed inconstant colours of emotion and soul vibrations, bad and good, happy and unhappy, satisfied and unsatisfied, troubled and calm, intense and dull. Thus agitated and invaded it is unacquainted with any real peace, incapable of a steady perfection of all its powers. By purification, by equality, by the light of knowledge, by a harmonising of the will it can be brought to a tranquil intensity and perfection. The first two elements of this perfection are on one side a high and large sweetness, openness, gentleness, calm, clarity, on the other side a strong and ardent force and intensity. In the divine no less than in ordinary human character and action there are always two strands, sweetness and strength, mildness and force, *saumya* and *raudra*, the force that bears and harmonises, the force that imposes itself and compels, Vishnu and Ishana, Shiva and Rudra. The two are equally necessary to a perfect world-action. The perversions of the Rudra power in the heart are stormy passion, wrath and fierceness and harshness, hardness, brutality, cruelty, egoistic ambition and love of violence and domination. These and other human perversions have to be got rid of by the flowering of a calm, clear and sweet psychical being.

But on the other hand incapacity of force is also an imperfection. Laxity and weakness, self-indulgence, a certain flabbiness and limpness or inert passivity of the psychical being are the last result of an emotional and psychic life in which energy and power of assertion have been quelled, discouraged or killed. Nor is it a total perfection to have only the strength that endures or to cultivate only a heart of love, charity, tolerance, mildness, meekness and forbearance. The other side of perfection is a self-contained and calm and unegoistic Rudra-power armed with psychic force, the energy of the strong heart which is capable of supporting without shrinking an insistent, an outwardly austere or even, where need is, a violent action. An unlimited light of energy, force, puissance harmonised with sweetness of heart and clarity, capable of being one with it in action, the lightning of Indra starting from the orb of the nectarous moon-rays of Soma is the double perfection. And these two things *saumyatva, tejas*, must base their presence and action on a firm equality of the temperament and of the psychical soul delivered from all crudity and all excess or defect of the heart's light or the heart's power.

Another necessary element is a faith in the heart, a belief in and will to the universal good, an openness to the universal Ananda. The pure psychic being is of the essence of Ananda, it comes from the delight-soul in the universe; but the superficial heart of emotion is overborne by the conflicting appearances of the world and suffers many reactions of grief, fear, depression, passion, short-lived and partial joy. An equal heart is needed for perfection, but not only a passive equality; there must be the sense of a divine power making for good behind all experiences, a faith and will which can turn the poisons of the world to nectar, see the happier spiritual intention behind adversity, the mystery of love behind suffering, the flower of divine strength and joy in the seed of pain. This faith, *kalyāṇa-śraddhā*, is needed in order that the heart and the whole overt psychic being may respond to the secret divine Ananda and change itself into this true original essence. This faith and will must be accompanied by and open into an illimitable widest and intensest capacity for love. For the main business of the heart, its true function is love. It is our destined instrument of complete union and oneness; for to see oneness in the world by the understanding is not enough unless we also feel it with the heart and in the psychic being, and this means a delight in the One and in all existences in the world in him, a love of God and all beings. The heart's faith and will in good are founded on a perception of the one Divine immanent in all things and leading the world. The universal love has to be founded on the heart's sight and psychical and emotional sense of the one Divine, the one Self in all existence. All four elements will then form a unity and even the Rudra power to do battle for the right and the good proceed on the basis of a power of universal love. This is the highest and the most characteristic perfection of the heart, *prema-sāmarthya*.

The last perfection is that of the intelligence and thinking mind, *buddhi*. The first need is the clarity and the purity of the intelligence. It must be freed from the claims of the vital being which seeks to impose the desire of the mind in place of the truth, from the claims of the troubled emotional being which strives to colour, distort, limit and falsify the truth with the hue and shape of the emotions. It must be free too from its own defect, inertia of the thought-power, obstructive narrowness and un-willingness to open to knowledge, intellectual unscrupulousness in thinking, prepossession and preference, self-will in the reason and false determination of the will to knowledge. Its sole will must be to make itself an unsullied mirror of the truth, its essence and its forms and measures and relations, a clear mirror, a just measure, a fine and subtle instrument of harmony, an integral intelligence. This clear and pure intelligence can then become a serene thing of light, a pure and strong radiance emanating from the sun of Truth. But, again, it must become not merely a thing of concentrated dry or white light, but capable of all variety of understanding, supple, rich, flexible, brilliant with all the flame and various with all the colours of the manifestation of the Truth, open to all its forms. And so equipped it will get rid of limitations, not be shut up in this or that faculty or form or working of knowledge, but an instrument ready and capable for whatever work is demanded from it by the Purusha. Purity, clear radiance, rich and flexible variety, integral capacity are the fourfold perfection of the thinking intelligence, *viśuddhi, prakāśa, vicitra-bodha, sarva-jñāna-sāmarthya.*

The normal instruments thus perfected will act each in its own kind without undue interference from each other and serve the unobstructed will of the Purusha in a harmonised totality of our natural being. This perfection must rise constantly in its capacity for action, the energy and force of its working and a certain greatness of the scope of the total nature. They will then be ready for the transformation into their own supra-mental action in which they will find a more absolute, unified and luminous spiritual truth of the whole perfected nature. The means of this perfection of the instruments we shall have to consider later on; but at present it will be enough to say that the principal conditions are will, self-watching and self-knowledge and a constant practice, *abhyāsa*, of self-modification and transformation. The Purusha has that capacity; for the spirit within can always change and perfect the working of its nature. But the mental being must open the way by a clear and a watchful introspection, an opening of itself to a searching and subtle self-knowledge which will give it the understanding and to an increasing extent the mastery of its natural instruments, a vigilant and insistent will of self-modification and self-transformation — for to that will the Prakriti must with whatever difficulty and whatever initial or prolonged resistance eventually respond, — and an unfailing practice which will constantly reject all defect and perversion and replace it by right state and a right and enhanced working. Askesis, tapasya, patience and faithfulness and rectitude of knowledge and will are the things required until a greater Power than our mental selves directly intervenes to effect a more easy and rapid transformation.

Chapter XV

Soul-Force and the Fourfold Personality

THE PERFECTING of the normal mind, heart, prana and body gives us only the perfection of the psycho-physical machine we have to use and creates certain right instrumental conditions for a divine life and works lived and done with a purer, greater, clearer power and knowledge. The next question is that of the Force which is poured into the instruments, *karaṇa*, and the One who works it for his universal ends. The force at work in us must be the manifest divine Shakti, the supreme or the universal Force unveiled in the liberated individual being, *parā prakṛtir jīvabhūtā*, who will be the doer of all the action and the power of this divine life, *kartā*. The One behind this force will be the Ishwara, the Master of all being, with whom all our existence will be in our perfection a Yoga at once of oneness in being and of union in various relations of the soul and its nature with the Godhead who is seated within us and in whom too we live, move and have our being. It is this Shakti with the Ishwara in her or behind her whose divine presence and way we have to call into all our being and life. For without this divine presence and this greater working there can be no siddhi of the power of the nature.

All the action of man in life is a nexus of the presence of the soul and the workings of Nature, Purusha and Prakriti. The presence and influence of the Purusha represents itself in nature as a certain power of our being which we may call for our immediate purpose soul-force; and it is always this soul-force which supports all the workings of the powers of the reason, the mind, life and body and determines the cast of our conscious being and the type of our nature. The normal ordinarily developed man possesses it in a subdued, a modified, a mechanised, submerged form as temperament and character; but that is only its most outward mould in which Purusha, the conscious soul or being, seems to be limited, conditioned and given some shape by the mechanical Prakriti. The soul flows into whatever moulds of intellectual, ethical, aesthetic, dynamic, vital and physical mind and type the developing nature takes and can act only in the way this formed Prakriti lays on it and move in its narrow groove or relatively wider circle. The man is then sattwic, rajasic or tamasic or a mixture of these qualities and his temperament is only a sort of subtler soul-colour which has been given to the major prominent operation of these fixed modes of his nature. Men of a stronger force get more of the soul-power to the surface and develop what we call a strong or great personality, they have in them something of the Vibhuti as described by the Gita, *vibhūtimat sattvaṁ śrīmad ūrjitam eva vā*, a higher power of being often touched with or sometimes full of some divine afflatus or more than ordinary manifestation of the Godhead which is indeed present in all, even in the weakest or most clouded living being, but here some special force of it begins to come out from behind the veil of the average humanity, and there is something beautiful, attractive, splendid or powerful in these exceptional persons which shines out in their personality, character, life and work. These men too work in the type of their nature-force according to its gunas, but there is something evident in them and yet not easily analysable which is in reality a direct power of the Self and spirit using to strong purpose the mould and direction of the nature. The nature itself thereby rises to or towards a higher grade of its being. Much in the working of the Force may seem egoistic or even perverse, but it is still the touch of the Godhead behind, whatever Daivic, Asuric or even Rakshasic form it may take, which drives the Prakriti and uses it for its own greater purpose. A still more developed power of the being will bring out the real character of this spiritual presence and it will then be seen as something impersonal and self-existent and self-empowered, a sheer soul-force which is other than the mind-force, life-force, force of intelligence, but drives them and, even while following to a certain extent their mould of working, guna, type of nature, yet puts its stamp of an initial transcendence, impersonality, pure fire of spirit, a something beyond the gunas of our normal nature. When the spirit in us is free, then what was behind this soul-force comes out in all its light, beauty and greatness, the Spirit, the Godhead who makes the nature and soul of man his foundation and living representative in cosmic being and mind, action and life.

The Godhead, the spirit manifested in Nature appears in a sea of infinite quality, Ananta-guna. But the executive or mechanical Prakriti is of the threefold guna, sattwa, rajas, tamas, and the Ananta-guna, the spiritual play of infinite quality, modifies itself in this mechanical nature into the type of these three gunas. And in the soul-force in man this Godhead in Nature represents itself as a fourfold effective Power, *catur-vyūha*, a Power for knowledge, a Power for strength, a Power for mutuality and active and productive relation and interchange, a Power for works and labour and service, and its presence casts all human life into a nexus and inner and outer operation of these four things. The ancient thought of India conscious of this fourfold type of active human personality and nature built out of it the four types of the Brahmana, Kshatriya, Vaishya and Shudra, each with its spiritual turn, ethical ideal, suitable upbringing, fixed function in society and place in the evolutionary scale of the spirit. As always tends to be the case when we too much externalise and mechanise the more subtle truths of our nature, this became a hard and fast system inconsistent with the freedom and variability and complexity of the finer developing spirit in man. Nevertheless the truth behind it exists and is one of some considerable importance in the perfection of our power of nature; but we have to take it in its inner aspects, first, personality, character, temperament, soul-type, then the soul-force which lies behind them and wears these forms, and lastly the play of the free spiritual Shakti in which they find their culmination and unity beyond all modes. For the crude external idea that a man is born as a Brahmana, Kshatriya, Vaishya or Shudra and that alone, is not a psychological truth of our being. The psychological fact is that there are these four active powers and tendencies of the Spirit and its executive Shakti within us and the predominance of one or the other in the more well-formed part of our personality gives us our main tendencies, dominant qualities and capacities, effective turn in action and life. But they are more or less present in all men, here manifest, there latent, here developed, there subdued and depressed or subordinate, and in the perfect man will be raised up to a fullness and harmony which in the spiritual freedom will burst out into the free play of the infinite quality of the spirit in the inner and outer life and in the self-enjoying creative play of the Purusha with his and the world's Nature-Power.

The most outward psychological form of these things is the mould or trend of the nature towards certain dominant tendencies, capacities, characteristics, form of active power, quality of the mind and inner life, cultural personality or type. The turn is often towards the predominance of the intellectual element and the capacities which make for the seeking and finding of knowledge and an intellectual creation or formativeness and a preoccupation with ideas and the study of ideas or of life and the information and development of the reflective intelligence. According to the grade of the development there is produced successively the make and character of the man of active, open, inquiring intelligence, then the intellectual and, last, the thinker, sage, great mind of knowledge. The soul-powers which make their appearance by a considerable development of this temperament, personality, soul-type, are a mind of light more and more open to all ideas and knowledge and incomings of Truth; a hunger and passion for knowledge, for its growth in ourselves, for its communication to others, for its reign in the world, the reign of reason and right and truth and justice and, on a higher level of the harmony of our greater being, the reign of the spirit and its universal unity and light and love; a power of this light in the mind and will which makes all the life subject to reason and its right and truth or to the spirit and spiritual right and truth and subdues the lower members to their greater law; a poise in the temperament turned from the first to patience, steady musing and calm, to reflection, to meditation, which dominates and quiets the turmoil of the will and passions and makes for high thinking and pure living, founds the self-governed sattwic mind, grows into a more and more mild, lofty, impersonalised and universalised personality. This is the ideal character and soul-power of the Brahmana, the priest of knowledge. If it is not there in all its sides, we have the imperfections or perversions of the type, a mere intellectuality or curiosity for ideas without ethical or other elevation, a narrow concentration on some kind of intellectual activity without the greater needed openness of mind, soul and spirit, or the arrogance and exclusiveness of the intellectual shut up in his intellectuality, or an ineffective idealism without any hold on life, or any other of the characteristic incompletenesses and limitations of the intellectual, religious, scientific or philosophic mind. These are stoppings short on the way or temporary exclusive concentrations, but a fullness of the divine soul and power of truth and knowledge in man is the perfection of this Dharma or Swabhava, the accomplished Brahminhood of the complete Brahmana.

On the other hand the turn of the nature may be to the predominance of the will-force and the capacities which make for strength, energy, courage, leadership, protection, rule, victory in every kind of battle, a creative and formative action, the will-power which lays its hold on the material of life and on the wills of other men and compels the environment into the shapes which the Shakti within us seeks to impose on life or acts powerfully according to the work to be done to maintain what is in being or to destroy it and make clear the paths of the world or to bring out into definite shape what is to be. This may be there in lesser or greater power or form and according to its grade and force we have successively the mere fighter or man of action, the man of self-imposing active will and personality and the ruler, conqueror, leader of a cause, creator, founder in whatever field of the active formation of life. The various imperfections of the soul and mind produce many imperfections and perversities of this type, — the man of mere brute force of will, the worshipper of power without any other ideal or higher purpose, the selfish, dominant personality, the aggressive violent rajasic man, the grandiose egoist, the Titan, Asura, Rakshasa. But the soul-powers to which this type of nature opens on its higher grades are as necessary as those of the Brahmana to the perfection of our human nature. The high fearlessness which no danger or difficulty can daunt and which feels its power equal to meet and face and bear whatever assault of man or fortune or adverse gods, the dynamic audacity and daring which shrinks from no adventure or enterprise as beyond the powers of a human soul free from disabling weakness and fear, the love of honour which would scale the heights of the highest nobility of man and stoop to nothing little, base, vulgar or weak, but maintains untainted the ideal of high courage, chivalry, truth, straightforwardness, sacrifice of the lower to the higher self, helpfulness to men, unflinching resistance to injustice and oppression, self-control and mastery, noble leading, warriorhood and captainship of the journey and the battle, the high self-confidence of power, capacity, character and courage indispensable to the man of action, — these are the things that build the make of the Kshatriya. To carry these things to their highest degree and give them a certain divine fullness, purity and grandeur is the perfection of those who have this Swabhava and follow this Dharma.

A third turn is one that brings out into relief the practical arranging intelligence and the instinct of life to produce, exchange, possess, enjoy, contrive, put things in order and balance, spend itself and get and give and take, work out to the best advantage the active relations of existence. In its outward action it is this power that appears as the skilful devising intelligence, the legal, professional, commercial, industrial, economical, practical and scientific, mechanical, technical and utilitarian mind. This nature is accompanied at the normal level of its fullness by a general temperament which is at once grasping and generous, prone to amass and treasure, to enjoy, show and use, bent upon efficient exploitation of the world or its surroundings, but well capable too of practical philanthropy, humanity, ordered benevolence, orderly and ethical by rule but without any high distinction of the finer ethical spirit, a mind of the middle levels, not straining towards the heights, not great to break and create noble moulds of life, but marked by capacity, adaptation and measure. The powers, limitations and perversions of this type are familiar to us on a large scale, because this is the very spirit which has made our modern commercial and industrial civilisation. But if we look at the greater inner capacities and soul-values, we shall find that here also there are things that enter into the completeness of human perfection. The Power that thus outwardly expresses itself on our present lower levels is one that can throw itself out in the great utilities of life and at its freest and widest makes, not for oneness and identity which is the highest reach of knowledge or the mastery and spiritual kingship which is the highest reach of strength, but still for something which is also essential to the wholeness of existence, equal mutuality and the exchange of soul with soul and life with life. Its powers are, first, a skill, *kauśala*, which fashions and obeys law, recognises the uses and limits of relations, adapts itself to settled and developing movements, produces and perfects the outer technique of creation and action and life, assures possession and proceeds from possession to growth, is watchful over order and careful in progress and makes the most of the material of existence and its means and ends; then a power of self-spending skilful in lavishness and skilful in economy, which recognises the great law of interchange and amasses in order to throw out in a large return, increasing the currents of interchange and the fruitfulness of existence; a power of giving and ample creative liberality, mutual helpfulness and utility to others which becomes the source in an open soul of just beneficence, humanitarianism, altruism of a practical kind; finally, a power of enjoyment, a productive, possessive, active opulence luxurious of the prolific Ananda of existence. A largeness of mutuality, a generous fullness of the relations of life, a lavish self-spending and return and ample interchange between existence and existence, a full enjoyment and use of the rhythm and balance of fruitful and productive life are the perfection of those who have this Swabhava and follow this Dharma.

The other turn is towards work and service. This was in the old order the dharma or soul-type of the Shudra and the Shudra in that order was considered as not one of the twice-born, but an inferior type. A more recent consideration of the values of existence lays stress on the dignity of labour and sees in its toil the bed-rock of the relations between man and man. There is a truth in both attitudes. For this force in the material world is at once in its necessity the foundation of material existence or rather that on which it moves, the feet of the creator Brahma in the old parable, and in its primal state not uplifted by knowledge, mutuality or strength a thing which reposes on instinct, desire and inertia. The well-developed Shudra soul-type has the instinct of toil and the capacity of labour and service; but toil as opposed to easy or natural action is a thing imposed on the natural man which he bears because without it he cannot assure his existence or get his desires and he has to force himself or be forced by others or circumstances to spend himself in work. The natural Shudra works not from a sense of the dignity of labour or from the enthusiasm of service, — though that comes by the cultivation of his dharma, — not as the man of knowledge for the joy or gain of knowledge, not from a sense of honour, nor as the born craftsman or artist for love of his work or ardour for the beauty of its technique, nor from an ordered sense of mutuality or large utility, but for the maintenance of his existence and gratification of his primal wants, and when these are satisfied, he indulges, if left to himself, his natural indolence, the indolence which is normal to the tamasic quality in all of us, but comes out most clearly in the uncompelled primitive man, the savage. The unregenerated Shudra is born therefore for service rather than for free labour and his temperament is prone to an inert ignorance, a gross unthinking self-indulgence of the instincts, a servility, an unreflective obedience and mechanical discharge of duty varied by indolence, evasion, spasmodic revolt, an instinctive and uninformed life. The ancients held that all men are born in their lower nature as Shudras and only regenerated by ethical and spiritual culture, but in their highest inner self are Brahmanas capable of the full spirit and godhead, a theory which is not far perhaps from the psychological truth of our nature.

And yet when the soul develops, it is in this Swabhava and

Dharma of work and service that there are found some of the most necessary and beautiful elements of our greatest perfection and the key to much of the secret of the highest spiritual evolution. For the soul powers that belong to the full development of this force in us are of the greatest importance, — the power of service to others, the will to make our life a thing of work and use to God and man, to obey and follow and accept whatever great influence and needful discipline, the love which consecrates service, a love which asks for no return, but spends itself for the satisfaction of that which we love, the power to bring down this love and service into the physical field and the desire to give our body and life as well as our soul and mind and will and capacity to God and man, and, as a result, the power of complete self-surrender, *ātma-samarpaṇa*, which transferred to the spiritual life becomes one of the greatest most revealing keys to freedom and perfection. In these things lies the perfection of this Dharma and the nobility of this Swabhava. Man could not be perfect and complete if he had not this element of nature in him to raise to its divine power.

None of these four types of personality can be complete even in its own field if it does not bring into it something of the other qualities. The man of knowledge cannot serve Truth with freedom and perfection, if he has not intellectual and moral courage, will, audacity, the strength to open and conquer new kingdoms, otherwise he becomes a slave of the limited intellect or a servant or at most a ritual priest of only an established knowledge,[1] — cannot use his knowledge to the best advantage unless he has the adaptive skill to work out its truths for the practice of life, otherwise he lives only in the idea, — cannot make the entire consecration of his knowledge unless he has the spirit of service to humanity, to the Godhead in man and the Master of his being. The man of power must illumine and uplift and govern his force and strength by knowledge, light of reason or religion or the spirit, otherwise he becomes the mere forceful

---

[1] That perhaps is why it was the Kshatriya bringing his courage, audacity, spirit of conquest into the fields of intuitive knowledge and spiritual experience who first discovered the great truths of Vedanta.

Asura, — must have the skill which will help him best to use and administer and regulate his strength and make it creative and fruitful and adapted to his relations with others, otherwise it becomes a mere drive of force across the field of life, a storm that passes and devastates more than it constructs, — must be capable too of obedience and make the use of his strength a service to God and the world, otherwise he becomes a selfish dominator, tyrant, brutal compeller of men's souls and bodies. The man of productive mind and work must have an open inquiring mind and ideas and knowledge, otherwise he moves in the routine of his functions without expansive growth, must have courage and enterprise, must bring a spirit of service into his getting and production, in order that he may not only get but give, not only amass and enjoy his own life, but consciously help the fruitfulness and fullness of the surrounding life by which he profits. The man of labour and service becomes a helpless drudge and slave of society if he does not bring knowledge and honour and aspiration and skill into his work, since only so can he rise by an opening mind and will and understanding usefulness to the higher dharmas. But the greater perfection of man comes when he enlarges himself to include all these powers, even though one of them may lead the others, and opens his nature more and more into the rounded fullness and universal capacity of the fourfold spirit. Man is not cut out into an exclusive type of one of these dharmas, but all these powers are in him at work at first in an ill-formed confusion, but he gives shape to one or another in birth after birth, progresses from one to the other even in the same life and goes on towards the total development of his inner existence. Our life itself is at once an inquiry after truth and knowledge, a struggle and battle of our will with ourselves and surrounding forces, a constant production, adaptation, application of skill to the material of life and a sacrifice and service.

These things are the ordinary aspects of the soul while it is working out its force in nature, but when we get nearer to our inner selves, then we get too a glimpse and experience of something which was involved in these forms and can disengage itself and stand behind and drive them, as if a general Presence or Power brought to bear on the particular working of this living and thinking machine. This is the force of the soul itself presiding over and filling the powers of its nature. The difference is that the first way is personal in its stamp, limited and determined in its action and mould, dependent on the instrumentation, but here there emerges something impersonal in the personal form, independent and self-sufficient even in the use of the instrumentation, indeterminable though determining both itself and things, something which acts with a much greater power upon the world and uses particular power only as one means of communication and impact on man and circumstance. The Yoga of self-perfection brings out this soul-force and gives it its largest scope, takes up all the fourfold powers and throws them into the free circle of an integral and harmonious spiritual dynamis. The godhead, the soul-power of knowledge rises to the highest degree of which the individual nature can be the supporting basis. A free mind of light develops which is open to every kind of revelation, inspiration, intuition, idea, discrimination, thinking synthesis; an enlightened life of the mind grasps at all knowledge with a delight of finding and reception and holding, a spiritual enthusiasm, passion, or ecstasy; a power of light full of spiritual force, illumination and purity of working manifests its empire, *brahma-tejas*, *brahma-varcas*; a bottomless steadiness and illimitable calm upholds all the illumination, movement, action as on some rock of ages, equal, unperturbed, unmoved, *acyuta*.

The godhead, the soul-power of will and strength rises to a like largeness and altitude. An absolute calm fearlessness of the free spirit, an infinite dynamic courage which no peril, limitation of possibility, wall of opposing force can deter from pursuing the work or aspiration imposed by the spirit, a high nobility of soul and will untouched by any littleness or baseness and moving with a certain greatness of step to spiritual victory or the success of the God-given work through whatever temporary defeat or obstacle, a spirit never depressed or cast down from faith and confidence in the power that works in the being, are the signs of this perfection. There comes too to fulfilment a large godhead, a soul-power of mutuality, a free self-spending and spending of gift and possession in the work to be done, lavished for the production, the creation, the achievement, the possession, gain, utilisable return, a skill that observes the law and adapts the relation and keeps the measure, a great taking into oneself from all beings and a free giving out of oneself to all, a divine commerce, a large enjoyment of the mutual delight of life. And finally there comes to perfection the godhead, the soul-power of service, the universal love that lavishes itself without demand of return, the embrace that takes to itself the body of God in man and works for help and service, the abnegation that is ready to bear the yoke of the Master and make the life a free servitude to Him and under his direction to the claim and need of his creatures, the self-surrender of the whole being to the Master of our being and his work in the world. These things unite, assist and enter into each other, become one. The full consummation comes in the greatest souls most capable of perfection, but some large manifestation of this fourfold soul-power must be sought and can be attained by all who practise the integral Yoga.

These are the signs, but behind is the soul which thus expresses itself in a consummation of nature. And this soul is an outcoming of the free self of the liberated man. That self is of no character, being infinite, but bears and upholds the play of all character, supports a kind of infinite, one, yet multiple personality, *nirguṇo guṇī*, is in its manifestation capable of infinite quality, *anantaguṇa*. The force that it uses is the supreme and universal, the divine and infinite Shakti pouring herself into the individual being and freely determining action for the divine purpose.

Chapter XVI

The Divine Shakti

THE RELATION between the Purusha and Prakriti which emerges as one advances in the Yoga of self-perfection is the next thing that we have to understand carefully in this part of the Yoga. In the spiritual truth of our being the power which we call Nature is the power of being, consciousness and will and therefore the power of self-expression and self-creation of the self, soul or Purusha. But to our ordinary mind in the ignorance and to its experience of things the force of Prakriti has a different appearance. When we look at it in its universal action outside ourselves, we see it first as a mechanical energy in the cosmos which acts upon matter or in its own created forms of matter. In matter it evolves powers and processes of life and in living matter powers and processes of mind. Throughout its operations it acts by fixed laws and in each kind of created thing displays varying properties of energy and laws of process which give its character to the genus or species and again in the individual develops without infringing the law of the kind minor characteristics and variations of a considerable consequence. It is this mechanical appearance of Prakriti which has preoccupied the modern scientific mind and made for it its whole view of Nature, and so much so that science still hopes and labours with a very small amount of success to explain all phenomena of life by laws of matter and all phenomena of mind by laws of living matter. Here soul or spirit has no place and nature cannot be regarded as power of spirit. Since the whole of our existence is mechanical, physical and bounded by the biological phenomenon of a brief living consciousness and man is a creature and instrument of material energy, the spiritual self-evolution of Yoga can be only a delusion, hallucination, abnormal state of mind or self-hypnosis. In any case it cannot be what it represents itself to be, a discovery of the eternal truth of our being and a passing above the limited truth of the mental, vital and physical to the full truth of our spiritual nature.

But when we look, not at external mechanical Nature to the exclusion of our personality, but at the inner subjective experience of man the mental being, our nature takes to us a quite different appearance. We may believe intellectually in a purely mechanical view even of our subjective existence, but we cannot act upon it or make it quite real to our self-experience. For we are conscious of an I which does not seem identical with our nature, but capable of a standing back from it, of a detached observation and criticism and creative use of it, and of a will which we naturally think of as a free will; and even if this be a delusion, we are still obliged in practice to act as if we were responsible mental beings capable of a free choice of our actions, able to use or misuse and to turn to higher or lower ends our nature. And even we seem to be struggling both with our environmental and with our own present nature and striving to get mastery over a world which imposes itself on and masters us and at the same time to become something more than we now are. But the difficulty is that we are only in command, if at all, over a small part of ourselves, the rest is subconscient or subliminal and beyond our control, our will acts only in a small selection of our activities; the most is a process of mechanism and habit and we must strive constantly with ourselves and surrounding circumstances to make the least advance or self-amelioration. There seems to be a dual being in us; Soul and Nature, Purusha and Prakriti, seem to be half in agreement, half at odds, Nature laying its mechanical control on the soul, the soul attempting to change and master nature. And the question is what is the fundamental character of this duality and what the issue.

The Sankhya explanation is that our present existence is governed by a dual principle. Prakriti is inert without the contact of Purusha, acts only by a junction with it and then too by the fixed mechanism of her instruments and qualities; Purusha, passive and free apart from Prakriti, becomes by contact with her and sanction to her works subject to this mechanism, lives in her limitation of ego-sense and must get free by withdrawing the sanction and returning to its own proper principle. Another explanation that tallies with a certain part of our experience is that there is a dual being in us, the animal and material, or more widely the lower nature-bound, and the soul or spiritual being entangled by mind in the material existence or in world-nature, and freedom comes by escape from the entanglement, the soul returning to its native planes or the self or spirit to its pure existence. The perfection of the soul then is to be found not at all in, but beyond Nature.

But in a higher than our present mental consciousness we find that this duality is only a phenomenal appearance. The highest and real truth of existence is the one Spirit, the supreme Soul, Purushottama, and it is the power of being of this Spirit which manifests itself in all that we experience as universe. This universal Nature is not a lifeless, inert or unconscious mechanism, but informed in all its movements by the universal Spirit. The mechanism of its process is only an outward appearance and the reality is the Spirit creating or manifesting its own being by its own power of being in all that is in Nature. Soul and Nature in us too are only a dual appearance of the one existence. The universal energy acts in us, but the soul limits itself by the ego-sense, lives in a partial and separate experience of her workings, uses only a modicum and a fixed action of her energy for its self-expression. It seems rather to be mastered and used by this energy than to use it, because it identifies itself with the ego-sense which is part of the natural instrumentation and lives in the ego experience. The ego is in fact driven by the mechanism of Nature of which it is a part and the ego-will is not and cannot be a free will. To arrive at freedom, mastery and perfection we have to get back to the real self and soul within and arrive too thereby at our true relations with our own and with universal nature.

In our active being this translates itself into a replacement of our egoistic, our personal, our separatively individual will and energy by a universal and a divine will and energy which determines our action in harmony with the universal action and reveals itself as the direct will and the all-guiding power of the Purushottama. We replace the inferior action of the limited, ignorant and imperfect personal will and energy in us by the action of the divine Shakti. To open ourselves to the universal energy is always possible to us, because that is all around us and always flowing into us, it is that which supports and supplies all our inner and outer action and in fact we have no power of our own in any separately individual sense, but only a personal formulation of the one Shakti. And on the other hand this universal Shakti is within ourselves, concentrated in us, for the whole power of it is present in each individual as in the universe, and there are means and processes by which we can awaken its greater and potentially infinite force and liberate it to its larger workings.

We can become aware of the existence and presence of the universal Shakti in the various forms of her power. At present we are conscious only of the power as formulated in our physical mind, nervous being and corporeal case sustaining our various activities. But if we can once get beyond this first formation by some liberation of the hidden, recondite, subliminal parts of our existence by Yoga, we become aware of a greater life force, a pranic Shakti, which supports and fills the body and supplies all the physical and vital activities, — for the physical energy is only a modified form of this force, — and supplies and sustains too from below all our mental action. This force we feel in ourselves also, but we can feel it too around us and above, one with the same energy in us, and can draw it in and down to aggrandise our normal action or call upon and get it to pour into us. It is an illimitable ocean of Shakti and will pour as much of itself as we can hold into our being. This pranic force we can use for any of the activities of life, body or mind with a far greater and effective power than any that we command in our present operations, limited as they are by the physical formula. The use of this pranic power liberates us from that limitation to the extent of our ability to use it in place of the body-bound energy. It can be used so to direct the prana as to manage more powerfully or to rectify any bodily state or action, as to heal illness or to get rid of fatigue, and to liberate an enormous amount of mental exertion and play of will or knowledge. The exercises of Pranayama are the familiar mechanical means of freeing and getting control of the pranic energy. They heighten too and set free the psychic, mental and spiritual energies which ordinarily depend for their opportunity of action on the pranic force. But the same thing can be done by mental will and practice or by an increasing opening of ourselves to a higher spiritual power of the Shakti. The pranic Shakti can be directed not only upon ourselves, but effectively towards others or on things or happenings for whatever purposes the will dictates. Its effectivity is immense, in itself illimitable, and limited only by defect of the power, purity and universality of the spiritual or other will which is brought to bear upon it; but still, however great and powerful, it is a lower formulation, a link between the mind and body, an instrumental force. There is a consciousness in it, a presence of the spirit, of which we are aware, but it is encased, involved in and preoccupied with the urge to action. It is not to this action of the Shakti that we can leave the whole burden of our activities; we have either to use its lendings by our own enlightened personal will or else call in a higher guidance; for of itself it will act with greater force, but still according to our imperfect nature and mainly by the drive and direction of the life-power in us and not according to the law of the highest spiritual existence.

The ordinary power by which we govern the pranic energy is that of the embodied mind. But when we get clear above the physical mind, we can get too above the pranic force to the consciousness of a pure mental energy which is a higher formulation of the Shakti. There we are aware of a universal mind consciousness closely associated with this energy in, around and above us, — above, that is to say, the level of our ordinary mind status, — giving all the substance and shaping all the forms of our will and knowledge and of the psychic element in our impulses and emotions. This mind force can be made to act upon the pranic energy and can impose upon it the influence, colour, shape, character, direction of our ideas, our knowledge, our more enlightened volition and thus more effectively bring our life and vital being into harmony with our higher powers of being, ideals and spiritual aspirations. In our ordinary state these two, the mental and the pranic being and energies, are very much mixed up and run into each other, and we are not able clearly to distinguish them or get a full hold of the one on the other and so control effectively the lower by the higher and more understanding principle. But when we take our station above the physical mind, we are able then to separate clearly the two forms of energy, the two levels of our being, disentangle their action and act with a clearer and more potent self-knowledge and an enlightened and a purer will-power. Nevertheless the control is not complete, spontaneous, sovereign so long as we work with the mind as our chief guiding and controlling force. The mental energy we find to be itself derivative, a lower and limiting power of the conscious spirit which acts only by isolated and combined seeings, imperfect and incomplete half-lights which we take for full and adequate light, and with a disparity between the idea and knowledge and the effective will-power. And we are aware soon of a far higher power of the Spirit and its Shakti concealed or above, superconscient to mind or partially acting through the mind, of which all this is an inferior derivation.

The Purusha and Prakriti are on the mental level as in the rest of our being closely joined and much involved in each other and we are not able to distinguish clearly soul and nature. But in the purer substance of mind we can more easily discern the dual strain. The mental Purusha is naturally able in its own native principle of mind to detach itself, as we have seen, from the workings of its Prakriti and there is then a division of our being between a consciousness that observes and can reserve its will-power and an energy full of the substance of consciousness that takes the forms of knowledge, will and feeling. This detachment gives at its highest a certain freedom from the compulsion of the soul by its mental nature. For ordinarily we are driven and carried along in the stream of our own and the universal active energy partly floundering in its waves, partly maintaining and seeming to guide or at least propel ourselves by a collected thought and an effort of the mental will muscle; but now there is a part of ourselves, nearest to the pure essence of self, which is free from the stream, can quietly observe and to a certain extent decide its immediate movement and course and to a greater extent its ultimate direction. The Purusha can at last act upon the Prakriti from half apart, from behind or from above her as a presiding person or presence, *adhyakṣa*, by the power of sanction and control inherent in the spirit.

What we shall do with this relative freedom depends on our aspiration, our idea of the relation we must have with our highest self, with God and Nature. It is possible for the Purusha to use it on the mental plane itself for a constant self-observation, self-development, self-modification, to sanction, reject, alter, bring out new formulations of the nature and establish a calm and disinterested action, a high and pure sattwic balance and rhythm of its energy, a personality perfected in the sattwic principle. This may amount only to a highly mentalised perfection of our present intelligence and the ethical and the psychic being or else, aware of the greater self in us, it may impersonalise, universalise, spiritualise its self-conscious existence and the action of its nature and arrive either at a large quietude or a large perfection of the spiritualised mental energy of its being. It is possible again for the Purusha to stand back entirely and by a refusal of sanction allow the whole normal action of the mind to exhaust itself, run down, spend its remaining impetus of habitual action and fall into silence. Or else this silence may be imposed on the mental energy by rejection of its action and a constant command to quietude. The soul may through the confirmation of this quietude and mental silence pass into some ineffable tranquillity of the spirit and vast cessation of the activities of Nature. But it is also possible to make this silence of the mind and ability to suspend the habits of the lower nature a first step towards the discovery of a superior formulation, a higher grade of the status and energy of our being and pass by an ascent and transformation into the supramental power of the spirit. And this may even, though with more difficulty, be done without resorting to the complete state of quietude of the normal mind by a persistent and progressive transformation of all the mental into their greater corresponding supramental powers and activities. For everything in the mind derives from and is a limited, inferior, groping, partial or perverse translation into mentality of something in the supermind. But neither of these movements can be successfully executed by the sole individual unaided power of the mental Purusha in us, but needs the help, intervention and guidance of the divine Self, the Ishwara, the Purushottama. For the supermind is the divine mind and it is on the supramental plane that the individual arrives at his right, integral, luminous and perfect relation with the supreme and universal Purusha and the supreme and universal Para Prakriti.

As the mind progresses in purity, capacity of stillness or freedom from absorption in its own limited action, it becomes aware of and is able to reflect, bring into itself or enter into the conscious presence of the Self, the supreme and universal Spirit, and it becomes aware too of grades and powers of the spirit higher than its own highest ranges. It becomes aware of an infinite of the consciousness of being, an infinite ocean of all the power and energy of illimitable consciousness, an infinite ocean of Ananda, of the self-moved delight of existence. It may be aware of one or other only of these things, for the mind can separate and feel exclusively as distinct original principles what in a higher experience are inseparable powers of the One, or it may feel them in a trinity or fusion which reveals or arrives at their oneness. It may become aware of it on the side of Purusha or on the side of Prakriti. On the side of Purusha it reveals itself as Self or Spirit, as Being or as the one sole existent Being, the divine Purushottama, and the individual Jiva soul can enter into entire oneness with it in its timeless self or in its universality, or enjoy nearness, immanence, difference without any gulf of separation and enjoy too inseparably and at one and the same time oneness of being and delight-giving difference of relation in active experiencing nature. On the side of Prakriti the power and Ananda of the Spirit come into the front to manifest this Infinite in the beings and personalities and ideas and forms and forces of the universe and there is then present to us the divine

Mahashakti, original Power, supreme Nature, holding in herself infinite existence and creating the wonders of the cosmos. The mind grows conscious of this illimitable ocean of Shakti or else of her presence high above the mind and pouring something of herself into us to constitute all that we are and think and will and do and feel and experience, or it is conscious of her all around us and our personality a wave of the ocean of power of spirit, or of her presence in us and of her action there based on our present form of natural existence but originated from above and raising us towards the higher spiritual status. The mind too can rise towards and touch her infinity or merge itself in it in trance of samadhi or can lose itself in her universality, and then our individuality disappears, our centre of action is then no longer in us, but either outside our bodied selves or nowhere; our mental activities are then no longer our own, but come into this frame of mind, life and body from the universal, work themselves out and pass leaving no impression on us, and this frame of ourselves too is only an insignificant circumstance in her cosmic vastness. But the perfection sought in the integral Yoga is not only to be one with her in her highest spiritual power and one with her in her universal action, but to realise and possess the fullness of this Shakti in our individual being and nature. For the supreme Spirit is one as Purusha or as Prakriti, conscious being or power of conscious being, and as the Jiva in essence of self and spirit is one with the supreme Purusha, so on the side of Nature, in power of self and spirit it is one with Shakti, *parā prakṛtir jīvabhūtā*. To realise this double oneness is the condition of the integral self-perfection. The Jiva is then the meeting-place of the play of oneness of the supreme Soul and Nature.

To reach this perfection we have to become aware of the divine Shakti, draw her to us and call her in to fill the whole system and take up the charge of all our activities. There will then be no separate personal will or individual energy trying to conduct our actions, no sense of a little personal self as the doer, nor will it be the lower energy of the three gunas, the mental, vital and physical nature. The divine Shakti will fill us and preside over and take up all our inner activities, our outer life, our Yoga. She will take up the mental energy, her own lower formation, and raise it to its highest and purest and fullest powers of intelligence and will and psychic action. She will change the mechanical energies of the mind, life and body which now govern us into delight-filled manifestations of her own living and conscious power and presence. She will manifest in us and relate to each other all the various spiritual experiences of which the mind is capable. And as the crown of this process she will bring down the supramental light into the mental levels, change the stuff of mind into the stuff of supermind, transform all the lower energies into energies of her supramental nature and raise us into our being of gnosis. The Shakti will reveal herself as the power of the Purushottama, and it is the Ishwara who will manifest himself in his force of supermind and spirit and be the master of our being, action, life and Yoga.

Chapter XVII

The Action of the Divine Shakti

THIS IS the nature of the divine Shakti that it is the timeless power of the Divine which manifests itself in time as a universal force creating, constituting, maintaining and directing all the movements and workings of the universe. This universal Power is apparent to us first on the lower levels of existence as a mental, vital and material cosmic energy of which all our mental, vital and physical activities are the operations. It is necessary for our sadhana that we should thoroughly realise this truth in order to escape from the pressure of the limiting ego view and universalise ourselves even on these lower levels where ordinarily the ego reigns in full force. To see that we are not the originators of action but that it is rather this Power that acts in ourselves and in all others, not I and others the doers, but the one Prakriti, which is the rule of the Karmayoga, is also the right rule here. The ego sense serves to limit, separate and sharply differentiate, to make the most of the individual form and it is there because it is indispensable to the evolution of the lower life. But when we would rise above to a higher divine life we must loosen the force of the ego and eventually get rid of it — as for the lower life the development of ego, so for the higher life this reverse movement of elimination of the ego is indispensable. To see our actions as not our own but those of the divine Shakti working in the form of the lower Prakriti on the inferior levels of the conscious being, helps powerfully towards this change. And if we can do this, then the separation of our mental, vital and physical consciousness from that of other beings thins and lessens; the limitations of its workings remain indeed, but they are broadened and taken up into a large sense and vision of the universal working; the specialising and individualising differentiations of Nature abide for their own proper purpose, but are no longer a prison. The individual feels his mind, life and physical existence to be one with that of others amid all differences and one with the total power of the spirit in Nature.

This however is a stage and not the whole perfection. The existence, however comparatively large and free, is still subject to the inferior nature. The sattwic, rajasic and tamasic ego is diminished but not eliminated; or if it seems to disappear, it has only sunk in our parts of action into the universal operation of the gunas, remains involved in them and is still working in a covert, subconscient fashion and may force itself to the front at any time. The sadhaka has therefore first to keep the idea and get the realisation of a one self or spirit in all behind all these workings. He must be aware behind Prakriti of the one supreme and universal Purusha. He must see and feel not only that all is the self-shaping of the one Force, Prakriti or Nature, but that all her actions are those of the Divine in all, the one Godhead in all, however veiled, altered and as it were perverted — for perversion comes by a conversion into lower forms — by transmission through the ego and the gunas. This will farther diminish the open or covert insistence of the ego and, if thoroughly realised, it will make it difficult or impossible for it to assert itself in such a way as to disturb or hamper the farther progress. The ego-sense will become, so far as it interferes at all, a foreign intrusive element and only a fringe of the mist of the old ignorance hanging on to the outskirts of the consciousness and its action. And, secondly, the universal Shakti must be realised, must be seen and felt and borne in the potent purity of its higher action, its supramental and spiritual workings. This greater vision of the Shakti will enable us to escape from the control of the gunas, to convert them into their divine equivalents and dwell in a consciousness in which the Purusha and Prakriti are one and not separated or hidden in or behind each other. There the Shakti will be in its every movement evident to us and naturally, spontaneously, irresistibly felt as nothing else but the active presence of the Divine, the shape of power of the supreme Self and Spirit.

The Shakti in this higher status reveals itself as the presence or potentiality of the infinite existence, consciousness, will, delight, and when it is so seen and felt, the being turns towards it in whatever way, with its adoration or its will of aspiration or some kind of attraction of the lesser to the greater, to know it, to be full of and possessed by it, to be one with it in the sense and action of the whole nature. But at first while we still live in the mind, there is a gulf of division or else a double action. The mental, vital and physical energy in us and the universe is felt to be a derivation from the supreme Shakti, but at the same time an inferior, separated and in some sense another working. The real spiritual force may send down its messages or the light and power of its presence above us to the lower levels or may descend occasionally and even for a time possess, but it is then mixed with the inferior workings and partially transforms and spiritualises them, but is itself diminished and altered in the process. There is an intermittent higher action or a dual working of the nature. Or we find that the Shakti for a time raises the being to a higher spiritual plane and then lowers it back into the inferior levels. These alternations must be regarded as the natural vicissitudes of a process of transformation from the normal to the spiritual being. The transformation, the perfection cannot for the integral Yoga be complete until the link between the mental and the spiritual action is formed and a higher knowledge applied to all the activities of our existence. That link is the supramental or gnostic energy in which the incalculable infinite power of the supreme being, consciousness, delight formulates itself as an ordering divine will and wisdom, a light and power in the being which shapes all the thought, will, feeling, action and replaces the corresponding individual movements.

This supramental Shakti may form itself as a spiritualised intuitive light and power in the mind itself, and that is a great but still a mentally limited spiritual action. Or it may transform altogether the mind and raise the whole being to the supramental level. In any case this is the first necessity of this part of the Yoga, to lose the ego of the doer, the ego idea and the sense of one's own power of action and initiation of action and control of the result of action and merge it in the sense and vision of the universal Shakti originating, shaping, turning to its ends the action of ourselves and others and of all the persons and forces of the world. And this realisation can become absolute and complete in all the parts of our being only if we can have that sense and vision of it in all its forms, on all the levels of our being and the world being, as the material, vital, mental and supramental energy of the Divine, but all these, all the powers of all the planes must be seen and known as self-formulations of the one spiritual Shakti, infinite in being, consciousness and Ananda. It is not the invariable rule that this power should first manifest itself on the lower levels in the lower forms of energy and then reveal its higher spiritual nature. And if it does so come, first in its mental, vital or physical universalism, we must be careful not to rest content there. It may come instead at once in its higher reality, in the might of the spiritual splendour. The difficulty then will be to bear and hold the Power until it has laid powerful hands on and transformed the energies of the lower levels of the being. The difficulty will be less in proportion as we have been able to attain to a large quiet and equality, *samatā*, and either to realise, feel and live in the one tranquil immutable self in all or else to make a genuine and complete surrender of ourselves to the divine Master of the Yoga.

It is necessary here to keep always in mind the three powers of the Divine which are present and have to be taken account of in all living existences. In our ordinary consciousness we see these three as ourselves, the Jiva in the form of the ego, God — whatever conception we may have of God, and Nature. In the spiritual experience we see God as the supreme Self or Spirit, or as the Being from whom we come and in whom we live and move. We see Nature as his Power or God as Power, Spirit in Power acting in ourselves and the world. The Jiva is then himself this Self, Spirit, Divine, *so 'ham*, because he is one with him in essence of his being and consciousness, but as the individual he is only a portion of the Divine, a self of the Spirit, and in his natural being a form of the Shakti, a power of God in movement and action, *parā prakṛtir jīvabhūtā*. At first, when we become conscious of God or of the Shakti, the difficulties of our relation with them arise from the ego consciousness which we bring into the spiritual relation. The ego in us makes claims on the Divine other than the spiritual claim, and these claims are in a sense legitimate, but so long as and in proportion as they take the egoistic form, they are open to much grossness and great perversions, burdened with an element of falsehood, undesirable reaction and consequent evil, and the relation can only be wholly right, happy and perfect when these claims become part of the spiritual claim and lose their egoistic character. And in fact the claim of our being upon the Divine is fulfilled absolutely only then when it ceases at all to be a claim and is instead a fulfilment of the Divine through the individual, when we are satisfied with that alone, when we are content with the delight of oneness in being, content to leave the supreme Self and Master of existence to do whatever is the will of his absolute wisdom and knowledge through our more and more perfected Nature. This is the sense of the self-surrender of the individual self to the Divine, *ātma-samarpaṇa*. It does not exclude a will for the delight of oneness, for participation in the divine consciousness, wisdom, knowledge, light, power, perfection, for the satisfaction of the divine fulfilment in us, but the will, the aspiration is ours because it is his will in us. At first, while there is still insistence on our own personality, it only reflects that, but becomes more and more indistinguishable from it, less personal and eventually it loses all shade of separateness, because the will in us has grown identical with the divine Tapas, the action of the divine Shakti.

And equally when we first become aware of the infinite Shakti above us or around or in us, the impulse of the egoistic sense in us is to lay hold on it and use this increased might for our egoistic purpose. This is a most dangerous thing, for it brings with it a sense and some increased reality of a great, sometimes a titanic power, and the rajasic ego, delighting in this sense of new enormous strength, may instead of waiting for it to be purified and transformed throw itself out in a violent and impure action and even turn us for a time or partially into the selfish and arrogant Asura using the strength given him for his own and not for the divine purpose: but on that way lies, in the end, if it is persisted in, spiritual perdition and material ruin. And even to regard oneself as the instrument of the Divine is not a perfect remedy; for when a strong ego meddles in the matter, it falsifies the spiritual relation and under cover of making itself an instrument of the Divine is really bent on making instead God its instrument. The one remedy is to still the egoistic claim of whatever kind, to lessen persistently the personal effort and individual straining which even the sattwic ego cannot avoid and instead of laying hold on the Shakti and using it for its purpose rather to let the Shakti lay hold on us and use us for the divine purpose. This cannot be done perfectly at once — nor can it be done safely if it is only the lower form of the universal energy of which we are aware, for then, as has already been said, there must be some other control, either of the mental Purusha or from above, — but still it is the aim which we must have before us and which can be wholly carried out when we become insistently aware of the highest spiritual presence and form of the divine Shakti. This surrender too of the whole action of the individual self to the Shakti is in fact a form of real self-surrender to the Divine.

It has been seen that a most effective way of purification is for the mental Purusha to draw back, to stand as the passive witness and observe and know himself and the workings of Nature in the lower, the normal being; but this must be combined, for perfection, with a will to raise the purified nature into the higher spiritual being. When that is done, the Purusha is no longer only a witness, but also the master of his prakriti, *īśvara*. At first it may not be apparent how this ideal of active self-mastery can be reconciled with the apparently opposite ideal of self-surrender and of becoming the assenting instrument of the divine Shakti. But in fact on the spiritual plane there is no difficulty. The Jiva cannot really become master except in proportion as he arrives at oneness with the Divine who is his supreme Self. And in that oneness and in his unity with the universe he is one too in the universal self with the will that directs all the operations of Nature. But more directly, less transcendentally, in his individual action too, he is a portion of the Divine and participates in the mastery over his nature of that to which he has surrendered himself. Even as instrument, he is not a mechanical but a conscious instrument. On the Purusha side of him he is one with the Divine and participates in the divine mastery of the Ishwara. On the nature side of him he is in his universality one with the power of the Divine, while in his individual natural being he is an instrument of the universal divine Shakti, because the individualised power is there to fulfil the purpose of the universal Power. The Jiva, as has been seen, is the meeting-place of the play of the dual aspect of the Divine, Prakriti and Purusha, and in the higher spiritual consciousness he becomes simultaneously one with both these aspects, and there he takes up and combines all the divine relations created by their interaction. This it is that makes possible the dual attitude.

There is however a possibility of arriving at this result without the passage through the passivity of the mental Purusha, by a more persistently and predominantly kinetic Yoga. Or there may be a combination of both the methods, alternations between them and an ultimate fusion. And here the problem of spiritual action assumes a more simple form. In this kinetic movement there are three stages. In the first the Jiva is aware of the supreme Shakti, receives the power into himself and uses it under her direction, with a certain sense of being the subordinate doer, a sense of minor responsibility in the action, — even at first, it may be, a responsibility for the result; but that disappears, for the result is seen to be determined by the higher Power, and only the action is felt to be partly his own. The sadhaka then feels that it is he who is thinking, willing, doing, but feels too the divine Shakti or Prakriti behind driving and shaping all his thought, will, feeling and action: the individual energy belongs in a way to him, but is still only a form and an instrument of the universal divine Energy. The Master of the Power may be hidden from him for a time by the action of the Shakti, or he may be aware of the Ishwara sometimes or continually manifest to him. In the latter case there are three things present to his consciousness, himself as the servant of the Ishwara, the Shakti behind as a great Power supplying the energy, shaping the action, formulating the results, the Ishwara above determining by his will the whole action.

In the second stage the individual doer disappears, but there is not necessarily any quietistic passivity; there may be a full kinetic action, only all is done by the Shakti. It is her power of knowledge which takes shape as thought in the mind; the sadhaka has no sense of himself thinking, but of the Shakti thinking in him. The will and the feelings and action are also in the same way nothing but a formation, operation, activity of the Shakti in her immediate presence and full possession of all the system. The sadhaka does not think, will, act, feel, but thought, will, feeling, action happen in his system. The individual on the side of action has disappeared into oneness with universal Prakriti, has become an individualised form and action of the divine Shakti. He is still aware of his personal existence, but it is as the Purusha supporting and observing the whole action, conscious of it in his self-knowledge and enabling by his participation the divine Shakti to do in him the works and the will of the Ishwara. The Master of the power is then sometimes hidden by the action of the power, sometimes appears governing it and compelling its workings. Here too there are three things present to the consciousness, the Shakti carrying on all the knowledge, thought, will, feeling, action for the Ishwara in an instrumental human form, the Ishwara, the Master of existence governing and compelling all her action, and ourself as the soul, the Purusha of her individual action enjoying all the relations with him which are created by her workings. There is another form of this realisation in which the Jiva disappears into and becomes one with the Shakti and there is then only the play of the Shakti with the Ishwara, Mahadeva and Kali, Krishna and Radha, the Deva and the Devi. This is the intensest possible form of the Jiva's realisation of himself as a manifestation of Nature, a power of the being of the Divine, *parā prakṛtir jīva-bhūtā.*

A third stage comes by the increasing manifestation of the Divine, the Ishwara in all our being and action. This is when we are constantly and uninterruptedly aware of him. He is felt in us as the possessor of our being and above us as the ruler of all its workings and they become to us nothing but a manifestation of him in the existence of the Jiva. All our consciousness is his consciousness, all our knowledge is his knowledge, all our thought is his thought, all our will is his will, all our feeling is his Ananda and form of his delight in being, all our action is his action. The distinction between the Shakti and the Ishwara begins to disappear; there is only the conscious activity in us of the Divine with the great self of the Divine behind and around and possessing it; all the world and Nature is seen to be only that, but here it has become fully conscious, the Maya of the ego removed, and the Jiva is there only as an eternal portion of his being, *aṁśa sanātana*, put forth to support a divine individualisation and living now fulfilled in the complete presence and power of the Divine, the complete joy of the Spirit manifested in the being. This is the highest realisation of the perfection and delight of the active oneness; for beyond it there could be only the consciousness of the Avatara, the Ishwara himself assuming a human name and form for action in the Lila.

Chapter XVIII

Faith and Shakti

THE THREE parts of the perfection of our instrumental nature of which we have till now been reviewing the general features, the perfection of the intelligence, heart, vital consciousness and body, the perfection of the fundamental soul powers, the perfection of the surrender of our instruments and action to the divine Shakti, depend at every moment of their progression on a fourth power that is covertly and overtly the pivot of all endeavour and action, faith, *śraddhā*. The perfect faith is an assent of the whole being to the truth seen by it or offered to its acceptance, and its central working is a faith of the soul in its own will to be and attain and become and its idea of self and things and its knowledge, of which the belief of the intellect, the heart's consent and the desire of the life mind to possess and realise are the outward figures. This soul faith, in some form of itself, is indispensable to the action of the being and without it man cannot move a single pace in life, much less take any step forward to a yet unrealised perfection. It is so central and essential a thing that the Gita can justly say of it that whatever is a man's *śraddhā*, that he is, *yo yacchraddhaḥ sa eva saḥ*, and, it may be added, whatever he has the faith to see as possible in himself and strive for, that he can create and become. There is one kind of faith demanded as indispensable by the integral Yoga and that may be described as faith in God and the Shakti, faith in the presence and power of the Divine in us and the world, a faith that all in the world is the working of one divine Shakti, that all the steps of the Yoga, its strivings and sufferings and failures as well as its successes and satisfactions and victories are utilities and necessities of her workings and that by a firm and strong dependence on and a total self-surrender to the Divine and to his Shakti in us we can attain to oneness and freedom and victory and perfection.

The enemy of faith is doubt, and yet doubt too is a utility and necessity, because man in his ignorance and in his progressive labour towards knowledge needs to be visited by doubt, otherwise he would remain obstinate in an ignorant belief and limited knowledge and unable to escape from his errors. This utility and necessity of doubt does not altogether disappear when we enter on the path of Yoga. The integral Yoga aims at a knowledge not merely of some fundamental principle, but a knowing, a gnosis which will apply itself to and cover all life and the world action, and in this search for knowledge we enter on the way and are accompanied for many miles upon it by the mind's unregenerated activities before these are purified and transformed by a greater light: we carry with us a number of intellectual beliefs and ideas which are by no means all of them correct and perfect and a host of new ideas and suggestions meet us afterwards demanding our credence which it would be fatal to seize on and always cling to in the shape in which they come without regard to their possible error, limitation or imperfection. And indeed at one stage in the Yoga it becomes necessary to refuse to accept as definite and final any kind of intellectual idea or opinion whatever in its intellectual form and to hold it in a questioning suspension until it is given its right place and luminous shape of truth in a spiritual experience enlightened by supramental knowledge. And much more must this be the case with the desires or impulsions of the life mind, which have often to be provisionally accepted as immediate indices of a temporarily necessary action before we have the full guidance, but not always clung to with the soul's complete assent, for eventually all these desires and impulsions have to be rejected or else transformed into and replaced by impulsions of the divine will taking up the life movements. The heart's faith, emotional beliefs, assents are also needed upon the way, but cannot be always sure guides until they too are taken up, purified, transformed and are eventually replaced by the luminous assents of a divine Ananda which is at one with the divine will and knowledge. In nothing in the lower nature from the reason to the vital will can the seeker of the Yoga put a complete and permanent faith, but only at last in the spiritual truth, power, Ananda which become in the spiritual reason his sole guides and luminaries and masters of action.

And yet faith is necessary throughout and at every step because it is a needed assent of the soul and without this assent there can be no progress. Our faith must first be abiding in the essential truth and principles of the Yoga, and even if this is clouded in the intellect, despondent in the heart, outwearied and exhausted by constant denial and failure in the desire of the vital mind, there must be something in the innermost soul which clings and returns to it, otherwise we may fall on the path or abandon it from weakness and inability to bear temporary defeat, disappointment, difficulty and peril. In the Yoga as in life it is the man who persists unwearied to the last in the face of every defeat and disillusionment and of all confronting, hostile and contradicting events and powers who conquers in the end and finds his faith justified because to the soul and Shakti in man nothing is impossible. And even a blind and ignorant faith is a better possession than the sceptical doubt which turns its back on our spiritual possibilities or the constant carping of the narrow pettily critical uncreative intellect, *asūyā*, which pursues our endeavour with a paralysing incertitude. The seeker of the integral Yoga must however conquer both these imperfections. The thing to which he has given his assent and set his mind and heart and will to achieve, the divine perfection of the whole human being, is apparently an impossibility to the normal intelligence, since it is opposed to the actual facts of life and will for long be contradicted by immediate experience, as happens with all far-off and difficult ends, and it is denied too by many who have spiritual experience but believe that our present nature is the sole possible nature of man in the body and that it is only by throwing off the earthly life or even all individual existence that we can arrive at either a heavenly perfection or the release of extinction. In the pursuit of such an aim there will for long be plenty of ground for the objections, the carpings, *asūyā*, of that ignorant but persistent criticising reason which founds itself plausibly on the appearances of the moment, the stock of ascertained fact and experience, refuses to go beyond and questions the validity of all indices and illuminations that point forward; and if he yields to these narrow suggestions, he will either not arrive or be seriously hampered and long delayed in his journey. On the other hand ignorance and blindness in the faith are obstacles to a large success, invite much disappointment and disillusionment, fasten on false finalities and prevent advance to greater formulations of truth and perfection. The Shakti in her workings will strike ruthlessly at all forms of ignorance and blindness and all even that trusts wrongly and superstitiously in her, and we must be prepared to abandon a too persistent attachment to forms of faith and cling to the saving reality alone. A great and wide spiritual and intelligent faith, intelligent with the intelligence of that larger reason which assents to high possibilities, is the character of the *śraddhā* needed for the integral Yoga.

This *śraddhā* — the English word faith is inadequate to express it — is in reality an influence from the supreme Spirit and its light a message from our supramental being which is calling the lower nature to rise out of its petty present to a great self-becoming and self-exceeding. And that which receives the influence and answers to the call is not so much the intellect, the heart or the life mind, but the inner soul which better knows the truth of its own destiny and mission. The circumstances that provoke our first entry into the path are not the real index of the thing that is at work in us. There the intellect, the heart, or the desires of the life mind may take a prominent place, or even more fortuitous accidents and outward incentives; but if these are all, then there can be no surety of our fidelity to the call and our enduring perseverance in the Yoga. The intellect may abandon the idea that attracted it, the heart weary or fail us, the desire of the life mind turn to other objectives. But outward circumstances are only a cover for the real workings of the spirit, and if it is the spirit that has been touched, the inward soul that has received the call, the *śraddhā* will remain firm and resist all attempts to defeat or slay it. It is not that the doubts of the intellect may not assail, the heart waver, the disappointed desire of the life mind sink down exhausted on the wayside. That is almost inevitable at times, perhaps often, especially with us, sons of an age of intellectuality and scepticism and a materialistic denial of spiritual truth which has not yet lifted its painted clouds from the face of the sun of a greater reality and is still opposed to the light of spiritual intuition and inmost experience. There will very possibly be many of those trying obscurations of which even the Vedic Rishis so often complained, "long exiles from the light", and these may be so thick, the night on the soul may be so black that faith may seem utterly to have left us. But through it all the spirit within will be keeping its unseen hold and the soul will return with a new strength to its assurance which was only eclipsed and not extinguished, because extinguished it cannot be when once the inner self has known and made its resolution.[1] The Divine holds our hand through all and if he seems to let us fall, it is only to raise us higher. This saving return we shall experience so often that the denials of doubt will become eventually impossible and, when once the foundation of equality is firmly established and still more when the sun of the gnosis has risen, doubt itself will pass away because its cause and utility have ended.

Moreover not only a faith in the fundamental principle, ideas, way of the Yoga is needed, but a day to day working faith in the power in us to achieve, in the steps we have taken on the way, in the spiritual experiences that come to us, in the intuitions, the guiding movements of will and impulsion, the moved intensities of the heart and aspirations and fulfilments of the life that are the aids, the circumstances and the stages of the enlarging of the nature and the stimuli or the steps of the soul's evolution. At the same time it has always to be remembered that we are moving from imperfection and ignorance towards light and perfection, and the faith in us must be free from attachment to the forms of our endeavour and the successive stages of our realisation. There is not only much that will be strongly raised in us in order to be cast out and rejected, a battle between the powers of ignorance and the lower nature and the higher powers that have to replace them, but experiences, states of thought

---

[1] *saṅkalpa, vyavasāya.*

and feeling, forms of realisation that are helpful and have to
be accepted on the way and may seem to us for the time to be
spiritual finalities, are found afterwards to be steps of transition,
have to be exceeded and the working faith that supported them
withdrawn in favour of other and greater things or of more full
and comprehensive realisations and experiences, which replace
them or into which they are taken up in a completing transformation. There can be for the seeker of the integral Yoga no
clinging to resting-places on the road or to half-way houses; he
cannot be satisfied till he has laid down all the great enduring
bases of his perfection and broken out into its large and free
infinities, and even there he has to be constantly filling himself
with more experiences of the Infinite. His progress is an ascent
from level to level and each new height brings in other vistas and
revelations of the much that has still to be done, *bhūri kartvam*,
till the divine Shakti has at last taken up all his endeavour and he
has only to assent and participate gladly by a consenting oneness
in her luminous workings. That which will support him through
these changes, struggles, transformations which might otherwise
dishearten and baffle, — for the intellect and life and emotion
always grasp too much at things, fasten on premature certitudes
and are apt to be afflicted and unwilling when forced to abandon
that on which they rested, — is a firm faith in the Shakti that is
at work and reliance on the guidance of the Master of the Yoga
whose wisdom is not in haste and whose steps through all the
perplexities of the mind are assured and just and sound, because
they are founded on a perfectly comprehending transaction with
the necessities of our nature.

The progress of the Yoga is a procession from the mental
ignorance through imperfect formations to a perfect foundation
and increasing of knowledge and in its more satisfyingly positive
parts a movement from light to greater light, and it cannot cease
till we have the greatest light of the supramental knowledge. The
motions of the mind in its progress must necessarily be mixed
with a greater or lesser proportion of error, and we should not
allow our faith to be disconcerted by the discovery of its errors
or imagine that because the beliefs of the intellect which aided

us were too hasty and positive, therefore the fundamental faith in the soul was invalid. The human intellect is too much afraid of error precisely because it is too much attached to a premature sense of certitude and a too hasty eagerness for positive finality in what it seems to seize of knowledge. As our self-experience increases, we shall find that our errors even were necessary movements, brought with them and left their element or suggestion of truth and helped towards discovery or supported a necessary effort and that the certitudes we have now to abandon had yet their temporary validity in the progress of our knowledge. The intellect cannot be a sufficient guide in the search for spiritual truth and realisation and yet it has to be utilised in the integral movement of our nature. And while, therefore, we have to reject paralysing doubt or mere intellectual scepticism, the seeking intelligence has to be trained to admit a certain large questioning, an intellectual rectitude not satisfied with half-truths, mixtures of error or approximations and, most positive and helpful, a perfect readiness always to move forward from truths already held and accepted to the greater corrective, completing or transcending truths which at first it was unable or, it may be, disinclined to envisage. A working faith of the intellect is indispensable, not a superstitious, dogmatic or limiting credence attached to every temporary support or formula, but a large assent to the successive suggestions and steps of the Shakti, a faith fixed on realities, moving from the lesser to the completer realities and ready to throw down all scaffolding and keep only the large and growing structure.

A constant *śraddhā*, faith, assent of the heart and the life too are indispensable. But while we are in the lower nature the heart's assent is coloured by mental emotion and the life movements are accompanied by their trail of perturbing or straining desires, and mental emotion and desire tend to trouble, alter more or less grossly or subtly or distort the truth, and they always bring some limitation and imperfection into its realisation by the heart and life. The heart too when it is troubled in its attachments and its certitudes, perplexed by throw-backs and failures and convictions of error or involved in the wrestlings which attend a call to move forward from its assured positions, has its draggings, wearinesses, sorrowings, revolts, reluctances which hamper the progress. It must learn a larger and surer faith giving in the place of the mental reactions a calm or a moved spiritual acceptance to the ways and the steps of the Shakti which is in its nature the assent of a deepening Ananda to all necessary movements and a readiness to leave old moorings and move always forward towards the delight of a greater perfection. The life mind must give its assent to the successive motives, impulsions, activities of the life imposed on it by the guiding power as aids or fields of the development of the nature and to the successions also of the inner Yoga, but it must not be attached or call a halt anywhere, but must always be prepared to abandon old urgency and accept with the same completeness of assent new higher movements and activities, and it must learn to replace desire by a wide and bright Ananda in all experience and action. The faith of the heart and the life mind, like that of the intelligence, must be capable of a constant correction, enlarging and transformation.

This faith is essentially the secret *śraddhā* of the soul, and it is brought more and more to the surface and there satisfied, sustained and increased by an increasing assurance and certainty of spiritual experience. Here too the faith in us must be unattached, a faith that waits upon Truth and is prepared to change and enlarge its understanding of spiritual experiences, to correct mistaken or half-true ideas about them and receive more enlightening interpretations, to replace insufficient by more sufficient intuitions, and to merge experiences that seemed at the time to be final and satisfying in more satisfying combinations with new experience and greater largenesses and transcendences. And especially in the psychical and other middle domains there is a very large room for the possibility of misleading and often captivating error, and here even a certain amount of positive scepticism has its use and at all events a great caution and scrupulous intellectual rectitude, but not the scepticism of the ordinary mind which amounts to a disabling denial. In the integral Yoga psychical experience, especially of the kind associated with what is often called occultism and savours of the miraculous, should be altogether subordinated to spiritual truth and wait upon that for its own interpretation, illumination and sanction. But even in the purely spiritual domain, there are experiences which are partial and, however attractive, only receive their full validity, significance or right application when we can advance to a fuller experience. And there are others which are in themselves quite valid and full and absolute, but if we confine ourselves to them, will prevent other sides of the spiritual truth from manifestation and mutilate the integrality of the Yoga. Thus the profound and absorbing quietude of impersonal peace which comes by the stilling of the mind is a thing in itself complete and absolute, but if we rest in that alone, it will exclude the companion absolute, not less great and needed and true, of the bliss of the divine action. Here too our faith must be an assent that receives all spiritual experience, but with a wide openness and readiness for always more light and truth, an absence of limiting attachment and no such clinging to forms as would interfere with the forward movement of the Shakti towards the integrality of the spiritual being, consciousness, knowledge, power, action and the wholeness of the one and the multiple Ananda.

The faith demanded of us both in its general principle and its constant particular application amounts to a large and ever increasing and a constantly purer, fuller and stronger assent of the whole being and all its parts to the presence and guidance of God and the Shakti. The faith in the Shakti, as long as we are not aware of and filled with her presence, must necessarily be preceded or at least accompanied by a firm and virile faith in our own spiritual will and energy and our power to move successfully towards unity and freedom and perfection. Man is given faith in himself, his ideas and his powers that he may work and create and rise to greater things and in the end bring his strength as a worthy offering to the altar of the Spirit. This spirit, says the Scripture, is not to be won by the weak, *nāyam ātmā balahīnena labhyaḥ*. All paralysing self-distrust has to be discouraged, all doubt of our strength to accomplish, for that is a false assent to impotence, an imagination of weakness and a denial of the omnipotence of the spirit. A present incapacity, however heavy may seem its pressure, is only a trial of faith and a temporary difficulty and to yield to the sense of inability is for the seeker of the integral Yoga a non-sense, for his object is a development of a perfection that is there already, latent in the being, because man carries the seed of the divine life in himself, in his own spirit, the possibility of success is involved and implied in the effort and victory is assured because behind is the call and guidance of an omnipotent power. At the same time this faith in oneself must be purified from all touch of rajasic egoism and spiritual pride. The sadhaka should keep as much as possible in his mind the idea that his strength is not his own in the egoistic sense but that of the divine universal Shakti and whatever is egoistic in his use of it must be a cause of limitation and in the end an obstacle. The power of the divine universal Shakti which is behind our aspiration is illimitable, and when it is rightly called upon it cannot fail to pour itself into us and to remove whatever incapacity and obstacle, now or later; for the times and durations of our struggle while they depend at first, instrumentally and in part, on the strength of our faith and our endeavour, are yet eventually in the hands of the wisely determining secret Spirit, alone the Master of the Yoga, the Ishwara.

The faith in the divine Shakti must be always at the back of our strength and when she becomes manifest, it must be or grow implicit and complete. There is nothing that is impossible to her who is the conscious Power and universal Goddess all-creative from eternity and armed with the Spirit's omnipotence. All knowledge, all strengths, all triumph and victory, all skill and works are in her hands and they are full of the treasures of the Spirit and of all perfections and siddhis. She is Maheshwari, goddess of the supreme knowledge, and brings to us her vision for all kinds and widenesses of truth, her rectitude of the spiritual will, the calm and passion of her supramental largeness, her felicity of illumination: she is Mahakali, goddess of the supreme strength, and with her are all mights and spiritual force and severest austerity of tapas and swiftness to the battle and the victory and the laughter, the *aṭṭahāsya*, that makes light of defeat and death and the powers of the ignorance: she is Mahalakshmi, the goddess of the supreme love and delight, and her gifts are the spirit's grace and the charm and beauty of the Ananda and protection and every divine and human blessing: she is Mahasaraswati, the goddess of divine skill and of the works of the Spirit, and hers is the Yoga that is skill in works, *yogaḥ karmasu kauśalam*, and the utilities of divine knowledge and the self-application of the spirit to life and the happiness of its harmonies. And in all her powers and forms she carries with her the supreme sense of the masteries of the eternal Ishwari, a rapid and divine capacity for all kinds of action that may be demanded from the instrument, oneness, a participating sympathy, a free identity, with all energies in all beings and therefore a spontaneous and fruitful harmony with all the divine will in the universe. The intimate feeling of her presence and her powers and the satisfied assent of all our being to her workings in and around it is the last perfection of faith in the Shakti.

And behind her is the Ishwara and faith in him is the most central thing in the *śraddhā* of the integral Yoga. This faith we must have and develop to perfection that all things are the workings under the universal conditions of a supreme self-knowledge and wisdom, that nothing done in us or around us is in vain or without its appointed place and just significance, that all things are possible when the Ishwara as our supreme Self and Spirit takes up the action and that all that has been done before and all that he will do hereafter was and will be part of his infallible and foreseeing guidance and intended towards the fruition of our Yoga and our perfection and our life work. This faith will be more and more justified as the higher knowledge opens, we shall begin to see the great and small significances that escaped our limited mentality and faith will pass into knowledge. Then we shall see beyond the possibility of doubt that all happens within the working of the one Will and that that will was also wisdom because it develops always the true workings in life of the self and nature. The highest state of the assent, the *śraddhā* of the being will be when we feel the presence of the Ishwara and feel all our existence and consciousness and thought and will and action in his hand and consent in all things and with every part of our self and nature to the direct and immanent and occupying will of the Spirit. And that highest perfection of the *śraddhā* will also be the opportunity and perfect foundation of a divine strength: it will base, when complete, the development and manifestation and the works of the luminous supramental Shakti.

Chapter XIX

The Nature of the Supermind

THE OBJECT of Yoga is to raise the human being from the consciousness of the ordinary mind subject to the control of vital and material Nature and limited wholly by birth and death and Time and the needs and desires of the mind, life and body to the consciousness of the spirit free in its self and using the circumstances of mind, life and body as admitted or self-chosen and self-figuring determinations of the spirit, using them in a free self-knowledge, a free will and power of being, a free delight of being. This is the essential difference between the ordinary mortal mind in which we live and the spiritual consciousness of our divine and immortal being which is the highest result of Yoga. It is a radical conversion as great as and greater than the change which we suppose evolutionary Nature to have made in its transition from the vital animal to the fully mentalised human consciousness. The animal has the conscious vital mind, but whatever beginnings there are in it of anything higher are only a primary glimpse, a crude hint of the intelligence which in man becomes the splendour of the mental understanding, will, emotion, aesthesis and reason. Man elevated in the heights and deepened by the intensities of the mind becomes aware of something great and divine in himself towards which all this tends, something he is in possibility but which he has not yet become, and he turns the powers of his mind, his power of knowledge, his power of will, his power of emotion and aesthesis to seek out this, to seize and comprehend all that it may be, to become it and to exist wholly in its greater consciousness, delight, being and power of highest becoming. But what he gets of this higher state in his normal mind is only an intimation, a primary glimpse, a crude hint of the splendour, the light, the glory and divinity of the spirit within him. A complete conversion of all the parts of his being into moulds and instruments of the spiritual consciousness is demanded of him before he can make quite real, constant, present to himself this greater thing that he can be and entirely live in what is now to him at the best a luminous aspiration. He must seek to develop and grow altogether into a greater divine consciousness by an integral Yoga.

The Yoga of perfection necessary to this change has, so far as we have been considering it, consisted in a preparatory purification of the mental, vital and physical nature, a liberation from the knots of the lower Prakriti, a consequent replacement of the egoistic state always subject to the ignorant and troubled action of the desire soul by a large and luminous static equality which quiets the reason, the emotional mind, the life mind and the physical nature and brings into us the peace and freedom of the spirit, and a dynamical substitution of the action of the supreme and universal divine Shakti under the control of the Ishwara for that of the lower Prakriti, — an action whose complete operation must be preceded by the perfection of the natural instruments. And all these things together, though not as yet the whole Yoga, constitute already a much greater than the present normal consciousness, spiritual in its basis and moved by a greater light, power and bliss, and it might be easy to rest satisfied with so much accomplished and think that all has been done that was needed for the divine conversion.

A momentous question however arises as light grows, the question through what medium is the divine Shakti to act in the human being? Is it to be always through the mind only and on the mind plane or in some greater supramental formulation which is more proper to a divine action and which will take up and replace the mental functions? If the mind is to be always the instrument, then although we shall be conscious of a diviner Power initiating and conducting all our inner and outer human action, yet it will have to formulate its knowledge, will, Ananda and all things else in the mental figure, and that means to translate them into an inferior kind of functioning other than the supreme workings native to the divine consciousness and its Shakti. The mind spiritualised, purified, liberated, perfected within its own limits may come as near as possible to a faithful mental translation, but we shall find that this is after all a relative fidelity and an imperfect perfection. The mind by its very nature cannot render with an entirely right rightness or act in the unified completeness of the divine knowledge, will and Ananda because it is an instrument for dealing with the divisions of the finite on the basis of division, a secondary instrument therefore and a sort of delegate for the lower movement in which we live. The mind can reflect the Infinite, it can dissolve itself into it, it can live in it by a large passivity, it can take its suggestions and act them out in its own way, a way always fragmentary, derivative and subject to a greater or less deformation, but it cannot be itself the direct and perfect instrument of the infinite Spirit acting in its own knowledge. The divine Will and Wisdom organising the action of the infinite consciousness and determining all things according to the truth of the spirit and the law of its manifestation is not mental but supramental and even in its formulation nearest to mind as much above the mental consciousness in its light and power as the mental consciousness of man above the vital mind of the lower creation. The question is how far the perfected human being can raise himself above mind, enter into some kind of fusing union with the supramental and build up in himself a level of supermind, a developed gnosis by the form and power of which the divine Shakti can directly act, not through a mental translation, but organically in her supramental nature.

It is here necessary in a matter so remote from the ordinary lines of our thought and experience to state first what is the universal gnosis or divine supermind, how it is represented in the actual movement of the universe and what are its relations to the present psychology of the human being. It will then be evident that though the supermind is suprarational to our intelligence and its workings occult to our apprehension, it is nothing irrationally mystic, but rather its existence and emergence is a logical necessity of the nature of existence, always provided we grant that not matter or mind alone but spirit is the fundamental reality and everywhere a universal presence. All things are a manifestation of the infinite spirit out of its own being, out of its own consciousness and by the self-realising, self-determining, self-fulfilling power of that consciousness. The Infinite, we may say, organises by the power of its self-knowledge the law of its own manifestation of being in the universe, not only the material universe present to our senses, but whatever lies behind it on whatever planes of existence. All is organised by it not under any inconscient compulsion, not according to a mental fantasy or caprice, but in its own infinite spiritual freedom according to the self-truth of its being, its infinite potentialities and its will of self-creation out of those potentialities, and the law of this self-truth is the necessity that compels created things to act and evolve each according to its own nature. The Intelligence — to give it an inadequate name — the Logos that thus organises its own manifestation is evidently something infinitely greater, more extended in knowledge, compelling in self-power, large both in the delight of its self-existence and the delight of its active being and works than the mental intelligence which is to us the highest realised degree and expression of consciousness. It is to this intelligence infinite in itself but freely organising and self-determiningly organic in its self-creation and its works that we may give for our present purpose the name of the divine supermind or gnosis.

The fundamental nature of this supermind is that all its knowledge is originally a knowledge by identity and oneness and even when it makes numberless apparent divisions and discriminating modifications in itself, still all the knowledge that operates in its workings, even in these divisions, is founded upon and sustained and lit and guided by this perfect knowledge by identity and oneness. The Spirit is one everywhere and it knows all things as itself and in itself, so sees them always and therefore knows them intimately, completely, in their reality as well as their appearance, in their truth, their law, the entire spirit and sense and figure of their nature and their workings. When it sees anything as an object of knowledge, it yet sees it as itself and in itself, and not as a thing other than or divided from it about which therefore it would at first be ignorant of the nature, constitution and workings and have to learn about them, as the mind is at first ignorant of its object and has to learn about it because the mind is separated from its object and regards and senses and meets it as something other than itself and external to its own being. The mental awareness we have of our own subjective existence and its movements, though it may point to, is not the same thing as this identity and self-knowledge, because what it sees are mental figures of our being and not the inmost or the whole and it is only a partial, derivative and superficial action of our self that appears to us while the largest and most secretly determining parts of our own existence are occult to our mentality. The supramental Spirit has, unlike the mental being, the real because the inmost and total knowledge of itself and of all its universe and of all things that are its creations and self-figurings in the universe.

This is the second character of the supreme Supermind that its knowledge is a real because a total knowledge. It has in the first place a transcendental vision and sees the universe not only in the universal terms, but in its right relation to the supreme and eternal reality from which it proceeds and of which it is an expression. It knows the spirit and truth and whole sense of the universal expression because it knows all the essentiality and all the infinite reality and all the consequent constant potentiality of that which in part it expresses. It knows rightly the relative because it knows the Absolute and all its absolutes to which the relatives refer back and of which they are the partial or modified or suppressed figures. It is in the second place universal and sees all that is individual in the terms of the universal as well as in its own individual terms and holds all these individual figures in their right and complete relation to the universe. It is in the third place, separately with regard to individual things, total in its view because it knows each in its inmost essence of which all else is the resultant, in its totality which is its complete figure and in its parts and their connections and dependences, — as well as in its connections with and its dependences upon other things and its nexus with the total implications and the explicits of the universe.

The mind on the contrary is limited and incapable in all these directions. Mind cannot arrive at identity with the Absolute even when by a stretch of the intellect it conceives the idea, but can only disappear into it in a swoon or extinction: it can only have a kind of sense or an intimation of certain absolutes which it puts by the mental idea into a relative figure. It cannot grasp the universal, but only arrives at some idea of it through an extension of the individual or a combination of apparently separate things and so sees it either as a vague infinite or indeterminate or a half-determined largeness or else only in an external scheme or constructed figure. The indivisible being and action of the universal, which is its real truth, escapes the apprehension of the mind, because the mind thinks it out analytically by taking its own divisions for units and synthetically by combinations of these units, but cannot seize on and think entirely in the terms, though it may get at the idea and certain secondary results, of the essential oneness. It cannot, either, know truly and thoroughly even the individual and apparently separate thing, because it proceeds in the same way, by an analysis of parts and constituents and properties and a combination by which it erects a scheme of it which is only its external figure. It can get an intimation of the essential inmost truth of its object, but cannot live constantly and luminously in that essential knowledge and work out on the rest from within outward so that the outward circumstances appear in their intimate reality and meaning as inevitable result and expression and form and action of the spiritual something which is the reality of the object. And all this which is impossible for the mind to do, but possible only to strive towards and figure, is inherent and natural to the supramental knowledge.

The third characteristic of the supermind arising from this difference, which brings us to the practical distinction between the two kinds of knowledge, is that it is directly truth-conscious, a divine power of immediate, inherent and spontaneous knowledge, an Idea holding luminously all realities and not depending on indications and logical or other steps from the known to the unknown like the mind which is a power of the Ignorance. The supermind contains all its knowledge in itself, is in its highest divine wisdom in eternal possession of all truth and even in its lower, limited or individualised forms has only to bring the latent truth out of itself, — the perception which the old thinkers tried to express when they said that all knowing was in its real origin and nature only a memory of inwardly existing knowledge. The supermind is eternally and on all levels truth-conscious and exists secretly even in mental and material being, surveys and knows the things, even obscurest, of the mental ignorance and understands and is behind and governs its processes, because everything in the mind derives from the supermind — and must do so because everything derives from the spirit. All that is mental is but a partial, a modified, a suppressed or half-suppressed figure of the supramental truth, a deformation or a derived and imperfect figure of its greater knowledge. The mind begins with ignorance and proceeds towards knowledge. As an actual fact, in the material universe, it appears out of an initial and universal inconscience which is really an involution of the all-conscient spirit in its own absorbed self-oblivious force of action; and it appears therefore as part of an evolutionary process, first a vital feeling towards overt sensation, then an emergence of a vital mind capable of sensation and, evolving out of it, a mind of emotion and desire, a conscious will, a growing intelligence. And each stage is an emergence of a greater suppressed power of the secret supermind and spirit.

The mind of man, capable of reflection and a coordinated investigation and understanding of itself and its basis and surroundings, arrives at truth but against a background of original ignorance, a truth distressed by a constant surrounding mist of incertitude and error. Its certitudes are relative and for the most part precarious certainties or else are the assured fragmentary certitudes only of an imperfect, incomplete and not an essential experience. It makes discovery after discovery, gets idea after idea, adds experience to experience and experiment to experiment, — but losing and rejecting and forgetting and having to recover much as it proceeds, — and it tries to establish a relation between all that it knows by setting up logical and other sequences, a series of principles and their dependences, generalisations and their application, and makes out of its devices a structure in which mentally it can live, move and act and enjoy and labour. This mental knowledge is always limited in extent: not only so, but in addition the mind even sets up other willed barriers, admitting by the mental device of opinion certain parts and sides of truth and excluding all the rest, because if it gave free admission and play to all ideas, if it suffered truth's infinities, it would lose itself in an unreconciled variety, an undetermined immensity and would be unable to act and proceed to practical consequences and an effective creation. And even when it is widest and most complete, mental knowing is still an indirect knowledge, a knowledge not of the thing in itself but of its figures, a system of representations, a scheme of indices, — except indeed when in certain movements it goes beyond itself, beyond the mental idea to spiritual identity, but it finds it extremely difficult to go here beyond a few isolated and intense spiritual realisations or to draw or work out or organise the right practical consequences of these rare identities of knowledge. A greater power than the reason is needed for the spiritual comprehension and effectuation of this deepest knowledge.

This is what the supermind, intimate with the Infinite, alone can do. The supermind sees directly the spirit and essence, the face and body, the result and action, the principles and dependences of the truth as one indivisible whole and therefore can work out the circumstantial results in the power of the essential knowledge, the variations of the spirit in the light of its identities, its apparent divisions in the truth of its oneness. The supermind is a knower and creator of its own truth, the mind of man only a knower and creator in the half light and half darkness of a mingled truth and error, and creator too of a thing which it derives altered, translated, lessened from something greater than and beyond it. Man lives in a mental consciousness between a vast subconscient which is to his seeing a dark inconscience and a vaster superconscient which he is apt to take for another but a luminous inconscience, because his idea of consciousness is confined to his own middle term of mental sensation and intelligence. It is in that luminous superconscience that there lie the ranges of the supermind and the spirit.

The supermind is again, because it acts and creates as well as knows, not only a direct truth-consciousness, but an illumined, direct and spontaneous truth-will. There is not and cannot be in the will of the self-knowing spirit any contradiction, division or difference between its will and its knowledge. The spiritual will is the Tapas or enlightened force of the conscious being of the spirit effecting infallibly what is there within it, and it is this infallible operation of things acting according to their own nature, of energy producing result and event according to the force within it, of action bearing the fruit and event involved in its own character and intention which we call variously in its different aspects law of Nature, Karma, Necessity and Fate. These things are to mind the workings of a power outside or above it in which it is involved and intervenes only with a contributory personal effort which partly arrives and succeeds, partly fails and stumbles and which even in succeeding is largely overruled for issues different from or at any rate greater and more far-reaching than its own intention. The will of man works in the ignorance by a partial light or more often flickerings of light which mislead as much as they illuminate. His mind is an ignorance striving to erect standards of knowledge, his will an ignorance striving to erect standards of right, and his whole mentality as a result very much a house divided against itself, idea in conflict with idea, the will often in conflict with the ideal of right or the intellectual knowledge. The will itself takes different shapes, the will of the intelligence, the wishes of the emotional mind, the desires and the passion of the vital being, the impulsions and blind or half-blind compulsions of the nervous and the subconscient nature, and all these make by no means a harmony, but at best a precarious concord among discords. The will of the mind and life is a stumbling about in search of right force, right Tapas which can wholly be attained in its true and complete light and direction only by oneness with the spiritual and supramental being.

The supramental nature on the contrary is just, harmonious and one, will and knowledge there only light of the spirit and power of the spirit, the power effecting the light, the light illumining the power. In the highest supramentality they are intimately fused together and do not even wait upon each other but are one movement, will illumining itself, knowledge fulfilling itself, both together a single jet of the being. The mind knows only the present and lives in an isolated movement of it though it tries to remember and retain the past and forecast and compel the future. The supermind has the vision of the three times, *trikāladṛṣṭi*; it sees them as an indivisible movement and sees too each containing the others. It is aware of all tendencies, energies and forces as the diverse play of unity and knows their relation to each other in the single movement of the one spirit. The supramental will and action are therefore a will and action of the spontaneous self-fulfilling truth of the spirit, the right and at the highest the infallible movement of a direct and total knowledge.

The supreme and universal Supermind is the active Light and Tapas of the supreme and universal Self as the Lord and Creator, that which we come to know in Yoga as the divine Wisdom and Power, the eternal knowledge and will of the Ishwara. On the highest planes of Being where all is known and all manifests as existences of the one existence, consciousnesses of the one consciousness, delight's self-creations of the one Ananda, many truths and powers of the one Truth, there is the intact and integral display of its spiritual and supramental knowledge. And in the corresponding planes of our own being the Jiva shares in the spiritual and supramental nature and lives in its light and power and bliss. As we descend nearer to what we are in this world, the presence and action of this self-knowledge narrows but retains always the essence and character when not the fullness of the supramental nature and its way of knowing and willing and acting, because it still lives in the essence and body of the spirit. The mind, when we trace the descent of the self towards matter, we see as a derivation which travels away from the fullness of self, the fullness of its light and being and which lives in a division and diversion, not in the body of the sun, but first in its nearer and then in its far-off rays. There is a highest intuitive mind which receives more nearly the supramental truth, but even this is a formation which conceals the direct and greater real knowledge. There is an intellectual mind which is a luminous half-opaque lid which intercepts and reflects in a radiantly distorting and suppressively modifying atmosphere the truth known to the supermind. There is a still lower mind built on the foundation of the senses between which and the sun of knowledge there is a thick cloud, an emotional and a sensational mist and vapour with here and there lightnings and illuminations. There is a vital mind which is shut away even from the light of intellectual truth, and lower still in submental life and matter the spirit involves itself entirely as if in a sleep and a night, a sleep plunged in a dim and yet poignant nervous dream, the night of a mechanical somnambulist energy. It is a re-evolution of the spirit out of this lowest state in which we find ourselves at a height above the lower creation having taken it up all in us and reaching so far in our ascent only the light of the well-developed mental reason. The full powers of self-knowledge and the illumined will of the spirit are still beyond us above the mind and reason in supramental Nature.

If the spirit is everywhere, even in matter — in fact matter itself is only an obscure form of the spirit — and if the supermind is the universal power of the spirit's omnipresent self-knowledge organising all the manifestation of the being, then in matter and everywhere there must be present a supramental action and, however concealed it may be by another, lower and obscurer kind of operation, yet when we look close we shall find that it is really the supermind which organises matter, life, mind and reason. And this actually is the knowledge towards which we are now moving. There is even a quite visible intimate action of the consciousness, persistent in life, matter and mind, which is clearly a supramental action subdued to the character and need of the lower medium and to which we now give the name of intuition from its most evident characteristics of direct vision and self-acting knowledge, really a vision born of some secret identity with the object of the knowledge. What we call the intuition is however only a partial indication of the presence of the supermind, and if we take this presence and power in its widest character, we shall see that it is a concealed supramental force with a self-conscient knowledge in it which informs the whole action of material energy. It is that which determines what we call law of nature, maintains the action of each thing according to its own nature and harmonises and evolves the whole, which would otherwise be a fortuitous creation apt at any moment to collapse into chaos. All the law of nature is a thing precise in its necessities of process, but is yet in the cause of that necessity and of its constancy of rule, measure, combination, adaptation, result a thing inexplicable, meeting us at every step with a mystery and a miracle, and this must be either because it is irrational and accidental even in its regularities or because it is suprarational, because the truth of it belongs to a principle greater than that of our intelligence. That principle is the supramental; that is to say, the hidden secret of Nature is the organisation of something out of the infinite potentialities of the self-existent truth of the spirit the nature of which is wholly evident only to an original knowledge born of and proceeding by a fundamental identity, the spirit's constant self-perception. All the action of life too is of this character and all the action of mind and reason, — reason which is the first to perceive everywhere the action of a greater reason and law of being and try to render it by its own conceptional structures, though it does not always perceive that it is something other than a mental Intelligence which is at work, other than an intellectual Logos. All these processes are actually spiritual and supramental in their secret government, but mental, vital and physical in their overt process.

The outward matter, life, mind do not possess this occult action of the supermind, even while possessed and compelled by the necessity it imposes on their workings. There is what we are sometimes moved to call an intelligence and will operating in the material force and the atom (although the words ring false because it is not actually the same thing as our own will and intelligence), — let us say, a covert intuition of self-existence at work, — but the atom and force are not aware of it and are only the obscure body of matter and of power created by its first effort of self-manifestation. The presence of such an intuition becomes more evident to us in all the action of life because that is nearer to our own scale. And as life develops overt sense and mind, as in the animal creation, we can speak more confidently of a vital intuition which is behind its operations and which emerges in the animal mind in the clear form of instinct, — instinct, an automatic knowledge implanted in the animal, sure, direct, self-existent, self-guided, which implies somewhere in its being an accurate knowing of purpose, relation and the thing or object. It acts in the life force and mind, but yet the surface life and mind do not possess it and cannot give an account of what it does or control or extend the power at its will and pleasure. Here we observe two things, first, that the overt intuition acts only for a limited necessity and purpose, and that in the rest of the operations of the nature there is a double action, one uncertain and ignorant of the surface consciousness and the other subliminal implying a secret subconscient direction. The surface consciousness is full of a groping and seeking which increases rather than diminishes as life rises in its scale and widens in the scope of its conscious powers; but the secret self within assures in spite of the groping of the vital mind the action of the nature and the result needed for the necessity, the purpose and the destiny of the being. This continues on a higher and higher scale up to the human reason and intelligence.

The being of man also is full of physical, vital, emotional, psychical and dynamic instincts and intuitions, but he does not rely on them as the animal does, — though they are capable in him of a far larger scope and greater action than in the animal and lower creation by reason of his greater actual evolutionary development and his yet greater potentiality of development of the being. He has suppressed them, discontinued their full and overt action by atrophy, — not that these capacities are destroyed but rather held back or cast back into the subliminal consciousness, — and consequently this lower part of his being is much less sure of itself, much less confident of the directions of his nature, much more groping, errant and fallible in its larger scope than that of the animal in his lesser limits. This happens because man's real dharma and law of being is to seek for a greater self-aware existence, a self-manifestation no longer obscure and governed by an ununderstood necessity, but illumined, conscious of that which is expressing itself and able to give it a fuller and more perfect expression. And finally his culmination must be to identify himself with his greatest and real self and act or rather let it act (his natural existence being an instrumental form of the expression of the spirit) in its spontaneous perfect will and knowledge. His first instrument for this transition is the reason and the will of the rational intelligence and he is moved to depend upon that to the extent of its development for his knowledge and guidance and give it the control of the rest of his being. And if the reason were the highest thing and the greatest all-sufficient means of the self and spirit, he could by it know perfectly and guide perfectly all the movements of his nature. This he cannot do entirely because his self is a larger thing than his reason and if he limits himself by the rational will and intelligence, he imposes an arbitrary restriction both in extent and in kind on his self-development, self-expression, knowledge, action, Ananda. The other parts of his being demand too a complete expression in the largeness and perfection of the self and cannot have it if their expression is changed in kind and carved, cut down and arbitrarily shaped and mechanised in action by the inflexible machinery of the rational intelligence. The godhead of the reason, the intellectual Logos, is only a partial representative and substitute for the greater supramental Logos, and its function is to impose a preliminary partial knowledge and order upon the life of the creature, but the real, final and integral order can only be founded by the spiritual supermind in its emergence.

The supermind in the lower nature is present most strongly as intuition and it is therefore by a development of an intuitive mind that we can make the first step towards the self-existent spontaneous and direct supramental knowledge. All the physical, vital, emotional, psychic, dynamic nature of man is a surface seizing of suggestions which rise out of a subliminal intuitive self-being of these parts, and an attempt usually groping and often circuitous to work them out in the action of a superficial embodiment and power of the nature which is not overtly enlightened by the inner power and knowledge. An increasingly intuitive mind has the best chance of discovering what they are seeking for and leading them to the desired perfection of their self-expression. The reason itself is only a special kind of application, made by a surface regulating intelligence, of suggestions which actually come from a concealed, but sometimes partially overt and active power of the intuitive spirit. In all its action there is at the covered or half-covered point of origination something which is not the creation of the reason, but given to it either directly by the intuition or indirectly through some other part of the mind for it to shape into intellectual form and process. The rational judgment in its decisions and the mechanical process of the logical intelligence, whether in its more summary or in its more developed operations, conceals while it develops the true origin and native substance of our will and thinking. The greatest minds are those in which this veil wears thin and there is the largest part of intuitive thinking, which often no doubt but not always brings with it a great accompanying display of intellectual action. The intuitive intelligence is however never quite pure and complete in the present mind of man, because it works in the medium of mind and is at once seized on and coated over with a mixed stuff of mentality. It is as yet not brought out, not developed and perfected so as to be sufficient for all the operations now performed by the other mental instruments, not trained to take them up and change them into or replace them by its own fullest, most direct, assured and sufficient workings. This can indeed only be done if we make the intuitive mind a transitional means for bringing out the secret supermind itself of which it is a mental figure and forming in our frontal consciousness a body and instrument of supermind which will make it possible for the self and spirit to display itself in its own largeness and splendour.

It must be remembered that there is always a difference between the supreme Supermind of the omniscient and omnipotent Ishwara and that which can be attained by the Jiva. The human being is climbing out of the ignorance and when he ascends into the supramental nature, he will find in it grades of its ascension, and he must first form the lower grades and limited steps before he rises to higher summits. He will enjoy there the full essential light, power, Ananda of the infinite self by oneness with the Spirit, but in the dynamical expression it must determine and individualise itself according to the nature of the self-expression which the transcendent and universal Spirit seeks in the Jiva. It is God-realisation and God-expression which is the object of our Yoga and more especially of its dynamic side, it is a divine self-expression in us of the Ishwara, but under the conditions of humanity and through the divinised human nature.

Chapter XX

The Intuitive Mind

THE ORIGINAL nature of supermind is the self-conscience and all-conscience of the Infinite, of the universal Spirit and Self in things, organising on the foundation and according to the character of a direct self-knowledge its own wisdom and effective omnipotence for the unfolding and the regulated action of the universe and of all things in the universe. It is, we might say, the gnosis of the Spirit master of its own cosmos, *ātmā jñātā īśvaraḥ*. As it knows itself, so too it knows all things — for all are only becomings of itself — directly, totally and from within outward, spontaneously in detail and arrangement, each thing in the truth of itself and its nature and in its relation to all other things. And it knows similarly all action of its energy in antecedent or cause and occasion of manifestation and effect or consequence, all things in infinite and in limited potentiality and in selection of actuality and in their succession of past, present and future. The organising supermind of a divine being in the universe would be a delegation of this omnipotence and omniscience for the purpose and within the scope of his own action and nature and of all that comes into its province. The supermind in an individual would be a similar delegation on whatever scale and within whatever province. But while in the god this would be a direct and an immediate delegation of a power illimitable in itself and limited only in action, but otherwise unaltered in operation, natural to the being and full and free always, in man any emergence of the supermind must be a gradual and at first an imperfect creation and to his customary mind the activity of an exceptional and supernormal will and knowledge.

In the first place it will not be for him a native power always enjoyed without interruption, but a secret potentiality which has to be discovered and one for which there are no organs in his present physical or mental system: he has either to evolve a new organ for it or else to adopt or transform existing ones and make them utilisable for the purpose. He has not merely to uncover the hidden sun of the supermind in the subliminal cavern of his secret being or remove the cloud of his mental ignorance from its face in the spiritual skies so that it shall at once shine out in all its glory. His task is much more complex and difficult because he is an evolutionary being and by the evolution of Nature of which he is a part he has been constituted with an inferior kind of knowledge, and this inferior, this mental power of knowledge forms by its persistent customary action an obstacle to a new formation greater than its own nature. A limited mental intelligence enlightening a limited mind of sense and the capacity not always well used of a considerable extension of it by the use of the reason are the powers by which he is at present distinguished from all other terrestrial creatures. This sense mind, this intelligence, this reason, however inadequate, are the instruments in which he has learned to put his trust and he has erected by their means certain foundations which he is not over willing to disturb and has traced limits outside of which he feels all to be confusion, uncertainty and a perilous adventure. Moreover the transition to the higher principle means not only a difficult conversion of his whole mind and reason and intelligence, but in a certain sense a reversal of all their methods. The soul climbing above a certain critical line of change sees all its former operations as an inferior and ignorant action and has to effect another kind of working which sets out from a different starting-point and has quite another kind of initiation of the energy of the being. If an animal mind were called upon to leave consciently the safe ground of sense impulse, sense understanding and instinct for the perilous adventure of a reasoning intelligence, it might well turn back alarmed and unwilling from the effort. The human mind would here be called upon to make a still greater change and, although self-conscious and adventurous in the circle of its possibility, might well hold this to be beyond the circle and reject the adventure. In fact the change is only possible if there is first a spiritual development on our present level of consciousness and

it can only be undertaken securely when the mind has become
aware of the greater self within, enamoured of the Infinite and
confident of the presence and guidance of the Divine and his
Shakti.

The problem of this conversion resolves itself at first into
a passage through a mediary status and by the help of the one
power already at work in the human mind which we can recognise as something supramental in its nature or at least in its
origin, the faculty of intuition, a power of which we can feel
the presence and the workings and are impressed, when it acts,
by its superior efficiency, light, direct inspiration and force, but
cannot understand or analyse it as we understand or analyse the
workings of our reason. The reason understands itself, but not
what is beyond it, — of that it can only make a general figure or
representation; the supermind alone can discern the method of
its own workings. The power of intuition acts in us at present for
the most part in a covert manner secret and involved in or mostly
veiled by the action of the reason and the normal intelligence; so
far as it emerges into a clear separate action, it is still occasional,
partial, fragmentary and of an intermittent character. It casts a
sudden light, it makes a luminous suggestion or it throws out
a solitary brilliant clue or scatters a small number of isolated
or related intuitions, lustrous discriminations, inspirations or
revelations, and it leaves the reason, will, mental sense or intelligence to do what each can or pleases with this seed of succour
that has come to them from the depths or the heights of our
being. The mental powers immediately proceed to lay hold on
these things and to manipulate and utilise them for our mental
or vital purposes, to adapt them to the forms of the inferior
knowledge, to coat them up in or infiltrate them with the mental
stuff and suggestion, often altering their truth in the process and
always limiting their potential force of enlightenment by these
accretions and by this subdual to the exigencies of the inferior
agent, and almost always they make at once too little and too
much of them, too little by not allowing them time to settle and
extend their full power for illumination, too much by insisting
on them or rather on the form into which the mentality casts

them to the exclusion of the larger truth that the more consistent use of the intuitive faculty might have given. Thus the intuition intervening in the ordinary mental operations acts in lightning flashes that make lustrous a space of truth, but is not a steady sunlight illumining securely the whole reach and kingdom of our thought and will and feeling and action.

It appears at once that there are two necessary lines of progress which we must follow, and the first is to extend the action of the intuition and make it more constant, more persistent and regular and all-embracing until it is so intimate and normal to our being that it can take up all the action now done by the ordinary mind and assume its place in the whole system. This cannot wholly be done so long as the ordinary mind continues to assert its power of independent action and intervention or its habit of seizing on the light of the intuition and manipulating it for its own purposes. The higher mentality cannot be complete or secure so long as the inferior intelligence is able to deform it or even to bring in any of its own intermixture. And either then we must silence altogether the intellect and the intellectual will and the other inferior activities and leave room only for the intuitive action or we must lay hold on and transform the lower action by the constant pressure of the intuition. Or else there must be an alternation and combination of the two methods if that be the most natural way or at all possible. The actual process and experience of Yoga manifests the possibility of several methods or movements none of which by itself produces the entire result in practice, however it may seem at first sight that logically each should or might be adequate. And when we learn to insist on no particular method as exclusively the right one and leave the whole movement to a greater guidance, we find that the divine Lord of the Yoga commissions his Shakti to use one or the other at different times and all in combination according to the need and turn of the being and the nature.

At first it might seem the straight and right way to silence the mind altogether, to silence the intellect, the mental and personal will, the desire mind and the mind of emotion and sensation, and to allow in that perfect silence the Self, the Spirit, the Divine to disclose himself and leave him to illuminate the being by the supramental light and power and Ananda. And this is indeed a great and powerful discipline. It is the calm and still mind much more readily and with a much greater purity than the mind in agitation and action that opens to the Infinite, reflects the Spirit, becomes full of the Self and awaits like a consecrated and purified temple the unveiling of the Lord of all our being and nature. It is true also that the freedom of this silence gives a possibility of a larger play of the intuitive being and admits with less obstruction and turmoil of mental groping and seizing the great intuitions, inspirations, revelations which emerge from within or descend from above. It is therefore an immense gain if we can acquire the capacity of always being able at will to command an absolute tranquillity and silence of the mind free from any necessity of mental thought or movement and disturbance and, based in that silence, allow thought and will and feeling to happen in us only when the Shakti wills it and when it is needful for the divine purpose. It becomes easier then to change the manner and character of the thought and will and feeling. Nevertheless it is not the fact that by this method the supramental light will immediately replace the lower mind and reflective reason. When the inner action proceeds after the silence, even if it be then a more predominatingly intuitive thought and movement, the old powers will yet interfere, if not from within, then by a hundred suggestions from without, and an inferior mentality will mix in, will question or obstruct or will try to lay hold on the greater movement and to lower or darken or distort or minimise it in the process. Therefore the necessity of a process of elimination or transformation of the inferior mentality remains always imperative, — or perhaps both at once, an elimination of all that is native to the lower being, its disfiguring accidents, its depreciations of value, its distortions of substance and all else that the greater truth cannot harbour, and a transformation of the essential things our mind derives from the supermind and spirit but represents in the manner of the mental ignorance.

A second movement is one which comes naturally to those who commence the Yoga with the initiative that is proper to the way of Bhakti. It is natural to them to reject the intellect and its action and to listen for the voice, wait for the impulsion or the command, the *ādeśa*, obey only the idea and will and power of the Lord within them, the divine Self and Purusha in the heart of the creature, *īśvaraḥ sarvabhūtānāṁ hṛddeśe*. This is a movement which must tend more and more to intuitivise the whole nature, for the ideas, the will, the impulsions, the feelings which come from the secret Purusha in the heart are of the direct intuitive character. This method is consonant with a certain truth of our nature. The secret Self within us is an intuitive self and this intuitive self is seated in every centre of our being, the physical, the nervous, the emotional, the volitional, the conceptual or cognitive and the higher more directly spiritual centres. And in each part of our being it exercises a secret intuitive initiation of our activities which is received and represented imperfectly by our outer mind and converted into the movements of the ignorance in the external action of these parts of our nature. The heart or emotional centre of the thinking desire mind is the strongest in the ordinary man, gathers up or at least affects the presentation of things to the consciousness and is the capital of the system. It is from there that the Lord seated in the heart of all creatures turns them mounted on the machine of Nature by the Maya of the mental ignorance. It is possible then by referring back all the initiation of our action to this secret intuitive Self and Spirit, the ever-present Godhead within us, and replacing by its influences the initiations of our personal and mental nature to get back from the inferior external thought and action to another, internal and intuitive, of a highly spiritualised character. Nevertheless the result of this movement cannot be complete, because the heart is not the highest centre of our being, is not supramental nor directly moved from the supramental sources. An intuitive thought and action directed from it may be very luminous and intense but is likely to be limited, even narrow in its intensity, mixed with a lower emotional action and at the best excited and troubled, rendered unbalanced or exaggerated by a miraculous or abnormal character in its action or at least in many of its accompaniments which is injurious to the harmonised perfection of the being. The aim of our effort at perfection must be to make the spiritual and supramental action no longer a miracle, even if a frequent or constant miracle, or only a luminous intervention of a greater than our natural power, but normal to the being and the very nature and law of all its process.

The highest organised centre of our embodied being and of its action in the body is the supreme mental centre figured by the yogic symbol of the thousand-petalled lotus, *sahasradala*, and it is at its top and summit that there is the direct communication with the supramental levels. It is then possible to adopt a different and a more direct method, not to refer all our thought and action to the Lord secret in the heart-lotus but to the veiled truth of the Divinity above the mind and to receive all by a sort of descent from above, a descent of which we become not only spiritually but physically conscious. The siddhi or full accomplishment of this movement can only come when we are able to lift the centre of thought and conscious action above the physical brain and feel it going on in the subtle body. If we can feel ourselves thinking no longer with the brain but from above and outside the head in the subtle body, that is a sure physical sign of a release from the limitations of the physical mind, and though this will not be complete at once nor of itself bring the supramental action, for the subtle body is mental and not supramental, still it is a subtle and pure mentality and makes an easier communication with the supramental centres. The lower movements must still come, but it is then found easier to arrive at a swift and subtle discrimination telling us at once the difference, distinguishing the intuitional thought from the lower intellectual mixture, separating it from its mental coatings, rejecting the mere rapidities of the mind which imitate the form of the intuition without being of its true substance. It will be easier to discern rapidly the higher planes of the true supramental being and call down their power to effect the desired transformation and to refer all the lower action to the superior power and light that it may reject and eliminate, purify and transform and select among them its right material for the Truth that has to be organised within us. This opening up of a higher level and of higher and higher planes of it and the consequent re-formation of our whole consciousness and its action into their mould and into the substance of their power and luminous capacity is found in practice to be the greater part of the natural method used by the divine Shakti.

A fourth method is one which suggests itself naturally to the developed intelligence and suits the thinking man. This is to develop our intellect instead of eliminating it, but with the will not to cherish its limitations, but to heighten its capacity, light, intensity, degree and force of activity until it borders on the thing that transcends it and can easily be taken up and transformed into that higher conscious action. This movement also is founded on the truth of our nature and enters into the course and movement of the complete Yoga of self-perfection. That course, as I have described it, included a heightening and greatening of the action of our natural instruments and powers till they constitute in their purity and essential completeness a preparatory perfection of the present normal movement of the Shakti that acts in us. The reason and intelligent will, the buddhi, is the greatest of these powers and instruments, the natural leader of the rest in the developed human being, the most capable of aiding the development of the others. The ordinary activities of our nature are all of them of use for the greater perfection we seek, are meant to be turned into material for them, and the greater their development, the richer the preparation for the supramental action.

The intellectual being too has to be taken up by the Shakti in the Yoga and raised to its fullest and its most heightened powers. The subsequent transformation of the intellect is possible because all the action of the intellect derives secretly from the supermind, each thought and will contains some truth of it however limited and altered by the inferior action of the intelligence. The transformation can be brought about by the removal of the limitation and the elimination of the distorting or perverting element. This however cannot be done by the heightening and greatening of the intellectual activity alone; for that must always be limited by the original inherent defects of the mental intelligence. An intervention of the supramental energy is needed that can light up and get rid of its deficiencies of thought and will and feeling. This intervention too cannot be completely effective unless the supramental plane is manifested and acts above the mind no longer from behind a lid or veil, however thin the veil may have grown, but more constantly in an open and luminous action till there is seen the full sun of Truth with no cloud to moderate its splendour. It is not necessary, either, to develop the intellect fully in its separateness before calling down this intervention or opening up by it the supramental levels. The intervention may come in earlier and at once develop the intellectual action and turn it, as it develops, into the higher intuitive form and substance.

The widest natural action of the Shakti combines all these methods. It creates, sometimes at first, sometimes at some later, perhaps latest stage, the freedom of the spiritual silence. It opens the secret intuitive being within the mind itself and accustoms us to refer all our thought and our feeling and will and action to the initiation of the Divine, the Splendour and Power who is now concealed in the heart of its recesses. It raises, when we are ready, the centre of its operations to the mental summit and opens up the supramental levels and proceeds doubly by an action from above downward filling and transforming the lower nature and an action from below upwards raising all the energies to that which is above them till the transcendence is completed and the change of the whole system integrally effected. It takes and develops the intelligence and will and other natural powers, but brings in constantly the intuitive mind and afterwards the true supramental energy to change and enlarge their action. These things it does in no fixed and mechanically invariable order, such as the rigidity of the logical intellect might demand, but freely and flexibly according to the needs of its work and the demand of the nature.

The first result will not be the creation of the true supermind, but the organisation of a predominantly or even a completely intuitive mentality sufficiently developed to take the place of the ordinary mentality and of the logical reasoning intellect of the developed human being. The most prominent change will be the transmutation of the thought heightened and filled by that substance of concentrated light, concentrated power, concentrated joy of the light and the power and that direct accuracy which are the marks of a true intuitive thinking. It is not only primary suggestions or rapid conclusions that this mind will give, but it will conduct too with the same light, power, joy of sureness and direct spontaneous seeing of the truth the connecting and developing operations now conducted by the intellectual reason. The will also will be changed into this intuitive character, proceed directly with light and power to the thing to be done, *kartavyaṁ karma*, and dispose with a rapid sight of possibilities and actualities the combinations necessary to its action and its purpose. The feelings also will be intuitive, seizing upon right relations, acting with a new light and power and a glad sureness, retaining only right and spontaneous desires and emotions, so long as these things endure, and, when they pass away, replacing them by a luminous and spontaneous love and an Ananda that knows and seizes at once on the right *rasa* of its objects. All the other mental movements will be similarly enlightened and even too the pranic and sense movements and the consciousness of the body. And usually there will be some development also of the psychic faculties, powers and perceptions of the inner mind and its senses not dependent on the outer sense and the reason. The intuitive mentality will be not only a stronger and a more luminous thing, but usually capable of a much more extensive operation than the ordinary mind of the same man before this development of the Yoga.

This intuitive mentality, if it could be made perfect in its nature, unmixed with any inferior element and yet unconscious of its own limitations and of the greatness of the thing beyond it, might form another definite status and halting place like the instinctive mind of the animal or the reasoning mind of man. But the intuitive mentality cannot be made abidingly perfect and self-sufficient except by the opening power of the supermind above it and that at once reveals its limitations and makes of it a secondary action transitional between the intellectual mind and the true supramental nature. The intuitive mentality is still mind and not gnosis. It is indeed a light from the supermind, but modified and diminished by the stuff of mind in which it works, and stuff of mind means always a basis of ignorance. The intuitive mind is not yet the wide sunlight of truth, but a constant play of flashes of it keeping lighted up a basic state of ignorance or of half-knowledge and indirect knowledge. As long as it is imperfect, it is invaded by a mixture of ignorant mentality which crosses its truth with a strain of error. After it has acquired a larger native action more free from this intermixture, even then so long as the stuff of mind in which it works is capable of the old intellectual or lower mental habit, it is subject to accretion of error, to clouding, to many kinds of relapse. Moreover the individual mind does not live alone and to itself but in the general mind and all that it has rejected is discharged into the general mind atmosphere around it and tends to return upon and invade it with the old suggestions and many promptings of the old mental character. The intuitive mind, growing or grown, has therefore to be constantly on guard against invasion and accretion, on the watch to reject and eliminate immixtures, busy intuitivising more and still more the whole stuff of mind, and this can only end by itself being enlightened, transformed, lifted up into the full light of the supramental being.

Moreover, this new mentality is in each man a development of the present power of his being and, however new and remarkable its developments, its organisation is within a certain range of capacity. Adventuring beyond that border — it may indeed limit itself to the work in hand and its present range of realised capacity, but the nature of a mind opened to the infinite is to progress and change and enlarge — it there becomes liable to a return, however modified by the new intuitive habit, of the old intellectual seeking in the ignorance, — unless and until it is constantly overtopped and led by the manifested action of a fuller supramental luminous energy. This is indeed its nature that it is a link and transition between present mind and the supermind and, so long as the transition is not complete, there is sometimes a gravitation downward, sometimes a tendency upward, an oscillation, an invasion and attraction from below, an invasion and attraction from above, and at best an uncertain and limited status between the two poles. As the higher intelligence of man is situated between his animal and customary human mind below and his evolving spiritual mind above, so this first spiritual mind is situated between the intellectualised human mentality and the greater supramental knowledge.

The nature of mind is that it lives between half-lights and darkness, amid probabilities and possibilities, amid partly grasped aspects, amid incertitudes and half certitudes: it is an ignorance grasping at knowledge, striving to enlarge itself and pressing against the concealed body of true gnosis. The supermind lives in the light of spiritual certitudes: it is to man knowledge opening the actual body of its own native effulgence. The intuitive mind appears at first a lightening up of the mind's half-lights, its probabilities and possibilities, its aspects, its uncertain certitudes, its representations, and a revealing of the truth concealed or half concealed and half manifested by these things, and in its higher action it is a first bringing of the supramental truth by a nearer directness of seeing, a luminous indication or memory of the spirit's knowledge, an intuition or looking in through the gates of the being's secret universal self-vision and knowledge. It is a first imperfect organisation of that greater light and power, imperfect because done in the mind, not based on its own native substance of consciousness, a constant communication, but not a quite immediate and constant presence. The perfect perfection lies beyond on the supramental levels and must be based on a more decisive and complete transformation of the mentality and of our whole nature.

Chapter XXI

The Gradations of the Supermind

THE INTUITIVE mind is an immediate translation of truth into mental terms half transformed by a radiant supramental substance, a translation of some infinite self-knowledge that acts above mind in the superconscient spirit. That spirit becomes conscient to us as a greater self at once above and in and around us of which our present self, our mental, vital and physical personality and nature, is an imperfect portion or a partial derivation or an inferior and inadequate symbol, and as the intuitive mind grows in us, as our whole being grows more moulded to an intuitive substance, we feel a sort of half transformation of our members into the nature of this greater self and spirit. All our thought, will, impulse, feeling, even in the end our more outward vital and physical sensations become more and more direct transmissions from the spirit and are of another and a more and more pure, untroubled, powerful and luminous nature. This is one side of the change: the other is that whatever belongs still to the lower being, whatever still seems to us to come from outside or as a survival of the action of our old inferior personality, feels the pressure of the change and increasingly tends to modify and transform itself to the new substance and nature. The higher comes down and largely takes the place of the lower, but also the lower changes, transforms itself into material of the action and becomes part of the substance of the higher being.

The greater spirit above the mind appears at first as a presence, a light, a power, a source, an infinite, but all that is knowable to us in it is at first an infinite identity of being, consciousness, power of consciousness, Ananda. The rest comes from it, but takes no determinate shape of thought, will or feeling above us, but only in the intuitive mind and on its level. Or we feel and are manifoldly aware of a great and infinite Purusha who is the eternally living truth of that being and presence, a great and infinite knowledge which is the potency of that light and consciousness, a great and infinite will which is the potency of that power of consciousness, a great and infinite love which is the potency of that Ananda. But all these potencies are only known to us in any definite manner, apart from the strong reality and effect of their essential presence, in so far as they are translated to our intuitive mental being and on its level and within its limits. As however we progress or as we grow into a more luminous and dynamic union with that spirit or Purusha, a greater action of knowledge and will and spiritual feeling manifests and seems to organise itself above the mind and this we recognise as the true supermind and the real native play of the infinite knowledge, will and Ananda. The intuitive mentality then becomes a secondary and inferior movement waiting upon this higher power, responding and assenting to all its illuminations and dictates, transmitting them to the lower members, and, when they do not arrive or are not in immediate evidence, often attempting to supply its place, imitate its action and do as best it can the works of the supramental nature. It takes in fact the same place and relation with regard to it as was taken with regard to itself by the ordinary intelligence at an earlier stage of the Yoga.

This double action on the two planes of our being at first strengthens the intuitive mentality as a secondary operation and assists it to expel or transform more completely the survivals or invasions or accretions of the ignorance. And more and more it intensifies the intuitive mentality itself in its light of knowledge and eventually transforms it into the image of the supermind itself, but at first, ordinarily, in the more limited action of the gnosis when it takes the form of what we might call a luminous supramental or divine reason. It is as this divine reason that the supermind itself at the beginning may manifest its action and then, when it has changed the mind into its own image, it descends and takes the place of the ordinary intelligence and reason. Meanwhile a higher supramental power of a much greater character has been revealing itself above which takes the supreme lead of the divine action in the being. The divine reason is of a more limited character because, although not of the mental stamp and although an operation of the direct truth and knowledge, it is a delegated power for a range of purposes greater in light, but still to a certain extent analogous to those of the ordinary human will and reason; it is in the yet greater supermind that there comes the direct, altogether revealed and immediate action of the Ishwara in the human being. These distinctions between the intuitive mind, the divine reason and the greater supermind, and others within these gradations themselves, have to be made because eventually they become of great importance. At first the mind takes all that comes from beyond it without distinction as the sufficient spiritual illumination and accepts even initial states and first enlightenments as a finality, but afterwards it finds that to rest here would be to rest in a partial realisation and that one has to go on heightening and enlarging till at least there is reached a certain completeness of divine breadth and stature.

It is difficult for the intellect to grasp at all what is meant by these supramental distinctions: the mental terms in which they can be rendered are lacking or inadequate and they can only be understood after a certain sight or certain approximations in experience. A number of indications are all that at present it can be useful to give. And first it will be enough to take certain clues from the thinking mind; for it is there that some of the nearest keys to the supramental action are discoverable. The thought of the intuitive mind proceeds wholly by four powers that shape the form of the truth, an intuition that suggests its idea, an intuition that discriminates, an inspiration that brings in its word and something of its greater substance and a revelation that shapes to the sight its very face and body of reality. These things are not the same as certain movements of the ordinary mental intelligence that look analogous and are easily mistaken for the true intuition in our first inexperience. The suggestive intuition is not the same thing as the intellectual insight of a quick intelligence or the intuitive discrimination as the rapid judgment of the reasoning intellect; the intuitive inspiration is not the same as the inspired action of the imaginative intelligence, nor the intuitive revelation as the strong light of a purely mental close seizing and experience.

It would perhaps be accurate to say that these latter activities are mental representations of the higher movements, attempts of the ordinary mind to do the same things or the best possible imitations the intellect can offer of the functionings of the higher nature. The true intuitions differ from these effective but insufficient counterfeits in their substance of light, their operation, their method of knowledge. The intellectual rapidities are dependent on awakenings of the basic mental ignorance to mental figures and representations of truth that may be quite valid in their own field and for their own purpose but are not necessarily and by their very nature reliable. They are dependent for their emergence on the suggestions given by mental and sense data or on the accumulation of past mental knowledge. They search for the truth as a thing outside, an object to be found and looked at and stored as an acquisition and, when found, scrutinise its surfaces, suggestions or aspects. This scrutiny can never give a quite complete and adequate truth idea. However positive they may seem at the time, they may at any moment have to be passed over, rejected and found inconsistent with fresh knowledge.

The intuitive knowledge on the contrary, however limited it may be in its field or application, is within that scope sure with an immediate, a durable and especially a self-existent certitude. It may take for starting-point or rather for a thing to light up and disclose in its true sense the data of mind and sense or else fire a train of past thought and knowledge to new meanings and issues, but it is dependent on nothing but itself and may leap out of its own field of lustres, independent of previous suggestion or data, and this kind of action becomes progressively more common and adds itself to the other to initiate new depths and ranges of knowledge. In either case there is always an element of self-existent truth and a sense of absoluteness of origination suggestive of its proceeding from the spirit's knowledge by identity. It is the disclosing of a knowledge that is secret but already existent in the being: it is not an acquisition, but something that was always there and revealable. It sees the truth from within and illumines with that inner vision the outsides and it harmonises, too, readily — provided we keep intuitively awake — with whatever fresh truth has yet to arrive. These characteristics become more pronounced and intense in the higher, the proper supramental ranges: in the intuitive mind they may not be always recognisable in their purity and completeness, because of the mixture of mental stuff and its accretion, but in the divine reason and greater supramental action they become free and absolute.

The suggestive intuition acting on the mental level suggests a direct and illumining inner idea of the truth, an idea that is its true image and index, not as yet the entirely present and whole sight, but rather of the nature of a bright memory of some truth, a recognition of a secret of the self's knowledge. It is a representation, but a living representation, not an ideative symbol, a reflection, but a reflection that is lit up with something of the truth's real substance. The intuitive discrimination is a secondary action setting this idea of the truth in its right place and its relation to other ideas. And so long as there is the habit of mental interference and accretion it works also to separate the mental from the higher seeing, to discrete the inferior mental stuff that embarrasses with its alloy the pure truth substance, and labours to unravel the mingled skein of ignorance and knowledge, falsehood and error. As the intuition is of the nature of a memory, a luminous remembering of the self-existent truth, so the inspiration is of the nature of truth hearing: it is an immediate reception of the very voice of the truth, it readily brings the word that perfectly embodies it and it carries something more than the light of its idea; there is seized some stream of its inner reality and vivid arriving movement of its substance. The revelation is of the nature of direct sight, *pratyakṣa-dṛṣṭi*, and makes evident to a present vision the thing in itself of which the idea is the representation. It brings out the very spirit and being and reality of the truth and makes it part of the consciousness and the experience.

In the actual process of the development of the supramental nature, supposing it to follow a regular gradation, it may be seen

that the two lower powers come out first, though not necessarily
void of all action of the two higher powers, and as they increase
and become a normal action, they make a sort of lower intuitive
gnosis. The combination of the two together is necessary for
its completeness. If the intuitive discrimination works by itself,
it creates a sort of critical illumination that acts on the ideas
and perceptions of the intellect and turns them on themselves
in such a way that the mind can separate their truth from their
error. It creates in the end in place of the intellectual judgment
a luminous intuitive judgment, a sort of critical gnosis: but it is
likely to be deficient in fresh illuminative knowledge or to create
only so much extension of truth as is the natural consequence
of the separation of error. On the other hand, if the suggestive
intuition works by itself without this discrimination, there is indeed a constant accession of new truths and new lights, but they
are easily surrounded and embarrassed by the mental accretions
and their connections and relation or harmonious development
out of each other are clouded and broken by the interference. A
normalised power of active intuitive perception is created, but
not any complete and coherent mind of intuitive gnosis. The
two together supply the deficiencies of each other's single action
and build up a mind of intuitive perception and discrimination
which can do the work and more than the work of the stumbling
mental intelligence and do it with the greater light, surety and
power of a more direct and unfaltering ideation.

The two higher powers in the same way make a higher intuitive gnosis. Acting as separate powers in the mentality they too
are not in themselves sufficient without the companion activities.
The revelation may indeed present the reality, the identities of
the thing in itself and add something of great power to the experience of the conscious being, but it may lack the embodying word,
the out-bringing idea, the connected pursuit of its relations and
consequences and may remain a possession in the self but not
a thing communicated to and through the members. There may
be the presence of the truth but not its full manifestation. The
inspiration may give the word of the truth and the stir of its
dynamis and movement, but this is not a complete thing and sure

in its effect without the full revelation of all that it bears in itself and luminously indicates and the ordering of it in its relations. The inspired intuitive mind is a mind of lightnings lighting up many things that were dark, but the light needs to be canalised and fixed into a stream of steady lustres that will be a constant power for lucidly ordered knowledge. The higher gnosis by itself in its two sole powers would be a mind of spiritual splendours living too much in its own separate domain, producing perhaps invisibly its effect on the outside world, but lacking the link of a more close and ordinary communication with its more normal movements that is provided by the lower ideative action. It is the united or else the fused and unified action of the four powers that makes the complete and fully armed and equipped intuitive gnosis.

A regular development would at first, allowing for some simultaneous manifestation of the four powers, yet create on a sufficiently extensive scale the lower suggestive and critical intuitive mind and then develop above it the inspired and the revelatory intuitive mentality. Next it would take up the two lower powers into the power and field of the inspiration and make all act as one harmony doing simultaneously the united — or, at a higher intensity, indistinguishably as one light the unified — action of the three. And last it would execute a similar movement of taking up into and fusion with the revelatory power of the intuitive gnosis. As a matter of fact in the human mind the clear process of the development is likely always to be more or less disturbed, confused and rendered irregular in its course, subjected to relapses, incomplete advances, returns upon things unaccomplished or imperfectly accomplished owing to the constant mixture and intervention of the existing movements of the mental half-knowledge and the obstruction of the stuff of the mental ignorance. In the end however a time can come when the process, so far as it is possible in the mind itself, is complete and a clear formation of a modified supramental light is possible composed of all these powers, the highest leading or absorbing into its own body the others. It is at this point, when the intuitive mind has been fully formed in the mental being and is strong enough to dominate if not yet wholly to occupy the various mental activities, that a farther step becomes possible, the lifting of the centre and level of action above the mind and the predominance of the supramental reason.

The first character of this change is a complete reversal, a turning over, one might almost say, upside down of the whole activity. At present we live in the mind and mostly in the physical mind, but still not entirely involved like the animal in the physical, vital and sensational workings. On the contrary we have attained to a certain mental elevation from which we can look down on the action of the life, sense and body, turn the higher mental light on them, reflect, judge, use our will to modify the action of the inferior nature. On the other hand we look up too from that elevation more or less consciously to something above and receive from it either directly or through our subconscient or subliminal being some secret superconscient impulsion of our thought and will and other activities. The process of this communication is veiled and obscure and men are not ordinarily aware of it except in certain highly developed natures: but when we advance in self-knowledge, we find that all our thought and will originate from above though formed in the mind and there first overtly active. If we release the knots of the physical mind which binds us to the brain instrument and identifies us with the bodily consciousness and can move in the pure mentality, this becomes constantly clear to the perception.

The development of the intuitive mentality makes this communication direct, no longer subconscient and obscure; but we are still in the mind and the mind still looks upward and receives the supramental communication and passes it on to the other members. In doing so it no longer wholly creates its own form for the thought and will that come down to it, but still it modifies and qualifies and limits them and imposes something of its own method. It is still the receiver and the transmitter of the thought and will, — though not formative of them now except by a subtle influence, because it provides them or at least surrounds them with a mental stuff or a mental setting and framework and atmosphere. When however the supramental reason develops, the Purusha rises above the mental elevation and now looks down on the whole action of mind, life, sense, body from quite another light and atmosphere, sees and knows it with quite a different vision and, because he is no longer involved in the mind, with a free and true knowledge. Man is at present only partly liberated from the animal involution, — for his mind is partially lifted above, partially immerged and controlled by the life, sense and body, — and he is not at all liberated from the mental forms and limits. But after he rises to the supramental elevation, he is delivered from the nether control and governor of his whole nature — essentially and initially only at first and in his highest consciousness, for the rest remains still to be transformed, — but when or in proportion as that is done, he becomes a free being and master of his mind, sense, life and body.

The second character of the change is that the formation of the thought and will can take place now wholly on the supramental level and therefore there is initiated an entirely luminous and effective will and knowledge. The light and the power are not indeed complete at the beginning because the supramental reason is only an elementary formulation of the supermind and because the mind and other members have yet to be changed into the mould of the supramental nature. The mind, it is true, no longer acts as the apparent originator, formulator or judge of the thought and will or anything else, but it still acts as the transmitting channel and therefore in that degree as a recipient and to a certain extent an obstructor and qualifier in transmission of the power and light that comes from above. There is a disparateness between the supramental consciousness in which the Purusha now stands, thinks and wills and the mental, vital and physical consciousness through which he has to effectuate its light and knowledge. He lives and sees with an ideal consciousness, but he has yet in his lower self to make it entirely practical and effective. Otherwise he can only act with a greater or less spiritual effectiveness through an internal communication with others on the spiritual level and on the higher mental level that is most easily affected by it, but the effect is diminished and is retarded by the inferiority or lack of the integral play of the being. This can only be remedied by the supermind taking hold of and supramentalising the mental, the vital and the physical consciousness, — transforming them, that is to say, into moulds of the supramental nature. This is much more easily done if there has been that Yogic preparation of the instruments of the lower nature of which I have already spoken; otherwise there is much difficulty in getting rid of the discord or disparateness between the ideal supramentality and the mental transmitting instruments, the mind channel, the heart, the sense, the nervous and the physical being. The supramental reason can do the first and a fairly ample, though not the entire work of this transformation.

The supramental reason is of the nature of a spiritual, direct, self-luminous, self-acting will and intelligence, not mental, *mānasa buddhi*, but supramental, *vijñāna buddhi*. It acts by the same four powers as the intuitive mind, but these powers are here active in an initial fullness of body not modified by the mental stuff of the intelligence, not concerned mainly with an illumining of the mind, but at work in their own proper manner and for their own native purpose. And of these four the discrimination here is hardly recognisable as a separate power, but is constantly inherent in the three others and is their own determination of the scope and relations of their knowledge. There are three elevations in this reason, one in which the action of what we may call a supramental intuition gives the form and the predominant character, one in which a rapid supramental inspiration and one in which a large supramental revelation leads and imparts the general character, and each of these raises us to a more concentrated substance and a higher light, sufficiency and scope of the truth will and the truth knowledge.

The work of the supramental reason covers and goes beyond all that is done by the mental reason, but it starts from the other end and has a corresponding operation. The essential truths of self and the spirit and the principle of things are not to the spiritual reason abstract ideas or subtle unsubstantial experiences to which it arrives by a sort of overleaping of limits, but a constant reality and the natural background of all its ideation and experience. It does not like the mind arrive at, but discloses directly both the general and total and the particular truths of being and consciousness, of spiritual and other sensation and Ananda and of force and action, — reality and phenomenon and symbol, actuality and possibility and eventuality, that which is determined and that which determines, and all with a self-luminous evidence. It formulates and arranges the relations of thought and thought, of force and force, of action and action and of all these with each other and throws them into a convincing and luminous harmony. It includes the data of sense, but gives to them another meaning in the light of what is behind them, and treats them only as outermost indications: the inner truth is known to a greater sense which it already possesses. And it is not dependent on them alone even in their own field of objects or limited by their range. It has a spiritual sense and sensation of its own and it takes and relates to that the data too of a sixth sense, the inner mind sense. And it takes also the illuminations and the living symbols and images familiar to the psychic experience and relates these too to the truths of the self and spirit.

The spiritual reason takes also the emotions and psychic sensations, relates them to their spiritual equivalents and imparts to them the values of the higher consciousness and Ananda from which they derive and are its modifications in an inferior nature and it corrects their deformations. It takes similarly the movements of the vital being and consciousness and relates them to the movements and imparts to them the significances of the spiritual life of the self and its power of Tapas. It takes the physical consciousness, delivers it from its darkness and tamas of inertia and makes it a responsive recipient and a sensitive instrument of the supramental light and power and Ananda. It deals with life and action and knowledge like the mental will and reason, but not starting from matter, life and sense and their data and relating to them through the idea the truth of higher things, but it starts on the contrary from truth of self and spirit and relates to that through a direct spiritual experience assuming all other experience as its forms and instruments the things of mind and soul and life and sense and matter. It commands a far vaster range than the ordinary embodied mind shut up in the prison of the physical senses and vaster too than the pure mentality, even when that is free in its own ranges and operates with the aid of the psychical mind and inner senses. And it has that power which the mental will and reason do not possess, because they are not truly self-determined and originally determinative of things, the power of transforming the whole being in all its parts into a harmonious instrument and manifestation of the spirit.

At the same time the spiritual reason acts mainly by the representative idea and will in the spirit, though it has a greater and more essential truth as its constant source and supporter and reference. It is, then, a power of light of the Ishwara, but not the very self-power of his immediate presence in the being; it is his *sūrya-śakti*, not his whole *ātma-śakti* or *parā svā prakṛti*, that works in the spiritual reason. The immediate self-power begins its direct operation in the greater supermind, and that takes up all that has hitherto been realised in body, life and mind and in the intuitive being and by the spiritual reason and shapes all that has been created, all that has been gathered, turned into stuff of experience and made part of the consciousness, personality and nature by the mental being, into a highest harmony with the high infinite and universal life of the spirit. The mind can have the touch of the infinite and the universal and can reflect and even lose itself in them, but the supermind alone can enable the individual to be completely one in action with the universal and transcendent spirit.

Here the one thing that is always and constantly present, that which one has grown to and in which one lives always, is infinite being and all that is is seen, felt, known, existed in as only substance of the one being; it is infinite consciousness and all that is conscious and acts and moves is seen, felt, received, known, lived in as self-experience and energy of the one being; it is infinite Ananda and all that feels and is felt is seen and felt and known, received and lived in as forms of the one Ananda. Everything else is only manifestation and circumstance of this one truth of our existence. This is no longer merely the seeing or knowing, but the very condition of the self in all and all in the self, God in all and all in God and all seen as God, and that condition is now not a thing offered to the reflecting spiritualised mind but held and lived by an integral, always present, always active realisation in the supramental nature. There is thought here and will and sensation and everything that belongs to our nature, but it is transfigured and elevated into a higher consciousness. All thought is here seen and experienced as a luminous body of substance, a luminous movement of force, a luminous wave of Ananda of the being; it is not an idea in the void air of mind, but experienced in the reality and as the light of a reality of the infinite being. The will and impulsions are similarly experienced as a real power and substance of the Sat, the Chit, the Ananda of the Ishwara. All the spiritualised sensation and emotion are experienced as pure moulds of the consciousness and Ananda. The physical being itself is experienced as a conscious form and the vital being as an outpouring of the power and possession of the life of the spirit.

The action of the supermind in the development is to manifest and organise this highest consciousness so as to exist and act no longer only in the infinite above with some limited or veiled or lower and deformed manifestations in the individual being and nature, but largely and totally in the individual as a conscious and self-knowing spiritual being and a living and acting power of the infinite and universal spirit. The character of this action, so far as it can be expressed, may be spoken of more fitly afterwards when we come to speak of the Brahmic consciousness and vision. In the succeeding chapters we shall only deal with so much of it as concerns the thought, will and psychic and other experience in the individual nature. At present all that is necessary to note is that here too there is in the field of the thought and the will a triple action. The spiritual reason is lifted and broadened into a greater representative action that formulates to us mainly the actualities of the existence of the self in and around us. There is then a higher interpretative action of the supramental knowledge, a greater scale less insistent on actualities, that opens out yet greater potentialities in time and space and beyond. And lastly there is a highest knowledge by identity that is a gate of entrance to the essential self-awareness and the omniscience and omnipotence of the Ishwara.

It must not however be supposed that these superimposed stages are shut off in experience from each other. I have placed them in what might be a regular order of ascending development for the better possibility of understanding in an intellectual statement. But the infinite even in the normal mind breaks through its own veils and across its own dividing lines of descent and ascension and gives often intimations of itself in one manner or another. And while we are still in the intuitive mentality, the things above open and come to us in irregular visitations, then form as we grow a more frequent and regularised action above it. These anticipations are still more large and frequent the moment we enter on the supramental level. The universal and infinite consciousness can always seize on and surround the mind and it is when it does so with a certain continuity, frequency or persistence that the mind can most easily transform itself into the intuitive mentality and that again into the supramental movement. Only as we rise we grow more intimately and integrally into the infinite consciousness and it becomes more fully our own self and nature. And also, on the other, the lower side of existence which it might seem would then be not only beneath but quite alien to us, even when we live in the supramental being and even when the whole nature has been formed into its mould, that need not cut us off from the knowledge and feeling of others who live in the ordinary nature. The lower or more limited may have a difficulty in understanding and feeling the higher, but the higher and less limited can always, if it will, understand and identify itself with the lower nature. The supreme Ishwara too is not aloof from us; he knows, lives in, identifies himself with all and yet is not subjugated by the reactions or limited in his knowledge, power and Ananda by the limitations of the mind and life and physical being in the universe.

Chapter XXII

The Supramental Thought and Knowledge

THE TRANSITION from mind to supermind is not only the substitution of a greater instrument of thought and knowledge, but a change and conversion of the whole consciousness. There is evolved not only a supramental thought, but a supramental will, sense, feeling, a supramental substitute for all the activities that are now accomplished by the mind. All these higher activities are first manifested in the mind itself as descents, irruptions, messages or revelations of a superior power. Mostly they are mixed up with the more ordinary action of the mind and not easily distinguishable from them in our first inexperience except by their superior light and force and joy, the more so as the mind greatened or excited by their frequent coming quickens its own action and imitates the external characteristics of the supramental activity: its own operation is made more swift, luminous, strong and positive and it arrives even at a kind of imitative and often false intuition that strives to be but is not really the luminous, direct and self-existent truth. The next step is the formation of a luminous mind of intuitive experience, thought, will, feeling, sense from which the intermixture of the lesser mind and the imitative intuition are progressively eliminated: this is a process of purification, *śuddhi*, necessary to the new formation and perfection, *siddhi*. At the same time there is the disclosure above the mind of the source of the intuitive action and a more and more organised functioning of a true supramental consciousness acting not in the mind but on its own higher plane. This draws up into itself in the end the intuitive mentality it has created as its representative and assumes the charge of the whole activity of the consciousness. The process is progressive and for a long time chequered by admixture and the necessity of a return upon the lower movements in order to correct and transform them. The higher and the lower power act sometimes alternately, — the consciousness descending back from the heights it had attained to its former level but always with some change, — but sometimes together and with a sort of mutual reference. The mind eventually becomes wholly intuitivised and exists only as a passive channel for the supramental action; but this condition too is not ideal and presents, besides, still a certain obstacle, because the higher action has still to pass through a retarding and diminishing conscious substance, — that of the physical consciousness. The final stage of the change will come when the supermind occupies and supramentalises the whole being and turns even the vital and physical sheaths into moulds of itself, responsive, subtle and instinct with its powers. Man then becomes wholly the superman. This is at least the natural and integral process.

It would be to go altogether outside present limits to attempt anything like an adequate presentation of the whole character of the supermind; and it would not be possible to give a complete presentation, since the supermind carries in it the unity, but also the largeness and multiplicities of the infinite. All that need now be done is to present some salient characters from the point of view of the actual process of the conversion in the Yoga, the relation to the action of mind and the principle of some of the phenomena of the change. This is the fundamental relation that all the action of the mind is a derivation from the secret supermind, although we do not know this until we come to know our higher self, and draws from that source all it has of truth and value. All our thoughts, willings, feelings, sense representations have in them or at their roots an element of truth, which originates and sustains their existence, however in the actuality they may be perverted or false, and behind them a greater ungrasped truth, which if they could grasp it, would make them soon unified, harmonious and at least relatively complete. Actually, however, such truth as they have is diminished in scope, degraded into a lower movement, divided and falsified by fragmentation, afflicted with incompleteness, marred by perversion. Mental knowledge is not an integral but always a partial knowledge. It adds constantly detail to detail, but has a difficulty in relating them aright; its wholes too are not real but incomplete wholes which it tends to substitute for the more real and integral knowledge. And even if it arrived at a kind of integral knowledge, it would still be by a sort of putting together, a mental and intellectual arrangement, an artificial unity and not an essential and real oneness. If that were all, the mind might conceivably arrive at some kind of half reflection half translation of an integral knowledge, but the radical malady would still be that it would not be the real thing, but only at best an intellectual representation. That the mental truth must always be, an intellectual, emotional and sensational representation, not the direct truth, not truth itself in its body and essence.

The supermind can do all that the mind does, present and combine details and what might be called aspects or subordinate wholes, but it does it in a different way and on another basis. It does not like the mind bring in the element of deviation, false extension and imposed error, but even when it gives a partial knowledge, gives it in a firm and exact light, and always there is behind implied or opened to the consciousness the essential truth on which the details and subordinate wholes or aspects depend. The supermind has also a power of representation, but its representations are not of the intellectual kind, they are filled with the body and substance of light of the truth in its essence, they are its vehicles and not substituted figures. There is such an infinite power of representation of the supermind and that is the divine power of which the mental action is a sort of fallen representative. This representative supermind has a lower action in what I have called the supramental reason, nearest to the mental and into which the mental can most easily be taken up, and a higher action in the integral supermind that sees all things in the unity and infinity of the divine consciousness and self-existence. But on whatever level, it is a different thing from the corresponding mental action, direct, luminous, secure. The whole inferiority of the mind comes from its being the action of the soul after it has fallen into the nescience and the ignorance and is trying to get back to self-knowledge but doing it still on the basis of the nescience and the ignorance. The mind is the ignorance attempting to know or it is the ignorance receiving a derivative knowledge: it is the action of Avidya. The supermind is always the disclosure of an inherent and self-existent knowledge; it is the action of Vidya.

A second difference that we experience is a greater and a spontaneous harmony and unity. All consciousness is one, but in action it takes on many movements and each of these fundamental movements has many forms and processes. The forms and processes of the mind consciousness are marked by a disturbing and perplexing division and separateness of the mental energies and movements in which the original unity of the conscious mind does not at all or only distractedly appears. Constantly we find in our mentality a conflict or else a confusion and want of combination between different thoughts or a patched up combination and the same phenomenon applies to the various movements of our will and desire and to our emotions and feelings. Again our thought and our will and our feeling are not in a state of natural harmony and unison with each other, but act in their separate power even when they have to act together and are frequently in conflict or to some degree at variance. There is too an unequal development of one at the expense of another. The mind is a thing of discords in which some kind of practical arrangement rather than a satisfying concord is established for the purposes of life. The reason tries to arrive at a better arrangement, aims at a better control, a rational or an ideal harmony, and in this attempt it is a delegate or substitute of the supermind and is trying to do what only the supermind can do in its own right: but actually it is not able wholly to control the rest of the being and there is usually a considerable difference between the rational or ideal harmony we create in our thoughts and the movement of the life. Even at the best the arrangement made by the reason has always in it something of artificiality and imposition, for in the end there are only two spontaneous harmonic movements, that of the life, inconscient or largely subconscient, the harmony that we find in the animal creation and in lower Nature, and that of the spirit. The human condition is a stage of transition, effort and imperfection between the one and the other, between the natural and the ideal or spiritual life and it is full of uncertain seeking and disorder. It is not that the mental being cannot find or rather construct some kind of relative harmony of its own, but that it cannot render it stable because it is under the urge of the spirit. Man is obliged by a Power within him to be the labourer of a more or less conscious self-evolution that shall lead him to self-mastery and self-knowledge.

The supermind in its action is on the contrary a thing of unity and harmony and inherent order. At first when the pressure from above falls on the mentality, this is not realised and even a contrary phenomenon may for a time appear. That is due to several causes. First, there may be a disturbance, even a derangement created by impact of the greater hardly measurable power on an inferior consciousness which is not capable of responding to it organically or even perhaps of bearing the pressure. The very fact of the simultaneous and yet uncoordinated activity of two quite different forces, especially if the mind insists on its own way, if it tries obstinately or violently to profit by the supermind instead of giving itself up to it and its purpose, if it is not sufficiently passive and obedient to the higher guidance, may lead to a great excitation of power but also an increased disorder. It is for this reason that a previous preparation and long purification, the more complete the better, and a tranquillising and ordinarily a passivity of the mind calmly and strongly open to the spirit are necessities of the Yoga.

Again the mind, accustomed to act in limits, may try to supramentalise itself on the line of any one of its energies. It may develop a considerable power of intuitive half-supramentalised thought and knowledge, but the will may remain untransformed and out of harmony with this partial half-supramental development of the thinking mind, and the rest of the being too, emotional and nervous, may continue to be equally or more unregenerate. Or there may be a very great development of intuitive or strongly inspired will, but no corresponding uplifting of the thought mind or the emotional and psychic being, or only at most so much as is specially needed in order not wholly to obstruct the will action. The emotional or psychic mind may try to intuitivise and supramentalise itself and to a great extent succeed, and yet the thinking mind remain ordinary, poor in stuff and obscure in its light. There may be a development of intuitivity in the ethical or aesthetic being, but the rest may remain very much as it was. This is the reason of the frequent disorder or one-sidedness which we mark in the man of genius, poet, artist, thinker, saint or mystic. A partially intuitivised mentality may present an appearance of much less harmony and order outside its special activity than the largely developed intellectual mind. An integral development is needed, a wholesale conversion of the mind; otherwise the action is that of the mind using the supramental influx for its own profit and in its own mould, and that is allowed for the immediate purpose of the Divine in the being and may even be considered as a stage sufficient for the individual in this one life: but it is a state of imperfection and not the complete and successful evolution of the being. If however there is an integral development of the intuitive mind, it will be found that a great harmony has begun to lay its own foundations. This harmony will be other than that created by the intellectual mind and indeed may not be easily perceptible or, if it is felt, yet not intelligible to the logical man, because not arrived at or analysable by his mental process. It will be a harmony of the spontaneous expression of the spirit.

As soon as we arise above mind to the supermind, this initial harmony will be replaced by a greater and a more integral unity. The thoughts of the supramental reason meet together and understand each other and fall into a natural arrangement even when they have started from quite opposite quarters. The movements of will that are in conflict in the mind, come in the supermind to their right place and relation to each other. The supramental feelings also discover their own affinities and fall into a natural agreement and harmony. At a higher stage this harmony intensifies towards unity. The knowledge, will, feeling and all else become a single movement. This unity reaches its greatest completeness in the highest supermind. The harmony, the unity are inevitable because the base in the supermind is knowledge and characteristically self-knowledge, the knowledge of the self in all its aspects. The supramental will is the dynamic expression of this self-knowledge, the supramental feeling the expression of the luminous joy of the self and all else in supermind a part of this one movement. At its highest range it becomes something greater than what we call knowledge; there it is the essential and integral self-awareness of the Divine in us, his being, consciousness, Tapas, Ananda, and all is the harmonious, unified, luminous movement of that one existence.

This supramental knowledge is not primarily or essentially a thought knowledge. The intellect does not consider that it knows a thing until it has reduced its awareness of it to the terms of thought, not, that is to say, until it has put it into a system of representative mental concepts, and this kind of knowledge gets its most decisive completeness when it can be put into clear, precise and defining speech. It is true that the mind gets its knowledge primarily by various kinds of impression beginning from the vital and the sense impressions and rising to the intuitive, but these are taken by the developed intelligence only as data and seem to it uncertain and vague in themselves until they have been forced to yield up all their content to the thought and have taken their place in some intellectual relation or in an ordered thought sequence. It is true again that there is a thought and a speech which are rather suggestive than definitive and have in their own way a greater potency and richness of content, and this kind already verges on the intuitive: but still there is a demand in the intellect to bring out in clear sequence and relation the exact intellectual content of these suggestions and until that is done it does not feel satisfied that its knowledge is complete. The thought labouring in the logical intellect is that which normally seems best to organise the mental action and gives to the mind a sense of sure definiteness, security and completeness in its knowledge and its use of knowledge. Nothing of this is at all true of the supramental knowledge.

The supermind knows most completely and securely not by thought but by identity, by a pure awareness of the self-truth of things in the self and by the self, *ātmani ātmānam ātmanā.* I get the supramental knowledge best by becoming one with the truth, one with the object of knowledge; the supramental satisfaction and integral light is most there when there is no further division between the knower, knowledge and the known, *jñātā, jñānam, jñeyam.* I see the thing known not as an object outside myself, but as myself or a part of my universal self contained in my most direct consciousness. This leads to the highest and completest knowledge; thought and speech being representations and not this direct possession in the consciousness are to the supermind a lesser form and, if not filled with the spiritual awareness, thought becomes in fact a diminution of knowledge. For it would be, supposing it to be a supramental thought, only a partial manifestation of a greater knowledge existing in the self but not at the time present to the immediately active consciousness. In the highest ranges of the infinite there need be no thought at all because all would be experienced spiritually, in continuity, in eternal possession and with an absolute directness and completeness. Thought is only one means of partially manifesting and presenting what is hidden in this greater self-existent knowledge. This supreme kind of knowing will not indeed be possible to us in its full extent and degree until we can rise through many grades of the supermind to that infinite. But still as the supramental power emerges and enlarges its action, something of this highest way of knowledge appears and grows and even the members of the mental being, as they are intuitivised and supramentalised, develop more and more a corresponding action upon their own level. There is an increasing power of a luminous vital, psychic, emotional, dynamic and other identification with all the things and beings that are the objects of our consciousness and these transcendings of the separative consciousness bring with them many forms and means of a direct knowledge.

The supramental knowledge or experience by identity carries in it as a result or as a secondary part of itself a supramental vision that needs the support of no image, can concretise what is to the mind abstract and has the character of sight though its object may be the invisible truth of that which has form or the truth of the formless. This vision can come before there is any identity, as a sort of previous emanation of light from it, or may act detached from it as a separate power. The truth or the thing known is then not altogether or not yet one with myself, but an object of my knowledge: but still it is an object subjectively seen in the self or at least, even if it is still farther separated and objectivised to the knower, by the self, not through any intermediate process, but by a direct inner seizing or a penetrating and enveloping luminous contact of the spiritual consciousness with its object. It is this luminous seizing and contact that is the spiritual vision, *dṛṣṭi*, — "*paśyati*", says the Upanishad continually of the spiritual knowledge, "he sees"; and of the Self conceiving the idea of creation, where we should expect "he thought", it says instead "he saw". It is to the spirit what the eyes are to the physical mind and one has the sense of having passed through a subtly analogous process. As the physical sight can present to us the actual body of things of which the thought had only possessed an indication or mental description and they become to us at once real and evident, *pratyakṣa*, so the spiritual sight surpasses the indications or representations of thought and can make the self and truth of all things present to us and directly evident, *pratyakṣa*.

The sense can only give us the superficial image of things and it needs the aid of thought to fill and inform the image; but the spiritual sight is capable of presenting to us the thing in itself and all truth about it. The seer does not need the aid of thought in its process as a means of knowledge, but only as a means of representation and expression, — thought is to him a lesser power and used for a secondary purpose. If a further extension of knowledge is required, he can come at it by new seeing without the slower thought processes that are the staff of support of the mental search and its feeling out for truth, — even as we scrutinise with the eye to find what escaped our first observation. This experience and knowledge by spiritual vision is the second in directness and greatness of the supramental powers. It is something much more near, profound and comprehensive than mental vision, because it derives direct from the knowledge by identity, and it has this virtue that we can proceed at once from the vision to the identity, as from the identity to the vision. Thus when the spiritual vision has seen God, Self or Brahman, the soul can next enter into and become one with the Self, God or Brahman.

This can only be done integrally on or above the supramental level, but at the same time the spiritual vision can take on mental forms of itself that can help towards this identification each in its own way. A mental intuitive vision or a spiritualised mental sight, a psychic vision, an emotional vision of the heart, a vision in the sense mind are parts of the Yogic experience. If these seeings are purely mental, then they may but need not be true, for the mind is capable of both truth and error, both of a true and of a false representation. But as the mind becomes intuitivised and supramentalised, these powers are purified and corrected by the more luminous action of the supermind and become themselves forms of a supramental and a true seeing. The supramental vision, it may be noted, brings with it a supplementary and completing experience that might be called a spiritual hearing and touch of the truth, — of its essence and through that of its significance, — that is to say, there is a seizing of its movement, vibration, rhythm and a seizing of its close presence and contact and substance. All these powers prepare us to become one with that which has thus grown near to us through knowledge.

The supramental thought is a form of the knowledge by identity and a development, in the idea, of the truth presented to the supramental vision. The identity and the vision give the truth in its essence, its body and its parts in a single view: the thought translates this direct consciousness and immediate power of the truth into idea-knowledge and will. It adds or need add otherwise nothing new, but reproduces, articulates, moves round the body of the knowledge. Where, however, the identity and the vision are still incomplete, the supramental thought has a larger office and reveals, interprets or recalls as it were to the soul's memory what they are not yet ready to give. And where these greater states and powers are still veiled, the thought comes in front and prepares and to a certain extent effects a partial rending or helps actively in the removal of the veil. Therefore in the development out of the mental ignorance into the supramental knowledge this illumined thought comes to us often though not always first, to open the way to the vision or else to give first supports to the growing consciousness of identity and its greater knowledge. This thought is also an effective means of communication and expression and helps to an impression or fixation of the truth whether on one's own lower mind and being or on that of others. The supramental thought differs from the intellectual not only because it is the direct truth idea and not a representation of truth to the ignorance, — it is the truth consciousness of the spirit always presenting to itself its own right forms, the *satyam* and *ṛtam* of the Veda, — but because of its strong reality, body of light and substance.

The intellectual thought refines and sublimates to a rarefied abstractness; the supramental thought as it rises in its height increases to a greater spiritual concreteness. The thought of the intellect presents itself to us as an abstraction from something seized by the mind sense and is as if supported in a void and subtle air of mind by an intangible force of the intelligence. It has to resort to a use of the mind's power of image if it wishes to make itself more concretely felt and seen by the soul sense and soul vision. The supramental thought on the contrary presents always the idea as a luminous substance of being, luminous stuff of consciousness taking significative thought form and it therefore creates no such sense of a gulf between the idea and the real as we are liable to feel in the mind, but is itself a reality, it is real-idea and the body of a reality. It has as a result, associated with it when it acts according to its own nature, a phenomenon of spiritual light other than the intellectual clarity, a great realising force and a luminous ecstasy. It is an intensely sensible vibration of being, consciousness and Ananda.

The supramental thought, as has already been indicated, has three elevations of its intensity, one of direct thought vision, another of interpretative vision pointing to and preparing the greater revelatory idea-sight, a third of representative vision recalling as it were to the spirit's knowledge the truth that is called out more directly by the higher powers. In the mind these things take the form of the three ordinary powers of the intuitive mentality, — the suggestive and discriminating intuition, the inspiration and the thought that is of the nature of revelation. Above they correspond to three elevations of the supramental being and consciousness and, as we ascend, the lower first calls down into itself and is then taken up into the higher, so that on each level all the three elevations are reproduced, but always there predominates in the thought essence the character that belongs to that level's proper form of consciousness and spiritual substance. It is necessary to bear this in mind; for otherwise the mentality, looking up to the ranges of the supermind as they reveal themselves, may think it has got the vision of the highest heights when it is only the highest range of the lower ascent that is being presented to its experience. At each height, *sānoḥ sānum āruhat*, the powers of the supermind increase in intensity, range and completeness.

There is also a speech, a supramental word, in which the higher knowledge, vision or thought can clothe itself within us for expression. At first this may come down as a word, a message or an inspiration that descends to us from above or it may even seem a voice of the Self or of the Ishwara, *vāṇī*, *ādeśa*. Afterwards it loses that separate character and becomes the normal form of the thought when it expresses itself in the form of an inward speech. The thought may express itself without the aid of any suggestive or developing word and only — but still quite completely, explicitly and with its full contents — in a luminous substance of supramental perception. It may aid itself when it is not so explicit by a suggestive inward speech that attends it to bring out its whole significance. Or the thought may come not as silent perception but as speech self-born out of the truth and complete in its own right and carrying in itself its own vision and knowledge. Then it is the word revelatory, inspired or intuitive or of a yet greater kind capable of bearing the infinite intention or suggestion of the higher supermind and spirit. It may frame itself in the language now employed to express the ideas and perceptions and impulses of the intellect and the sense mind, but it uses it in a different way and with an intense bringing out of the intuitive or revelatory significances of which speech is capable. The supramental word manifests inwardly with a light, a power, a rhythm of thought and a rhythm of inner sound that make it the natural and living body of the supramental thought and vision and it pours into the language, even though the same as that of mental speech, another than the limited intellectual, emotional or sensational significance. It is formed and heard in the intuitive mind or supermind and need not at first except in certain highly gifted souls come out easily into speech and writing, but that too can be freely done when the physical consciousness and its organs have been made ready, and this is a part of the needed fullness and power of the integral perfection.

The range of knowledge covered by the supramental thought, experience and vision will be commensurate with all that is open to the human consciousness, not only on the earthly but on all planes. It will however act increasingly in an inverse sense to that of the mental thinking and experience. The centre of mental thinking is the ego, the person of the individual thinker. The supramental man on the contrary will think more with the universal mind or even may rise above it, and his individuality will rather be a vessel of radiation and communication to which the universal thought and knowledge of the Spirit will converge than a centre. The mental man thinks and acts in a radius determined by the smallness or largeness of his mentality and of its experience. The range of the supramental man will be all the earth and all that lies behind it on other planes of existence. And finally the mental man thinks and sees on the level of the present life, though it may be with an upward aspiration, and his view is obstructed on every side. His main basis of knowledge and action is the present with a glimpse into the past and ill-grasped influence from its pressure and a blind look towards the future. He bases himself on the actualities of the earthly existence, first on the facts of the outward world, —

to which he is ordinarily in the habit of relating nine tenths if not the whole of his inner thinking and experience, — then on the changing actualities of the more superficial part of his inner being. As he increases in mind, he goes more freely beyond these to potentialities which arise out of them and pass beyond them; his mind deals with a larger field of possibilities: but these for the most part get to him a full reality only in proportion as they are related to the actual and can be made actual here, now or hereafter. The essence of things he tends to see, if at all, only as a result of his actualities, in a relation to and dependence on them, and therefore he sees them constantly in a false light or in a limited measure. In all these respects the supramental man must proceed from the opposite principle of truth vision.

The supramental being sees things from above in large spaces and at the highest from the spaces of the infinite. His view is not limited to the standpoint of the present but can see in the continuities of time or from above time in the indivisibilities of the Spirit. He sees truth in its proper order first in the essence, secondly in the potentialities that derive from it and only last in the actualities. The essential truths are to his sight self-existent, self-seen, not dependent for their proof on this or that actuality; the potential truths are truths of the power of being in itself and in things, truths of the infinity of force and real apart from their past or present realisation in this or that actuality or the habitual surface forms that we take for the whole of Nature; the actualities are only a selection from the potential truths he sees, dependent on them, limited and mutable. The tyranny of the present, of the actual, of the immediate range of facts, of the immediate urge and demand of action has no power over his thought and his will and he is therefore able to have a larger will-power founded on a larger knowledge. He sees things not as one on the levels surrounded by the jungle of present facts and phenomena but from above, not from outside and judged by their surfaces, but from within and viewed from the truth of their centre; therefore he is nearer the divine omniscience. He wills and acts from a dominating height and with a longer movement in time and a larger range of potencies, therefore he is nearer to the divine omnipotence. His being is not shut into the succession of the moments, but has the full power of the past and ranges seeingly through the future: not shut in the limiting ego and personal mind, but lives in the freedom of the universal, in God and in all beings and all things; not in the dull density of the physical mind, but in the light of the self and the infinity of the spirit. He sees soul and mind only as a power and a movement and matter only as a resultant form of the spirit. All his thought will be of a kind that proceeds from knowledge. He perceives and enacts the things of the phenomenal life in the light of the reality of the spiritual being and the power of the dynamic spiritual essence.

At first, at the beginning of the conversion into this greater status, the thought will continue to move for a shorter or a longer time to a greater or a less extent on the lines of the mind but with a greater light and increasing flights and spaces and movements of freedom and transcendence. Afterwards the freedom and transcendence will begin to predominate; the inversion of the thought view and the conversion of the thought method will take place in different movements of the thought mind one after the other, subject to whatever difficulties and relapses, until it has gained on the whole and effected a complete transformation. Ordinarily the supramental knowledge will be organised first and with the most ease in the processes of pure thought and knowledge, *jñāna*, because here the human mind has already the upward tendency and is the most free. Next and with less ease it will be organised in the processes of applied thought and knowledge because there the mind of man is at once most active and most bound and wedded to its inferior methods. The last and most difficult conquest, because this is now to his mind a field of conjecture or a blank, will be the knowledge of the three times, *trikāladṛṣṭi*. In all these there will be the same character of a spirit seeing and willing directly above and around and not only in the body it possesses and there will be the same action of the supramental knowledge by identity, the supramental vision, the supramental thought and supramental word, separately or in a united movement.

This then will be the general character of the supramental thought and knowledge and these its main powers and action. It remains to consider its particular instrumentation, the change that the supermind will make in the different elements of the present human mentality and the special activities that give to the thought its constituents, motives and data.

Chapter XXIII

The Supramental Instruments — Thought-Process

THE SUPERMIND, the divine gnosis, is not something entirely alien to our present consciousness: it is a superior instrumentation of the spirit and all the operations of our normal consciousness are limited and inferior derivations from the supramental, because these are tentatives and constructions, that the true and perfect, the spontaneous and harmonious nature and action of the spirit. Accordingly when we rise from mind to supermind, the new power of consciousness does not reject, but uplifts, enlarges and transfigures the operations of our soul and mind and life. It exalts and gives to them an ever greater reality of their power and performance. It does not limit itself either to the transformation of the superficial powers and action of the mind and psychic parts and the life, but it manifests and transforms also those rarer powers and that larger force and knowledge proper to our subliminal self that appear now to us as things occult, curiously psychic, abnormal. These things become in the supramental nature not at all abnormal but perfectly natural and normal, not separately psychic but spiritual, not occult and strange, but a direct, simple, inherent and spontaneous action. The spirit is not limited like the waking material consciousness, and the supermind when it takes possession of the waking consciousness, dematerialises it, delivers it from its limits, converts the material and the psychic into the nature of the spiritual being.

The mental activity that can be most readily organised is, as has been already indicated, that of pure ideative knowledge. This is transformed on the higher level to the true *jñāna*, supramental thought, supramental vision, the supramental knowledge by identity. The essential action of this supramental knowledge has been described in the preceding chapter. It is necessary however to see also how this knowledge works in outward application and how it deals with the data of existence. It differs from the action of the mind first in this respect that it works naturally with those operations that are to the mind the highest and the most difficult, acting in them or on them from above downward and not with the hampered straining upward of the mind or with its restriction to its own and the inferior levels. The higher operations are not dependent on the lower assistance, but rather the lower operations depend on the higher not only for their guidance but for their existence. The lower mental operations are therefore not only changed in character by the transformation, but are made entirely subordinate. And the higher mental operations too change their character, because, supramentalised, they begin to derive their light directly from the highest, the self-knowledge or infinite knowledge.

The normal thought-action of the mind may for this purpose be viewed as constituted of a triple motion. First and lowest and most necessary to the mental being in the body is the habitual thought mind that founds its ideas upon the data given by the senses and by the surface experiences of the nervous and emotional being and on the customary notions formed by the education and the outward life and environment. This habitual mind has two movements, one a kind of constant undercurrent of mechanically recurrent thought always repeating itself in the same round of physical, vital, emotional, practical and summarily intellectual notion and experience, the other more actively working upon all new experience that the mind is obliged to admit and reducing it to formulas of habitual thinking. The mentality of the average man is limited by this habitual mind and moves very imperfectly outside its circle.

A second grade of the thinking activity is the pragmatic idea mind that lifts itself above life and acts creatively as a mediator between the idea and the life-power, between truth of life and truth of the idea not yet manifested in life. It draws material from life and builds out of it and upon it creative ideas that become dynamic for farther life development: on the other side it receives new thought and mental experience from the mental plane or more fundamentally from the idea power of the Infinite and immediately turns it into mental idea force and a power for actual being and living. The whole turn of this pragmatic idea mind is towards action and experience, inward as well as outward, the inward casting itself outward for the sake of a completer satisfaction of reality, the outward taken into the inward and returning upon it assimilated and changed for fresh formations. The thought is only or mainly interesting to the soul on this mental level as a means for a large range of action and experience.

A third gradation of thinking opens in us the pure ideative mind which lives disinterestedly in truth of the idea apart from any necessary dependence on its value for action and experience. It views the data of the senses and the superficial inner experience, but only to find the idea, the truth to which they bear witness and to reduce them into terms of knowledge. It observes the creative action of mind in life in the same way and for the same purpose. Its preoccupation is with knowledge, its whole object is to have the delight of ideation, the search for truth, the effort to know itself and the world and all that may lie behind its own action and the world action. This ideative mind is the highest reach of the intellect acting for itself, characteristically, in its own power and for its own purpose.

It is difficult for the human mind to combine rightly and harmonise these three movements of the intelligence. The ordinary man lives mainly in the habitual, has a comparatively feeble action of the creative and pragmatic and experiences a great difficulty in using at all or entering into the movement of the pure ideative mentality. The creative pragmatic mind is commonly too much occupied with its own motion to move freely and disinterestedly in the atmosphere of pure ideative order and on the other hand has often an insufficient grasp on the actualities imposed by the habitual mentality and the obstacles it imposes as also on other movements of pragmatic thought and action than that which it is itself interested in building. The pure ideative mentality tends to construct abstract and arbitrary systems of truth, intellectual sections and ideative edifices, and either misses the pragmatic movement necessary to life and lives only or mainly in ideas, or cannot act with sufficient power and directness in the life field and is in danger of being divorced from or weak in the world of the practical and habitual mentality. An accommodation of some kind is made, but the tyranny of the predominant tendency interferes with the wholeness and unity of the thinking being. Mind fails to be assured master even of its own totality, because the secret of that totality lies beyond it in the free unity of the self, free and therefore capable of an infinite multiplicity and diversity, and in the supramental power that can alone bring out in a natural perfection the organic multiple movement of the self's unity.

The supermind in its completeness reverses the whole order of the mind's thinking. It lives not in the phenomenal, but in the essential, in the self, and sees all as being of the self and its power and form and movement, and all the thought and the process of the thought in the supermind must also be of that character. All its fundamental ideation is a rendering of the spiritual knowledge that acts by identity with all being and of the supramental vision. It moves therefore primarily among the eternal, the essential and the universal truths of self and being and consciousness and infinite power and delight of being (not excluding all that seems to our present consciousness non-being), and all its particular thinking originates from and depends upon the power of these eternal verities; but in the second place it is at home too with infinite aspects and applications, sequences and harmonies of the truths of being of the Eternal. It lives therefore at its heights in all that which the action of the pure ideative mind is an effort to reach and discover, and even on its lower ranges these things are to its luminous receptivity present, near or easily grasped and available.

But while the highest truths or the pure ideas are to the ideative mind abstractions, because mind lives partly in the phe-nomenal and partly in intellectual constructions and has to use the method of abstraction to arrive at the higher realities, the supermind lives in the spirit and therefore in the very substance of what these ideas and truths represent or rather fundamentally are and truly realises them, not only thinks but in the act of thinking feels and identifies itself with their substance, and to it they are among the most substantial things that can be. Truths of consciousness and of essential being are to the supermind the very stuff of reality, more intimately and, as one might almost say, densely real than outward movement and form of being, although these too are to it movement and form of the reality and not, as they are to a certain action of the spiritualised mind, an illusion. The idea too is to it real-idea, stuff of the reality of conscious being, full of power for the substantial rendering of the truth and therefore for creation.

And again, while the pure ideative mind tends to build up arbitrary systems which are mental and partial constructions of the truth, the supermind is not bound by any representation or system, though it is perfectly able to represent and to arrange and construct in the living substance of the truth for the pragmatic purposes of the Infinite. The mind when it gets free from its exclusivenesses, systematising, attachment to its own constructions, is at a loss in the infiniteness of the infinite, feels it as a chaos, even if a luminous chaos, is unable any longer to formulate and therefore to think and act decisively because all, even the most diverse or contradictory things, point at some truth in this infinity and yet nothing it can think is entirely true and all its formulations break down under the test of new suggestions from the infinite. It begins to look on the world as a phantasmagory and thought as a chaos of scintillations out of the luminous indefinite. The mind assailed by the vastness and freedom of the supramental loses itself and finds no firm footing in the vastness. The supermind on the contrary can in its freedom construct harmonies of its thought and expression of being on the firm ground of reality while still holding its infinite liberty and rejoicing in its self of infinite vastness. All that it thinks, as all that it is and does and lives, belongs to the truth, the right, the vast, *satyam, ṛtam, bṛhat.*

The result of this wholeness is that there is no division or incompatibility between the free essential ideation of the supermind corresponding to the mind's pure ideation, free, disinterested, illimitable, and its creative, pragmatic ideation purposeful and determinative. The infinity of being results naturally in a freedom of the harmonies of becoming. The supermind perceives always action as a manifestation and expression of the Self and creation as a revelation of the Infinite. All its creative and pragmatic thought is an instrument of the self's becoming, a power of illumination for that purpose, an intermediary between the eternal identity and infinite novelty and variety of illimitable Being and its self-expression in the worlds and life. It is this that the supermind constantly sees and embodies and while its ideative vision and thought interpret to it the illimitable unity and variety of the Infinite, which it is by a perpetual identity and in which it lives in all its power of being and becoming, there is constantly too a special creative thought, associated with an action of the infinite will, Tapas, power of being, which determines what it shall present, manifest or create out of the infinite in the course of Time, what it shall make — here and now or in any range of Time or world — of the perpetual becoming of the self in the universe.

The supermind is not limited by this pragmatic movement and does not take the partial motion or the entire stream of what it so becomes and creates in its thought and life for the whole truth of its self or of the Infinite. It does not live only in what it is and thinks and does selectively in the present or on one plane only of being; it does not feed its existence only on the present or the continual succession of moments to whose beats we give that name. It does not see itself only as a movement of Time or of the consciousness in time or as a creature of the perpetual becoming. It is aware of a timeless being beyond manifestation and of which all is a manifestation, it is aware of what is eternal even in Time, it is aware of many planes of existence; it is aware of past truth of manifestation and of much truth of being yet to be manifested in the future, but already existing in the self-view of the Eternal. It does not mistake the pragmatic reality which is the truth of action and mutation for the sole truth, but sees it as a constant realisation of that which is eternally real. It knows that creation whether on the plane of matter or of life or of mind or of supermind is and can be only a self-determined presentation of eternal truth, a revelation of the Eternal, and it is intimately aware of the pre-existence of the truth of all things in the Eternal. This seeing conditions all its pragmatic thought and its resultant action. The maker in it is a selective power of the seer and thinker, the self-builder a power of the self-seer, the self-expressing soul a power of the infinite spirit. It creates freely, and all the more surely and decisively for that freedom, out of the infinite self and spirit.

It is therefore not prisoned in its special becoming or shut up in its round or its course of action. It is open, in a way and a degree to which the mind cannot attain, to the truth of other harmonies of creative becoming even while in its own it puts forth a decisive will and thought and action. When it is engaged in action that is of the nature of a struggle, the replacing of past or other thought and form and becoming by that which it is appointed to manifest, it knows the truth of what it displaces and fulfils even in displacing as well as the truth of what it substitutes. It is not bound by its manifesting, selecting, pragmatic conscious action, but it has at the same time all the joy of a specially creative thought and selective precision of action, the Ananda of the truth of the forms and movements equally of its own and of others' becoming. All its thought and will of life and action and creation, rich, manifold, focussing the truth of many planes, is liberated and illumined with the illimitable truth of the Eternal.

This creative or pragmatic movement of the supramental thought and consciousness brings with it an action which corresponds to that of the habitual or mechanical mentality but is yet of a very different character. The thing that is created is the self-determination of a harmony and all harmony proceeds upon seen or given lines and carries with it a constant pulsation and rhythmic recurrence. The supramental thought, organising the harmony of manifested existence of the supramental being, founds it on eternal principles, casts it upon the right lines of the truth that is to be manifested, keeps sounding as characteristic notes the recurrence of the constant elements in the experience and the action which are necessary to constitute the harmony. There is an order of the thought, a cycle of the will, a stability in the motion. At the same time its freedom prevents it from being shut up by the recurrence into a groove of habitual action turning always mechanically round a limited stock of thinking. It does not like the habitual mind refer and assimilate all new thought and experience to a fixed customary mould of thinking, taking that for its basis. Its basis, that to which all is referred, is above, *upari budhne*, in the largeness of the self, in the supreme foundation of the supramental truth, *budhne ṛtasya*. Its order of thought, its cycle of will, its stable movement of action does not crystallise into a mechanism or convention, but is always alive with the spirit, does not live by exclusiveness or hostility to other coexistent or possible order and cycle, but absorbs sustenance from all that it contacts and assimilates it to its own principle. The spiritual assimilation is practicable because all is referred to the largeness of the self and its free vision above. The order of the supramental thought and will is constantly receiving new light and power from above and has no difficulty in accepting it into its movement; it is, as is proper to an order of the Infinite, even in its stability of motion indescribably supple and plastic, capable of perceiving and rendering the relation of all things to each other in the One, capable of expressing always more and more of the Infinite, at its fullest of expressing in its own way all that is actually expressible of the Infinite.

Thus there is no discord, disparity or difficulty of adjustment in the complex motion of the supramental *jñāna*, but a simplicity in the complexity, an assured ease in a many-sided abundance that comes from the spontaneous sureness and totality of the self-knowledge of the spirit. Obstacle, inner struggle, disparity, difficulty, discord of parts and movements continues in the transformation of mind to supermind only so long as the action, influence or pressure of the mind insisting on its own methods of construction continues or its process of building knowledge or thought and will of action on the foundation of a primal ignorance resists the opposite process of supermind organising all as a luminous manifestation out of the self and its inherent and eternal self-knowledge. It is thus that the supermind acting as a representative, interpretative, revealingly imperative power of the spirit's knowledge by identity, turning the light of the infinite consciousness freely and illimitably into substance and form of real-idea, creating out of power of conscious being and power of real-idea, stabilising a movement which obeys its own law but is still a supple and plastic movement of the infinite, uses its thought and knowledge and a will identical in substance and light with the knowledge to organise in each supramental being his own right manifestation of the one self and spirit.

The action of the supramental *jñāna* so constituted evidently surpasses the action of the mental reason and we have to see what replaces the reason in the supramental transformation. The thinking mind of man finds its most clear and characteristic satisfaction and its most precise and effective principle of organisation in the reasoning and logical intelligence. It is true that man is not and cannot be wholly governed either in his thought or his action by the reason alone. His mentality is inextricably subjected to a joint, mixed and intricate action of the reasoning intelligence with two other powers, an intuition, actually only half luminous in the human mentality, operating behind the more visible action of the reason or veiled and altered in the action of the normal intelligence, and the life-mind of sensation, instinct, impulse, which is in its own nature a sort of obscure involved intuition and which supplies the intelligence from below with its first materials and data. And each of these other powers is in its own kind an intimate action of the spirit operating in mind and life and has a more direct and spontaneous character and immediate power for perception and action than the reasoning intelligence. But yet neither of these powers is capable of organising for man his mental existence.

His life-mind — its instincts, its impulses, — is not and cannot be self-sufficient and predominant as it is in the lower creation. It has been seized upon by the intelligence and profoundly altered by it even where the development of the intelligence is imperfect and itself most insistent in its prominence. It has lost most of its intuitive character, is indeed now infinitely richer as a supplier of materials and data, but no longer quite itself or at ease in its action because half rationalised, dependent at least on some infused element however vague of reasoning or intelligent activity and incapable of acting to good purpose without the aid of the intelligence. Its roots and place of perfection are in the subconscient from which it emerges and man's business is to increase in the sense of a more and more conscient knowledge and action. Man reverting to a governance of his being by the life mind would become either irrational and erratic or dull and imbecile and would lose the essential character of manhood.

The intuition on the other hand has its roots and its place of perfection in the supramental which is now to us the superconscient, and in mind it has no pure and no organised action, but is immediately mixed with the action of the reasoning intelligence, is not quite itself, but limited, fragmentary, diluted and impure, and depends for the ordered use and organisation of its suggestions on the aid of the logical reason. The human mind is never quite sure of its intuitions until they have been viewed and confirmed by the judgment of the rational intelligence: it is there that it feels most well founded and secure. Man surmounting reason to organise his thought and life by the intuitive mind would be already surpassing his characteristic humanity and on the way to the development of supermanhood. This can only be done above: for to attempt it below is only to achieve another kind of imperfection: there the mental reason is a necessary factor.

The reasoning intelligence is an intermediate agent between the life mind and the yet undeveloped supramental intuition. Its business is that of an intermediary, on the one side to enlighten the life mind, to make it conscient and govern and regulate as much as may be its action until Nature is ready to evolve the supramental energy which will take hold of life and illumine and perfect all its movements by converting its obscurely intuitive motions of desire, emotion, sensation and action into a spiritually and luminously spontaneous life manifestation of the self and spirit. On the other higher side its mission is to take the rays of light which come from above and translate them into terms of intelligent mentality and to accept, examine, develop, intellectually utilise the intuitions that escape the barrier and descend into mind from the superconscience. It does this until man, becoming more and more intelligently conscient of himself and his environment and his being, becomes also aware that he cannot really know these things by his reason, but can only make a mental representation of them to his intelligence.

The reason, however, tends in the intellectual man to ignore the limitations of its power and function and attempts to be not an instrument and agent but a substitute for the self and spirit. Made confident by success and predominance, by the comparative greatness of its own light, it regards itself as a thing primary and absolute, assures itself of its own entire truth and sufficiency and endeavours to become the absolute ruler of mind and life. This it cannot do successfully, because it depends on the lower life intuition and on the covert supermind and its intuitive messages for its own real substance and existence. It can only appear to itself to succeed because it reduces all its experience to rational formulas and blinds itself to half the real nature of the thought and action that is behind it and to the infinite deal that breaks out of its formulas. The excess of the reason only makes life artificial and rationally mechanical, deprives it of its spontaneity and vitality and prevents the freedom and expansion of the spirit. The limited and limiting mental reason must make itself plastic and flexible, open itself to its source, receive the light from above, exceed itself and pass by an euthanasia of transformation into the body of the supramental reason. Meanwhile it is given power and leading for an organisation of thought and action on the characteristically human scale intermediate between the subconscient power of the spirit organising the life of the animal and the superconscient power of the spirit which becoming conscient can organise the existence and life of a spiritual supermanhood.

The characteristic power of the reason in its fullness is a logical movement assuring itself first of all available materials and data by observation and arrangement, then acting upon them for a resultant knowledge gained, assured and enlarged by a first use of the reflective powers, and lastly assuring itself of the correctness of its results by a more careful and formal action, more vigilant, deliberate, severely logical which tests, rejects or confirms them according to certain secure standards and processes developed by reflection and experience. The first business of the logical reason is therefore a right, careful and complete observation of its available material and data. The first and easiest field of data open to our knowledge is the world of Nature, of the physical objects made external to it by the separative action of mind, things not ourself and therefore only indirectly knowable by an interpreting of our sense perceptions, by observation, accumulated experience, inference and reflective thinking. Another field is our own internal being and its movements which one knows naturally by an internally acting mental sense, by intuitive perception and constant experience and by reflective thought on the evidences of our nature. The reason with regard even to these inner movements acts best and knows them most correctly by detaching itself and regarding them quite impersonally and objectively, a movement which in the Yoga of knowledge ends in viewing our own active being too as not self, a mechanism of Nature like the rest of the world-existence. The knowledge of other thinking and conscious beings stands between these two fields, but is gained, too, indirectly by observation, by experience, by various means of communication and, acting on these, by reflection and inference largely founded on analogy from our knowledge of our own nature. Another field of data which the reason has to observe is its own action and the action of the whole human intelligence, for without that study it cannot be assured of the correctness of its knowledge or of right method and process. Finally, there are other fields of knowledge for which the data are not so easily available and which need the development of abnormal faculties, — the discovery of things and ranges of existence behind the appearances of the physical world and the discovery of the secret self or principle of being of man and of Nature. The first the logical reason can attempt to deal with, accepting subject to its scrutiny whatever data become available, in the same way as it deals with the physical world, but ordinarily it is little disposed to deal with them, finding it more easy to question and deny, and its action here is seldom assured or effective. The second it usually attempts to discover by a constructive metaphysical logic founded on its analytic and synthetic observation of the phenomena of life, mind and matter. The operation of the logical reason is the same in all these fields of its data. At first the intelligence amasses a store of observations, associations, percepts, recepts, concepts, makes a more or less obvious arrangement and classification of relations and of things according to their likenesses and differences, and works upon them by an accumulating store and a constant addition of ideas, memories, imaginations, judgments; these make up primarily the nature of activity of our knowledge. There is a kind of natural enlargement of this intelligent activity of the mind progressing by its own momentum, an evolution aided more and more by a deliberate culture, the increase of faculties gained by the culture becoming in its turn a part of the nature as they settle into a more spontaneous action, — the result a progression not of the character and essential power of the intelligence, but of its degree of power, flexibility, variety of capacity, fineness. There is a correction of errors, an accumulating of assured ideas and judgments, a reception or formation of fresh knowledge. At the same time a necessity arises for a more precise and assured action of the intelligence which will get rid of the superficiality of this ordinary method of the intelligence, test every step, scrutinise severely every conclusion and reduce the mind's action to a well-founded system and order.

This movement develops the complete logical mind and raises to its acme the acuteness and power of the intelligence. The rougher and more superficial observation is replaced or supplemented by a scrutinising analysis of all the process, properties, constituents, energies making up or related to the object and a synthetic construction of it as a whole which is added to or in great part substituted for the mind's natural conception of it. The object is more precisely distinguished from all others and at the same time there is a completer discovery of its relations with others. There is a fixing of sameness or likeness and kinship and also of divergences and differences resulting on one side in the perception of the fundamental unity of being and Nature and the similarity and continuity of their processes, on the other in a clear precision and classification of different energies and kinds of beings and objects. The amassing and ordering of the materials and data of knowledge are carried to perfection as far as is possible to the logical intelligence.

Memory is the indispensable aid of the mind to preserve its past observations, the memory of the individual but also of the race, whether in the artificial form of accumulated records or the general race memory preserving its gains with a sort of constant repetition and renewal and, an element not sufficiently appreciated, a latent memory that can under the pressure of various kinds of stimulation repeat under new conditions past movements of knowledge for judgment by the increased information and intelligence. The developed logical mind puts into order the action and resources of the human memory and trains it to make the utmost use of its materials. The human judgment naturally works on these materials in two ways, by a more or less rapid and summary combination of observation, inference, creative or critical conclusion, insight, immediate idea — this is largely an attempt of the mind to work in a spontaneous manner with the directness that can only be securely achieved by the higher faculty of the intuition, for in the mind it produces much false confidence and unreliable certitude, — and a slower but in the end intellectually surer seeking, considering and testing judgment that develops into the careful logical action.

The memory and judgment are both aided by the imagination which, as a function of knowledge, suggests possibilities not actually presented or justified by the other powers and opens the doors to fresh vistas. The developed logical intelligence uses the imagination for suggesting new discovery and hypothesis, but is careful to test its suggestions fully by observation and a sceptical or scrupulous judgment. It insists too on testing, as far as may be, all the action of the judgment itself, rejects hasty inference in favour of an ordered system of deduction and induction and makes sure of all its steps and of the justice, continuity, compatibility, cohesion of its conclusions. A too formalised logical mind discourages, but a free use of the whole action of the logical intelligence may rather heighten a certain action of immediate insight, the mind's nearest approach to the higher intuition, but it does not place on it an unqualified reliance. The endeavour of the logical reason is always by a detached, disinterested and carefully founded method to get rid of error, of prejudgment, of the mind's false confidence and arrive at reliable certitudes.

And if this elaborated method of the mind were really sufficient for truth, there would be no need of any higher step in the evolution of knowledge. In fact, it increases the mind's hold on itself and on the world around it and serves great and undeniable utilities: but it can never be sure whether its data supply it with the frame of a real knowledge or only a frame useful and necessary for the human mind and will in its own present form of action. It is more and more perceived that the knowledge of phenomena increases, but the knowledge of reality escapes this laborious process. A time must come, is already coming when the mind perceives the necessity of calling to its aid and developing fully the intuition and all the great range of powers that lie concealed behind our vague use of the word and uncertain perception of its significance. In the end it must discover that these powers can not only aid and complete but even replace its own proper action. That will be the beginning of the discovery of the supramental energy of the spirit.

The supermind, as we have seen, lifts up the action of the mental consciousness towards and into the intuition, creates an intermediate intuitive mentality insufficient in itself but greater in power than the logical intelligence, and then lifts up and transforms that too into the true supramental action. The first well-organised action of the supermind in the ascending order is the supramental reason, not a higher logical intellect, but a directly luminous organisation of intimately subjective and intimately objective knowledge, the higher *buddhi*, the logical or rather the logos Vijnana. The supramental reason does all the work of the reasoning intelligence and does much more, but with a greater power and in a different fashion. It is then itself taken up into a higher range of the power of knowledge and in that too nothing is lost, but all farther heightened, enlarged in scope, transformed in power of action.

The ordinary language of the intellect is not sufficient to describe this action, for the same words have to be used, indicating a certain correspondence, but actually to connote inadequately a different thing. Thus the supermind uses a certain sense action, employing but not limited by the physical organs, a thing which is in its nature a form consciousness and a contact consciousness, but the mental idea and experience of sense can give no conception of the essential and characteristic action of this supramentalised sense consciousness. Thought too in the supramental action is a different thing from the thought of the mental intelligence. The supramental thinking is felt at its basis as a conscious contact or union or identity of the substance of being of the knower with the substance of being of the thing known and its figure of thought as the power of awareness of the self revealing through the meeting or the oneness, because carrying in itself, a certain knowledge form of the object's content, action, significance. Therefore observation, memory, judgment too mean each a different thing in the supermind from what it is in the process of the mental intelligence.

The supramental reason observes all that the intelligence observes — and much more; it makes, that is to say, the thing to be known the field of a perceptual action, in a certain way objective, that causes to emerge its nature, character, quality, action. But this is not that artificial objectivity by which the reason in its observation tries to extrude the element of personal or subjective error. The supermind sees everything in the self and its observation must therefore be subjectively objective and much nearer to, though not the same as the observation of our own internal movements regarded as an object of knowledge. It is not in the separatively personal self or by its power that it sees and therefore it has not to be on guard against the element of personal error: that interferes only while a mental substratum or environing atmosphere yet remains and can still throw in its influence or while the supermind is still acting by descent into the mind to change it. And the supramental method with error is to eliminate it, not by any other device, but by an increasing spontaneity of the supramental discrimination and a constant heightening of its own energy. The consciousness of supermind is a cosmic consciousness and it is in this self of universal consciousness, in which the individual knower lives and with which he is more or less closely united, that it holds before him the object of knowledge.

The knower is in his observation a witness and this relation would seem to imply an otherness and difference, but the point is that it is not an entirely separative difference and does not bring an excluding idea of the thing observed as completely not self, as in the mental seeing of an external object. There is always a basic feeling of oneness with the thing known, for without this oneness there can be no supramental knowledge. The knower carrying the object in his universalised self of consciousness as a thing held before his station of witness vision includes it in his own wider being. The supramental observation is of things with which we are one in the being and consciousness and are capable of knowing them even as we know ourselves by the force of that oneness: the act of observation is a movement towards bringing out the latent knowledge.

There is, then, first a fundamental unity of consciousness that is greater or less in its power, more or less completely and immediately revelatory of its contents of knowledge according to our progress and elevation and intensity of living, feeling and seeing in the supramental ranges. There is set up between the knower and the object of knowledge, as a result of this fundamental unity, a stream or bridge of conscious connection — one is obliged to use images, however inadequate — and as a consequence a contact or active union enabling one to see, feel, sense supramentally what is to be known in the object or about it. Sometimes this stream or bridge of connection is not sensibly felt at the moment, only the results of the contact are noted, but it is always really there and an after memory can always make us aware that it was really all the time present: as we grow in supramentality, it becomes an abiding factor. The necessity of this stream or this bridge of connection ceases when the fundamental oneness becomes a complete active oneness. This process is the basis of what Patanjali calls *samyama*, a concentration, directing or dwelling of the consciousness, by which, he says, one can become aware of all that is in the object. But the necessity of concentration becomes slight or nil when the active oneness grows; the luminous consciousness of the object and its contents becomes more spontaneous, normal, facile.

There are three possible movements of this kind of supramental observation. First, the knower may project himself in consciousness on the object, feel his cognition in contact or enveloping or penetrating it and there, as it were in the object itself, become aware of what he has to know. Or he may by the contact become aware of that which is in it or belongs to it, as for example the thought or feeling of another, coming from it and entering into himself where he stands in his station of the witness. Or he may simply know in himself by a sort of supramental cognition in his own witness station without any such projection or entrance. The starting-point and apparent basis of the observation may be the presence of the object to the physical or other senses, but to the supermind this is not indispensable. It may be instead an inner image or simply the idea of the object. The simple will to know may bring to the supramental consciousness the needed knowledge — or, it may be, the will to be known or communicate itself of the object of knowledge.

The elaborate process of analytical observation and synthetical construction adopted by the logical intelligence is not the method of the supermind and yet there is a corresponding action. The supermind distinguishes by a direct seeing and without any mental process of taking to pieces the particularities of the thing, form, energy, action, quality, mind, soul that it has in view, and it sees too with an equal directness and without any process of construction the significant totality of which these particularities are the incidents. It sees also the essentiality, the Swabhava, of the thing in itself of which the totality and the particularities are the manifestation. And again it sees, whether apart from or through the essentiality or swabhava, the one self, the one existence, consciousness, power, force of which it is the basic expression.

It may be observing at the time only the particularities, but the whole is implied, and *vice versa*, — as for an example, the total state of mind out of which a thought or a feeling arises, — and the cognition may start from one or the other and proceed at once by immediate suggestion to the implied knowledge. The essentiality is similarly implied in the whole and in each or all of the particulars and there may be the same rapid or immediate alternative or alternate process. The logic of the supermind is different from that of the mind: it sees always the self as what is, the essentiality of the thing as a fundamental expression of the being and power of the self, and the whole and particulars as a consequent manifestation of this power and its active expression. In the fullness of the supramental consciousness and cognition this is the constant order. All perception of unity, similarity, difference, kind, uniqueness arrived at by the supramental reason is consonant with and depends on this order.

This observing action of supermind applies to all things. Its view of physical objects is not and cannot be only a surface or outward view, even when concentrated on the externals. It sees the form, action, properties, but it is aware at the same time of the qualities or energies, *guṇa*, *śakti*, of which the form is a translation, and it sees them not as an inference or deduction from the form or action, but feels and sees them directly in the being of the object and quite as vividly, — one might say, with a subtle concreteness and fine substantiality, — as the form or sensible action. It is aware too of the consciousness that manifests itself in quality, energy, form. It can feel, know, observe, see forces, tendencies, impulsions, things abstract to us quite as directly and vividly as the things we now call visible and sensible. It observes in just the same way persons and beings. It can take as its starting-point or first indication the speech, action, outward signs, but it is not limited by or dependent on them. It can know and feel and observe the very self and consciousness of another, can either proceed to that directly through the sign or can in its more powerful action begin with it and at once, instead of seeking to know the inner being through the evidence of the outer expression, understand rather all the outer expression in the light of the inner being. Even so, completely, the supramental being knows his own inner being and nature. The supermind can too act with equal power and observe with direct experience what is hidden behind the physical order; it can move in other planes than the material universe. It knows the self and reality of things by identity, by experience of oneness or contact of oneness and a vision, a seeing and realising ideation and knowledge dependent on or derived from these things, and its thought presentation of the truths of the spirit is an expression of this kind of sight and experience.

The supramental memory is different from the mental, not a storing up of past knowledge and experience, but an abiding presence of knowledge that can be brought forward or, more characteristically, offers itself, when it is needed: it is not dependent on attention or on conscious reception, for the things of the past not known actually or not observed can be called up from latency by an action which is yet essentially a remembrance. Especially on a certain level all knowledge presents itself as a remembering, because all is latent or inherent in the self of supermind. The future like the past presents itself to knowledge in the supermind as a memory of the preknown. The imagination transformed in the supermind acts on one side as a power of true image and symbol, always an image or index of some value or significance or other truth of being, on the other as an inspiration or interpretative seeing of possibilities and potentialities not less true than actual or realised things. These are put in their place either by an attendant intuitive or interpretative judgment or by one inherent in the vision of the image, symbol or potentiality, or by a supereminent revelation of that which is behind the image or symbol or which determines the potential and the actual and their relations and, it may be, overrides and overpasses them, imposing ultimate truths and supreme certitudes.

The supramental judgment acts inseparably from the supramental observation or memory, inherent in it as a direct seeing or cognition of values, significances, antecedents, consequences, relations, etc.; or it supervenes on the observation as a luminous disclosing idea or suggestion; or it may go before, independent of any observation, and then the object called up and observed confirms visibly the truth of the idea. But in each case it is sufficient in itself for its own purpose, is its own evidence and does not really depend for its truth on any aid or confirmation. There is a logic of the supramental reason, but its function is not to test or scrutinise, to support and prove or to detect and eliminate error. Its function is simply to link knowledge with knowledge, to discover and utilise harmonies and arrangement and relations, to organise the movement of the supramental knowledge. This it does not by any formal rule or construction of inferences but by a direct, living and immediate seeing and placing of connection and relation. All thought in the supermind is in the nature of intuition, inspiration or revelation and all deficiency of knowledge is to be supplied by a farther action of these powers; error is prevented by the action of a spontaneous and luminous discrimination; the movement is always from knowledge to knowledge. It is not rational in our sense but suprarational, — it does sovereignly what is sought to be done stumblingly and imperfectly by the mental reason.

The ranges of knowledge above the supramental reason, taking it up and exceeding it, cannot well be described, nor is it necessary here to make the endeavour. It is sufficient to say that the process here is more sufficient, intense and large in light, imperative, instantaneous, the scope of the active knowledge larger, the way nearer to the knowledge by identity, the thought more packed with the luminous substance of self-awareness and all-vision and more evidently independent of any other inferior support or assistance.

These characteristics, it must be remembered, do not fully apply even to the strongest action of the intuitive mentality, but are there seen only in their first glimpses. Nor can they be entirely or unmixedly evident so long as supramentality is only forming with an undercurrent, a mixture or an environment of mental action. It is only when mentality is overpassed and drops away into a passive silence that there can be the full disclosure and the sovereign and integral action of the supramental gnosis.

Chapter XXIV

The Supramental Sense

ALL THE instruments, all the activities of the mind have their corresponding powers in the action of the supramental energy and are there exalted and transfigured, but have there a reverse order of priority and necessary importance. As there is a supramental thought and essential consciousness, so too there is a supramental sense. Sense is fundamentally not the action of certain physical organs, but the contact of consciousness with its objects, *samjñāna*.

When the consciousness of the being is withdrawn wholly into itself, it is aware only of itself, of its own being, its own consciousness, its own delight of existence, its own concentrated force of being, and of these things not in their forms but in their essence. When it comes out of this self-immersion, it becomes aware of or it releases or develops out of its self-immersion its activities and forms of being, of consciousness, of delight and force. Then too, on the supramental plane, its primary awareness still remains of a kind native to and entirely characteristic of the self-awareness of the spirit, the self-knowledge of the one and infinite; it is a knowledge that knows all its objects, forms and activities comprehensively by being aware of them in its own infinite self, intimately by being aware in them as their self, absolutely by being aware of them as one in self with its own being. All its other ways of knowledge are projected from this knowledge by identity, are parts or movements of it, or at the lowest depend on it for their truth and light, are touched and supported by it even in their own separate way of action and refer back to it overtly or implicitly as their authority and origin.

The activity which is nearest to this essential knowledge by identity is the large embracing consciousness, especially characteristic of the supramental energy, which takes into itself all truth and idea and object of knowledge and sees them at once in their essence, totality and parts or aspects, — *vijñāna*. Its movement is a total seeing and seizing; it is a comprehension and possession in the self of knowledge; and it holds the object of consciousness as a part of the self or one with it, the unity being spontaneously and directly realised in the act of knowledge. Another supramental activity puts the knowledge by identity more into the background and stresses more the objectivity of the thing known. Its characteristic movement, descending into the mind, becomes the source of the peculiar nature of our mental knowledge, intelligence, *prajñāna*. In the mind the action of intelligence involves, at the outset, separation and otherness between the knower, knowledge and the known; but in the supermind its movement still takes place in the infinite identity or at least in the cosmic oneness. Only, the self of knowledge indulges the delight of putting the object of consciousness away from the more immediate nearness of the original and eternal unity, but always in itself, and of knowing it again in another way so as to establish with it a variety of relations of interaction which are so many minor chords in the harmony of the play of the consciousness. The movement of this supramental intelligence, *prajñāna*, becomes a subordinate, a tertiary action of the supramental for the fullness of which thought and word are needed. The primary action, because it is of the nature of knowledge by identity or of a comprehensive seizing in the consciousness, is complete in itself and has no need of these means of formulation. The supramental intelligence is of the nature of a truth seeing, truth hearing and truth remembering and, though capable of being sufficient to itself in a certain way, still feels itself more richly fulfilled by the thought and word that give it a body of expression.

Finally, a fourth action of the supramental consciousness completes the various possibilities of the supramental knowledge. This still farther accentuates the objectivity of the thing known, puts it away from the station of experiencing consciousness and again brings it to nearness by a uniting contact effected either in a direct nearness, touch, union or less closely across the bridge or through the connecting stream of consciousness of which there has already been mention. It is a contacting of existence, presences, things, forms, forces, activities, but a contacting of them in the stuff of the supramental being and energy, not in the divisions of matter and through the physical instruments, that creates the supramental sense, *saṁjñāna*.

It is a little difficult to make the nature of the supramental sense understood to a mentality not yet familiar with it by enlarged experience, because our idea of sense action is governed by the limiting experience of the physical mind and we suppose that the fundamental thing in it is the impression made by an external object on the physical organ of sight, hearing, smell, touch, taste, and that the business of the mind, the present central organ of our consciousness, is only to receive the physical impression and its nervous translation and so become intelligently conscious of the object. In order to understand the supramental change we have to realise first that the mind is the only real sense even in the physical process: its dependence on the physical impressions is the result of the conditions of the material evolution, but not a thing fundamental and indispensable. Mind is capable of a sight that is independent of the physical eye, a hearing that is independent of the physical ear, and so with the action of all the other senses. It is capable too of an awareness, operating by what appears to us as mental impressions, of things not conveyed or even suggested by the agency of the physical organs, — an opening to relations, happenings, forms even and the action of forces to which the physical organs could not have borne evidence. Then, becoming aware of these rarer powers, we speak of the mind as a sixth sense; but in fact it is the only true sense organ and the rest are no more than its outer conveniences and secondary instruments, although by its dependence on them they have become its limitations and its too imperative and exclusive conveyors. Again we have to realise — and this is more difficult to admit for our normal ideas in the matter — that the mind itself is only the characteristic instrument of sense, but the thing itself, sense in its purity, *saṁjñāna*, exists behind and beyond the mind it uses and is a movement of the self, a direct and original activity of the infinite power of its consciousness.

The pure action of sense is a spiritual action and pure sense is itself a power of the spirit.

The spiritual sense is capable of knowing in its own characteristic way, which is other than that of supramental thought or of the intelligence or spiritual comprehension, *vijñāna*, or knowledge by identity, all things whatsoever, things material and what is to us immaterial, all forms and that which is formless. For all is spiritual substance of being, substance of consciousness and force, substance of delight; and the spiritual sense, pure *saṁjñāna*, is the conscious being's contactual, substantial awareness of its own extended substance of self and in it of all that is of the infinite or universal substance. It is possible for us not only to know by conscious identity, by a spiritual comprehension of self, of principles and aspects, force, play and action, by a direct spiritual, supramental and intuitive thought knowledge, by the heart's spiritually and supramentally illumined feeling, love, delight, but also to have in a very literal significance the sense — sense-knowledge or sensation — of the spirit, the self, the Divine, the Infinite. The state described by the Upanishad in which one sees, hears, feels, touches, senses in every way the Brahman and the Brahman only, for all things have become to the consciousness only that and have no other, separate or independent existence, is not a mere figure of speech, but the exact description of the fundamental action of the pure sense, the spiritual object of the pure *saṁjñāna*. And in this original action, — to our experience a transfigured, glorified, infinitely blissful action of the sense, a direct feeling out inward, around, everywhere of the self to embrace and touch and be sensible of all that is in its universal being, — we can become aware in a most moving and delightful way of the Infinite and of all that is in it, cognizant, by intimate contact of our being with all being, of whatever is in the universe.

The action of the supramental sense is founded on this true truth of sense; it is an organisation of this pure, spiritual, infinite, absolute *saṁjñāna*. The supermind acting through sense feels all as God and in God, all as the manifest touch, sight, hearing, taste, perfume, all as the felt, seen, directly experienced substance and power and energy and movement, play, penetration, vibration, form, nearness, pressure, substantial interchange of the Infinite. Nothing exists independently to its sense, but all is felt as one being and movement and each thing as indivisible from the rest and as having in it all the Infinite, all the Divine. This supramental sense has the direct feeling and experience, not only of forms, but of forces and of the energy and the quality in things and of a divine substance and presence which is within them and round them and into which they open and expand themselves in their secret subtle self and elements, extending themselves in oneness into the illimitable. Nothing to the supramental sense is really finite: it is founded on a feeling of all in each and of each in all: its sense definition, although more precise and complete than the mental, creates no walls of limitation; it is an oceanic and ethereal sense in which all particular sense knowledge and sensation is a wave or movement or spray or drop that is yet a concentration of the whole ocean and inseparable from the ocean. Its action is a result of the extension and vibration of being and consciousness in a supra-ethereal ether of light, ether of power, ether of bliss, the Ananda Akasha of the Upanishads, which is the matrix and continent of the universal expression of the Self, — here in body and mind experienced only in limited extensions and vibrations, — and the medium of its true experience. This sense even at its lowest power is luminous with a revealing light that carries in it the secret of the thing it experiences and can therefore be a starting-point and basis of all the rest of the supramental knowledge, — the supramental thought, spiritual intelligence and comprehension, conscious identity, — and on its highest plane or at its fullest intensity of action it opens into or contains and at once liberates these things. It is strong with a luminous power that carries in it the force of self-realisation and an intense or infinite effectiveness, and this sense-experience can therefore be the starting-point of impulsion for a creative or fulfilling action of the spiritual and supramental will and knowledge. It is rapturous with a powerful and luminous delight that makes of it, makes of all sense and sensation a key to or a vessel of the divine and infinite Ananda.

The supramental sense can act in its own power and is independent of the body and the physical life and outer mind and it is above too the inner mind and its experiences. It can be aware of all things in whatever world, on whatever plane, in whatever formation of universal consciousness. It can be aware of the things of the material universe even in the trance of samadhi, aware of them as they are or appear to the physical sense, even as it is of other states of experience, of the pure vital, the mental, the psychical, the supramental presentation of things. It can in the waking state of the physical consciousness present to us the things concealed from the limited receptivity or beyond the range of the physical organs, distant forms, scenes and happenings, things that have passed out of physical existence or that are not yet in physical existence, scenes, forms, happenings, symbols of the vital, psychical, mental, supramental, spiritual worlds and all these in their real or significant truth as well as their appearance. It can use all the other states of sense consciousness and their appropriate senses and organs adding to them what they have not, setting right their errors and supplying their deficiencies: for it is the source of the others and they are only inferior derivations from this higher sense, this true and illimitable *saṁjñāna*.

*
* *

The lifting of the level of consciousness from the mind to the supermind and the consequent transformation of the being from the state of the mental to that of the supramental Purusha must bring with it to be complete a transformation of all the parts of the nature and all its activities. The whole mind is not merely made into a passive channel of the supramental activities, a channel of their downflow into the life and body and of their outflow or communication with the outward world, the material existence, — that is only the first stage of the process, — but is itself supramentalised along with all its instruments. There is accordingly a change, a profound transformation in the physical sense, a supramentalising of the physical sight, hearing, touch, etc., that creates or reveals to us a quite different view, not merely of life and its meaning, but even of the material world and all its forms and aspects. The supermind uses the physical organs and confirms their way of action, but it develops behind them the inner and deeper senses which see what are hidden from the physical organs and farther transforms the new sight, hearing, etc. thus created by casting it into its own mould and way of sensing. The change is one that takes nothing from the physical truth of the object, but adds to it its supraphysical truth and takes away by the removal of the physical limitation the element of falsehood in the material way of experience.

The supramentalising of the physical sense brings with it a result similar in this field to that which we experience in the transmutation of the thought and consciousness. As soon as the sight, for example, becomes altered under the influence of the supramental seeing, the eye gets a new and transfigured vision of things and of the world around us. Its sight acquires an extraordinary totality and an immediate and embracing precision in which the whole and every detail stand out at once in the complete harmony and vividness of the significance meant by Nature in the object and its realisation of the idea in form, executed in a triumph of substantial being. It is as if the eye of the poet and artist had replaced the vague or trivial unseeing normal vision, but singularly spiritualised and glorified, — as if indeed it were the sight of the supreme divine Poet and Artist in which we were participating and there were given to us the full seeing of his truth and intention in his design of the universe and of each thing in the universe. There is an unlimited intensity which makes all that is seen a revelation of the glory of quality and idea and form and colour. The physical eye seems then to carry in itself a spirit and a consciousness which sees not only the physical aspect of the object but the soul of quality in it, the vibration of energy, the light and force and spiritual substance of which it is made. Thus there comes through the physical sense to the total sense consciousness within and behind the vision a revelation of the soul of the thing seen and of the universal spirit that is expressing itself in this objective form of its own conscious being.

There is at the same time a subtle change which makes the sight see in a sort of fourth dimension, the character of which is a certain internality, the seeing not only of the superficies and the outward form but of that which informs it and subtly extends around it. The material object becomes to this sight something different from what we now see, not a separate object on the background or in the environment of the rest of Nature, but an indivisible part and even in a subtle way an expression of the unity of all that we see. And this unity that we see becomes not only to the subtler consciousness but to the mere sense, to the illumined physical sight itself, that of the identity of the Eternal, the unity of the Brahman. For to the supramentalised seeing the material world and space and material objects cease to be material in the sense in which we now on the strength of the sole evidence of our limited physical organs and of the physical consciousness that looks through them receive as our gross perception and understand as our conception of matter. It and they appear and are seen as spirit itself in a form of itself and a conscious extension. The whole is a unity — the oneness unaffected by any multitudinousness of objects and details — held in and by the consciousness in a spiritual space and all substance there is conscious substance. This change and this totality of the way of seeing comes from the exceeding of the limitations of our present physical sense, because the power of the subtle or psychical eye has been infused into the physical and there has again been infused into this psycho-physical power of vision the spiritual sight, the pure sense, the supramental *saṁjñāna*.

All the other senses undergo a similar transformation. All that the ear listens to, reveals the totality of its sound body and sound significance and all the tones of its vibration and reveals also to the single and complete hearing the quality, the rhythmic energy, the soul of the sound and its expression of the one universal spirit. There is the same internality, the going of the sense into the depths of the sound and the finding there of that which informs it and extends it into unity with the harmony of all sound and no less with the harmony of all silence, so that the ear is always listening to the infinite in its heard expression and the voice of its silence. All sounds become to the supramentalised ear the voice of the Divine, himself born into sound, and a rhythm of the concord of the universal symphony. And there is too the same completeness, vividness, intensity, the revelation of the self of the thing heard and the spiritual satisfaction of the self in hearing. The supramentalised touch also contacts or receives the touch of the Divine in all things and knows all things as the Divine through the conscious self in the contact: and there is too the same totality, intensity, revelation of all that is in and behind the touch to the experiencing consciousness. There comes a similar transformation of the other senses.

There is at the same time an opening of new powers in all the senses, an extension of range, a stretching out of the physical consciousness to an undreamed capacity. The supramental transformation extends too the physical consciousness far beyond the limits of the body and enables it to receive with a perfect concreteness the physical contact of things at a distance. And the physical organs become capable of serving as channels for the psychic and other senses so that we can see with the physical waking eye what is ordinarily revealed only in the abnormal states and to the psychical vision, hearing or other sense knowledge. It is the spirit or the inner soul that sees and senses, but the body and its powers are themselves spiritualised and share directly in the experience. The entire material sensation is supramentalised and it becomes aware, directly and with a physical participation and, finally, a unity with the subtler instrumentation, of forces and movements and the physical, vital, emotional, mental vibrations of things and beings and feels them all not only spiritually or mentally but physically in the self and as movements of the one self in these many bodies. The wall that the limitations of the body and its senses have built around us is abolished even in the body and the senses and there is in its place the free communication of the eternal oneness. All sense and sensation becomes full of the divine light, the divine power and intensity of experience, a divine joy, the delight of the Brahman. And even that which is now to us discordant and jars on the senses takes its place in the universal concord of the universal movement, reveals its *rasa,* meaning, design and, by delight in its intention in the divine consciousness and its manifestation of its law and dharma, its harmony with the total self, its place in the manifestation of the divine being, becomes beautiful and happy to the soul experience. All sensation becomes Ananda.

The embodied mind in us is ordinarily aware only through the physical organs and only of their objects and of subjective experiences which seem to start from the physical experience and to take them alone, however remotely, for their foundation and mould of construction. All the rest, all that is not consistent with or part of or verified by the physical data, seems to it rather imagination than reality and it is only in abnormal states that it opens to other kinds of conscious experience. But in fact there are immense ranges behind of which we could be aware if we opened the doors of our inner being. These ranges are there already in action and known to a subliminal self in us, and much even of our surface consciousness is directly projected from them and without our knowing it influences our subjective experience of things. There is a range of independent vital or pranic experiences behind, subliminal to and other than the surface action of the vitalised physical consciousness. And when this opens itself or acts in any way, there are made manifest to the waking mind the phenomena of a vital consciousness, a vital intuition, a vital sense not dependent on the body and its instruments, although it may use them as a secondary medium and a recorder. It is possible to open completely this range and, when we do so, we find that its operation is that of the conscious life force individualised in us contacting the universal life force and its operations in things, happenings and persons. The mind becomes aware of the life consciousness in all things, responds to it through our life consciousness with an immediate directness not limited by the ordinary communication through the body and its organs, records its intuitions, becomes capable of experiencing existence as a translation of the universal Life or Prana. The field of which the vital consciousness and the vital sense are primarily aware is not that of forms but, directly, that of forces: its world is a world of the play of energies, and form and event are sensed only secondarily as a result and embodiment of the energies. The mind working through the physical senses can only construct a view and knowledge of this nature as an idea in the intelligence, but it cannot go beyond the physical translation of the energies, and it has therefore no real or direct experience of the true nature of life, no actual realisation of the life force and the life spirit. It is by opening this other level or depth of experience within and by admission to the vital consciousness and vital sense that the mind can get the true and direct experience. Still, even then, so long as it is on the mental level, the experience is limited by the vital terms and their mental renderings and there is an obscurity even in this greatened sense and knowledge. The supramental transformation supravitalises the vital, reveals it as a dynamics of the spirit, makes a complete opening and a true revelation of all the spiritual reality behind and within the life force and the life spirit and of all its spiritual as well as its mental and purely vital truth and significance.

The supermind in its descent into the physical being awakens, if not already wakened by previous yogic sadhana, the consciousness — veiled or obscure in most of us — which supports and forms there the vital sheath, the *prāṇa koṣa*. When this is awakened, we no longer live in the physical body alone, but also in a vital body which penetrates and envelops the physical and is sensitive to impacts of another kind, to the play of the vital forces around us and coming in on us from the universe or from particular persons or group lives or from things or else from the vital planes and worlds which are behind the material universe. These impacts we feel even now in their result and in certain touches and affectations, but not at all or very little in their source and their coming. An awakened consciousness in the pranic body immediately feels them, is aware of a pervading vital force other than the physical energy, and can draw upon it to increase the vital strength and support the physical energies, can deal directly with the phenomena and causes of health and disease by means of this vital influx or by directing pranic currents, can be aware of the vital and the vital-emotional atmosphere of others and deal with its interchanges, along with a host of other phenomena which are unfelt by or obscure to our outward consciousness but here become conscient and sensible. It is acutely aware of the life soul and life body in ourself and others. The supermind takes up this vital consciousness and vital sense, puts it on its right foundation and transforms it by revealing the life-force here as the very power of the spirit dynamised for a near and direct operation on and through subtle and gross matter and for formation and action in the material universe.

The first result is that the limitations of our individual life being break down and we live no longer with a personal life force, or not with that ordinarily, but in and by the universal life energy. It is all the universal Prana that comes consciently streaming into and through us, keeps up there a dynamic constant eddy, an unseparated centre of its power, a vibrant station of storage and communication, constantly fills it with its forces and pours them out in activity upon the world around us. This life energy, again, is felt by us not merely as a vital ocean and its streams, but as the vital way and form and body and outpouring of a conscious universal Shakti, and that conscient Shakti reveals itself as the Chit Shakti of the Divine, the Energy of the transcendent and universal Self and Purusha of which — or rather of whom — our universalised individuality becomes an instrument and channel. As a result we feel ourselves one in life with all others and one with the life of all Nature and of all things in the universe. There is a free and conscious communication of the vital energy working in us with the same energy working in others. We are aware of their life as of our own or, at the least, of the touch and pressure and communicated movements of our life being on them and theirs upon us. The vital sense in us becomes powerful, intense, capable of bearing all the small or large, minute or immense vibrations of this life world on all its planes physical and supraphysical, vital and supravital, thrills with all its movement and Ananda and is aware of and open to all forces. The supermind takes possession of all this great range of experience, and makes it all luminous, harmonious, experienced not obscurely and fragmentarily and subject to the limitations and errors of its handling by the mental ignorance, but revealed, it and each movement of it, in its truth and totality of power and delight, and directs the great and now hardly limitable powers and capacities of the life dynamis on all its ranges according to the simple and yet complex, the sheer and spontaneous and yet unfalteringly intricate will of the Divine in our life. It makes the vital sense a perfect means of the knowledge of the life forces around us, as the physical of the forms and sensations of the physical universe, and a perfect channel too of the reactions of the active life force through us working as an instrument of self-manifestation.

*
* *

The phenomena of this vital consciousness and sense, this direct sensation and perception of and response to the play of subtler forces than the physical, are often included without distinction under the head of psychical phenomena. In a certain sense it is an awakening of the psyche, the inner soul now hidden, clogged wholly or partially covered up by the superficial activity of the physical mind and senses that brings to the surface the submerged or subliminal inner vital consciousness and also an inner or subliminal mental consciousness and sense capable of perceiving and experiencing directly, not only the life forces and their play and results and phenomena, but the mental and psychical worlds and all they contain and the mental activities, vibrations, phenomena, forms, images of this world also and of establishing a direct communication between mind and mind without the aid of the physical organs and the limitations they impose on our consciousness. There are however two different kinds of action of these inner ranges of the consciousness. The first is a more outer and confused activity of the awakening subliminal mind and life which is clogged with and subject to the grosser desires and illusions of the mind and vital being and vitiated in spite of its wider range of experience and powers and capacities by an enormous mass of error and deformations of the will and knowledge, full of false suggestions and images, false and distorted intuitions and inspirations and impulses, the latter often even depraved and perverse, and vitiated too by the interference of the physical mind and its obscurities. This is an inferior activity to which clairvoyants, psychists, spiritists, occultists, seekers of powers and siddhis are very liable and to which all the warnings against the dangers and errors of this kind of seeking are more especially applicable. The seeker of spiritual perfection has to pass as quickly as possible, if he cannot altogether avoid, this zone of danger, and the safe rule here is to be attached to none of these things, but to make spiritual progress one's sole real objective and to put no sure confidence in other things until the mind and life soul are purified and the light of the spirit and supermind or at least of the spiritually illumined mind and soul are shed on these inner ranges of experience. For when the mind is tranquillised and purified and the pure psyche liberated from the insistence of the desire soul, these experiences are free from any serious danger, — except indeed that of limitation and a certain element of error which cannot be entirely eliminated so long as the soul experiences and acts on the mental level. For there is then a pure action of the true psychical consciousness and its powers, a reception of psychical experience pure in itself of the worse deformations, although subject to the limitations of the representing mind, and capable of a high spiritualisation and light. The complete power and truth, however, can only come by the opening of the supermind and the supramentalising of the mental and psychical experience.

The range of the psychic consciousness and its experiences is almost illimitable and the variety and complexity of its phenomena almost infinite. Only some of the broad lines and main features can be noted here. The first and most prominent is the activity of the psychic senses of which the sight is the most developed ordinarily and the first to manifest itself with any largeness when the veil of the absorption in the surface consciousness which prevents the inner vision is broken. But all the physical senses have their corresponding powers in the psychical being, there is a psychical hearing, touch, smell, taste: indeed the physical senses are themselves in reality only a projection of the inner sense into a limited and externalised operation in and through and upon the phenomena of gross matter. The psychical sight receives characteristically the images that are formed in the subtle matter of the mental or psychical ether, *cittākāśa*. These may be transcriptions there or impresses of physical things, persons, scenes, happenings, whatever is, was or will be or may be in the physical universe. These images are very variously seen and under all kinds of conditions; in samadhi or in the waking state, and in the latter with the bodily eyes closed or open, projected on or into a physical object or medium or seen as if materialised in the physical atmosphere or only in a psychical ether revealing itself through this grosser physical atmosphere; seen through the physical eyes themselves as a secondary instrument and as if under the conditions of the physical vision or by the psychical vision alone and independently of the relations of our ordinary sight to space. The real agent is always the psychical sight and the power indicates that the consciousness is more or less awake, intermittently or normally and more or less perfectly, in the psychical body. It is possible to see in this way the transcriptions or impressions of things at any distance beyond the range of the physical vision or the images of the past or the future.

Besides these transcriptions or impresses the psychical vision receives thought images and other forms created by constant activity of consciousness in ourselves or in other human beings, and these may be according to the character of the activity images of truth or falsehood or else mixed things, partly true, partly false, and may be too either mere shells and representations or images inspired with a temporary life and consciousness and, it may be, carrying in them in one way or another some kind of beneficent or maleficent action or some willed or unwilled effectiveness on our minds or vital being or through them even on the body. These transcriptions, impresses, thought images, life images, projections of the consciousness may also be representations or creations not of the physical world, but of vital, psychic or mental worlds beyond us, seen in our own minds or projected from other than human beings. And as there is this psychical vision of which some of the more external and ordinary manifestations are well enough known by the name of clairvoyance, so there is a psychical hearing and psychical touch, taste, smell — clairaudience, clairsentience are the more external manifestations, — with precisely the same range each in its own kind, the same fields and manner and conditions and varieties of their phenomena.

These and other phenomena create an indirect, a representative range of psychical experience; but the psychical sense has also the power of putting us in a more direct communication with earthly or supraterrestrial beings through their psychical selves or their psychical bodies or even with things, for things also have a psychical reality and souls or presences supporting them which can communicate with our psychical consciousness. The most notable of these more powerful but rarer phenomena are those which attend the power of exteriorisation of our consciousness for various kinds of action otherwise and elsewhere than in the physical body, communication in the psychical body or some emanation or reproduction of it, oftenest, though by no means necessarily, during sleep or trance and the setting up of relations or communication by various means with the denizens of another plane of existence.

For there is a continuous scale of the planes of consciousness, beginning with the psychical and other belts attached to and dependent on the earth plane and proceeding through the true independent vital and psychical worlds to the worlds of the gods and the highest supramental and spiritual planes of existence. And these are in fact always acting upon our subliminal selves unknown to our waking mind and with considerable effect on our life and nature. The physical mind is only a little part of us and there is a much more considerable range of our being in which the presence, influence and powers of the other planes are active upon us and help to shape our external being and its activities. The awakening of the psychical consciousness enables us to become aware of these powers, presences and influences in and around us; and while in the impure or yet ignorant and imperfect mind this unveiled contact has its dangers, it enables us too, if rightly used and directed, to be no longer their subject but their master and to come into conscious and self-controlled possession of the inner secrets of our nature. The psychical consciousness reveals this interaction between the inner and the outer planes, this world and others, partly by an awareness, which may be very constant, vast and vivid, of their impacts, suggestions, communications to our inner thought and conscious being and a capacity of reaction upon them there, partly also through many kinds of symbolic, transcriptive or representative images presented to the different psychical senses. But also there is the possibility of a more direct, concretely sensible, almost material, sometimes actively material communication — a complete though temporary physical materialisation seems to be possible — with the powers, forces and beings of other worlds and planes. There may even be a complete breaking of the limits of the physical consciousness and the material existence.

The awakening of the psychical consciousness liberates in us the direct use of the mind as a sixth sense, and this power may be made constant and normal. The physical consciousness can only communicate with the minds of others or know the happenings of the world around us through external means and signs and indications, and it has beyond this limited action only a vague and haphazard use of the mind's more direct capacities, a poor range of occasional presentiments, intuitions and messages. Our minds are indeed constantly acting and acted upon by the minds of others through hidden currents of which we are not aware, but we have no knowledge or control of these agencies. The psychical consciousness, as it develops, makes us aware of the great mass of thoughts, feelings, suggestions, will impacts, influences of all kinds that we are receiving from others or sending to others or imbibing from and throwing into the general mind atmosphere around us. As it evolves in power, precision and clearness, we are able to trace these to their source or feel immediately their origin and transit to us and direct consciously and with an intelligent will our own messages. It becomes possible to be aware, more or less accurately and discerningly, of the activities of minds whether near to us physically or at a distance, to understand, feel or identify ourselves with their temperament, character, thoughts, feelings, reactions, whether by a psychic sense or a direct mental perception or by a very sensible and often intensely concrete reception of them into our mind or on its recording surface. At the same time we can consciously make at least the inner selves and, if they are sufficiently sensitive, the surface minds of others aware of our own inner mental or psychic self and plastic to its thoughts, suggestions, influences or even cast it or its active image in influence into their subjective, even into their vital and physical being to work there as a helping or moulding or dominating power and presence.

All these powers of the psychic consciousness need have and often have no more than a mental utility and significance, but it can also be used with a spiritual sense and light and intention in it and for a spiritual purpose. This can be done by a spiritual meaning and use in our psychical interchange with others, and it is largely by a psycho-spiritual interchange of this kind that a master in Yoga helps his disciple. The knowledge of our inner subliminal and psychic nature, of the powers and presences and influences there and the capacity of communication with other planes and their powers and beings can also be used for a higher than any mental or mundane object, for the possession and mastering of our whole nature and the overpassing of the intermediate planes on the way to the supreme spiritual heights of being. But the most direct spiritual use of the psychic consciousness is to make it an instrument of contact, communication and union with the Divine. A world of psycho-spiritual symbols is readily opened up, illuminating and potent and living forms and instruments, which can be made a revelation of spiritual significances, a support for our spiritual growth and the evolution of spiritual capacity and experience, a means towards spiritual power, knowledge or Ananda. The mantra is one of these psycho-spiritual means, at once a symbol, an instrument and a sound body for the divine manifestation, and of the same kind are the images of the Godhead and of its personalities or powers used in meditation or for adoration in Yoga. The great forms or bodies of the Divine are revealed through which he manifests his living presence to us and we can more easily by their means intimately know, adore and give ourselves to him and enter into the different lokas, worlds of his habitation and presence, where we can live in the light of his being. His word, command, Adesha, presence, touch, guidance can come to us through our spiritualised psychic consciousness and, as a subtly concrete means of transmission from the spirit, it can give us a close communication and nearness to him through all our psychic senses. These and many more are the spiritual uses of the psychic consciousness and sense and, although capable of limitation and deformation, — for all secondary instruments can be also by our mental capacity of exclusive self-limitation means of a partial but at the same time hindrances to a more integral realisation, — they are of the greatest utility on the road to the spiritual perfection and afterwards, liberated from the limitation of our minds, transformed and supramentalised, an element of rich detail in the spiritual Ananda.

As the physical and vital, the psychical consciousness and sense also are capable of a supramental transformation and receive by it their own integral fullness and significance. The supermind lays hold on the psychical being, descends into it, changes it into the mould of its own nature and uplifts it to be a part of the supramental action and state, the supra-psychic being of the Vijnana Purusha. The first result of this change is to base the phenomena of the psychical consciousness on their true foundation by bringing into it the permanent sense, the complete realisation, the secure possession of the oneness of our mind and soul with the minds and souls of others and the mind and soul of universal Nature. For always the effect of the supramental growth is to universalise the individual consciousness. As it makes us live, even in our individual vital movement and its relations with all around us, with the universal life, so it makes us think and feel and sense, although through an individual centre or instrument, with the universal mind and psychical being. This has two results of great importance.

First, the phenomena of the psychical sense and mind lose the fragmentariness and incoherence or else difficult regulation and often quite artificial order which pursues them even more than it pursues our more normal mental activities of the surface, and they become the harmonious play of the universal inner mind and soul in us, assume their true law and right forms and relations and reveal their just significances. Even on the mental plane one can get by the spiritualising of the mind at some realisation of soul oneness, but it is never really complete, at least in its application, and does not acquire this real and entire law, form, relation, complete and unfailing truth and accuracy of its significances. And, secondly, the activity of the psychical consciousness loses all character of abnormality, of an exceptional, irregular and even a perilously supernormal action, often bringing a loss of hold upon life and a disturbance or an injury to other parts of the being. It not only acquires its own right order within itself but its right relation with the physical life on one side and with the spiritual truth of being on the other and the whole becomes a harmonious manifestation of the embodied spirit. It is always the originating supermind that contains within itself the true values, significances and relations of the other parts of our being and its unfolding is the condition of the integral possession of our self and nature.

The complete transformation comes on us by a certain change, not merely of the poise or level of our regarding conscious self or even of its law and character, but also of the whole substance of our conscious being. Till that is done, the supramental consciousness manifests above the mental and psychical atmosphere of being — in which the physical has already become a subordinate and to a large extent a dependent method of our self's expression, — and it sends down its power, light, and influence into it to illumine it and transfigure. But only when the substance of the lower consciousness has been changed, filled potently, wonderfully transformed, swallowed up as it were into the greater energy and sense of being, *mahān, bṛhat,* of which it is a derivation and projection, do we have the perfected, entire and constant supramental consciousness. The substance, the conscious ether of being in which the mental or psychic consciousness and sense live and see and feel and experience is something subtler, freer, more plastic than that of the physical mind and sense. As long as we are dominated by the latter, psychical phenomena may seem to us less real, hallucinatory even, but the more we acclimatise ourselves to the psychical and to the ether of being which it inhabits, the more we begin to see the greater truth and to sense the more spiritually concrete substance of all to which its larger and freer mode of experience bears witness. Even, the physical may come to seem to itself unreal and hallucinatory — but this is an exaggeration and new misleading exclusiveness due to a shifting of the centre and a change of action of the mind and sense — or else may seem at any rate less powerfully real. When, however, the psychical and physical experiences are well combined in their true balance, we live at once in two complementary worlds of our being each with its own reality, but the psychical revealing all that is behind the physical, the soul view and experience taking precedence and enlightening and explaining the physical view and experience. The supramental transformation again changes the whole substance of our consciousness; it brings in an ether of greater being, consciousness, sense, life, which convicts the psychical also of insufficiency and makes it appear by itself an incomplete reality and only a partial truth of all that we are and become and witness.

All the experiences of the psychical are accepted and held up indeed in the supramental consciousness and its energy, but they are filled with the light of a greater truth, the substance of a greater spirit. The psychical consciousness is first supported and enlightened, then filled and occupied with the supramental light and power and the revealing intensity of its vibrations. Whatever exaggeration, whatever error born of isolated incidence, insufficiently illumined impression, personal suggestion, misleading influence and intention or other cause of limitation or deformation interferes in the truth of the mental and psychical experience and knowledge, is revealed and cured or vanishes, failing to stand in the light of the self-truth — *satyam, ṛtam* — of things, persons, happenings, indications, representations proper to this greater largeness. All the psychical communications, transcriptions, impresses, symbols, images receive their true value, take their right place, are put into their proper relations. The psychical intelligence and sensation are lit up with the supramental sense and knowledge, their phenomena, intermediate between the spiritual and material worlds, begin to reveal automatically their own truth and meaning and also the limitations of their truth and significance. The images presented to the inner sight, hearing, sensation of all kinds are occupied by or held in a larger and more luminous mass of vibrations, a greater substance of light and intensity which brings into them the same change as in the things of the physical sense, a greater totality, precision, revealing force of sense knowledge carried in the image. And finally all is lifted up and taken into the supermind and made a part of the infinitely luminous consciousness, knowledge and experience of the supramental being, the Vijnana Purusha.

The state of the being after this supramental transformation will be in all its parts of consciousness and knowledge that of an infinite and cosmic consciousness acting through the universalised individual Purusha. The fundamental power will be an awareness of identity, a knowledge by identity, — an identity of being, of consciousness, of force of being and consciousness, of delight of being, an identity with the Infinite, the Divine, and with all that is in the Infinite, all that is the expression and manifestation of the Divine. This awareness and knowledge will use as its means and instruments a spiritual vision of all that the knowledge by identity can found, a supramental real idea and thought of the nature of direct thought vision, thought hearing, thought memory that reveals, interprets or represents to the awareness the truth of all things, and an inner truth speech that expresses it, and finally a supramental sense that provides a relation of contact in substance of being with all things and persons and powers and forces in all the planes of existence.

The supramental will not depend on the instrumentation, for example, of the sense, as the physical mind is dependent on the evidence of our senses, although it will be capable of making them a starting-point for the higher forms of knowledge, as it will also be capable of proceeding directly through these higher forms and making the sense only a means of formation

and objective expression. The supramental being will transform
at the same time and take up into itself the present thinking
of the mind transfigured into an immensely larger knowledge
by identity, knowledge by total comprehension, knowledge by
intimate perception of detail and relation, all direct, immediate,
spontaneous, all the expression of the self's already existent
eternal knowledge. It will take up, transform, supramentalise
the physical sense, the sixth sense capacities of the mind and the
psychic consciousness and senses and use them as the means of
an extreme inner objectivisation of experience. Nothing will be
really external to it, for it will experience all in the unity of the
cosmic consciousness which will be its own, the unity of being
of the infinite which will be its own being. It will experience
matter, not only gross matter but the subtle and the most subtle,
as substance and form of the spirit, experience life and all kinds
of energy as the dynamics of the spirit, supramentalised mind as
a means or channel of knowledge of the spirit, supermind as the
infinite self of knowledge and power of knowledge and Ananda
of knowledge of the spirit.

Chapter XXV

Towards the Supramental
Time Vision

A LL BEING, consciousness, knowledge moves, secretly
for our present surface awareness, openly when we rise
beyond it to the spiritual and supramental ranges, between two states and powers of existence, that of the timeless
Infinite and that of the Infinite deploying in itself and organising all things in time. These two states are opposed to and
incompatible with each other only for our mental logic with its
constant embarrassed stumbling around a false conception of
contradictions and a confronting of eternal opposites. In reality,
as we find when we see things with a knowledge founded on
the supramental identity and vision and think with the great,
profound and flexible logic proper to that knowledge, the two
are only coexistent and concurrent status and movement of the
same truth of the Infinite. The timeless Infinite holds in itself,
in its eternal truth of being, beyond this manifestation, all that
it manifests in Time. Its time consciousness too is itself infinite
and maintains in itself at once in a vision of totalities and of
particularities, of mobile succession or moment sight and of
total stabilising vision or abiding whole sight what appears to
us as the past of things, their present and their future.

The consciousness of the timeless Infinite can be brought
home to us in various ways, but is most ordinarily imposed on
our mentality by a reflection of it and a powerful impression or
else made present to us as something above the mind, something
of which it is aware, towards which it lifts, but into which it
cannot enter because itself lives only in the time sense and in the
succession of the moments. If our present mind untransformed
by the supramental influence tries to enter into the timeless, it
must either disappear and be lost in the trance of Samadhi or

else, remaining awake, it feels itself diffused in an Infinite where there is perhaps a sense of supra-physical space, a vastness, a boundless extension of consciousness, but no time self, time movement or time order. And if then the mental being is still mechanically aware of things in time, it is yet unable to deal with them in its own manner, unable to establish a truth relation between the timeless and things in time and unable to act and will out of its indefinite Infinite. The action that then remains possible to the mental Purusha is the mechanical action of the instruments of the Prakriti continuing by force of old impulsion and habit or continued initiation of past energy, *prārabdha*, or else an action chaotic, unregulated, uncoordinated, a confused precipitate from an energy which has no longer a conscious centre.

The supramental consciousness on the other hand is founded upon the supreme consciousness of the timeless Infinite, but has too the secret of the deployment of the infinite Energy in time. It can either take its station in the time consciousness and keep the timeless infinite as its background of supreme and original being from which it receives all its organising knowledge, will and action, or it can, centred in its essential being, live in the timeless but live too in a manifestation in time which it feels and sees as infinite and as the same Infinite, and can bring out, sustain and develop in the one what it holds supernally in the other. Its time consciousness therefore will be different from that of the mental being, not swept helplessly on the stream of the moments and clutching at each moment as a stay and a swiftly disappearing standpoint, but founded first on its eternal identity beyond the changes of time, secondly on a simultaneous eternity of Time in which past, present and future exist together for ever in the self-knowledge and self-power of the Eternal, thirdly, in a total view of the three times as one movement singly and indivisibly seen even in their succession of stages, periods, cycles, last — and that only in the instrumental consciousness — in the step by step evolution of the moments. It will therefore have the knowledge of the three times, *trikāladṛṣṭi*, — held of old to be a supreme sign of the seer and the Rishi, — not as an abnormal power, but as its normal way of time knowledge.

This unified and infinite time consciousness and this vision and knowledge are the possession of the supramental being in its own supreme region of light and are complete only on the highest levels of the supramental nature. But in the ascent of the human consciousness through the uplifting and transmuting evolutionary — that is to say, self-unveiling, self-developing, progressively self-perfecting — process of Yoga, we have to take account of three successive conditions all of which have to be overpassed before we are able to move on the highest levels. The first condition of our consciousness, that in which we now move, is this mind of ignorance that has arisen out of the inconscience and nescience of material Nature, — ignorant but capable of seeking for knowledge and finding it at least in a series of mental representations which may be made clues to the true truth and, more and more refined and illuminated and rendered transparent by the influence, the infiltration and the descent of the light from above, prepare the intelligence for opening to the capacity of true knowledge. All truth is to this mind a thing it originally had not and has had to acquire or has still to acquire, a thing external to it and to be gathered by experience or by following certain ascertained methods and rules of enquiry, calculation, application of discovered law, interpretation of signs and indices. Its very knowledge implies an antecedent nescience; it is the instrument of Avidya.

The second condition of consciousness is potential only to the human being and gained by an inner enlightening and transformation of the mind of ignorance; it is that in which the mind seeks for its source of knowledge rather within than without and becomes to its own feeling and self-experience, by whatever means, a mind, not of original ignorance, but of self-forgetful knowledge. This mind is conscious that the knowledge of all things is hidden within it or at least somewhere in the being, but as if veiled and forgotten, and the knowledge comes to it not as a thing acquired from outside, but always secretly there and now remembered and known at once to be true, — each thing in its own place, degree, manner and measure. This is its attitude to knowledge even when the occasion of knowing is some external experience, sign or indication, because that is to it only the occasion and its reliance for the truth of the knowledge is not on the external indication or evidence but on the inner confirming witness. The true mind is the universal within us and the individual is only a projection on the surface, and therefore this second state of consciousness we have either when the individual mind goes more and more inward and is always consciously or subconsciously near and sensitive to the touches of the universal mentality in which all is contained, received, capable of being made manifest, or, still more powerfully, when we live in the consciousness of universal mind with the personal mentality only as a projection, a marking board or a communicating switch on the surface.

The third state of consciousness is that of the mind of knowledge in which all things and all truths are perceived and experienced as already present and known and immediately available by merely turning the inner light upon it, as when one turns the eye upon things in a room already known and familiar, — though not always present to the vision because that is not attentive, — and notes them as objects of a pre-existent knowledge. The difference from the second self-forgetful state of consciousness is that there is here no effort or seeking needed but simply a turning or opening of the inner light on whatever field of knowledge, and therefore it is not a recalling of things forgotten and self-hidden from the mind, but a luminous presentation of things already present, ready and available. This last condition is only possible by a partial supramentalising of the intuitive mentality and its full openness to any and every communication from the supramental ranges. This mind of knowledge is in its essentiality a power of potential omnipotence, but in its actual working on the level of mind it is limited in its range and province. The character of limitation applies to the supermind itself when it descends into the mental level and works in the lesser substance of mentality, though in its own manner and body of power and light, and it persists even in the action of the supramental reason. It is only the higher supramental Shakti acting on its own ranges whose will and knowledge work always in a boundless light or with a free capacity of illimitable extension of knowledge subject only to such limitations as are self-imposed for its own purposes and at its own will by the spirit.

The human mind developing into supermind has to pass through all these stages and in its ascent and expansion it may experience many changes and various dispositions of the powers and possibilities of its time consciousness and time knowledge. At first man in the mind of ignorance can neither live in the infinite time consciousness nor command any direct and real power of the triple time knowledge. The mind of ignorance lives, not in the indivisible continuity of time, but successively in each moment. It has a vague sense of the continuity of self and of an essential continuity of experience, a sense of which the source is the deeper self within us, but as it does not live in that self, also it does not live in a true time continuity, but only uses this vague but still insistent awareness as a background, support and assurance in what would otherwise be to it a constant baseless flux of its being. In its practical action its only support other than its station in the present is the line left behind by the past and preserved in memory, the mass of impressions deposited by previous experience and, for the future, an assurance of the regularity of experience and a power of uncertain forecast founded partly upon repeated experience and well-founded inference and partly on imaginative construction and conjecture. The mind of ignorance relies on a certain foundation or element of relative or moral certainties, but for the rest a dealing with probabilities and possibilities is its chief resource.

This is because the mind in the Ignorance lives in the moment and moves from hour to hour like a traveller who sees only what is near and visible around his immediate standpoint and remembers imperfectly what he has passed through before, but all in front beyond his immediate view is the unseen and unknown of which he has yet to have experience. Therefore man in his self-ignorance moving in time exists, as the Buddhists saw, only in the succession of thoughts and sensations and of the external forms present to his thought and sense. His present momentary self is alone real to him, his past self is dead or vanishing or only preserved in memory, result and impression, his future self is entirely non-existent or only in process of creation or preparation of birth. And the world around him is subject to the same rule of perception. Only its actual form and sum of happenings and phenomena is present and quite real to him, its past is no longer in existence or abides only in memory and record and in so much of it as has left its dead monuments or still survives into the present, the future is not yet at all in existence.

It must be noted however that if our knowledge of the present were not limited by our dependence on the physical mind and sense, this result would not be altogether inevitable. If we could be aware of all the present, all the action of physical, vital, mental energies at work in the moment, it is conceivable that we would be able to see their past too involved in them and their latent future or at least to proceed from present to past and future knowledge. And under certain conditions this might create a sense of real and ever present time continuity, a living in the behind and the front as well as the immediate, and a step farther might carry us into an ever present sense of our existence in infinite time and in our timeless self, and its manifestation in eternal time might then become real to us and also we might feel the timeless Self behind the worlds and the reality of his eternal world manifestation. In any case the possibility of another kind of time consciousness than we have at present and of a triple time knowledge rests upon the possibility of developing another consciousness than that proper to the physical mind and sense and breaking our imprisonment in the moment and in the mind of ignorance with its limitation to sensation, memory, inference and conjecture.

Actually man is not content solely with living in the present, though it is that he does with the most pressing vividness and insistence: he is moved to look before and after, to know as much as he can of the past and try to penetrate as far as he can, however obscurely, into the future. And he has certain aids towards this endeavour of which some depend on his surface mind, while others open to intimations from another subliminal or superconscient self which has a greater, subtler and more certain knowledge. His first aid is that of the reason proceeding forward from cause to effect and backward from effect to cause, discovering the law of energies and their assured mechanic process, assuming the perpetual sameness of the movements of Nature, fixing her time measures and thus calculating on the basis of a science of general lines and assured results the past and the future. A certain measure of limited but sufficiently striking success has been gained by this method in the province of physical Nature and it might seem that the same process might eventually be applied to the movements of mind and life and that at any rate this alone is man's one reliable means in any field of looking with precision back and forwards. But as a matter of fact the happenings of vital and still more of mental nature escape to a very great degree the means of inference and calculation from assured law that apply in the field of physical knowledge: it can apply there only to a limited range of regularised happenings and phenomena and for the rest leaves us where we were amid a mixed mass of relative certainties, uncertain probabilities and incalculable possibilities.

This is because mind and life bring in a great subtlety and intricacy of movement, each realised movement carries in it a complex of forces, and even if we could disengage all these, all, that is to say, that are simply actualised and on or near the surface, we should still be baffled by all the rest that is obscure or latent, — concealed and yet potent contributory causes, hidden motion and motive force, undeployed possibilities, uncalculated and incalculable chances of variation. It ceases to be practicable here for our limited intelligence to calculate accurately and with certitude as in the physical field from precise cause to precise effect, that is to say, from a given apparent set of existing conditions to an inevitable resultant of subsequent or a necessary precedence of antecedent conditions. It is for this reason that the predictions and previsions of the human intelligence are constantly baffled and contradicted by the event, even when largest in their view of the data and most careful in their survey of possible consequence. Life and mind are a constant flux of possibles intervening between spirit and matter and at each step bring in, if not an infinite, at least an indefinite of possibles, and this would be enough to make all logical calculation uncertain and relative. But in addition there reigns behind them a supreme factor incalculable by human mind, the will of the soul and secret spirit, the first indefinitely variable, fluid and elusive, the second infinite and inscrutably imperative, bound, if at all, only by itself and the Will in the Infinite. It is therefore only by going back from the surface physical mind to the psychic and spiritual consciousness that a vision and knowledge of the triple time, a transcendence of our limitation to the standpoint and view range of the moment, can be wholly possible.

Meanwhile there are certain doors opening from the inner on to the outer consciousness which make an occasional but insufficient power of direct retro-vision of the past, circumvision of the present, prevision of the future even in the physical mind at least potentially feasible. First, there are certain movements of the mind sense and the vital consciousness that are of this character — of which one kind, that which has most struck our perceptions, has been called presentiment. These movements are instinctive perceptions, obscure intuitions of the sense mind and the vital being, and like all that is instinctive in man have been suppressed, rendered rare or discredited as unreliable by the engrossing activity of the mental intelligence. If allowed a free scope, these could develop and supply data not available to the ordinary reason and the senses. But still they would not be of themselves perfectly useful or reliable indices unless their obscurity were enlightened by an interpretation and guidance which the ordinary intelligence cannot give, but a higher intuition could provide. Intuition, then, is the second and more important possible means available to us, and actually intuition can and does sometimes give us in this difficult field an occasional light and guidance. But acting in our present mentality it is subject to the disadvantage that it is uncertain in operation, imperfect in its functioning, obscured by false imitative movements of the imagination and fallible mental judgment and continually seized on and alloyed and distorted by the normal action of mind with its constant liability to error. The formation of an organised intuitive mentality purified from these deficiencies would be needed to enlarge and assure this possibility of the functioning of a higher luminous intelligence.

Man, confronted by this incapacity of the intelligence and yet avid of the knowledge of the future, has fallen back on other and external means, omens, sortileges, dreams, astrology and many other alleged data for a past and future knowledge that have been in less sceptical times formulated as veridical sciences. Challenged and discredited by the sceptical reason these still persist in attracting our minds and hold their own, supported by desire and credulity and superstition, but also by the frequent though imperfect evidence we get of a certain measure of truth in their pretensions. A higher psychical knowledge shows us that in fact the world is full of many systems of correspondences and indices and that these things, however much misused by the human intelligence, can in their place and under right conditions give us real data of a supraphysical knowledge. It is evident, however, that it is only an intuitive knowledge that can discover and formulate them, — as it was in fact the psychical and intuitive mind that originally formulated these ways of veridical knowledge, — and it will be found in practice that only an intuitive knowledge, not the mere use either of a traditional or a haphazard interpretation or of mechanical rule and formula, can ensure a right employment of these indices. Otherwise, handled by the surface intelligence, they are liable to be converted into a thick jungle of error.

The true and direct knowledge or vision of past, present and future begins with the opening of the psychical consciousness and the psychical faculties. The psychical consciousness is that of what is now often called the subliminal self, the subtle or dream self of Indian psychology, and its range of potential knowledge, almost infinite as has been pointed out in the last chapter, includes a very large power and many forms of insight into both the possibilities and the definite actualities of past, present and future. Its first faculty, that which most readily attracts attention, is its power of seeing by the psychical sense images of all things in time and space. As exercised by clairvoyants, mediums and others this is often, and indeed usually, a specialised faculty limited though often precise and accurate in action, and implies no development of the inner soul or the spiritual being or the higher intelligence. It is a door opened by chance or by an innate gift or by some kind of pressure between the waking and the subliminal mind and admitting only to the surface or the outskirts of the latter. All things in a certain power and action of the secret universal mind are represented by images — not only visual but, if one may use the phrase, auditory and other images, — and a certain development of the subtle or psychical senses makes it possible, — if there is no interference of the constructing mind and its imaginations, if, that is to say, artificial or falsifying mental images do not intervene, if the psychical sense is free, sincere and passive, — to receive these representations or transcriptions with a perfect accuracy and not so much predict as see in its correct images the present beyond the range of the physical sense, the past and the future. The accuracy of this kind of seeing depends on its being confined to a statement of the thing seen and the attempt to infer, interpret or otherwise go beyond the visual knowledge may lead to much error unless there is at the same time a strong psychical intuition fine, subtle and pure or a high development of the luminous intuitive intelligence.

A completer opening of the psychical consciousness leads us far beyond this faculty of vision by images and admits us not indeed to a new time consciousness, but to many ways of the triple time knowledge. The subliminal or psychic self can bring back or project itself into past states of consciousness and experience and anticipate or even, though this is less common, strongly project itself into future states of consciousness and experience. It does this by a temporary entering into or identification of its being or its power of experiencing knowledge with either permanences or representations of the past and the future that are maintained in an eternal time consciousness behind our mentality or thrown up by the eternity of supermind into an indivisible continuity of time vision. Or it may receive the impress of these things and construct a transcriptive experience of them in the subtle ether of psychical being. Or it may call up the past from the subconscious memory where it is always latent and give it in itself a living form and a kind of renewed memorative existence, and equally it may call up from the depths of latency, where it is already shaped in the being, and similarly form to itself and experience the future. It may by a kind of psychical thought vision or soul intuition — not the same thing as the subtler and less concrete thought vision of the luminous intuitive intelligence — foresee or foreknow the future or flash this soul intuition into the past that has gone behind the veil and recover it for present knowledge. It can develop a symbolic seeing which conveys the past and the future through a vision of the powers and significances that belong to supraphysical planes but are powerful for creation in the material universe. It can feel the intention of the Divine, the mind of the gods, all things and their signs and indices that descend upon the soul and determine the complex movement of forces. It can feel too the movement of forces that represent or respond to the pressure — as it can perceive the presence and the action — of the beings of the mental, vital and other worlds who concern themselves with our lives. It can gather on all hands all kinds of indications of happenings in past, present and future time. It can receive before its sight the etheric writing, *ākāśa lipi*, that keeps the record of all things past, transcribes all that is in process in the present, writes out the future.

All these and a multitude of other powers are concealed in our subliminal being and with the waking of the psychical consciousness can be brought to the surface. The knowledge of our past lives, — whether of past soul states or personalities or scenes, occurrences, relations with others, — of the past lives of others, of the past of the world, of the future, of present things that are beyond the range of our physical senses or the reach of any means of knowledge open to the surface intelligence, the intuition and impressions not only of physical things, but of the working of a past and present and future mind and life and soul in ourselves and others, the knowledge not only of this world but of other worlds or planes of consciousness and their manifestations in time and of their intervention and workings and effects on the earth and its embodied souls and their destinies, lies open to our psychical being, because it is close to the intimations of the universal, not engrossed only or mainly with the immediate and not shut up into the narrow circle of the purely personal and physical experience.

At the same time these powers are subject to this disadvantage that they are not by any means free from liability to confusion and error, and especially the lower ranges and more outer workings of the psychical consciousness are subject to dangerous influences, strong illusions, misleading, perverting and distorting suggestions and images. A purified mind and heart and a strong and fine psychical intuition may do much to protect from perversion and error, but even the most highly developed psychical consciousness cannot be absolutely safe unless the psychical is illumined and uplifted by a higher force than itself and touched and strengthened by the luminous intuitive mind and that again raised towards the supramental energy of the spirit. The psychical consciousness does not derive its time knowledge from a direct living in the indivisible continuity of the spirit and it has not to guide it a perfect intuitive discrimination or the absolute light of the higher truth consciousness. It receives its time perceptions, like the mind, only in part and detail, is open to all kinds of suggestions, and as its consequent range of truth is wider, more manifold too are its sources of error. And it is not only that which was but that which might have been or tried and failed to be that comes to it out of the past, not only that which is but that which may be or wishes to be that crowds on it from the present and not only things to be but suggestions, intuitions, visions and images of many kinds of possibility that visit it from the future. And always too there is the possibility of mental constructions and mental images interfering with the true truth of things in the presentations of the psychical experience.

The coming of the intimations of the subliminal self to the surface and the activity of the psychical consciousness tend to

turn the mind of ignorance, with which we begin, increasingly though not perfectly into a mind of self-forgetful knowledge constantly illuminated with intimations and upsurgings from the inner being, *antarātman*, rays from the still concealed awareness of its whole self and infinite contents and from the awareness — representing itself here as a sort of memory, a recalling or a bringing out — of an inherent and permanent but hidden knowledge of past, present and future that is always carried within itself by the eternal spirit. But embodied as we are and founded on the physical consciousness, the mind of ignorance still persists as a conditioning environment, an intervening power and limiting habitual force obstructing and mixing with the new formation or, even in moments of large illumination, at once a boundary wall and a strong substratum, and it imposes its incapacities and errors. And to remedy this persistence the first necessity would seem to be the development of the power of a luminous intuitive intelligence seeing the truth of time and its happenings as well as all other truth by intuitive thought and sense and vision and detecting and extruding by its native light of discernment the intrusions of misprision and error.

All intuitive knowledge comes more or less directly from the light of the self-aware spirit entering into the mind, the spirit concealed behind mind and conscious of all in itself and in all its selves, omniscient and capable of illumining the ignorant or the self-forgetful mind whether by rare or constant flashes or by a steady instreaming light, out of its omniscience. This all includes all that was, is or will be in time and this omniscience is not limited, impeded or baffled by our mental division of the three times and the idea and experience of a dead and no longer existent and ill-remembered or forgotten past and a not yet existent and therefore unknowable future which is so imperative for the mind in the ignorance. Accordingly the growth of the intuitive mind can bring with it the capacity of a time knowledge which comes to it not from outside indices, but from within the universal soul of things, its eternal memory of the past, its unlimited holding of things present and its prevision or, as it has been paradoxically but suggestively called, its memory of the future. But this capacity works at first sporadically and uncertainly and not in an organised manner. As the force of intuitive knowledge grows, it becomes more possible to command the use of the capacity and to regularise to a certain degree its functioning and various movements. An acquired power can be established of commanding the materials and the main or the detailed knowledge of things in the triple time, but this usually forms itself as a special or abnormal power and the normal action of the mentality or a large part of it remains still that of the mind of ignorance. This is obviously an imperfection and limitation and it is only when the power takes its place as a normal and natural action of the wholly intuitivised mind that there can be said to be a perfection of the capacity of the triple time knowledge so far as that is possible in the mental being.

It is by the progressive extrusion of the ordinary action of the intelligence, the acquiring of a complete and total reliance on the intuitive self and a consequent intuitivising of all the parts of the mental being that the mind of ignorance can be, more successfully, if not as yet wholly, replaced by the mind of self-contained knowledge. But, — and especially for this kind of knowledge, — what is needed is the cessation of mental constructions built on the foundation of the mind of ignorance. The difference between the ordinary mind and the intuitive is that the former, seeking in the darkness or at most by its own unsteady torchlight, first, sees things only as they are presented in that light and, secondly, where it does not know, constructs by imagination, by uncertain inference, by others of its aids and makeshifts things which it readily takes for truth, shadow projections, cloud edifices, unreal prolongations, deceptive anticipations, possibilities and probabilities which do duty for certitudes. The intuitive mind constructs nothing in this artificial fashion, but makes itself a receiver of the light and allows the truth to manifest in it and organise its own constructions. But so long as there is a mixed action and the mental constructions and imaginations are allowed to operate, this passivity of the intuitive mind to the higher light, the truth light, cannot be complete or securely dominate and there cannot therefore be a firm organisation of the triple time knowledge. It is because of this obstruction and mixture that that power of time vision, of back-sight and around-sight and foresight, which sometimes marks the illuminated mind, is not only an abnormal power among others rather than part of the very texture of the mental action, but also occasional, very partial and marred often by an undetected intermixture or a self-substituting intervention of error.

The mental constructions that interfere are mainly of two kinds, and the first and most powerfully distorting are those which proceed from the stresses of the will claiming to see and determine, interfering with knowledge and not allowing the intuition to be passive to the truth light and its impartial and pure channel. The personal will, whether taking the shape of the emotions and the heart's wishes or of vital desires or of strong dynamic volitions or the wilful preferences of the intelligence, is an evident source of distortion when these try, as they usually do try with success, to impose themselves on the knowledge and make us take what we desire or will for the thing that was, is or must be. For either they prevent the true knowledge from acting or if it at all presents itself, they seize upon it, twist it out of shape and make the resultant deformation a justifying basis for a mass of will-created falsehood. The personal will must either be put aside or else its suggestions must be kept in their place until a supreme reference has been made to the higher impersonal light and then must be sanctioned or rejected according to the truth that comes from deeper within than the mind or from higher above. But even if the personal will is held in abeyance and the mind passive for reception, it may be assailed and imposed on by suggestions from all sorts of forces and possibilities that strive in the world for realisation and come representing the things cast up by them on the stream of their will-to-be as the truth of past, present or future. And if the mind lends itself to these impostor suggestions, accepts their self-valuations, does not either put them aside or refer them to the truth light, the same result of prevention or distortion of the truth is inevitable. There is a possibility of the will element being entirely excluded and the mind being made a silent and passive register of a higher luminous knowledge, and in that case a much more accurate reception of time intuitions becomes possible. The integrality of the being demands however a will action and not only an inactive knowing, and therefore the larger and more perfect remedy is to replace progressively the personal by a universalised will which insists on nothing that is not securely felt by it to be an intuition, inspiration or revelation of what must be from that higher light in which will is one with knowledge.

The second kind of mental construction belongs to the very nature of our mind and intelligence and its dealing with things in time. All is seen here by mind as a sum of realised actualities with their antecedents and natural consequences, an indeterminate of possibilities and, conceivably, although of this it is not certain, a determining something behind, a will, fate or Power, which rejects some and sanctions or compels others out of many possibles. Its constructions therefore are made partly of inferences from the actual, both past and present, partly of a volitional or an imaginative and conjectural selection and combining of possibilities and partly of a decisive reasoning or preferential judgment or insistent creative will-intelligence that tries to fix among the mass of actuals and possibles the definitive truth it is labouring to discover or determine. All this which is indispensable to our thought and action in mind, has to be excluded or transformed before the intuitive knowledge can have a chance of organising itself on a sound basis. A transformation is possible because the intuitive mind has to do the same work and cover the same field, but with a different handling of the materials and another light upon their significance. An exclusion is possible because all is really contained in the truth consciousness above and a silencing of the mind of ignorance and a pregnant receptivity is not beyond our compass in which the intuitions descending from the truth consciousness can be received with a subtle or strong exactitude and all the materials of the knowledge seen in their right place and true proportion. As a matter of practice it will be found that both methods are used alternatively or together to effect the transition from the one kind of mentality to the other.

The intuitive mind dealing with the triple time movement

has to see rightly in thought sense and vision three things, actualities, possibles and imperatives. There is first a primary intuitive action developed which sees principally the stream of successive actualities in time, even as the ordinary mind, but with an immediate directness of truth and spontaneous accuracy of which the ordinary mind is not capable. It sees them first by a perception, a thought action, a thought sense, a thought vision, which at once detects the forces at work on persons and things, the thoughts, intentions, impulsions, energies, influences in and around them, those already formulated in them and those in process of formation, those too that are coming or about to come into or upon them from the environment or from secret sources invisible to the normal mind, distinguishes by a rapid intuitive analysis free from seeking or labour or by a synthetic total view the complex of these forces, discerns the effective from the ineffective or partly effective and sees too the result that is to emerge. This is the integral process of the intuitive vision of actualities, but there are others that are less complete in their character. For there may be developed a power of seeing the result without any previous or simultaneous perception of the forces at work or the latter may be seen only afterwards and the result alone leap at once and first into the knowledge. On the other hand there may be a partial or complete perception of the complex of forces, but an incertitude of the definitive result or only a slowly arriving or relative certitude. These are stages in the development of the capacity for a total and unified vision of actualities.

This kind of intuitive knowledge is not an entirely perfect instrument of time knowledge. It moves normally in the stream of the present and sees rightly from moment to moment only the present, the immediate past and the immediate future. It may, it is true, project itself backward and reconstruct correctly by the same power and process a past action or project itself forward and reconstruct correctly something in the more distant future. But this is for the normal power of the thought vision a more rare and difficult effort and usually it needs for a freer use of this self-projection the aid and support of the psychical seeing.

Moreover it can see only what will arrive in the undisturbed process of the actualities and its vision no longer applies if some unforeseen rush of forces or intervening power comes down from regions of a larger potentiality altering the complex of conditions, and this is a thing that constantly happens in the action of forces in the time movement. It may help itself by the reception of inspirations that illumine to it these potentialities and of imperative revelations that indicate what is decisive in them and its sequences and by these two powers correct the limitations of the intuitive mind of actuality. But the capacity of this first intuitive action to deal with these greater sources of vision is never quite perfect, as must always be the case with an inferior power in its treatment of the materials given to it from a greater consciousness. A considerable limitation of vision by its stress on the stream of immediate actualities must be always its character.

It is possible however to develop a mind of luminous inspiration which will be more at home among the greater potentialities of the time movement, see more easily distant things and at the same time take up into itself, into its more brilliant, wide and powerful light, the intuitive knowledge of actualities. This inspired mind will see things in the light of the world's larger potentialities and note the stream of actuality as a selection and result from the mass of forceful possibles. It will be liable, however, if it is not attended with a sufficient revelatory knowledge of imperatives, to a hesitation or suspension of determining view as between various potential lines of the movement or even to a movement away from the line of eventual actuality and following another not yet applicable sequence. The aid of imperative revelations from above will help to diminish this limitation, but here again there will be the difficulty of an inferior power dealing with the materials given to it from the treasury of a higher light and force. But it is possible to develop too a mind of luminous revelation which taking into itself the two inferior movements sees what is determined behind the play of potentialities and actualities and observes these latter as its means of deploying its imperative decisions. An intuitive mind thus constituted and aided by an active psychic consciousness may be in command of a very remarkable power of time knowledge.

At the same time it will be found that it is still a limited instrument. In the first place it will represent a superior knowledge working in the stuff of mind, cast into mental forms and still subject to mental conditions and limitations. It will always lean chiefly on the succession of present moments as a foundation for its steps and successions of knowledge, however far it may range backward or forward, — it will move in the stream of Time even in its higher revelatory action and not see the movement from above or in the stabilities of eternal time with their large ranges of vision, and therefore it will always be bound to a secondary and limited action and to a certain dilution, qualification and relativity in its activities. Moreover, its knowing will be not a possession in itself but a reception of knowledge. It will at most create in place of the mind of ignorance a mind of self-forgetful knowledge constantly reminded and illumined from a latent self-awareness and all-awareness. The range, the extent, the normal lines of action of the knowledge will vary according to the development, but it can never be free from very strong limitations. And this limitation will give a tendency to the still environing or subconsciously subsisting mind of ignorance to reassert itself, to rush in or up, acting where the intuitive knowledge refuses or is unable to act and bringing in with it again its confusion and mixture and error. The only security will be a refusal to attempt to know or at least a suspension of the effort of knowledge until or unless the higher light descends and extends its action. This self-restraint is difficult to mind and, too contentedly exercised, may limit the growth of the seeker. If on the other hand the mind of ignorance is allowed again to emerge and seek in its own stumbling imperfect force, there may be a constant oscillation between the two states or a mixed action of the two powers in place of a definite though relative perfection.

The issue out of this dilemma is to a greater perfection towards which the formation of the intuitive, inspired and revelatory mind is only a preparatory stage, and that comes by a constant instreaming and descent of more and more of the supramental light and energy into the whole mental being and a constant raising of the intuition and its powers towards their source in the open glories of the supramental nature. There is then a double action of the intuitive mind aware of, open to and referring its knowledge constantly to the light above it for support and confirmation and of that light itself creating a highest mind of knowledge, — really the supramental action itself in a more and more transformed stuff of mind and a less and less insistent subjection to mental conditions. There is thus formed a lesser supramental action, a mind of knowledge tending always to change into the true supermind of knowledge. The mind of ignorance is more and more definitely excluded, its place taken by the mind of self-forgetful knowledge illumined by the intuition, and the intuition itself more perfectly organised becomes capable of answering to a larger and larger call upon it. The increasing mind of knowledge acts as an intermediary power and, as it forms itself, it works upon the other, transforms or replaces it and compels the farther change which effects the transition from mind to supermind. It is here that a change begins to take place in the time consciousness and time knowledge which finds its base and complete reality and significance only on the supramental levels. It is therefore in relation to the truth of supermind that its workings can be more effectively elucidated: for the mind of knowledge is only a projection and a last step in the ascent towards the supramental nature.

and imperatively compels into manifestation the truth it sees and dwells on and evolves its play, combinations, sequences, not a limited mental will and power like ours, but a conscious force supramental and illimitable, Tapas, Chit-shakti, not bound to this or that movement and result of energy, but ordering out of the infinite truth of self-existence the movement and result of all possible energies. And it is finally an Ananda of the being that deploys itself, that ranges at will among the infinities of consciousness and of its power of manifestation, not a limited mental joy or pleasure like our chequered delight of being and action and feeling, but supramental and illimitable, not subject to a given set of reactions, but embracing and taking a free and sovereign and compelling delight of all that is possible in the truth of the infinite consciousness and existence.

[Version B]

It is necessary in order to understand the phenomena of the supramental time consciousness to realise very firmly certain truths which are strange to our ordinary mentality or presented to it only as constructions of the metaphysical intellect, intelligible but unsubstantial abstractions as all mere philosophical statements must be, but to the supermind are realised experience and the normal and natural truth of the consciousness in which it lives, moves, acts and manifests its being. It is only in their light that we can grasp the truth and reality and the manifestation of things in time, otherwise only an illusion or else a flux of transient, inexplicable and incalculable actualities, and the law, source and order of their manifestation, otherwise only a process of inscrutable Law or else a play of chance and probabilities and possibilities. The truths that reveal the inner meaning and way of the universe are of a spiritual and supramental order. It is difficult however to express them at all in a language adapted to the mental intellect and one can at most try to indicate.

The first of the truths that thus becomes real to the consciousness is the truth of infinite being, a thing abstract to

Appendix to Part IV

Sri Aurobindo began another chapter of "The Yoga of Self-Perfection" before deciding to discontinue the publication of the *Arya*. He wrote two versions of the opening of this chapter, which are reproduced here from his typescript.

Chapter XXVI

The Supramental Time Consciousness

[Version A]

The supermind in its supreme status is the truth-consci⟨ous⟩
of the Infinite, the inherent light and power of self-kno⟨wledge⟩
and all-knowledge of the Supreme who is the self of ⟨the⟩
living eternal truth of all that is and of whom all obje⟨cts⟩
beings, all the universe and motion of things and hap⟨penings⟩
in time is a partial continually proceeding manifestati⟨on he⟩
Supreme organises through the power of self-realisati⟨on and⟩
self-manifestation that resides in this self-knowledge ⟨and all-⟩
knowledge all truth of his being that he has the will and d⟨elight to⟩
put forth in his universal existence, — to create, as we s⟨ay from⟩
our standpoint. But this creation is not a making or bring⟨ing into⟩
being of that which was non-existent, neither is it a c⟨rea-⟩
tion of illusory phenomena in a self of dream, but a re⟨lease⟩
in condition of being, substance of consciousness, move⟨ment,⟩
force, name, form, idea, significance, of the truths of bei⟨ng of the⟩
Eternal. All that manifests itself in time, is the coming i⟨nto⟩
effective disclosure, result, form, power, evolution, m⟨anifestation⟩
of some truth of being, a truth of Sat, of the eternal exi⟨stence of⟩
the Supreme and Eternal.

The power that brings it into play is the infinite c⟨onscious-⟩
ness of the Supreme aware of itself and all that is i⟨n it, not⟩
a limited mental consciousness like ours but suprame⟨ntal,⟩
illimitable, not bound by this or that condition, but det⟨ermining⟩
out of an infinite truth of self-existence its own condit⟨ions⟩
by this or that relation or step and sequence, but capa⟨ble of all⟩
possible relations and steps and sequences. It is a powe⟨r⟩
inherent in that consciousness which spontaneously, s⟨o⟩

our present sense and intelligence to which only phenomena are concrete and real, but to the supramental being always and absolutely and intimately present and real. This indeed is that which to its knowledge, sense, vision, idea, feeling is most concretely real and the phenomena which are now so close and all-important to us, are to it less concrete, not self-existent at all but dependent on the support of the infinite consciousness and its force of presentation: there is thus a complete reversal of the order in the conception of realities. It is not that the phenomena in their turn become abstract, unreal, unsubstantial creations of consciousness, — that is only the result of a certain exclusive realisation, when there is an identification with the essence of absolute being to the exclusion of its power, — but that they are felt as existing here only in a certain movement of the infinite, real only because they are made, as it were, out of the substance of infinite being. That which determines them, the truth of their essence and nature, *svarūpa, svabhāva*, that which gives them the power to be, is not originally here, but above in the supreme being and consciousness of the infinite. All their true truth, all their real reality is there in that supreme consciousness and here only hidden in the inmost heart of their existence, *guhāyām*, but not fully expressed in their overt outward phenomena. Therefore to know them only through the externals or through superficial inner movements which is all that our mind now does, is to miss their true truth and reality and to know them only with a partial and mistaken knowledge subject to the limitations, errors, incapacities of the mental ignorance. All that determines their manifestation in our time and space is also beyond and here only in the hidden secrecy within them, and therefore the mind following their line of manifestation misses that which determines them and can only see a part of the actually present outward executive play of forces that help to give them their immediate character and direction. It is only the consciousness that reigns above, that of the supreme Ishwara, and is present in their secret heart, *hṛddeśe tiṣṭhati*, that knows and determines all their true truth and their manifestation in eternal time.

This supreme of infinite being is supreme in the sense of being above the manifestation in time, its eternal origin, support, control, itself beyond time and space. It is this of which the supermind, itself a luminous power of this supreme of infinite being, is always and fundamentally conscious.

Note on the Text

Note on the Text

THE SYNTHESIS OF YOGA first appeared in seventy-seven monthly instalments in the philosophical review *Arya*, beginning with its first issue, August 1914, and continuing until its last, January 1921. The *Arya* text of the *Synthesis* consisted of five introductory chapters numbered I–V and seventy-two other chapters numbered I–II and IV–LXXIII (the number III was inadvertently omitted). Each of the instalments was written immediately before its publication.

In the *Arya* the division of the main series of chapters into four parts, corresponding to the yogas of Works, Knowledge, Devotion and Self-Perfection, was not marked explicitly until the fifth year, when the heading "The Yoga of Self-Perfection" began to be added above the chapter numbers.

The Synthesis of Yoga was left incomplete when the *Arya* ceased publication in January 1921. Before abandoning the work, Sri Aurobindo wrote part of a chapter entitled "The Supramental Time Consciousness", which was meant to follow the last published chapter of "The Yoga of Self-Perfection". He never completed this chapter and never published the portion that he had written.

A letter that Sri Aurobindo wrote in 1936 gives some idea of his purpose in writing *The Synthesis of Yoga* and his overall plan for the work:

> *The Synthesis of Yoga* was not meant to give a method for all to follow. Each side of the Yoga was dealt with separately with all its possibilities, and an indication [was given] as to how they meet so that one starting from knowledge could realise Karma and Bhakti also and so with each path. It was intended when the Self-Perfection was finished, to suggest a way in which all could be combined, but this was never written.

One can gauge how much of *The Synthesis of Yoga* remained to be written by comparing the actually completed chapters of "The Yoga of Self-Perfection" with the outline of this part found in chapter X of Part IV. The "elements and requisites of perfection, *siddhi*" which are set forth discursively in that chapter are listed more explicitly in *Sapta Chatusthaya*, a text of 1913 published along with *Record of Yoga* in volume 10 of THE COMPLETE WORKS OF SRI AUROBINDO. The system of seven (*sapta*) sets of four elements (*catuṣṭaya*) evidently underlies the structure of Part IV of *The Synthesis of Yoga*. The last and most general *catuṣṭaya*, the *siddhi catuṣṭaya*, is taken up first, in chapters I to IX. Chapters XI to XVIII correspond to the *śānti* and *samatā catuṣṭayas*, the first two of the seven. Chapters XIX to XXV, and the incomplete chapter "The Supramental Time Consciousness", correspond to the first two elements of the third or *vijñāna catuṣṭaya*. By breaking off at this point, Sri Aurobindo left untreated the rest of the third and all of the fourth *catuṣṭayas*. He had covered the fifth and sixth *catuṣṭayas* to some degree in the rest of the *Synthesis*, but undoubtedly intended to deal with them in more depth before concluding.

When Sri Aurobindo turned his attention to *The Synthesis of Yoga* during the 1930s after a gap of more than a decade, he made no effort to complete "The Yoga of Self-Perfection". Instead he applied himself to the revision of already existing chapters.

THE REVISION OF *The Synthesis of Yoga*

Sri Aurobindo revised the text of *The Synthesis of Yoga* during three distinct periods, referred to below as Period 1, Period 2, and Period 3.

Period 1. At various times after the printed text of the *Arya* began to appear, perhaps up to the end of the 1920s, Sri Aurobindo made corrections to certain chapters of *The Synthesis of Yoga* while reading over his own copies of the journal. Most of these chapters received only sporadic and minor revision; two chapters of Part II, however, were substantially altered.

Period 2. During 1932, and possibly somewhat before and after, Sri Aurobindo undertook a full-scale revision of *The Synthesis of Yoga* with a view to publishing it as a book. At this time he revised all the chapters of what became Part I, "The Yoga of Divine Works", and nine chapters of what became Part II, "The Yoga of Integral Knowledge" (the addition of part-titles was part of the revision). He began this work by marking up pages torn from the *Arya* and then continued on copies handwritten or typed by disciples.

Period 3. During the early 1940s, Sri Aurobindo did further work on the later chapters of Part I, using typed copies of the pages from the *Arya* revised during Period 2. At the same time he began to write two new chapters, which he apparently intended to add to this part, but which he abandoned before completion.

During the later part of the 1940s, Sri Aurobindo lightly revised the entire first part of the *Synthesis* while preparing it for publication.

What follows is a brief part-by-part description of the revision.

Introduction: The Conditions of the Synthesis

Sri Aurobindo made sporadic minor changes to these five chapters during Period 1 and possibly also Period 2 of the revision. His alterations and additions, marked in issues of the *Arya* and a set of pages torn from the journal, were not discovered until the 1970s, and appear as part of the text for the first time in the present edition.

Part I: The Yoga of Divine Works

The twelve chapters of this part correspond to eleven *Arya* chapters: I–II and IV–XII. (There was no chapter numbered III in the *Arya*; the present chapters V and VI correspond to *Arya* chapter VI.) Sri Aurobindo revised each of these chapters during Period 2. The work done ranges from the light retouching of some pages to the rewriting or new-writing of long passages. During Period 3 he continued the work of revision begun in Period 2, concentrating on the last six chapters, and prepared the entire part for publication.

Chapter I. Moderately revised during Period 2.

Chapters II–IV. Heavily revised during Period 2. Sri Aurobindo added the entire second half of chapter IV at this time. He also made stylistic changes and added new material to all three chapters, but did not fundamentally alter their structure.

Chapters V and VI. Completely rewritten during Period 2 on the basis of *Arya* chapter VI, little of which remains in the final text.

Chapters VII–XII. Extensively revised during Periods 2 and 3. The typed sheets containing the later stages of the Period 2 revision of chapters VII and VIII were misplaced before the start of Period 3, obliging Sri Aurobindo to work on transcripts of the *Arya* pages containing only the earlier stages of the revision. The unused versions from Period 2 have since been found, and are reproduced in the reference volume (volume 35).

Appendix: Chapter XIII. During Period 3, Sri Aurobindo wrote this draft of a chapter meant to follow the last complete chapter of Part I, but did not prepare it for publication in the 1948 edition of the *Synthesis*. Found among his papers after his passing, it was published for the first time in the 1955 edition of the book.

Around the same time that Sri Aurobindo worked on the chapter published as "Appendix: Chapter XIII", he produced several drafts of a chapter entitled "The Yogic Consciousness and Works", which he also intended to place at the end of Part I. None of these drafts are sufficiently well worked out to be published as part of the text of *The Synthesis of Yoga*. The most important of them are reproduced in the reference volume (volume 35).

Part II: The Yoga of Integral Knowledge

These twenty-eight chapters correspond to *Arya* chapters XIII–XL. Sri Aurobindo revised eleven of these chapters during Periods 1 and 2, but did not prepare any of them for publication. The Period 2 revision was incorporated into the text of the 1955 edition; the Period 1 revision was not discovered until the 1970s and appears in print for the first time in the present edition.

Chapter I. Extensively revised during Period 2.
Chapter II. First four paragraphs revised significantly during Period 2.
Chapters III–VIII. Never revised.
Chapter IX. Extensively revised during Period 2.
Chapters X–XIV. Never revised.
Chapter XV. Moderately revised during Period 1.
Chapter XVI. One page lightly revised during Period 1.
Chapter XVII. Some of the later paragraphs revised significantly during

Period 1; the first paragraph separately revised during Period 2. The present text includes both sets of revision, which do not overlap.
Chapters XVIII–XX. Never revised.
Chapters XXI–XXIV. Extensively revised during Period 2.
Chapter XXV. Never revised.
Chapter XXVI. Lightly revised during Period 2.
Chapters XXVII and XXVIII. Never revised.

Part III: The Yoga of Divine Love

No chapter in this part was ever revised by Sri Aurobindo. The texts of these eight chapters are identical to those of *Arya* chapters XLI–XLVIII. They were renumbered I–VIII and the part-title was added by the editors of the 1955 edition.

Part IV: The Yoga of Self-Perfection

No chapter in this part was ever revised by Sri Aurobindo. The texts of these twenty-five chapters are identical to those of *Arya* chapters XLIX–LXXIII. They were renumbered I–XXV by the editors of the 1955 edition. The Appendix consists of two incomplete versions of a chapter Sri Aurobindo began to write in 1920 or 1921, just before he discontinued the *Arya*.

PUBLISHING HISTORY

The revised versions of chapters VII–XII of Part I of *The Synthesis of Yoga* were published in the quarterly review *Advent* between August 1946 and April 1948. The entire first part was published by the Sri Aurobindo Library, Madras, in October 1948. In 1950, and again in 1953, the same text was brought out by the Sri Aurobindo Library, New York. In each of these editions, the title of the book was given as *The Synthesis of Yoga*. A half-title specified that the contents consisted only of Part I ("Book One" in the American edition) of the complete work. Separate publication of the other parts had been planned, but this plan was never carried out.

In 1955, the *Arya* text of the Introduction, the 1948 text of Part I, a text of Part II incorporating Sri Aurobindo's revisions from Period 2, and the *Arya* texts of the chapters comprising Part III and Part IV, were published by the Sri Aurobindo International University Centre as *On Yoga I: The Synthesis of Yoga.* (*On Yoga II*, published in 1958, consisted of a selection of Sri Aurobindo's letters on yoga.) The incomplete chapter "The Supermind and the Yoga of Works" appeared in this edition for the first time as chapter XIII of Part I. The SAIUC edition was reprinted, with corrections, in 1957. The same publisher (under the new name Sri Aurobindo International Centre of Education) issued a new edition of the same text in 1965.

In 1970 *The Synthesis of Yoga* was published as volumes 20 and 21 of the Sri Aurobindo Birth Centenary Library. This edition was reprinted many times.

The present edition has been thoroughly checked against all related manuscripts and printed texts. Many typographical and other errors have been corrected. The edition includes for the first time Sri Aurobindo's scattered revisions in the Introduction and substantial revision of chapters XV–XVII of Part II. It is the first edition of the book to include the text of "The Supramental Time Consciousness", the incomplete chapter Sri Aurobindo wrote for Part IV before setting aside "The Yoga of Self-Perfection".

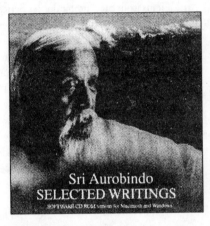

OTHER TITLES BY SRI AUROBINDO

Bases of Yoga (New US edition)	p	6.95
Bhagavad Gita and Its Message	p	15.95
Dictionary of Sri Aurobindo's Yoga (compiled)	p	11.95
Essays on the Gita (new US edition)	p	19.95
Gems from Sri Aurobindo, 1st Series (compiled)	p	8.95
Gems from Sri Aurobindo, 2nd Series (compiled)	p	12.95
Gems from Sri Aurobindo, 3rd Series (compiled)	p	10.95
Gems from Sri Aurobindo, 4th Series (compiled)	p	8.95
Growing Within	p	9.95
Human Cycle: Psychology of Social Development (new US edition)	p	14.95
Hymns to the Mystic Fire (new US edition)	p	17.95
Ideal of Human Unity (new US edition)	p	17.95
Integral Yoga: Sri Aurobindo's Teaching and Method of Practice (compiled)	p	14.95
The Life Divine (new US edition)	p	29.95
	hb	39.95
Lights on Yoga	p	2.95
Living Within (compiled)	p	8.95
Looking from Within (compiled)	p	6.95
The Mother (new US edition)	p	2.95
A Practical Guide to Integral Yoga (compiled)	p	7.95
The Psychic Being: Soul in Evolution (compiled)	p	8.95
Rebirth and Karma (new US edition)	p	9.95
Savitri: A Legend and a Symbol (new US edition)	p	24.95
The Secret of the Veda (new US edition)	p	19.95
The Synthesis of Yoga (new US edition)	p	29.95
	hb	34.95
The Upanishads (new US edition)	p	17.95
Vedic Symbolism (compiled)	p	9.95
Wisdom of the Gita, 2nd Series (compiled)	p	10.95
Wisdom of the Upanishads (compiled)	p	7.95

available from your local bookseller or
LOTUS PRESS, Box 325, Twin Lakes, WI 53181 USA
262/889-8561 • www. lotuspress.com
email: lotuspress@lotuspress.com

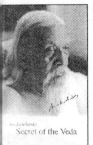

Secret of the Veda

SECRET OF THE VEDA by Sri Aurobindo

In this ground-breaking book, Sri Aurobindo has revealed the secret of the Veda and illustrated his method with numerous translations of the ancient hymns. *Secret of the Veda* has been acclaimed by scholars and yogins as the ultimate key to revealing the hidden sense and secret inner meanings of the original spiritual revelation of the Veda. The Rig Veda provides an inner spiritual and psychological practice to achieve realization. It is the foundation upon which the Upanishads were later developed.
Now in it first US edition.

LOTUS PRESS   ISBN 0-914955-19-5 581p pb $19.95

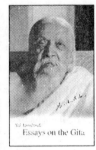

Essays on the Gita

ESSAYS ON THE GITA by Sri Aurobindo

The Bhagavad Gita stands alone in the spiritual tradition of humanity by being at the same time a Scripture, a teaching , a poetic utterance and a practical guidebook to the problems of life in the world. For this reason, the Gita is a powerful aid to anyone who wants to integrate the life of the Spirit with the issues of life in the world. It does not "cut the knot" but systematically works to untie it. In so doing, it helps us clarify the issues alive within ourselves. Sri Aurobindo understood these issues and in his famous *Essays on the Gita* he was able to reveal many subtle and hidden aspects of the teaching of the Gita. He entered into the spirit of the original and created a commentary that has stood the test of time in its lucidity and value for anyone wishing to truly understand the Bhagavad Gita. *Essays on the Gita* has been widely acclaimed for opening up the deeper sense of the Bhagavad Gita.
Now in its first US edition

LOTUS PRESS   ISBN 0-914955-18-7 588p pb $19.95

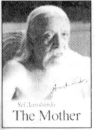

The Mother

THE MOTHER by Sri Aurobindo

Sri Aurobindo has created, in this small book, a powerful guide to the practice of spirituality in life. To discover this gem is to gain a constant companion whose guidance remains forever meaningful. Its power of expression and meaning are so concentrated and far reaching that many have called it "Matri Upanishad", the Upanishad of the Mother. Sri Aurobindo's Matri Upanishad is the text which reveals this power and energy of creation in its universal and personal sense, providing both truth of philosophy and truth of yogic experience at one and the same time.
Now in its first US edition

LOTUS PRESS   ISBN 0-941524-79-5 62p pb $2.95

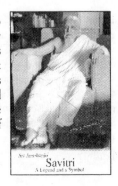

Savitri
A Legend and a Symbol

SAVITRI: A LEGEND AND A SYMBOL by Sri Aurobindo

Savitri is an inner guidebook for the soul. These mantric verses imbue even the body with potent spiritual resonance. In this epic spiritual poem, Sri Aurobindo reveals his vision of mankind's destiny within the universal evolution. He sets forth the optimistic view that life on earth has a purpose, and he places our travail within the context of this purpose: to participate in the evolution of consciousness that represents the secret thread behind life on earth. Sri Aurobindo's verses describe the origin of the universe, the appearance of sentient beings and the stages of evolution, as well as speak to many of mankind's unanswered questions concerning pain and death.
Now in its first US edition

LOTUS PRESS   ISBN 0-941524-80-9 816p pb $24.95

available from your local bookseller or
Lotus Press, PO Box 325, Twin Lakes, WI 53181 • 262-889-8561
www.lotuspress.com • email: lotuspress@lotuspress.com

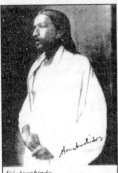
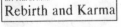

REBIRTH AND KARMA by Sri Aurobindo
In depth study of the concepts of rebirth, karma and the higher lines of karma. One of the best introductions to this area we've ever found.

LOTUS PRESS   ISBN 0-941524-63-9   190p   pb $9.95

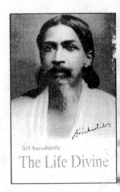

THE LIFE DIVINE by Sri Aurobindo
The Life Divine is Sri Aurobindo's major philosophical exposition, spanning more than a thousand pages and integrating the major spiritual directions of mankind into a coherent picture of the growth of the spiritual essence of man through diverse methods, philosophies and spiritual practices.

LOTUS PRESS   ISBN 0-941524-61-2   1113p   pb $29.95

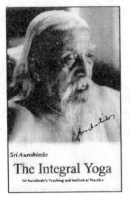

THE INTEGRAL YOGA
Sri Aurobindo's Teaching and Method of Practice
by Sri Aurobindo (compilation)
> "These carefully selected excerpts from the writings of Sri Aurobindo provide a wonderfully accessible entre into the writings of one of the great masters of spiritual synthesis."
> Ram Dass

LOTUS PRESS   ISBN 0-941524-76-0   416p   pb $14.95

SYNTHESIS OF YOGA, US EDITION by Sri Aurobindo
In *The Synthesis of Yoga* Sri Aurobindo unfolds his vision of an integral yoga embracing all the powers and activities of man. First, he reviews the three great yogic paths of Knowledge, Works and Love, along with Hatha Yoga, Raja Yoga and Tantra, and then integrates them all into a great symphony. "Truth of philosophy is of a merely theoretical value unless it can be lived, and we have therefore tried in the *The Synthesis of Yoga* to arrive at a synthetical view of the principles and methods of the various lines of spiritual self-discipline and the way in which they can lead to an integral divine life in the human existence".

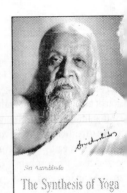

LOTUS PRESS   ISBN 0-941524-66-3   899p   hb $34.95
LOTUS PRESS   ISBN 0-941524-65-5   899p   pb $29.95

available from your local bookseller or
Lotus Press, PO Box 325, Twin Lakes, WI 53181 • 262-889-8561
www.lotuspress.com • email: lotuspress@lotuspress.com